MW00323835

Differential Diagnosis by Laboratory Medicine
A Quick Reference for Physicians

Springer

Berlin
Heidelberg
New York
Hong Kong
London
Milan
Paris
Tokyo

Vincent Marks
Thomas Cantor
Dusan Mesko
Rudolf Pullmann
Gabriela Nosalova

Differential Diagnosis by Laboratory Medicine

A Quick Reference for Physicians

Editor-in-Chief: Dusan Mesko

With a Foreword by Alexander Schirger

Springer

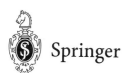

Library of Congress Cataloguing-in-Publication Data
Differential diagnosis by laboratory medicine : a quick reference for physicans /
editor-in-chief, Vincent Marks ; Thomas Cantor ; Dusan Mesko ... [et al.] (eds.).
    p. ; cm
  ISBN 3540430571 (alk. paper)
    1. Diagnosis, Laboratory–Handbooks, manuals etc. 2. Diagnosis,
    Differential–Handbooks, manuals etc. I. Mesko, Dusan, 1956- II. Marks,Vincent.
    [DNLM: Diagnosis, Differential–Handbooks. 2. Laboratory Techniques and
    Procedures–Handbooks. WB 39 D569 2002]
  RB38.2 .D545 2002
  616.07'56–dc21

ISBN 3-540-43057-1   Springer Verlag Berlin Heidelberg New York

Springer-Verlag Berlin Heidelberg New York
a member of BertelsmannSpringer Science+Business Media GmbH

http://www.springer.de/medizin

© Springer-Verlag Berlin Heidelberg 2002
Printed in Germany

Cover Design: Erich Kirchner, Heidelberg
Production: Frank Krabbes, Heidelberg
Typesetting: Hilger VerlagsService, Heidelberg
Printed on acid free paper   SPIN 10839663   14/3109 – 5 4 3 2 1 0

List of Contributors

Thomas Cantor, BA
SCANTIBODIES Laboratory, Inc.
9336 Abraham Way
Santee
CA 92071
USA

Prof. Vincent Marks, BA, BCh,
MA, DM, FRCP
Oriel House
Derby Road
Haslemere
Surrey GU27 1BP
United Kingdom

Prof. Dusan Mesko, M.D., Ph.D.
Clinic of Sports Medicine
University Hospital
Kollarova 2
036 59 Martin
Slovak Republic

Prof. Gabriela Nosalova, M.D., Ph.D.
Dept. of Pharmacology
Comenius University
Jessenius Faculty of Medicine
Sklabinska 26
037 53 Martin
Slovak Republic

Prof. Rudolf Pullmann, M.D., Ph.D.
Dept. of Clinical Biochemistry
University Hospital
Kollarova 2
036 59 Martin
Slovak Republic

Prof. Alexander Schirger, M.D., Ph.D.
Mayo Clinic
Hypertension, Cardiovascular Diseases
and Internal Medicine Unit
200 First Street SW
Rochester, MN 55904
USA

Foreword

I have been asked to write a foreword to the next edition of the Vademecum of Clinical Biochemistry renamed to Differential Diagnosis by Laboratory Medicine. The Editor in-Chief, Professor Dusan Mesko, conceived the idea of the Vademecum during a very intensely, intellectually active period as a visiting Olga Havel Fellow from Slovak Republic at the Mayo Clinic in Rochester. It was here during his study stay that much of the conceptual planning and detailed realization was being completed. It was with much interest that I observed Professor Mesko in his effort, and I know while here he has gained admiration of those who had the privilege of interacting with him. When the first edition of the Vademecum appeared and we received the copy for the Mayo Library and for myself, I was overcome with a genuine sense of joy. In this era of rapid information and the need to access usable information book such as this cannot be but judged extremely useful. It is my hope that this work, which attests to the thoroughness of Professor Mesko's and his co-workers efforts will prove to be fruitful for the students quick reference, for clinicans and house officers lightening of burdens, particularly of on-call nights, and for the teaching staff as well to quickly access needed information. With these sentiments, we wish the authors and the book well and also hope that the potential widening circle of readers and users will benefit from the work presented.

Alexander Schirger

Preface

In everyday clinical practice physicians cope with all kinds of problems while establishing precise diagnosis and adequate treatment. Longevity and hi-tech technologies promote the use of sensitive tests to monitor all clients' well-being and to make specific diagnoses. It makes them not only mobilize their medical knowledge and skills, but also to analyze and synthesize their knowledge and compare it with the latest achievements in clinical biochemistry and laboratory medicine. The same type of "processing" is experienced by the medical student who is struggling with orientation, needs and problems posed by the latest clinical and biochemical diagnosis. Laboratory tests are an increasing part of most patient-physician relationships and contribute greatly to the selection of additional diagnostic procedures and ultimately to diagnosis, differential diagnosis and treatment. In this respect, "Differential Diagnosis by Laboratory Medicine" tries to provide help and wants to fill the existing gap in the market of medical books.

The book gives quick, pertinent information about parameters, tests and their purposes, clinical conditions associated with disease and drugs related to abnormal test results. We offer this book to medical doctors of most areas, to laboratory medicine, pathologiy, dentistry, laboratory technology, biochemistry, pharmacy staffs as well as to medical and nursing students. Its unique, easy to use and easy-to-understand format has been developed to provide help in undergraduate and postgraduate studies, in laboratory and clinical practice, in emergency rooms and within the field of diagnosis/differential diagnosis. Some of the clinical-biochemical/laboratory parameters presented in the book enhance value of the book because they might still be more common in basic research and not yet in current use. Parameters which are also employed by clinical biochemistry departments are included because of apparatus availability, work organization or other reasons, although they do not fall directly within their competency. The book fully considers the wide range experience of medical doctors.

The introductory chapter of the book deals with technical and organizational questions that are connected with clinical-biochemical diagnosis and introduces laboratory medicine. The second part provides alphabetically ordered passwords of more than 850 biochemical/laboratory parameters and laboratory tests in 17 biological materials. Each password definition starts with brief clinical, biochemical, and physiological characteristics, test purposes followed by pathological units or other conditions that are accompanied by increased or decreased levels of biochemical/laboratory parameters in question. Medicamentous interfering factors are also noted. Mentioned are not only "direct" parameters, but also "borderline" and derived items. Inspite of the enormously varied medical terminology, the authors utilized more uniform versions.

The authors provide the reader with the latest lexicon-type information on clinical units/conditions and with a parameter spectrum that may deviate from the reference range in a particular disease, condition, or physiological circumstance. Data of more than 1950 diseases/conditions are given for all age groups. The findings more frequently described in the literature are printed in bold letters. To enable an easy and fast orientation, single clinical units/conditions are presented in an alphabetical order.

A separate part of the book is devoted to drug interference and parameters reflecting the conditions of human organs/systems (inner circumstances/milieu of the human organism) in more than 1200 drugs and medicine groups. The authors have used drug names which are not protected by copyright (INN) and are recommended by WHO, thereby improving the quality and ensuring a wider range of data acceptance.

The final part of the book provides a summary of the international reference values of clinical-biochemical/laboratory parameters in biological samples/materials. Reference values may differ among institutions. Values mentioned are guidelines and users should check with their institution the laboratory policies and reference values for the tests. The book uses Système International (SI) units, a table to convert SI units into conventional units is included. The book comprises a detailed parameter register, synonymous terms/names, dictionary terminology and a list of most abbreviations currently in use.

The book does not provide special technical issues and directions, selected referral laboratory, bibliographic references for individual tests. Most of the data are not original but have been adopted from hundreds of regional and literature sources worldwide over the years.

The innovative concept, the contents as well as the structure and format of the book resulted from the needs and requirements of medical practice.

The book was written to intermediate and improve the laboratory-clinical linkage by making it simpler for both sides to select and interpret the biochemical/laboratory tests and parameters.

The authors together with the Publishing House Springer-Verlag hope that the book "Differential Diagnosis by Laboratory Medicine" meets your expectations and becomes a helpful advisory that offers solutions in the everyday clinical practice and study.

The authors

Acknowledgements

We thank colleagues and students for their inspirations, remarks, ideas, corrections and support. Our thanks to Executive Editor, Developmental Editor, Supervising Editor, Production editor, Manufacturing Manager, Content and Cover Designers, Compositor, Printer for their diligent work on this project as well as to all the other people behind the scenes at Springer-Verlag who where helpful.

We are sincerely grateful to Prof. N. Tryding, MD., (Kristianstad, Sweden) for kind permission of PC Database use: Drug Effects in Clinical Chemistry. (Software). Polydata Ltd., PharmaSoft SWEDIS AB, 1996.

For comments, suggestions and cooperation in the book preparation we are grateful namely to the following colleagues: Prof. A. Kallner, MD. (Karolinska Sjughuset, Stockholm, Sweden), Prof. Dr. H. Wisser (Robert-Bosch Krankenhaus, Stuttgart, Germany), Prof. Ing. M. Ferencik, Ph.D. (Faculty of Medicine, Comenius University, Bratislava, Slovak Republic), Prof. P. Kubisz, M.D., Ph.D., Prof. J. Danko, M.D., Ph.D., Prof. S. Straka, M.D., Ph.D., Ing. A. Hutko, PhDr. M. Bujalkova, Ph.D., R. Vysehradsky, M.D., Ph.D., PhDr. A. Jureckova (Jessenius Faculty of Medicine, Comenius University, Martin, Slovak Republic), Assoc. Prof. M. Dobrotova, M.D., Ph.D., J. Rickova, M.D. (Martin University Hospital, Martin, Slovak Republic), the Computer Center of Jessenius Faculty of Medicine in Martin. For partial technical assistance we are grateful to Mrs. L. Ferjancova, Mrs. J. Hubacova (Martin University Hospital, Martin, Slovak Republic).

Notes

Translation of notions/abbreviations was done on the basis of those found in sources/literature available. We cannot provide all possible abbreviations and their translations, it was not our goal. When we found alternative versions of some notions/abbreviations, we offered them.

In the book are used some synonymous expressions for abbreviated terms as well as for pathological and other conditions, as they are found in literature. The dynamic development and fast changes in pathological terminology makes it difficult to give only the latest one. The findings mentioned in the book (pathological/other units/conditions, biochemical/laboratory parameters) are written as found in the majority of the literature available. For the use of the clinical handbook a dynamic attitude of the reader towards individual data is needed, in order to connect them with own clinical experience.

Some parameters are commonly written in one word or with a hyphen. Written in bold are pathological/other units/conditions whose parameters are frequently presented in the literature as either increased or decreased, e.g. bronchitis – (acute b., chronic b.), as well as the biochemical/laboratory parameters whose levels are often either increased/decreased, e.g. cirrhosis – (AST). An asterisk (*) is used to mark parameters/tests that are diagnostic/suggestive/supportive for the disease. Parameters/tests that left unmarked indicate that such test results may occur and are non-specific. They may, however, provide useful additional information in the differential diagnosis of an individual patient/situation.

Names of single parameters/tests, common abbreviation and pathological and other conditions are listed in alphabetical order. Numerical prefixes or prefixes of the Greek alphabet have been ignored.

The chapter "Blood – plasma – serum" contains the section "tumor markers". Here, we have put together all tumor markers. In the chapter "Biochemical/laboratory findings in clinical units and conditions", in the section "disease/s" all conditions named "disease/diseases" were put together, under the section 'infectious diseases' all infectious diseases (e.g. anthrax, morbilli) were assembled and in the section "tumors" all tumor types are listed. If the section within this chapter does not specify the biological material, either increased or decreased parameter levels in the blood – plasma – serum apply.

Alphabetical order as used in dictionaries/registers has been employed in this book, e.g. acute pancreatitis, bronchitis. For practical reasons, British-American English has been used throughout.

Contents

Abbreviations Used

AAP	alanine aminopeptidase
5-NT	5-nucleotidase
A2MG (AMG)	alpha-2-macroglobulin
AA	amino acids
AAT (A1AT)	alpha-1-antitrypsin
AB	actual bicarbonates
Ab (AB)	antibody, antibodies
ABG	arterial blood gases
ACA (ACAb)	anticentromere antibodies
ACE	angiotensin-converting enzyme
ACH (Ach)	acetylcholine
ACHE (AChE, ACHS)	(acetyl) cholinesterase
ACLA (ACLAb)	anticardiolipin antibodies
ACLRA	anti-acetylcholine receptor antibodies
ACP	acid phosphatase
ACPA	antineutrophil cytoplasmic antibodies
ACTH	adrenocorticotropic hormone
AD (ADH)	alcohol dehydrogenase
ADA	adenosine deaminase
ADF	adult T-cell leukemia-derived factor
ADH	antidiuretic hormone
ADM	adrenomedullin
ADNase	antideoxyribonuclease
ADP	adenosine diphosphate
AFP	alpha-1-fetoprotein
Ag (AG)	antigen
AGA	antigliadin antibodies
AGBMA (AGBMAb)	antiglomerular basement membrane antibodies
AGP	alpha-1 acid glycoprotein (orosomucoid)
AGT	angiotensinogen
AHA (AHAb)	antihistone antibodies
AHBD (AHBDH)	alpha-hydroxybutyrate dehydrogenase
AHF	antihemophilic factor (f. VIII)
AHG	antihemophilic globulin (f. VIII)
Al	aluminum
ALA	aminolevulinic acid (delta-aminolevulic acid)
Ala	alanine
ALD	aldolase
ALG	antilymphocyte globulin
ALP	alkaline phosphatase
ALT (ALAT)	alanine aminotransferase

AMA (AMAb)	antimitochondrial antibodies
AMF	autocrine motility factor
AMP	adenosine monophosphate
AMS	amylase
AMS (P)	pancreatic isoenzyme of amylase
AMS (S)	salivary isoenzyme of amylase
ANA (ANAb)	antinuclear antibodies
ANCA (ANCAb)	antineutrophil cytoplasm antibodies
ANF	atrial natriuretic factor (antinuclear factor)
ANH	atrial natriuretic hormone
ANP	atrial natriuretic peptide
ANP-B	atrial natriuretic peptide (B-type)
anti-ACHR	anti-acetylcholine receptor antibodies
anti-CMV	anti-cytomegalovirus antibodies
anti-DNA	antideoxyribonucleic acid antibodies
anti-DNAase	anti-deoxyribonuclease antibodies
anti-DNP	antideoxyribonucleoprotein antibodies
anti-ds-DNA	anti-double stranded DNA antibodies
anti-EBV	anti-Epstein-Barr virus antibodies
anti-EBV-VCA	antibodies against Epstein-Barr virus viral capsid antigen
anti-EJ	anti-glycyl-tRNA synthetase antibodies
anti-EN	anti-extractable nuclear antibodies
anti-GAD	glutamic acid decarboxylase antibodies
anti-GBM	anti-glomerular basement membrane antibodies
anti-HAV	anti-hepatitis A virus antibodies
anti-HAV (IgG)	anti-hepatitis A virus IgG antibodies
anti-HAV (IgM)	anti-hepatitis A virus IgM antibodies
anti-HBc	anti-hepatitis B core antigen antibodies
anti-HBc (IgG)	anti-hepatitis B core antigen IgG antibodies
anti-HBc (IgM)	anti-hepatitis B core antigen IgM antibodies
anti-HBe	anti-hepatitis B e antigen antibodies
anti-HBs	anti-hepatitis B surface antigen antibodies
anti-HCV	anti-hepatitis C virus antibodies
anti-HDV	anti-hepatitis D virus antibodies
anti-HEV	anti-hepatitis E virus antibodies
anti-HPV	anti-human papillomavirus antibodies
anti-HSP	anti-heat shock proteins antibodies
anti-HSV	anti-herpes simplex virus antibodies
anti-IF	intrinsic factor antibodies
anti-Jo-1	anti-histidyl-tRNA synthetase antibodies
anti-La/SSB (anti-La, Ha/SSB)	antibodies against small nuclear ribonucleoproteins (SnRNPs, La, Ha particles)
anti-LCA	antilymphocytotoxic antibodies
anti-LKM-1	liver-kidney-microsome antibodies
anti-MPO (MPOA)	antimyeloperoxidase antibodies
anti-NE	antinuclear envelope antibodies
anti-NOR 90	antinucleolar organizing region antibodies
anti-nuclear-RNP	antinuclear ribonucleoprotein antibodies
anti-OJ	anti-isoleucyl-tRNA synthetase antibodies (OJ)
anti-p53	antibodies against protein 53
anti-PCNA	anti-proliferating cell nuclear antigen antibodies

anti-PL-7	anti-threonyl-tRNA synthetase antibodies
anti-PLT	antiplatelet antibodies
anti-RBC	anti-red blood cells antibodies
anti-RNA	antiribonucleic acid antibodies
anti-RNP	antiribonucleoprotein antibodies
anti-Ro/SSA	antibodies against small nuclear ribonucleoproteins (SnRNPs, Ro particle)
anti-SLA	anti-soluble liver antigen antibodies
anti-Sm	anti-Smith antibodies
anti-SRP	anti-signal recognition particle antibodies
anti-ss-DNA	anti-single stranded DNA antibodies
anti-TPO	antithyroid peroxidase antibodies
anti-TSH-receptors	antibodies against thyrotropin receptors
anti-tTG	anti-tissue transglutaminase autoantibodies
anti-U1-RNP	anti-uridyl-1-ribonucleo-protein antibodies
anti-VZV	anti-varicella–zoster virus antibodies
anti-Yo	antibodies against Purkinje cells (Yo)
AP (Ap)	alkaline phosphatase
APA (APAb)	antiparietal cell antibodies
APC	antigen presenting cell
APF	antiperinuclear factor
APLA (APLAb)	antiphospholipid antibodies
Apo	apolipoprotein
Apo A	apolipoprotein A
Apo B	apolipoprotein B
Apo C	apolipoprotein C
Apo E	apolipoprotein E
Apo-LPs	apolipoproteins
APP	amyloid precursor protein
APR	acute-phase reactants
APTT (aPTT)	activated partial thromboplastin time
AR	amphiregulin
ARA	antireticulin antibodies
Arg	arginine
ARDS	adult respiratory distress syndrome
ARS-A	arylsulfatase A
As	arsenic
ASAL	argininosuccinate lyase
ASCA	antibodies against Saccharomyces cerevisiae
ASGP-R	hepatic asialoglycoprotein receptor
ASH	antistreptococcal hyaluronidase
ASK	antistreptokinase
ASLO (ASO)	antistreptolysin O
ASMA (ASMAb)	anti-smooth muscle antibodies
AST (ASAT)	aspartate aminotransferase
AT I	angiotensin I
AT II	angiotensin II
AT III	antithrombin III
ATBMA (ATBMAb)	antitubular basement membrane antibodies
ATG	antithymocyte globulin
ATGA (ATGAb)	antithyroglobulin antibodies

ATP	adenosine triphosphate
ATPase	adenosinetriphosphatase
BALF (BAL)	bronchoalveolar lavage fluid
BALP	bone specific alcaline phosphatase
bas (baso)	basophils
BB	buffer base
BCF	basophil chemotactic factor
BCG	Bacillus Calmette-Guérin
BCGF	B-cell growth factor
BCM	breast cancer mucin
BCSF	B-cell stimulating factor
BDNF	brain-derived neutrophic factor
BE	base excess
bFGF (BFGF)	basic fibroblast growth factor
BGG	bovine gamma globulin
BGP	bone Gla-protein (osteocalcin)
BHBA (BOHB)	beta-hydroxybutyric acid
Bil (Bili)	bilirubin
B-lym	B-lymphocytes
B2M	beta-2-microglobulin
BNP	brain natriuretic peptide
BSP	bromo-sulfophthalein test
BT	bleeding time
BTA	bladder tumor antigen
BUN	blood urea nitrogen
$C1, 2, 3$ $(C_{1,2,3})$	complement
C1-INH	C1-esterase inhibitor
Ca	calcium
CA	carbonic anhydrase, cancer antigen, carbohydrate antigen
CAC	circulating anticoagulant
CAM	cell adhesion molecules
cAMP (3´5´-AMP)	cyclic adenosine monophosphate
CAP-37	cationic antimicrobial protein-37
CASA	cancer associated serum
cAST	cytosolic aspartate aminotransferase
CBG	corticosteroid-binding globulin
CBS	cystathione beta-synthetase
CCK	cholecystokinin
CCK-PZ	cholecystokinin-pancreozymin
CD	cluster of differentiation
CEA	carcinoembryonic antigen
CER	ceruloplasmin
CgA, B	chromogranin A, B
CGRP	calcitonin gene related peptide
CHS (ChE)	cholinesterase
CIC	circulating immune complexes
CIPD	chronic inflammatory demyelinating polyneuropathy
CK	creatine kinase
CK-BB	creatine kinase BB isoenzyme
CK-MB	creatine kinase MB isoenzyme
CK-MM	creatine kinase MM isoenzyme

CMV	cytomegalovirus
CNTF	ciliary neurotrophic factor
Co	cobalt
CO	carbon monoxide
CO_2	carbon dioxide
CoA	coenzyme A
COHb	carboxyhemoglobin
CP	coproporphyrins
CPK (CP)	creatine phosphokinase
Cr	chromium
CRDGF	colorectum cell-derived growth factor
CRH	corticotropin-releasing hormone
CRP	C-reactive protein
CSF	colony stimulating factor, cerebrospinal fluid
CSIF	cytokine synthesis inhibitory factor
CT	calcitonin
CTGF	connective tissue growth factor
CTL	cytotoxic T-lymphocyte
cTnI	cardiac specific troponin I
cTnT	cardiac specific troponin T
Cu	copper
Cys	cysteine
DAF	decay accelerating factor
DHAA	dehydroascorbic acid
DHEA	dehydroepiandrosterone
DHEAS	dehydroepiandrosterone sulfate
DHT	dihydrotestosterone
DIA	differentiation inhibitory activity
DIF	differentiation inhibitory factor
DOC	deoxycorticosterone
DPD	deoxypyridinoline
2,3-DPG	2,3-diphosphoglycerate
DRF	differentiation retarding factor
ds-DNA	double-stranded DNA
DSF	differentiating stimulating factor
DST	dexamethasone suppression test
ds-RNA	double-stranded RNA
EBNA	Epstein–Barr nuclear antigen
EBV	Epstein–Barr virus
EBV-VCA	Epstein–Barr virus viral capsid antigen
ECF	eosinophilic chemotactic factor
ECF-A	eosinophil chemotactic factor of anaphylaxis
ECGF	endothelial cell growth factor
ECP	eosinophil cationic protein
EDF	eosinophil differentiation factor
EDRF	endothelial derived relaxing factor
EDTA	ethylene-diaminotetra-acetic acid
EGF	epidermal growth factor
EMA (EMAb)	endomysial antibodies
EMF	erythrocyte maturation factor
ENA (ENAb)	extractable nuclear antigen antibodies

beta-END	beta-endorphins
eos	eosinophils
EPO	erythropoietin
ERCP	endoscopic retrograde cholangio-pancreatography
ESR	erythrocyte sedimentation rate
ET-1	endothelin-1
ETAF	epidermal T-cell activating factor
F	females
FA	fatty acids
FAD	flavin adenine dinucleotide
Fas-L	Fas-ligand
FBS	fasting blood sugar
FDP	fibrin degradation products
Fe	iron
FFA	free fatty acids
FGF	fibroblast growth factor
FMN	flavin mononucleotide
FN	fibronectin
FPA	fibrinopeptide A
FSH	follicle-stimulating hormone
FT3	free triiodothyronine
FT4	free thyroxine
FTI	free thyroxine index
G	glucose
G6Pase (G-6-Pase)	glucose-6-phosphatase
G6PD (G-6-PD)	glucose-6-phosphate dehydrogenase
GABA	gamma-aminobutyric acid
GAD	glutamic acid decarboxylase
GADA	glutamic acid decarboxylase antibodies
GAG	glycosaminoglycans
GCP-2	granulocyte chemotactic protein
G-CSF	granulocyte colony stimulating factor
GD (GDH)	glutamate dehydrogenase
GDF	growth and differential factor
GDNF	glial-derived neurotropic factor
GG	gamma globulin
GGTP	gamma-glutamyl transpeptidase
GH-RH	growth hormone releasing hormone
GH-RIH	growth hormone-release inhibiting hormone, somatostatin
GIP	gastric inhibitory peptide (polypeptide)
GLD (GLDH)	glutamate dehydrogenase
Gln	glutamine
Glu	glutamic acid
Gly	glycine
GM-CSF	granulocyte–macrophage colony stimulating factor
GMD	glutamate dehydrogenase
GMP	guanosine monophosphate
GMT (GGT)	gamma-glutamyltransferase
GnRH (GRH)	gonadotropin releasing hormone
GOT	glutamic-oxaloacetic transaminase
GP-BB	glycogenphosphorylase, isoenzyme BB

GPT (SGPT)	glutamic-pyruvic transaminase
GPUT	galactose-1-phosphate uridyl transferase
GPx	glutathione peroxidase
GRO	growth-related oncogene
GRP	gastrin releasing peptide, bombesin
GRPs	glucose regulated proteins
GST	glutathione S-transferase
HA	hepatitis A
HAA	hepatitis-associated antigen
HAAg	hepatitis A antigen
HAV	hepatitis A virus
HB	hepatitis B
Hb (Hgb, Hg)	hemoglobin
HbA$_{1c}$	glycated hemoglobin A$_{1c}$
HbAc (GHb)	total glycated hemoglobin Ac, glycosylated hemoglobin
HBc	hepatitis B core (antigen)
HBcAg	hepatitis B core antigen
HBD (HBDH)	hydroxybutyrate dehydrogenase
HBe	hepatitis B e (antigen)
HBeAg	hepatitis B e antigen
HBGF	heparin binding growth factor
HbO$_2$	oxyhemoglobin
HBs	hepatitis B surface (antigen)
HBsAg	hepatitis B surface antigen
HBV	hepatitis B virus
HC	hepatitis C
hCG (HCG, b-hCG)	human chorionic gonadotropin
HCl	hydrochloric acid
HCO$_3^-$	bicarbonate
hCS (HCS)	human chorionic somatomammotropin
hCT	human calcitonin
HCT (Hct)	hematocrit
HCV	hepatitis C virus
Hcys	homocysteine
HD	hepatitis D
HDAg	hepatitis D antigen (delta)
HDL-C	high-density lipoprotein cholesterol
HDV	hepatitis D virus (delta)
HE	hepatitis E
HEAg	hepatitis E antigen
HER-2	human epidermal growth factor receptor 2
HEV	hepatitis E virus
H-FABP	heart fatty acid binding protein
Hg	mercury
HGF	hepatocyte growth factor, hyperglycemic-glycogenolytic factor
hGH (HGH)	human growth hormone
HHPMA	human hepatocyte plasma membrane antigen
5-HIAA	5-hydroxyindoleacetic acid
His	histidine
HIV	human immunodeficiency virus

HLA	human leukocyte antigen
HMA (HMAb)	heart-mitochondrial antibodies
HMMA	4-hydroxy-3-methylmandelic acid
HMWK	high-molecular weight kininogen
HMW-NCF	high-molecular weight neutrophil chemotactic factor
HNANB	hepatitis non A, non B
hNE	human neutrophil elastase
hNGF	human nerve growth factor
hPL (HPL)	human placental lactogen
HPV	human papilloma virus
HRFs	histamine-releasing factors
h-sELAM-1	human soluble endothelial cell leukocyte adhesion molecule-1
h-sICAM-1	human soluble intercellular adhesion molecule-1
HSP	heat shock proteins
h-sPLA2	human soluble phospholipase A2
HSV	herpes simplex virus
h-sVCAM-1	human soluble vascular cell adhesion molecule-1
5-HT	5-hydroxytryptamine
HTLV	human T-lymphotrophic virus, human T-lymphotrophic virus
HVA	homovanillic acid
Hyp	hydroxyproline
I	iodine
IAA	insulin autoantibodies
IAP	immunosuppressive acidic protein
IAPP	insular amyloid polypeptide
ICA	islet cell antibodies
ICAM	intercellular adhesion molecules
ICD (ICDH)	isocitrate dehydrogenase
ICE	interleukin 1 converting enzyme
ICSA	islet cell surface antibodies
ICSH	interstitial cells stimulating hormone
ICTP	C-terminal telopeptide type I
IDL-C	intermediate-density lipoprotein cholesterol
IFN	interferon
Ig	immunoglobulin
IGFBP-1, 2, 3, 4, 5, 6	insulin-like growth factor binding protein
IL	interleukin
Ile	isoleucine
ILGF-I, II	insulin-like growth factor
INTP	N-terminal telopeptide type I
IRI	immunoreactive insulin
I-alpha-TI	inter-alpha-trypsin inhibitor
K	potassium, kalium
KGF	keratinocyte growth factor
17-KGS	17-ketogenic steroids
KS	ketosteroids
17-KS	17-ketosteroids
LA	lactic acid, lactate
LAA	leucine aryl-amidase

LAF	leukocyte-activating factor
LAM	leukocyte adhesion molecule
LAP	leucine aminopeptidase
LASA	lipid associated sialic acid
LATS	long-acting thyroid stimulator
LAV	lymphadenopathy-associated virus
LCA (LCAb)	lymphocytotoxic antibodies
LCA-1	liver cytosolic antigen-1
LCAT	lecithin-cholesterol acyltransferase
LD (LDH)	lactate dehydrogenase
LDL-C	low-density lipoprotein cholesterol
LEK	leucine-enkephalin
Leu	leucine
LFA	leukocyte function antigen
LH (ICSH)	luteinizing hormone
LH-RH	luteinizing hormone-releasing hormone
LIF	leukemia inhibitory factor
LMA	liver membrane antibodies
LMF	lymphocyte mitogen factor
LMIF	leukocyte migration inhibiting factor
LMW-BCGF	low-molecular weight B-cell growth factor
beta-LP	beta-lipoproteins
LP lipase	lipoprotein lipase
Lp(a)	lipoprotein (a)
LPA	liver-pancreas antigen
LPs	lipoproteins
LPS	lipase(s)
LP-X	lipoprotein-X
LSA	lipid bound sialic acid
LSP	liver-specific membrane lipoprotein
LT	leukotriene
lym	lymphocytes
Lys	lysine
M	males
MAC	metabolic acidosis
MAdCAM-1	mucosal addressin cell adhesion molecule-1
MAF	macrophages activating factor
MAG	myelin-associated glycoprotein
MAL	metabolic alkalosis
mAST	mitochondrial aspartate aminotransferase
Mb	myoglobin
MBP	myelinic basic protein
MCA	mucin-like carcinoma-associated antigen
MCAF	monocyte chemotactic and activating factor
MCF	macrophage chemotactic factor
MCH	mean corpuscular hemoglobin
MCHC	mean corpuscular hemoglobin concentration
MCP	membrane cofactor protein
MCP-1	monocyte chemoattractant protein-1 (peptide)
M-CSF	macrophage colony-stimulating factor
MCV	mean corpuscular volume

MD (MDH)	malate dehydrogenase
MDA	malone dialdehyde
MDGF	megakaryocyte development and growth factor
MDGI	mammary-derived growth inhibitor
MEK	methionine-enkephalin
Met	methionine
Mg	magnesium
MGSA	melanoma growth stimulating activity
MHb	methemoglobin
MHC	main/major histocompatibility complex
MIA	melanoma inhibiting activity
MIF	migration inhibition factor
MIG	monokine induced by interferon gamma
MIP	macrophage inflammatory protein
MIS	Müllerian inhibiting substance
MLC	myosin light chains
MMIF	macrophage migration inhibiting factor
MMPs	matrix metalloproteinases
Mn	manganese
Mn-SOD	manganese-superoxide dismutase
Mo	molybdenum
mono	monocytes
MPO	myeloperoxidase
MPOA	antimyeloperoxidase antibodies
MPV	mean platelet volume
m-RNA	messenger RNA
MSA	multiplication stimulation activity
MSH	melanocyte stimulating hormone
MTHFR	methylene-tetrahydrofolate reductase
Na	natrium
NAD	nicotinamide adenine dinucleotide
NADH$_2$	reduced nicotinamide adenine dinucleotide
NADP	nicotinamide adenine dinucleotide phosphate
NADPH	reduced nicotinamide adenine dinucleotide phosphate
NAG	N-acetylglucosaminidase
NANA	N-acetyl neuraminic acid
NAP	neutrophil activating protein
NBBs	normal buffer bases
N-CAM	neural cell adhesion molecule
neu	neutrophils
NGF	nerve growth factor
NH$_3$	ammonia
Ni	nickel
NK	natural killers
NMP 22	nuclear matrix protein 22
NPN	non-protein nitrogen
NSE	neuron-specific enolase
NT-pro-ANP	N-terminal atrial natriuretic pro-peptide
OAF	osteoclast activating factor
OCT	ornithine carbamoyltransferase
OGTT	oral glucose tolerance test

11-OHCS	11-hydroxycorticosteroids
17-OHCS	17-hydroxycorticosteroids
1,25-(OH)$_2$D3	1,25-dihydroxycholecalciferol, vitamin D3
18-OH DOC	18-hydroxy-deoxycorticosterone
17-OHP	17-hydroxyprogesterone
Orn	ornithine
OSM	oncostatin M
P	phosphorus (PO$_4$, phosphate)
PA	prealbumin
PABA	para-aminobenzoic acid
PAF	platelet activating factor
PAG	pregnancy-associated glycoprotein
PAI	plasminogen activator inhibitor
PAP	prostatic acid phosphatase
PAPP-A	pregnancy-associated plasma protein A
Pb	plumbum, lead
PBG	porphobilinogen
PBG-S	porphobilinogen synthase
PBP	platelet basic protein
PCA (PCAb)	parietal cell antibodies
PCNA	proliferating cell nuclear antigen
pCO$_2$	partial pressure of carbon dioxide
PCR	polymerase chain reaction
PCT	procalcitonin
PD-ECGF	platelet derived endothelial cell growth factor
PDGF	platelet-derived growth factor
PECAM-1	platelet-endothelial cell adhesion molecule-1
PF	platelet factor
PG(s)	prostaglandin(s)
PGA2	prostaglandin A2
PGD2	prostaglandin D2
PGE1	prostaglandin E1
PGE2	prostaglandin E2
PGF2-alpha	prostaglandin F2-alpha
PGG2	prostaglandin G2
PGH2	prostaglandin H2
PGI2	prostaglandin I2, prostacyclin
Phe	phenylalanine
PICP	procollagen I C-terminal propeptide
PINP	procollagen I N-terminal propeptide
PK	pyruvate kinase
PL	phospholipids
PLP	pyridoxal phosphate
PLT	platelets
PMN	polymorphonuclear leukocytes
pO$_2$	partial pressure of oxygen
POMC	proopiomelanocortin
PP	pancreatic polypeptide
PRA	plasma renin activity
PRIH	prolactin-release inhibiting hormone
PRL	prolactin

Pro	proline
PSA	prostate-specific antigen
PSG	pepsinogen
PT (PCT)	prothrombin time (prothrombin consumption time)
PTCA	percutaneous transluminal coronary angioplasty
PTH	parathormone
PTHrP	parathormone related protein
PTT	partial thromboplastin time
PZP	pregnancy zone protein
RAC	respiratory acidosis
RAL	respiratory alkalosis
RANA (RANAb)	rheumatoid-associated nuclear antigen, antirheumatoid arthritis nuclear antigen antibodies
RANTES	regulated on activation, normal T-cell expressed and secreted, beta chemokin
RAST	radioallergosorbent analysis
RBC	red blood cells
RBP	retinol-binding protein
RIA	radioimmunologic analysis, radioimmunoassay
RIST	radioimmunosorbent analysis
RF	rheumatoid factor
RIF	release-inhibiting factor
RMSF Ab	Rocky Mountain spotted fever antibodies
RNA	ribonucleic acid
RPTA	renal percutaneous transluminal angioplasty
rT3	reverse triiodothyronine
RTC	reticulocytes
SAA	serum amyloid A
SACE	serum angiotensin converting enzyme
SBG	sterkobilinogen
SCCA	squamous cell carcinoma antigen
SCF	stem cell factor
SD (SDH)	sorbitol dehydrogenase
SDF-1	stromal cell-derived factor-1
Se	selen, selenium
Ser	serine
sGM-CSFR	soluble granulocyte macrophage colony stimulating factor receptor
SGPT	serum glutamic-pyruvic transaminase
SHBG	sex hormone binding globulin
sIL-2R	soluble interleukin 2 receptor
sIL-6R	soluble interleukin 6 receptor
sLA	soluble liver antigen
Sm-C	somatomedin C
SOD	superoxide dismutase
SRSA	slow-reacting substance of anaphylaxis
sTfR	soluble transferrin receptor
STH (GH)	somatotropic hormone, somatotropin, growth hormone
StMA (StMAb)	anti-striated muscle antibodies
T3	triiodothyronine
T4	thyroxine

TAA	tumor-associated antigen
TAF	tumor angiogenesis factors
TAG	triacylglycerols
TAM	tumor-associated macrophages
TATA	tumor-associated transplantation antigen
Tau	taurine
TBG	thyroxine-binding globulin
TBPA	thyroxine-binding prealbumin
TC	transcobalamin
TCGF	T-cell growth factor
TCR	T-cell receptor
TCT	thyrocalcitonin
TdT	terminal deoxynucleotidyl transferase
TeBG	testosterone-binding globulin
Tf	transferrin
TF	transfer factor
Tg	thyroglobulin
TG	thromboglobulin, (triglycerides)
TGF	transforming growth factor
TGT	thromboplastin generation time
THF	thymic humoral factor
T_H-lym	T-helper lymphocytes
Thr	threonine
TIBC	total iron-binding capacity
TIMP	tissue inhibitor of metalloproteinases
Tl	thallium
T-lym	T-lymphocytes
TM	tumor marker/s
TNF	tumor necrosis factor
TPA	tissue polypeptide antigen
tPA	tissue plasminogen activator
TPO	thrombopoietin
TPOA	antithyroid peroxidase antibodies
TPS	tissue polypeptide substance
TRH	thyrotropin releasing hormone, thyroliberin
Trp	tryptophan
TSH	thyroid-stimulating hormone, thyrotropin
TSI	thyroid-stimulating immunoglobulin
Ts-lym	T-supressor lymphocytes
TT	thrombin time
TT3	total triiodothyronine
TT4	total thyroxine
TTR	transthyretin
TXA2	thromboxane A2
Tyr	tyrosine
U	urine
UBBC	unsaturated vitamin B_{12}-binding capacity
UBG	urobilinogen
UDPGT	uridine diphosphate glucuronyl transferase
Val	valine
VCA	viral capsid antigen

VCAM	vascular cell adhesion molecule
VDBP	vitamin D-binding protein
VDRL	veneral disease research laboratory
VEGF	vascular endothelial growth factor
VIP	vasoactive intestinal polypetide
VLA-3	very large antigen 3
VLA-4	very late activation antigen 4
VLDL-C	very-low density lipoprotein cholesterol
VMA	vanilmandelic acid
VPF	vascular permeability factor
vWf	von Willebrand's factor
VZV	varicella–zoster virus
WBC	white blood cells, leukocytes
Zn	zinc
ZPP	zinc protoporphyrin

Introduction to Laboratory Medicine

V. Marks, T. Cantor, R. Pullmann, D. Mesko

The essential feature of basic laboratory medicine is reliability that is achieved through a system of controls that include internal/external quality assessment, laboratory competency and certification.

A laboratory test that will lead to a correct clinical diagnosis begins with the appropriate test selection → a clear written order and specimen/test specifications → patient preparation → specimen acquisition → sample delivery → specimen preparation → specimen processing – laboratory analysis (measurement + calculations) → results reporting and interpretation.

Laboratory tests usually are ordered: 1) to confirm a clinical impression, to discover an occult disease or to make a diagnosis (e.g. blood glucose for diabetes mellitus, hemoglobin for anemia), 2) to prevent irreparable damage (e.g. phenylalanine screening to prevent phenylketonuria), 3) to determine the disease stage (e.g. amylase activity in pancreatitis, or tumor markers in cancer follow-up), 4) to rule out a condition, disease or diagnosis (e.g. beta-hCG – pregnancy test to rule out an ectopic pregnancy or to provide amylase activity in acute abdominal pain with negative test values), 5) to provide differential diagnosis of various possible diseases, 6) to provide prognostic and disease activity information (e.g. aspartate aminotransferase and alanine aminotransferase serum levels to determine liver injury severity), 7) to guide and monitor therapy (e.g. prothrombin time prolongation in anticoagulation therapy, medicament concentration determination), 8) to screen for and prevent disease, 9) to aid in genetic counseling in familial conditions, 10) to manage and monitor disease progression, including determining the long-term risk, recurrence, prognosis and therapy, 11) to detect disease complications, 12) to provide epidemiologic information, 13) to provide forensic information for medico-legal problems (e.g. to detect semen on the body/clothing in suspected rape or elsewhere at a crime scene), 14) to provide information for scientific-research activities, including the establishment of disease management guidelines, 15) to improve understanding of disease, 16) to provide information for quality assurance and audit purposes.

Before a test is ordered, particular regard should be given to Asher's criteria: 1) why do I order this test, 2) what am I going to look for in the results, 3) if I find it, will it affect my diagnosis, therapy, 4) how will this affect my management of the case, 5) will this ultimately benefit the patient?

The ever increasing range of laboratory investigations for diagnosis, differential diagnosis and treatment of disease must be kept in mind. The state of the art clinician should use important resources to practice scientifically sound, evidence based medicine. It is not possible for the clinician to be knowledgeable in all aspects of laboratory investigations, but some basic concepts are important if laboratory medicine is to be scientific and cost effective in patient care.

Uncertainty is an unfortunate inherent part of health care provision, mainly in the area of diagnostic process and procedures, a concept which also needs to be understood and accepted by patients, their relatives, the community, lawyers, insurance companies, bureaucrats and politicians. It is the role of good laboratory medicine to recommend the appropriate test to order, competently perform the test and carefully interpret the results in order to reduce this clinical uncertainty. It is particularly important for the clinician to realize the limitations of laboratory tests (including reasons for false positives and false negatives) to not inappropriately over-rely on test results.

Laboratory tests have greater specificity and sensitivity than the physical examination for many disorders. But there is no test that is 100% sensitive or specific. A negative test result does not necessarily rule out a clinical condition. The good diagnostician performs the appropriate test with competence, on the right patient, at the right time, in the right lab and knows what to do with the result. But the test can only be as good as the gold standard, not better.

Pre-Test Analytic Phase

Pre-Analytic Phase
- The correct test selection for diagnosis, therapy and prevention. The good test means – the results should be accurate, precise, timely and easily available. The test should discriminate disease from non-disease condition. The results should be interpretable and practicable, providing a clear course of follow up action. The test should offer maximum useful information at minimum cost and minimal potential for harm.
- Test order specifying when results are required.
- Patient preparation including advising. The preparation aim/goal is informed/co-operating patient consent (ethical criteria).
- Specimen sampling and material handling (specified sampling containers, controlled sample storage, confirmed labeling, transport to laboratory under correct temperature conditions). Blood samples must be collected with the minimum of correct and patient trauma and venous stasis. Testing accuracy is inherently dependent upon careful attention to the collection technique, sample storage, and specimen preparation. Precise practice ensures the safety of individuals sampling/transporting/receiving specimens to avoid degradation of analyte, leakage or breakage during specimen transition from patient to laboratory.

Basic Rules
- do not routinely order laboratory tests without a good reason
- know the proper choice/order of tests and the implication of individual/population/diagnosis related reference values/ranges
- know the testing purpose (especially the suspected clinical condition), procedures, special methods and abbreviations used
- know the admission test results
- clinical strategy is developed or modified on the basis of the test results
- know institutional policy about appropriate reporting and filling of results (e.g. patient privacy)
- know how to easily and quickly retrieve diagnostic information from the charts
- first review the most recent laboratory data to determine the current status, then work backward in the chart to note trends to track disease progression
- state the disease probability before ordering laboratory tests and interpret the results accordingly
- minimalize the risk of false-positive results by restricting screening tests in patients with risk factors or other findings, which can increase the probability of disease

- restrict the use of screening tests in these situations – if it is important to reveal a disease, if it is needed to immediately start therapy, if the test has high sensitivity and specificity and if it is possible to distinguish false-positive results from truly positive results or false-negative results from truly negative results
- question yourself, if test results will not influence your diagnostic algorithm or therapy, do not order the test.

Proper Patient Preparation

After obtaining his/her consent (a signed consent is best). How well the patient is prepared may well affect the test outcomes. Educate the patient and family about the tests. The patient needs both sensory and objective information about the test purpose and procedure. Sensory information helps interpret a situation that is completely different from anything he/she has experienced in the past. Sensation reactions during the tests should be discussed with the patient, then the person is less apt to misinterpret.

Patient Preparation Advice

- Explain what the test/procedure detects/evaluates and why the test was ordered/what you expect from the test (e.g. the test helps determine the salt and water balance in the body or the test assesses the fluid space around the lungs if pleural fluid analysis is needed).
- If needed, inform him/her about the test itself, by whom and when will the test be performed, where will it take place and approximately how much time the procedure will take (e.g. tumor marker analysis).
- If needed, explain, that some other studies may precede the actual test (e.g. chest radiography to help locate fluid in pleural cavity before pleural puncture).
- If needed, explain the test technique (e.g. the gastric acid stimulation test requires passing a tube through the nose, into the stomach and giving a pentagastrin subcutaneous injection).
- If possible/needed, withhold drugs before the test (e.g. in the aspartate aminotransferase testing codeine, methyldopa).
- If needed, warn, that he/she may feel some sensations during some procedures (e.g. sting, when anesthetic is injected).
- If needed, ask him/her not to cough, breathe deeply or move.
- Inform when he/she should/should not maintain normal/special diet or about any restrictions (e.g. rhubarb and spinach 1 week before urine oxalate examination; meat restriction in some urine samples, e.g. in osteoporosis).
- Inform when he/she needs/need not restrict fluids (e.g. restrict fluids 8 hours before the basal gastric secretion test).
- If needed, inform him/her about other restrictions (e.g. smoking, drinking alcohol).
- Tell him/her if the test requires sample collection (e.g. urine), and if the specimen is to be collected at home, instruct the patient on proper collection techniques, and tell the patient not to contaminate the specimen (e.g. with toilet tissue, stool).
- If needed, advise him/her that strenuous physical exercise before test/collecting period should be avoided (e.g. in the urine creatinine evaluation).
- If needed, encourage him/her to be as active as possible before test (e.g. microalbuminuria, calcium/phosphates examination in urine).
- Tell the patient when the results will be generally available, if needed provide psychological support to alleviate anxiety and assure him/her that complications are rare (e.g. in screening/prenatal diagnosis examinations).

- If needed, inform the patient what the procedure will influence (e.g. peritoneal fluid evacuation will relieve his/her discomfort and allow him/her to breathe more easily).
- If needed, tell the patient that normal test results cannot guarantee normal health condition (e.g. a normal fetus because some fetal disorders are undetectable; screening method restriction).

Proper Activity Co-ordination
- Co-ordinate patient activities and testing to avoid conflicts with meal times, medications, lengthy treatments and other diagnostic tests.
- Be ever aware of patients who are not allowed to receive anything orally.
- Take action to minimize stress and anxiety, fear, nausea and vomiting.

Correct Procedures
- Correctly order test. Requests should be submitted on appropriate forms, information should be complete, accurate and legible (date, collection time, full patient identification, sex, birth date, full identification of physician and department should be noted, kind of material, specimen type and site, clinic/provisional diagnosis and medicaments used – antibiotics, investigations required, urgency of investigation, address of the facility to which the results will be sent). Follow the formal insurance company requirements properly.
- Label if the sample carries a high risk of infection.
- Ensure that all specimens are dependably handled, labeled and delivered to the appropriate departments.
- Make it part of your regular reliable algorithm check during pre-analytic phase.

Analytic Test Phase

Analytic Phase
- Sample laboratory processing including pipetting and storage.
- Examination of the materials for both the sample and proper control groups.

Universally blood and certain body fluids/secretions are considered biohazardous and potentially infectious, i.e. of Human Immunodeficiency Virus (HIV), hepatitis viruses, Epstein-Barr virus, cytomegalovirus, oncogenic viruses, Helicobacter pylori and other blood-borne pathogens.

General Rules for Infectious Diseases Prevention During Sampling
- Each biological material must be considered as potentially dangerous.
- Infection entrance site is usually impaired/unimpaired skin or the oral and ocular mucous membranes.
- Be careful when sampling (where it is possible use gloves, sometimes necessary).
- Be careful when opening/shaking samples (aerosol creation).
- Never perform mouth pipetting and never blow out pipettes.
- Do not mix potentially infectious material by bubbling air through the liquid.
- Always wash hands or use antiseptic hand cleaner after/between sampling.
- It is forbidden to eat/drink/smoke during sampling/handling specimens.
- Facial protection should be used if there is significant chance of blood or body fluids spattering.
- Try to prevent accidental injuries.
- Keep your hands away from your mouth, nose, eyes and any other mucous membranes, this will reduce the possibility of self-inoculation.

- Never leave discarded tubes or infected materials open, unattended or unlabeled.
- Do not speak in open-system sampling.

Investigations are performed to reduce uncertainty of diagnostic process, but ultimately a final diagnosis may not be definitive, nor can disease always be excluded. Individuals with disease may not be totally separable from individuals without disease. To be a successful diagnostician, appreciation of uncertainty, its quantitation, reduction and communication is basic. It does not matter how skillfully specimens are requested and obtained for diagnosis, if they are not appropriately transported and studied in the laboratory, the whole process is pointless.

   Many patient factors may affect/interfere with accurate test results: age, race, sex, environment, posture, diurnal, cyclic biorhythms and other chronobiologic influences, diet preparation, current illness, plasma volume, fasting or postprandial state (non-fasting, time since patient ate last, recent food ingestion), foods eaten, current drug history, position/activity at the time a specimen was obtained, level of exercise/physical fitness, pregnancy, stress, smoking, sampling time, temperature of body/environment, seasonal cycles, nourishment, menstruation, menopause, pregnancy, lactation and somatotype.
Each laboratory result is loaded with some variability regarding clinical reliability.

Sources of variability

Erroneous results (laboratory error) can be caused by: the venipuncture technique, prolonged tourniquet application, incorrect specimen collection/handling/storage and transport temperature, insufficient specimen quantity, improper tube sequencing, analyzing a specimen from the wrong patient, wrong preservative/fixative or lack of the necessary preservative, culture media, ice – refrigeration, delayed specimen delivery to the laboratory (old specimens may contain destroyed cells and may increase/decrease test results), incorrect/incomplete patient preparation or collection, inaccurate 24 hour urine specimen collection, concentration variations of the randomly collected urine specimen, blood sample hemolysis, inappropriate anticoagulant addition, contaminated glassware/other apparatus, specimen mislabeling, delayed specimen processing/analyzing in the laboratory, inappropriate laboratory processing (human/machine error), use of expired or contaminated test reagents, sample contamination, transcriptional mistakes, incorrect test or calculation, manual vs. automated processing, hardcopy vs. verbal report, (patient is a victim of statistics).

Causes of possible abnormal results (interfering factors) – examples
- **Hospitalization/immobilization – serum/plasma:** ↑ HCT, CK (early), ↓ plasma volume, proteins, albumin, AST, CK (later), K. Urine: ↑ Ca, Na, K, P, ↓ H$^+$
- **Exercise:** 1) moderate – serum/plasma: ↑ G, lactate, creatinine, uric acid, AST, LD, CK, aldolase, urea, ↓ pH, pCO_2, cholesterol, TG, 2) strenuous: ↑ glycoproteins, transferrin, alpha-2-macroglobulin, fibrinolytic activity, plasma renin activity, cortisol, chloride, ACP, ALT, aldosterone, GH, PRL, catecholamines, FFA, creatinine, urea, ↓ albumin, bilirubin, Fe, LD, K, Na, total lipids. Urine: ↑ free cortisol, catecholamines, pH
- **Circadian variation:**
  - AM > PM – serum/plasma: K, cortisol, PRA, TSH, insulin. Urine: volume, creatinine
  - AM < noon – urine: 17-KS, 17-OHCS, catecholamines
  - PM > AM – serum/plasma: testosterone, prolactin, GH. Urine: Ca, Mg
  - noon > AM – urine: K, Na
- **Recent food ingestion – serum/plasma:** ↑ ALT, AST, G, P, K, uric acid
- **Seasonal effect:**
  - spring – serum/plasma: ↑ AST, TG, ↓ ALT, G, thyroidal hormones, urea
  - summer – serum/plasma: ↑ creatinine, LD, uric acid, ↓ ALT, albumin, urea

- fall – serum/plasma: ↑ albumin, Ca, G, urea, ↓ AST, TG
- winter – serum/plasma: ↑ ALT, ↓ Ca, creatinine, LD, uric acid, total antioxidants
■ **Vegetarianism – serum/plasma:** ↑ Bil, ↓ LDL-C, VLDL-C, total lipids, phospholipids, cholesterol, TAG, vitamin B_{12}, Ca, G, Hb, urea, uric acid, methylmalonic acid. Urine: ↓ pH
■ **Starvation – serum/plasma:** ↑ aldosterone, ↓ K, Mg, Ca, P, T3. Urine: ↑ K, Mg, Ca
■ **Medications/herbal remedies/vitamins**

During pregnancy the following abnormal blood test results may occur – examples

Increased Values
alkaline phosphatase (from the placenta from 4th month to 4th week postpartum), glucose (intolerance caused by ovarian and placental hormones), chloride (through bicarbonate decrease secondary to respiratory alkalosis especially during labor), cholesterol (through increased hepatic synthesis), creatine kinase (during last weeks of pregnancy), lactate dehydrogenase, leukocytes (late pregnancy, labor), erythrocyte sedimentation rate (from the third month to 3rd week postpartum because of increased fibrinogen)

Decreased Values
albumin (expanded intravascular space), AST (by pyridoxine decrease levels during pregnancy), bicarbonate (respiratory alkalosis), phosphorus, hemoglobin/hematocrit (by increased plasma volume that can be aggravated by iron deficiency anemia), creatine kinase (from 8th to 12th week), creatinine, pCO_2 (respiratory alkalosis during uterus enlargement and a stimulated respiration by pregnancy hormones), natrium (expanded intravascular space), urea (expanded intravascular space and increased glomerular filtration), calcium (insufficient calcium, phosphorus and vitamin D intake)

Other factors: drugs/medicaments used, growing child, pregnancy, alcohol, smoking, unrecognized disease.

Errors in ordering and interpretation of laboratory tests can include
■ incorrect selection of laboratory tests
■ frequent ordering/misuse of statim tests
■ ordering of laboratory tests without looking at the previous test results
■ unnecessary duplication of laboratory testing
■ forgetting indicated laboratory test
■ inability to distinguish between the test profit for the patient and clinical interest
■ inability to link test results to a clinical condition
■ frequent repetition of entrance and monitoring test sets
■ inability to evaluate clinical meaning of positive/negative/abnormal test result correctly
■ inability to determine and to interpret the false-positive/negative test results
■ inability to state a working diagnosis correctly and then choose the most appropriate economical advantageous test for confirmation/elimination (e.g. molecular diagnosis method misuse)
■ inability to evaluate the possible risks after diagnosis determination on the basis of laboratory test results
■ incorrect clinical examinations leading to laboratory test results misinterpretation
■ incorrect determination of a non-existing disease, based on an isolated non-specific laboratory test

Reference ranges

Reference ranges are customarily defined as limits within 2 standard deviations from the mean, thus some results in healthy individuals (about 2.5%) are either above or below the normal range in the absence of disease. Reference ranges vary from lab to another one. They represent collected statistical data based upon the statistical definition of normal as 95% range of values. Values outside of these ranges do not necessarily mean disease. By convention, limits are determined by assuming an underlying gaussian distribution even though this often is not the case. How the clinicians cope with "error" (or abnormal test results from a healthy individual) is to repeat the test or doubled result reliability (the reliability is increased 1.4-times in other sample examination e.g. with other name use).

Precision of the test tells us into what range the test will fall if repeated by the same method in the same laboratory on the same sample, i.e. the standard deviation of a series of repeated measurements. This random scattering from the true value is referred to random error.

Reference values can vary with the collection method employed/laboratory/conditions and specimen storage/preservation/transport. Influences include: 1) reference population and how it was chosen, 2) the environmental and physiological conditions under which the specimens were obtained, 3) the specimen collection techniques, timing, transport, preparation and storage, 4) analytical methods i.e. specificity, precision and standardization, 5) data collection and methods used to derive the reference range.

So-called diagnosis-related reference ranges also exist (e.g. cholesterol, TAG, Apo in patients with hereditary hyperlipoproteinemia, minerals in non-treated patients with osteoporosis). From the point of clinical usage these values are well comparable with population reference range in relatively big diagnosis group. There are also recommended reference ranges/limits as a professional consensus result, which are the results of other theoretical bases (e.g. WHO, EASD, world society for atherosclerosis recommendations); they define desired limits quite often without age/sex stratification.

It is recommended to use so-called critical difference in result evaluation which can be reached in co-operation with laboratory; a calculation depends on method variation coefficient which is used in particular laboratory.

Post-Test Phase

Post-Test Phase
- Results processing.
- Analytic and medical findings check – longitudinal/transversal evaluation, extreme value/trend check.
- Test results formulation/release and implementation into patient chart.
- Findings interpretation (both positive and negative) connected with clinical picture, decision making.

Post-Test Care

The primary-care physician needs to be alert to critical laboratory test values that have immediate life threatening significance to the patient.

As long as the result is accurate and precise the further interpretation of the result, in terms of its predictive value in diagnosing disease, rests with the clinician. It can thus be seen, that the likelihood of an abnormal laboratory result being clinically significant, increases or decreases when interpreted in the light of the clinical information. "Abnormal" multiple test results are more likely to be significant than single test result abnormality.

What is a "normal" result of a test? 1) qualitative normality – when the parameter/s in question cannot be quantified with any degree of objective accuracy, the result is dependent on the observer's opinion and subjective and observer dependent. As most disease is a continuum from "not got it yet" to "got it real bad", the point in time at which the diagnosis is made depends on numerous other factors than just observations at one point of time. 2) quantitative normality – when the result of the investigation can be numerically quantitated, the interpretation of normality depends on statistics and the knowledge of a reference range which may or may not be appropriate to the patient in question. Clinically significant test result which represents a real condition/disease is frequently based on the greater abnormality degree of a test result. 3) molecular normality – is absolute and statistical methods are not needed for interpretation. Unfortunately, molecular biology is not the hoped „gold standard" in diagnosis. Not only do the techniques require a high level of laboratory quality control, but many so called molecular abnormalities do not represent disease and may only be a manifestation of genetic polymorphism or insignificant mutations. Detection of molecular abnormalities in the diagnosis of disease are most valuable when the disease entity has been confirmed or there is compelling evidence. Such diseases usually have a single gene abnormality (e.g. hemochromatosis, cystic fibrosis) and in such circumstances the molecular tests are no so much of value in the diagnosing the patient in question but for genetic screening and antenatal diagnosis. In other diseases which have multifactorial pathogenesis (e.g. malignancy, vascular disease) molecular biology is only one of the tools for identifying patients with disease and risk groups for disease.

It is important to recognize the accuracy of the test. Accuracy is the measure of how close the result is to the true value as determined by comparison with known reference standard. A test with poor accuracy is one in which there is a systematic deviation from the true value, referred to as bias. The predictive value of a positive test is the percentage of all positive results that represent disease. The predictive value of negative test is the percentage of all negative results that exclude disease. The predictive value of a test is determined by the sensitivity, the specificity and the prevalence of the disease in the population tested.

It is important to recognize abnormal test results, the meaning and the possible effects on the patient and to distinguish test results that are markedly abnormal from those that are minimally abnormal. Recognize false-positive and false-negative results. If the disease seems to be highly improbable, the positive test result is usually false-positive, if the disease seems highly probable, the negative test result is usually false-negative. To eliminate the disease, negative test results with high sensitivity are needed, i.e. with a low false-negative results frequency. To confirm the disease, positive test results with a high specificity are needed, i.e. with a low false-positive results frequency. The most sensitive tests are used to rule out a suspected condition/disease. If the test result interpretation requires other laboratory tests, consider if the test is sensitive for presymptomatic or minimally symptomatic patients. The sensitivity is "inversely" related to specificity, i.e. the more likely a test is to detect patients with the disease, the more likely is it to produce false positives in patients without disease. The most specific tests are used to confirm a suspected condition/disease. Sensitivity measures the capacity of a test to identify people with disease, i.e. the percentage of patients with disease who have a positive test. Specificity measures the capacity of a test to identify people who do not have the disease, i.e. the percentage of patients without the disease having a negative test. Also consider, how often the test results can be false-positive in patients with other diseases manifesting similar symptoms, especially in very similar diseases. A healthy person with a false-positive test results has been called the Ulysses syndrome, like Ulysses, the patient must pass through a long investigative journey before returning to the previous health state. A slightly abnormal test result which does not fit with the patient's clinical condition and other laboratory findings, may represent a statistical outlier that lies just outside the reference range (more than 2 but less than 3 standard deviations) and may be ignored. The effective use of laboratory data can be understood only in the context of the clinical decisions which are influenced.

The likelihood of the patient having the disease in question is known as the pre-test probability of disease. Following the performance of the investigations the results will either support or refute the diagnosis by raising or lowering probability, resulting in post-test probability of disease.

Test results in the elderly must be evaluated and interpreted carefully taking into account some specific factors (aging, age based biological variability, atypical symptoms/signs, chronic multimorbidity, chronic multimedication).

Document the diagnostic process. The physician is the responsible person he/she must inform the patient of a serious disease diagnosis. Be able to wisely use crisis intervention skills if findings indicate a very serious disease.

A general approach for verifying unexplained laboratory results

Check the pre-analytic phase. Consider possible interferences. Repeat the measurement if needed.

- Prepare the patient properly.
- Obtain a proper sample.
- Ensure correct and appropriate specimen handling.
- Use the best laboratory method available.
- Use the proper reference range/critical difference for the age and sex of the patient.
- Repeat the measurement.

Biological materials

Blood, urine, cerebrospinal fluid, sputum, stool, synovial fluid, cavitary fluids – (amniotic, ascitic = peritoneal, pericardial, pleural), gastroenteric fluid, biopsy specimens, breast milk, smear – (fistulas, genitals, throat, lesions, nose, wound, conjunction), sweat, secretions – (nasal, saliva, tears, spermatic, vaginal), tissues, hair, nails, broncho-alveolar lavage fluid, vomitus.

Blood – Plasma – Serum

Full native blood = blood cells + plasma (serum after coagulation = cellular elements clotting).

Collection procedures – blood sampling

- arterial → artery puncture
- venous → venipuncture (usually from v. cubiti) with syringe, evacuated blood tube, or i.v. line
- capillary → skin puncture (fingerprick, pricking of the skin):
  - arterialized from the finger-tip or from the ear-lobe in adults
  - from the great toe or heel in infants under 1 year old
  - from the finger-tip in infants over 1 year old

Precautions

Never draw blood for any laboratory test from the same extremity that is being used for i.v. medications, i.v. fluids or blood. If difficulty is encountered in obtaining blood, slightly warm the extremity and allow it to remain in a hanging position for some time. Avoid intensive extremity exercise, extreme warm-up, squeezing and intensive finger-belly massage to obtain blood, because doing this will alter the blood composition (misinterpretation of results). Pumping the fist before venipuncture → causes e.g. ↑ K, P, lactate concentrations, ↓ Ca concentration.

Sampling
■ Patient usually should be fasting.
■ Blood
  ■ → coagulated
  ■ → uncoagulated – with anticoagulants (oxalates, citrates, heparin)
■ Draw sufficient blood with the indicated anticoagulant to yield the required volume of plasma.
■ Specimens containing a preservative should be mixed thoroughly.
■ Avoid hemolysis, if possible, as some tests are invalidated by hemolysis.

Basic sampling rules
■ The blood sampling usually following fasting (8–12 hours).
■ Exception: water is usually permitted as desired.

Infusion Therapy and Biological Material Sampling

Infusion type	Time between infusion end and sampling (hours)
electrolytes	1
saccharides	1
amino acids and hydrolyzates	1
protein	1–1.5
fat emulsions	7–8

Additives and Anticoagulant Character and Colour Code for Blood Containers

Colour	Character	Additive	Note
lavender	KE	K₂EDTA	routine hematological work
	NE	Na₂EDTA	
blue	9NC (I)	Na₃citrate	(blood : anticoagulant 9:1) blood coagulation
black	4NC (I)	Na₃citrate	(blood : anticoagulant 4:1) ESR
gray	FX	fluoride/oxalate	glucose, ethanol
green	NH	natrium heparinate ammonium heparinate	plasma chemistry
green LH		lithium heparinate	routine chemistry, electrolytes
	AKX	ammonium/potassium oxalate	
jeltoro yellow	ACD	citric acid (dextrose)	blood transfusion purpose
red	Z	no additives	routine chemistry
red/black	S	medium for serum isolation	
red/gray		medium for serum isolation	

Note: above mentioned colours are valid for Becton-Dickinson → system (Vacutainer →) which can be different from other systems (e.g. Sarstedt).

Blood Storage Sampled to K₂EDTA and Blood Count Parameters (1.5 mg EDTA/ml blood)

Temperature	hours	Examination
room	2	blood count, differential count, platelets, glucose
room	8	leukocytes, erythrocytes
2–8 °C	24	hemoglobin, hematocrit

Concentration Gradient Erythrocytes: Plasma

Parameter	Coefficient
iron	550
LD	160
ACP	67
potassium	24
AST	20
ALT	5
Mg	2.5
urea	1.5
glucose, cholesterol, uric acid, chloride	1.1
Na, Ca, P, triacylglycerols	1.03

Differences Between Serum and Plasma Analyte Levels

■ **No differences:** ALT, Bi, Ca, CK, pCO₂, urea
■ **Serum<Plasma:** albumin, ALP, glucose, uric acid, Na, phosphate, proteins, triacylglycerols
■ **Serum>Plasma:** aldosterone, AST, Cu, coagulation factors, hemoglobin, K, LD, ACP

Because plasma and serum contain about 92–93 % water when compared to blood, plasma and serum analyte concentrations are about 10–12% higher.

Differences Between Capillary and Venous Blood (capillary blood = 100%)

Parameter	Differences	%	SI
free hemoglobin	400	4	
pO₂	350	3.5	
thrombocytes	125	1.25	
potassium	95	0.95	
calcium	95	0.95	
protein	90–92	0.90–0.92	
bilirubin	90–92	0.90–0.92	
lactate dehydrogenase	90–92	0.90–0.92	
pH	90–92	0.90–0.92	
cholesterol	90–92	0.90–0.92	
triacylglycerols	90–92	0.90–0.92	
glucose	90–92	0.90–0.92	
pCO₂	85	0.85	
lactate	50	0.50	
ammonia	50	0.50	

Organ-Associated Enzymes – Examples

- **liver:** 1) conjugation and liver transport of organic anions testing: total + direct bilirubin, bilirubin – urine, urobilinogen – urine, 2) hepatocytes injury markers: AST, ALT, glutathione-S-transferase, LD, LD5, 3) biliary ways obstruction markers: ALP, GMT, 5'-nucleotidase, leucine aminopeptidase, lipoprotein X, 4) liver synthesis function markers: albumin, prealbumin, cholinesterase, lecithin-cholesterol acyltransferase, prothrombin time, partial prothrombin time
- **heart:** CK-MB, LD1,2
- **skeletal muscle:** aldolase, CK-MM, LD5
- **bone:** ALP (+ isoenzyme), acid ACP
- **prostate:** ACP
- **pancreas:** AMS (+ isoenzyme), lipase, elastase
- **brain:** CK-BB
- **granulocytes:** PMN-elastase
- **lungs:** ACE

Interference of Diagnostic and Therapeutic Procedures

Intervention	Parameter	Note	
Allergyc diagnostics	eosinophils	↑	
	granulocytes	↑	
Blood (sampling)	reticulocytes	↑	
	iron	↓	
Blood transfusion	hematocrit	↑↑	
	hemoglobin		
	potassium		
Dialysis	proteins of acute phase	↑	
	glucose	↓	
	amino acids	↓	
	leukocytes	↓↑	
Ergometry	creatine kinase	↑	CK-MB
	myoglobin	↑↑	
ERCP	amylase	↑↑	3–8 x (within 48 hrs)
	lipase	↑↑	12 x (within 72 hrs)
Endoscopic rectoscopy	occult blood	↑	
Oral glucose tolerance test	insulin	↑↑	
	C-peptide	↑	
	potassium, magnesium	↑	
	natrium, calcium	↓	
	pyruvate	↑	
	phosphorus/phosphate	↑	
Ionization	malone dialdehyde	↑	
	uric acid	↑	
	leukocytes	↓	
	thrombocytes	↓	
Labor (cesarean section)	creatine kinase	↑	2 days
	myoglobin	↑	
	troponin T	↑	

Intervention	Parameter	Note	
Breast palpation	prolactin	↑	10 x
Prostate palpation (puncture)			
	prostate specific antigen	↑	1–2 days
	prostatic acid phosphatase	↑	
	chromogranin A	↑	
Injection/needle biopsy	aspartate aminotransferase	↑	
(also laparoscopy, puncture)	creatine kinase	↑	
	myoglobin	↑	
	haptoglobin	↑	
	fibrinogen	↑	
	lactate dehydrogenase	↑	
	C-reactive protein	↑	
Surgery	acute phase proteins	↑	depends on localization/
	(CRP, haptoglobin)	↑	extent/duration
	aspartate aminotransferase	↑	AST > ALT
	alanine aminotransferase	↑	
	lactate dehydrogenase	↑	
	aldosterone	↑	
	prolactin	↑	
	plasma renin activity	↑	
	alpha-2-globulins (ELPHO)	↑	2–5 x
	bilirubin	↑	
	creatine kinase	↑	
	ESR	↑	
	free fatty acids	↑	
	fibrinogen	↑	
	uric acid	↑	
	urea	↑	surgery extent
	lactate	↑	
	myoglobin	↑	
	leukocytes	↑	
	non-protein nitrogen	↑	
	albumin	↓	
	hematocrit	↓	
	hemoglobin	↓	mostly with
	beta globulins	↓	normal creatinine
	transferrin	↓	
	plasminogen	↓	
Resuscitation	pH	↓	
	pO_2	↓	
	pCO_2	↑	
	BE	↓	
	HCO_3^-	↓	
	lactate	↑	
	creatine kinase	↑	
	troponin T	↑	

Sex Differences in Some Analytes

Analyte	% (M > F)	SI
TAG	60 – 80	0.60 – 0.80
CK, GMT, ferritin	50 – 60	0.50 – 0.60
ALT, ALP, ammonia, iron (Fe), creatinine uric acid, ACP, urea aldolase, AST, cholinesterase, albumin, cholesterol,	30 – 40	0.30–0.40
erythrocytes (RBC)	10–15	0.10–0.15
Ca, phosphorus/phosphate	10	0.10

Analyte	% (F > M)	SI
ESR, HDL-C, copper, reticulocytes (RTC), TSH, prolactin (PRL)	20–25	0.20–0.25

Changes of Different Analytes During Pregnancy

Increase (%)	Decrease (%)
ALP (42), WBC (50), free fatty acids (50), cholesterol (63), triacyl-glycerols (100), leucine arylamidase (400), ceruloplasmin, transferrin, AFP, hCG, SP-1-GP, thyroxine (50), T3 (50), PSA, aldosterone (300), prolactin (2000)	calcium (5), erythrocytes (7), hemoglobin (8), hematocrit (8), total proteins (12), magnesium (16), iron (18), cholinesterase (21), albumin (10), ferritin, urea

Influence of Body Position on Parameters
(upright position > supine position)

Parameter	%	SI
alanine aminotransferase	+ 15	+ 0.15
apolipoprotein A-I	+ 15	+ 0.15
aldosterone	+ 15 – 50	+ 0.15–0.50
albumin	+ 10	+ 0.10
aspartate aminotransferase	+ 11	+ 0.11
acid phosphatase	+ 11	+ 0.11
alkaline phosphatase	+ 11	+ 0.11
apolipoprotein B	+ 11	+ 0.11
calcium	+ 4	+ 0.04
catecholamines (norepine-phrine)	+ 120	+ 1.2
cholesterol (LDL-C, HDL-C)	+ 8	+ 0.08
creatinine	+ 5	+ 0.05
erythrocytes	+ 5	+ 0.05
hemoglobin	+ 6	+ 0.06
hematocrit	+ 6	+ 0.06

Parameter	%	SI
iron	+ 7	+ 0.07
leukocytes	+ 8	+ 0.08
lipase	+ 9	+ 0.09
inorganic phosphorus/phosphate	+ 11	+ 0.11
plasma renin activity	+ 80 – 160	+ 0.8 – 1.6
protein total	+ 9	+ 0.09
T3, T4, FT4, FT3	+ 8 – 10	+ 0.08 – 0.10
immunoglobulin A, G	+ 7	+ 0.07
uric acid	– 4	– 0.04
triacylglycerols	+ 12 – 24	+ 0.12–0.24
chloride	+ 5	+ 0.05
bilirubin	+ 5	+ 0.05

Smoking and Analyte Levels

Parameter	%	SI
alkaline phosphatase	+	
amylase (secretin stimulation)	+	
carcinoembryonic antigen	+ 20–60	+ 0.20–0.60 + 100 and more (inductors)
C-reactive protein	+	
cholesterol	+ 2–5	+ 0.02–0.05
alpha-1-antitrypsin	+	
ceruloplasmin	+ 30–50	+ 0.30–0.50
copper	+ 20	+ 0.20
free fatty acids	+ 50–500	+ 0.50–5.00
haptoglobin	+	
glucose	+	
hemoglobin	+	
hematocrit	+ 5	
leukocytes	+ 30–40	+ 0.30–0.40
lipase (secretin stimulation)	+	
carboxyhemoglobin	+ 100–1500	+ 1.00–1500
endothelial PLT aggregation	+	
cadmium, lead	+ 30	+ 0.30
malone dialdehyde	+	
cAMP	+	
GIT hormones (e.g. insulin, gastrin)	+	
low-density lipoprotein cholesterol	+ 5	+ 0.05
fibrinogen	+ 15–20	+ 0.15–0.20
lymphocytes	+ 30	+ 0.30
lipoprotein (a)	– 40–60	– 0.40–0.60
angiotensin-converting enzyme	– 40–60	– 0.40–0.60
prolactin	– 20	– 0.20
beta-carotene	– 20	– 0.20
ascorbic acid	– 20	– 0.20

Parameter	%	SI
selen	– 10	– 0.10
high-density lipoprotein cholesterol	– 10	– 0.10
tocopherols	– 5	– 0.05
bilirubin	–	
triacylglycerols	–	
vitamin B_{12}	–	

Drug Biological Influence on Some Analytes

hashis-canabis	↑ Na, K, urea, chloride, insulin
	↓ creatinine, glucose, uric acid
heroin	↑ pCO_2, FT4, cholesterol, K, Mg
	↓ pO_2, albumin, TSH
morphine	↑ AMS, lipase, AST, ALT, bilirubin, ALP, gastrin, TSH, PRL
	↓ insulin, norepinephrine, neurotensin, chromogranin A
amphetamine	↑ VMK, catecholamines

Alcohol Biological Influence on Some Analytes

acute influence	↑ glucose, HCO_3^-, lactate, aldosterone (150%), triacyl-glycerols (30–50%), uric acid, osmolality
	↓ cholesterol (10%), ADH, cortisol, prolactin, osteocalcin, ANF (40–50%)
chronic influence	↑ GMT (1000%), AST (260%), catecholamines (200%), estradiol (50–80%), ALT, cortisol, MCV, triacylglycerols
	↓ LDL-C

Diurnal Variations of Some Analytes

	Maximum (hours)	Minimum (hours)	Amplitude (%)
ACTH	6–10	0–4	150–200
cortisol	5–8	21–30	180–200
testosterone	2–4	20–24	30–50
TSH	20–24	7–13	5–15
FT4	8–12	23–30	10–20
growth hormone	21–23	1–21	300–400
prolactin	5–7	10–12	80–100
aldosterone	2–4	12–14	60–80
plasma renin activity	0–6	10–12	120–140
epinephrine	9–12	2–5	30–50
norepinephrine	9–12	2–5	50–120
hemoglobin	6–18	22–24	8–15
eosinophils	4–6	18–20	30–40
iron	14–18	2–4	50–70
kalium	14–16	23–28	5–10
natrium	4–6	12–16	60–80
phosphorus/phosphates	2–4	8–12	30–40

Analyte Biological Half-Time

	Minutes	Hours	Days
Proteins			
albumin			19–20
alpha-1-antitrypsin			4–5
free haptoglobin			3
bound haptoglobin		3–5	
free hemopexin			3–7
bound hemopexin		3–7	
IgA			6
IgM			10
IgG			23–25
IgE			2
IgD			3
alpha-2-macroglobulin			5
transferrin			7
complement C3			1
complement C4			1
ceruloplasmin			7
CRP			2
alpha-fetoprotein			6
alpha-1-acid glycoprotein			5
myoglobin		15	
plasminogen			2.5
prealbumin			3
retinol-binding protein			8

	Minutes	Hours	Days
Enzymes			
ALT			2
AST		18	
ALP (bone, liver isoenzyme)			5
ALP (intestinal isoenzyme)		8	
AMS		10	
cholinesterase			10
creatine kinase CK-MB		12	
creatine kinase CK-MM		18	
creatine kinase CK-BB		5	
glutamate dehydrogenase		16	
GMT			3
LD1			5
LD5		10	
lipase		8	

	Minutes	Hours	Days
Substrates			
cholesterol		6	
chylomicrons	10		
VLDL	20		
LDL			3
ferritin	30		

	Minutes	Hours	Days
Hormones			
insulin	10		
prolactin	15		
growth hormone	25		
testosterone	4		
thyroxine			8
estrogens	5		
parathormone	15		
human placental			
lactogen	15		
ACTH	7–15		

Immunoassay Interference from Heterophilic Antibodies

Most immunoassays operate on the sandwich principle where a labelled antibody becomes indirectly bound to a solid phase (via a capture antibody or an affixed antigen) when the analyte forms the sandwich. Sandwich assays bring improved sensitivity and specificity, but they have the significant disadvantage of being susceptible to heterophilic antibody interference. Although, heterophilic antibodies can cause false negative interference the most typical observation of heterophilic antibody interference is a false positive. A false positive is defined as a laboratory result indicating that the analyte is present, although the analyte is not present. The most typical way in which a heterophilic antibody causes a false positive is by forming a sandwich by creating an "antibody-cross-bridge" between the capture antibody and the labelled antibody. Four obvious questions arise about false positive causing heterophilic antibodies: What is their prevalence? What causes them? How can they be identified? How can a correct test value be obtained?

The exact prevalence of heterophilic antibodies is difficult to determine. The College of American Pathologists has warned that more than 10% of patients may have heterophilic antibodies. A recent study using known heterophilic antibody containing samples found between 5% to 7% of immunoassays showed some interference. Good laboratory medicine cannot ignore the problem of heterophilic antibody false positive interference. Some individuals have developed heterophilic antibodies after they have experienced: rheumatoid arthritis, vaccinations, influenza, contact with animals, allergies, autoimmune diseases and severe bacterial infections. There are three basic methods to identify a false positive sample: the blocker method, the alternate assay method and the dilution recovery method. To use the blocker method, heterophilic antibody blockers (these are commercially available as mouse immunoglobulin or specific blockers) are added to the sample and it is re-assayed to see if the test value is different from the unblocked sample. Since heterophilic antibody interference is usually assay method specific the use of an alternate assay method may both identify a false positive sample and provide the correct test value. Since the test values of a diluted false positive sample will not be in linear correlation with the dilution factor, the dilution-recovery method is useful to identify a false positive. In this method the sample is diluted with an equal volume of the assay diluent (provided as part of the assay reagents) and the diluted sample is re-tested. If the diluted sample test value is not within 40%–60% of the undiluted sample test value then the sample test value is considered to be false and must be further assayed by alternate methods or by adding an adequate quantity of blockers. Whenever misdiagnosis or mistreatment have occurred it is not uncommon for the patient to blame the doctor for not confirming the diagnosis and for the doctor to blame the laboratory for giving the false test value and for the laboratory to blame the manufacturer of the test reagents for poor product quality and for the manufacturer to blame the patient for being part of an unusually rare part of society. The most common and unfortunate occurrences of mistreatment due to false positive test results occur for diseases without many symptoms as in cancer and cardiac disease. In these cases tumor marker and cardiac marker test results are heavily relied upon to base a diagnosis. Unfortunately, the mistreatment that can occur for cancer and cardiac disease can be serious for the patient. Therefore, good laboratory medicine is to be proactive to avoid misdiagnosis and mistreatment from false positive heterophilic antibody interference. This is part of the reason for the laboratory to work closely with the primary care physician so that together a diagnosis can be reached. This communication means that the laboratory must ask the primary care physician to advise the laboratory when a test result is not in agreement with other clinical indicators. Moreover, good laboratory medicine is to advise the primary care physician of test limitations, false positive heterophilic antibody interference possibility and options available for confirming test results that do not agree with other clinical indicators.

Examination Sets

Basic Biochemical Set (Screening)

Analyte	
urea	kidney
creatinine	
uric acid	purines, antioxidatives
ALT	liver
GMT	biliary ways
ALP	
AST	myocardium
LD	
cholesterol	lipid metabolism
TAG	
glucose	glycide metabolism
proteins	hydratation
albumin	proteosynthesis status
Ca	parathyroid, bone metabolism
phosphate	
mucoproteins	inflammatory activity
circulating immune complexes	
Urine:	urinary system, kidney
proteins	
blood	
pH	
leukocytes	

Preoperation and Postoperation Set
- **I – basic**
  - Hb, HCT, WBC, RBC, PLT, ESR, blood group, PTT, thrombin time, fibrinogen, HBsAg, glucose, proteins, creatinine, bilirubin, AST, GMT, cholesterol, Na, K, Cl, Ca
  - *Urine*: protein, blood, glucose, nitrites, urobilinogen
  - **endoscopy** – Quick time fibrinogen, thrombin time

- **II – enhanced**
  - ALT, AMS, CK, CRP, cholinesterase, osmolality, urea, ionized calcium, PO_4^- albumin, LDL-C, TAG, pH, pCO_2, pO_2, BE, HCO_3^- sat. O_2, BWR
  - *Urine*: creatinine, urea, Na, K, sediment
  - **diabetic patient** – glycemic profile
- **III – additional:** CK-MB, uric acid
  - **Other:**
  - **thyroid:** TSH, FT4
  - **gynecologic:** chlamydia, HIV
  - **biliary ways:** ALP, AMS, protein electrophoresis, immunoglobulins
  - **urologic:** sediment, ACP, cortisol, PSA
  - **ophthalmologic:** CIC, MDA
  - **ENT:** IgA, IgE, IgG, IgM, cationic eosinophil protein, specific IgE

Inflammatory Process Activity Determination Set
- **I – basic:** ESR, mucoproteins, fibrinogen, protein ELPHO, CRP
- **II – enhanced:** alpha-2-macroglobulin, alpha-1-antitrypsin, haptoglobin, orosomucoid, ceruloplasmin, serum amyloid A, C3, C4 complement, IgA, IgG, IgM, anti-DNP, procalcitonin, neopterin
- **III – additional:** elastase (PMN), procollagen III peptide, Mg, fibronectin, alpha-1-antichymotrypsin

Diabetic Set
- **I – basic**
  - glucose (fasting, 1–2 hrs after meal)
  - *Urine*: glucose, ketobody
- **II – enhanced**
  - glycemic profile, LDL-C, fructosamine, cholesterol, MDA, IRI, glycated hemoglobin, TAG, uric acid, HDL2/HDL3
  - *Urine*: glucose, microalbuminuria, osmolality
- **III – additional:** insulin, glucagon, ICA, IAA antibodies, anti-GAD, amylin, Apo B, Apo A-I, leptin

Atherosclerosis Risk – Lipid Set
- **I – basic:** cholesterol, TAG, HDL-C, LDL-C, lipoprotein, ELPHO, fibrinogen, uric acid
- **II – enhanced:** Lp(a), Apo B, Apo A-I, Apo E, Apo C-III, MDA, total antioxidative status, HDL2/HDL3, von Willebrand's factor, t-PAi, AT III, ANP, plasma viscosity
- **III – additional I:** lipoprotein lipase, SOD, GPx, phospholipids, homocysteine, Apo E phenotypes, fatty acid spectrum, endothelin-1, conjugated dienes, tocopherols, beta-carotene
- **IV – additional II:** DNA diagnosis, D/D ACE polymorphism, LDL receptors, Lp(a) phenotypes, Apo B polymorphism*, beta-fibrinogen polymorhism, thrombocytase GIIIb polymorphism, factor V (Leiden) mutation, prothrombin mutation (alele 20210), LP-lipase polymorphism, von Willebrand's factor phenotypes, tetrahydrofolate reductase phenotypes, cystathione synthase phenotype

*   XbaI, ins/del, familiar defect Apo B 3500

Thrombophilia Set
- **I – basic:** activated protein C resistance, protein C, protein S, antithrombin III, lupus anticoagulant, F II 20210A, homocysteine
- **II – enhanced:** heparin II co-factor, plasminogen, reptilase time, F XII

- **III – additional**
  - **Immunologic:** AT III, protein C, protein S, heparin II co-factor, plasminogen, fibrinogen
  - **Specific tests:** lupus anticoagulant, antiplasmin
  - **Molecular-biological tests:** factor V Leiden, MTHFR, CBS, methionine synthase, F II 20210A, beta-fibrinogen (455 G/A), glycoprotein IIIa, m-RNA (Ia, Ib, IIb, IX), protein C, protein S

Urolithiasis Metaphylaxia Set
- **I – basic**
  - Ca, uric acid, inorganic phosphorus
  - *Urine:* Ca (24 hrs), creatinine, pH profile, nitrites, proteins, leukocytes, sediment, **Quantitative:** Ca, Mg, inorganic phosphorus, uric acid, oxalate, citrate
- **II – enhanced**
  - glycosaminoglycans, cystine, sulfate
  - **Loading tests:** Ca, purines, NH_4Cl, risk and saturation indices
- **III – additional**
  - **Urine:** uromucoid, mineralogic calculus analysis*
  - If possible, perform metaphylaxia in connection with calculus analysis.

* Note: mineralogic calculus analysis, not chemical.

Oncological Set
- **I – basic:** Hb, HCT, RBC, PLT, WBC, ESR, creatinine, urea, proteins, albumin, protein ELPHO, GMT, LD, mucoproteins, CRP
- **II – enhanced:** ALP, ACP, beta-2-microglobulin, haptoglobin, orosomucoid, tumour markers
- **III – additional:** polyamines, ferritin

Oncologic patient monitoring: 1/ nutrition status, 2/ side and adverse effects of radiation/cytostatics (hepatic, renal, cardiac, immunological, inflammatory profile), 3/ tumour markers and peripheral paraneoplastic secretion markers change dynamics.

Nutrition Status Set
- **I – basic:** proteins, albumin, creatinine, urea, glucose, inorganic P, Ca
- **II – enhanced:** transferrin, RBP, prealbumin, Mg, Fe, TAG
  - *Urine:* urea, creatinine, alpha-aminonitrogen
- **III – additional**
  - Zn, amino acids, fatty acids, 3-methylhistidine
  - *Urine:* amino acids

Purine Metabolism Set
- **I – basic**
  - uric acid
  - *Urine:* uric acid, pH, volume
- **II – enhanced**
  - uric acid after purine loading, TAG, glucose, total antioxidative status
  - *Urine:* uric acid, uric acid and creatinine clearance
- **III – additional**
  - hypoxanthine guaninephosphoribosyltransferase adenosine deaminase (DNA analysis of enzymes)
  - *Urine:* urea

Liver Set

- ■ **I – basic:**
  - ■ ALT, AST, GMT, AST/ALT, GMT/AST, ALP, bilirubin, MCV, prothrombin, thrombocytes
  - ■ *Urine*: urobilin, bilirubin
- ■ **II – enhanced:** protein ELFO, IgA, IgG, IgM, prealbumin, LpX, cholinesterase, GMT/CHS, GMD, LD, oGTT, bromsulfophthalein – retention, porphyrins, HBsAg, anti-HBc, anti-HAV
- ■ **III – additional:** Fe, Cu, ceruloplasmin, alpha-1-antitrypsin, HBeAg, anti-HBe, anti-HAV IgM, anti-HCV, anti-CMV, anti-EBV, ammonia, biliary acids, 5-nucleotidase, autoantibodies (LSP, LMA, ASGP, SLA, LCA-1, LPA, HHPMA)

Cardiologic Set (myocardial infarction diagnosis)

- ■ **I – basic:** CK, CK-MB, LD, HBD, myoglobin, AST
- ■ **II – enhanced:**
  - ■ troponin T, troponin I, K, Na, Ca, Mg, ALT, GMT, BNP, APC resistance
  - ■ *Urine*: K, Na
- ■ **III – additional:** LD isoenzymes, FA-binding protein, 2,3-DPG

Hereditary Metabolic Disorder Suspicion Set

- ■ **A. I – basic**
  - ■ Hb, HCT, RBC, PLT, WBC, bilirubin, AST, acid-base balance, glucose, urea, Ca, P, uric acid
  - ■ *Urine*: pH, glucose, ketobodies, proteins, urobilinogen, reducing substances
- ■ **A. II – enhanced:**
  - ■ galactose, lactate/pyruvate, ammonia, TSH, CK
  - ■ *Urine*: glycosaminoglycans, meconium test, porphobilinogen
- ■ **A. III – additional:** carnitine, biotinidase
- ■ **B.** *Urine*: disulfides, phenylpyruvate, thiosulfates, SAICAR, orotic acid, methylmalonic acid
- ■ **C.** *Urine*: saccharide screening (fructoses, pentoses), mucopolysaccharide fractions
- ■ **D.** amino acids, fatty acids
- ■ **E.** organic acid screening

A., B. (partially) examinations are statim, B.–D. until 24 hrs (in some laboratories), E. gas chromatography, HPLC, also mass spectrometry is often needed.

Renal Set

- ■ **I – basic**
  - ■ creatinine, urea
  - ■ *Urine*: pH, protein, blood, leukocytes, nitrites, sediment, quantitative proteinuria
- ■ **II – enhanced**
  - ■ Na, K, Cl, protein ELPHO, cholesterol, uric acid, Ca, inorganic phosphorus, cystatine C
  - ■ *Urine*: Na, K, Cl, Ca, inorganic phosphorus, creatinine, urea, osmolality, cystatine (clearance), creatinine clearance, concentration test, pH, hippuric acid, alpha-amino-nitrogen, transferrin, IgG, protein fraction ELPHO
- ■ **III – additional**
  - ■ C3 complement, C4 complement

■ *Urine*: protein SDS-PAGE (ELPHO), selectivity index, beta-2-microglobulin, N-acetylglucosaminidase, lysozyme, ammonia, alpha-1-microglobulin, RBP

Thyroid Gland Set
■ I – **basic:** TSH (ultrasensitive), fT4
■ II – **enhanced:** FT3, TBG, T3, T4, cortisol, antithyroglobulin Ab, anti-TPO, anti-TSH-receptor Ab, creatine kinase, cholesterol, LDL-C
■ III – **additional**
  ■ rT3, indices rT3/T4, calcitonin
  ■ **Tests:** TRH, multiaxial

Immunological Set
■ I – **basic:** IgA, IgE, IgG, IgM, Hb, HCT, RBC, PLT, WBC + differential count, total T-lymphocytes, T_H-, T_S-lymphocytes, NK-cells, CIC, CH50, C3-complement, cool antibodies, rosettes
■ II – **enhanced:** BTL test, immunoelectrophoresis, B-lymphocytes (CD19), T-lymphocytes (CD3+, CD4+, CD8+), skin tests, phagocytic activity (MSH particles, Candida albicans), C1-inhibitor, C4-complement, antilymphocyte antibodies
■ III – **additional:** amyloid, flow cytometry, HLA typization

Gastroenterologic Set
■ I – **basic**
  ■ *Stool:* occult bleeding
■ II – **enhanced**
  ■ gastrin, Helicobacter pylori (serol.), insulin, 5-HIT, C-peptide
  ■ *Gastric Juice:* BAO, MAO
  ■ *Duodenal Fluid:* giardia
  ■ *Stool:* elastase-1, parasites, residuum, proteins, fatty acids
  ■ **Resorption Tests:** beta-carotene, vitamin A, vitamin B_{12}, xylose
  ■ **Functional Tests:** protein, glucagon, gastrozepin, secretin, calcium infusion, food
■ III – **additional**
  ■ antimitochondrial Ab, GIP, VIP, pancreatic polypeptide, glucagon, proinsulin, chromogranin A
  ■ **Tests:** I-polyvinylpyrolide resorption, chromium-albumin, serotonin, reserpine provocation, somatostatin-tolbutamine
  ■ **Viruses:** Herpes simplex, Varicella zoster, cytomegalovirus, HIV, fungi, fungi (yeasts) (candida)

Pancreatic Set
■ I – **basic**
  ■ AMS, glucose, acid-base balance, creatinine, Hb, HCT, thrombocytes, WBC, Na, K, chloride, Ca, Ca^{2+}
  ■ *Urine:* AMS
■ II – **enhanced**
  ■ lipase, AST, ALT, GMT, ALP, LD, albumin, TAG, cholesterol, prothrombin, elastase
  ■ *Stool:* elastase-1, chymotrypsin
■ III – **additional**
  ■ methemalbumin, trypsin, GMT (isoenzymes), CA 242, CA 19-9, CEA, CA 50
  ■ **Functional Tests:** secretin-pancreozymin (enzymes, lactoferrin), NBT-PABA

Autoimmune Diseases Set I

- **I – basic**
  - ESR, Hb, HCT, thrombocytes, WBC + differential count, complement (CH50, C3), CIC, CRP, fibrinogen, cryoglobulins, immunoglobulins, protein ELPHO, VDRL, direct Coombs' test, anti-ds-DNA, ANA, APTT
  - *Urine:* proteins, N-acetylglucosaminidase, microalbumin
- **II – enhanced**
  - HLA typing, complement C2, C4, anti-Sm, anti-SSA, anti-SSB, anti-Scl-70, ANCA, ENA (U1-RNP), soluble receptor IL-2, h-sICAM-1, CD 19, CD 71, IL-1, IL-6, TNF-alpha, anti-EBV, anti-toxocara Ab, anti-HSV, anti-CMV, antibodies against borrelia
  - *Urine:* alpha-1-microglobulin, beta-2-microglobulin
- **III – additional:** anti-TPO, anti-TSH-receptor Ab, antithyroglobulin Ab, anti-LKM, anti-SLA, antimitochondrial Ab, amyloid A (SAA), viral hepatitis markers and viral RNA, NAG (isoenzyme), ACE (D/D polymorphism)

Autoimmune Diseases Set II

		HLA	Allergy type reaction
Liver			
chronic active hepatitis	Non-specific: ANA, ANCA, anti-NE, SMA, anti-LKM, AMA	DR3, DR4	
	Specific: LSP, LMA, ASGP-R, LCA-1, LPA, SLA, HHPMA, HLA B8		
primary biliary cirrhosis	AMA-M2		
primary sclerosing cholangitis	p-ANCA		
Myasthenia Gravis	antiacetylcholin receptor Ab	DR3	
Blood			
hemolytic anemia	antibodies against RBC membrane, cryoglobulins		II
thrombocytopenia	anti-PLT Ab, GIIb/IIIa polymorphism		II
granulocytes	antineutrophil Ab, ANCA		II
Skin			
bullous pemphigoid			
pemphigus vulgaris		DR4	
Endocrinopathies			
thyroiditis	antithyroglobulin Ab, anti-TPO	DR5	II, IV
M. Basedow	anti-TSH-receptor Ab	B8/DR3	V
primary myxedema	LATS, anti-TSH-receptor Ab		
diabetes mellitus	ICA, IAA, antireceptor Ab, GAD	DR3, DR4	IV, II
M. Addison	antimicrosomal Ab	DR3	IV, II
hypoparathyroidism			IV, II

	HLA	Allergy type reaction
male sterility	antispermatozoa Ab	V, IV
female sterility	anti-FSH-receptor Ab, antimicrosomal Ab	IV, V
CNS		
sclerosis multiplex	anti-MBP Ab	
Eyes	MDA, CIC, ACE, antibody against – (borrelia, toxocara, HSV, CMV)	
Kidney		
Goodpasture's syndrome	anti-GBM Ab	DR2	II

Adrenal Cortex Set
- ■ **I – basic:** Na, K, chloride, cortisol
- ■ **II – enhanced**
- ■ **IIa:** plasma renin activity, aldosterone, K (intracelullar), granulocyte Mg
  - ■ *Urine:* free cortisol, 17-OHCS
  - ■ **Tests:** ACTH
- ■ **IIb**
  - ■ **Tests:** dexamethasone suppression (DST), enhanced DST
- ■ **III – additional**
- ■ **IIIa:** ACTH, cortisol, antimicrosomal Ab
  - ■ **Tests:** CRH, multiaxial
- ■ **IIIb:** gastrin, calcitonin, catecholamines, STH, prolactin, chromogranin A, B, VIP, somatostatin, 5-HIT
  - ■ **Tests:** enhanced DST, metopyrone, CRH

Hematologic Set
- ■ **I – basic**
  - ■ ESR, Hb, HCT, RBC, RTC, PLT, WBC + differential count, blood group, CT, BT, PT, thromboplastin time, factors (V, VII, VIII, IX, XI), Fe, transferrin, TIBC
  - ■ *Urine:* basic
  - ■ *Stool:* occult bleeding
- ■ **II – enhanced:** AST, ALT, bil, creatinine, urea, LD, ferritin, anti-HIV, plasma Hb, RBC autohemolysis, haptoglobin, MCV, MCH, MCHC, PLT aggregation/adhesion, HLA, vitamin B_{12}, RBC osmotic, resistance, folic acid
- ■ **III – additional**
  - ■ B2M, Hb ELPHO, anti-RBC Ab, MHb, total blood volume, anti-intrinsic factor Ab, CIC, ANCA, LE cells, HZV, HCV, HBsAg
  - ■ *Gastric Fluid:* intrinsic factor

Hematologic Subsets
- ■ **Coagulation Subset:** prothrombin time, activated partial thromboplastin time, bleeding time, thrombin time
- ■ **Coagulation Factors Subset:** beta-thromboglobulin, fibrinogen, factors – (II, V, VII, VIII, IX, X, XI, XII, XIII), ristocetin cofactor assay, von Willebrand's factor
- ■ **Platelet Kinetics Subset:** platelet survival, sites of platelet organ sequestration, platelet turnover

- **Fibrinolysis Subset:** fibrinogen degradation products, D-dimers, fibrin monomer screening, PAI-1, euglobulin lysis time
- **Lupus Anticoagulant Subset:** kaolin clotting time, partial thromboplastin time, platelet neutralization procedure, tissue thromboplastin inhibition test, diluted Russel viper venom test
- **Hemolytic Condition Subset:** hemoglobin electrophoresis, hemosiderin (U), Ham test, haptoglobin, cryoglobulins, screening test for hereditary spherocytosis, methemoglobin, Schumm's test, full blood count, sulph-hemoglobin, reticulocytes, bilirubin, lactate dehydrogenase, methemalbumin, hemopexin
- **Hemoglobinopathy Subset:** hemoglobin column chromatography, hemoglobin electrophoresis, hemoglobin H, methemoglobin, unstable hemoglobin
- **Platelet Metabolism Subset:** arachidonic acid metabolism, platelet fatty acid content, platelet membrane phospholipid content
- **Platelet Subset:** platelet aggregation, platelet antibodies, platelet factor 3, platelet factor 4, beta-thromboglobulin
- **Thrombophilia Subset:** activated partial thromboplastin time, activated protein C resistance, alpha-2-antiplasmin, anticardiolipin antibodies, antithrombin III, factor V Leiden, factors – (VII, VIII, X), fibrinogen, lupus anticoagulant, plasminogen, plasminogen activator, plasminogen activator inhibitor, protein C, protein S, tissue plasminogen activator, von Willebrand's factor, MTHFR mutation
- **Red Blood Cell Enzyme Defects Subset:** glucose-6-phosphate dehydrogenase, glutathione reductase, pyruvate kinase

Osteoporosis Set
- **I – basic**
  - ESR, Hb, HCT, PLT, WBC + differential count, Ca, P (phosphate), chloride, creatinine, uric acid, albumin, (protein ELPHO, AST, GMT), ALP, ACP (tartrate-resistant), TSH
  - *Urine:* Ca/creatinine, deoxypyridinoline/creatinine, phosphate, chloride
- **II – enhanced**
  - ALP (isoenzymes), osteocalcin, Ca^{2+}, FSH, PTH, FT4, prothrombin time
  - *Urine:* hydroxyproline/creatinine, telopeptide fragments (NTx, cross-labs)
- **III – additional**
  - 1,25-$(OH)_2$D3, 25-hydroxycholecalciferol, immunoelectrophoresis, carboxy-terminal propeptide procollagen I, decarboxylated osteocalcin
  - *Urine:* free cortisol

Recommended parameters in minimal enhanced screening program: tartrate resistant ACP, bone isoenzyme ALP, creatinine, URINE: creatinine, Ca, P + at least one of osteoresorption markers (ICTP, NTx, CTx, cross-labs, urine – hydroxyproline, deoxypyridinoline, pyridinoline) + least one of osteoformation markers (osteocalcin, urine – procollagen I peptides – PICP, PINP)

Abortion Set
- **I – basic**
  - blood group, Rh factor, BWR, HBsAg, anti-HCV, hCG
  - *Urine:* uricult
- **II – enhanced:** lupus anticoagulant, HCV (quantit.), HSV, brucella, toxoplasma, homocysteine
- **III – additional:** methylene-tetrahydrofolate reductase (MTHFR), cystathione-beta-synthase (CBS), cellular immunity

Anovulation Set (WHO)

- ■ **I – basic:** PRL, FSH, LH, estrogens, progesterone, 17-OH progesterone, testosterone, androstenedione, DHEAS, TSH, fT4
- ■ **II – enhanced**
  - ▪ antiphospholipid Ab, karyotype
- ■ **Functional Tests:** gestagen test, estrogen-gestagen test, clomiphene test, ACTH test, GnRH test
- ■ **III – additional:** molecular genetic examination

Anorchia Set (WHO)

- ■ **I – basic:** testosterone, LH, FSH, SHBG
- ■ **II – enhanced**
  - ▪ **Functional Tests:** hCG test, GnRH test
- ■ **III – additional:** chromosome examination, molecular examination

Azoospermia Set (WHO)

- ■ **I – basic:** LH, FSH, PRL, PSA, testosterone, estrogens, SHBG
- ■ **II – enhanced**
  - ▪ **Functional Tests:** MAR test (mixed antiglobulin reaction), TAT test (tray agglutination test)
- ■ **III – additional**
  - ▪ **Molecular-Biological Tests:** receptors, KALIG gene, CFTR gene, Y-chromosome: AZF (azoospermia factor), DAZ (deleted in azoospermia)

Chronic Fatigue Syndrome Set

- ■ **I – basic**
  - ▪ ESR, fibrinogen, CRP, mucoproteins, glucose, creatinine, bilirubin, cholesterol, TAG, AST, ALT, GMT, CK, LD, Na, K, chloride, Ca + ionized, FT4, TSH, cortisol, Fe, transferrin, CIK, immunoglobulins, phagocytic activity, complete blood count, CMV, TB, HIV, borrelia, brucella, HBsAg, anti-HCV, EBV, anti-DNA, ASLO, RF
  - ▪ *Urine:* proteins, albumin, phosphate, protein ELPHO, drugs, caffeine
  - ▪ *Stool:* occult blood, parasites
  - ▪ *Cerebrospinal Fluid:* proteins, immunoglobulins, glucose, chloride, protein ELPHO
- ■ **II – enhanced**
  - ▪ aldosterone, FSH, LH, PRL, carbohydrate deficient protein, soluble transferrin receptor, ANP, BNP, TM (CEA, PSA, CA 125, CA 15-3, SCCA, TPS), MDA, conjugated di-enes, PMN-elastase, neopterin, procalcitonin, anti-HHV-6, anti-HTLV1, anti-HTLV2, antibodies against circulating enteroviral antigen, antibodies against chlamydia
  - ▪ *Urine:* drug + medicament identification, glycosaminoglycans
  - ▪ *Cerebrospinal Fluid:* oligoclonal bands + proteins
  - ▪ **Functional Tests:** dexamethasone suppression test
  - ▪ **Cellular Immunity:** CD antigens, esp. CD 20, CD 5, T-helper/T-suppressor cells index, p-ANCA, c-ANCA
  - ▪ **Skin Tests:** mitogen stimuli, antigen stimuli
- ■ **III – additional**
  - ▪ **Molecular-Biological Tests:** retroviruses, herpes viruses, EBV, CMV, rubella

Electrophoresis Fractions and Specific Serum Proteins

	Typical fractions	Atypical fractions	Findings
prealbumin	prealbumins		
albumin	albumin, post-albumin	– double fraction	– familial bisalbumin-emia
		– missing	– familial analbumin-emia
alpha-1-globulins	alpha-1-antitrypsin, alpha-1 acid glyco-protein, HDL-C	almost missing (< 1 %)	AAT defect
alpha-2-globulins	alpha-2-macroglo-bulin, haptoglobin, C-1 esterase inhi-bitor	extragradient alpha	IgA plasmocytoma
beta-1-globulins	transferrin, hemo-pexin		
beta-2-globulins	C3-complement, CRP, IgA part	extragradient beta	IgA plasmocytoma, lymphomas and leukemia
	IgG, IgM part, fibrinogen part	extragradient beta-gamma	IgA, IgM plasmocy-toma, chronic lym-phatic leukemia
gamma globulins	IgM, IgA, IgG, CRP part	extragradient gamma	IgG plasmocytoma, Waldenström's macroglobulinemia, chronic leukemias

Action Values for Immediate Information

Test results may indicate the need for immediate clinical intervention.

Blood

Analyte	Warning limits Hospitalization	Outpatient	Unit	Note
alanine amino-transferase (ALT)	>6.0	>3.0	µkat/l	
alcohol	>0.002	>0.002	g/l	
alkaline phosphatase (ALP)		>10.0	µkat/l	
ammonia	>50		µmol/l	
amylase (AMS)	>15		µkat/l	
aspartate amino-transferase (AST)	>6.0	>3.0	µkat/l	
bilirubin	>170	>100	µmol/l	
bilirubin (newborns)	>240		µmol/l	
calcium (Ca)	<1.3 >3.0	<1.5 >3.0	mmol/l	
ionized calcium	<0.85 >1.55	<0.8 >1.55	mmol/l	
cardiac troponin T	>0.1		µg/l	

Analyte	Warning limits		Unit	Note
	Hospitalization	Outpatient		
cardiac troponin I	>1.6		µg/l	
chloride	<90	<90	mmol/l	
creatinine	>500	>350	µmol/l	
creatine kinase (CK)	>15.0	>8.0	µkat/l	
glucose	<2.2	<3.0	mmol/l	fasting
	>20.0	>16.0	mmol/l	
	>25.0	>18.0	mmol/l	postprandial
natrium (Na)	<125 >155	<125 >155	mmol/l	
potassium (K)	<2.8 >6.0	<3.0 >6.0	mmol/l	
blood gases				
pH	<7.20 >7.55			
pCO$_2$	<3.00 >8.00		kPa	
BE	<-8 >8		mmol/l	
pO$_2$	<7.0 >20.0		kPa	

Hematology

Analyte	Warning limits		Unit	Note
activated partial thromboplastin time	>60	>60	s	
carboxyhemoglobin	>0.1	>0.1		non-smokers
fibrinogen	<1.0	<1.0	g/l	
hematocrit (HCT)	<0.20	<0.25		
	>0.60	>0.60		
hemoglobin (Hb)	<64 >165	<80 >165	g/l	
leukocytes (WBC)	<1.5 >20	<2 >15	x 10^9/l	
methemoglobin	>0.02	>0.02		
thrombin time (TT)	>50		s	
thrombocytes (PLT)	<50 >700	<50 >700	x 10^9/l	
thrombocytes (PLT)– pediatric	<20 >1000	<40 >700	x 10^9/l	

Cerebrospinal Fluid

Analyte	Warning Limits	Unit	Note
Glucose	<80% of blood level		
Leukocytes	>10	ml	
Proteins	>0.45	g/l	

Other critical values/results

■ **Blood:** positive tests – (fibrin degradation products, protamine sulfate), high heparin level, new diagnosis – (leukemia, aplastic crisis, sickle cell anemia), positive findings – (sickle cells, blast cells).

■ **Cerebrospinal fluid:** positive bacterial stain (Gram's, acid-fast), antigen detection, culture. Presence of malignant cells or blasts, other body fluid.

- **Microbiology:** positive blood culture, positive Gram's stain or culture from any body fluid, positive acid-fast stain or culture from any site, positive culture or isolate – (Corynebacterium diphtheriae, Cryptococcus neoformans, Bordetella pertussis, Neisseria gonorrhoeae, Histoplasma, Coccidioides, Blastomyces, Paracoccidioides), presence of blood parasites, positive antigen detection. Stool culture positive for Salmonella, Shigella, Campylobacter, Vibrio, Yersinia.
- **Urine:** strongly positive test for glucose, ketones and leukocytes. Presence of reducing sugars in infants. Presence of pathological crystals (urate, cysteine, leucine, tyrosine).
- **Serology:** Incompatible cross match. Positive direct/indirect antiglobulin (Coombs') test on routine specimens. Positive direct antiglobulin (Coombs') test on cord blood. Titers of significant RBC alloantibodies during pregnancy. Transfusion reaction workup showing incompatible unit of transfused blood. Positive confirmed test for hepatitis (especially hepatitis C), syphilis, acquired immunodeficiency syndrome (AIDS). Increased blood antibody levels for infectious agents (mainly infectious mononucleosis, cytomegalovirus infection, herpes simplex virus infection, toxoplasmosis).
- Laboratory announces the test result by telephone as soon as possible.

Urine

Urinalysis – sampling
- single fresh urine sampling – (random specimen, early morning collection of the sample before ingestion of any fluid, or taken at any time of day)
- urine time-sampling (1–3 hrs) – (timed, short-term specimen)
- urine time-sampling (12–24 hrs) – (timed, long-term specimen)

An important factor is the interval of time which elapses from collection to examination in the laboratory. Changes, which occur with time after collection include: 1/ decreased clarity due to crystallization of solutes, 2/ rising pH, 3/ loss of ketone bodies, 4/ loss of bilirubin, 5/ dissolution of cells and casts, 6/ overgrowth of contaminating microorganisms. Generally, urinalysis may not reflect the findings of absolutely fresh urine if the sample is >1 hour old. Therefore, get the urine to the laboratory as quickly as possible.

Collection of urine
- from spontaneous urination (voiding, voided urine)
- from middle stream (clean-catch mainstream specimen) for urine culture/cytological analyses
- from percutaneous suprapubic puncture of urinary bladder in specific indications (i.e. infants and small children, when done under ideal conditions, this provides the purest sampling of bladder urine)
- from single catheterization of urinary bladder (namely in special circumstances – i.e. in a comatose or confused patient)
- from urine time-sampling
- from permanent catheter-sampling (catheterized specimen, specimen from an indwelling catheter)
- from double-voided specimens: test for sugar and acetone

Urinalysis can reveal some unnoticed conditions because they do not always accompany clear signs/symptoms (diseases of kidney, urinary tract infections, diabetes mellitus). The most cost-effective device used to screen urine is a paper/plastic dipstick. This is a microchemistry system which allows qualitative and semiquantitative analysis within a short time by simple and careful observation. On the contrary, a careless evaluating staff can misread or misinterpret the results. Random specimens may be dilute, isotonic, hypertonic, and may contain white cells, bacteria, and squamous epithelium as contaminants. In females, the specimen may contain vaginal contaminants such as trichomonads, yeast, and during menses, RBC's. In the urine collection, one of the methods is clean catch, midstream specimen collected after cleansing the external urethral meatus. A midstream urine is one in which the first half of the bladder urine is discharded and the collection vessel is introduced into the urinary stream to catch the last half. The first half of stream serves to flush contaminating cells and microbes from the outer urethra prior to collection. This sounds easy, but it is not (try it yourself, before criticizing the patient). Procedure of bladder catheterization through urethra for urine collection risks introducing infection and traumatizing the urethra and bladder, thus producing iatrogenic infection or hematuria.

24-hour urine collection: patients should receive precise instructions for obtaining a complete 24-hour urine sample. Specimen containers should be labeled with the type of preservative added. Patients should avoid alcoholic beverages and vitamins for at least 24 hours before starting to collect urine and during the collection period. Patients should not discontinue medications unless instructed to do so by physician.

Methods of Examination
- **physical**: volume, colour, odour, opacity = turbidity, specific gravity, settled sediment
- **biochemical**: pH, minerals, proteins, carbohydrates
- **microbiological**: bacteria
- **microscopic**: organ particles, crystals, cells, casts, bacteria, epithelia

Macroscopic examination. The first part of urinalysis is a direct visual observation. Normal, fresh urine is pale to dark yellow or amber in color and clear. Normal urine volume is 650 – 2200 ml/24 hr. Turbidity or cloudiness may be caused by excessive cellular material/protein in the urine or may develop from crystallization/precipitation of salts upon standing at room temperature or in the refrigerator. Clearing of the specimen after addition of a small amount of acid indicates that precipitation of salts is the probable cause of turbidity.

Chemical analysis. Routine chemical urine analysis generally includes testing for pH (acidity), protein, reducing sugars, glucose, ketones, blood, bilirubin, urobilinogen and nitrate (as an infection indicator). In some special instances other tests may be required – e.g. tests for phenylketones, chloride. Usually it is sufficient to obtain semiquantitative or even qualitative estimates of urinary components. Strip tests (dipsticks) for pH, proteins, glucose, ketones, blood, bilirubin, urobilinogen and nitrite are available, often singly, or in various combinations on multiple-test strips. When using any strip test, it is important to exactly follow the instructions for use and for product preservation, and to check that the product is within its labeled expiration date (expired strip usage does not apologize). Screening spot tests are used in genetic diagnosis.

Microscopic examination. Normally the urine contains small amount of: casts and epithelial cells from the nephron/pelvis/ureters/bladder/urethra, mucous threads, spermatozoa from the prostate as well as some white and red blood cells. A sample of well-mixed urine (usually 5–15 ml) is centrifuged in a test tube at a relatively low speed. The supernate is decanted and a volume of 0.2–0.5 ml is left inside the tube. The sediment is resuspended in the remaining supernate by flicking the bottom of the tube several times. A drop of resuspended sediment is poured onto a glass slide and coverslipped. The sediment is first examined under low power to identify most crystals, casts, squamous cells and other large objects. Since the number of elements found in each field may vary considerably from one field to another, several fields are averaged. Next, examination is carried out at high power to identify crystals, cells and bacteria. Any disruption in the blood-urine barrier, whether at the glomerular or tubular level, will cause RBC's to enter the urine. RBC's may appear normally shaped, swollen by dilute urine (in fact, only cell ghosts and free hemoglobin may remain) or crenated by concentrated urine. Both swollen, partly hemolyzed and crenated RBC's are sometimes difficult to distinguish from WBC's in the urine. Red cell ghosts may simulate yeasts. The presence of dysmorphic RBC's in urine suggests a glomerular diseases. Dysmorphic RBC's have odd shapes as a consequence of being distorted via passage through the abnormal glomerular structure. Renal tubular epithelial cells, usually larger than granulocytes, contain a large round or oval nucleus and normally slough into the urine in small numbers.

Microscopic urinary sediment
- **formed elements:** bacteria, red cells, red cell casts, granular casts, hemoglobin casts, yeasts, white blood cells, tumour cells, parasites – (Enterobius vermicularis – pin worm ova, Schistosoma haematobium, Trichomonas vaginalis), spermatozoa, waxy casts
- **crystals:** amorphous urates, cystine, calcium phosphates, calcium carbonate, calcium oxalate, uric acid, leucine, sodium urates, tyrosine

General instructions for reagent strip (dipstick) handling
- completely immerse all strip reagent areas in fresh, well-mixed uncentrifuged urine and remove immediately
- tap strip edge against urine container to remove excess urine, hold the strip horizontally to prevent possible hand soiling with urine or chemical mix from adjacent reagent areas, and make sure that the test areas face upwards
- compare test areas closely with corresponding colour charts on the bottle label at the times specified; hold strip close to colour blocks and match carefully and read at the prescribed time.

Urine Preservation

Agent	Amount	Indication
Thymol	5 ml (10% solution in 2-propanol)	most parameters
HCl (alternative boric acid)	6N (25 ml)	hormones (steroids), Mg, Ca, VMA, 5-HIT
Natrium azid (to add in first urine portion)	0.5 g/dU	glucose
	1.0 g/dU	Bence Jones protein, specific proteins, selective proteinuria, hCG, cAMP, uric acid
Natrium carbonate	25–30 g	porphyrins, urobilinogen quantitatively
Urine sampling in about 0 °C		free cortisol, cAMP

Urine Sampling and Examination Indications
- **spontaneous urine sample:** most of qualitative and quantitative samples (chemical and microbiological examination), urine should be sent within 2 hours of urination to microbiological examination, if urine is stored in room temperature

- **first morning urine:** as above mentioned; more useful for sediment examination (cells and casts)
- **second morning urine (7.–10. AM):** for all quantitative determination referred for creatinine (functional test part), osteoporosis diagnosis test part (NTx)
- **urine after physical exertion:** microalbuminuria in hypertension, glomerulonephritis, diabetes, parasite determination
- **24-hour urine:** quantitative determination, functional loading tests (galactose, caffeine etc.)

Minimal Sampling Time in Some Urine Parameters

Analyte	Hours	Indication
calcium, phosphorus, creatinine, cAMP, NTx	>2	differential diagnosis of hyperkalciuria and fast-turn-over osteoporosis
amylase	2	differential diagnosis of hyperamylasemia in acute pancreatitis suspicion – spontaneous urine
leukocytes, erythrocytes	2	mainly in childhood infections
Functional tests – Ca, P, osmolality, pH	2	test with DDAVP, differential diagnosis in renal tubular acidosis
pH	2	sleep apnea differential diagnosis
uric acid, pH	2	hyperuricosuria differential diagnosis
cortisol (17-OHCS)	2 x 10	ACTH-stimulation, dexamethasone-suppression test
fructose	6	fructose-resorption test
galactose	5	galactose-tolerance test
xylose	5	xylose-tolerance test
parasites (Schistosoma hemolyticum)	2	afternoon urine after physical exertion
dela-aminolevulic acid	5–10	industrial intoxication
lead	4–5	industrial intoxication
trichloracetic acid	4–5	industrial intoxication
trichlorethanol	4–5	industrial intoxication

Cerebrospinal Fluid

Cerebrospinal Fluid Sampling

	Adults	Children	Note
I. fraction	do not use first 200–500 µl		special analysis can be used if minimum CSF after spectrophotometry
II. fraction microbiological and virologic examination	2 ml	1 ml	if possible 36 hours after therapy end
III. fraction cytology and clinical-biochemical parameters	10 ml	1–1.5 ml	tumorous cells, leukocytes, supernatant for clinical-biochemical parameters

CSF transport for all fractions
- ■ if examination is within 1 hour (native): room temperature
- ■ if examination is within 3 hours: on ice, do not refrigerate, do not fix, do not preserve

Note: valid for all sampling localization (spinal, suboccipital, ventricular).

Microbiology – Virology

Biological Material Sampling Basic Rules

Material Sampling and Transport Conditions for Viral Infection Determination

Material	Time sample	Method	Transport temperature
Nasal, throat swab	1–7 days	a) tampon with culture medium	4 °C
		b) dry cotton + transport medium	
Lavage fluid	1–7 days	5 ml of sterile physiological solution into each nostril	4 °C
Nasal secretion Sputum	1–7 days		
Bronchial brush swab	as required	sterile tube with 1 ml transport medium (immediately)	4 °C
Bronchoalveolar lavage fluid	as required	sterile tube with 1 ml transport medium (immediately)	ice transport
Pleural fluid	as required	without transport medium (sample into sterile tube)	4 °C
Synovial fluid	as required	without transport medium (sample into sterile tube)	4 °C
Cerebrospinal fluid	as required	without transport medium (sample into sterile tube), do not sample first 0.5 ml	ice transport, observe sample order
Stool	1–14 days	a) into special sample container	room temperature
		b) into boiled medicine bottle	
		c) stool swab	
Urine	1–28 d		4 °C
Urogenital swab	as required	a) sterile cotton stick	4 °C
		b) special tampon	
Urogenital secretion	as required	a) sterile syringe aspirate + 1 ml transport medium	4 °C
		b) aspirated material in syringe	
Cutaneous swab	as required	a) crusts in transport medium	4 °C
		b) swab with special tampon	
Conjunctival swab	as required	a) special tampon	4 °C

Material	Time sample	Method	Transport temperature
		b) dry cotton tampon in medium	
Heparinized blood ev. leukoprep-tube	as required	virus isolation, lymphocyte isolation, DNA, RNA determination, for molecular-biologic analysis	4 °C, heparinized blood is less suitable, transport immediately
Amniotic fluid	as required	10 ml without transport medium	ice transport

Sampling and Awaited Infection Verification

Clinical picture	Etiological agent	Suspect finding		Prove (cultivation and sensitivity)	Serology	Note
		micro-biological	culti-vation			
Diarrhea	Campylobacter jejuni/coli	1 day	3 days	5 days		MB – molecular biology
	salmonellae, shigellae, yersinia, Escherichia coli (pathog.)		2 days	3 days		
	Clostridium difficile		3 days	5 days		
Phlegmon	Clostridium perfringens, Clostridium novyi	1 day	2 days	5 days		
Tetanus	Clostridium tetani	1 day		2 days		experimental animal, 5 days
Botulism	Clostridium botulinum			8–10 hrs		MB experimental animal, 6 days
Purulent septic anaerobic infections	bacteroides, peptostreptococci	1 day	3 days	6 days		
Venerologic infections	neisseriae, chlamydiae,	1 day		5 days		
	HSV	1 day		3 days		MB
Tuberculosis	Mycobacterium TB,	1 day		3–6 weeks		2 d MB

Clinical picture	Etiological agent	Suspect finding		Prove (cultivation and sensitivity)	Serology	Note
		micro-biological	cultivation			
	Mycobacterium bovis	1 day				
Enteroviral infections	enteroviruses			tissue culture, 3 days	3 weeks	
Enteritis	rotaviruses	1–2 days		1–2 days	2 days, 3 weeks	serological subtypes
Hepatitis viruses	HAV, HBV, HCV, HDV, HEV, HGV				1 day	MB (especially HCV RNA, HGV, HEV RNA, HDV RNA)
Rubella					IgM 1 day	MB
Morbilli					3 days	MB
Parotitis					3 days	
Ornithosis	Chlamydia psittaci				3 days	MB
Toxoplasmosis	Toxoplasma gondii				1 day	MB
Legionella infection	Legionella				3 days	
Listeriosis	Listeria monocytogenes				2 days	
Septic conditions, bacteremia	streptococci, staphylococci, klebsiellae, proteus, fungi		2 days	3 days		
Uropoietic system infections	bacteria	1 day	2 days	3 days		
Bacterial menigitides	Neisseria meningitidis	1 day		2 days		
ENT infections	bacteria	1 day	2 days	3 days		
Respiratory system infections			2 days	3 days	3 weeks (2 samples)	subtypes evidence
	influenza viruses, adenoviruses, mycoplasma, chlamydia			3 days chicken germ; 3 days cell culture		

Material for Viral Infection Verification by Clinical Syndromes

System/clinical syndrome	Routine sampling	Additional sampling	Etiologic agent
Respiratory airways			
upper	HN swab, washout,	urine	CMV, Pneumocys.
lower	brush swab	pleural fluid	carinii
CNS			
meningitis	CSF, HN swab, stool	urine	EBV
encephalitis	CSF, HN swab, stool	blood, (biopsy)	HSV, arboviruses, borreliae, rickett-siae
polyradiculitis	CSF, HN swab, stool	heparinized blood,	
subacute sclerosing	CSF, urine		
panencephalitis		lymphocyte isolation	
GIT			
gastroenteritis	stool, rectal swab		
hepatitides	stool, serum	urine	HCV, HDV, HEV
pancreatitis	stool, urine	serum	EBV, coxsackie
Urogenital system			
fluor	swab, secretion		neisseriae
vulva/penis lesions	swab, lesion content	blood	HSV1/2, HSV6
condyloma	swab	biopsy	
acute hemorrhagic			
cystitis	urine	swab, stool	
Skin			
maculopapular lesions	swab, blood, lesion content	urine, stool	
vesicular lesions			
hemorrhagic lesions			
Lymphadenopathies	throat swab	blood, urine	
Eye			
conjunctival infections	secretion, swab	blood	
keratitis	swab	throat swab, serum, blood	
CV system			
myocarditis	throat swab	blood (DNA)	streptococci
Locomotor system			
arthritis	throat swab, blood, stool, puncture fluid	blood (DNA)	yersiniae, borre-liae, campylobac-ter, salmonellae, listeria, shigellae, citrobacter, strepto-cocci
Septic condition	throat swab, urine, CSF, stool, secretion	duodenal juice	

Remarks Concerning Medical Ethics

The patient's consent is required for every investigation. If you plan to use the material for the next investigations or for research in dependence on the results of the previous investigation, patient should be informed about your intention and signed informed consent obtained. All the examinations designed in terms of the prenatal diagnostics should be confirmed at every step by the patient. She has the right to cancel her consent and must not be sanctioned (by the following behaviour of the physician, insurance company or by the others). The written patient consent is required for every investigation as a part of the clinical trial. When testing the drug effects and their influence on the clinical and laboratory picture in clinical trials, always make sure that you have the institutional ethical committee consent. This holds true also for the general practitioners. In some drugs or procedures the patient insurance by the firm is required (possible adverse effects or permanent disorders). If you have suspicion of the ethical norms not being kept (most common ethical conflict – patient autonomy versus social goodness versus scientific and professional contribution – economical contribution, literature, foreign congresses participation etc.) do not hesitate to stop your participation in the clinical trial until the particular questions are satisfactorily answered.

The patient has full rights to his/her own DNA (but also for the sample of his/her own when checked up routinely in the lab) and that is why it is not possible to use his/her DNA neither for the polymorphism assessment (frequency and prevalence) nor for the other investigations without his/her consent or compensated consent. Compensated consent, even if the compensation is small, is preferable from a legal standpoint.

As far as the result of the examination seems conflicting (positive results in STD investigation, HIV or genetic investigation); autonomy and contribution versus social goodness – please be careful to solve it. When necessary, do not hesitate to consult the approved method for patient informing and resolution of the conflict.

I

Biochemical/Laboratory Parameters in Biological Materials

Blood – Plasma – Serum

D. Mesko, R. Pullmann

Acetoacetic Acid

(syn: acetoacetate) Ketone body which is produced in fat metabolism – fat oxidation end product in liver + fat oxidation intermediary product in muscles.

Increased Values
active acromegaly, anorexia nervosa, **branched-chain ketonuria, catecholamines excess,** conditions – (**febrile c., post-anesthesia c.**), **diabetic ketoacidosis, exercise in untrained subjects, glycogenoses** (glycogen storage disease), **hyperglycemia,** hyperinsulinism, **increased fat intake, methylmalonic aciduria, persistent vomiting,** pregnancy, **prolonged excessive insulin administration in diabetics, prolonged fasting** (most common in children 1 to 6 years old), **severe carbohydrate restriction with normal fat intake, severe thyrotoxicosis, stress, weight-reducing diets**
    Interfering Factors: medicaments – (acetylsalicylic acid, ACTH, ethanol, glucocorticoids, growth hormone, levodopa, streptozocin)

Analyte	Age/Gender	Reference Range	SI Units	Note
Acetoacetic Acid	0–3 y	0–310	µmol/l	
	4 – 15 y	0–270	µmol/l	
	Adults	5–75	µmol/l	

Acetaminophen

Test Purpose. 1) to confirm suspected acetaminophen toxicity from patient history or clinical observations, 2) to monitor detoxification treatment with i.v. acetylcysteine.

Increased Values
acetaminophen overdose
    Interfering Factors: alcohol, medicaments – (barbiturates)

Acetone

Ketobody produced in fat metabolism. Acetone is the end product of liver fat oxidation + an intermediary product of muscle fat oxidation, originating from acetoacetic acid decarboxylation.
Test Purpose. 1) diagnosis of ketonemia resulting from diabetes mellitus, intestinal disorders, glycogen storage diseases and alcohol consumption.

acetonemic vomiting in children, **alcoholism**, **intestinal diseases**, ketoacidosis – (**diabetic k.**, fasting k.), severe carbohydrate intake restriction, **starvation**

Analyte	Age/Gender	Reference Range	SI Units	Note
Acetone				
semiquantitative		neg.		
quantitative		0.05–0.34	mmol/l	

Acetylcholine

(ACH) A reversible acetic acid ester of choline. It is a cholinergic agonist.

Production. Synthesized from choline and mitochondrially derived acetylcoenzyme A by the enzyme choline acetyltransferase. ACH is released at a motor neuron end-plate by an electrical impulse travelling down the nerve toward a muscle.

Function. The major neurotransmitter of: a) motoneurons (mediates impulse transfer from motoric nerve fibre to striated muscle), b) postganglionic parasympathetic fibers, c) vegetative sympathetic and parasympathetic ganglia of nerve system, d) CNS cholinergic neurons (basal ganglia, motor cortex). ACH acts through muscarine (M) and nicotine (N) receptors. There are 5 types M receptors; M_1 receptors are localized on parasympathetic nerve endings. Their activation lead to IP3 and DAG production increase with subsequent intracellular Ca^{2+} level increase leading to gastrointestinal tract secretion and motility increase, as well as CNS excitation. M_2 receptors are in myocardium and smooth muscles. They decrease cAMP production and open K^+ channels resulting in bradycardia, increased ureter and bladder peristalsis. M_3 receptors are in exocrine glands, smooth muscles and vascular endothelium. They cause bronchial smooth muscle and uterus contraction and bronchial, salivary, lacrimal, and sweat glands secretion increase by intracellular Ca^{2+} concentration increase. ACH acts on vessels directly with subsequent contraction (after high doses) and secondly indirectly with subsequent dilation (by EDRF release). M_4 and M_5 receptors are in CNS, their function is not clear yet. Nicotine N_N receptors are localized at the vegetative ganglia level. Na^+ and K^+ channel openings are active effect mechanisms. Nicotine N_M receptors are in skeletal muscles and mediate nerve-muscular transfer from motoric fibre onto skeletal muscle. Acetylcholine levels are regulated by the activity of choline acetyltransferase which hydrolyzes ACH to choline and acetate ion. Choline is back uptaken and enters with acetylcoenzyme A into ACH synthesis cycle.

Increased Values

intoxication by – (mushrooms, snake venom, organophosphates), myasthenia gravis

Decreased Values

botulism

N-Acetyl-Beta-D-Glucosaminidase

(NAG) Materials: serum, fibroblasts

Test Purpose. 1) diagnosis of acute tubular injury, 2) to monitor tubulopathies.

Increased Values

acute tubular necrosis, chronic glomerulonephrosis, chronic pyelonephritis, renal allotransplant rejection, toxic renal injury – (poisons, medicaments)

Acid Phosphatase

(syn: AP, total ACP)

Function. Enzyme important in the absorption/metabolism of carbohydrates, nucleotides, phospholipids and in bone calcification. Involved in breakdown of own cellular compounds and cell invading compounds.

Occurrence. Prostate, liver, bones (bone marrow), milk, erythrocytes, leucocytes, spleen, thrombocytes, reticuloendothelial system, lysosomes, kidney.

Isoenzymes. Serum ACP activity is based on isoenzyme activity mixture that come from prostate (PAP), liver (reticuloendothelial system), bones, RBC, PLT. Isoenzyme PAP is not identical with tartrate-labile phosphatase. RBC and PLT isoenzymes have 200-times higher activity which results in increased values in thrombosis. Highest values are in PM, lowest in AM. Within-day concentrations variation is 25–50%, day-to-day variation 50–100%.

Test Purpose. 1) parameter which aids in prostatic cancer diagnosis, 2) to monitor response prostate cancer therapy, 3) to help diagnose bone tumours and tumours metastasing into bones, 4) to help diagnose Gaucher's disease, 5) non-specific parameter in osteoporosis.

Increased Values

benign prostate hyperplasia, bone metastases from – (**prostate, mammary gland**), acute/chronic renal failure, colonoscopy, decreased blood flow to prostate, disease – (**Gaucher's d., Niemann–Pick d., Paget's d.**), diseases – (kidney d., biliary d., febrile d., **bone d., hepatic d.,** reticuloendothelial system d., infectious d.), **disseminated intravascular coagulation,** embolism, excessive platelet destruction, **hemolysis,** cirrhosis – (**hepatic c.,** cardiac c.), acute hepatitis – (type A, type B, type D, type E), **hyperparathyroidism, myocardial infarction,** megaloblastic anemia, **obstructive jaundice, osteogenesis imperfecta,** osteoporosis, **polycythemia vera,** pregnancy, **primary thrombocythemia,** prostate – (**p. biopsy, p. infarction, p. massage, p. injury**), **prostatitis,** renal insufficiency, renal osteopathy, sickle cell crisis, **thromboembolic disease,** idiopathic thrombocytopenic purpura, thrombosis, thrombophlebitis, transurethral prostatic resection, tumours – (**bone t.,** chronic lymphatic leucemia, acute/chronic myeloid leucemia, **myeloproliferative t., plasmocytoma** – incl. multiple myeloma, **t. of prostate,** lung t., **t. of breast**), prostate calculus

    Interfering Factors: children, medicaments – (androgens in women, clofibrate)

Decreased Values

castration, ethanol, hormonal therapy of prostate hyperplasia, oxalates

    Interfering Factors: medicaments – (fluorides, heparin)

Analyte	Age/Gender	Reference Range	SI Units	Note
Acid Phosphatase (ACP)				
Total ACP	F	<92	nkat/l	
	M	<108	nkat/l	
Prostatic ACP	M	<43	nkat/l	
Total ACP	F + M	75–215	nkat/l	See ref.
Prostatic ACP	M	<68	nkat/l	ranges note

Activin A

Activins (activin A, activin B, activin AB) are present in the testis and some areas of adult brain.

Production. Normal bone marrow cells and myelomonocytic cells lines. Synthesis enhancement in monocytes by: GM-CSF and IFN gamma. Synthesis in bone marrow stromal cells is induced by TNF alpha, IL-1-alpha and bacterial endotoxins.

Function. Originally activin A was described as a protein stimulating in vitro the release of FSH. Activin A controls the expression and secretion of hormones (FSH, prolactin, ACTH, oxytocin). Activin A acts as a neuronal survival factor and inhibits neuronal differentiation, influences the development of granulosa cells, supports the proliferation of a number of cells lines. Also stimulates the synthesis of GRH receptors and inhibits the release of GH. The biological activities of activin A can be inhibited by follistatin. Possible activin A clinical significance: a growth inhibitory and an erythroid differentiation factor in the treatment of erythroleukemia.

Acute-Phase Reactants

(APRs, syn: acute phase proteins) Acute phase reactants is the generic name given to a group of approximately 30 different biochemically and functionally unrelated proteins. The levels of acute phase proteins in the serum are either increased (positive acute phase reactants) or reduced (negative APR). Plasma constituents that appear or increase acutely in response to inflammation (infection, trauma, burns, surgery, tissue necrosis) approximately 90 minutes after the onset. They are produced in hepatocytes (each hepatocyte possessing the capacity to produce the entire spectrum of these proteins) after IL-6 stimulation (main mediator of the APR). Following stimulation of single hepatocytes within individual lobules one observes a stimulation of further hepatocytes and this process continues until almost all hepatocytes produce these proteins and release them into the circulation. Reactants synthesis is followed by decrease of so-called anti-reactants synthesis (prealbumin, albumin, transferrin). Acute phase reactants are glycoproteins, with exception of CRP and serum amyloid A. They include: ESR, CRP, serum mucoproteins, alpha/gamma globulins, complement components, transferrin, ferritin, alpha-1-acid glycoprotein, WBC, AAT, ceruloplasmin, haptoglobin, fibrinogen. These agents can be also mediators associated with inflammation: chemotactic protein ECF-A, ECF-oligopeptide, neutral proteinases (PMN-elastase, cathepsin G, collagenases), lysosome glycosidases (lysozyme, hexosaminidases), cytokines, IL-1, IL-2, TNF-alpha, fibronectin, alpha-1 antichymotrypsinogen, alpha-1 antitrypsin. The term acute phase response summarizes a number of very complex endocrine and metabolic or neurological changes observed in an organism, either locally or systematically, a short time after injuries or the onset of infections, immunological reactions and inflammatory processes. Development/effects of acute-phase response: 1) injuring agents (surgery and burns, bacterial or parasitic infection, ischemic necrosis, chemical irritants, tumor growth) → 2) local reaction (dilation and blood vessels leakage, platelet aggregation and clot formation, accumulation of neutrophils and macrophages, proteases and other lysosomal enzymes release, mediators formation, fibroblasts stimulation. Local reaction leads to systemic reaction (fever, pain, leukocytosis, increased secretion of certain hormones, activation of complement and clotting cascades, decreased serum iron and zinc, amino acids transfer from muscles to liver, increased synthesis of acute-phase proteins); reactions mediated by: interleukin 1, prostaglandins, histamine, serotonin, kinines. Local reaction can lead also to acute-phase response → a) reparative processes, b) systemic reaction, or c) cell death and necrosis.

Inflammatory mediators. CRP (phosphorylcholine binding, complement activation and opsonization), plasminogen (complement activation, clotting, fibrinolysis), factors VII, VIII + prothrombin + fibrinogen + fibronectin (clotting, fibrin matrix formation for repair), kininogenase (kallikrein) + kininogen (vascular permeability and dilatation), complement components (opsonization, chemotaxis, mast cell degranulation), kallikreins (vascular permeability and dilatation), haptoglobin, ceruloplasmin, fibrinopeptides

Inhibitors. AAT (serine proteinase inhibition, resolution of emphysema), alpha-1-anti-chymotrypsin (cathepsin G inhibition, protease inhibition), thiol protease inhibitor (cysteine protease inhibition), haptoglobin (cathepsins inhibition), AT III + C1 INH + factor B + factor I + factor H (mediator pathways control), alpha-2-antiplasmin (modulation of coagulation cascade), heparin-co-factor II (proteinase inhibitor), plasminogen activator inhibitor I (protease inhibitor), alpha-2-macroglobulin

Complement proteins. C2, C3, C4, C5, C9, C1-inhibitor (negative control of complement cascade), C4-binding protein, factor B

Hemocoagulation proteins. Fibrinogen, von Willebrand's factor (coagulation protein), alpha-2 antiplasmin (modulation of coagulation cascade), factor VIII (clotting formation of fibrin matrix for repair), prothrombin (clotting formation of fibrin matrix for repair), antithrombin 3 (modulation of coagulation cascade), plasminogen (proteolytic activation of complement, clotting, fibrinolysis), fibronectin (fibrin clot formation)

Miscellaneous. Haptoglobin, serum amyloid A (cholesterol and HDL scavenger), serum amyloid P (formation of IgG immune complexes), CRP (binding to membrane phosphorylcholine, complement activation and opsonization, interaction with T- and B-cells), ceruloplasmin, heme oxygenase (heme degradation), mannose binding protein (serum lectin), leukocyte protein I, lipoprotein (a), lipopolysaccharide binding protein (macrophage cell activation), apolipoprotein E

Cellular immune regulation. CRP, alpha-1-acid glycoprotein (interaction with collagen, promotion of fibroblasts growth, binding of certain steroids), fibrinogen, amyloid P (formation of IgG immune complexes), haptoglobin

Metal binding proteins. Albumin, haptoglobin (hemoglobin scavenger), hemopexin (heme binding and transport protein), alpha-1-acid glycoprotein, ceruloplasmin (copper transport protein), ferritin (iron transport protein), manganese containing superoxide dismutase (copper zinc binding protein, formation of reactive oxygen species), transferrin, macroglobulins

Repair and resolution. Alpha-1-acid glycoprotein, AAT, alpha-1-antichymotrypsin

Time and quantitative profile of selected inflammation reactants

Half-time	Parameter	Increase
very short half-time 6–10 hrs	CRP, serum amyloid A, alpha-1-antichymotrypsin	10–500 x
short half-time 24–48 hrs	alpha-1-acid glycoprotein, alfa-1-antitrypsin, haptoglobin, fibrinogen	2–3 x
medium half-time 48–72 hrs	C3, C4, ceruloplasmin	less 2 x

Increased Values – during inflammation
alpha-1-antitrypsin, alpha-2-macroglobulin, ceruloplasmin, fibrinogen, haptoglobin, C3 complement, orosomucoid, C-reactive protein

Decreased Values – during inflammation
albumin, alpha-lipoprotein, prealbumin, transferrin

Adenosine Deaminase

(ADA) An enzyme of the hydrolase class that catalyzes the adenosine deamination to form inosin, a reaction of purine metabolism. Adenosine deaminase is found in erythrocytes and leukocytes, as well as in the liver, stomach, genitourinary tract and serum.

Increased Values
autoimmune diseases, gout (uratic arthritis), heart failure, hemochromatosis, hemolytic anemia, hepatic cirrhosis, hepatitis, infectious mononucleosis, myeloid leukemia, obstructive jaundice, rheumatic fever, thalassaemia major, tuberculosis, tumors of – (bladder, prostate), typhoid fever

Adhesive Molecules

Adhesive molecules mediate cell adhesion to extracelullar matrix and reciprocal intercellular contacts. Soluble molecule forms can inhibit leukocyte and tumorous cells adhesion to endothelial cells. Adhesive molecules are involved in immune system cells communication, angiogenesis, and metastases. They are divided to integrins (beta-1, beta-2), selectins (L, E, P), and adhesion immunoglobulin molecules (ICAM-1, 2, 3, VCAM-1, PECAM-1, MAdCAM-1, CD2, CD31, LFA-3).

Adrenocorticotropic Hormone

(ACTH, syn: corticotropin, adrenocorticotropin)
Production. Anterior pituitary (adenohypophysis) hormone. Apart from its production in the pituitary authentic ACTH has been found to be produced also by macrophages and lymphocytes.
Target organ. Adrenal gland.
Function. Regulates adrenal cortex growth, adrenal steroids (glucocorticoids) synthesis and release, partially mineralocorticoids and androgens. Inhibits antibody production, IFN-gamma production, and stimulates NK-cells activity and B-lymphocytes mitogenesis. In supraphysiologic concentrations activates adenylate cyclase in adipose cells, which results in a cAMP-mediated lipase activation and increased lipolysis in fatty tissue (fatty acids). In supraphysiologic concentrations stimulates insulin release from the pancreas → insulin-secretion influence in Langerhans' islands → ↓ blood glucose. ACTH levels typically manifest circadian rhythm and pulsatile secretion (maximum shortly before awaking and 9AM, minimum occurs before midnight). Secretion is stimulated by serotonin and acetylcholine, viral infections, bacterial lipopolysaccharides, corticotropin releasing factor, antidiuretic hormone, IL-1, IL-6 and inhibited by gamma-aminobutyric acid.
Hypothalamic hormone. Corticotropin releasing hormone (CRH, corticoliberin).
Test Purpose. 1) to facilitate differential diagnosis of primary and secondary adrenal hypofunction, 2) to aid differential diagnosis of Cushing's sy (indirectly also obesity), 3) assisting diagnosis of adrenogenital sy.

Increased Values
Addison's disease, adrenal autoimmune diseases, adrenal tuberculosis, adrenoleukodystrophy, **congenital adrenal hyperplasia, ectopic production of ACTH,** pseudo-Cushing's states, syndrome – (**adrenogenital sy, Cushing's sy,** empty sella sy, Nelson's sy), tumours of – (hypophysis, lung)

Interfering Factors: exercise, hemoconcentration, hypoglycemia, neonates, pregnancy, stress, medicaments – (amphetamines, calcium gluconate, corticosteroids, desipramine, erythropoietin, estrogens, ethanol, insulin, ketoconazole, levodopa, lithium, metoclopramide, metyrapone, mifepristone, vasopressin)

Decreased Values
adrenal adenoma, adrenal tumors, central hypocorticism, Cushing's sy related to adrenal tumor, exogenous Cushing's sy, **Sheehan's syndrome**, empty sella sy, hypopituitarism, pan-hypopituitarism, **secondary insufficiency of adrenal cortex in pituitary insufficiency**
Interfering Factors: breast feeding, weight loss, medicaments – (clonidine, corticosteroids, dexamethasone, glucocorticoids, heparin)

Analyte	Age/ Gender	Reference Range	SI Units	Note
Adrenocortico-tropic Hormone (ACTH)	Umbilicus	130–160	µg/l	
	1–7 d	100–140	µg/l	
	Adults			
	8 AM	4.4–22	pmol/l	
	6 PM	11	pmol/l	

Adrenomedullin

(ADM) ADM is a peptide isolated from extracts of human pheochromocytomas arising from adrenal medulla.
Production. Synthesized by columnar epithelium, some glands, neurons of the pulmonary parasympathetic nervous system, vascular endothelial cells, chondrocytes, alveolar macrophages and vascular smooth muscle cells. ADM expression has been observed in most of the non-small cell lung carcinomas and small cell lung carcinomas. The protein is found also in human plasma.
Function. High concentrations of ADM in the brain suggests that it may act as a neurotransmitter, neuromodulator or neurohormone. ADM was detected initially by its stimulating activity of platelet cAMP.
Production. ADM is a potent vasorelaxant. Can also suppress mitogenesis in renal glomerular mesangial cells and may function as an endogenous paracrine suppressor of cell proliferation.

Adult T-Cell Leukemia-Derived Factor

(ADF, syn: ATL-derived factor)
Production. ADF is constitutively produced and secreted by T-cells. Produced also by HTLV-I-transformed T-cells.
Function. Induces the synthesis and expression of high affinity receptors for IL-2 in various lymphoid cell types. It thus indirectly promotes the autocrine growth of T-cells that depend on the presence of IL-2. ADF synergizes with IL-1 and IL-2 and allows virus-infected cells to respond to suboptimal doses of growth factors. Factor can protect cells against the cytotoxic actions of TNF. Also plays a role in the immortalization of lymphocytes by viruses such as HTLV-I and EBV. Acts as a growth factor for hepatoma cell lines. ADF has been

shown to regulate eosinophil migration. A loss of ADF-producing cells has been observed to occur in patients undergoing HIV infections. Down-regulation of ADF production by HIV-1 may play a role in the pathophysiology of HIV-infected individuals.

Alanine

(Ala) A nonessential amino acid, alpha-aminopropanoic acid, occurring in proteins and free in plasma. It is synthesized from pyruvate.

Increased Values – hyperalaninemia
citrullinemia, Cushing's disease, **histidinemia, hyperornithinemia, kwashiorkor,** parenteral nutrition, **pyruvate carboxylase deficiency,** septicemia, uratic arthritis (gout), **urea cycle enzyme defects**
    Interfering Factors: medicaments – (glucose, glutamic acid, histidine, valproic acid)

Decreased Values – hypoalaninemia
chronic renal diseases, Huntington's chorea, ketotic hypoglycemia
    Interfering Factors: medicaments – (ethanol, oral contraceptives, progesterone)

Beta-Alanine

An amino acid, beta-aminopropionic acid, not found in proteins but occurring both free and in several peptides, it is a precursor of acetyl coenzyme A, several related compounds, an intermediate in uracil and cytosine catabolism. Enzyme defect: beta-alanine alpha-ketoglutarate aminotransferase.

Increased Values
beta-alaninemia

Alanine Aminopeptidase

(AAP, syn: microsomal aminopeptidase) Elevation parallels ALP levels.

Increased Values
diseases – (**pancreas d., hepatobiliary tract d.**), pregnancy (3rd trimester)

Decreased Values
abortion

Alanine Aminotransferase

(syn: alanine transaminase – ALT, serum glutamic-pyruvic transaminase – SGPT, serum glutamate pyruvate transaminase, glutamate pyruvate transaminase – GPT)
Function. Intracellular cytoplasmic enzyme (of the transferase class) involved in amino acid/carbohydrate metabolism. Transports (reversibly) the amino acid part from alanine to alpha-ketoglutaric acid → glutamic acid and pyruvic acid (transamination), with pyridoxal phosphate as a co-factor.

Occurrence. Cytoplasm and mitochondria of the liver, then skeletal muscles, myocardium and kidney. ALT is located in the microsomal portion of the hepatic cell. ALT test is specific for liver malfunction. Concentration gradient intracellular space to plasma = $10^4{:}1$. Level increase starts at 2% liver parenchyma necrosis and damage.

Test Purpose. 1) to detect especially acute hepatic disease (hepatitis, cirrhosis, toxic/medicamentous liver damage) and evaluate acute hepatic disease treatment, 2) to distinguish between myocardial and hepatic tissue damage, 3) to help in differential diagnosis of hepatobiliary system and pancreatic diseases, 4) to help in chronicity detection of hepatitis.

Increased Values

incomplete abortion, AIDS, abscess – (brain a., liver a., pancreas a.), **amebiasis**, secondary amyloidosis, **giant cell arteritis**, aspergillosis, **primary biliary atresia, acute**/chronic **pancreatitis, acute viral hepatitis (A, B, C, D, E)**, anemia – (sickle cell a., microangiopathic hemolytic a., acquired hemolytic a., hereditary spherocytic hemolytic a., thalassemia major, thalassemia minor), angina pectoris, babesiosis, biliary tract obstruction, cerebrovascular accident, **cholecystitis, choledocholithiasis, cholelithiasis, chronic alcohol abuse**, hepatitis – (**chronic h.**, drug-induced h., **autoimmune h., alcoholic h.**, chemical-induced h., peliosis h.), conditions – (hemolytic c., **acute hypoxic c.**, postsurgery c., **shock c.**), cor pulmonale chronicum, coronary insufficiency, crush injuries, **delirium tremens, dermatomyositis**, diabetic ketoacidosis, disease – (Gaucher's d., **adult Still's d.**, graft-versus-host d., legionnaire's d., Graves' d., Crohn's d., Letterer–Siwe d., cytomegalic inclusion d., Niemann–Pick d., Brill-Zinsser d., Whipple's d., **Wilson's d.**), dysrhythmias, encephalitis – (St. Louis e., Japanese B e., e. lethargica), Wernicke's encephalopathy, acute bacterial endocarditis, congenital hepatic fibrosis, encephalomyelitis – (epidemic myalgic e., necrotizing hemorrhagic e., acute disseminated e.), fever – (Q f., lassa f., yellow f., rheumatic f., typhoid f., Rocky Mountain spotted f.), cystic fibrosis, **galactosemia**, gangrene – (penis g., diabetic g.), Wegener's granulomatosis, extensive hematoma, glycogen storage disease – (type I, type III, type VI), **extra/intrahepatic cholestasis**, hemochromatosis – (secondary h., **idiopathic h.**), hemorrhage, hepatic cirrhosis – (**alcoholic h. c., biliary h. c., primary biliary h. c.**, posthepatitic h. c.), alcoholic cardiomyopathy, coma – (**hepatic c.**, non-ketotic hyperosmolar c., **myxedema c.**), passive liver congestion, hepatic ischemia, ulcerative colitis, hepatic lesions – (**acute h. l., toxic medicamentous h. l.**), hepatic necrosis, malignant histiocytosis, **acute fatty liver of pregnancy, hepatic steatosis**, infarction – (intestine i., myocard i., liver i., kidney i., lung i.), intramuscular injections, lesions of skeletal muscle by – (electroshock, infections, seizure, trauma), metachromatic leukodystrophy, systemic lupus erythematosus, primary amebic meningoencephalitis, muscular gangrene, mycosis fungoides, myocarditis – (bacterial m., metabolic m., rheumatic m., viral m.), **myodystrophy**, myoglobinuria, myotonia – (atrophic m., congenital m.), **myositis, obesity, obstructive icterus**, pericarditis – (constrictive p., purulent p.), perihepatitis, pleural effusion, poisoning by – (aflatoxin, alcohol, antimony, arsenic, cadmium, carbon disulfide, carbon tetrachloride, chromates, cocaine, copper, DDT, herbicides, iron, lead, methyl bromide, mushrooms, naphthalene, nitrobenzene, opioid, phosphorus, solvents/trichlorethylene, vinyl chloride), **polyarteritis nodosa**, polymyalgia rheumatica, polymyositis, polytrauma, portal hypertension, **pre/eclampsia, pregnancy**, porphyria – (acute intermittent p., p. cutanea tarda), pulmonary embolism, pyoderma gangrenosum, reactive hepatitis after – (filariasis, cryptococcosis, **fascioliasis**, herpes zoster, echinococcosis, histoplasmosis, brucellosis, **leptospirosis**, malaria, **infectious mononucleosis**, ornithosis, toxoplasmosis, **schistosomiasis**, trichinosis, endemic typhus, tularemia, poliomyelitis), sarcoidosis, cholangitis – (**secondary ch., primary sclerosing ch.**), severe burns, thrombotic thrombocytopenic purpura, tropical sprue, shock – (cardiogenic s., septic s.), heat stroke, syndrome – (crush sy, Dubin–Johnson sy, chronic fatigue sy, **HELLP sy**, postcholecystectomy sy, Hand–Schueller–Christian sy, **eosinophilia-myalgia sy**, hepatorenal sy, toxic shock sy, Sezary's sy, **Reye's sy**), thrombosis – (pulmonary artery t., portal vein t.), tumors – (brain t., Burkitt's lymphoma, carcinoid, male breast t., breast t., renal t., **gallbladder t.**, melanoma, **leukemia, liver t.**, Hodgkin's d., prostate t., lung t., leukemic reticuloendotheliosis, pancreas t., ovarian t., stomach t.), thyrotoxic crisis, tumour metastases, tetanus, miliary tuberculosis, withdrawal – (acute alcohol w., opioid w.), failure – (**cardiac f., acute liver f.**), inborn error of amino acid metabolism

Interfering Factors: medicaments – (abacavir, acarbose, acetaminophen, acetylsalicylic acid, aciclovir, ajmaline, aldesleukin, allopurinol, alosetron, aminosalicylic acid, amiodarone, amlodipine, amoxicillin, amphotericin B, aminoglutethimide, amiodarone, amitriptyline, ampicillin, anabolics, anagrelide, androgens, antiepileptics, antihemophilic factor, aprindine, ardeparin, argatroban, asparaginase, atenolol, atorvastatin, atovaquone, azapropazone, azathioprine, aztreonam, BCG, benazepril, bexarotene, bicalutamide, bismuth salts, bisoprolol, bromfenac, bromocriptine, busulfan, candesartan, capecitabine, captopril, carbamazepine, carbenicillin, carbidopa, carbimazole, carboplatin, carbutamide, carmustine, cefalexin, cefalosporins, cefalotin, cefamandole, cefazolin, cefepime, cefoperazone, cefoxitin, cefradine, ceftizoxime, celecoxib, cerivastatin, chenodeoxycholic acid, chenodiol, chloramphenicol, chlorpromazine, chlorpropamide, chlorzoxazone, cimetidine, cisplatin, clarithromycin, clindamycin, clofazimine, clofibrate, clometacin, clomiphene, clomipramine, clonidine, clotrimazole, cloxacillin, codeine, cortisone, coumarin, cyclofenil, cyclophosphamide, cycloserine, cyclosporine, cytarabine, dacarbazine, dactinomycin, danazol, dantrolene, dapsone, delavirdine, demeclocycline, desmopressin, dexmedetomidine, diazepam, diclofenac, dicloxacillin, didanosine, diethylstilbestrol, diflunisal, dihydralazine, diltiazem, disopyramide, disulfiram, docetaxel, dofetilide, dolasetron, doxorubicin, doxycycline, efavirenz, enalapril, enflurane, eprosartan, erythromycin, estradiol, estramustine, estrogens, ethacrynic acid, ethambutol, ethanol, ethinylestradiol, ethionamide, ethosuximide, etodolac, etretinate, felbamate, fenofibrate, floxuridine, flucloxacillin, fluconazole, flucytosine, fluphenazine, flurazepam, flurbiprofen, flutamide, fluvastatin, fluvoxamine, fomivirsen, fosinopril, fosphenytoin, gemcitabine, gemtuzumab, glibenclamide, granisetron, griseofulvin, haloperidol, halothane, heparin, hydantoines, hydralazine, hydrochlorothiazide, hydrocodone, ibuprofen, idarubicin, imipramine, inamrinone, indomethacin, infliximab, interferon, interleukin 2, irinotecan, isocarboxazid, isoflurane, isoniazid, isotretinoin, itraconazole, ketoconazole, ketoprofen, ketorolac, labetalol, lamivudine, lansoprazole, leflunomide, levodopa, levonorgestrel, lincomycin, linezolid, loracarbef, losartan, lovastatin, mebendazole, meclofenamate, medroxyprogesterone, mefloquine, megestrol, meloxicam, menotropins, mephenytoin, meropenem, mesalamine, mestranol, metandienone, metaxalone, methimazole, methotrexate, methoxyflurane, methyldopa, methyltestosterone, metolazone, metoprolol, mexiletine, mezlocillin, minocycline, mirtazapine, mitoxantrone, modafinil, moexipril, moricizine, morphine, moxifloxacin, nabumetone, nafcillin, nalidixic acid, naltrexone, nandrolone, naproxen, nefazodone, nevirapine, niacin, nifedipine, nilutamide, nisoldipine, nitrofurantoin, nizatidine, norethindrone, norethisterone, norgestrel, olanzapine, olsalazine, omeprazole, ondasetron, oral contraceptives, oxacillin, oxaprozin, oxazepam, paclitaxel, palivizumab, pantoprazole, papaverine, paracetamol, paramethadione, pemoline, penicillamine, penicillin G, pentamidine, perazine, phenobarbital, phenothiazines, phenylbutazone, phenytoin, pindolol, piperacillin, piroxicam, plicamycin, prasterone, pravastatin, probenecid, probucol, procainamide, progesterone, propoxyphene, propranolol, propylthiouracil, protriptyline, pyrazinamide, quetiapine, quinacrine, quinidine, quinine, rabeprazole, ranitidine, retinol, rifabutin, rifampicin, rifapentine, riluzole, ritodrine, ritonavir, rofecoxib, salicylates, sertraline, sibutramine, simvastatin, sotalol, stavudine, streptokinase, streptozocin, sulfamethoxazole, sulfasalazine, sulfonamides, sulfonylureas, sulindac, tacrine, tamoxifen, terbinafine, testosterone, tetracycline, thioguanine, thiopental, thioridazine, thiothixene, tizanidine, tocainide, tolazamide, tolbutamide, tolcapone, tolmetin, toremifene, trandolapril, tranylcypromine, tretinoin, trimethoprim, trimetrexate, troglitazone, trovafloxacin, valerian, valproic acid, valsartan, verapamil, verteporfin, warfarin, zafirlukast, zalcitabine, zidovudine, zileuton, zimeldine, zonisamide)

Decreased Values
alcoholic liver disease, genitourinary tract infectious diseases, hemodialysis patients, malnutrition, pregnancy, pyridoxal phosphate deficiency, **pyridoxine deficiency** (vitamin B₆), renal failure, **tumors**
> **Interfering Factors:** medicaments – (oral contraceptives, phenothiazines)

Analyte	Age/Gender	Reference Range	SI Units	Note
Alanine Aminotransferase (ALT)	1 d	<0.52	µkat/l	
Glutamate pyruvate transaminase (GPT)	2–5 d	<0.87	µkat/l	
	6 d–6 m	<1.00	µkat/l	
	7–12 m	<0.95	µkat/l	
	1–3 y	<0.65	µkat/l	
	4–6 y	<0.48	µkat/l	
	7–12 y	<0.65	µkat/l	
	13–17 y F	<0.38	µkat/l	
	13–17 y M	<0.43	µkat/l	
	Adults F	<0.52	µkat/l	
	Adults M	<0.68	µkat/l	

Albumin

Production. Albumin is synthesized in the liver, representing 55–65% of the total protein.
Function. Albumin creates a protein reserve and presents low-affinity hormone binding activity. Osmotic function: a main determinant of plasma oncotic pressure and the maintenance of normal distribution body water = colloidal-osmotic pressure (oncotic pressure). Transports bilirubin, enzymes, heme, ions, pigments, steroid hormones, thyroxine, drugs, copper, cystine, fatty acids. Albumin is a source of amino acids for various tissues.
Test Purpose. 1) to aid in hepatic diseases, protein deficiency, renal disorders, gastrointestinal and neoplastic diseases diagnosis, 2) to detect protein metabolism disorders.

Increased Values – hyperalbuminemia
dehydration – (**exsicosis**, pseudohyperalbuminemia without absolute increase of albumin), diabetes insipidus, diarrhea, **hemoconcentration**, hemorrhagic diathesis, hypoglobulinemia, i.v. albumin infusions, metastatic carcinomatosis, meningitis, myasthenia gravis, plasmocytoma (incl. multiple myeloma), pneumonia, polyarteritis nodosa, shock, systemic lupus erythematosus, tumors
> **Interfering Factors:** medicaments – (ampicillin, chlorpropamide, colchicine, corticosteroids, furosemide, progesterone, thyroxine)

Decreased Values – hypoalbuminemia
acute/chronic glomerulonephritis, septic abortion, AIDS, abscess – (tubo-ovarian a., **liver a.,** lung a., appendix a., omentum a., pancreas t., pelvis a.), actinomycosis, amebiasis, renal tubular acidosis, anemia – (posthemorrhagic a., sickle-cell a.), hypersensitivity angiitis, arteritis – (giant cell a., Takayasu's a.), **rheumatoid arthritis,** allergic pulmonary aspergillosis, **acute/chronic hepatitis, acute cholecystitis,** acute phase reactions, **acute polyarthritis, amyloidosis, ascites,** blastomycosis, brucellosis, cachexia, coccidioidomycosis, **colitis ulcerosa, collagenoses,** conditions – (febrile c., edematous c., postoperative c.), constrictive pericarditis, cor pulmonale chronicum, cryoglobulinemia, dermatomyositis, diabetic nephropathy/sclerosis, disease – (**Crohn's d.,** Cushing's d., **Whipple's d.,** Gaucher's d., Ménétrier's d., Brill-Zinsser d., Wilson's d., adult Still's d., Graves' d., **IgG/IgM heavy chain d.,** cytomegalic inclusion d., pelvic inflammatory d., duodenal ulcer d., **celiac d.),** diseases – (cardiac valvular d., **hepatic d.,** pleural d., rheumatic d., congenital heart d., **acute/chronic inflammatory d.),** eclampsia, encephalitis – (cytomegalovirus e.), echinococcosis, endocarditis, enterocolitis – (pseudomembranous e., tuberculous e.), **protein-losing enteropathy,** dermatitis – (**exfoliative d.,** d. herpetiformis), **exudative enteropathy,** eosinophilic gastroenteritis, **fatty liver, cystic fibrosis,** galactosemia, glycogen storage disease (type V), Wegener's granulomatosis, eosinophilic granuloma, hemochromatosis – (secondary h., idiopathic h.), familial idiopathic hypoproteinemia, fever – (**rheumatic f.,** Rocky Mountain spotted f.), fistula – (gastrointestinal f., lymphatic f.), **hemorrhage,** cholangitis – (secondary ch., primary sclerosing ch.), **hepatic cirrhosis together with other symptoms of dysproteinemia,** malignant histiocytosis, histoplasmosis, hepatic encephalopathy, hepatic insufficiency – (**acute/chronic h. i.,** irreversible stage of h. i.), **hereditary analbuminemia,** hypersplenism, hyperhydration, hypertension – (malignant h., portal h.), hypervitaminosis A, **hyperthyroidism,** hypocalcemia, hypogammaglobulinemia, infectious diseases – (**bacterial i. d., parasitic i. d., viral i. d.),** inflammatory bowel disease, intake – (excessive administration of i.v. glucose, decreased iron i.), intestinal capillariasis, hepatic coma, leprosy, leptospirosis, kwashiorkor, leishmaniasis, intestinal lymphangiectasia, loss of proteins in – (diarrhea, **burns, nephrosis,** transudation, **exudates),** Waldenström's macroglobulinemia, malaria, **malnutrition, metastatic tumours,** infectious mononucleosis, mycosis fungoides, myocardial infarction, endocardium myxoma, necrosis – (**hepatocellular n.,** tissue n.), malignant nephrosclerosis, **nephritis,** sickle cell nephropathy, pyogenic osteomyelitis, ornithosis, pancreatitis – (acute p., acute necrotizing p.), peptic gastric ulcer, constrictive pericarditis, **pneumonia,** poisoning by – (alkali, DDT, vinyl chloride), intestine perforation, polyarteritis nodosa, polycythemia vera, polymyalgia rheumatica, polymyositis, acute idiopathic polyneuritis, polytrauma, poor nutrition, porphyria cutanea tarda, **preeclampsia, pregnancy,** prolonged immobility, proteinosis – (alveolar lung p., lipoid p.), **protein-losing enteropathy,** purpura – (thrombocytopenic thrombotic p., Henoch-Schoenlein p.), pyelitis, **pyelonephritis,** rapid intravenous hydration, **renal vein thrombosis,** repeated thoracentesis, repeated paracentesis, leukemic reticuloendotheliosis, acute fatty liver of pregnancy, **sarcoidosis,** septicemia, schistosomiasis, scleroderma, scurvy, shock – (septic s., hypovolemic s., cardiogenic s.), **sprue,** starvation, steatohepatitis, tricuspid valve stenosis, strongyloidiasis, syndrome – (hepatorenal sy, **malabsorption sy, nephrotic sy,** dumping sy, Goodpasture's sy, Fanconi's sy, Felty's sy, Kawasaki's sy, eosinophilia-myalgia sy, vena cava inferior obstruction sy, blind loop sy, toxic shock sy, Sjögren's sy, Sezary's sy, Zollinger-Ellison sy, SIADH), syphilis, **systemic lupus erythematosus,** hereditary hemorrhagic teleangiectasia, thrombosis – (renal vein t., portal vein t.), acute suppurative thyroiditis, thyrotoxic crisis, toxoplasmosis, trichinosis, thyrotoxicosis, **tuberculosis,** tumours – (**leukemia,** breast t., male breast t., Hodgkin's d., colorectal t., melanoma,

gallbladder t., pancreas t., kidney t., liposarcoma, osteosarcoma, rhabdomyosarcoma, liver t., lung t., intestine t., prostate t., thymoma, Wilm's t., Burkitt's lymphoma, **plasmocytoma** incl. multiple myeloma, Kaposi's sarcoma, stomach t., uterus t.), typhus – (endemic t., epidemic t.), vasculitis, **Waldenström's macroglobulinemia, water intoxication,** failure – (**heart f.,** chronic kidney f., acute liver f.)

> Interfering Factors: medicaments – (aldesleukin, allopurinol, amiodarone, antiepileptics, antimetabolites, asparaginase, azathioprine, chlorpropamide, cisplatin, clofibrate, dapsone, denileukin, dextran, estrogens, follitropin, heparin, ibuprofen, isoniazid, kava kava, menotropins, mestranol, nitrofurantoin, oral contraceptives, phenylbutazone, phenytoin, prednisone, sulindac, valproic acid)

Analyte	Age/Gender	Reference Range	SI Units	Note
Albumin	Neonates	38–42	g/l	
	Adults	33–50	g/l	See ref. ranges note
		37–53	g/l	See ref. ranges note

Alcohol Dehydrogenase

(AD, ADH) An oxidoreductase enzyme that catalyzes reversible oxidation of primary/secondary alcohols to aldehydes using NAD^+ as an electron acceptor. The reaction is the first step in the alcohol metabolism by the liver. Alcohol dehydrogenase is a hepatic cytoplasmic enzyme predominantly located in the centrilobular region. Alcohol dehydrogenase isoenzymes specific for the liver, gastric mucosa and kidney have been identified.

Function. Activity of this enzyme is responsible for methanol and ethylene glycol metabolic conversion to toxic compounds. Such conversion is inhibited by the ethanol administration. Alcohol dehydrogenase is claimed to be a highly sensitive marker for liver anoxia with centrilobular damage.

Increased Values
diseases – (infectious d., **inflammatory d.**), drug hepatotoxicity, **hepatocellular damage, tumors**

> Interfering Factors: medicaments – (thiourea)

Decreased Values
> Interfering Factors: oxalate, heavy metals

Aldolase

(syn: aldehydelyase)
Function. Glycolytic enzyme (lyase) that catalyzes the fructose-1,6-diphosphate breakdown into the triase phosphates, it is a part of glycolytic glucose breakdown into lactate.
Occurrence. Aldolase is found throughout most tissues of the body, mainly in the skeletal muscles, heart, brain and kidney.
Test Purpose. 1) differential diagnosis of cellular necrosis, cartilage disorders, myocardial infarction, pancreatitis, 2) activity determination useful in indicating muscular or hepatic cellular injury, 3) tumor marker.

Increased Values – hyperaldolasemia

acute psychoses, anemia – (hemolytic a., macrocytic a., **megaloblastic a.**), **burns,** congenital heart failure, decompensated heart defects, **delirium tremens, dermatomyositis,** diabetes mellitus, epilepsy, erythroblastosis fetalis, furunculosis, **gangrene,** glycogenosis (type V), hemorrhagic pericarditis, **hepatic cirrhosis,** hepatic necrosis, hepatitis – (**acute h., chronic h., viral h.**), hepatoma, malignant hyperthermia, hyperthyroidism, disease – (McArdle's d., Niemann-Pick d.), diseases – (viral diseases of upper respiratory tract in children, **liver d., muscular infectious d.**), infarction – (**myocardial i.**, pulmonary i.), **infectious mononucleosis,** injuries – (crush i., **muscular i.**), leptospirosis, metastases into the liver, muscular dystrophy – (**Duchenne's m. d.,** Erb's m. d.), myoglobinuria, myopathy, inclusion body myositis, **obstructive jaundice,** osteomyelitis, pancreatitis – (acute p., hemorrhagic p.), paroxysmal myoglobinemia, pneumonia, poisoning by – (chlorate hydrocarbonates, lead), burns, polycythemia vera, **polymyositis, rhabdomyolysis,** schizophrenia, surgery, syndrome – (eosinophilia-myalgia sy, toxic shock sy), tetanus, **trichinosis,** tuberculosis, tumors – (**CNS t., leukemia,** lymphoma, melanoma, colorectal t., stomach t., **liver t., lung t., pancreas t., prostate t., breast t., gastrointestinal tract t., genitourinary system t.**)

    Interfering Factors: medicaments – (ACTH, cortisone)

Decreased Values – hypoaldolasemia
hereditary fructose intolerance, late muscular dystrophy, loss of muscle mass

Analyte	Age/Gender	Reference Range	SI Units	Note
Aldolase	10–24 m	3.4–11.8	U/l	
	25 m–16 y	1.2–8.8	U/l	
	Adults	<135	nkat/l	

Aldosterone

Production. Adrenal cortex steroid hormone (21-C-corticosteroid) is the most potent suprarenal mineralocorticoid, produced exclusively in the zona glomerulosa. Almost all aldosterone circulates freely or weakly non-specifically bound to albumin, action occurrs after binding to mineralocorticoid receptors in the kidney and brain. Aldosterone is metabolized rapidly by the liver and excreted as tetrahydroaldosterone, it is also metabolized by the kidney and excreted as aldosterone glucuronide.

Function. Increases renal tubular resorption of natrium and chloride = retention, decreases tubular resorption of kalium and hydrogen = elimination. Renin-aldosterone-angiotensin system share body fluid balance maintenance, in the blood pressure support. Aldosterone levels are affected (production stimulated) by the: renin-angiotensin system, plasma potassium and natrium concentrations, adrenocorticotropic hormone, beta-melanotropin and serotonin. Inhibited by the: dopamine and atrial natriuretic hormone. While supine, aldosterone levels decrease during day, upright position increases aldosterone levels progressively. Position reactivity and total synthesis of aldosterone decrease occurs in the elderly. Day-to-day variation can be 40%.

Test Purpose. 1) to aid in diagnosis of primary aldosteronism and potential disorders causes, including adrenal adenoma and adrenal hyperplasia, 2) to aid diagnosis of secondary hyperaldosteronism and commonly related conditions, such as salt-losing sy, potassium excess, congestive heart failure with ascites, or other conditions that characteristically increase the renin-angiotensin system activity and especially in the differential diagnosis of hypertension.

Increased Values – hyperaldosteronemia
adrenal cortical hyperplasia, adrenal enzymopathy, anorexia nervosa, burns, cardiac failure, chronic obstructive pulmonary disease, eclampsia, cirrhosis – (congenital hepatic c., liver c.), Conn's disease (primary hyperaldosteronism), secondary hyperaldosteronism, diabetes mellitus, edema – (renal e., hepatic e., cardiac e.), hemorrhage, hyperkalemia, hyperthyroidism, hyponatremia, hypovolemia, malignant hypertension, menstruation, nephrosis, pheochromocytoma, renal artery stenosis, renal ischemia, salt depletion, secondary hyperaldosteronism, syndrome – (Bartter's sy, Cushing's sy, nephrotic sy, postsurgical sy), pregnancy, transudation, tumours producing – (aldosterone, renin)
  Interfering Factors: change of posture, dehydration, diet, starvation, neonates, obesity, pregnancy, strenuous exercise, stress, medicaments – (ACTH, amiloride, angiotensin, captopril, chlortalidone, contraceptives, diazoxide, diuretics, estrogens, furosemide, hydralazine, laxatives, lithium, metoclopramide, nifedipine, nitroprusside, potassium, spironolactone, steroids, thiazides, triamterene, verapamil)

Decreased Values – hypoaldosteronemia
acute alcoholic intoxication, bilateral nephrectomy, congenital 17-hydroxylase defect, deficiency of – (aldosterone, renin, aldosterone synthetase), diabetes mellitus, excessive secretion of deoxycorticosterone, high-sodium diet, hypernatremia, hyporeninemic hypoaldosteronism, hypoaldosteronism – (primary h., secondary h.), hypokalemia, insufficiency – (pituitary i., adrenal cortex i.), PIH (pregnancy induced hypertension), renal impairment, septic states, stress, syndrome – (adrenogenital sy, Turner's sy, salt-losing sy)
  Interfering Factors: alcohol, high altitude, intense weight loss in obesity, over age 60, medicaments – (ACE inhibitors, antihypertensives, captopril, cisplatin, deoxycorticosterone, enalapril, etomidate, heparin, indomethacin, non-steroidal anti-inflammatory agents, prazosin, propranolol, ranitidine, saralazine)

Alkaline Phosphatase

(total ALP, AP, syn: alkaline optimum, orthophosphoric monoester phosphohydrolase)
Function. Hydrolytic enzyme splitting esters of phosphoric acid. ALP catalyzes hydrolysis of phosphate esters and transports it through cellular membrane. ALP exits from the hepatic cell directly to the biliary tree lumen.
Occurrence. Bones – osteoblasts, liver and biliary tract, intestine, kidneys – proximal tubules, leukocytes, placenta, bile, lactating mammary glands and in nearly all body cells that are rapidly dividing or are otherwise metabolically active. Liver ALP is localized in the hepatic cell sinusoidal membrane, microvillus of the bile canaliculus and portal, central vein endothelial cells and in Kupffer's cells (these cells line the biliary collecting system).
Isoenzymes. Intestinal, placental, vascular endothelium, tissue non-specific – (bone, hepatic, renal, reticuloendothelial system). Tumorous and biliary ducts ALP do not belong to isoenzymes because they are not produced under genetic control. ALP is an enzymatic tumor marker. Day-to-day variation is 5–10%. No diurnal variation.
Test Purpose. 1) to detect/identify skeletal diseases, primarily characterized by marked osteoblastic and chondroblastic activity, 2) to detect focal hepatic lesions causing biliary obstruction and cholestasis, such as tumor/abscesses, 3) to assess response to vitamin D in the rickets treatment, 4) to supplement information from other liver function studies and gastrointestinal enzyme tests, 5) to help in diagnosis of tumor diseases with metastases – tumor marker, 6) to monitor placental function in threatened 3rd trimester pregnancy.

Increased Values

abortion – (threatened a., septic a.), **acromegaly, active tuberculosis, acute fatty liver**, acute gastritis, **acute hypotension**, acute hypoxia, **acute pancreatitis**, alcoholism, amebiasis, primary/secondary amyloidosis, **amyloid liver infiltrate**, anemia – (sickle cell a., **hemolytic a., acute hemolytic a.**, myelophthisic a., thalassemia major), angina pectoris, argininosuccinic aciduria, ascariasis, babesiosis, blastomycosis, **bone metastases**, bowel perforation, brucellosis, **cardiac catheterization/angiography/angioplasty, cholangitis**, cholecystitis – (**acute ch., chronic ch.**), **choledocholithiasis**, chronic hemodialysis, **hepatic coma**, coccidioidomycosis, congenital hepatic fibrosis, **congenital atresia of intrahepatic bile ducts, congestive hepatomegalia**, cor pulmonale chronicum, coronary insufficiency, cryoglobulinemia, cryptococcosis, cystic fibrosis, **cytomegalovirus infection, dermatomyositis, diabetes mellitus,** diabetic gangrene, dialysis dementia, disease – (**celiac d.**, adult Still's d., Caroli's d., graft-versus-host d., **Boeck's d.**, light chain d., Brill-Zinsser d., Crohn's d., legionnaire's d., **Graves' d.**, Gaucher's d., Lyme d., **Paget's d.**, Whipple's d., Wilson's d.), diseases – (**acute renal d., hepatocellular d., bone d.**, lung destructive d.), drug induced liver disease, duodenal ulcer, echinococcosis, embolism – (systemic arterial e., pulmonary e.), encephalitis – (cytomegalovirus e.), endocarditis, enteritis regionalis, Epstein-Barr virus infection, erosive ulcerative lesions – (colon e. u. l., small intestine e. u. l.), failure – (**cardiac f.**, acute liver f., acute renal f.), familial osteoectasia, fever – (Q f., Rocky Mountain spotted f., typhoid f.), giant cell arteritis, granulomatous colitis, **healing fractures**, hemochromatosis – (secondary h., idiopathic h.), hepatic cirrhosis – (portal h. c., **postnecrotic h. c., primary biliary h. c.**), hepatic congestion, hepatic granuloma, hepatitis – (**alcoholic h.**, autoimmune h., drug cholestatic h., peliosis h., chronic active h., **toxic h., viral h.**), malignant histiocytosis, histoplasmosis, hypercalcemia of malignancy, hyperphosphatemia – (familial h., idiopathic h.), **hyperparathyroidism, hyperthyroidism,** hypervitaminosis – (h. D, h. A), infarction – (**small intestine i.,** myocardial i., renal i., **lung i.,** spleen i.), intestinal obstruction, intestinal ischemia, **involvement of skeletal system in other diseases, infective mononucleosis** (glandular fever), leptospirosis, **liver abscess/cyst**, malaria, march fracture, multiple endocrine neoplasia (type I, type II), mycosis fungoides, myelofibrosis, myositis ossificans, hepatocellular necrosis, nodular vasculitis, obstruction of efferent biliary ways by – (**cholelithiasis, intrahepatic cholestasis, primary sclerosing cholangitis**), ornithosis, osteitis fibrosa cystica, renal osteodystrophy, **osteogenesis imperfecta, osteomalacia, osteomyelitis**, papillary stenosis, parasitic liver diseases, parenteral hyperalimentation of glucose, passive liver congestion, peptic gastric ulcer, peptic chronic esophagitis, peritonitis, **physiologically in children** (normal bone growth), pituitary gigantism, poisoning by – (cadmium, phosphorus, vinyl chloride), polyarteritis nodosa, polycythemia vera, polyostotic fibrous dysplasia, porphyria – (acute intermittent p., p. cutanea tarda), portal hypertension, portal vein thrombosis, pre-/eclampsia, pregnancy – (2nd–3rd trimester, early postpartum), pregnancy induced hypertension, pulmonary aspergillosis, pyoderma gangrenosum, renal insufficiency, **rhachitis** (rickets), **rheumatoid arthritis**, schistosomiasis, **sepsis**, severe malabsorption, shock – (septic s.), steatohepatitis, syndrome – (Albright's sy, **Cushing's sy**, Kawasaki sy, Sezary's sy, Reye's sy, chronic fatigue sy, milk-alkali sy, toxic shock sy), syphilis, thyrotoxicosis, thyrotoxic crisis, toxoplasmosis, transient hyperphosphatasemia of infancy, tularemia, tumors – (**pancreas head t., bone t., leukemia**, kidney t., osteosarcoma, **liver t.**, melanoma, plasmocytoma incl. multiple myeloma, **Hodgkin's lymphoma, lung t., breast t.**, male breast t., cervical t., gastrointestinal tract t., **ovary t.**, prostate t., seminoma, testes t., trophoblast t., gallbladder t., colorectal t.), endemic typhus, **ulcerative colitis**, vitamin D intoxication, Wegener's granulomatosis

Interfering Factors: diurnal/seasonal rhythms, sample standing at room/refrigerator temperature, total parenteral nutrition, medicaments – (acetylsalicylic acid, ajmaline, albumin, allopurinol, amantadine, aminoglutethimide, amiodarone, amitriptyline, amphotericin B, anabolic steroids, antibiotics, antiepileptics, aprindine, ascorbic acid, asparaginase, azathioprine, benoxaprofen, bromocriptine, captopril, carbamazepine, carbenicillin, carbimazole, carbutamide, cefalexin, cefaloridine, cefamandole, cefazolin, cefoperazone, cefoxitin, ceftizoxime, cephalosporins, chloramphenicol, chlordiazepoxide, chlorpromazine, chlorpropamide, cholestatics, cimetidine, clindamycin, clofibrate, clotrimazole, cloxacillin, colchicine, cyclofenil, cyclophosphamide, cyclosporine, cytarabine, dantrolene, dapsone, desipramine, diazepam, dicumarol, dihydralazine, disulfiram, disopyramide, enalapril, ergosterol, erythromycin, estradiol, estrogens, estron, ethambutol, ethotoin, etretinate, flucloxacillin, fluorides, fluoxymesterone, fluphenazine, flurazepam, gentamicin, gestagens, glibenclamide, gold salts, haloperidol, halothane, hydantoines, hydralazine, ibuprofen, imipramine, indomethacin, interferon, isoniazid, isotretinoin, ketoconazole, labetalol, levamisol, lincomycin, lithium, magnesium salts, mebendazole, mepacrine, mephenytoin, metandienone, methotrexate, methoxyflurane, methyldopa, methyltestosterone, meticillin, morphine, nafcillin, nandrolone, naproxen, nicotinic acid, nifedipine, nitrofurantoin, norethisterone, oral contraceptives, oxacillin, oxazepam, oxymetholone, papaverine, paracetamol, paramethadione, penicillamine, penicillins, phenobarbital, phenothiazines, phenylbutazone, phenytoin, plicamycin, practolol, probenecid, prochlorperazine, progesterone, propoxyphene, propranolol, propylthiouracil, protionamide, protriptyline, pyrazinamide, quinidine, quinine, retinol, rifampicin, manganese salts, streptokinase, streptozocin, sulfafurazole, sulfamethizole, sulfamethoxazole, sulfasalazine, sulfonamides, sulfonylurea, sulindac, tetracyclines, thiamazole, thiopental, thiabendazole, ticlopidine, thioguanine, tolazamide, tolbutamide, trimethadione, trimethoprim, verapamil, zalcitabine, zimeldine)

Increased isoenzymes

■ **biliary ways:** cholestasis, biliary obstruction
■ **hepatic:** parenchymal cell diseases, hepatic congestion, hepatic parenchyma lesion, pregnancy, vasculitis, hepatitis, chronic alcohol ingestion
■ **intestinal:** hepatic cirrhosis, intrahepatic cholestasis, inflammatory/ulcerative intestinal diseases, severe malabsorption, chronic hemodialysis
■ **bone:** hyperparathyroidism, hyperthyroidism, Gaucher's disease, Niemann-Pick disease, **Paget's disease**, bone metastases, renal osteodystrophy, **osteomalacia**, osteoporosis, postmenopausal osteoporosis, osteosarcoma, **rickets**, physiological bone growth, malabsorption sy, healing bone fractures, osteoblastic bone cancers
■ **placental** (physiologically in the 2nd half of pregnancy, disappears 3–6 days after placenta delivery): pregnancy induced hypertension, pre-/eclampsia
■ **tumorous:** tumors – (bronchial t., leukemia, hypernephroma, gastrointestinal t.)

Decreased Values

achondroplasia, alcoholism, **anemia**, cardiac surgery with cardiopulmonary bypass pump, **celiac disease**, cretinism, Cushing's disease, deficiency – (growth hormone d., **magnesium d.**, vitamin B$_{12}$ d., protein intake d., zinc d.), growth retardation in children, **hypervitaminosis D**, **hypophosphatasia**, **hypoparathyroidism**, hypophyseous nanism, hypothyroidism – (**primary h.**, juvenile h., hypothalamic h., iodine h.), intoxication by – (arsenate, beryllium, carbon disulfide, EDTA, fluoride, phosphorus, cyanide, manganese, oxalate, vitamin D), kwashiorkor, leukemia – (lymphatic l., chronic myeloid l.), lymphomas, **malnutrition**, myxedema, toxic liver disorders, increased intake of – (protein, vitamin B), placental insufficiency, pregnancy, pubertas praecox (precocious puberty), acute pyelonephritis, rheumatoid arthritis, **scorbutus** (scurvy), syndrome – (chronic malabsorption sy, **milk-alkali sy**), irradiation, poor nutrition

   Interfering Factors: rhythms – (diurnal r., seasonal r.), collection of blood in – (EDTA, fluoride, oxalate anticoagulant), medicaments – (ACTH, arsenicals, azathioprine, calcitonin, citrates, clofibrate, corticoids, danazol, estrogens, fenofibrate, fluorides, nitrofurantoin, oral contraceptives, penicillamine, sucralfate, tamoxifen, theophylline, thiocompounds, trifluoperazine, zinc salts)

Decreased isoenzymes

■ **bone:** pernicious anemia, chronic nutritional deficiency of – (magnesium, vitamin B_{12}, zinc, protein), hypothyroidism, osteopenia due to genetic hypophosphatasemia, poor nutrition

Analyte	Age/Gender	Reference Range	SI Units	Note
Alkaline Phosphatase (ALP)				
Total	1 d	<10.00	µkat/l	
	2–5 d	<9.22	µkat/l	
	6 d–6 m	<17.94	µkat/l	
	7 m–1 y	<18.45	µkat/l	
	2–3 y	<11.22	µkat/l	
	4–6 y	<10.74	µkat/l	
	7–12 y	<12.00	µkat/l	
	13–17 y F	<7.47	µkat/l	
	13–17 y M	<15.60	µkat/l	
	Adults F	<4.00	µkat/l	
	Adults M	<4.50	µkat/l	
	Adults F	0.74–2.1	µkat/l	
	Adults M	0.9–2.29	µkat/l	
Bone ALP	Adults F	<2.00	µkat/l	
	Adults M	<2.50	µkat/l	
	Adults F	<0.83	µkat/l	
	Adults M	<1.00	µkat/l	

Alpha-Aminonitrogen

(syn: nitrogen of amino acids)
Test Purpose. 1) renal glycosuria, phosphaturia diagnosis, 2) diagnosis of suspect aminoaciduria, 3) diagnosis of suspect Fanconi's sy, 4) proximal tubules disorders.

Increased Values

aminoaciduria – (prerenal a., renal a.), cardiac decompensation, diabetes mellitus, eclampsia, chronic hepatitis, PIH, hyperthyroidism, hypothyroidism, acute infections, hepatic insufficiency, poisoning by – (arsenic, phosphorus, chloroform, tetrachlormethane), myeloid leukemia, nephritis, severe parenchymatous hepatic lesions – (acute dystrophy of the liver, poisoning, hepatotoxic agents), pregnancy, uremia

Decreased Values

nephrosis, pneumonia

Aluminium

(Al, syn: aluminum) Aluminium is ubiquitous in our environment, the third most prevalent element in the earth's crust. Tends to form very stable oxides. Human exposure resulting in pathology has been reported for aluminium containing dusts, domestic water supplies and medications. The gastrointestinal tract is relatively impervious to aluminum, absorption normally is only about 2%. Aluminium is absorbed by a mechanism related to calcium. Gastric acidity and oral citrate favours absorption, H_2-blockers reduce absorption. Transferrin is the primary protein binder and an aluminium carrier in the plasma, where 80% is protein bound and 20% is free or complexed in small molecules. Important target organs for pathology are bone and brain. Accumulations may be also found in lungs, bone and muscle. The predominant excretory pathway is the kidney. $Al(OH)_3$ is used medically as a gastric antacid and phosphate-binding agent in dialysis patients. Aluminium toxicity in chronical renal failure, associated with exposure to the metal's compounds during treatment, is the most commonly reported incident. Recommended specimens: serum, dialysis fluid, urine, cerebrospinal fluid.

Test Purpose. 1) patients on parenteral nutrition, 2) burn patients through administration of intravenous albumin particularly with coexisting renal failure, 3) adult or pediatric patients with chronic renal failure who accumulate aluminium readily from medications or dialysate, 4) patients with industrial exposure.

Increased Values – hyperaluminemia
dialysis dementia, industrial aluminium exposure, cystic fibrosis, diseases – (**hepatic d., bile ducts d.**), leukemias, Alzheimer's disease, Hodgkin's disease, pregnancy, total parenteral nutrition, **renal failure**

Decreased Values – hypoaluminemia
pernicious anemia, diabetes mellitus, gastric ulcer disease, skin diseases (except psoriasis)

Analyte	Age/Gender	Reference Range	SI Units	Note
Aluminium		<0.11	µmol/l	

Amino Acid Profile

Test includes: alanine, amino-guanidino-propionic acid, amino-N-butyric acid, aminoadipic acid, aminobutyric acid, aminoisobutyric acid, anserine, arginine, asparagine, aspartic acid, beta-alanine, carnosine, citrulline, cystathionine, cystine, glutamic acid, glutamine, glycine, histidine, homocystine, hydroxylysine, hydroxyproline, isoleucine, leucine, lysine, methionine, 1-methylhistidine, 3-methylhistidine, ornithine, phenylalanine, phosphoethanolamine, phosphoserine, proline, sarcosine, serine, taurine, threonine, tyrosine, tryptophan, valine

Amino Acids

(AA) Any organic compound containing an amino ($-NH_2$) and a carboxyl ($-COOH$) group. The nine essential alpha-amino acids required for protein synthesis that cannot be synthesized by humans and must be obtained in the diet are histidine, isoleucine, leucine, lysine, methionine, phenylalanine, threonine, tryptophan and valine. Nonessential amino acids include the eleven alpha-amino acids required for protein synthesis, that are synthesized by humans but are not specifically required in the diet: alanine, arginine, asparagine, cysteine, glutamic acid, aspartic acid, glutamate, glycine, proline, serine and tyrosine. Increased amino acid concentrations in plasma may reflect inherited metabolic abnormalities. The usual approach is to test urine for amino acids. However, urinary levels are variable, plasma is more definitive. In all cases where an amino acid is elevated in blood, it will also be elevated in urine.

Increased Values – hyperaminoacidemia

acidemia – (methylmalonic a., propionic a.), alkaptonuria, **specific aminoacidemias**, aminoaciduria – (dibasic a., dicarboxylic a.), argininemia, citrullinemia, cystathioninuria, cystinuria, diabetes mellitus with ketosis, eclampsia, hemolysis, histidinemia, homocystinuria, hyperphenylalaninemia, hyperglycinemia, hyperornithinemia, hyperprolinemia, maple syrup urine disease, iminoglycinuria, hereditary fructose intolerance, intoxication by bismuth salts, carnosinemia, Hartnup disease, malabsorption, burns, severe liver damage, Reye's sy, shock, tyrosinemia, renal failure – (acute r. f., chronic r. f.)

> **Interfering Factors:** medicaments – (EDTA, glucocorticoids, heparin, levarterenol, sulfonamides, testosterone)

Decreased Values – hypoaminoacidemia

rheumatoid arthritis, glomerulonephritis, **adrenocortical hyperfunction**, Huntington's chorea, polycystic kidney disease, **Hartnup disease**, **acute pancreatitis**, syndrome – (carcinoid sy, **nephrotic sy**)

Ammonia

(NH$_3$)

Production. End product (by-product) of protein metabolism from the bacteria action on the proteins in the intestines and from the glutamine hydrolysis in the kidneys (catabolism of amino acids results in the free ammonia production, which is highly toxic to the central nervous system). In the liver most of the ammonia is detoxified – converted to urea (urea cycle = Krebs-Henseleit cycle) → excretion by the kidney and within skeletal muscles and brain by combining with glutamate → glutamine. Ammonia is a non-protein nitrogen compound that helps maintain acid-base balance.

Test Purpose. 1) to help monitor the severe hepatic disease progression and the therapy effectiveness, 2) to recognize impending or established hepatic coma, 3) to test the renal presence in acid-base balance maintenance.

Increased Values – hyperammonemia

acidemia – (**isovaleric a., methylmalonic a., propionic a.**), aciduria – (glutaric a. – type II, argininosuccinic a.), **portocaval anastomosis** (portal-systemic shunting of blood), **azotemia**, acute bronchitis, elevated intake of proteins, cardiac cirrhosis, **hepatic cirrhosis** (far advanced), **citrullinemia**, cor pulmonale, **deficiency of the urea cycle enzymes, pulmonary emphysema**, encephalopathy – (**neonatal/infantile e., hepatic e.**), hepatectomy, hereditary enzymopathy, hepatitis – (acute h. D, chronic active h., autoimmune h., acute h. B, alcoholic h., chemical induced h.), **hereditary hyperammonemia**, hyperalimentation, hyperglycinemia, portal hypertension, **hyperornithinemia, erythroblastosis fetalis**, diseases – (renal d., **chronic liver d., infectious genitourinary tract d.**), insufficiency – (**renal i., hepatic i.**), lysine intolerance, intoxication by fluorides, renal ischemia, diabetic ketoacidosis, coma – (diabetic c., **hepatic c.**), bleeding – (**into the bowels, from the esophageal varices**), leukemia – (lymphatic l., myelocytic l.), **acute hepatic necrosis**, fatty liver, acute fatty liver of pregnancy, premature infants, **pericarditis**, pneumonia, steatohepatitis, syndrome – (**Reye's sy**, HELLP sy), shock, uremia, parenteral nutrition, transient hyperammonemia in newborn, moribund children, failure – (**renal f.**, **fulminant hepatic f.**, **cardiac f.**, congenital heart f.)

Interfering Factors: physical exertion, medicaments – (acetazolamide, ammonium chloride, asparaginase, barbiturates, chlorothiazide, diuretics, ethanol, furosemide, heparin, methicillin, narcotic analgesics, neomycin, oxalate, polymyxin B, thiazides, valproic acid)

Decreased Values – hypoammonemia

hyperornithinemia, smoking, hypertension – (essential h., malignant h.), **renal failure**

Interfering Factors: medicaments – (antibiotics, cephalotin, kanamycin, lactobacillus acidophilus, lactulose, levodopa, neomycin, potassium salts, tetracycline)

Analyte	Age/Gender	Reference Range	SI Units	Note
Ammonia	1 d	<144	µmol/l	
	5–6 d	<134	µmol/l	
	Children	<48	µmol/l	
	Adults F	6–48	µmol/l	
	Adults M	10–55	µmol/l	

Amphiregulin

(AR, syn: colorectum cell-derived growth factor, CRDGF, keratinocyte-derived autocrine factor, KAF) Amphiregulin can be isolated from placenta, testes, ovaries and a number of tumor cell lines. Inhibits the growth of various human carcinoma cell lines in vitro. The proliferation of some tumor cell lines and also of fibroblasts and other normal cells is enhanced by amphiregulin. Acts in an autocrine manner on some human, colon carcinomas.

Amylase

(AMS, syn: alpha-amylase, diastase) Excretory enzyme.

Production. Secreted from 1) salivary glands, 2) pancreatic acinar cells into the pancreatic duct and then into the duodenum.

Function. Salivary amylase starts digestion → hydrolyzes carbohydrate alpha-1,4 linking to give maltose, maltotriose and dextrans. Digestive enzyme → splits (hydrolyzes) starch (carbohydrates) to simple sugar (oligosaccharides, maltose, maltotriose) in the intestine.

Occurrence. Pancreas, salivary glands, placenta, lungs, liver, milk, sweat, fallopian tubes. Inflammatory diseases of these glands or duct obstructions result in enzyme regurgitation into the blood and increased excretion via the kidney. Macroamylasemia indicates complexes of AMS and IgA (70%) or IgG (30%), can include albumin and alpha-1-antitrypsin.

Isoenzymes. 1) pancreatic (P), 2) salivary (S) – salivary glands, fallopian tube, lung, liver.

Test Purpose. 1) to diagnose acute pancreatitis, acute relapse of chronic pancreatitis, 2) to distinguish between acute pancreatitis and other causes of abdominal pain requiring immediate surgery, 3) to evaluate possible pancreatic injury caused by abdominal trauma or surgery, 4) to help in the diagnosis of epidemic and alcoholic parotitides.

Increased Values – hyperamylasemia

acidosis (S), abscess – (pancreas a., appendix a., parotid gland a.), **acute alcoholism** (P, S), amyloidosis, aortic aneurysm with dissection, anorexia nervosa, **acute appendicitis**, ascariasis, ascites (P), brain contusion, bulimia, cyst – (**pancreatic c.** – P, **ovarian c.** – S), delirium tremens, diabetes mellitus (S), partial gastrectomy, endoscopic retrograde choledochopancreatography (ERCP), heroin addiction (S), cholelithiasis, **acute cholecystitis**, cholecysto-pathy, **choledocholithiasis** (P), disease – (Crohn's d., polycystic kidney d.), diseases – (**liver d.**, duodenal ulcer d., biliary tract d., intestinal d., genitourinary tract d., lung d., breast d., prostate d., CNS d., tubo-ovarian d.), subdural intracranial empyema, Wernicke's encepha-lopathy, fascioliasis, eosinophilic granuloma, subdural intracranial hematoma, hepatitis – (acute h. B, alcoholic h., acute h. A, acute h. D, acute h. E), hyperlipoproteinemia (type I, type IV), benign familial hypocalcemia, infarction – (**mesenteric i.** – P, **pulmonary i.**), renal **insufficiency** (P, S), obstructive jaundice, alcoholic cardiomyopathy, **diabetic ketoacidosis** (P, S), non-ketotic hyperosmolar coma, diabetic coma (S), **macroamylasemia**, myoglobinuria, tumors – (**esophageal t., colon t.** – S, P; **pancreas t.**– P, S; **lung t.** – S, prostate t. – S, plasmo-cytoma, **breast t.** – P, **ovary t.** – S, stomach t.), lupus nephritis, chronic lead nephropathy, alcoholic neuropathy, intestinal obstruction (P), obstruction of pancreatic ducts by (P) – (stone, tumor, morphine, duct sphincter spasm, stricture), pancreatitis (P) – (**acute p., chronic obstructive p., acute necrotizing p.**), renal osteodystrophy, paraneoplasia, parotitis (S), **parotitis epidemica** (parotiditis) (S), perforated – (**bowels** – P, **peptic ulcer** – P, **gallblad-der** – P, esophagus), **peritonitis** (P, S), pneumonia (S), poisoning by – (alkali, arsenic, opioid, salicylate, mushroom, cocaine), sigmoid colon volvulus, burns (P, S), placental/ovarian dis-orders, **acute relapse of chronic pancreatitis** (P), **renal failure**, rupture – (aortic aneurysm r., ectopic pregnancy r., spleen r., esophageal r.), sarcoidosis, scleroderma, sialadenitis, **sia-lolithiasis** (S), steatohepatitis, syndrome – (CREST sy, Mallory–Weiss sy, Mikulicz sy, Zol-linger–Ellison sy), conditions – (postoperative abdominal/heart surgery c. – P, S; shock c.), intestinal strangulation, pregnancy, graviditas extrauterina (ectopic pregnancy), **renal trans-plantation** (S), trauma – (skull t., cerebral t., pancreatic t. – P), **mesenteric thrombosis** (P), tuberculosis (S), typhoid fever (S), pancreas pseudocyst (P), pancreas abscess (P), salivary gland inflammation, failure – (acute liver f., kidney f.)

Interfering Factors: medicaments – (aminosalicylic acid, asparaginase, azathioprine, captopril, cholinergics, cimetidine, codeine, corticosteroids, estrogens, ethacrynic acid, ethyl alcohol, fluorides, furosemide, glucocorticoids, histamine, ibuprofen, indometh-acin, iodine-containing contrast media, meperidine, methyldopa, methylprednisolone, morphine, narcotics, nitrofurantoin, opioids, oral contraceptives, oxyphenbutazone, pancreozymin, pentamidine, pentazocine, phenformin, phenylbutazone, prednisolone, prednisone, salicylates, steroids, sulfonamides, sulindac, tetracyclines, thiazides, thia-bendazole, valproic acid)

Decreased Values – hypoamylasemia

hepatic abscess, acute alcoholism, acute/chronic bronchitis, hepatic cirrhosis, **severe des-truction of hepatic/pancreatic tissue**, eclampsia, bacterial endocarditis, **cystic fibrosis of pancreas**, **hepatitis**, **pregnancy induced hypertension**, hyperthyroidism, liver diseases – (al-coholic l. d., severe l. d.), **pancreatic insufficiency**, cachexia, lung metastases, tumors – (liver t., pancreas t.), pancreatic ways obstruction, pancreatectomy, pancreatitis – (**acute fulmi-nant p.**, acute necrotizing p., **chronic advanced p.**), **severe burns**, acute intermittent porphy-ria, tuberculosis, **severe thyrotoxicosis**, hepatic necrosis, acute liver failure

Interfering Factors: medicaments – (anabolic steroids, barbiturates, citrates, glucose, metandienone, narcotics, oxalates)

Analyte	Age/Gender	Reference Range	SI Units	Note
Amylase (AMS)				
Total	Adults	0.50–3.67	µkat/l	
Pancreatic	1–5 d	<0.03	µkat/l	
	6 d–6 m	<0.27	µkat/l	
	7 m–1 y	<0.75	µkat/l	

Analyte	Age/Gender	Reference Range	SI Units	Note
	2–3 y	<1.02	μkat/l	
	4–6 y	<1.10	μkat/l	
	7–12 y F	<1.22	μkat/l	
	7–12 y M	<1.08	μkat/l	
	13–17 y	<1.28	μkat/l	
	Adults	<1.92	μkat/l	

Amylin

(IAPP, syn: insular amyloid polypeptide) Short 37 amino acid polypeptide synthesized as precursor proamylin (93 amino acids). Gene contains three exones and has 50% homology with CGRP (calcitonin gene-related peptide), from this can be partially explained its biological effect on calcium concentration → hypocalcemia (similar to calcium antagonist effect) and influences also a blood pressure → BP decrease. It appears with insulin secretion in the same time and responses on endo/exogenous stimuli. In prolonged secretory granules accumulation amylin decreases beta-cells reactivity by unknown mechanism and later also their structure, C-peptide and insulin secretion. Two main effects are phase and stoichiometrically shifted. Amylin concentration evaluation is a sensitive diabetic nephropathy development marker in microalbuminuria starting stage. Increased lactate concentration are often causative manifestation of IAPP increased concentration in pancreas tumors. It is also a major component of islet amyloid in patients with non-insulin dependent diabetes. Amylin inhibits insulin-stimulated glycogen synthesis in isolated skeletal muscle and inhibits insulin-induced glucose utilization in vivo.

Test Purpose. 1) diabetes mellitus type I and II differential diagnosis, 2) differential diagnosis of hyperinsulinism and nesidioma, 3) diabetic nephropathy development follow up.

Increased Values – hyperamylinemia
diabetes mellitus type II with multiple secretory granules in beta-cells, chronic renal diseases, renal insufficiency

Decreased Values – hypoamylinemia
pancreatoprive diabetes mellitus, IDDM caused by autoimmune process

Analyte	Age/Gender	Reference Range	SI Units	Note
Amylin		2.90–3.40	pmol/l	

3-Alpha-Androstanediol Glucuronide

(3-alpha-diol G) It is a metabolite of dihydrotestosterone formed in the peripheral tissues.
Test Purpose. Useful in a differential diagnosis of hirsutism and peripheral androgen activity evaluation.

Increased Values
acne in females, hirsutism – (idiopathic h., h. associated with polycystic ovary sy)

Decreased Values
men with disorders of androgen action, male pseudohermaphroditism

Androstenedione

Androstenedione is a major precursor of adrenal androgens biosynthesis produced in the ovaries, and to a lesser extent in the adrenal glands. Synthesis is stimulated by ACTH and is suppressed by exogenous glucocorticoid administration. Some androstenedione is secreted into the plasma and the remainder is converted to estrogen in ovarian granulosa cells or to testosterone in the interstitium. In the peripheral tissues, this hormone also can be converted to testosterone and estrogens. Highest levels are found in AM, lowest in PM. In women highest levels are at midcycle. Day-to-day variation is 30–50%.

Test Purpose. To aid in determining the cause of gonadal dysfunction, menstrual or menopausal irregularities, and premature sexual development.

Increased Values – hyperandrostenedionemia

hirsutism, **congenital adrenal hyperplasia**, **polycystic ovarian disease**, tumors of – (**adrenals**, testes, **ovary**), **ectopic ACTH-producing tumors**, osteoporosis in females, syndrome – (**Cushing's sy, Stein-Leventhal sy**)

Interfering Factors: exercise, **smoking**, obesity, postprandial, pregnancy, medicaments – (cimetidine, clomiphene, metyrapone)

Decreased Values – hypoandrostenedionemia

hypogonadism, Addison's disease, failure – (**adrenal f.**, ovarian f.)

Interfering Factors: medicaments – (carbamazepine, ketoconazole, norplant)

Analyte	Age/Gender	Reference Range	SI Units	Note
Androstenedione		2.9–9.4	nmol/l	
	F postmenopause	<6.3	nmol/l	

Angiogenin

Belongs to cytokines.

Production. Fibroblasts, lymphocytes, colon epithelium, carcinoma cells.

Function. Can serve as a substrate for endothelial and fibroblast cell adhesion. It is a member of the pancreatic ribonuclease superfamily. Very likely the biological activity of angiogenin is due to the activation of accessory cells induced to secrete a cytokine or cytokines activating endothelial cells. Also promotes the adhesion of endothelial cells and fibroblasts. Angiogenin activates phospholipase C and induces the rapid incorporation of fatty acid into cholesterol esters in vascular smooth muscle cells.

Angiopoietin-1

Angiopoietin-1 is chemotactic for endothelial cells. Belongs to the group of angiopoietins (angiopoietin 1, 2, 3, 4). Promotes angiogenesis. The physiological roles of angiopoietin-1 and its receptor are limited to angiogenic processes that occur subsequent to the earlier vasculogenic and angiogenic actions of the VEGF (vascular endothelial growth factor) family and their receptors. Angiopoietins can potentiate the effects of other angiogenic cytokines.

Angiotensin I

(AT I) A decapeptide cleaved from renin substrate by the enzyme renin. It has some biological activities but serves mainly as a precursor to angiotensin II.

Increased Values
    Interfering Factors: neonates, during sleep, upright position, medicaments – (oral contraceptives)

Angiotensin II

(AT II) Angiotensin II is an active hormone of the renin-angiotensin system. An octapeptide hormone formed from angiotensin I by angiotensin-converting enzyme action on angiotensin I, chiefly in the lungs but also at other sites such as in blood vessel walls, the uterus and the brain. It is a powerful vasopressor and aldosterone secretion stimulator by the adrenal cortex, functioning also as a neurotransmitter. Its vasopressor action raises blood pressure and diminishes fluid loss in the kidney by restricting the blood flow. Smooth muscle effects: renal vasoconstriction, glomerular filtration rate decrease, renal tubular sodium reabsorption decrease. Cerebral effects: vasopressin and oxytocin release increase, pituitary secretion increase of ACTH, LH and PRL. Miscellaneous effects: stimulation of catecholamine production from nerve endings and adrenal medulla, glucagon hepatic effects inhibition, angiogenic factor, growth factor, and ovulation regulation. AT II possesses also activities of cytokines. It has been described as a factor promoting growth in several cellular systems and shares many signal transduction mechanisms with growth factors. Appears to be a bifunctional vascular smooth muscle cell growth modulator. It stimulates a hypertrophied growth response in vascular smooth muscle cells characterized by increases in cell size and protein synthesis, but not cell number. Locally produced AT II can act in an autocrine or paracrine fashion to alter the growth of human mesangial and neuroblastoma cells.

Increased Values
hepatic cirrhosis, volume depletion, **hypertension, renin-secreting juxtaglomerular renal tumors**, congestive heart failure
    Interfering Factors: neonates, upright position, **pregnancy** (1st trimester), medicaments – (estrogens, oral contraceptives)

Decreased Values
primary aldosteronism, patients – (**anephric p., p. after nephrectomy**), Cushing sy
    Interfering Factors: medicaments – (ACE inhibitors)

Angiotensin-I-Converting Enzyme

(ACE, syn: serum angiotensin-converting enzyme SACE)
Function. Glycoprotein (dipeptidyl carboxypeptidase), that catalyzes the angiotensin I conversion to the vasoactive peptide angiotensin II (a potent vasoconstrictor). Conversion occurs primarily within the lung. It functions also to split dipeptides from the free carboxy end of a variety of polypeptides. A primary function of ACE is arterial pressure regulation. Thyroid hormone may modulate ACE activity.

Occurrence. Vascular endothelium – lungs, kidneys, macrophages, epitheloid cells. Day-to-day variation is 10%.

Test Purpose. 1) to aid sarcoidosis diagnosis, especially pulmonary sarcoidosis, 2) to monitor response to therapy in sarcoidosis and prognostic indicator, 3) to help confirm Gaucher's disease or leprosy.

Increased Values

AIDS, **fibrosing cryptogenic alveolitis, amyloidosis**, rheumatoid arthritis, **asbestosis, berylliosis**, chronic bronchitis, hepatic cirrhosis – (**alcoholic c., primary biliary c.**), **diabetes mellitus, pulmonary embolism**, hyperparathyroidism, **hyperthyroidism**, diseases – (chronic hepatic d., chronic renal d., connective tissue d.), infectious diseases – (coccidioidomycosis, **histoplasmosis**, atypical mycobacterial infection, **leprosy**, fungal i. d., **tuberculosis**), Lennert's lymphoma, disease – (**Gaucher's d., Hodgkin's d.**), **plasmocytoma** (incl. multiple myeloma), Melkersson–Rosenthal sy, oncogenic hypercalcemia, paraquat poisoning, osteoarthritis, **multisystem sarcoidosis**, alpha-1-antitrypsin variants (MZ, ZZ, MS Pi types), diabetic retinopathy, **pulmonary sarcoidosis** (Boeck's disease), **silicosis, scleroderma**

Interfering Factors: **young people under 20 years of age**, newborn

Decreased Values

anorexia nervosa, diabetes mellitus, smoking, **hypothyroidism**, severe illnesses, coccidioidomycosis, acute/chronic leukemia, **tumors of the lung**, plasmocytoma (incl. multiple myeloma), farmers lung, adult respiratory distress sy (ARDS), pulmonary tuberculosis, pregnancy, **starvation**

Interfering Factors: medicaments – (angiotensin converting enzyme inhibitors, corticosteroids, prednisone, steroids)

Analyte	Age/Gender	Reference Range	SI Units	Note
Angiotensin Converting Enzyme (ACE)	2–9 y	250–440	U/l	
	10–20 y	280–450	U/l	
	21–50 y	252–360	U/l	
	51–80 y	233–314	U/l	
	Adults	6.1–21.1	U/l	
		133–867	nkat/l	

Annexin V

(apoptosis assay, syn: calcimedin, anchorin, calphobindin, endonexin, lipocortin V) Annexin V is a member of a highly conserved family of proteins that bind acidic phospholipids in a calcium-dependent manner. The protein has been shown to possess a high affinity for phosphatidylserine. Phosphatidylserine is translocated from the inner side of the plasma membrane to the outer layer when cells undergo death by apoptosis or cell necrosis and serves as one of several signals by which cell destined for death are recognized by phagocytic cells. Cell death by apoptosis and necrosis differ from each other in that cell membranes maintain their integrity during the initial stages of apoptosis, while they become leaky during necrotic cells death. If annexin V binds to the cell surface this indicates that cell death is imminent.

Anti-Acetylcholine Receptor Antibodies

(anti-ACHR, ACLRA, syn: AChR binding antibodies, acetylcholine modulating antibodies, receptor blocking antibodies, anti-AChR antibody, myasthenia gravis antibody, receptor modulating antibodies) Antibodies against acetylcholine membrane receptors bound at the skeletal muscle motor endplate → block neuromuscular transmission by interfering with ACHR binding sites on the muscle membrane (receptor blocking antibodies) → thereby preventing muscle contraction. These antibodies bind to a site different from that which binds acetylcholine and receptor injury may be mediated by complement.
Test Purpose. To contribute to myasthenia gravis diagnosis.

Increased Values
false positive values – (amyotrophic lateral sclerosis treated with cobra venom, penicilla-mine-induced myasthenia-like symptoms), snake venom, **myasthenia gravis**
  Interfering Factors: medicaments – (succinylcholine)

Analyte	Age/Gender	Reference Range	SI Units	Note
Anti-Acetylcholine Receptor Ab		<0.5	nmol/l	

Anti-Adrenal Antibodies

(syn: anti-adrenal cortex antibodies)
Test Purpose. To evaluate adrenal insufficiency.

Increased Values – positive
adrenals destruction – (metastatic a. d., fungal a. d., tuberculous a. d.), idiopathic hypopar-athyroidism, **idiopathic Addison's disease**, autoimmune hypoadrenalism – Hashimoto's thy-roiditis

Anti-Alanyl-tRNA Synthetase Antibodies

(anti-PL-12, syn: anti-PL-12 antibodies) Belongs to extractable nuclear antigens (ENA) auto-antibodies. Their interpretation should always be made in association with the clinical find-ings.
Test Purpose. To help in diagnosis of polymyositis.

Increased Values – positive
dermatomyositis, polymyositis

Anti-Arbovirus Antibodies

Test Purpose. To aid in arbovirus infectious diseases diagnosis.

Increased Values
encephalitis – (Ross River e., dengue, Sindbis e., Barmah Forest e., Australian e., Japanese e., Chikugunyah e., O'nyong-nyong e., Eastern, Western and Venezuelan equine e.), **yellow fever**

Antiarrhythmics

There is a narrow margin of safety between therapeutic and toxic levels of antiarrhythmics. Quantitative test monitors high and low drug concentrations to determine safe therapeutic range.

Test Purpose. 1) to determine most effective dose of antiarrhythmics, 2) to check for suspected toxicity of antiarrhythmic drugs, as determined from patient history or clinical observations.

Increased Values
antiarrhythmic drug overdose
> **Interfering Factors:** medicaments – (acetazolamide, antacids, barbiturates, disopyramide, lidocaine, N-acetyl procainamide, phenytoin, procainamide, propranolol, quinidine, sodium bicarbonate, verapamil)

Antibodies Against Bartonella Henselae

(syn: Cat scratch disease antibodies)
Test Purpose. To establish the diagnosis of cat scratch fever (infection with Bartonella henselae) in patients with a suggestive clinical syndrome. A four-fold rise in titre between acute and convalescent samples supports the clinical diagnosis of cat scratch disease.

Increased Values
cat scratch disease

Antibodies Against Bordetella Pertussis

Test Purpose. To investigate suspected pertussis, early in the course of the illness, in conjunction with culture. Serum antibody test may be useful for retrospective diagnosis. Serum IgA antibodies do not become positive until later and can remain positive for several years. IgA antibodies are not stimulated by vaccination, so a positive result in a vaccinated patient indicates past or current infection.

Increased Values
pertussis

Antibodies Against Borrelia Burgdorferi Sensu Lato

Lyme borreliosis is complex multisystem disease caused by spirochete Borrelia burgdorferi sensu lato. Laboratory diagnosis does not respond to clinical practice needs yet. Significant divergence can be seen between isolates in different monoclonal/plasmid antibodies reactivity and mainly in clinical manifestation. Recent immunoblotting studies (flagellin gene sequence detemination, DNA hybridization, plasmid profiles) have revealed four spirochete species (B. burgdorferi sensu lato, B. garinii, B. afzelii, B. japonica). Specificity and sensitivity is increased by recombinant B. burgdorferi antigens selection; these antigens are: antigen p100, outer surface antigen (Osp-A, Osp-C), antigen p41-p41/i specific subunit (inner part) and flagellar antigen p41. Class IgM and IgG antibodies against these antigens are evaluated separately.

Finding positivity. Reaction against two of five antigens minimally.

Finding negativity. No reactant in class IgM, no reactant in class IgG or reactant p41 only.

Borderline findings. In all other cases. Serological technique (sandwich hybridization system) against specific Osp-A gene epitope was used recently. Immunoblotting usage increases IgG specificity to 86% and IgM to 90%. IgM antibody becomes positive 2–3 weeks after onset of disease, IgG levels peak after some months. Presence represents early Lyme disease, persists in prolonged Lyme disease, reappears in late Lyme disease exacerbation. The antibodies cross react with other spirochetes, but patients with Lyme disease do not usually have a positive VDRL.

Test Purpose. 1) B. burgdorferi infection evidence in serum and cerebrospinal fluid in typical signs of different location, 2) bilateral facial nerve paralysis, 3) sclerosis multiplex diagnosis, 4) cardiomyopathy and carditis diagnosis, 5) monoarthritis diagnosis.

Increased Values – positive

Lyme borreliosis, patients with autoantibodies – (antiphospholipid, antinuclear), patients with rheumatoid factors positivity, cross-reacting antibodies against – (non-pathogenic borrelia which are the physiological microflora constituents, leptospira, spirochete, phylogenetically distant microbes which contain highly preserved HSP, Treponema pallidum, yaws), polyclonal stimulation (EBV, VZV, HSV)

Antibodies Against Brucella

A bacterial agglutination of >160 suggests past or recent infection; a fourfold rise in titre between acute and convalescent samples is evidence of recent infection. Blocking antibodies can lead to false negative results at low dilutions of serum.

Increased Values
brucellosis

Antibodies Against Burkholderia Pseudomallei

Test Purpose. The diagnosis of suspected melioidosis (pseudomalleus) in patients who have lived in, or visited endemic areas and have presented with pneumonia, secondary abscesses or unexplained acute septicemic episodes. Culture of Burkholderia pseudomallei from blood, sputum, or tissue is a more rapid and reliable means of diagnosing infection than is serology.

Increased Values
pseudomalleus

Antibodies Against Chlamydia

Test detects antibodies against a group antigen (LGV-1) shared by Chlamydia psittaci and Chlamydia trachomatis. Test detects both live and dead organisms. A four-fold rise in IgG, or the presence of IgM, indicates recent psittacosis or lymphogranuloma venereum. Chlamydia antibodies are of no real value in the diagnosis of genital tract infection or trachoma caused by non-LGV-1 strains of Chl. trachomatis. The presence of IgM antibodies supports the diagnosis of Chl. trachomatis pneumonia in neonates although negative results do not exclude the possibility.

Test Purpose. 1) to detect atypical pneumonia, pneumonia in the first 6 months of life, 2) to detect lymphogranuloma venereum (LGV).

Increased Values

atypical pneumonia, arteriosclerosis, atherosclerosis, **infectious diseases caused by chlamydia, lymphogranuloma venereum, psittacosis, Chlamydia trachomatis pneumonia in neonates, trachoma**

Antibodies Against Coccidioides Immitis

The detection of IgM antibodies (appear 1–3 weeks after onset of symptoms) is very helpful test in identifying recent infection. IgG antibody becomes positive after IgM Ab. Serological cross-reactions occur with Histoplasma capsulatum and Blastomyces dermatitidis.

Test Purpose. To help in diagnosis and management of coccidioidomycosis.

Increased Values – positive
Coccidioidomycosis

Antibodies Against Coxiella Burnetii

(syn: Coxiella burnetii antibodies, anti-Q-fever Ab). Coxiella burnetii stimulates antibodies to both phase I and phase II antigens. In acute Q fever, antibodies to phase II antigen are detectable 1–2 weeks after onset of the illness and peak between 4 and 12 weeks. Recent infection is confirmed by a four fold rise in titre or a positive IgM test. Antibodies to phase I antigen are only present in significant titre in chronic Q fever (e.g. endocarditis or granulomatous liver disease).

Test Purpose. 1) to help diagnosis of suspected Q fever, atypical pneumonia, hepatitis of unknown cause, blood culture-negative endocarditis, 2) to help in differential diagnosis for Q fever.

Increased Values – positive
Q fever

Antibodies Against Fasciola Hepatica

Test Purpose. To support the diagnosis of Fasciola hepatica infection.

Increased Values – positive
Fasciola hepatica infection

Antibodies Against Filaria

Test Purpose. To investigate recurrent fever, unexplained chronic edema, chyluria, chylous effusions in a patient from endemic area. A positive result indicates infection at some time, but does not distinguish between previous and current infection. A low titer or a negative result may be found in the presence of parasitemia.

Increased Values – positive
infections caused by Filaria

Antibodies Against Francisella Tularensis

(syn: tularemia agglutinins). Test is used as a serological aid for the diagnosis of tularemia. Antibodies to Francisella tularensis develop 2–3 week after infection and peak in 4–5 weeks. Although antibodies may cross react with Brucella, those titers will generally be much lower. Rising titers over 2-week interval are the best indicator of recent infection.

Increased Values – positive
tularemia

Antibodies Against Beta-2 Glycoprotein I

(beta-2 GP I) Beta-2 glycoprotein I is a plasmatic protein with anticoagulant activity. It inhibits hemostasis reactions in vitro, which are catalysed by phospholipids (prothrombin to thrombin change, factor XII activation). Beta-2 GP I is needed for the bond of autoimmune anticardiolipin antibodies onto cardiolipin. Anti-beta-2 GP I antibodies (IgG, IgA, IgM) have higher value in vascular complication evaluation in comparison to anticardiolipin antibodies. But anti-beta-2 GP I antibodies have higher specificity and lower sensitivity in comparison to anticardiolipin antibodies, so both tests are used in diagnostic procedure.

Increased Values – positive
antiphospholipid syndrome, myocardial infarction, recurrent miscarriages, systemic lupus erythematosus, thrombocytopenia, venous thrombosis, stroke

Antibodies Against Helicobacter Pylori

Helicobacter pylori pathogenesis discovery belongs to the biggest discoveries in medicine. Most of patients infected with H. pylori create a massive specific antibody response which is complex and highly variable. H. pylori positive patients create antibodies directed against 61 kD and 28 kD polypeptides; these are the urease subunits which are characteristically created by H. pylori. The third important anti-120 kD polypeptide antibody is directed against body proteins. Unlike of above mentioned antibodies the 3rd one is in body also after infection eradication and correlates with infection severity. Cytotoxic vacuolated antigen is placed on H. pylori surface, its expression/polymorphism is probably connected with H. pylori oncogenicity. During H. pylori infection also other antibodies are produced but are not specific. Antibody specificity difference is characterized mainly by host immune system and less by antigen differences. No antigen was isolated till now which is able to react exclusively, definitely, and specifically with all positive examined sera; this means that this is a patient immune system function or antigen used in test does not contain antigen determinants against which the antibodies are produced. In H. pylori infection suspicion and negative serological examination it is needed to order other tests. Molecular-biological methods reveal infection in teeth plaques, saliva, stool, and water.

Test Purpose. H. pylori infection evidence in gastroduodenal ulcer, dyspepsia, and malignant stomach tumors, but probably also in other symptoms (cardiovascular, neurological and systemic).

Increased Values – positive
Helicobacter pylori infection

Antibodies Against Histoplasma Capsulatum

Test Purpose. To investigate suspected acute, chronic or disseminated histoplasmosis.

Increased Values – positive
histoplasmosis

Antibodies Against Influenza Virus

A four-fold rise in titre between acute and convalescent samples is considered diagnostic. Serology does not usually assist with management, as diagnostic antibody levels are not present until the infection has resolved. A single high titre in a convalescent sample does not necessarily indicate recent infection.

Test Purpose. To investigate serious respiratory infection and atypical pneumonia.

Increased Values – positive
influenza, severe respiratory infectious diseases, acute viral infectious diseases, atypical pneumonia

Antibodies Against Legionella

Test detect antibodies to Legionella pneumophila (L. longbeachae, L. micdadei) and support the clinical diagnosis of legionnaires' disease. A four-fold rise in titer >1:128 from the acute to convalescent phase provides evidence of recent infection. A single titer 1:256 is evidence of infection at an undetermined time. Seroconversion may take up to 6 weeks.

Test Purpose. To help in diagnosis of legionnaires' disease.

Increased Values
legionnaires' disease

Antibodies Against Leptospira

(syn: Canicola fever, Ft Bragg fever, leptospira species antibodies, Leptospirosis antibodies, Weil's disease).

Test Purpose. To help in diagnosis of acute, febrile systemic illnesses as well as other milder manifestations caused by leptospiral infections.

Increased Values
leptospirosis

Antibodies Against Mumps Virus

A four-fold rise in titre between acute and convalescent specimens is suggestive, in the presence of an appropriate clinical picture. IgM assays have better specificity and sensitivity than do IgG assays.
Test Purpose. To help in diagnosis of infection with mumps virus (paramyxovirus).

Increased Values – positive
epidemic parotitis

Antibodies Against Mycoplasma Pneumoniae Antibodies

(syn: atypical pneumonia antibodies, pleuropneumonia-like organism antibodies). Belong to IgG and IgM antibodies. A positive result indicates prior exposure to Mycoplasma. A single positive IgG result may be present in the absence of any clinical symptoms as specific IgG antibodies may remain elevated long after initial infection. Low IgM positive results are presumptive evidence of acute or recent infection. Specific IgM may persist for several months after initial infection or be absent during reinfection.
Test Purpose. To aid in the diagnosis of atypical pneumonia and Stevens–Johnson sy.

Increased Values – positive
atypical pneumonia, Stevens-Johnson sy, meningoencephalitis, Guillain-Barré syndrome, acute pancreatitis, pericarditis, erythema nodosum, cold hemagglutinin-mediated hemolytic anemia

Antibodies Against Parainfluenza Virus

Test is used to aid in the diagnosis of parainfluenza viral infections. A four-fold increase in titre between acute and convalescent sera indicates recent infection.

Increased Values – positive
parainfluenza viral infections

Antibodies Against Parvovirus B19

IgM antibodies provide evidence of recent infection. IgG levels fluctuate, so rising titres may not indicate recent exposure. Diagnosis of persistent infection requires detection of virus by nucleic acid probe after PCR amplification.
Test Purpose. 1) to investigate aplastic crisis in chronic hemolysis, 2) to assess anemia with or without neutropenia in immunosuppressed patients, 3) to assess maternal infection associated with hydrops fetalis, subacute polyarthritis or suspected fifth disease (erythema infectiosum).

Increased Values – positive
parvovirus infections

Antibodies Against Purkinje Cells

(Anti-Yo, anti-Hu antibodies) IgG anti-Yo antibodies are associated with cerebellar syndromes, most commonly in females with gynecologic neoplasms. Anti-Hu antibodies may be found in paraneoplastic encephalomyelitis and in sensory neuropathy. A negative test result does not exclude the possibility of a paraneoplastic syndrome.
Test Purpose. To help in investigation of suspected paraneoplastic syndromes affecting the central nervous system.

Increased Values – positive
cerebellar syndromes, paraneoplastic syndromes, sensory neuropathy

Antibodies Against Rabies Virus

Antibodies can be detected in most patients with clinical rabies within two weeks of onset. Much higher titres are found in patients with clinical rabies than in immunised subjects.
Test Purpose. 1) to support a clinical diagnosis of rabies, 2) to determine immune status in an individual wishing to live or work in a high risk endemic setting.

Increased Values – positive
rabies virus infection

Antibodies Against Respiratory Syncytial Virus

Titres of antibody may take up to 4 weeks to rise after onset of illness. Infants in the first 6 months of life often do not have an adequate antibody response. Older patients with repeated infections may not have a rise in titre. A four-fold rise in titre between acute and convalescent sera provides a retrospective diagnosis. Rapid antigen detection is the preferred test for the diagnosis of severe infant respiratory infection.
Test Purpose. To aid in establishing the diagnosis of respiratory syncytial virus infection.

Increased Values – positive
respiratory syncytial virus infection

Antibodies Against Rickettsia Species

The diagnosis of rickettsial infection is confirmed by a four-fold rise in antibody titre between acute and convalescent samples.
Test Purpose. To help in confirmation of a clinical diagnosis of typhus (murine or scrub) or spotted fever.

Increased Values – positive
rickettsial infectious diseases

Antibodies Against Rickettsia Ricketsii

(syn: RMSF IgM antibodies) Test is used to aid in a diagnosis of Rocky Mountain spotted fever (Rickettsia rickettsii).

Increased Values – positive
Rocky Mountain spotted fever

Antibodies Against Rubella Virus

(syn: German measles IgG, IgM antibodies) Rubella virus is the cause of German measles (rubella). Recent infection – a four-fold rise in IgG titre between acute and convalescent samples. The role of serologic testing for IgG antibodies to rubella is different in different clinical settings. The simplest application is in premarital assessment of immunity. If a woman has IgG antibodies against rubella, even of low titer, she need not worry about infection during subsequent pregnancy. If she is not immune, and is not pregnant, she can receive rubella vaccine. IgM antibodies are associated with acute viral infections. IgM detection is useful in the following situations: evidence of infection can be obtained from only one acute phase specimen if the IgM results are positive. IgM antibodies in maternal serum indicate high fetal risk, particularly in the first and second trimester. The absence of IgM at birth does not rule out congenital rubella since the frequency of IgM detection in cord blood decreases as the time between conception and fetal infection increases. Acquired rubella infection in infants is rare but must be considered if the blood is positive for IgM but was not obtained during the immediate postnatal period.

Test Purpose. 1) to support a clinical diagnosis of rubella, 2) to determine immune status, especially before or during pregnancy and after vaccination, 3) to help in diagnosis of congenital infection, 4) to differentiate between primary infection and re-exposure.

Increased Values – positive
rubella

Antibodies Against Rubeola Virus

(syn: measles antibodies). Test is used to determine status or, with paired sera, to aid in the diagnosis of recent infection.

Increased Values – positive
measles

Antibodies Against Saccharomyces Cerevisiae

(ASCA, syn: anti Saccharomyces cerevisiae antibodies) Antibodies (IgG, IgA) are specific against oligomannose remnants, which are localized on the yeast cellular membrane (Saccharomyces cerevisiae). These antibodies do not correlate with disease extent and activity, they are marker of immunoregulatory disorder, which is characteristic for Crohn's disease. ASCA antibodies are highly specific (92%) for this disease.

Test Purpose. 1) to help in differential diagnosis of intestinal diseases (inflammatory bowel disease), 2) to evaluate genetic susceptibility for Crohn's disease in non-manifest conditions.

Increased Values – positive
Crohn's disease, ulcerative colitis

Antibodies Against Salivary Duct

Test Purpose. To help in diagnosis of Sjögren's syndrome.

Increased Values – positive
Sjögren's syndrome, rheumatoid arthritis

Antibodies Against Schistosoma Species

In countries where schistosomiasis is endemic, the test can only be used to demonstrate exposure. Demonstration of ova in tissue, feces or urine provides a more specific proof of active infection.
Test Purpose. To support the diagnosis of past or present infection with Schistosoma species, when suspected because of exposure in an endemic area and hematuria or other clinical features.

Increased Values – positive
schistosomal infectious diseases

Antibodies Against St. Louis Encephalitis Virus

Test is used to support the diagnosis of St. Louis encephalitis virus infection through IgG antibodies detection.

Increased Values – positive
St. Louis encephalitis

Antibodies Against Thermoactinomyces Candidus

(syn: hypersensitivity pneumonitis profile, farmer's lung) Test is used to confirm the presence of precipitating antibodies to Thermoactinomyces candidus. A positive test does not establish the diagnosis of hypersensitivity pneumonitis, nor does the absence of precipitins rule out the diagnosis. There must be careful correlation of clinical and laboratory results.

Increased Values – positive
allergic exogenous alveolitis

Antibodies Against Thermomonospora Viridis

(syn: hypersensitivity pneumonitis profile, farmer's lung) Test is used to confirm the presence of precipitating antibodies to Thermomonospora viridis. There must be careful correlation of clinical and laboratory results.

Increased Values – positive
allergic exogenous alveolitis

Anti-Cardiolipin Antibodies

(ACLA, ACLAb, syn: cardiolipin antibodies) Belong to antiphospholipid antibodies.

Increased Values – positive
AIDS, dermatomyositis, myocardial infarction, spontaneous abortion, recurrent miscarriages, polymyositis, scleroderma, **systemic lupus erythematosus**, thrombocytopenia, syphilitic arthritis, syndrome – (**autoimmune lymphoproliferative sy**, primary antiphospholipid sy, Sjögren's sy, Cogan's sy), venous thrombosis, stroke, **secondary syphilis**

Analyte	Age/ Gender	Reference Range	SI Units	Note
Anti-Cardiolipin Ab				
IgG		<8.5	*	See ref.
IgA		10.5–100	**	ranges note
IgM		9.0–100	***	

Anti-Centromere Antibodies

(ACA, ACAb)
Test Purpose. 1) investigation of systemic rheumatic disease, 2) diagnosis of CREST syndrome.

Increased Values – positive
rheumatoid arthritis, dermatosclerosis, **progressive systemic sclerosis** (scleroderma), **CREST sy** (calcinosis cutis + Raynaud's phenomenon + esophageal dysfunction + sclerodactyly + teleangiectasia), Raynaud's sy

Alpha-1-Antichymotrypsin

Very sensitive acute phase protein and inhibitor of serine proteases, it is most active against leukocyte cathepsin G or prostate-specific antigen, and inactive against trypsin or plasmin.

Increased Values
cystic fibrosis, diseases – (**infectious d., rheumatic d., inflammatory d.**), malnutrition, **tumors, tissue necrosis**, surgery, **trauma**

Anticonvulsants

Test Purpose. 1) to monitor therapeutic levels of anticonvulsants, 2) to confirm suspected toxicity as determined from patient history or clinical observations.

Increased Values
anticonvulsants overdose

Decreased Values
less than therapeutic levels

Anti-Cytomegalovirus Antibodies IgM, IgA, IgG

(anti-CMV) CMV infection course is asymptomatic/non-characteristic during childhood. Primary infection is shifted to later decades in western civilizations, this lead to pregnancy infections (child risk), post-transfusion infection (infectious mononucleosis induced by CMV), post-immunosuppressive therapy infection (organ/bone marrow transplantation). CMV infection diagnosis cannot be determined without laboratory evidence: 1) virus isolation, 2) virus DNA evidence, 3) significant changes of specific antibody concentrations evidence. CMV persists latent in glands and kidney. Significant IgG antibody increase does not signify active viral infection and is a recent antigen stimulation evidence only. 400% IgG antibody fluctuation is seen in healthy persons. The presence of specific IgM antibody in a neonate indicates intrauterine infection. In other patients, a four-fold rise in titre suggests recent infection. IgM antibody can indicate recent infection, but as it can persist over long periods, it is not a reliable indicator of recent infection. DNA diagnosis or virus cultivation is indicated in risk/clinical cases (immunodeficient conditions).
Test Purpose. 1) primary infection evidence, 2) reactivation evidence, 3) pregnancy infection diagnosis, possible congenital CMV infection, 4) diagnosis of infection after organ transplantation, 5) severe infectious diseases and septic conditions, 6) chronic fatigue syndrome, 7) to screen of blood transfusion donors, 8) to screen donor and recipient before transplantation, 9) to evaluate patients with HIV infection.

Increased Values – positive
cytomegalovirus infection

Analyte	Age/ Gender	Reference Range	SI Units	Note
Anti-Cytomegalo-	negative	<0.80		
virus Antibodies	borderline	0.81–0.99		
IgM	positive	>1.00		

Anti-Decorin Antibodies

(BJ antigen) IgM antibodies to Decorin (BJ antigen) occur in myopathies with proximal weakness and a moderately high CK. 50% of such patients have an associated serum M-protein or Waldenström's macroglobulinemia.

Increased Values – positive
myopathies

Anti-Deoxyribonuclease B

(ADNase-B, syn: anti-DNase-B titer, antistreptococcal DNase-B titer, streptodornase) Test detects antigens produced by group A streptococci. The titre peaks at 4–6 weeks.

Increased Values
poststreptococcal glomerulonephritis, severe streptococcal skin infections, necrotising fasciitis, **acute rheumatic fever**

Analyte	Age/Gender	Reference Range	SI Units	Note
Antideoxyribonu-clease B Titre		<170	U/l	A

Antidepressants

Test Purpose. 1) to check toxicity of antidepressant drugs, 2) to monitor therapeutic levels, 3) to detect presence of antidepressant for medical-legal purposes.

Increased Values
antidepressants overdose
> **Interfering Factors:** alcohol, medicaments – (aminophylline, antihistamines, barbiturates, diuretics, hypnotics, methylphenidate, narcotics, phenothiazines, tranquilizers)

Antidiuretic Hormone

(ADH, syn: vasopressin, arginine vasopressin, adiuretin, vasotocin, pituitrin P, pitressin)
Production. Hypothalamic hormone → stored in posterior pituitary (neurohypophysis) in the supraoptic and paraventricular nuclei nerve bodies. ADH has been found also in other tissues, including testis, ovary, uterus, adrenal gland, superior cervical ganglion and thymus. ADH is derived from a larger prepro-protein precursor, prepro-arginine-vasopressin-neurophysin-2. Synthesized and released mainly under plasma osmolality influence (hypothalamic osmoreceptors stimulation), circulatory blood volume and blood pressure, atrial receptors stimulation, aortic cardiovascular baroreceptors of sinus caroticus. ADH is bound to basolateral cell membrane receptors of cortical and medullary collecting kidney ducts. After the series of events, the luminal cell membrane is transformed and water, urea, sodium and other solutes permeability is strikingly increased. The synthesis and secretion of ADH can be induced by IL-1 and IL-2.
Function. It has direct antidiuretic activity in the kidney, mediated by the antidiuretic receptor V2. Decreases diuresis → antidiuretic effect, controls the water amount reabsorbed by the kidney, maintains the body water volume. With low ADH levels, water is allowed to be excreted, thereby producing hemoconcentration and very diluted urine. Causes vasoconstriction of peripheral small blood vessels in the gastrointestinal tract, kidney, uterus, myocardium, skin. Significantly increases anti-hemophilic factor VIII plasma levels. Besides circulation failure, ADH decreases the sympathetic baroreceptor system activity and the renin-angiotensin-aldosterone system reciprocally. ADH has been shown to play an impor-

tant role in the modulation of the stress response. It directly stimulates the release of ACTH and affects ACTH levels indirectly by enhancing production of corticotropin releasing factor. ADH also plays an important role in the regulation of IFN-gamma production by providing a helper signal. Other stimuli for ADH release: pain, stress, sleep, exercise, catecholamines, angiotensin II, prostaglandins. ADH levels increase during night to the maximum upon rising and fall during the day. In women peaking at ovulation time.

Test Purpose. To aid in the differential diagnosis of pituitary diabetes insipidus, nephrogenic diabetes insipidus and syndrome of inappropriate antidiuretic hormone secretion (SIADH) and some tumors.

Increased Values

pulmonary abscess, pulmonary aspergillosis, bronchial asthma, hepatic cirrhosis, pulmonary emphysema, encephalitis, infectious hepatitis, **isovolemic hypotonic hyponatremia,** hypopituitarism, hypothyroidism, diseases – (**CNS d., endocrine d.,** infectious d., pulmonary d.), hemorrhage – (subarachnoid h., severe h.), **Addison's disease,** meningitis, **myxedema,** tumors – (bronchial t., **CNS t.,** duodenal t., lung small cell carcinoma, adrenal cortex t., colon t., intestine t., leukemia, lymphomas, pancreas t., prostate t., thymoma), nephrogenic diabetes insipidus, **pneumonia,** pneumothorax, **acute intermittent porphyria,** ectopic production of ADH, acute psychosis, conditions – (painful c., **postoperative c.**), syndrome – (Guillain-Barré sy, **SIADH sy, Schwartz-Bartter sy**), circulatory shock, **tuberculosis,** head injuries, prolonged mechanical ventilation, CNS infectious diseases, post-surgery fluid imbalance

> **Interfering Factors:** dehydration, hypotension, hypovolemia, stress, medicaments – (acetaminophen, amitriptyline, narcotic analgesics, tricyclic antidepressants, barbiturates, bromocriptine, carbamazepine, chlorothiazides, chlorpropamide, cholinergic agents, cisplatin, clofibrate, cyclophosphamide, estrogens, furosemide, haloperidol, lithium, morphine, nicotine, oral hypoglycemic agents, oxytocin, phenothiazines, thiazide diuretics, tolbutamide, vasopressin, vincristine)

Decreased Values

diabetes insipidus – (**central** d. i., hereditary d. i., pituitary d. i., nephrogenous d. i., acquired d. i.), surgical ablation of the pituitary gland, viral infections, malignant tumor metastases, tumors of – (hypothalamus, neurohypophysis), neuroborreliosis, neurosyphilis, psychogenic polydipsia, sarcoidosis, nephrotic sy, tuberculosis, head trauma, neurosurgical procedures, damage to the pituitary gland

> **Interfering Factors:** overhydration, hypervolemia, hypoosmolality, recumbency, medicaments – (alcohol, beta-adrenergics, carbamazepine, lithium, morphine antagonists, phenytoin)

Analyte	Age/Gender	Reference Range	SI Units	Note
Antidiuretic Hormone (ADH), plasma osmolality				
270–280 mOsm/kg		<1.38	pmol/l	
281–285 mOsm/kg		<2.38	pmol/l	
286–290 mOsm/kg		0.92–4.81	pmol/l	
291–295 mOsm/kg		1.84–6.45	pmol/l	
296–300 mOsm/kg		3.7–11.1	pmol/l	

Anti-DNA Antibodies

(anti-ds-DNA, anti-ss-DNA, n-DNA, syn: antideoxyribonucleic acid antibodies, antibodies to single and double-stranded DNA, anti-double-stranded DNA, DNA antibodies, native double-stranded DNA, anti-single-stranded DNA) Autoantibodies can be divided into 3 groups: a) against phosphoribosome chain, b) against helical conformation structures, c) against bases or base sequentions.

Test Purpose. Anti-ds-DNA 1) confirmatory test for systemic lupus erythematosus, 2) to monitor clinical disease course and treatment response, 3) collagenoses differential diagnosis. Anti-ds-DNA IgM and IgG can be also determined.

2-Fibre DNA – Double Stranded, anti-ds-DNA

Increased Values – positive
rheumatoid arthritis, **dermatomyositis**, hepatitis – (chronic active h. B, autoimmune h., drug-induced h.), biliary cirrhosis, Epstein–Barr virus infection, cytomegalovirus infection, mixed connective tissue disease, autoimmune diseases, ulcerative colitis, collagenoses, lupus erythematosus – (discoid l. e., drug-induced l. e., **systemic l. e.**), **lupus nephritis**, lupus CNS involvement, **myasthenia gravis**, polyarteritis nodosa, polymyositis, syndrome – (CREST sy, Sharp's sy, **Sjögren's sy**), **scleroderma**, thyrotoxicosis, Hashimoto's thyroiditis
   Interfering Factors: healthy people, medicaments – (hydralazine, procainamide)

Analyte	Age/Gender	Reference Range	SI Units	Note
Anti-ds-DNA Ab		6.3–20.0	IU/ml	

Test Purpose. Anti-ss-DNA 1) diagnosis of medicament induced lupus erythematosus, juvenile rheumatoid arthritis, 2) to help in clinical suspect systemic lupus erythematosus diagnosis in negative indirect immunofluorescence test (IIF), 3) collagenoses differential diagnosis, 4) to help diagnose clinical suspected MEN I, MEN II polyendocrinopathies.

1-Fibre DNA – Single Stranded, anti-ss-DNA

Increased Values – positive
rheumatoid arthritis, juvenile rheumatoid arthritis, **biliary cirrhosis**, **chronic aggressive hepatitis**, **mixed connective tissue disease**, **collagenoses**, leukemia – (lymphatic l., acute/chronic myeloid l.), lupus erythematosus – (induced by medicaments, **systemic l. e.**), **infective mononucleosis**, lupus nephritis, polyendocrinopathies – (MEN I, MEN II), scleroderma, polymyositis, **Sjögren's sy**

Anti-Endomysial Antibodies

(IgA-EMA, EMA, EMAb, syn: endomysial antibodies) Anti-endomysial antibodies have a specificity of >90% for the diagnosis of celiac disease.
Test Purpose. 1) to help in differential diagnosis of unclear bulous dermatitides and dermatitis herpetiformis, 2) to help in diagnosis of celiac disease.

Increased Values – positive
celiac disease (gluten-sensitive enteropathy), **dermatitis herpetiformis**

Anti-Enterovirus Antibodies

The enterovirus group includes Coxsackieviruses A and B and echoviruses with numerous serotypes. Viral isolation (nasopharyngeal aspirate, CSF) is more satisfactory.
Test Purpose. To help in diagnosis of myocarditis, encephalitis, aseptic meningitis, pleurodynia.

Increased Values – positive
aseptic meningitis, encephalitis, myocarditis, pleurodynia

Anti-Epstein-Barr Virus Antibodies

(anti-EBV) Immunoassay for IgM and IgG antibodies to viral capsid antigen (VCA IgM, VCA IgG) and Epstein-Barr nuclear antigen (EBNA). VCA IgM antibodies indicate recent infection, VCA IgG antibodies or EBNA antibodies indicate past infection.
Test Purpose. 1) to provide laboratory diagnosis of infectious mononucleosis heterophile-negative cases, 2) to determine the EBV antibody condition of immunosuppressed patients with lymphoproliferative processes.

Increased Values – positive
Epstein–Barr virus infection, hereditary sex-linked lymphadenopathy, heterophil-negative mononucleosis

Anti-Ga1NAc-GD1a Antibodies

Antibodies against Ga1NAc-GD1a often cross-react with GM2 ganglioside. IgG anti-Ga1NAc-GD1a antibodies are associated with acute motor neuropathies having distal predominant weakness and sparing of the cranial nerves. IgM anti-Ga1NAc-GD1a antibodies are associated with a GBS-variant syndrome (gay bowel sy).

Increased Values – positive
acute motor neuropathies, chronic axonal motor neuropathies, GBS-variant syndrome, chronic demyelinating polyneuropathy

Ki-1 Antigen

T-cell type immune response can be seen in atopic disease, bronchial asthma and allergic rhinoconjunctivitis. CD30 (Ki-1) antigen is a T-cell activity marker with a strong B-cell helping activity (IL-5 and IFN-gamma are produced) and CD4+ and CD8+ T-cell activity with cytokine $T_H 2$ profile. Soluble sCD30 (Ki-1) is released by CD30+ cells in vivo. Antigen Ki-1 concentrations do not correlate with IgE. It is used also as a tumor marker in rare lymphomatoid papulosis, in differential diagnosis of Ki-1-ALCL (anaplastic large-cell lymphoma) and in Hodgkin's disease mainly with HIV infection immunodeficient patient. To soluble and blood antigens currently belong: a) inflammatory – CD1a, CD4, CD8, CD11b, b) proliferatory – proliferating cell nuclear antigen, Ki-67, c) differentiation – transglutaminase, IG cytokeratin, involucrin.

Test Purpose. 1) lymphoma differential diagnosis, 2) atopic disease diagnosis.

Analyte	Age/Gender	Reference Range	SI Units	Note
Ki-1 Antigen (CD30)		<6	U/ml	

p24 Antigen

(syn: HIV core antigen) It is a protein product of the HIV "gag" gene. As a viral rather than host product, it appears concomitant with initial infection, and then generally becomes undetectable during viral latency period. It reappears with renewed viral replication. The reappearance of p24 antigen in serum generally heralds progression of clinical disease in AIDS. p24 antigen belongs to early indicator of HIV-1 infection. A negative results does not exclude HIV viremia.

Test Purpose. To diagnose recent acute infection with HIV, therapeutic response monitoring it may also be of prognostic significance in AIDS.

Increased Values – positive
HIV infection

Anti-GM1 Ganglioside Antibodies

Measurement of anti-GM1 IgM antibodies helps to distinguish multifocal motor neuropathy from other immune demyelinating polyneuropathies. IgG testing screens for antibodies that occur with acute and chronic lower motor neuron syndromes. IgG antibodies that bind to GM1 but not to sulfatide occur in acute, usually axonal motor neuropathies that are associated with preceding Campylobacter jejuni infection.

Increased Values – positive
multifocal motor neuropathy, lower motor neuron syndrome, chronic axonal lower motor neuron syndromes

Anti-GD1a Antibodies

IgM anti-GD1a ganglioside antibodies are unusual. High titers are associated with demyelinating motor neuropathies and lower motor neuron syndromes. Most serums with this IgM reactivity also show binding to GM1 ganglioside. IgG anti-GD1a antibodies are associated with Guillain–Barré-like syndromes, that are predominantly motor and axonal neuropathies.

Increased Values – positive
demyelinating motor neuropathies, lower motor neuron syndromes, Guillain–Barré-like syndromes

Anti-GD1b Antibodies

IgM antibodies that bind to GD1b ganglioside, but not GM1 ganglioside, are associated with axonal sensory neuropathy syndromes (CANOMAD – Chronic Ataxic Neuropathy, Ophthalmoplegia, M-protein, Agglutination, Disialosyl antibody).

Increased Values – positive
sensory neuropathy syndromes

Anti-Glomerular Basement Membrane Antibodies

(AGBM, AGBMA, AGBMAb, anti-GBM, syn: anti-GBM antibodies, glomerular basement antibodies, Goodpasture's antibodies)

Increased Values – positive
glomerulonephritis (anti-GBM), **tubulointerstitial nephritis**, **Goodpasture's sy** (anti-GBM), acute nephritic syndrome

Analyte	Age/Gender	Reference Range	SI Units	Note
Anti-Glomerular Basement Membrane Ab (IgG)		<3	U/ml	

Anti-Glycyl-tRNA Synthetase Antibodies

(anti-EJ, syn: anti-EJ antibodies) Belongs to extractable nuclear antigens (ENA) autoantibodies. Their interperation should always be made in association with the clinical findings.
Test Purpose. To help in diagnosis of polymyositis.

Increased Values – positive
dermatomyositis, polymyositis

Anti-GQ1b Antibodies

IgG anti-GQ1 antibodies often occur with ophthalmoplegia and ataxia as part of Miller–Fisher syndrome.

Increased Values – positive
Miller–Fisher syndrome, ataxic Guillain–Barré sy in Japan

Anti-Heparan Sulfate Antibodies

IgM and IgG antibodies to heparan sulfate occur in 35% of patients with Guillain–Barré syndrome.

Increased Values – positive
Guillain–Barré syndrome, patients with IgM anti-MAG M-proteins

Anti-Herpes Simplex Virus 1, 2 Antibodies

(anti-HSV 1, 2) Herpes virus family consists of two morphologically identical members (type 1 and 2); about 40% DNA homology is common. Viruses have a lot of common antigens and present identical skin and mucous membrane lesions. Viruses can be distinguished on the basis of antigens, biological, molecular-biological, clinical, and epidemiological signs. HSV-1 is joined with oral infections, generally lesions "above waist"; HSV-2 with genital infections and lesions "bellow waist". Most of people are infected before 20. Antigenic cross reactivity occurs between HSV-1 and HSV-2. Specific IgM antibodies determination is important for primary infection detection (IgM levels decrease to low values after infection) and for reinfection detection (with identical/homologous type). A four-fold rise in titre between acute and convalescent samples supports the diagnosis of primary herpes infection. Anti-HSV-1 IgG antibodies do not protect from HSV-2 infection (mitigation of disease course). Unambiguous results also after test repetition should be re-checked with alternative method in a new sample.

Test Purpose. 1) primary infection detection in clinical suspicion and recurrent infections, 2) infection differential diagnosis in immunodeficient conditions and tumors, mainly in gynecological tumors and lymphomas, 3) septic condition differential diagnosis, 4) infection diagnosis in patient after transplantation.

Increased Values – positive
herpes simplex infection

Anti-Histidyl-tRNA Synthetase Antibodies

(anti-Jo-1, syn: Jo-1 antibodies) Belongs to extractable nuclear antigens (ENA) autoantibodies. Their interpreration should always be made in association with the clinical findings. **Test Purpose.** To help in diagnosis of polymyositis.

Increased Values – positive
dermatomyositis, **polymyositis**, **overlap syndrome** (systemic lupus erythematosus + dermatomyositis + scleroderma), interstitial lung disease, Raynaud's phenomenon

Anti-Histone Antibodies

(AHA, AHAb, syn: histone antibody) Histones are a group of nucleus proteins that contain high lysine and arginine concentrations, these substances are released into surrounding tissues by cell death/autolysis. Histones have direct antimicrobial activity.
Test Purpose. 1) used for the differential diagnostics of collagen vascular autoimmune diseases, 2) diagnosis of lupus erythematosus induced by medicaments (mainly after procainamide, hydralazine, chlorpromazine, D-penicillamine, alpha-methyldopa, contraceptives), systemic lupus erythematosus, ANA-positive seropositive rheumatoid arthritis, ANA-positive progressive systemic scleroderma, juvenile rheumatoid arthritis, juvenile chronic arthritis, Felty's sy.

rheumatoid arthritis, juvenile rheumatoid arthritis, lupus erythematosus induced by medicaments – (**alpha-methyldopa, hydralazine, chlorpromazine, D-penicillamine, oral contraceptives, procainamide**), **systemic lupus erythematosus,** scleroderma, Felty's sy

Interfering Factors: medicaments – (hydralazine, procainamide)

Anti-Hu Antibodies

Belong to Purkinje cell antibodies. Patients with anti-Hu IgG antibodies in serum and CSF often have a pure sensory syndrome (gangliopathy) associated with small cell neoplasms (especially lung).

Increased Values – positive
gangliopathy, limbic encephalitis, cerebellar disorders, gastrointestinal dysfunction

Anti-Human Papilloma Virus Antibodies

(anti-HPV, syn: human papilloma virus testing, HVP testing) Human papilloma viruses belong to Papovaviridae virus family; they contain circular two-chain DNA, more than 66 genotypes were determined. There are evidences of connection among some genotypes with uterus column malignant tumor development and pre-carcinomatous intraepithelial uterus cervix tumors. Viruses are divided to two groups according oncogene potential: low risk group (HPV genotypes 6 and 11) and high risk group (HPV genotypes 16, 18, 31, 33, 35). Viral DNA is incorporated into female host genome in uterus cervix malignant tumor samples. This integration signifies an early oncogenesis stage; it is not a sufficient transformation condition. HPV DNA detection is considered to be a serious malignant tumor risk factor. Incorporation prevalence is about 90% in pathological samples and 1.5% in normal samples. Current laboratory techniques are able to determine HPV 16, 18, 33 isotypes in samples.

Test Purpose. 1) to detect presence of papilloma virus infection when it is suspected but is not evident clinically, 2) to type of virus infection to determine relative risk of developing cancer.

Increased Values – Positive
papilloma virus infections, genital cancer

Anti-IgA Antibodies

Test Purpose. 1) in patients with IgA deficiency to determine the risk of transfusion associated anaphylaxis.

Increased Values – Positive
subgroup of IgA deficient patients

Anti-Insulin Antibodies

(IAA, insulin autoantibodies) Diabetics may form antibodies to the insulin they are given → larger insulin doses are required, since insulin is partially bound to antibodies. The most common anti-insulin antibody type is IgG. IgE may be responsible for insulin-allergic manifestations, IgM may cause insulin resistance.

Increased Values – positive
pre-type I diabetes mellitus (before insulin treatment), first-step relatives, **allergic reactions to insulin, insulin resistance**

Anti-Intrinsic Factor Antibodies

(anti-IF, IF antibodies, anti-intrinsic factor antibody) There are two antibody types. Type I – blocking antibodies, more common, prevent vitamin B_{12} and intrinsic factor binding, but will not react with complexed intrinsic factor; they distinguish vitamin B_{12} binding places on intrinsic factor. Type I – blocking antibodies are in 75% of patients with pernicious anemia and in 5–10% of patients with autoimmune thyroiditis. Type I Ab prevents the attachment of vitamin B_{12} to intrinsic factor. Type II – binding/precipitating antibodies, react with either free or complexed intrinsic factors; they are directed against other epitops than vitamin B_{12} epitop. Type II Ab prevents attachment of the vitamin B_{12}-intrinsic factor complex to ileal receptors. Blocking antibodies are extremely specific for pernicious anemia, more sensitive than binding antibodies. Chronic type A gastritis is typical autoimmune disease, type B followed with mucous membrane atrophy and achlorhydria is often in Helicobacter pylori infection. Malignant stomach tumor risk patients are: 1) if they suffer from autoimmune disease (adrenalitis, Hashimoto's thyroiditis, Basedow's disease, vitiligo), 2) relatives who suffer from above mentioned diseases, mainly pernicious anemia. Population antibody incidence increases with ageing. Vitamin B_{12} deficiency is determined after positive antibody determination. Gastric mucous membrane pro-ton pump antibodies are in 95% of patients with pernicious anemia and in 5% of patients with thyroid autoimmune disease.
Test Purpose. 1) to differentiate pernicious anemia from other megaloblastic anemias, 2) risk patient detection (stomach tumors).

Increased Values – positive
pernicious anemia, hyperthyroidism, insulin-dependent diabetes mellitus

Analyte	Age/Gender	Reference Range	SI Units	Note
Anti-Intrinsic Factor Antibodies	negative	>0.9		
	borderline	0.9–1.1		
	positive	>1.1		

Anti-Isoleucyl-tRNA Synthetase Antibodies

(anti-OJ, syn: anti-OJ antibodies) Belong to extractable nuclear antigens (ENA) autoantibodies. Their interpreration should always be made in association with the clinical findings.
Test Purpose. To help in diagnosis of polymyositis.

Increased Values – positive
dermatomyositis, polymyositis

Anti-Ku Antibodies

Increased Values – positive
systemic lupus erythematosus, polymyositis, dermatomyositis, scleroderma

Anti-LKM Antibodies

(syn: liver-kidney-microsomal antibodies – anti-LKM-1, anti-LKM-2, anti-LKM-3, antibodies against endoplasmic reticulum) Antibodies are directed against cytochromes.
Test Purpose. 1) diagnosis of chronic active hepatitis (mainly in children and adolescents), cryptogenic cirrhosis, hepatitis induced by medicaments, 2) non-HBV hepatitis differential diagnosis.

Increased Values – positive
autoimmune hepatitis, hepatitis C, cryptogenic cirrhosis, chronic active hepatitis (mainly in children and adolescents), hepatitis induced by medicaments, non-HBV hepatitis

Anti-MAG Antibodies

IgM anti-MAG testing screens for antibodies associated with sensory-motor neuropathies that often have demyelinating features.

Increased Values – positive
sensory-motor neuropathies

Anti-Mi2 Antibodies

Increased Values – positive
dermatomyositis, polymyositis, muscular inflammatory diseases

Anti-Microsomal Antibodies

(syn: antithyroid microsomal antibodies, microsomal antibodies, thyroid autoantibodies, thyroid antimicrosomal antibodies) Belong to antithyroid antibody group. Microsomes are normally within the epithelial cell cytoplasm surrounding the thyroid follicle, acting as antigens after the escape → specific antibodies production with cytotoxic effects on these follicular cells.
Test Purpose. 1) to differentiate autoimmune cause for thyroid disease, 2) to reveal predisposition to autoimmune thyroid disease, 3) to distinguish subacute thyroiditis from Hashimoto's thyroiditis.

Increased Values – positive
anemia – (**autoimmune hemolytic a., pernicious a.**), **rheumatoid arthritis,** dermatitis herpetiformis, hepatitis – (h. induced by medicaments, autoimmune h.), **systemic lupus erythematosus,** Graves' disease, myasthenia gravis, myxedema coma, **myxedema, thyroid tumors,** goiter – (**adenomatous g., non-toxic nodular g.**), **Sjögren's sy,** thyroiditis – (**granulomatous t., Hashimoto's t.,** juvenile lymphocytic t.), elder people

Anti-Mitochondrial Antibodies

(AMA, AMAb) Non-organ antibodies directed against inner mitochondrial membrane lipoproteins. AMA are predominantly of IgG class.
Test Purpose. 1) to aid in primary biliary cirrhosis diagnosis, 2) to distinguish between extrahepatic jaundice and biliary cirrhosis, 3) chronic active hepatitis differential diagnosis.

Increased Values – positive
renal tubular acidosis, fibrosing cryptogenic alveolitis, **pernicious anemia, rheumatoid arthritis,** celiac disease, cirrhosis – (**primary biliary c., cryptogenic c.**), dermatomyositis, hepatitis – (**chronic aggressive h. B, autoimmune-induced h., h. induced by medicaments, viral h.,** chronic h. C), diseases – (autoimmune d., thyroid d.), **collagenoses, systemic lupus erythematosus,** lymphomas, **idiopathic Addison's disease,** Crohn's disease, infectious mononucleosis, myasthenia gravis, **tumors, chronic long-standing hepatic obstruction,** polymyositis, syndrome – (CREST sy, Sjögren's sy), **scleroderma, syphilis, thyroiditis**
    Interfering Factors: medicaments – (chlorpromazine, halothane, oxyphenisatine)

Decreased Values
sclerosing cholangitis, drug-induced cholestatic jaundice, extrahepatic biliary ways obstruction

Analyte	Age/Gender	Reference Range	SI Units	Note
Anti-Mitochondrial Ab		<1:20		

Antimony

(Sb) Antimony is not an abundant metal, but is present in many minerals typically as the sulphide. Antimony is used in alloy industry, semi-conductor, paint, glass and weapons industries. Organoantimonials are used to treat parasitic disease. Normal environmental sources of the metal are very small with the exception of cigarette smoke and some dental materials. Under normal conditions antimony distributes to lung, liver and kidney. Antimony may cross the placenta but does not seem to be preferentially excreted in breast milk. Antimony is excreted in urine and bile.

Increased Values
industrial exposure – (lead i., paint i., glass i., weapons i.)

Anti-Myelin Antibodies

Increased Values – positive
peripheral neuropathy, healthy persons

Anti-Myeloperoxidase Antibodies

(anti-MPO) Myeloperoxidase is a neutrophil lysosomal enzyme (oxidoreductase) that catalyzes the reaction of hydrogen peroxide and halide ions to produce cytotoxic acids and other intermediates. These play a role in oxygendependent killing of microorganisms and tumor cells. The enzyme is a hemoprotein found in the azurophil granules of neutrophils and the primary lysosomes of monocytes and it has the green color seen in pus. MPO is associated with two subtypes of antineutrophil cytoplasmic antibodies: c-ANCA and p-ANCA. c-ANCA is in cytoplasm (C) and is of diagnostic value in Wegener's granulomatosis. p-ANCA is located perinuclearly (P). Anti-MPO is necrotizing vasculitides and glomerulonephritis diagnostic marker. Anti-MPO antibodies are represented mainly with P subtype; they can be determined semiquantitatively in IgM, IgA, and IgG classes.

Test Purpose. 1) necrotizing vasculitides, polyarteritis nodosa and Churg–Strauss sy diagnosis, 2) glomerulonephritis diagnosis.

Increased Values – positive
glomerulonephritis – (segmental necrotizing g., g. with antiglomerular basement antibodies), systemic lupus erythematosus, polyarteritis nodosa, Churg–Strauss sy, necrotizing vasculitides

Analyte	Age/Gender	Reference Range	SI Units	Note
Anti-Myeloperoxidase Ab (IgG)		<9.0	U/ml	

Anti-Myocardial Antibodies

(syn: heart mitochondrial antibodies – HMA, HMAb) Antibodies are directed against sarcolemma, myolemma or other contractile elements (actin, myosin, tropomyosin, troponins) as well as against mitochondrial antigens. Test has a very low specificity.

Increased Values – positive
endocarditis, endomyocardial fibrosis, **rheumatic fever**, chronic rheumatic diseases, **myocardial infarction**, streptococcal infections, **cardiomyopathies**, systemic lupus erythematosus, idiopathic myocarditis, idiopathic pericarditis, perimyocarditis, after heart transplantation conditions, syndrome – (**Dressler's sy**, **post-cardiotomic sy**, post-thoracotomic sy)

Anti-Neutrophil Antibodies

(syn: granulocyte antibodies, neutrophil antibodies)
Test Purpose. 1) to investigate possible immune neutropenia origins, 2) to detect antibodies against granulocyte-specific antigens in evaluating neonatal alloimmune neutropenia, autoimmune neutropenia and transfusion reactions.

Increased Values – positive
idiopathic neutropenia, **immune neutropenia**, transfusion reactions
    Interfering Factors: medicaments – (cephalosporins, penicillins, vancomycin)

Anti-Neutrophil Cytoplasmic Antibodies

(ANCA, ANCAb, ACPA, syn: neutrophil cytoplasmic antibody) Antibodies directed against selected cytoplasmic polymorphonuclears and monocytes antigens. There are two main types – cytoplasmic ANCA and perinuclear ANCA, the third type is atypical ANCA. Cytoplasmic staining (c-ANCA, azurophilic granules in neutrophils) is associated with anti-proteinase 3 antibody and is of diagnostic value in Wegener's granulomatosis. Proteinase 3 enzyme possesses some proteolytic properties against elastin, fibronectin, laminin, collagen type IV and antimicrobial activities against E. coli, C. albicans. Neutrophil granulocytes contain many enzymes in azurophilic granules (proteinase 3, myeloperoxidase, cathepsin G, elastase, lysozyme, beta-glucuronidase, bactericid permeability increasing protein, cationic proteins). In specific granules they contain collagenase, lactoferrin, gelatinase, vitamin B_{12} binding protein. p-ANCA is located perinuclearly (perinuclear staining). p-ANCA is associated with number of antibodies, including antimyeloperoxidase antibody.

Test Purpose. 1) to aid in Wegener's granulomatosis diagnosis, 2) diagnosis of vasculitis, 3) diagnosis of renal disease, idiopathic necrotising glomerulonephritis, 4) diagnosis of microscopic polyarteritis.

Increased Values – positive

rheumatoid arthritis, primary biliary cirrhosis, glomerulonephritis – (**necrotizing g., rapidly progressive g.** – c-ANCA, p-ANCA, idiopathic g. – p-ANCA, sclerosing g., membranous g.), chronic active hepatitis B, **primary sclerosing cholangitis** (atypical-ANCA), lupus erythematosus – (**drug-induced l. e.** – p-ANCA, **systemic l. e.** – p-ANCA), **Wegener's disease** (c-ANCA, p-ANCA), temporal arteritis (p-ANCA), Henoch–Schönlein purpura (p-ANCA), **polyarteritis nodosa** (c-ANCA, p-ANCA), **Felty's sy**, vasculitides (c-ANCA, p-ANCA), **Churg–Strauss vasculitis** (c-ANCA, p-ANCA), microscopic polyangiitis (c-ANCA, p-ANCA), false positive results (c-ANCA) – (pneumonia, AIDS, endocarditis, **ulcerative colitis**, monoclonal gammopathies), peripheral polyneuropathies (c-ANCA), paresis of n. facialis (c-ANCA), cranial nerve polyneuritis (c-ANCA), secondary polychondritis (c-ANCA), chronic renal insufficiency (c-ANCA), scleroderma (p-ANCA), syndrome – (Sjögren's sy – p-ANCA, Goodpasture's sy – p-ANCA), false positive results (p-ANCA) – (collagenoses, chronic inflammatory bowel disease, **ulcerative colitis**, **Crohn's disease**, lupus hepatitis, Felty's syndrome), atypical-ANCA – (HIV infection, Felty's sy, chronic inflammatory bowel disease, Kawasaki sy, **Crohn's disease**, ulcerative colitis, endocarditis, cystic fibrosis)

Anti-Nuclear Antibodies

(ANA, ANAb, ANF, FANA, syn: antinuclear antibody, antinuclear factor) In some conditions, the body's immune system may perceive portions of its own cell nuclei as foreign → antibody production. ANA nomenclature is not still standardized, it corresponds with disease in which the antibodies are present (e.g. anti-SSA, anti-SSB in Sjögren's sy), with first described patient name abbreviation (anti-Sm, Smith) or according to chemical structure against which are the antibodies directed. Antibody testing against these nuclear antigens are used in clinical practice: Sm (Smith), Ro (SSA), La (SSB), RNP (ribonucleoprotein), Scl-70 (DNA-topoisomerase I), Jo-1 (histidyl-tRNA synthase), Rib.Po (ribosomal Po antigen); ANA-bioblot tast is used as test name. Tests are used only as **additional**; test results must be interpreted in clinical/history picture context. About 5% of the normal population have a positive antinuclear antibody. The percent with positive ANA increases with age, and in people, 70–80 years, up to 15% will have a positive low titre ANA. In the over 70 age group, the ANA's are usually antibodies to histone proteins. Higher titres usually have greater diagnostic significance, particularly in younger patients. Use of the ANA as a screening test should be avoided, as interpretation is difficult in the absence of features suggestive of a systemic disease. Titres often remain elevated in remission and do not necessarily reflect disease activity. If the clinical findings and the ANA result do not agree, believe the clinical findings.

Test Purpose. 1) to screen for systemic lupus erythematosus (SLE), 2) to monitor the effectiveness of immunosuppressive SLE therapy, 3) diagnosis of suspected connective tissue disease or any inflammatory disease.

- Nuclear antigens:
  - nuclear membrane: lamin, pure nuclear protein
  - chromatin: DNA, histones, Ku (non-histone proteins), centromere
  - ribonucleoproteins: U1 RNP, Rib.Po, Sm (U1-U6 RNP), SSA, SSB
  - cell cycle proteins: PCNA (cyclines)
  - enzymes: Scl-70 (DNA-topoisomerase-I), Jo-1 (histidyl-t-RNA synthase)
- Nucleolar antigens:
  - proteins: fibrillarin, nucleolin, PM/Scl
  - ribonucleoproteins: U3-RNP
  - enzymes: RNA-polymerase-I

ANA findings in connective tissue diseases:

Antigen	SLE	MCTD	RA	Sjögren's sy	Polymyositis	Scleroderma
Sm B/B´	+	(+)				
Sm D	+					
RNP 68 kD		+				
RNP A	(+)	+	(+)			
RNP C	+	+	+			
SSA/Ro 60 kD	+	+	+	+		
SSA/Ro 52 kD				+		
SSB/La	(+)			+		
Jo-1					+	
Scl-70						+
Rib. Po	+					

Systemic lupus erythematosus patients ANA

Test	Specificity
native DNA	SLE
denatured DNA (ss, single stranded)	high titres in SLE, low titres in other diseases
histones H1, H3-H4	SLE
histones H2A-H2B	(medicament induced SLE)
Sm	SLE (positive in 25–60%)
U1-RNP	SLE, in high titres also in MCTD
nucleolar antigens	scleroderma, Sjögren's sy, SLE
SSB	Sjögren's sy, SLE
SSA	Sjögren's sy, SLE
DNA-RNA hybrides, double stranded DNA	SLE
Rib. Po	SLE

Increased Values – positive

fibrosing cryptogenic alveolitis, anemia – (pernicious a., acquired hemolytic autoimmune a., **hemolytic a.**), Takayasu's arteritis, arthritis – (**rheumatoid a.**, parvovirus a., **juvenile rheumatoid a.**), cirrhosis – (**primary biliary c.**, **hepatic c.**), **dermatomyositis, diabetes mellitus,**

infective endocarditis, pulmonary fibrosis, ulcerative colitis, glomerulonephritis, hepatitis – (alcoholic h., autoimmune h., acute h. A, acute h. B, **chronic h.**, **chronic active h. B**, acute h. E, chronic h. C, acute h. D, lupoid h.), fever – (**rheumatic f.**, Q fever), pulmonary hypertension, disease – (Addison's d., Crohn's d., **Raynaud's d.**, Grave's d., rheumatoid heart d.), **mixed connective tissue disease** (MCTD), diseases – (**autoimmune d.**, infectious bacterial d., chronic liver d., gastrointestinal d., infectious viral d., **rheumatoid d.**), collagenoses, leprosy, leukemia – (acute lymphoblastic l., acute myeloblastic l.), lupus erythematosus – (chronic discoid l. e., **drug induced l. e.**, **systemic l. e.**), **Waldenström's macroglobulinemia,** malaria, **infectious mononucleosis, myasthenia gravis,** acute myocarditis, tumors – (**anaplastic t.**, melanoma, breast t., lung t., kidney t., ovarian t., **lymphomas**), lupus nephritis, **pneumoconiosis, atypical pneumonia, periarteritis nodosa, polymyositis, idiopathic thrombocytopenic purpura, healthy family member of systemic lupus erythematosus patients, scleroderma,** pemphigus, psoriasis, syndrome – (**CREST sy**, eosinophilia-myalgia sy, chronic fatigue sy, postcardiac injury sy, Felty's sy, **Sjögren's sy**, Schnitzler's sy, **Still's sy**), **tuberculosis,** thyroiditis, **Hashimoto's thyroiditis, necrotizing vasculitis,** vitiligo

Interfering Factors: healthy adults and elderly patients, medicaments – (acebutolol, acetazolamide, aminosalicylic acid, captopril, carbamazepine, chlorprothixene, chlorothiazides, chlorpromazine, dilantin, ethosuximide, griseofulvin, hydralazine, isoniazid, labetalol, mephenytoin, methyldopa, nitrofurantoin, penicillamine, penicillin, phenylbutazone, phenytoin sodium, pindolol, practolol, primidone, procainamide, propylthiouracil, quinidine, streptomycin, sulfasalazine, sulfonamides, tetracyclines, thiazides, trimethadione)

Positive Speckled Antinuclear Antibody Pattern
systemic lupus erythematosus, dermatomyositis, mixed connective tissue disease, scleroderma, polymyositis, **Sjögren's syndrome**

Decreased Values
Interfering Factors: false negative values – (steroids)

Analyte	Age/Gender	Reference Range	SI Units	Note
Anti-Nuclear Ab (ANA)		1:80		
		>1:160		

Anti-Nuclear Antigen Antibodies

Increased Values – positive
systemic lupus erythematosus, Sjögren's sy

Anti-Ovarian Antibodies

Test Purpose. To help in diagnosis of autoimmune ovarian dysfunction.

Increased Values – positive
polyglandular autoimmune syndrome, ovarian failure, Addison's disease, menstrual disorders

Anti-p53 Antibodies

Tumor-suppressant gene p53 is altered in about 50% of malignant tumors, the most frequent is point-mutation form (in 90%). Alterations lead to abnormal protein p53 accumulation in tumor cell nucleus, this accumulation signifies bad prognosis of malignant tumors. p53 presence can lead to chemotherapy resistance in some tumors. An early tumor sign – gene alteration – can be detected very early in oncogenesis. Anti-p53 serum antibodies can be determined via serological analysis in patients with immune response against abnormally high protein p53 concentration in tumor cells. These antibodies are the indirect marker of pointmutation, they are stable and independent on tumor heterogenity.

Test Purpose. 1) malignant tumor suspection assessment (tumor marker), 2) chemotherapy regimen choice assessment, 3) some tumors prognosis assessment.

Increased Values – positive
tumors

Analyte	Age/Gender	Reference Range	SI Units	Note
Anti-p53				
negative index		<0.9		
positive index		1.1		

Anti-Pancreatic Islet Cell Antibodies

(ICA, ICAb, syn: islet cell antibodies, pancreatic islet cell autoantibodies) Antibodies have been found to both cytoplasmic and islet cell surface antigens. Presence of antibody may precede onset of clinical disease in IDDM, but levels decline subsequently.

Increased Values – positive
ongoing B-cell destruction, diabetes mellitus – (**IDDM** – early diagnosis, **identifying patients with high IDDM risk**)

Analyte	Age/Gender	Reference Range	SI Units	Note
Anti-Pancreatic Islet Cell Ab (ICA)		<2.5	JDF U/ml	

Anti-Parathyroid Antibodies

Test Purpose. To assess patients with hypocalcemia or suspected hypoparathyroidism.

Increased Values – positive
idiopathic hypoparathyroidism

Anti-Parietal Cell Antibodies

(APA, APAb, syn: parietal cell antibodies – PCA, PCAb) Autoimmune antibodies against gastric parietal cells antigens (microsomal compounds). They do not correlate with malabsorption of vitamin B_{12}. However, they may participate in the early pathogenesis of parietal cell destruction. Less than 2% of the general population has test positive for antiparietal cell antibodies, but the percentage increases with age. In people over 60, up to 16% may have test positive.

Test Purpose. To aid in pernicious anemia and atrophic gastritis differential diagnosis.

Increased Values – positive
anemia – (autoimmune megaloblastic a., **autoimmune pernicious a.**, **iron deficiency a.**), **juvenile diabetes mellitus**, **asymptomatic/presymptomatic atrophic gastritis**, **gastric ulcer disease**, Addison's disease, myasthenia gravis, **stomach tumors**, positive antinuclear antibodies, Sjögren's sy, **autoimmune thyroiditis**, elder people, **thyroid diseases**

Anti-Phospholipid Antibodies

(APLA, APLAb) Antiphospholipid antibodies are heterogenous antibody group primarily directed against a negative charged phospholipids, or against protein-phospholipid complex (beta-2-glycoprotein I, prothrombin, annexin V, protein C, protein S, kallikrein and transmembrane thrombomodulin). They involve: 1) anticardiolipin antibodies (ACLA, ACLAb), immuno-globulins directed against beta-2-glycoprotein I bounded to anion lipid surface, 2) lupus anticoagulant (LA, lupus inhibitor) represents immunoglobulins which distinguish prothrombin-phospholipid complex, 3) reagins and antibodies against negative/neutral phospholipids. Antiphospholipid antibody isotypes are IgG, IgM, IgA or their mixture. They possess a high cross reactivity occurring in monoclonal form. Isotypes IgG 2 an IgG 4 are of a high clinical value.

Test Purpose. 1) to aid in diagnosis of cardiolipin antibody syndrome with/without lupus erythematosus experiencing recurrent spontaneous deep venous thrombosis episodes, thromboembolic accidents, thrombocytopenia, lupus-like syndromes, false-positive VDRL, or habitual abortions, 2) in recurrent myocardial infarction, ischemic cerebrovascular accident, chorea, migraine, amaurosis fugax, Libman-Sacks endocarditis, livedo reticularis, primary biliary cirrhosis, HIV infection.

Increased Values – positive
AIDS, amaurosis fugax, autoimmune disorders, primary biliary cirrhosis, Libman–Sacks endocarditis, pulmonary hypertension, chorea, infarction – (myocardial i., placental i.), livedo reticularis, **systemic lupus erythematosus**, migraine, abortion – (habitual a., spontaneous a.), preeclampsia, ischemic cerebrovascular accident, **primary antiphospholipid sy involving arterial/venous thromboses**, thrombocytopenia and recurrent spontaneous abortions, **secondary antiphospholipid sy**, fetal loss, idiopathic thrombocytopenia, **arterial/venous thrombosis**, syphilis, healthy individuals

---

Anti-Poliovirus Antibodies

(syn: enterovirus antibodies, poliomyelitis antibodies). Test supports diagnosis of poliovirus infection, documents previous exposure or immunization for poliovirus.

Increased Values – positive
poliomyelitis

Anti-Red Blood Cell Antibodies

(syn: DTT testing) Test is used to distinguish IgG and IgM red blood cell antibody. Only IgG antibodies are considered clinically significant during pregnancy.

Increased Values – positive
AIDS, neonatal isoerythrolysis

Anti-Reticulin Antibodies

(syn: reticulin antibodies, antigluten antibodies, celiac disease IgA, IgG antibodies) Molecular basis of antigen is not known currently; probably these are antigliadin antibodies reacting with reticulin.
Test Purpose. 1) to aid in the diagnosis of gluten-sensitive enteropathies including celiac disease and dermatitis herpetiformis, 2) to monitor patient compliance to a gluten-free diet.

Increased Values – positive
dermatitis herpetiformis, **gluten-sensitive enteropathy** (celiac disease), **Crohn's disease**, healthy persons

Anti-Ribonucleoprotein Antibodies

(anti-RNP, RNP, syn: ribonucleoprotein antibodies) Autoantibodies from antinuclear antibody group. Belong to the small extractable nuclear antigen antibodies.
Test Purpose. 1) to aid in autoimmune disease differential diagnosis, 2) to screen for anti-RNP antibodies, common in SLE, scleroderma and other rheumatic disorders, 3) to monitor therapy response in patients with autoimmune diseases.

Increased Values – positive
mixed connective tissue disease (MCTD), lupus erythematosus – (discoid l. e., drug induced l. e., **systemic l. e.**), **progressive systemic sclerosis** (scleroderma), **rheumatoid arthritis**, **Sjögren's sy**

Anti-Ribosomal Po Antibodies

Increased Values – positive
systemic lupus erythematosus

Anti-Scleroderma Antibodies

(anti-Scl-70, syn: Scl-70 antibodies, scleroderma antibodies, anti-topoisomerase-T, topoisomerase-T) Enzyme DNA-topoisomerase-T affects the transcription pre-step. Belong to autoantibodies against extractable nuclear antigens (ENA, ENAb). Their interpreration should always be made in association with the clinical findings.

Increased Values – positive
rheumatoid arthritis, mixed connective tissue disease (MCTD), systemic lupus erythematosus, **polymyositis**, **scleroderma** (progressive systemic sclerosis), syndrome – (**CREST sy**, Raynaud's sy, Sjögren's sy)
>   **Interfering Factors:** medicaments – (aminosalicylic acid, isoniazid, methyldopa, penicillin, streptomycin, tetracyclines)

Anti-Skin Antibodies

(interepithelial Ab, dermal-epidermal Ab)
Test Purpose. To help in diagnosis of pemphigus and bullous disease.

Increased Values – positive
pemphigus, bullous diseases

Anti-Sm Antibodies

(anti-Sm, syn: anti-Smith antibodies) Belong to autoantibodies against extractable nuclear antigens (ENA). Their interpreration should always be made in association with the clinical findings.
Test Purpose. 1) to aid in autoimmune disease differential diagnosis, 2) to screen for anti-Sm antibodies, a specific marker for SLE, 3) to monitor therapy response in patients with autoimmune diseases.

Increased Values – positive
autoimmune diseases, **systemic lupus erythematosus**, drug induced lupus erythematosus, lupus nephritis

Anti-Smooth Muscles Antibodies

(ASMA, ASMAb, syn: smooth muscle antibody, antiactin antibody) Autoantibodies (IgG, IgM type) associated with liver and bile duct autoimmune diseases. Presence of antinuclear antibody may interfere with the interpretation of smooth muscle antibody.
Test Purpose. 1) to aid in diagnosis of chronic active hepatitis and primary biliary cirrhosis, 2) to help to distinguish lupoid hepatitis from systemic lupus erythematosus.

Increased Values – positive
asthma bronchiale, **primary biliary cirrhosis**, **liver cirrhosis**, hepatitis – (**autoimmune chronic active h.**, lupoid h., chronic h., **chronic active h.**, **viral h.**), hepatoma, yellow fever, EB virus disease, cytomegalovirus disease, mixed connective tissue disease (MCTD), diseases – (viral infectious d., drug-induced liver d., rheumatic d.), **infectious mononucleosis**, systemic lupus erythematosus, **tumours**, syndrome – (postinfarction sy, postpericardectomy sy)
>   **Interfering Factors:** elder people, healthy people

Anti-Spermatozoa Antibodies

(syn: antispermatozoal antibodies, sperm agglutination and inhibition, spermatozoon antibodies, antisperm antibodies, infertility screen) Spermatozoa reabsorption from blocked ducts results in autoantibodies against spermatozoa formation.

Test Purpose. 1) sterility diagnosis in cases with suspect andrological history (parotitis, trauma, surgery, testes infections), 2) suspect spermiogram (asthenozoospermia, ejaculate agglutination), 3) abnormal spermatozoa findings (mucus interaction test), 4) artificial insemination indication.

Increased Values – positive

asthenozoospermia, male infertility caused by – (**infections, surgery, parotitis, testes trauma**), **vasectomy, blocked efferent ducts in the testes, women with primary infertility** (about 75% of them have anti-spermatozoa agglutinins)

Anti-SSA and Anti-SSB Antibodies

(anti-Ro/SSA, anti-La/SSB, anti-Ro, anti-La, syn: anti-La antibodies, anti-Sjögren's, Sjögren's antibodies) Belong to autoantibodies against extractable nuclear antigens (ENA). Their interpreration should always be made in association with the clinical findings.

Test Purpose. 1) to screen for systemic lupus erythematosus (SLE), 2) to detect SSB autoantibodies produced in Sjögren's sy, 3) to aid in the diagnosis of lupus patients with Sjögren's overlap sy, 4) to monitor therapy response in patients with autoimmune diseases.

Increased Values – positive Anti-Ro

keratoconjunctivitis sicca, systemic lupus erythematosus, neonatal lupus, scleroderma, Sjögren's sy, isolated xerostomia, lupus nephritis, rheumatoid arthritis, drug induced lupus erythematosus, mixed connective tissue disease

Increased Values – positive Anti-La

systemic lupus erythematosus, rheumatoid arthritis, drug induced lupus erythematosus, long-term phenothiazine use, plasmocytoma (inc. multiple myeloma), ulcerative colitis, postpartum, hemophilia, tumors, chronic inflammatory diseases

Antistreptolysin O

(ASLO, ASO, ASOT, syn: antistreptococcal antibody titers) ASO titers demonstrate the body reaction to infection caused by group A streptococci. The streptococcus organism produces an enzyme called streptolysin O, which has the ability to destroy (lyse) red blood cells. Because streptolysin O is antigenic (protein antigen), the body reacts by producing ASO (a neutralizing antibody). Streptolysin O antibodies are produced by group A beta-hemolytic streptococci. ASO determination is a serologic test segment for diagnosis and evaluation of the streptococcal infection course. Antibody appears as early as one week after infection, titer rises rapidly by 3–4 weeks, may remain elevated for months. Serial determinations are most desirable, a four-fold increase confirms immunologic response to streptococcal organisms. Other tests are: antideoxyribonuclease B (ADN-ase B) and antihyaluronidase.

Test Purpose. 1) to confirm recent/ongoing infection with beta-hemolytic streptococci, 2) to help diagnose rheumatic fever, poststreptococcal glomerulonephritis with clinical symptoms and Henoch-Schönlein pupura, 3) to distinguish between rheumatic fever and rheumatoid arthritis when joint pain is experienced, 4) to investigate a severe cellulitis, rarely in recurrent tonsillitis, 5) to confirm diagnosis of scarlet fever, erysipelas, 6) to detect subclinical streptococcal infection.

Increased Values
bacterial endocarditis, **acute poststreptococcal glomerulonephritis**, **active/inactive rheumatic fever**, collagen diseases, false positive results – (tuberculosis, liver diseases, bacterial contamination), rheumatoid arthritis, **streptococcal infection**, **scarlet fever**, Henoch–Schönlein purpura, severe cellulitis, tonsillitis, streptococcal pyoderma
   Interfering Factors: increased beta-lipoproteins

Decreased Values
   Interfering Factors: medicaments – (adrenocorticosteroids, antibiotics)

Analyte	Age/Gender	Reference Range	SI Units	Note
Antistreptolysin O (ASLO)				
	Children	$<150.10^3$	U/ml	
	Adults	$<200.10^3$	U/ml	

Anti-Striated Muscle Antibodies

(StMA, StMAb, syn: striational antibodies, striational antibodies to skeletal muscles). Test is used for diagnosis of myasthenia gravis and thymoma. Measurement of acetylcholine receptor antibodies and striational antibodies is useful for predicting risk of myasthenia gravis in patients with thymoma.

Increased Values – positive
myasthenia gravis, polymyositis, **thymoma**

Anti-Sulfatide Antibodies

Anti-sulfatide testing screens for antibodies that are associated with polyneuropathies having a prominent sensory component. Anti-sulfatide antibodies associated with a serum IgM M-protein are most commonly associated with a demyelinating neuropathy. Polyclonal anti-sulfatide antibodies are more commonly associated with an axonal neuropathy.

Increased Values – positive
polyneuropathies, axonal neuropathy, demyelinating neuropathy

Anti-Teichoic Acid Antibodies

Test is used in assessing therapy in chronic infections caused by Staphylococcus aureus.

Increased Values – positive
chronic infections caused by Staphylococcus aureus

Anti-Testicular Antibodies

(syn: testicular antibodies)
Test Purpose. To investigate male infertility associated with polyglandular syndromes.

Increased Values – positive
testicular failure, male infertility

Anti-Tetanus Toxin Antibodies

(syn: tetanus antitoxoid antibodies, tetanus antibodies, tetanus toxin antibodies) Test is used to assess immunity against tetanus by determining levels of circulating antibodies to tetanus toxin or to measure the immune response, postvaccination, in individuals suspected of immunodeficiency disorders.

Increased Values – positive
tetanus infection

Anti-Threonyl-tRNA Synthetase Antibodies

(anti-PL-7, syn: anti-PL-7 antibodies) Belongs to extractable nuclear antigens (ENA) autoantibodies. Their interpreration should always be made in association with the clinical findings.
Test Purpose. To help in diagnosis of polymyositis.

Increased Values – positive
dermatomyositis, polymyositis

Anti-Thyroglobulin Antibodies

(ATGA, ATGAb, syn: thyroglobulin antibody, anti-thyroglobulin autoantibodies) Thyroglobulin is quite a strong autoantigen. In healthy blood there are many B-lymphocytes with membrane-bounded IgM type thyroglobulin antibodies. IgG antibodies against thyroglobulin are Hashimoto's thyroiditis markers. The presence of autoantibodies to thyroglobulin can lead to the functional destruction of the thyroid gland.
Test Purpose. To detect and confirm autoimmune thyroiditis, Hashimoto's thyroiditis

Increased Values – positive
anemia – (**pernicious a.**, autoimmune hemolytic a.), **rheumatoid arthritis**, **autoimmune disorders**, granulomatosis, hyperthyroidism, **hypothyroidism**, **systemic lupus erythematosus**, **Graves' disease**, myasthenia gravis, **idiopathic myxedema**, myxedema coma, myxedema heart disease, **thyroid tumors**, syndrome – (Down sy, **Sjögren's sy**, Turner's sy), thyroiditis – (**Hashimoto's t.**, de Quervain's subacute t.), **thyrotoxicosis**, rheumatoid-collagen disease, non-toxic nodular goiter
    Interfering Factors: healthy people, medicaments – (amiodarone)

Analyte	Age/Gender	Reference Range	SI Units	Note
Anti-Thyroglobulin Antibodies (ATGA)		<150	U/ml	

Anti-Thyroid Antibodies

(syn: thyroid antibodies, thyroid autoantibodies) Antibodies are divided: 1) anti-TSH, 2) antimicrosomal, 3) antithyroid peroxidase, 4) antithyroglobulin, 5) anticolloid, 6) anti-T3, 7) anti-T4. Certain destructive thyroid diseases lead to thyroglobulin release, thus stimulates antibody formation. It seems, that thyroid peroxidase is a main part of microsome antigen so antithyroid peroxidase antibodies determination is of same value as antimicrosomal antibodies determination. Postmenopausal women produce mainly antimicrosomal and antithyroglobulin antibodies; there is a tendency to chronic thyroiditis development followed by thyroid atrophy and hypothyroidism (so called idiopathic myxedema is chronic atrophic thyroiditis end-stage). In younger individuals the harder thyroid and high antithyroglobulin/antimicrosomal antibody titres are the chronic lymphomonocytic Hashimoto's thyroiditis signs. Silent thyroiditis is the other form which affects women exclusively with the antimicrosomal antibodies presence; clinical picture is typical after labor with temporary hyperthyroidism and subsequent hypothyroidism. Antithyroid/antimicrosomal antibodies in Graves–Basedow disease testifies to chronic thyroidism and toxic goiter coexistency.

Test Purpose. To detect circulating antithyroglobulin antibodies when clinical evidence indicates Hashimoto's thyroiditis, Graves' disease or other thyroid diseases.

Increased Values – positive
anemia – (**autoimmune hemolytic a., pernicious a.**), **rheumatoid arthritis, hypothyroidism, active autoimmune diseases of the thyroid, systemic lupus erythematosus,** Graves' disease, **myxedema, thyroid tumors,** goiter – (adenomatous g., diffuse g., lymphadenoid g., nodular g.), **Sjögren's sy,** thyroiditis – (granulomatous t., **Hashimoto's t.**), **thyrotoxicosis**
    Interfering Factors: healthy individuals, elderly women

Anti-Thyroid Peroxidase Antibodies

(anti-TPO, TPOA, TPO antibodies) TPO antibodies are the main and possibly only autoantigenic microsome component. Anti-TPO antibodies belong to thyroid tissue antibodies and are a useful biochemical marker for autoimmune thyroid disease.
Test Purpose. To help in differential diagnosis of hypothyroidism and thyroiditis.

Increased Values – positive
autoimmune thyroid disease – (Graves' disease, idiopathic myxedema, **Hashimoto's thyroiditis**)
    Interfering Factors: healthy individuals, elderly women

Analyte	Age/Gender	Reference Range	SI Units	Note
Anti-Thyroperoxidase Antibodies (TPOA)		<20	U/ml	

Anti-Thyrotropin-Receptor Antibodies

(anti-TSHr, TRAb, syn: thyrotropin receptor antibody, thyroid stimulating hormone receptor antibodies, TSH receptor antibodies, TSH receptor binding inhibitory immunoglobulin) The family of autoantibodies known as TSH Receptor Antibodies is comprised of two members (TSI, TBII). Thyrotropin-receptor antibodies are a group of related heterogenous IgG immunoglobulins that bind to thyroid cell membranes at/near the TSH-receptor site. Thyroid Stimulating Immunoglobulins (TSI) cause stimulation of the gland to release thyroid hormones. TSI is characteristic of Graves–Basedow disease and is detected using an in vitro bioassay (using human TSH transfected host cells where bioactivity is measured). TBII (thyrotropin-binding inhibiting immunoglobulins) determination is based on TSH and anti-TSHr competition. These are antibodies that bind the TSH receptor but do not stimulate it. By binding to the TSH receptor they inhibit the binding of TSH. High titres means active disease phase, low titres are during disease remission. Positive anti-TSHr in patient with hyperthyroidism marks Basedow's disease even without extrathyroid clinical signs or other autoimmune antibodies.

Test Purpose. 1) Basedow's disease diagnosis, 2) hypothyroidism diagnosis, 3) to detect clinically latent thyropathies and other autoimmune diseases, 4) TSI – a prognostic marker in patients on antithyroid drugs since the presence of TSI is a strong predictor of relapse after drug withdrawal, 5) transplacental passage of TSI may lead to neonatal thyrotoxicosis and documenting high levels of TSI in the 3rd trimester of pregnancy predicts the risk of neonatal thyrotoxicosis, 6) unexplained eye disease.

Increased Values – positive
Graves' disease, non-specific goiter, neonatal thyrotoxicosis, autoimmune thyroiditis

Analyte	Age/Gender	Reference Range	SI Units	Note
Anti-Thyrotropin Receptor Ab		<0.140	U/ml	

Anti-Tissue Transglutaminase Autoantibodies

(anti-tTG autoantibodies) Tissue transglutaminase belongs to calcium dependent enzyme group which catalyzes protein cross-linking producing epsilon-(gamma-glutamyl)-lysine linking. tTG stabilizes short-lasting extracellular matrix in granulating tissue (injury). Increased secretion is present also during apoptosis. Gliadin, an alcohol soluble fraction of gluten, plays a causal role in coeliac disease pathogenesis. Gliadin is a preference substrate for tissue transglutaminase and gliadin cross-linked to high-molecular complexes (gliadin-gliadin and gliadin-tTG) is a cellular and humoral immune response trigger. In this way, tissue transglutaminase represents one of the main endomysial antigen with neoepitopes.

Test Purpose. To help in diagnosis and therapy monitoring of celiac disease.

Increased Values – positive
celiac disease

Anti-Toxocara Antibodies

(Toxocara antibodies) Toxocariasis (Toxocara canis) belongs to the most common parasitosis (after toxoplasmosis), there are two pathogenic human type, Toxocara canis and Toxocara cati. It is important to distinguish seropositivity and clinical picture. Most of infections proceed subclinically, serum to clinical prevalence is about 50:1. An antibody creation against excretory-secretory antigen (ES), is used in serological diagnosis, recently against Tcn2 antigen. IgM type antibodies are increasing in 6th to 8th week and last longer time, IgG are increasing two weeks after infection; increased concentrations last 6 to 9 months after single infection. A negative result does not exclude the diagnosis.

Test Purpose. 1) differential diagnosis of atypical asthmatic conditions with fever and eosinophilia, 2) differential diagnosis of unclear hepatosplenomegaly, 3) chorioretinitis differential diagnosis, 4) to help in diagnosis of Toxocara canis causing visceral larva migrans or ocular larva migrans.

Increased Values – positive
hepatosplenomegaly, chorioretinitis, **toxocariasis**

Anti-Toxoplasma Antibodies

(syn: toxoplasma antibodies) A four-fold rise in IgG titre between acute and convalescent samples is diagnostic for toxoplasmosis.

Test Purpose. To help in diagnosis of suspected toxoplasmosis (e.g. glandular fever-like syndromes, hepatitis, fever in immunosuppressed patients, retinitis, TORCH (toxoplasma, other agents, rubella, cytomegalovirus, herpes simplex) syndrome in neonates).

Increased Values – positive
toxoplasmosis, AIDS

Anti-Trichinella Antibodies

Demonstration of four-fold rise in titre between acute and convalescent sera is considered significant. A single positive titre does not differentiate between past and present infection but may support the diagnosis in an appropriate clinical context and justify proceeding to a muscle biopsy.

Test Purpose. To support the diagnosis of trichinosis or visceral larva migrans caused by Trichinella species.

Increased Values – positive
trichinellosis

Alpha-1-Antitrypsin

(AAT, alpha-1 AT, syn: alpha-1-trypsin inhibitor, alpha-1-proteinase inhibitor).
Production. Glycoprotein (main component of alpha-1-globulin fraction) is produced by the liver.

Function. Inhibitor of proteases (proteolytic enzymes) released into the body fluids by apoptotic cells as leukocyte protease, elastase, plasmin, thrombin, cathepsin, collagenase, trypsin, chymotrypsin. During the inflammation course there is release of proteolytic enzymes from leukocytes in the body tissues. Those enzymes would do extensive damage to the tissue protein structure. When AAT is deficient, unopposed activity of these enzymes result in emphysema. AAT is a protein of acute phase (acute phase reactant), it raises rapidly, but nonspecifically whenever there is tissue injury, necrosis, inflammation or infection. Phenotyping is desirable on patients with low values and on all patients being worked up for AAT-deficiency liver disease. Most pathologic is homozygous state ZZ. An M-null genotype will have phenotype as MM but low serum level.

Test Purpose. 1) non-specific test of inflammation, severe infections and necrosis diagnosis, 2) diagnosis of jaundice, hepatic cirrhosis, 3) diagnosis of pulmonary emphysema, 4) to detect hereditary decreases in the production of AAT, 5) to detect neoplastic conditions, 6) diagnosis of unexplained high ESR, 7) to monitor disease activity.

Increased Values

rheumatoid arthritis, hereditary angioneurotic edema, diabetes mellitus, acute hepatitis, diseases – **(infectious d., renal d., chronic pulmonary d., chronic liver d., rheumatic d.,** systemic d., **thyroid infectious/inflammatory d., acute/chronic inflammatory d.,** gastric d., **collagen vascular d.), acute myocardial infarction,** systemic lupus erythematosus, **tumours, tissue necrosis,** pneumopathy – (infective p., tumorous p.), **pancreatitis, postoperative states, stress conditions, trauma, vasculitis**

Interfering Factors: healthy persons, **pregnancy** (3rd trimester), medicaments – (androgens, estrogens, oral contraceptives, oxymetholone, steroids, streptokinase, tamoxifen)

Decreased Values

infected bronchiectasis, chronic bronchitis, **hepatic cirrhosis,** familial infantile cirrhosis, **congenital alpha-1-antitrypsin deficiency, children/adult pulmonary emphysema,** encephalopathy, exudative enteropathy, **hepatitis, neonatal hepatitis, hepatoma,** chronic obstructive pulmonary disease, diseases – (**chronic liver d.,** pulmonary d.), **malnutrition,** nephrosis, **hepatic injury,** syndrome – (**neonatal respiratory distress sy, nephrotic sy),** intravascular hemolysis, **hemorrhagic shock,** large hematomas, **obstructive jaundice, portal hypertension**

Interfering Factors: newborn at birth

Analyte	Age/Gender	Reference Range	SI Units	Note
Alpha-1-Anti-Trypsin (AAT)		0.9–2.0	g/l	
Trypsin-inhibitory capacity (Pi)		1.4–2.4	kIU/l	
phenotype		PiMM		

Alpha-1-Antitrypsin Phenotyping

(syn: AAT phenotype, Pi Phenotype, A1A phenotyping). Over 75 alleles are described. Biosynthesis of AAT is controlled at the Pi locus by a pair of genes. There is codominant expression. The phenotype is "Pi" for protease inhibitor, Z and S are mutant proteins. PiMM phenotype is normal, PiMZ is heterozygous, intermediate deficient and PiZZ is homozygous, severely deficient. The age of occurrence of emphysema varies with the type of deficiency, ZZ being most severe, ZS less severe, and SS least severe. Individuals with AAT deficiency have PAS-positive diastase-negative granules accumulated in the periportal hepatocytes. AAT serves to counter the effects of several serine proteases including elastase and trypsin.

Test Purpose. Definitive analysis of hereditary alpha-1-antitrypsin deficiency, which is associated with chronic obstructive pulmonary disease (panacinar emphysema), hepatic cirrhosis and hepatoma.

Anti-Tubulin Antibodies

Patients with IgM and IgG anti-tubulin antibodies often have CIDP-like syndromes (chronic inflammatory demyelinating polyneuropathy) with some asymmetry by history or on examination.

Increased Values – positive
CIDP-like syndromes, Leber's hereditary optic neuropathy

Anti-Typhoid Antibodies

(syn: typhoid antibodies) False positive and negative results are common. Increased titres are consistent with infection, the carrier state or immunisation. Culture is the definitive method for diagnosis of Salmonella typhi or Salmonella paratyphi infection. Antibodies to Vi antigen have been used for epidemiological purposes.

Test Purpose. 1) to support the diagnosis of enteric fever if cultures are negative, 2) to investigate pyrexia of unknown origin.

Increased Values – positive
sallmonelosis

Anti-Varicella-Zoster Virus Antibodies IgG and IgM

(anti-VZV) Varicella and herpes zoster are two main clinical infection manifestations by varicella-zoster virus. It is probably latent virus reactivation in special ganglia from primary child age infection than reinfection. In the rare case where the diagnosis is not clear from clinical findings and virus detection has not been successful, a positive antibody result indicates previous varicella infection and likely immunity. A four-fold rise in titre over a 2–4 weeks period supports the diagnosis of acute varicella infection.

Test Purpose. 1) skin lesion differential diagnosis in herpes zoster, 2) congenital infection evidence, 3) immunodefence assessment in high-risk patients exposed to varicella-zoster virus, 4) immunoglobulin varicella-zoster potential carrier screening.

Increased Values – positive
herpes zoster virus infections

Apolipoproteins

(Apo, syn: apoproteins) Apolipoproteins have been shown to have a significant role in lipo-protein and lipid metabolism, as well as in structural lipoproteins formations. Genetic poly-morphisms and variations have clinical significance. In the case of Apo E there are "athero-genic" alleles epsilon-2 and epsilon-4, in the case of Apo B it is polymorphism EcoRI and XbaI. Apo A: highest levels are present at 8 PM, lowest at 6 AM. Day-to-day variation is 7%. Apo B: day-to-day variation is 10%.

■ **Apo A** (Apo A-I, Apo A-II, Apo A-IV, Apo (a)) are the major components of HDL-C (60 to 70%), HDL-C are associated with the decreased risk of coronary heart disease. Decreased Apo A levels have a high atherogenic potential, mainly in coronary heart dis-ease and brain atherosclerosis. LCAT is activated by Apo A-I (promotes breakdown of cholesterol-containing lipoproteins) and inhibited by Apo A-II. LCAT is involved in the transport of cholesterol from peripheral tissues to the liver, where it is degraded. Apo A-I has been suggested as a better discrimination of coronary artery disease than HDL. Its levels also correlate with survival rates or risk factors for patients with myocardial infarction and peripheral vascular disease. Apo A-I is involved in lipid efflux, it is syn-thesized in the liver and intestine. Apo A-II is involved in lipid transport. Apo A-IV is involved in chylomicrons and TAG transport. It is synthesized in the intestine. Apo (a) as a Lp(a) part has a genetic polymorphism, it occurs at least in 6 isomorphs and other variants. Individual phenotypes are associated with certain Lp(a) levels.

■ **Apo B** (Apo B-48, Apo B-100) belong to LDL-C and chylomicrons remnants. They are associated with an increased risk of atherogenesis. Apo B-100 is synthesized in the liver, is the major Apo B protein in fasting plasma specimens, and is found in both LDL-C and VLDL-C. Apo B-100 serves as a receptor for uptake of these particles by target cells. It is involved in lipid transport. Apo B-48 found in chylomicrons is synthesized in the intes-tinal jejunum. It is involved in chylomicrons transport. Apo B synthesis and incorpora-tion into chylomicrons and VLDL-C is essential to the formation and release of these lipoproteins into the plasma.

■ **Apo C** (Apo C-I, Apo C-II, Apo C-III) has been found in all lipoproteins. Apo C-I and Apo C-II are activators (cofactors) for LCAT and lipoprotein lipase (LPL), which are synthe-sized in the liver. Apo C-II inhibits VLDL-C and chylomicrons binding to hepatic recep-tors, thereby targeting them for extrahepatic clearance. Apo C-III is thought to have a role in triacylglycerol hydrolysis, possibly as an inhibitor of lipoprotein lipase. Apo C from HDL-C is transferred to the newly secreted chylomicrons and VLDL-C, whereas chylomicron and VLDL-C hydrolysis results in movement of apolipoproteins, (especially C-II), from these lipoproteins to HDL-C.

■ **Apo D** – it is suggested, that Apo D may function as a transfer protein, assisting in the movement of cholesterol esters and triacylglycerols between the lipoprotein species, especially from VLDL-C to HDL-C and vice versa.

■ **Apo E** – is coded with 3 alleles epsilon (2, 3 and 4). It creates 6 E phenotypes (2/2, 3/2, 4/2, 4/4, 4/3 and 3/3). There exist also rare minor variants. Apo E play a significant role in lipoprotein metabolism (catabolism), in detection and uptake of chylomicron remnants, as well as IDL-C and VLDL-C remnants by the specific receptors on hepatic/extrahepatic cellular membranes. Apo E initially enters the plasma as part of nascent HDL-C. Under the influence of LCAT, HDL-C accumulates cholesterol, Apo E is rapidly transferred to VLDL-C and chylomicrons, where Apo E remains and the lipoprotein is catabolized to IDL-C by the lipoprotein lipase system. Apo E may exert a significant role in atherogen-esis, because of the high affinity of Apo E for macrophages. Apo E has the important paracrine, endocrine-like and immunological functions. Apo E is synthesized in the liver. Apo E genotyping is done in patients with type III hyperlipidemia. It may be used to identify some patients at risk of developing Alzheimer's disease, but the ethical implications of such testing remain controversial.

Increased Values Apo A
HDL-hyperlipoproteinemia (Apo A-I, Apo A-II), **familial hyper-alpha-lipoproteinemia** (Apo A-I, Apo A-II), chylomicron-hyperlipoproteinemia (Apo A-IV), pregnancy (Apo A-I, Apo (a)), postprandial lipemia (Apo A-IV), acute myocardial infarction (Apo (a))

Increased Values Apo B
angina pectoris (Apo B-100), anorexia nervosa, **atherosclerosis** (Apo B-100), cigarette smoking (Apo B-100), diabetes mellitus, familial combined hyperlipoproteinemia (Apo B-100), dysglobulinemia, infantile hypercalcemia, hyperlipoproteinemia – (type I, IIa, IIb, IV and V, chylomicron h., LDL h., VLDL h.) (Apo B-48, Apo B-100), hemodialysis (Apo B-100), hypothyroidism, **coronary artery disease** (Apo B-100), hepatic diseases, hepatic obstruction, biliary obstruction (Apo B-100), porphyrias, sphingolipodystrophies, emotional stress, syndrome – (Cushing's sy, nephrotic sy – Apo B-100, Warner's sy), **pregnancy** (Apo B-100), renal failure, myocardial infarction (Apo B-100), acquired hyperlipidemia (Apo B-100), apoprotein E deficiency (Apo B-48)

Increased Values Apo C
angina pectoris (Apo C-II), myocardial infarction (Apo C-II), hyperlipoproteinemia – (type I, III, IV, V) (Apo C-I, Apo C-II), hyperlipoproteinemia – (type III, IV, V) (Apo C-III)

Increased Values Apo E
IDL-hyperlipoproteinemia (Apo E-II), hyperlipoproteinemia – (types I, III, IV, V), pregnancy, multiple sclerosis (remission), cholestasis
   Interfering Factors: Apo A-I – (alcohol consumption, physical exercise, weight reduction in overweight individuals), Apo A-II – (alcohol consumption), Apo B – (alcohol abuse, high saturated fat and high cholesterol diets), medicaments (Apo A-I) – (carbamazepine, clofibrate, estrogens, ethanol, lovastatin, niacin, oral contraceptives, phenobarbital, phenytoin, pravastatin, progesterone, simvastatin), medicaments (Apo B) – (androgens, beta-blockers, catecholamines, cyclosporine, diuretics, etretinate, glucocorticoids, isotretinoin, progestins), medicaments (Apo E) – (dexamethasone)

Decreased Values Apo A
abetalipoproteinemia (Apo A-I, Apo A-IV), **alpha-lipoproteins deficiency** (Tangier disease, Apo A-I, Apo A-II), familial lecithin-cholesterol acyltransferase deficiency (Apo A-I), uncontrolled diabetes mellitus (Apo A-I), infectious diseases (Apo A-I), HDL-hypolipoproteinemia (Apo A-I, Apo A-II), **hypo-alpha-lipoproteinemia** (Apo A-I), cholestasis (Apo A-I, Apo A-II), coronary artery disease (Apo A-I), hepatocellular disorders (Apo A-I), nephrotic sy (Apo A-I), chronic renal failure (Apo A-I), type I and V hyperlipoproteinemia (Apo A-I), hemodialysis (Apo A-I), cigarette smoking (Apo A-II), acute hepatitis (Apo A-IV), chronic pancreatitis (Apo A-IV), malabsorption (Apo A-IV), obstructive jaundice (Apo A-IV), total parenteral nutrition (Apo A-IV)

Decreased Values Apo B
chronic anemias, lecithin-cholesterol acyltransferase deficiency, uncontrolled diabetes mellitus, severe hepatocellular dysfunction, hyperthyroidism, apo-/hypobetalipoproteinemia (Apo B-48, Apo B-100), LDL-hypolipoproteinemia, diseases – (inflammatory joint d.,

chronic pulmonary d.), infectious diseases (Apo B-100), intestinal malabsorption (Apo B-48), malnutrition, liver diseases (Apo B-48, Apo B-100), exercise (Apo B-100), plasmocytoma, severe burns, acute stress, Reye's sy, hyperlipoproteinemia type I (Apo B-100)

Decreased Values Apo C
lipoprotein lipase co-factor deficiency (Apo C-II), hypertriacylglycerolemia (Apo C-II), HDL-hypolipoproteinemia (Apo C-III), **familial apoprotein C-II deficiency**, Tangier disease (Apo C-I, Apo C-II, Apo C-III), hypo-alpha-lipoproteinemia (Apo C-II), nephrotic syndrome (Apo C-II), combined Apo C-III and Apo A-I hereditary deficiency

Decreased Values Apo E
IDL-hyperlipoproteinemia (Apo E-III, Apo E-IV)

Interfering Factors: Apo A-I – (diets high in carbohydrates or polyunsaturated fat, smoking), Apo B – (high polyunsaturated fatty acid and low cholesterol diets, postmenopausal women), medicaments (Apo A-I) – (androgens, beta-blockers, cyclosporine, diuretics, glucocorticoids, probucol, progestins), medicaments (Apo (a)) – (anabolic steroids, neomycin, nicotinic acid), medicaments (Apo B) – (cholestyramine, clofibrate, estrogens, lovastatin, neomycin, niacin, pindolol, pravastatin, probucol, simvastatin, thyroxine), medicaments (Apo E) – (ACTH)

Analyte	Age/Gender	Reference Range	SI Units	Note
Apolipoprotein A-I				
	Children	1.20–1.76	g/l	
	F	1.15–1.98	g/l	
	M	0.95–1.76	g/l	
	F	1.20–2.20	g/l	See ref.
	M	1.10–2.00	g/l	ranges note
Apolipoprotein A-II		300–500	mg/l	
Apolipoprotein A-IV		130–230	mg/l	
Apolipoprotein B	F	0.63–1.47	g/l	
	M	0.70–1.60	g/l	
	F	0.60–1.25	g/l	See ref.
	M	0.55–1.35	g/l	ranges note
Apolipoprotein				
C-I		30–110	mg/l	
C-II		10–70	mg/l	
C-III		30–230	mg/l	
Apolipoprotein D		<100	mg/l	
Apolipoprotein E		20–60	mg/l	

Arginine

(Arg) Non-essential amino acid produced by the hydrolysis/digestion of proteins. Involved in metabolism of creatine and ornithine.

Increased Values – hyperargininemia
argininemia, hyperlysinemia

Decreased Values – hypoargininemia
rheumatoid arthritis, following abdominal surgery (2–3 days), **sepsis**, chronic renal failure

Argininosuccinate Lyase

(ASAL, syn: argininosuccinase) A lyase enzyme that catalyzes the cleavage of argininosuccinate to form fumarate and arginine. The reaction is part of the urea cycle in the liver. ASAL is more sensitive than ALT and AST in detecting hepatocellular diseases.

Increased Values
hepatic cirrhosis, diabetes mellitus, gastrectomy, hepatitis – (**toxic h., acute viral h.**), cholecystectomy, diseases – (pulmonary d., d. with secondary hepatic involvement), **liver metastases,** tumors, congestive cardiac failure

Decreased Values
genetic deficiency of ASAL, **mentally deficient patients with argininosuccinic aciduria**

Arsenic

(As) A non-metallic element, arsenic is found in house and garden pesticides. It occurs naturally in the environment and in food. As^{3+} is more toxic than As^{5+}. Industrial exposure proceeds from brass, bronze, ceramics, dye, wood products, glass, semi-conductors and paint manufacturing. Trivalent compounds are most toxic, while marine organoarsenicals are essentially non-toxic. Arsenic can be concentrated in the natural environment leading to localised water and soil hazards. Arsenic absorption from the gastrointestinal tract is related to compound water solubility. Marine organo-arsenicals are readily absorbed and excreted over a period of days. Significant absorption of arsenic aerosols and fumes occurs directly from the lungs. More than 90% of an injected dose of arsenic is cleared from the blood within a few hours. Circulating arsenic is able to cross the placenta. Target organs include skin, hair, nails, kidney and liver. Inorganic arsenicals are rapidly methylated and excreted to the urine. Arsenic is examined in serum, urine, hair and nails.

Increased Values
arsenic exposure, arsenic poisoning, basal cell carcinoma

Arylsulfatase A

(ARS-A) Materials: leukocytes, fibroblasts, uzine
Test Purpose. 1) to aid in diagnosis of cancer (bladder, colorectal, granulocytic leukemia), 2) to aid in diagnosis of metachromatic leukodystrophy.

Increased Values
tumors – (**bladder t., colorectal t., myeloid leukemia**)

Decreased Values
metachromatic leukodystrophy

Aspartate Aminotransferase

(AST, syn: serum glutamic-oxaloacetic transaminase – SGOT, serum glutamate oxaloacetate transaminase, glutamic-oxaloacetic transaminase – GOT).

Occurrence. Cytoplasm – decreasing concentrations: in the heart, liver, skeletal muscle, kidney, brain, pancreas, spleen, lungs. AST is located in the microsomal and mitochondrial (40% of activity) portions of the hepatic cell. Cytosol fraction shows about 60% of activity.

Function. Intracellular enzyme involved in amino acid/carbohydrate metabolism. AST is released into the blood following injury/death of cells directly related to quantities. Transfers amino-group from asparagine acid to alpha-ketoglutaric acid $\rightarrow$ glutamic acid and oxaloacetic acid. Measuring AST activity is useful for identifying liver inflammation and necrosis.

Isoenzymes. 1) mitochondrial (normally not detectable in blood), 2) microsomal.

Test Purpose. 1) to aid detection and differential diagnosis of acute hepatic disease/damage, 2) to monitor patient progress and prognosis in cardiac and hepatic diseases, 3) to aid in diagnosing myocardial infarction correlated to creatine kinase and lactate dehydrogenase levels, 4) to aid in myopathies diagnosis, 5) to aid in differential diagnosis of hepatobiliary system and pancreatic diseases.

Increased Values

acute hypotension, liver abscess, acute hypoxia, **acute pancreatitis**, AIDS, aspergillosis – (allergic pulmonary a., invasive a.), amyloidosis, anemia – (**hemolytic a., acute hemolytic a.**, thalassemia minor, thalassemia major, hemolytic microangiopathic a., G6PD deficiency hemolytic a., hereditary spherocytic hemolytic a., pyruvate kinase deficiency hemolytic a., acquired infectious hemolytic a.), angina pectoris, giant cell arteritis, primary biliary atresia, spinal muscular atrophy, **cardiac catheterization/angiography/angioplasty**, babesiosis, brucellosis, benign familial recurrent cholestasis, **cirrhosis of the liver**, conditions – (septic c.), **congestive hepatomegalia**, coronary insufficiency, cystic fibrosis, **dermatomyositis**, disease – (Forbes' d., Brill-Zinsser d., Gaucher's d., Caroli's d., myxedema heart d., von Gierke's d., **Wilson's d., legionnaire's d.**, Lyme d., adult Still's d., graft-versus-host d., Niemann-Pick d., rheumatic heart d., Whipple's d.), diseases – (**acute renal d., liver d.**, primary muscle d.), dissecting aneurysm of aorta, **eclampsia**, embolism – (pulmonary e., paradoxical e.), echinococcosis, encephalitis – (echo-encephalitis, cytomegalovirus e., e. lethargica, Japanese e. B), encephalopathy, Wernicke's encephalopathy, encephalomyelitis, endocarditis, Epstein-Barr virus infection, ethanol, congenital hepatic fibrosis, failure – (**cardiac f.**, acute renal f.), fever – (Dengue f., rheumatic f., Q f., Lassa f., yellow f., Rocky Mountain spotted f.), fascioliasis, gangrene – (muscular g., diabetic g., gas g., scrotum g.), glycogen storage disease (type V, VII), Wegener's granulomatosis, granulomas, Hantavirus infection, heat stroke/exhaustion, hemochromatosis – (secondary h., idiopathic h.), hemolysis, hemophilia, coma – (**hepatic c.**, myxedema c.), hepatic ischemia, hepatic metastases, hepatitis – (**alcoholic h.**, autoimmune h., acute h. type B, acute h. type C, fulminant h., **chronic h., acute viral h.**), malignant histiocytosis, histoplasmosis, **hypothyroidism**, primary sclerosing cholangitis, i.m. injections, infarction – (**cerebral i.**, liver i., renal i., **pulmonary i., intestinal i.**), **infective mononucleosis**, influenza, injury/trauma – (**liver i., skeletal muscle i.**, brain i., **crush i.**, local irradiation i.), intestinal obstruction, cretinism – (endemic c., goitrous c.), cryoglobulinemia, cryptococcosis, intracranial hemorrhage, jaundice – (cholestatic j., **obstructive j.**), lactate acidosis, leprosy, leptospirosis, leukemia – (basophilic l., eosinophilic l., acute lymphoblastic l., monoblastic l, acute myeloblastic l., chronic myelocytic l., plasma cell l., stem cell l., megakaryocytic l., acute monocytic l., promyelocytic l.), angioimmunoblastic lymphadenopathy, **malignant hyperthermia**, passive liver congestion, malaria, malnutrition, primary amebic meningoencephalitis, mucopolysaccharidosis (type II), **multiple trauma**, mycosis fungoides, **myocardial infarction** (increase at 6–24 hours, peaking at 24–72 hours, decrease 3–7 days), myocarditis – (**bacterial m., metabolic m., rheumatic m., viral m.**), **myodystrophy, myositis**, myotonia – (atrophic m., congenital m.), necrosis – (pancreatic n., **hepatic n.**), radiation nephritis, obesity, ornithosis, acute pancreatitis, paramyotonia congenita, **paroxysmal myoglobinuria**, inclusion body myositis, perihepatitis, pericardial effusion, pericarditis – (constrictive p., purulent p., tuberculous p.), pneumonia – (pneumococcal p.), traumatic pneumocephalus, poisoning by – (aflatoxin, antimony, arsenic, cadmium, carbon tetrachloride, DDT, phosphorus, herbicides, methyl bromide, **mushrooms**, copper, naphthalene, nitrobenzene, lead, solvents – trichlorethylene, chromates, vinyl chloride, opioids, iron), acute fatty liver of pregnancy, poliomyelitis, polyarteritis nodosa, polymyalgia rheumatica, **polymyositis**, porphyria – (acute intermittent p., p. cutanea tarda), Korsakoff's psychosis, thrombotic thrombocytopenic purpura, pyoderma gangrenosum, **recent convulsions, rhabdomyolysis**, sarcoidosis, **severe burns**, schistosomiasis, shock liver, hemorrhagic shock, skeletal muscle lesion, tropical sprue, surgery – (musculoskeletal s., intestinal s., **cardiac s.**), postcardiotomy syndrome, syphilis, systemic lupus erythematosus, tetanus, thrombosis – (cerebral t., renal vein t., portal vein t., pulmonary artery t.), **toxic hepatic lesions**, syndrome – (toxic shock sy, eosinophilia–myalgia sy, septic shock sy, Dubin-Johnson sy, Kawasaki's sy, Reye's sy, HELLP sy, Sézary sy, vena cava inferior obstruction sy, postcholecystectomy sy), toxoplasmosis, trichinosis, tuberculosis, tularemia, tumors – (**hepatic t.**, lung t., Hodgkin's disease, pancreas t., male breast t., melanoma, stomach t., parathyroid t., gallbladder t., cerebral t., Burkitt's lymphoma), thyroiditis – (Hashimoto's t., acute suppurative t., chronic fibrous t.), typhoid fever, endemic typhus, vasculitis – (nodular v., cerebral v.), inborn error of amino acid metabolism, acute liver failure, liver vein occlusion

Interfering Factors: hemolysis, lipemia, exercise, medicaments – (abacavir, acarbose, acetaminophen, acetylsalicylic acid, aciclovir, ajmaline, aldesleukin, allopurinol, alosetron, aminoglutethimide, aminoglycosides, aminosalicylic acid, amiodarone, amitriptylin, amlodipine, amoxicillin, amphotericin B, ampicillin, anabolics, anagrelide, androgens, antibiotics, antiepileptics, antihemophilic factor, antihypertensives, aprindine, ardeparin, argatroban, asparaginase, atenolol, atorvastatin, atovaquone, azapropazone, azathioprine, aztreonam, BCG, benazepril, bexarotene, bicalutamide, bisoprolol, bromfenac, bromocriptine, candesartan, capecitabine, captopril, carbamazepine, carbenicillin, carbidopa, carbimazole, carboplatin, carbutamide, carmustine, cefalotin, cefamandole, cefazolin, cefepime, cefoperazone, cefoxitin, ceftizoxime, celecoxib, cephalexin, cephalosporins, cephradine, cerivastatin, chenodeoxycholic acid, chenodiol, chlorambucil, chlorpromazine, chloramphenicol, chlorzoxazone, cholinergic agents, cimetidine, cisplatin, clarithromycin, clindamycin, clofazimine, clofibrate, clometacin, clomiphene, clotrimazol, cloxacillin, codeine, cortisone, coumarin-type anticoagulants, cyclofenil, cyclophosphamide, cycloserine, cyclosporine, cytarabine, dacarbazine, dactinomycin, danazol, dantrolene, dapsone, delavirdine, demeclocycline, denileukin, desmopressin, dexmedetomidine, diazepam, diclofenac, dicoumarol, dicloxacillin, didanosine, dienestrol, diethylstilbestrol, diflunisal, digitalis, dihydralazine, diltiazem, disopyramide, disulfiram, docetaxel, dofetilide, dolasetron, doxorubicin, doxycycline, efavirenz, enalapril, enflurane, eprosartan, erythromycin, estradiol, estramustine, estrogens, ethacrynic acid, ethambutol, ethanol, ethinylestradiol, ethionamide, ethosuximide, ethotoin, etodolac, etoposide, etretinate, felbamate, felodipine, fenofibrate, floxuridine, flucloxacillin, fluconazole, flucytosine, fluoroquinolones, fluphenazine, flurazepam, flurbiprofen, flutamide, fluvastatin, fluvoxamine, fomivirsen, fosinopril, fosphenytoin, ganciclovir, gemcitabine, gemtuzumab, glibenclamide, gold salts, granisetron, griseofulvin, haloperidol, halothane, heparin, hydralazine, hydrochlorothiazide, hydrocodone, ibuprofen, idarubicin, imipramine, inamrinone, indomethacin, infliximab, interferon, interleukin 2,

irinotecan, isocarboxazid, isoflurane, isoniazid, isotretinoin, itraconazole, ketamine, ketoconazole, ketoprofen, ketorolac, labetalol, lamivudine, lansoprazole, latamoxef, leflunomide, levamisole, levodopa, levonorgestrel, lincomycin, linezolid, loracarbef, losartan,
lovastatin, mebendazole, meclofenamate, medroxyprogesterone, mefloquine, megestrol,
meloxicam, menotropins, mephenytoin, mercaptopurine, meropenem, mesalamine, mestranol, metandienone, metaxalone, methandriol, methimazole, methotrexate, methoxyflurane, methyldopa, methyltestosterone, metolazone, metoprolol, mexiletine, mezlocillin, morphine, moxifloxacin, nabumetone, nafcillin, naltrexone, nandrolone, naproxen,
narcotics, nefazodone, nevirapine, nicotinic acid, nifedipine, nilutamide, nisoldipine,
nitrofurantoin, nizatidine, nomifensine, norethindrone, norethisterone, norethynodrel,
norgestrel, olanzapine, olsalazine, omeprazole, ondansetron, opiates, oral contraceptives,
oxacillin, oxaprozin, oxazepam, oxymetholone, oxyphenbutazone, paclitaxel, palivizumab, pantoprazole, papaverine, paracetamol, paramethadione, pemoline, penicillamine,
penicillins, pentamidine, pentosan, pentostatin, perazine, perindopril, phenazopyridine, phenelzine, phenobarbital, phenothiazines, phenylbutazone, phenytoin, pindolol,
piperacillin, pirenzepine, piroxicam, plicamycin, prasterone, pravastatin, probenecid,
probucol, procainamide, prochlorperazine, progesterone, promazine, propoxyphene,
propranolol, propylthiouracil, protriptyline, pyrazinamide, pyridoxine, quetiapine, quinacrine, quinidine, quinine, rabeprazole, ranitidine, retinol, rifabutin, rifampicin, rifapentine, riluzole, ritodrine, ritonavir, rofecoxib, salicylates, sertraline, sibutramine, simvastatin, sotalol, stavudine, stilbol, streptokinase, streptozocin, sulfafurazole, sulfamethoxazole, sulfasalazine, sulfonamides, sulfonylureas, sulindac, suloctidil, tacrine,
tamoxifen, terbinafine, testosterone, tetracycline, thiabendazole, thiamazole, thioguanine, thiopental, thioridazine, thiothixene, ticarcillin, ticlopidine, timolol, tizanidine,
tobramycin, tocopherol, tolazamide, tolbutamide, tolcapone, tolmetin, toremifene, trandolapril, tranylcypromine, tretinoin, trimethoprim, trimetrexate, troglitazone, trovafloxacin, valerian, valproic acid, valsartan, verapamil, verteporfin, warfarin, zafirlukast,
zalcitabine, zidovudine, zileuton, zimeldine, zonisamide)

Decreased Values

alcoholic liver disease, azotemia, **beriberi, chronic hemodialysis**, diabetes mellitus, **diabetic
ketoacidosis**, intoxication by – (fluorides, formaldehyde, cyanide), malnutrition, **pregnancy**
(gravidity, graviditas), **pyridoxine deficiency** (vitamin B_6), **pyridoxal phosphate deficiency**,
renal insufficiency, **severe/terminal stages of liver diseases, uremia**
  Interfering Factors: medicaments – (isoniazid, ascorbic acid, leucine, metronidazole,
  penicillamine, oral contraceptives, tartrate)

Analyte	Age/Gender	Reference Range	SI Units	Note
Aspartate Amino-transferase (AST)	1 d	1.82	µkat/l	
	2–5 d	<1.62	µkat/l	
	6 d–6 m	<1.28	µkat/l	
Glutamate oxaloacetic transaminase (GOT)	7–12 m	<1.37	µkat/l	
	1–3 y	<0.80	µkat/l	
	4–6 y	<0.60	µkat/l	
	7–12 y	<0.78	µkat/l	
	13–17 y F	<0.42	µkat/l	
	13–17 y M	<0.48	µkat/l	
	Adults F	<0.52	µkat/l	
	Adults M	<0.62	µkat/l	

Aspergillus Precipitins

Strong precipitin bands suggest aspergillosis. Weak bands suggest early infection or hypersensitivity pneumonitis.
Test Purpose. To investigate suspected aspergillosis in patients with asthma.

Increased Values – positive
allergic bronchopulmonary aspergillosis, aspergilloma, allergic exogenous alveolitis

AST/ALT Ratio

Test Purpose. To help in differential diagnosis of diseases of hepatobiliary system and pancreas.

Increased Values – ratio >1.0
drug hepatotoxicity, alcoholic hepatitis, alcoholic cirrhosis, chronic hepatitis, liver congestion, metastatic tumors of the liver, intrahepatic cholestasis, hepatocellular carcinoma

Decreased Values – ratio < 1.0
acute hepatitis due to – (virus, drugs, toxins), infectious mononucleosis, extrahepatic cholestasis

Atrial Natriuretic Peptide

(ANP, syn: atrionatriuretic peptide, atrial natriuretic factor – ANF, atriopeptin, atrial natriuretic hormone – ANH) ANP is a member of the natriuretic peptide family of proteins. Other members are BNP (brain natriuretic peptide) and CNP (C-type natriuretic peptide).
Production. ANP is an endogenous antihypertensive agent secreted from cardiac atria. Found also in the central nervous system and the kidney. The release of ANP is stimulated by adrenaline, ADH, acetylcholine. Specific receptors for ANP have been found in blood vessels, kidney, in the thymic cortex, medulla, splenic white pulp and on astrocytes.
Function. ANP is an extremely potent natriuretic agent and vasodilator, which rapidly produces diuresis and increases the glomerular filtration rate. Regulates extracellular fluid volume, blood pressure, sodium metabolism. Other functions: blocks aldosterone and renin secretion, inhibits angiotensin II and vasopressin action, inhibits smooth muscle contraction. Apart from its pharmacological activities ANP also displays activities of cytokines. It functions as a negative growth factor for vascular smooth muscle cells and endothelial cells and also has significant antiproliferative effects on astrocytes. ANP is also a suppressor of chondrocyte proliferation. It also appears to enhance natural killer cell activity and has neuromodulatory effects. Day-to-day concentration variation is 10–20%.
Test Purpose. 1) to confirm congestive heart failure, 2) to identify asymptomatic cardiac volume overload.

Increased Values
ethanol, starvation, **cardiovascular diseases with elevated cardiac filling pressure, atrial pacing, asymptomatic cardiac volume overload, paroxysmal atrial tachycardia,** pregnancy, failure – (renal f., **congestive heart f.**)

Interfering Factors: supine position, medicaments – (catecholamines, glucocorticoids, mineralocorticoids)

Decreased Values
volume depletion
Interfering Factors: medicaments – (ACE inhibitors)

Atrial Natriuretic Peptide (B-Type)

(ANP-B) Atrial natriuretic peptide (ANP – secreted from cardiac atria) and B-type of natriuretic peptide (BNP – brain natriuretic peptide, secreted from cardiac ventricles) have similar properties. BNP concentration is increasing both in atria and ventricles during heart failure. BNP is more sensitive and specific indicator of cardiac ventricles overload and of left ventricle end-diastolic pressure increase in comparison to other natriuretic peptides. Physiologically ANP/BNP concentration ratio is more than 1.

Test Purpose. 1) to confirm congestive heart failure, 2) to identify asymptomatic cardiac volume overload, 3) to help to identify ventricular dysfunction after myocardial infarction, 4) to help in diagnosis of hypertrophic obstructive cardiomyopathy and dilation cardiomyopathy, 5) to help in diagnosis of left heart ventricle hypertrophy.

Increased Values
cor pulmonale, chronic obstructive pulmonary disease, conditions with cardiac volume overload, ventricular dysfunction after myocardial infarction, diseases – (renal d., liver d.), failure – (renal f., liver f., congestive heart f.), cardiovascular diseases with elevated cardiac filling pressure

Analyte	Age/Gender	Reference Range	SI Units	Note
Brain Natriuretic Peptide (BNP)		1.5–9.0	pmol/l	

Autoantibodies

acetylcholine receptor, adrenal, antineutrophil cytoplasmic, antinuclear, cardiolipin, centromere, DNA, endomysial, extractable nuclear antigen, gliadin, glomerular basement membrane, glutamic acid decarboxylase, histone, intrinsic factor, islet cell, Jo-1, liver/kidney microsomal, lymphocytotoxic, mitochondrial, myocardial, ovarian, parathyroid, parietal cell, pemphigoid, pemphigus, Purkinje cell, Ra 33, reticulin, rheumatoid factor, salivary duct, skeletal muscle, smooth muscle, sperm, thyroid, TSH receptor

IA2 Autoantibodies

(syn: IA2 antibodies, ICA512 autoantibodies, tyrosine phosphatase autoantibodies) Type 1 diabetes, commonly referred to as insulin-dependent diabetes, is caused by pancreatic beta-cell destruction that leads to an absolute insulin deficiency. The clinical onset of diabetes does not occur until 80 to 90% of these cells have been destroyed. Prior to clinical onset, type 1 diabetes is often characterized by circulating autoantibodies against a variety of islet cell antigens, including tyrosine phosphatase autoantibodies (IA2). The presence of these autoantibodies provides early evidence of autoimmune disease activity, and their measurement can be useful in assisting the physician with the prediction, diagnosis and management of patients with diabetes. Autoantibodies IA2, a tyrosine phosphatase-like protein, are found in 50 to 75% of type 1 diabetics at and prior to disease onset. These autoantibodies are generally more prevalent in younger onset diabetics. Because the risk of diabetes is increaseed with the presence of each additional autoantibody, the positive predictive value of the IA2 antibody test is enhanced when measured in conjuction with antibodies to GAD and insulin.

Increased Values
diabetes mellitus (type 1)

Autocrine Motility Factor

(AMF, syn: autotaxin, tumor autocrine motility factor) AMF is produced constitutively by various melanomas, hepatomas, leukemic cell lines and some metastasizing tumors.
Function. Enhances the directed chemotactic and random (chemokinetic) motility of those cells secreting it. This process is accompanied by an increased generation of pseudopodia and an increased methylation of phospholipids. A study of bladder carcinoma patients has shown that the concentration of urinary AMF correlates with the degree of invasive growth of the tumors.

Barbiturates

Test studies various barbiturates, including phenobarbital, amobarbital, pentobarbital and secobarbital.
Test Purpose. 1) to detect suspected barbiturate toxicity from patient history or clinical observations, 2) to monitor therapeutic barbiturate levels for people with legitimate uses, 3) to detect presence of barbiturates for medical-legal purposes.

Increased Values
barbiturates overdose

Bile acids

(syn: total bile acids)
Production. 1) the primary bile acids – cholic and chenodeoxycholic – are synthesized in the liver by cholesterol catabolism → they are conjugated with glycine and taurine → forming glycocholates and taurocholates before entering the gallbladder for storage, 2) the secondary bile acids are formed by bacterial deconjugation and chemical alteration of the conjugated bile salts → deoxycholic and lithocholic acids. Both primary/secondary bile acids are reabsorbed almost completely from the bowel by passive/active reabsorption into the enterohepatic pathway → where they are reextracted from the blood by hepatocytes → reexcreted by bile. Hepatic bile salt uptake and serum bile salt concentrations are sensitive hepatocellular dysfunction indicators.

Increased Values
biliary atresia, **hepatic cirrhosis,** cystic fibrosis, hepatitis – (acute h., **alcoholic h.,** chronic h., viral h.), primary hepatoma, **cholestasis,** drug induced liver injury, neonatal hepatitis sy
    Interfering Factors: medicaments – (cyclosporine, isoniazid, methotrexate, rifampicin)

Decreased Values
    Interfering Factors: medicaments – (cholestyramine)

Analyte	Age/Gender	Reference Range	SI Units	Note
Bile Acids, Total				
fasting		0.3–2.3	mg/l	
2 hrs after meals		1.8–3.2	mg/l	

Bilirubin

(bil, syn: total, direct + indirect bilirubin).
Production. By the liver reticuloendothelial system. End product of the hemoglobin disintegration, also a by-product of hemolysis. 1) **indirect bilirubin** (indirect reacting bilirubin = free bilirubin = prehepatic = insoluble = unconjugated = nonconjugated bilirubin) from heme of hemoglobin from senescent RBC, bone marrow normoblasts, myoglobin and cytochrome → transported in the plasma bound to albumin in circulation → to the liver (hepatic uptake). 2) **direct bilirubin** (direct reacting bilirubin = conjugated = soluble = posthepatic = bound bilirubin in the liver endoplasmic reticulum) → form bilirubin mono/diglucuronides → excreted into the bile to circulation or in the gut → bacterial flora deconjugate and reduce it to various compounds called 1) stercobilinogens → excreted in the feces and creates brown-colored stool and 2) urobilinogens → undergo oxidation to brown pigment urobilin → fecal excretion. Urobilinogen (UBG) is partially reabsorbed through the intestine → through the portal circulation picked up by the liver → re-excretion in bile. Since UBG is freely water soluble → it can also pass out through the urine if it reaches the kidney. Bilirubin accumulates in the plasma e.g. when liver insufficiency exists, biliary obstruction is present or hemolysis rate is increased → tissue → icterus (jaundice). Direct bilirubin elevation in serum for whatever reason permits water-soluble species to pass into the urine.
Test Purpose. 1) to evaluate hepatobiliary and erythropoietic functions, 2) to aid in a differential diagnosis of jaundice and monitor its progress, 3) to aid diagnosis of biliary obstruction and hemolytic anemia, 4) to determine whether a newborn requires exchange transfusion or phototherapy because of dangerously high unconjugated bilirubin levels (newborn hemolytic disease).

Increased Values – hyperbilirubinemia
anemia – (idiopathic aplastic a., idiopathic autoimmune hemolytic a., secondary aplastic a., **hemolytic a., sickle cell a., pernicious a.**), cirrhosis hepatis, **erythroblastosis fetalis, viral hepatitis,** starvation (1–2 days), **cholangitis,** cholangiocarcinoma, transient familial hyperbilirubinemia in infants, hyperlipidemia, **hyperproduction of the bile,** hepatic encephalopathy, hypothyroidism, **cholelithiasis,** cholestasis – (**extrahepatic ch., intrahepatic ch.**), diseases – (infectious d., gallbladder inflammatory d., **liver d.**), jaundice – (familial nonhemolytic j., **hemolytic j.,** hepatocellular j., **neonatal physiological j.,** obstructive j.), fructose

intolerance, gallstone, **hepatotoxic agents**, malaria, metastases of carcinoma, infectious mononucleosis, **tumours, obstruction of the efferent biliary ways, lesion of the hepatic tissue, transfusion reactions**, prolonged caloric restriction, conditions – (hemolytic c., postoperative c., septic c.), **hepatic steatosis**, syndrome – (**Crigler-Najjar sy, Dubin-Johnson sy**, breast milk jaundice sy), typhoid fever, **resolution of large hematoma**, Epstein-Barr virus infection, cytomegalovirus infection, **Gilberts' disease, congestive heart failure**, hepatic congestion, pulmonary infarction, pulmonary embolism, **thrombotic thrombocytopenic purpura, Wilson's disease**

Interfering Factors: medicaments – (acetalozamide, acetylsalicylic acid, ajmaline, aldesleukin, allopurinol, aminoglutethimide, aminosalicylic acid, amiodarone, amitriptyline, amphotericin B, anabolics, aprindine, ascorbic acid, asparaginase, atenolol, azathioprine, benazepril, benoxaprofen, bisoprolol, busulfan, capecitabine, captopril, carbamazepine, carbidopa, carbimazole, carbutamide, cefalexin, cefazolin, cefoxitin, cephalosporins, chenodeoxycholic acid, chloral hydrate, chlorambucil, chloramphenicol, chlordiazepoxide, chlorpromazine, chlorpropamide, cimetidine, cisplatin, clarithromycin, clindamycin, clofibrate, clometacin, clotrimazole, cloxacillin, corticosteroids, coumarin, cyclofenil, cyclophosphamide, cyclosporine, cytarabine, dalfopristin, dantrolene, dapsone, dextran, dextrose, diazepam, diclofenac, dienestrol, dihydralazine, diphenylhydantoin, disopyramide, disulfiram, docetaxel, dopamine, doxorubicin, drugs causing hemolysis, enalapril, enflurane, erythromycin, estramustine, ethacrynic acid, ethanol, ethotoin, etoposide, flucloxacillin, fluoxymesterone, fluphenazine, flutamide, fosinopril, fructose, gemtuzumab, gentamicin, glibenclamide, gold salts, haloperidol, halothane, hepatotoxic drugs, hydantoines, hydralazine, hydrochlorothiazide, ibuprofen, imipramine, indinavir, indomethacin, interferons, interleukin 2, irbesatran, isoniazid, kava kava, ketoconazole, labetalol, lamivudine, lansoprazole, levodopa, lincomycin, meloxicam, mepacrine, mercaptopurine, metamizole, metandienone, methandriol, methotrexate, methoxyflurane, methyldopa, methyltestosterone, morphine, nandrolone, naproxen, nelfinavir, nevirapine, nicotinic acid, nitrofurantoin, norethisterone, norethynodrel, omeprazole, oral contraceptives, oxacillin, oxazepam, oxymetholone, pantoprazole, papaverine, paracetamol, paramethadione, penicillamine, penicillin, phenazone, phenobarbital, phenothiazines, phenylbutazone, phenytoin, practolol, probenecid, procainamide, prochlorperazine, progesterone, propranolol, propylthiouracil, protionamide, pyrazinamide, quinidine, ranitidine, rifampicin, sorbitol, stilbol, streptozocin, sulfamethoxazole, sulfasalazine, sulfonamides, sulindac, tamoxifen, tetracyclines, thiabendazole, thiamazole, thioguanine, thiopental, thioridazine, thiothixene, ticlopidine, tocopherol, tolazamide, tolbutamide, trazodone, tretinoin, trimethadione, trimethoprim, valproic acid, verapamil, zafirlukast)

Increased Values – conjugated (direct) hyperbilirubinemia

hepatic amyloidosis, **liver abscess**, bile ascites, **biliary atresia, hepatic cirrhosis**, primary biliary cirrhosis, cystic fibrosis, hepatic granulomas, hepatitis – (**alcoholic h., viral h., neonatal h.**, toxic h., **drug related h.**), medicamentous hepatitis/cholestasis – (amphotericin B, cytostatics, phenazopyridine, phenobarbital, phenothiazines, chlorpromazine, carbamazepine, levodopa, methotrexate, nitrofurantoin, oral contraceptives, sulfasalazine, tuberculostatics), cholangitis, cholelithiasis, familial intrahepatic cholestasis, Gaucher's disease, diseases – (**hepatocellular d.**, infectious d.), stasis of the bile – (**intrahepatic s.**, medicamentous s.), severe infectious diseases, right heart ventricle insufficiency, acute intoxication by – (Amanita phalloides, tetrachlormethane), hepatic metastases, tumours of – (pancreas, **liver, gall-bladder**), **hepatocellular lesions**, pyelonephritis, septic conditions, **hepatic steatosis**, syndrome – (Crigler–Najjar sy, **Dubin–Johnson sy, Rotor's sy**), pregnancy, biliary tract obstruction by – (**choledochal cyst**, abdominal mass, annular pancreas), prolonged total parenteral nutrition, neonatal sepsis, intrauterine viral infections, trisomy 18, galactosemia, tyrosinemia, hypermethioninemia, alpha-1-antitrypsin deficiency, neonatal posthemolytic disease, children – (hypopituitarism, hypothyroidism)

> **Interfering Factors:** medicaments – (aminophenol, aminosalicylic acid, amphotericin B, anabolic steroids, ascorbic acid, carbamazepine, chlorpromazine, cytostatics, dextran, epinephrine, ethoxazene, histidine, isoproterenol, levodopa, methotrexate, methyldopa, nitrofurantoin, novobiocin, oral contraceptives, phenazopyridine, phenelzine, phenobarbital, phenothiazines, rifampin, sulfasalazine, tetracycline, theophylline, tuberculostatics, tyrosine)

Increased Values – nonconjugated (indirect, unconjugated) hyperbilirubinemia

autoimmune hemolysis, hepatic abscess, anemia – (**hemolytic a., megaloblastic a.**, pernicious a., sickle-cell a., spherocytosis, thalassemia), **liver cirrhosis**, disseminated intravascular coagulation, **erythroblastosis fetalis**, ecchymoses, erythrocytosis, glucuronyltransferase deficiency/absence, hereditary elliptocytosis, infantile pyknocytosis, **ineffective erythropoiesis**, galactosemia, **hemoglobinopathies, hemolysis, hepatitis,** starvation, **functional hyperbilirubinemia** (Crigler-Najjar sy), hypermethioninemia, hyperthyroidism, hypoperistalsis, **neonatal hypothyroidism, morbus hemolyticus neonatorum,** autoimmune diseases, meconium ileus, hemorrhagic pulmonary infarct, right heart ventricle insufficiency, x-ray contrast agents, **Gilbert's disease,** infectious diseases – (viral i. d, bacterial i. d., protozoal i. d.), **tumors,** Hirschprung's disease, hepatic congestion, **hepatic malignancy,** physiological jaundice in newborns, **breast-milk jaundice,** obstruction – (duodenal o., jejunal o.), polycythemia vera, **hemolytic disorders,** portocaval shunt, postoperatively, pyloric stenosis, congenital erythropoietic porphyria, rubella, toxoplasmosis, syphilis, hepatic steatosis, meconium plug sy, pregnancy, RBC enzyme deficiencies – (G6PD d., pyruvate d., hexokinase d.), **transfusion of old blood, the presence of a large hematoma in trauma,** tyrosinosis, **heart failure**

> **Interfering Factors:** medicaments – (acetylsalicylic acid, chloramphenicol, novobiocin, pregnanediol, rifampicin, steroids, sulfonamides)

Increased Values – conjugated + nonconjugated hyperbilirubinemia

hepatic abscess, liver cirrhosis, **hepatitis,** cholestasis secondary to drugs, lymphoma, hepatic metastases of malignant tumors, right heart ventricle insufficiency, hepatic steatosis, pregnancy

Decreased Values – hypobilirubinemia

anemia

> **Interfering Factors:** medicaments – (aminophenazone, antiepileptics, barbiturates, carbamazepine, clofibrate, corticosteroids, isotretinoin, oral contraceptives, penicillin, phenobarbital, sulfonamides, thioridazine, urea)

Analyte	Age/Gender	Reference Range	SI Units	Note
Bilirubin				
Total bilirubin	1 d	<85.5	µmol/l	
	2 d	<154	µmol/l	
	3–5 d	<205	µmol/l	
	Children	<25.7	µmol/l	
	Adults	<22.2	µmol/l	
Conjugated bilirubin		<5.1	µmol/l	

Delta Bilirubin

Delta bilirubin is bilirubin covalently bound to albumin. Delta bilirubin formation appears to require an active bilirubin conjugating process. As cholestasis improves, delta bilirubin increases in proportion to the total bilirubin because it has a longer half-life and slower clearance than bilirubin.

Increased Values
hemolytic anemia, extra/intrahepatic cholestasis, healthy individuals, neonates with physiologic jaundice, hemolytic conditions, syndrome – (Crigler-Najjar sy, Gilbert's sy)

Biotin

(syn: vitamin H, coenzyme R, protective factor X) Water-soluble monocarboxylic acid is considered to be a part of the vitamin B-complex.
Function. Biotin is a prosthetic group of carboxylases (co-factor for carboxylation): acetyl-coenzyme A, propionyl-CoA, pyruvate. Important in fatty acid biosynthesis, propionic acid oxidation, leucine metabolism and gluconeogenesis.

Decreased Values – hypobiotinemia
biotin metabolism inborn errors – (propionic acidemia, beta-methylcrotonylglycinuria), long-term parenteral nutrition

Bombesin

(syn: gastrin releasing peptide – GRP) Gastrointestinal tract hormone belonging to cytokines. Bombesin-like peptides are produced by neurons of the central and peripheral nervous system, and many other neuroendocrine cell types. Bombesin-like peptides are grouped into three families (bombesin family, ranatensin family and the phyllolitorin family). The factors known as neuromedins are members of the ranatensin subfamily.
Function. Stimulates release of various hormones, neuropeptides and pancreatic enzymes, smooth muscle contractions. Involved in cardiovascular system and renal functions. GRP functions as mitogen in many tissues; it is produced in high concentration in small-cellular lung cancer. In human mammary carcinomas it induces the synthesis of endothelins which act on stromal cells of the mammary gland in a paracrine manner. Bombesin is synthesized after electric stimulation of nerve cells and induces the release of gastrin and cholecystokinin in the intestines and the pancreas. It has been observed that bombesin can be used to increase the sensitivity of cisplatin-sensitive and resistant variants of human ovarian carcinoma cell lines to cisplatin.

Bone Morphogenetic Proteins

(BMP) BMP is the generic name of a family of proteins (BMP-1 through BMP-15), identified originally in extracts of demineralized bone that were capable of inducing bone formation at ectopic sites. Also can be isolated from osteosarcoma cells. They have been shown also to be expressed in a variety of epithelial and mesenchymal tissues in the embryo. BMPs are proteins which act to induce the differentiation of mesenchymaltype cells into chondrocytes and osteoblasts before initiating bone formation. They promote the differentiation of cartilage- and bone-forming cells near sites of fractures but also at ectopic locations.

Bradykinin

Bradykinin is the final product of the kinin system and is split from a serum alpha-2-globulin precursor by the kallikreins and also by trypsin or plasmin. Bradykinin reduces blood pressure by dilating blood vessels. In bronchial smooth muscles and also in the intestines and the uterus bradykinin leads to muscle contraction. It is also one of the most potent known substances inducing pain. Bradykinin stimulates the synthesis of prostaglandins and this activity is potentiated by haptoglobin. It acts on small-cell lung cancers in a paracrine manner. It inhibits the growth of mammary stromal cells. Bradykinin induces the synthesis of IL-6 and synergizes with IL-1 in the IL-1-induced resorption of bones.

Bronchodilators

Test Purpose. 1) to determine most-effective dose of drugs used to dilate bronchial ways, 2) to check toxicity of bronchodilators suspected from patient history or clinical observations.

Increased Values
bronchodilators overdose

Cadmium

(Cd) Trace metal element cadmium is used in alloys, pigments and batteries. Cadmium is present as a contaminant in some fertilisers. The metal and its soluble compounds are toxic. Normal exposure to cadmium is through air and food. The release of fumes can compromise the surrounding environment. Levels in foods such as liver and kidney from the mature mammals, and oysters can be high. Cigarettes contain significant amounts of Cd that is available for absorption. Its absorption is dependent upon the particle size and water solubility of the compound. Absorbed cadmium is carried to the liver as an albumin complex. In the liver cadmium induces the production of metallothionine. The kidneys absorb the cadmiummetallothionine complex after it is released from the liver and account for up to half the body burden of cadmium. The majority of Cd is excreted through urine or via the loss of cadmium containing intestinal mucosal cells. Cadmium accumulates continuously throughout an individuals life. Cadmium (Cd) accumulates in tissue, concentrating primarily in the kidneys and liver. More than 95% of blood Cd is in the erythrocytes.
Test Purpose. 1) Cd toxicity proof in industry exposure (vapours), 2) Cd toxicity proof in non-industry exposure (e.g. food and low pH fluids storage in metal can).

Increased Values
industrial exposure – (alloy i., battery i.), smoking

Calcitonin

(CT, syn: parathyroidal polypeptide, thyrocalcitonin – TCT, human calcitonin – hCT) Calcitonin gene codes also other peptide (calcitonin gene-related peptide, CGRP). As katacalcin (PDN 21) is known other peptide, which is placed on procalcitonin C-terminal end and is cleavaged in posttranslation process. Tumor marker and often a product of paraneoplastic secretion.

Production. Hormone of 32 amino acids secreted by the thyroid C-cells/parafollicular cells as a response to elevated serum calcium levels. Gastrointestinal tract hormone (pentagastrin) can also stimulate secretion; this is used in functional tests.

Function. Hypocalcemic/hypophosphatemic effects. Main functions: 1) inhibits bone resorption by regulating the osteoblasts number and activity, mobilizes Ca^{2+} and phosphate from bone, increases phosphate excretion by decreasing renal phosphate reabsorption, decreases renal H^+ secretion causing increased bicarbonate excretion and chloride retention, enhances renal vitamin D_3 hydroxylation and increases calcium absorption from the gut through effects on 1,25-$(OH)_2D_3$. 2) increases calcium excretion by the kidneys → decreasing serum calcium levels. Calcitonin and parathormone are inversely related in the function. Released by: increased calcium level, pentagastrin. Release inhibition: decreased calcium level.

Test Purpose. 1) to aid in the diagnosis of thyroid medullary tumors, 2) ectopic calcitonin-producing tumors diagnosis (paraneoplastic secretion), 3) to aid in the diagnosis of unexplained and therapeutically resistant diarrhea, 4) pheochromocytoma differential diagnosis (to rule out MEN II sy), 5) in genetical examination of patient family with medular cancer and MEN sy, 6) follow-up of patients with thyroid medullary carcinoma after surgery.

Increased Values – hypercalcitoninemia
pernicious anemia, alcoholic cirrhosis, C-cells hyperplasia of thyroid gland, hypercalcemia, hyperparathyroidism – (**primary h., secondary h.**), calcium infusion, Cushing's disease, Paget's disease, tumours – (**pheochromocytoma,** carcinoid sy, **pancreas t.,** liver t., **lung t., breast t., thyroid t., ovary t.,** APUD cells t.), **pancreatitis,** ectopic production of calcitonin, pseudohypoparathyroidism, syndrome – (**Zollinger–Ellison sy**), **thyroiditis,** uremia, **chronic renal failure**

> **Interfering Factors:** newborns, hemolytic conditions, **pregnancy,** medicaments – (cholecystokinin, epinephrine, estrogens, glucagon, oral contraceptives, pentagastrin)

Decreased Values – hypocalcitoninemia
exercise
> **Interfering Factors:** medicaments – (antiepileptics, phenytoin)

Analyte	Age/Gender	Reference Range	SI Units	Note
Calcitonin (hCT)	M	3–26	pg/ml	
	F	2–17	pg/ml	

Calcium

(Ca)
Function. Creates the bone/teeth frames, involved in hemocoagulation (factor IV), kinin generation, enzyme regulation, neuromuscular excitability, cell-membrane permeability, cardiac function, hormone release and effects. Regulates excitable tissues/plasma membrane

potential and contraction – (striated, cardiac and smooth muscles). Ca^{2+} is needed for transmitter release (Mg^{2+} competes with Ca^{2+}). In skeletal muscles Ca^{2+} activates troponin → moves tropomyosin, which exposes/activates actin. In smooth muscles Ca^{2+} activates contraction by binding to calmodulin. Intracellular calcium participates in action potentials, contraction, motility, cell division, structural integrity, and storage procedures. The physiologically active form is free ionized calcium, which makes up almost half of the total circulating calcium. About 50% of blood calcium is ionized, the rest is protein-bound (mainly to albumin), about 10–15% is weakly bound to phosphates, sulfates, lactate and the remainder is unbound. About 99% is placed in bones, 1% is freely changeable with extracellular fluid. Factors influencing calcium level: parathyroid hormone, calcitonin, vitamin D, estrogens, androgens, carbohydrates, lactose. Blood calcium level maintenance depends on food intake, calcium absorption in gastrointestinal tract, renal calcium excretion, and the status of bone calcium reservoir. In critically ill patients, increased total serum calcium levels usually indicates ionized hypercalcemia, and a normal total serum calcium levels is evidence against ionized hypocalcemia. Ionized calcium is the preferred measurement rather than total calcium because it is physiologically active and can be rapidly measured. Serum magnesium should always be measured in any patient with hypocalcemia. Calcium has circadian and seasonal variations: highest levels are at 8 PM, lowest are at 4 AM, lower in winter and higher in summer; ionized calcium is highest at 8 AM.

Test Purpose. 1) to aid diagnosis of neuromuscular, skeletal and endocrine disorders, dysrhythmias, blood-clotting deficiencies, and acid-base imbalance, 2) to help in diagnosis of parathyroid dysfunction, hypercalcemia of malignancy.

Increased Values – hypercalcemia

acidosis – (respiratory a., renal tubular a.), tuberculous arthritis, **acromegaly, berylliosis, dehydration**, fractures, pituitary gigantism, hemoconcentration, malignant histiocytosis, histoplasmosis, starvation, diarrhea, hyperalbuminemia, hyperalimentation, **familial hypocalciuric hypercalcemia, hypercalcemia of malignancy, idiopathic infant hypercalciuria, hyperparathyroidism**, hypernatremia, parathyroid hyperplasia, **hyperthyroidism, A/D hypervitaminosis**, hyperproteinemia, **hypophosphatasia**, hyponatremia, hypocorti-cism, hypothyroidism, disease – (duodenal/gastric ulcer d., **Addison's d., Paget's d.**, Graves' d., glycogen storage d. type V, VII, light-chain d.), diseases – (**endocrine d.**, chronic liver d., **granulomatous d.**), obstructive jaundice, immobilization – (people with osteoporosis, quadriplegia, paraplegia), insufficiency – (**adrenal cortex i.**, renal i.), intoxication by – (acute alcohol, aluminium, diuretics, lithium, magnesium, vitamin A, D), candidiasis, coccidioidomycosis, metastases – (bronchogenic tumor m., **pancreas tumor m.**), leprosy, meningitis, mycoses, myxedema, tumours – (colorectum t., bone t., adrenal cortex t., endometrium t., esophagus t., gallbladder t., **pheochromocytoma, leukemia**, lymphoma, bladder t., Hodgkin's/non-Hodgkin's lymphoma, kidney t., melanoma, **lung t., pancreas t.**, liver t., ovary adenocarcinoma, **parathyroid t., plasmocytoma** incl. multiple myeloma, Burkitt's lymphoma, adult T-cell lymphoma, **mammary gland t.**, prostate t., Fallopian tube t., fibrosarcoma, sarcoma, stomach t., testes t., thyroid t., tongue t., uterus t., squamous cell carcinoma, **t. producing VIP), nephrocalcinosis**, hypercalcemic nephropathy, osteitis fibrosa cystica, osteomalacia, constipation, acute pancreatitis, paracoccidioidomycosis, polycythemia vera, porphyria, increased calcium intake – (total parenteral nutrition), ectopic PTH production, **rhabdomyolysis**, organism growth, silicone granulomas, **sarcoidosis**, silicotuberculosis, renal transplant rejection, **postrenal transplantation states**, syndrome – (**milk–alkali sy**, preleukemic sy, Cushing's sy, MEN sy, Waterhouse-Friederichsen sy, Fanconi's sy, Zollinger-Ellison sy, ovarian hyperstimulation sy), **tuberculosis**, tuberculous enterocolitis, Hashimoto's thyroiditis, **thyrotoxicosis**, ureterolithiasis, calcium urolithiasis, vomiting, **acute/chronic renal failure**

Interfering Factors: prolonged application of tourniquet, medicaments – (alkaline antacids, aluminum hydroxide, anabolic steroids, androgens, asparaginase, atenolol, benazepril, bisoprolol, calcifediol, calcipotriene, calcitriol, calcium carbonate, Ca salts, calusterone, captopril, chlorothiazide, chlorpropamide, chlortalidone, danazol, diethylstilbestrol, dihydrotachysterol, doxercalciferol, edetate calcium disodium, enalapril, ergocalciferol, estrogens, ethacrynic acid, fosinopril, furosemide, goserelin, hydrochlorothiazide, indapamide, insulin, irbesartan, isotretinoin, letrozole, lithium, magnesium salts, megestrol, methyltestosterone, nandrolone, parathormone, paricalcitol, polythiazide, progesterone, progestins, retinol, secretin, stilbol, sucralfate, tamoxifen, testolactone, testosterone, theophylline, thiazide diuretics, toremifene, tretinoin, vitamin A, vitamin D)

Increased ionized calcium values
primary hyperparathyroidism, ectopic parathyroid hormone-producing tumours, tumors, decreased plasma pH, excess vitamin D intake
Interfering Factors: medicaments – (androgens, calcium carbonate, chlortalidone, diethylstilbestrol, hydrochlorothiazides, lithium, thiazides, vitamin D)

Decreased Values – hypocalcemia
alkalosis, **alcoholism**, celiac disease, **liver cirrhosis**, cystinosis, **vitamin D deficiency, magnesium depletion**, dialysis, diarrhea, **hyperphosphatemia, hypoalbuminemia**, hypomagnesemia, anterior pituitary hypofunction, **hypoparathyroidism**, diseases – (**renal d.**, hepatic d.), **acute/chronic renal insufficiency, lactation**, fluoride intoxication, leprosy, **osteoblastic metastases**, infiltration of parathyroids with – (sarcoidosis, amyloidosis, hemochromatosis, tumor), increased bone mineralization, **medullar thyroid tumors**, malabsorption, tumors, nephrosis, neonatal prematurity, **renal osteodystrophy, osteomalacia**, osteopathies, obstructive jaundice, osteoporosis, **acute**/chronic pancreatitis, **burns, calcium resorption disorders**, decreased intake of – (**calcium**, phosphorus, **vitamin D**), **pseudohypoparathyroidism, rhabdomyolysis, rickets**, resection of – (small intestine, stomach, thyroid), renal tubular acidosis, sepsis, sprue, starvation, steatorrhea, syndrome – (Fanconi's sy, Cushing's sy, **malabsorption sy, nephrotic sy, toxic shock sy, DiGeorge sy**, tumor lysis sy), **pregnancy, tetany, blood transfusion** (massive), newborn complications – (hyperbilirubinemia, respiratory distress, asphyxia, cerebral injuries, infants of diabetic mothers, prematurity, maternal hypoparathyroidism), increased bone formation, **acute/chronic renal failure**
Interfering Factors: phosphate enemas, hemodilution, medicaments – (aldesleukin, alendronate, amifostine, aminoglycozides, amphotericin B, anticonvulsants, antiepileptics, asparaginase, barbiturates, betamethasone, bumetanide, calcitonin, capreomycin, carbamazepine, carboplatin, chlorothiazide, cimetidine, cisplatin, corticosteroids, corticotropin, cortisone, cytosine arabinoside, dactinomycin, denileukin, dexamethasone, dextrose, diuretics, estrogens, ethacrynic acid, ethanol, ethinylestradiol, etidronate, fluorides, foscarnet, furosemide, gentamicin, glucagon, glucocorticoids, hydrocortisone, interferon, isoniazid, ketoconazole, laxatives, magnesium salts, mannitol, mercurial diuretics, methylprednisolone, mithramycin, pamidronate, pentamidine, phenobarbital, phenytoin, phosphorus salts, plicamycin, polymyxin, prednisolone, prednisone, propranolol, propylthiouracil, rimiterol, risedronate, salbutamol, sodium polystyrene, steroids, tetracycline, tretinoin, triamcinolone, trimetrexate, viomycin)

Decreased ionized calcium VALUES
metabolic alkalosis (alkalemia), deficiency of – (magnesium, **vitamin D**), **hemodialysis**, primary/secondary hypoparathyroidism, diabetic ketoacidosis, **acute pancreatitis**, severe burns, pseudohypoparathyroidism, acute myocardial infarction, hyperventilation, **sepsis**,

conditions after – (transfusion with blood containing anions that complex free calcium, major surgery), multiple organ failure, toxic shock syndrome, fat embolism

Interfering Factors: alcohol, calcium-binding agents – citrate, oxalate, EDTA, elder people, increased free fatty acids in serum, medicaments – (anticonvulsants, antiepileptics, carbamazepine, danazol, epinephrine, estrogens, fluorides, foscarnet, furosemide, glucocorticoids, heparin, isoproterenol, laxatives, norepinephrine, phenytoin, tetracyclines)

Analyte		Age/Gender	Reference Range	SI Units	Note
Calcium					
	Total calcium	1 d–4 w	1.8–2.8	mmol/l	
		2–12 m	2.1–2.7	mmol/l	
		>1 y	2.1–2.6	mmol/l	
		Adults	2.15–2.55	mmol/l	
	Free ionized calcium	Children	1.15–1.45	mmol/l	
		Adults	1.13–1.32	mmol/l	

Calgranulins

Calgranulins are intracellular calcium-binding proteins consisting of at least two different peptide chains (calgranulin A – CAGA, calgranulin B – CAGB). These proteins are biochemically related to S-100 proteins. Calgranulin A is identical with MRP-8–migration inhibition factor-related protein-8, calgranulin B is identical with MRP-14. Calgranulins are synthesized by peripheral blood neutrophil granulocytes and monocytes, and also by squamous cell epithelia and keratinocytes of patients with inflammatory dermatoses. They function as inflammatory cytokines. Elevated amounts of both calgranulins are found in the serum of patients with cystic fibrosis and clinically normal heterozygous carriers. MRP-8 and MRP-14 are found also in body fluids in inflammatory conditions and thus may be considered as a very sensitive marker of inflammation. MRP-8 and MRP-14 complexes are identical with the cystic fibrosis antigen (CFAG – consists of CAGA and CAGB) found to be elevated in the serum of cystic fibrosis homozygotes and heterozygous carriers.

Carbohydrate-Deficient Transferrin

(CDT) CDT represents two transferrin isomorphs (di-sialo isomorph, a-sialo isomorph), which have a defect glycosylation. CDT is a reliable marker of chronic alcohol abuse. Chronic alcohol abuse leads to N-bounded saccharide chains synthesis defect; this defect leads to the a-sialo and di-sialo transferrin isomorphs accummulation. Transferrin glycosylation is present during postprandial period through some glycosyltranspherases. It is assumed, that their activity is supressed by anti-aldehyde, which is produced during high and long-lasting alcohol consumption.

Test Purpose. 1) diagnosis of alcoholism, 2) diagnosis of carbohydrate-deficient glycoprotein syndromes. Patients with a genetic carbohydrate-deficient glycoprotein syndrome show decreased levels and abnormal structure of a number of plasma glycoproteins, including transferrin, haptoglobin, thyroxine-binding globulin, antithrombin III and protein C.

Increased Values
alcoholism, false positive results – (iron deficiency, pregnancy, oral contraceptives)

Decreased Values
carbohydrate-deficient glycoprotein syndrome, false negative results – (malnutrition, chronic infectious diseases, alcoholic liver cirrhosis)

Carbonic Anhydrase

(CA, syn: carbonate dehydratase, carbonate hydrolase) Lyase class enzyme that catalyzes dissolved carbon dioxide and carbonic acid equilibration, speeding the carbon dioxide movement from tissues to blood and to alveolar air. It is a zinc protein found in kidney tubule cells and red blood cells.

Increased Values
pregnancy

Decreased Values
renal tubular acidosis, hyperthyroidism

Carcinoembryonic Antigen

(CEA) Glycoprotein, belongs to heterogenous group with variable saccharide segment (which create a great miscellany of antigen) and remarkably constant protein segment. Four CEA genes have been cloned. Heterogenity is based also on the alternative mRNA-splitting mechanism and provokes analytic-interference problems (cross-reacting antigens). The CEA levels in 10% of breast cancers without metastases are increased, in metastases it is 50–60%. Predictive value is low (0.0061) as well in risk groups with high prevalence, this means that it cannot be used for screening purposes because of the low sensitivity and specificity. It is a tumour marker, oncofetal protein.
Occurrence. 1) physiologically in fetal period (first 6 months) in embryonic endodermal cells, intestine, liver, pancreas, 2) pathologically in children/adults in carcinomatous tissue – colon, pancreas, liver, lungs, stomach, breasts and in non-neoplastic conditions. Normally found also in small amounts in the blood of most healthy people. It is found also in fecal and pancreatobiliary secretions. CEA circulates in blood when there is rapid epithelial cells multiplication, especially in the digestive system. At birth, detectable serum levels disappear. Day-to-day variation show 35% in persons with elevated CEA.
Test Purpose. 1) to monitor the effectiveness of colorectal and breast cancer therapy, 2) to assist in preoperative colorectal cancer staging, to assess surgical resection and to test for colorectal cancer recurrence, 3) to help in pancreatic carcinoma diagnosis and paraneoplastic processes, 4) to help in cancer diagnosis (stomach, ovary, medullary thyroid tumors).

Increased Values – positive
chronic alcoholism, **bronchitis**, **hepatic cirrhosis**, **pulmonary emphysema**, **smokers**, gastritis, **hepatitis**, **cholecystitis**, disease – (chronic ischemic heart d., peptic ulcer d.), diseases – (**liver d.**, collagen vascular d., **inflammatory bowel d.**, **benign breast d.**), lung diseases – (chronic l. d., **infectious l. d.**, inflammatory l. d.), **colitis**, radiation therapy, **Crohn's disease**, monitoring after carcinoma resection, tumors – (**esophagus t.**, **head t.**, **chorion t.**, **colorectum t.**, **neck t.**, leukemia, **uterus t.**, **bladder t.**, **neuroblastoma**, **pancreas t.**, **liver t.**, **lung t.**, melanoma, lymphoma, renal t., **mammary gland t.**, **prostate t.**, **testes t.**, **ovary t.**, **stomach t.**,

thyroid gland t.), **pancreatitis**, paraneoplastic processes, pneumonia, precancerosis – (diverticulitis, **colitis ulcerosa**, rectal polyps), conditions after surgery, transfusion with CEA rich blood, trauma, **renal failure**

Interfering Factors: medicaments – (antineoplastics, hepatotoxic drugs)

Analyte	Age/Gender	Reference Range	SI Units	Note
Carcinoembryonic Antigen (CEA)				
Non-smokers		<3.7	µg/ml	
Smokers		<10.0	µg/ml	
Inductors		<40	µg/ml	

Cardiac Glycosides

Test Purpose. To monitor therapeutic levels of cardiac glycosides, 2) to check for suspected toxicity from patient history or onset of symptoms.

Increased Values
cardiac glycosides overdose

Decreased Values
less than therapeutic levels

Carnitine

(total, free L-carnitine). A betaine derivative found in skeletal muscle and liver. L-carnitine is a normal component of human serum. Carnitine is a co-factor involved in free fatty acids and acyl CoA compound transport across the mitochondrial membrane and hence to the site of fatty acid beta-oxidation for energy production from fat. In this capacity it also assists in the detoxification and excretion of these compounds.

Test Purpose. Investigation of carnitine-deficient states.

Increased Values – hypercarnitinemia
ethanol, acute muscular necrosis, **severe renal diseases**

Decreased Values – hypocarnitinemia
carnitine deficiency, diabetes mellitus, cardiomyopathy, myopathies

Interfering Factors: medicaments – (carbamazepine, phenobarbital, pivampicillin, valproic acid)

Analyte	Age/Gender	Reference Range	SI Units	Note
Carnitine				
free	Adults F	17–45	µmol/l	
	Adults M	24–51	µmol/l	
total	Adults F	23–53	µmol/l	
	Adults M	29–59	µmol/l	

Beta-Carotene and Carotenoids

Carotenoids are a family of approximately 600 pigments found in all photosynthesizing plants. Of these approximately 50 serve as precursors to mammalian vitamin A (retinol). Only beta-carotene, representing approximately 25% of serum carotenoids, can form two vitamin A molecules from one precursor. Most beta-carotene is converted to vitamin A in the small intestine; both vitamin A and beta-carotene are found in serum. Serum beta-carotene level determinants are numerous and including dietary uptake rate, gastrointestinal destruction, absorption efficiency, metabolism and tissue uptake. Once in the circulation, beta-carotene is transported by lipoproteins: 80% are bound to LDL-C, 8% bound to HDL-C and 12% to VLDL-C. Beta-carotene is an efficient antioxidant that inactivates potentially dangerous reactive chemicals within the tissues including the toxic free radicals. As such, beta-carotene has been postulated to reduce neoplasia risk. Serum levels reflect recent changes in dietary intake and intestinal function. Day-to-day variation is 5–10%, lowest levels are in spring, and highest in fall.

Test Purpose. 1) to investigate suspected vitamin A deficiency or toxicity, 2) to aid visual disturbance diagnosis, especially night blindness and xerophthalmia, 3) to aid in skin diseases diagnosis, e. g. as keratocytosis follicularis or ichthyosis, 4) to screen for malabsorption, 5) to evaluate the serum antioxidants status.

Increased Values
amenorrhea, anorexia nervosa, **diabetes mellitus**, hemoconcentration, hypercholesterolemia, essential hyperlipidemia, **hyperlipidemia**, hyperlipoproteinemia I, II, **hypothyroidism**, liver diseases, myxedema, chronic nephritis, pancreatitis, **high dietary carotene intake**, **meals**, nephrotic sy, **pregnancy**, subacute thyroiditis

Decreased Values
celiac disease, **low fat diet**, enteritis, ethanol, smoking, cystic fibrosis, infectious hepatitis, diseases – (small bowel d., liver d.), obstructive jaundice, pancreatic insufficiency, kwashiorkor, **malabsorption**, **malnutrition**, high fever conditions, steatorrhea, pregnancy

Interfering Factors: medicaments – (kanamycin, metformin, neomycin, oral contraceptives)

Analyte	Age/Gender	Reference Range	SI Units	Note
Beta-Carotene		0.95–3.7	µmol/l	

Caspases

(caspases 1 through 14) These aspartate-specific cystein proteases are synthesized as inactive polypeptide precursors (zymogen). These are composed of a prodomain plus large and small catalytic subunits. Active caspases are tetramers consisting of 2 large and 2 small subunits from the cleaved proenzymes. Different caspases are capable of activating each other. They play an important role in programmed cell death. They constitute the effector arm of the cell-death pathway and effect the proteolytic degradation of other cellular components. The activation of the cascade of proteolytic caspases has been identified as the final common pathway of apoptosis in diverse biological systems. A variety of proteins are capable of suppressing or promoting apoptosis by interacting with and functionally antagonizing each other. These interactions either prevent caspase activation in the case of apoptosis inhibition, or promote caspase activation in the case of apoptosis induction. Group 1 caspases (caspase 1, 4, 5) appear to function primarily as mediators of inflammation. Group 2 caspases (caspase 2, 3, 7) play important role as effectors of cell death by apoptosis. Group 3 caspases (caspase 6, 8, 9, 10) play a role in signaling apoptotic events.

Catalase

Enzyme, oxidoreductase, tetramer composed of identical subunits. Protoporphyrin with Fe^{3+} is the non-protein part of each subunit. It is situated in mitochondria, peroxisomes, leukocytes, plasma; it is soluble in erythrocytes. Catalyzes hydrogenperoxide removal → water + O_2 and so protecting cells.

Increased Values – hypercatalasemia
vitamin D deficiency, methemoglobinemia

Decreased Values – hypocatalasemia
brucellosis, diseases – (chronic cerebrovascular d., hepatic d., gastrointestinal tract d.), intoxication, tumors, cardiosurgery procedures

Catecholamines

Catecholamines is the name for hormones, including epinephrine = adrenaline, norepinephrine = noradrenaline, dopamine.
Production. Adrenal medulla hormones, peripheral postganglionic sympathetic fibres endings (predominantly noradrenaline), brain.
Function. Mediate carbohydrate/lipid metabolism (glycogenolysis, gluconeogenesis in liver – beta- and alpha-receptors, glycogenolysis, glycolysis in muscles – beta-2 receptors). **Alpha-1 receptors** intermediate: smooth muscle contraction. **Alpha-1, alpha-2 receptors:** vasoconstriction (subcutaneous, mucosal, splanchnic, renal). **Alpha-2 receptors:** platelet aggregation, insulin secretion decrease, lipolysis in fatty tissue, presynaptic inhibition of mediator release. **Beta-1 receptors:** myocardial contraction + positive chronotrophy, dromotrophy, bathmotrophy, coronary vessels dilation, gastrointestinal motility and tonus decrease, renin secretion increase, lipolysis in fatty tissue. **Beta-2 receptors** intermediate: smooth muscle trachea, bronchi, vessels and uterus dilation, insulin secretion increase, glucagon secretion of increase, thermogenic effect, glycogenolysis in muscles. Sympathetic and central nervous system neurotransmitters. Catecholamines enhance cardiac output by stimulating venoconstriction, enhancing venous return, increasing the atrial contraction force → augmenting diastolic volume → prolonging fiber length. Cardiac stimulation increases myocardial oxygen consumption. Catecholamines also accelerate fuel mobilization in the liver, adipose tissue, skeletal muscle → liberating substrates (glucose, free fatty acids, lactate) into the circulation. Norepinephrine stimulates sodium reabsorption (extracellular fluid volume defence), dopamine promotes sodium excretion, norepinephrine and epinephrine promote cellular potassium uptake (defence against the hyperkalemia). Lowest concentrations are at night.
Test Purpose. 1) to rule out pheochromocytoma in patients with hypertension, 2) to help identify neuroblastoma, ganglioneuroblastoma and ganglioneuroma, 3) to distinguish between adrenal medullary tumours and other catecholamine-producing tumors, 4) to aid autonomic nervous system dysfunction diagnosis, such as idiopathic orthostatic hypoten-

sion, 5) to help in the hypertension diagnosis. Catecholamines measurement in urine has higher value than measurement in plasma. Also in physiological plasma values in confirmed tumor, catecholamine urine excretion is pathological.

Increased Values

anaphylaxis, **adrenal medullary hyperplasia**, anoxia, asphyxia, **prolonged exposure to cold**, volume depletion, progressive muscular dystrophy, endotoxins, encephalopathy, CNS hemorrhage, CNS infarction, anger, **arterial hypertension**, hypoglycemia, **hypothyroidism**, diseases – (**kidney d.**, cardiac d., thyroid d.), **acute myocardial infarction**, **diabetic ketoacidosis**, alcohol intoxication, **hemorrhage**, electroshock therapy, myasthenia gravis, tumours – (adrenal medullary t., carcinoid, **pheochromocytoma**, ganglioblastoma, **ganglioneuroma**, **neuroblastoma**), paraganglioma, acute intermittent porphyria, acute psychosis, **conditions after surgery**, fear, **stress**, **shock**, Guillain–Barré syndrome, **thyrotoxicosis**, **physical exertion/ exercise**, drug withdrawal (alcohol, clonidine)

> Interfering Factors: contrast media, amine-rich foods/beverages, upright posture, medicaments – (acetylsalicylic acid, adrenaline, ajmaline, alcohol, aminophylline, amphetamines, ampicillin, alpha-1-blockers, beta-blockers, caffeine, calcium channel blockers, chloral hydrate, chlorpromazine, clonidine, diazoxide, disulfiram, dopamine, ephedrine, erythromycin, ether, hydralazine, imipramine, insulin, isoproterenol, labetalol, levodopa, MAO inhibitors, methenamine, methyldopa, methylxanthines, minoxidil, niacin, nicotinic acid, nifedipine, nitroglycerin, perphenazine, phenacetin, phenothiazines, phentolamine, promethazine, propranolol, quinidine, quinine, reserpine, riboflavin, sodium nitroprusside, sympathomimetics, tetracyclines, theophylline, tricyclic antidepressants, vasodilators)

Decreased Values

> Interfering Factors: medicaments – (acetylsalicylic acid, alpha-2-agonists, anileridine, bretylium, bromocriptine, calcium channel blockers, cimetidine, clofibrate, clonidine, chlorpromazine, dexamethasone, disulfiram, guanethidine, imipramine, isoproterenol, levodopa, MAO inhibitors, propranolol, mephenesin, methocarbamol, methyldopa, metyrosine, nalidixic acid, penicillin, phenazopyridine, reserpine, thyroxine)

Analyte	Age/Gender	Reference Range	SI Units	Note
Catecholamines				
Norepinephrine				
– recumbency		591–2364	pmol/l	
– standing		1773–5320	pmol/l	
Epinephrine				
– recumbency		<382	pmol/l	
– standing		<546	pmol/l	
Dopamine		<196	pmol/l	

Cationic Antimicrobial Protein-37

(CAP-37, syn: neutrophil-derived heparin-binding protein) Glycoprotein CAP-37 is found in azurophil granules, specialized lysosomes of the neutrophil. It is a specific and strong chemoattractant for monocytes and possesses antibacterial activity. CAP-37 released from neutrophils during phagocytosis and degranulation may mediate recruitment of monocytes in the second wave of inflammation.

Celiac Disease Antibody Profile

(syn: antigluten antibodies, endomysial antibodies, gliadin antibodies, reticulin antibodies)
Test includes quantitative results for antibodies to gliadin IgG, gliadin IgA, endomysial IgA, reticulin IgA, reticulin IgG. The presence of antibodies to any one or a combination of three serum markers associated with a history of gastrointestinal disorders is consistent with a diagnosis of celiac disease or dermatitis herpetiformis, which are caused by sensitivity to gluten. Strict avoidance of gluten in the diet will control disease activity, and antibodies to serum markers will disappear with time.
Test Purpose. 1) to aid in the diagnosis of gluten-sensitive enteropathies and dermatitis herpetiformis, 2) to follow up of dietary restriction and challenge.

Increased Values
celiac disease, **dermatitis herpetiformis**, normal population

Ceruloplasmin

(CER) Acute phase alpha-glycoprotein (acute phase reactant) with oxidase activity (polyfenol-oxidase), alpha-2-globulin, metalloprotein, copper-binding serum protein.
Production. Synthesized in the liver and released into the blood stream after incorporation of copper.
Function. Ceruloplasmin binds and transports about 95% of the copper; as additional copper is absorbed, CER is synthesized and avoids potential copper toxicity. Participates in change $Fe^{2+} \rightarrow Fe^{3+}$ during its uptake by transferrin. Inactivates neurogenic amines. Day-to-day variation is 10–15%.
Test Purpose. To aid diagnosis of Wilson's disease, Menkes' kinky hair sy, copper deficiency from total parenteral nutrition, and oxidative stress.

Increased Values – hyperceruloplasminemia
abscess of liver, aplastic anemia, **rheumatoid arthritis**, cirrhosis – (**hepatic c.**, **primary biliary c.**), **smoking**, **hepatitis**, hyperthyroidism, **cholestasis**, diseases – (**infectious d.**, hepatic d., **inflammatory d.**), **obstructive icterus**, **copper intoxication** (**chronic**), increased basal metabolism, tumours – (acute leucemia, **Hodgkin's disease**), nephrosis, tissue necrosis, **extra/intrahepatic biliary tract obstruction**, **stress**, **thyrotoxicosis**, trauma, **extreme exercise**
    Interfering Factors: **pregnancy**, IUD (intrauterine device), medicaments – (androgens, antiepileptics, carbamazepine, estrogens, ethinylestradiol, methadone, oral birth-control pills, phenobarbital, phenytoin, tamoxifen)

Decreased Values – hypoceruloplasminemia
anemia, hepatic cirrhosis, **hepatolenticular degeneration** (Wilson's disease), **inherited ceruloplasmin deficiency**, chronic hepatitis, hyperalimentation, infectious diseases, **idiopathic hypoceruloplasminemia**, congenital hemolytic icterus, **kwashiorkor**, **malabsorption**, **malnutrition**, tumours, **copper nutrition deficiency**, **nephrosis**, sclerosis multiplex, **sprue**, syndrome – (**Menke's sy**, **nephrotic sy**), **long-term parenteral nutrition**, **liver failure**
    Interfering Factors: **newborns up to 6 months**, medicaments – (asparaginase)

Analyte	Age/Gender	Reference Range	SI Units	Note
Ceruloplasmin		0.15–0.45	mg/l	

Chemokines

Generic name given to a family of pro-inflammatory activation-inducible cytokines. According to the chromosomal locations of individual genes two different subfamilies of chemokines are distinguished (alpha-chemokines, beta-chemokines). Gamma-chemokines differ from the other chemokines by the absence of a cysteine residue. Chemokines are essential mediators of normal leukocyte trafficking. They are multipotent cytokines that localize and enhance inflammation by inducing chemotaxis and cell activation of different types of inflammatory cells typically present at inflammatory sites. Chemokines and other mediators are secreted also by these cells. Many genes encoding chemokines are expressed strongly during the course of a number of pathophysiological processes including autoimmune diseases, cancer, atherosclerosis and chronic inflammatory diseases. Several chemokines have been shown to modulate the growth of hematopoietic progenitor cell types and may thus have functions in hematopoiesis. May play also a role in trafficking of hematopoietic progenitor cells in and out of the bone marrow in inflammatory conditions.

Chemokines. IL-8, MCP-1, 2, 3 (monocyte chemoattractant protein, monocyte chemotactic protein, monocyte chemotactic protein and activating factor), MIP-1 (macrophage inflammatory protein), MIP-2, MIP-3, MIP-4, MIP-5, NAP-2 (neutrophil activating protein), PF-4 (platelet factor), beta-TG (beta-thromboglobulin), GCP-2 (granulocyte chemotactic protein), SDF-1-alpha/beta (stromal cell-derived factors), lymphotactin, PBP (platelet basic protein), CTAP-III (connetive tissue-activating protein-3), eotaxin (eosinophil-active chemokine), ENA-78 (epithelial-derived neutrophil attractant 78), MGSA/GRO (melanoma growth-stimulating activity/growth-related oncogen alpha), monotactin 1, megakaryocyte-stimulatory factor, oncostatin A, neurotactin, endothelial cell growth inhibitor, heparin neutralizing protein, IP-10 (gamma interferon-inducible protein 10), MIG (monokine induced by interferon gamma), RANTES (regulated on activation, normal T-cell expressed and secreted)

Chemokines involved in hemopoiesis. MIP-1-alpha, MIP-1-beta, MIP-2-alpha, IL-8, IL-10, PF-4

Chloride

(Cl⁻, syn: plasma chloride, Cl anion) Principal inorganic anion of the extracellular fluid.
Function. Maintain acid-base and water balance and all body fluids component, e. g. gastric juice. When chloride (HCl, NH_4Cl) are lost → alkalosis follows, if Cl⁻ is retained/ingested → acidosis follows. Chloride with natrium play an important role in body fluids osmolality control.
Test Purpose. 1) to detect acid-base imbalance and to aid fluid status and extracellular cation-anion balance evaluation, 2) to monitor NaCl intake, 3) to monitor chloride loss, 4) to monitor potassium balance disorders.

Increased Values – hyperchloremia
acidosis – (metabolic a., hyperchloremic metabolic a., metabolic a. after salicylate poisoning, **renal tubular a.**), **respiratory alkalosis, uretero-sigmoid anastomosis, anemia,** hepatic cirrhosis, **dehydration,** cardiac decompensation, diabetes insipidus – (**central d. i.**, nephrogenic d. i.), diuresis – (osmotic d., postobstructive d.), **eclampsia, diarrhea,** hyperalimentation, **hyperparathyroidism**, intestinal fistulas, pregnancy induced hypertension, **hyperventilation**, endocrine diseases, **renal insufficiency**, nephrosis, plasmocytoma (incl. multiple

myeloma), burns, aldosterone/antidiuretic hormone secretion disorders, sweating (chloride skin loses), lost of pancreatic secretion, ileal loops, overtreatment with saline solution, **increased chloride intake, decreased water intake, hypernatremic conditions**, syndrome – (**Cushing's sy**, nephrotic sy), ureterosigmoidostomy, failure – (**cardiac f., renal f.**)

Interfering Factors: medicaments – (acetazolamide, ammonium chloride, androgens, boric acid, bromides, chlorothiazide, cholestyramine, corticosteroids, cortisone, cyclosporine, diuretics – carboanhydrase blockers, estrogens, guanethidine, heparin, methyldopa, nonsteroidal antiinflammatory drugs, phenylbutazone, streptozocin, triamterene)

Decreased Values – hypochloremia

acidosis – (**diabetic a.**, metabolic a., **chronic respiratory a.**), **metabolic alkalosis**, anesthesia, hepatic cirrhosis, kalium deficiency, **diabetes mellitus**, pulmonary edema, emphysema, small bowel fistulae, **diarrhea**, hyperglycemia, **overhydration**, hypothyroidism, secondary hypoventilation, acute infectious diseases, insufficiency – (**adrenal cortex i., renal i.**), **water intoxication**, colitis ulcerosa, hemorrhage, **Addison's disease**, interstitial nephritis, **salt losing nephropathy, pyloric obstruction, gastrointestinal suction**, pneumothorax, **pneumonia**, poliomyelitis, **burns, excessive sweating, insufficient chloride intake**, repeated ascites puncture, **kalium balance disorders**, organism overheating, pseudohyponatremia, increased intake of bicarbonates, conditions – (**edematous c., hyponatremic c.**), **prolonged gastric suction**, respiratory losses, excessive chloride loss, syndrome – (Bartter's sy, Cushing's sy, nephrotic sy, **SIADH**), **acid vomiting**, failure – (**cardiac f., renal f.**)

Interfering Factors: medicaments – (aldosterone, amiloride, barbiturates, bicarbonates, bromides, bumetanide, carbamazepine, chlorpromazine, chlortalidone, clofibrate, corticosteroids, cortisone, diuretics, ethacrynic acid, furosemide, gentamicin, hydrochlorothiazide, hypertonic infusions, indapamide, laxatives, mercurial diuretics, metolazone, morphine, polythiazide, prednisolone, steroids, thiazides, tolbutamide, triamterene, tricyclic antidepressants)

Analyte	Age/Gender	Reference Range	SI Units	Note
Chloride	1 d–4 w	95–116	mmol/l	
	2–12 m	93–112	mmol/l	
	>1 y	96–111	mmol/l	
	Adults	98–106	mmol/l	

Cholecystokinin-Pancreozymin

(CCK-PZ) Gastrointestinal tract peptide (small intestine I-cells) with neurocrine (neurotransmitter) and endocrine effects.

Production. Duodenum, jejunum, hypothalamus.

Function. Stimulates pancreatic amylases (major stimulus for zymogen release), bicarbonates, insulin, glucagon, pancreatic polypeptide secretion. Causes gallbladder contraction, Oddi's sphincter relaxation, gastric smooth musculature contraction, slows gastric emptying, increases intestinal peristalsis. Secretion is stimulated by food, fatty acids, calcium and amino acids in gastrointestinal tract.

Increased Values

celiac disease, disease – (irritable bowel d., gastric ulcer d.), **pancreatic exocrine insufficiency, chronic pancreatitis**, fatty food intolerance, response to meals abolished after vagotomy, postgastrectomy states

Decreased Values
response to meals abolished by atropine

Cholesterol

(syn: total cholesterol, lipid fraction) Steroid alcohol (sterol).

Metabolism. Dietary cholesterol is first hydrolyzed by cholesterol esterase → to free cholesterol before it is absorbed by intestinal mucosa. Absorption of free cholesterol requires bile salts and lecithin. Then cholesterol in the intestinal mucosal cells is incorporated into lipid protein macromolecular complexes known as chylomicrons, which enter into circulation via the lymphatic system. After undergoing certain catabolic processes, lipid and apo-protein components exchange, the chylomicron remnants containing mostly the cholesterol ester are taken up by the liver. When dietary cholesterol derived from the chylomicron remnants is insufficient → the liver synthesizes its own cholesterol by increasing the rate limi-ting enzymatic activities. Intrahepatic cholesterol, triacylglycerols and apoproteins are reassembled into lipoproteins called VLDL-C and released into circulation. In the circulation VLDL-C undergoes several compositional changes by interacting with lecithin cholesterol acyltransferase, HDL-C and lipoprotein lipase → VLDL-C is transferred into LDL-C after releasing/exchanging most of its triacylglycerols and apolipoproteins. LDL-C delivers cholesterol to all peripheral tissues and cells with LDL-C receptors. Once cholesterol enters the cells → the cholesterol esters are hydrolyzed → to free cholesterol by cholesterol esterases. When the free cholesterol supply exceeds cellular metabolic requirements → the enzyme acylcholesterol acyltransferase → is activated to esterify free cholesterol to cholesterol ester for storage.

Production. Synthesis occurs in nearly all cells. The liver, intestine, adrenal glands and gonads are the major cholesterol biosynthesis sites. Metabolization in liver → bile acids creation.

Function. Substrate for adrenal and gonadal hormones production and production of all membrane structures (essential cell membranes structural component). Concentration is determined by metabolic functions – influenced by heredity, nutrition, endocrine factors, integrity of vital organs – kidney, liver. Cholesterol metabolism is intimately associated with whole lipoprotein metabolism. Cholesterol is transported by the low-density lipoproteins (LDL-C) 60–75% and high-density lipoproteins (HDL-C) 15–35%. Day-to-day levels variation is 7%, 3–5% higher in winter and lowest in summer.

Test Purpose. 1) to assess coronary artery disease risk, 2) to evaluate fat metabolism, 3) to aid diagnosis of nephrotic sy, pancreatitis, hyperurikemia, hepatic diseases and hypo/hyperthyroidism, 4) general and genetic screening, 5) to assess the patients' atherosclerosis condition, 6) to assess the patients' state with xanthoma, xanthelasma, arcus lipoides, 7) to monitor hypertension, 8) to monitor patients in dialysis program.

Increased Values – hypercholesterolemia
metabolic acidosis, **alcoholism**, analbuminemia, aplastic anemia, inhalatory anesthesia, **angina pectoris**, **anorexia nervosa**, **atherosclerosis**, **primary biliary cirrhosis**, **diabetes mellitus**, **dialysis program**, **gout** (uratic arthritis), dysglobulinemia, **smoking**, pheochromocytoma, gammapathy, glomerulonephritis, **chronic hepatitis**, idiopathic hypercalcemia, **primary hyperlipoproteinemia**, **arterial hypertension**, hyperuricemia, hypoproteinemia, **hypothy-**

roidism, cholangitis, cholecystitis, cholecystopathy, cholelithiasis, **extra/intrahepatic cholestasis,** disease – (cholesteryl ester storage d., **von Gierke's disease, coronary artery d., ischemic heart d.**), **obstructive icterus,** acute cardiac infarction (the levels ↑ quickly from the 2nd day, it is possible to evaluate only after 3–4 months), cretinism, macroglobulinemia, myxedema, tumors – (t. of pancreas, plasmocytoma, t. of prostate, t. of biliary ways), nephritis, **nephrosis, obesity, bile duct blockage, pancreatitis,** total pancreatectomy, acute intermittent porphyria, peripheral artery circulatory disorders, increased cholesterol intake, strumectomy, syndrome – (**nephrotic sy,** Werner's sy), **gravidity,** thyropathy, xanthelasma, xanthoma, chronic renal failure

    Interfering Factors: medicaments – (acetylsalicylic acid, aminoglutethimide, aminopyrine, amiodarone, amprenavir, androgens, ascorbic acid, asparaginase, atenolol, benazepril, beta-blockers, betamethasone, bexarotene, bisoprolol, buserelin, captopril, catecholamines, chenodeoxycholic acid, chlorpromazine, chlortalidone, cholestatics, corticosteroids, cortisone, cyclosporine, danazol, dexamethasone, diclofenac, disulfiram, diuretics, enalapril, epinephrine, ergocalciferol, estrogens, ether, etretinate, fosinopril, furosemide, glucocorticoids, glutethimide, hepatotoxic medicaments, hydrochlorothiazide, hydrocortisone, imipramine, indapamide, indinavir, irbesartan, isotretinoin, letrozole, levobetaxolol, levodopa, lisinopril, losartan, methyltestosterone, metolazone, metoprolol, miconazole, moexipril, mycophenolate, nandrolone, nelfinavir, norethisterone, oral contraceptives, oxymetholone, phenothiazines, phenytoin, pindolol, prednisolone, prednisone, prochlorperazine, progestins, propranolol, ritonavir, rosiglitazone, salicylates, saquinavir, sirolimus, testosterone, thiazides, ticlopidine, tocopherol, torsemide, tretinoin, triamcinolone, triamterene, troglitazone, valsartan, viomycin, vitamin A, vitamin C, vitamin D)

Decreased Values – hypocholesterolemia

alpha-/beta-lipoproteinemia, anemia – (megaloblastic a., hemolytic a., pernicious a., thalassemia), arthritis – (chronic a., rheumatoid a.), avitaminosis A, **cirrhosis of liver, apolipoproteins deficiency, acute liver dystrophy,** endocarditis, pancreatic fibrosis, hemophilia, **viral hepatitis,** starvation, **hyperthyroidism,** hypolipoproteinemia, disease – (**chronic obstructive pulmonary d.,** Tangier d., Gaucher's d.), diseases – (infectious d., **hepatic d.,** acute inflammatory d., myeloproliferative d.), hemolytic icterus, ileus, poisoning by – (arsenic, phosphorus, chloroform, tetrachlormethane), **cachexia,** intestinal lymphangiectasis, **malnutrition,** myocarditis, **tumours,** hepatocellular necrosis, osteomyelitis, chronic interstitial pneumonia, undernutrition, polytrauma, severe burns, severe liver lesion by – (chemicals, medicaments), cerebral palsy, mental retardation, conditions – (postoperative c., septic c.), **steatorrhea, malabsorption sy,** thrombocytopathy, tuberculosis, thyrotoxicosis, **uremia,** heart failure

    Interfering Factors: medicaments – (acetylsalicylic acid, ACTH, allopurinol, aminosalicylic acid, amiodarone, androgens, antibiotics, ascorbic acid, asparaginase, azathioprine, bunitrolol, calcium channel blockers, carbutamide, chlorpropamide, cholestyramine, clofibrate, clomiphene, clonidine, cortisonoids, doxazosin, enalapril, erythromycin, estradiol, estrogens, ethinylestradiol, fenfluramine, fenyramidol, glibenclamide, guanfacine, haloperidol, hepatotoxic medicaments, hydralazine, interferon, isoniazid, kanamycin, ketoconazole, levothyroxine, lovastatin, mepindolol, metoprolol, metyrapone, neomycin, norgestrel, oral contraceptives, paromomycin, pentetrazol, phenformin, phenobarbital, pravastatin, prazosin, probucol, simvastatin, spironolactone, tamoxifen, tetracycline, thyroxine, tolbutamide)

Analyte	Age/Gender	Reference Range	SI Units	Note
Cholesterol				
Total	< 4 w	1.3–4.4	mmol/l	
	2–12 m	1.6–4.5	mmol/l	
	Adults	2.8–5.2	mmol/l	
HDL	F	>1.68	mmol/l	
	M	>1.45	mmol/l	
LDL	Adults	<3.2	mmol/l	
		<2.8	mmol/l	See ref. ranges note
VLDL		0.1–0.5	mmol/l	

HDL-Cholesterol

(HDL-C, syn: high-density lipoprotein – HDL) HDL-C is an important high-density lipo-proteins part.

Production. HDL-C is synthesized and secreted in the liver and intestine, contains 20–50% of circulating cholesterol. The nascent HDL-C complexes contain 50% proteins and 50% lipids. Lipid is composed mainly of phospholipids (25–30%), cholesterol esters (15–20%), cholesterol (5%) and triacylglycerols (3%).

Function. Reverse cholesterol transport between lipoproteins. HDL-C transports cholesterol esters from the peripheral cells/tissues to the liver, where the HDL-C is degraded and the cholesterol is released → bile excretion. A close negative relation between TAG and HDL-C exists. HDL-C inhibits cellular uptake of low-density lipoproteins and serves as a circulating reservoir of Apo C-II, Apo A-I, Apo A-II. Anti-atherogenic factor. It is necessary to evaluate it with total cholesterol (ideal ratio 1 : 3) and triacylglycerols. Borderline ratio is 4. 5; in higher values there is significantly rising ischemic heart disease risk regardless of total cholesterol concentration. 5–8% day-to-day concentration variation.

Test Purpose. 1) to assess ischemic heart disease risk, 2) to determine classification of dyslipoproteinemias, 3) in hypercholesterolemia screening or genetic screening.

Increased Values

alcoholism, primary biliary cirrhosis, **familial hyper-alpha-lipoproteinemia**, weight reduction, **moderate ethanol consumption** (up to 30 g a day), chronic liver disorders, pregnancy (2nd trimester), **nutrition** (polyunsaturated fatty acids), **regular endurance aerobic physical exercise**

Interfering Factors: medicaments – (androgens, antiepileptics, ascorbic acid, atenolol, carprazidil, carbamazepine, celiprolol, cimetidine, clofibrate, cyclofenil, doxazosin, estradiol, estrogens, ethanol, ethinylestradiol, gemfibrozil, glutethimide, hydrochlorothiazide, indapamide, insulin, isotretinoin, lovastatin, mepindolol, niacin, nicotinic acid, nisoldipine, norethisterone, oral contraceptives, phenobarbital, phenytoin, pindolol, pravastatin, prazosin, prednisone, salbutamol, simvastatin, terbutaline)

Decreased Values

abetalipoproteinemia, AIDS, **alcoholism**, chronic anemias, angina pectoris, atherosclerosis, primary biliary cirrhosis, deficiency – (**lipoprotein lipase co-factor (Apo C-II) d.**, LCAT d.), **diabetes mellitus** (untreated), diet high in carbohydrates, **smoking**, chronic hepatitis, starvation, hyperuricemia, arterial hypertension, **hypertriacylglycerolemia**, **hyperthyroidism**, familial hypo-alpha-lipoproteinemia, **hypothyroidism**, cholestasis, disease – (**ischemic heart d.**, **Tangier d.**, Niemann–Pick d.), diseases – (**acute infectious d.**, **myeloproliferative d.**, **liver d.**), **prolonged physical inactivity**, **myocardial infarction**, malabsorption, **malnutrition**, nephrosis, **obesity**, **surgery**, hepatocellular disorders, weight reduction in overweight individuals, acute stress, nephrotic sy, **trauma**, **uremia**, nutrition, xanthoma, chronic renal failure, menopause, puberty in male

> Interfering Factors: medicaments – (anabolic steroids, androgens, atenolol, beta-blockers, carbamazepine, chenodeoxycholic acid, chlorpropamide, chlortalidone, cimetidine, clofibrate, corticoids, cyclofenil, cyproterone, danazol, diuretics, doxazosin, estrogens, etretinate, furosemide, interferon, interleukin, isotretinoin, lovastatin, lynestrenol, methyldopa, metoprolol, nadolol, neomycin, nicotinic acid, norethisterone, norgestrel, oxprenolol, oral contraceptives, phenobarbital, phenothiazines, phenytoin, pravastatin, prazosin, prednisolone, probucol, progesterone, progestins, propranolol, ranitidine, simvastatin, sotalol, spironolactone, stanozolol, terbutaline, thiazides)

IDL-Cholesterol

(IDL-C, syn: intermediate-density lipoprotein – IDL, floating beta-lipoprotein) IDL-C is intermediate product of VLDL-C catabolism which contains about 15% proteins, 25% phospholipids, equal amounts (30%) of cholesterol and triacylglycerols, the protein component is composed of Apo B (6%), Apo E (30%) and Apo C (10%). IDL-C undergoes further catalytic conversions to LDL-C, containing almost pure cholesterol core esters and Apo B on the surface. IDL-cholesterol is not measured individually, but because new knowledge about lipoprotein interconversion and functional measurement significance, its time will come.

Increased Values
diabetes mellitus, gout, maintenance hemodialysis, **hyperlipoproteinemia** (type III), hypothyroidism, acute renal failure

LDL-Cholesterol

(LDL-C, syn: low-density lipoprotein – LDL, beta-lipoprotein) LDL-C consists of about 50% cholesterol, 10% triacylglycerols, 20% protein, 17% phospholipids. The protein component is composed of Apo B (96%) with only trace amounts of Apo C and Apo A.
Function. Originates by VLDL-C degradation. One of the most important ischemic heart disease risk factors, and an atherogenic factor; it is the major cholesterol-carrying lipoprotein in normal plasma. Transports cholesterol from liver to the peripheral tissues. LDL-C metabolism is in closed connection with LDL-receptors interaction in fibroblasts, vascular system smooth muscular cells and lymphocytes. LDL-C is catabolized in the liver and peripheral tissues. Excess free cholesterol accumulation gives these cells a "foam cell" appearance, a basic component of atherosclerotic plaques.
Test Purpose. 1) to assess the coronary artery disease risk, 2) to determine hyper/hypolipoproteinemia classification and to help differential diagnosis, 3) in genetic screening, 4) to assess atherogenic process biochemical activity, 5) to monitor hypertension therapy with beta-blockers and diuretics, 6) to help in insulin dependent diabetes mellitus and hyperuricemia diagnosis.

Increased Values

anorexia nervosa, arcus corneae, **atherosclerosis, diabetes mellitus, dysgammaglobulin-emia**, smoking, familial hypercholesterolemia, pheochromocytoma, **gammopathies**, glyco-genosis, viral hepatitis, **hereditary hyperlipoproteinemia**, arterial hypertension, hyperuric-emia, **hypothyroidism, coronary artery disease**, diseases – (renal d., **hepatic d.**), lipoidosis, **obesity, hepatic obstruction**, acute pancreatitis, **plasmocytoma** (incl. multiple myeloma), **porphyria**, increased food intake – (**fatty foods, animal fats**), stress, syndrome – (Cushing's sy, **nephrotic sy**), **pregnancy, xanthoma, chronic renal failure**, acute myocardial infarction

> **Interfering Factors:** medicaments – (androgens, atenolol, beta-blockers, carbamazepine, catecholamines, chenodeoxycholic acid, chlortalidone, corticoids, cyclosporine, danazol, diuretics, estrogens, ethanol, etretinate, furosemide, glutethimide, hydrochlorothiazide, isotretinoin, lynestrenol, norethisterone, oral contraceptives, progestins, stanozolol, thiazides)

Decreased Values

abetalipoproteinemia, chronic anemias, alpha-lipoprotein deficiency (Tangier disease), diet high in polyunsaturated fats, **severe hepatocellular dysfunction**, starvation, intravenous hyperalimentation, **hyperlipoproteinemia** (type I), **hyperthyroidism**, diseases – (chronic infectious d., inflammatory joint d., myeloproliferative d., chronic pulmonary d.), myocardial infarction, **malabsorption, malnutrition**, plasmocytoma (incl. multiple myeloma), burns, severe stress conditions, **Reye's sy**, trauma

> **Interfering Factors:** medicaments – (aminosalicylic acid, chlorpropamide, cholestyramine, cimetidine, clofibrate, colestipol, doxazosin, estradiol, estrogens, gemfibrosil, interferon, interleukin, ketoconazole, lovastatin, mepindolol, metoprolol, neomycin, nicotinic acid, pravastatin, prazosin, probucol, progesterone, propranolol, simvastatin, terazosin, thyroxine)

VLDL-Cholesterol

(VLDL-C, syn: very low-density lipoprotein – VLDL, pre-beta-lipoprotein).

Production. VLDL-C is synthesized in the liver and intestine. Contains about 44–60% tria-cylglycerols, 20–23% phospholipids, 11–14% cholesterol esters, 5–8% cholesterol, 4–11% apoproteins.

Function. VLDL-C is catabolized rapidly to IDL-C (intermediate-density lipoprotein) and later to LDL-C. VLDL-C transport endogeniously synthesized triacylglycerols from the liver and intestine to the peripheral tissues. In healthy individuals, VLDL-C represents about 22–33% of the total circulating lipoproteins.

Test Purpose. 1) to assess coronary artery disease risk, 2) a part of dyslipoproteinemias classification.

Increased Values

alcoholism, lecithin cholesterol acyltransferase deficiency, **juvenile diabetes mellitus**, dysproteinemia, **glycogenoses** (glycogen storage disease), **hyperprebetalipoproteinemia, hypothyroidism, systemic lupus erythematosus**, Gaucher's disease, Niemann–Pick disease, **obesity, pancreatitis, excessive food intake** (especially simple carbohydrate), **nephrotic sy, pregnancy** (3rd trimester), uremia

> **Interfering Factors:** nonfasting specimen, medicaments – (beta-blockers, cortico-steroids, estrogens, oral contraceptives, thiazide diuretics)

Cholinesterase

(CHS, syn: choline esterase, acetylcholinesterase, acylcholinesterase – ACHS, AChE, ACHE, CHE, acylhydrolase) CHS is a group of 13 genetically determined enzymes, which are splitting acetylcholine esters, 11- and butyrylcholine esters. Two specific isoenzymes are known as acetylcholinesterases, others are pseudocholine esterases. A cholinesterase test is used to measure 2 enzyme groups that hydrolyze acetylcholine: 1) acetylcholinesterase (cholinesterase I) – in spleen erythrocytes, gray matter of the brain, lungs and at nerve endings, 2) pseudocholine esterase (choline esterase II) – in plasma, produced primarily in the liver and appearing slightly in the pancreas, intestine, heart and white matter of the brain. Cholinesterase activity present in the serum/plasma hydrolyses both choline and aliphatic esters, has a broader range of esterolytic activity and is referred to as "pseudo-" or "nonspecific" cholinesterase. It hydrolyses acetylcholine only slowly. The systematic name for acetylcholinesterase is acetylcholine acetylhydrolase. Systematic name for cholinesterase (serum/plasma) is acylcholine acylhydrolase). Measurable choline esterase activity in serum belongs nearly exclusively to pseudocholine esterase activity produced in the liver. Because of a lower method specifity (67%) and sensitivity (49%), the tests are evaluated in combination with other activities. Choline esterase synthesis in the liver is connected with albumin synthesis.

Function. Enzyme, splits esters of choline and fatty acids. Enzyme responsible for prompt acetylcholine hydrolysis is released at the nerve endings to mediate neural impulses across the synapse to choline and acetate. CHS degradation is necessary to nerve repolarization so that it can be depolarized in the next conduction event. In the muscles cholinesterase inactivates acetylcholine released at motor nerves end fibres → relaxation of contracted muscles. Atypic choline esterase can induce neuromuscular blockage after anesthetics administration (succinylcholine), rapidly splitting in normal conditions. Although variants A and F are normal in serum, they hydrolyze anesthetics slowly. Variants S, J, K are present in low concentrations so hydrolysis is also disordered.

Test Purpose. 1) to assess liver function and aid in the diagnosis of liver disease, 2) to assess overexposure to insecticides containing organophosphate and carbamate compounds, 3) to detect those who may have adverse reactions to muscle relaxants, 4) to predict, before surgery or electroconvulsive therapy, the patient's response to succinylcholine, 5) to prevent or evaluate prolonged anesthetic effect, prolonged apnea after surgery, 6) to establish patient's baseline value before exposure.

Increased Values

sickle cell anemia, anxiety, diabetes mellitus (II. type), **exudative enteropathy**, hemochromatosis, **benign hyperbilirubinemia** (Gilbert's disease), **hyperthyroidism**, tumors of breast, **nephrosis, obesity**, obese diabetic patients, psychiatric states, **liver steatosis, nephrotic sy**, thyrotoxicosis

Decreased Values

hepatic amebiasis, **anemia, hepatic cirrhosis**, exfoliative dermatitis, **dermatomyositis**, progressive muscular dystrophy, pulmonary embolism, paroxysmal nocturnal hemoglobinuria, **acute/chronic hepatitis**, pregnancy induced hypertension (PIH), hypothyroidism, diseases – (skin d., **infectious d.**, renal d., **liver d., muscular d.**), obstructive jaundice, **cardiac infarction**, intoxication by – (fungi, **organophosphates**, heavy metals), cachexia, chemical military agents – (**sarin, tabun, trilon**), malabsorption, **malnutrition, tumor metastases**, monitoring of nutrition status, tumours, **congenital cholinesterase deficiency**, irradiation, plasmapheresis, undernutrition, severe burns, hepatocellular damage, decreased proteosynthesis, relapse of megaloblastic anemia, sepsis, **conditions after surgeries, trichinellosis, pregnancy** (3rd trimester), congestive heart failure

Interfering Factors: medicaments – (ACHE blockers, anabolic steroids, atropine, caffeine, chlorpromazine, cimetidine, codeine, cyclophosphamide, cytostatics, estrogens, glucocorticoids, iodide, lithium, MAO blockers, neuromuscular relaxants, neostigmine, oral contraceptives, phenothiazines, physiostigmine, procainamide, quinidine, ranitidine, streptokinase, testosterone, theophylline, vitamin K)

Analyte	Age/Gender	Reference Range	SI Units	Note
Cholinesterase (CHE)	Children, adults			
	(M, F >40y)	88–215	μkat/l	
	F 16–39 y	72–187	μkat/l	
	F 18–39 y	52–160	μkat/l	See ref. ranges note

Chromium

(Cr) Metal ultratrace element. Chromium compounds adopt three oxidation states, 3+, 4+ and 6+. The oxidation state determines toxicity, metabolism and excretion. Occupational exposure is related to the industry of steels, photography, pigments, leather tanning, wood preservation solutions, electroplating, plating chemicals and cement. Chromium is present in solutions used for total parenteral nutrition as a contaminant. Cutaneous absorption of hexavalent form has been demonstrated. Pulmonary absorption is related to water solubility. Very little chromium is absorbed in the gut. Trivalent chromium after absorption binds to the beta globulin fraction in serum proteins, specifically to transferrin. Chromium is distributed diffusely in the body with generally higher levels found in kidney, liver, spleen and blood. Chromium is primarily excreted in the urine.

Function. Glucose tolerance factor as part of a trivalent chromium – Cr^{3+} and nicotinic acid complex. Involved in lipid metabolism. Influences insulin action (Cr^{3+}) in peripheral tissues (action on the cell surface). Chromium is an essential micronutrient and is suspected of playing a role in glucose tolerance.

Sources. Meats and whole-grain products are the best chromium sources. Pure metallic chromium is nontoxic. Cr^{6+} is considerably more toxic than Cr^{3+}. Iron competetively inhibits the binding of Cr^{3+} to transferrin. Recommended specimens: serum, urine, hair.

Test Purpose. 1) to evaluate suspected chromium toxicity or exposure, 2) to follow patients who receive chromium for a long time in their parenteral nutrition, 3) to evaluate acquired glucose intolerance in refeeding programs, and in parenteral or enteral nutrition, 4) to evaluate insulin resistance in nonseptic patients during parenteral nutrition.

Increased Values
professional (occupational) **exposure** (Cr^{6+})

Decreased Values
diabetic children, **chromium intake deficiency, kwashiorkor, elder people,** breast feeding, gastrectomy, severe burns, severe injuries, **chronic severe diseases, postsurgery conditions,** alcohol abuse, **excessive stress conditions, malnutrition, insulin resistance in noninsulin-dependent diabetes mellitus** (NIDDM), **pregnancy, impaired glucose tolerance in undernourished children, total parenteral nutrition**

Chromogranin A, B, C

(CgA, CgB, CgC) Chromogranins are ubiquitary acid secretory proteins from the chromogranin/secreto-granin group. They are stored/released from many neuroendocrinous cells and organs creating a so-called disperse neuroendocrine system (DNS). Its activity is a part of tumorous and neurodegenerative processes in the adrenals, chromaffin tissue, thymus, stomach, GIT, pancreas, thyroid, parathyroid and prostate. Chromogranin A (known also as parathyroid secretory protein-1) is costored and coreleased with parathyroid hormone from storage granules in the parathyroid gland in response to hypocalcemia. CgA is also costored and co-released with catecholamines from storage granules in the adrenal medulla. It has been suggested that CgA may play an autocrine role as a glucocorticoid responsive inhibitor regulating the secretion of peptides derived from proopiomelanocortin (POMC). Chromogranin B (known also as secretogranin-1) is a tyrosine-sulfated protein found in a wide variety of peptidergic endocrine cells. Chromogranin B is main part of the prostatosomes. About 50% of prostate cancers contain neuroendocrine cells; less than 2% are of neuroendocrine origin. Similar situations occur with stomach cancer, mammary gland ductal cancer, intraductal papilloma of pancreas, anaplastic neuroendocrine lung cancer, and kidney cancer. Chronic atrophic gastritis type A is connected with fundus neuroendocrine cell stimulation and with CgA increase. Brain CgA is present in areas which are affected with neurodegenerative processes (Alzheimer's disease, Parkinson's disease, Pick's disease). These areas are infiltrated with active neuroglial cells, i. e. resident CNS macrophage population. CgA induces an active microglia phenotype, so involvement in disease pathogenesis is investigated. Urine catecholamines and plasmatic CgA determination is a pheochromocytoma operation radicality indicator (CgA decrease in 24 hrs, CgB in few days). CgA determination in mid-gut carcinoid is more sensitive than 5-HT; it serves as prognostic indicator in combination with the functional reserpine test. Chromogranin C is known as secretogranin-2 present in anterior pituitary and adrenal medulla. It is synthesized by most neuroendocrine cells.

Test Purpose. 1) diagnosis of a disperse neuroendocrine system, pheochromocytoma, neuroblast paraganglioma, medullary thyroid carcinoma, parathyroid carcinoma, thymus and intestinal carcinoid, endocrinous pancreas tumor, 2) diagnosis of prostate, stomach, lung and kidney carcinomas, 3) type A chronic gastritis diagnosis.

Increased Values

tumors – (pheochromocytoma – CgA, parathyroid adenoma – CgA, medullary thyroid t. – CgA, carcinoids – CgA, oat-cell lung t. – CgA, pancreatic islet-cell t. – CgA, aortic-body t. – CgA, stomach t. – CgB, mammary gland ductal t. – CgB, anaplastic neuroendocrine lung t. – CgB, intraductal papilloma of pancreas – CgB, kidney t. – CgB), chronic atrophic gastritis (CgA), diseases – (Alzheimer's d., Parkinson's d., Pick's d.)

Analyte	Age/Gender	Reference Range	SI Units	Note
Chromogranin A and B		10–53	µg/l	

Chylomicrons

Chylomicrons mediate dietary fat transport.
Production. Synthesized and released by the intestinal epithelial cells, they consist of: 7% cholesterol, 7% phospholipids, 84% triacylglycerols, 2% proteins. Chylomicrons do not enter the portal venous system, but traverse the lymphatics into the thoracic duct/or enter

directly into the jugular vein and main systemic circulation → after entry → chylomicrons meet with other triacylglycerol-rich lipoproteins. Action of lipoprotein lipases hydrolyze individual components onto glycerol and free fatty acids → which can then be taken up at the cellular level for energy metabolism or for triacylglycerol resynthesis and stored, or in cell membranes synthesis where they act in receptor and messenger functions or they serve as precursors of important biologically active agents (e. g. leukotrienes). Chylomicrons have 2 types of remnant particles: core remnants containing relatively more cholesterol esters and Apo E and surface remnants, which contain more phospholipids, free cholesterol, and Apo C. Core remnants are taking up by liver via receptor mechanism. Surface remnants are partially transferred onto HDL3 particles and big HDL2 particles are created. Chylomicronemia is physiologically present for a few hours after fatty food intake.

Increased Values – hyperchylomicronemia
- isolated chylomicrons increase: **apolipoprotein C-II defect, familial lipoprotein lipase defect,** dysglobulinemia, systemic lupus erythematosus
- isolated VLDL increase: diabetes mellitus, dysglobulinemia, **familial hypertriacylglycerolemia** (phenotype IR), nephrotic syndrome, uremia
- combined chylomicrons and VLDL increase: decompensated diabetes mellitus, dysglobulinemia, **familial hypertriacylglycerolemia** (phenotype V)
- abnormal VLDL: **familial dysbetalipoproteinemia,** hypothyroidism, systemic lupus erythematosus

---

Chymotrypsin

Serine protease.
Function. Chymotrypsin hydrolyzes peptide bonds which involve carboxyl groups of tryptophan, tyrosine, phenylalanine, leucine.
Production. Acinar cells of the pancreas synthesize two different chymotrypsins (I, II) in an inactive proenzyme form (chymotrypsinogens I, II) → which in the intestinal tract are converted → to chymotrypsin by the trypsin action. Chymotrypsin is plasma bound by alpha-1-antitrypsin and alpha-2-macroglobulin.

Increased Values – hyperchymotrypsinemia
fibrocystic disease, hepatobiliary diseases, tumors – (pancreas t., stomach t.), newborns, **acute pancreatitis,** renal failure

Decreased Values – hypochymotrypsinemia
total pancreatectomy

Circulating Immune Complexes

(CIC) An immune complexes are formed when antibodies combine with soluble antigens circulating in the intravascular space; these circulating immune complexes can be deposited in blood vessels or filtering membranes. Findings must be evaluated with complement levels (activity).

Test Purpose. 1) to demonstrate circulating immune complexes in serum, 2) to monitor therapy response, 3) to estimate disease severity.

Increased Values
medicamentous allergy, **allergic exogenous alveolitis**, arthritis – (Lyme a., **rheumatoid a.**, juvenile rheumatoid a.), allergic bronchial asthma, primary biliary cirrhosis, monoclonal gammopathy, **glomerulonephritis**, **Wegener's granulomatosis**, mixed connective tissue disease, rheumatic diseases, allergic complications, control of desensibilization, **cryoglobulinemia**, systemic lupus erythematosus, polyarteritis nodosa, progression of pulmonary tumours, psoriasis, conditions after – (infectious diseases, immunization, vaccination), syndrome – (Behcet's sy, **Felty's sy**, Reiter's sy, **Sjögren's sy**), scleroderma, ankylosing spondylitis, vasculitis

> **Interfering Factors:** protein denaturation, hypergammaglobulinemia, serum contamination

Decreased Values
agammaglobulinemia, hypogammaglobulinemia

Analyte	Age/Gender	Reference Range	SI Units	Note
Circulating Immune Complexes		<8.8	%	See ref. ranges note
		<0.035		
		<6.1	%	
		<12.8	%	
		<12	mg/l	

Citric Acid

A compound from citrus fruits and intermediate in the tricarboxylic acid Krebs cycle.

Increased Values
diabetes mellitus, hyperparathyroidism, hypervitaminosis D, healing fractures

Decreased Values
rhachitis, idiopathic tetany

Citrulline

Citrulline is formed from ornithine and is itself converted to arginine in the urea cycle. Enzyme defect: argininosuccinyl acid synthetase.

Increased Values – hypercitrullinemia
citrullinemia, pyruvate carboxylase deficiency, liver diseases, lysinuric protein intolerance, ammonia intoxication

Cobalt

(Co) Trace metal element. Human intestine microflora cannot utilize cobalt to synthesize physiologically active cobalamin.
Function. Vitamin B_{12} component.
Test Purpose. Intoxication and occupational exposure diagnosis.

Increased Values – hypercobaltemia
professional (occupational) exposure (hard-metal workers), cardiomyopathy, beer drinkers (cobalt foam stabilizer), renal failure (cobalt treatment as a erythropoietic agent)

Decreased Values – hypocobaltemia
anemia

Analyte	Age/Gender	Reference Range	SI Units	Note
Cobalt		80–170	µmol/l	

Cold Agglutinins

(syn: cool agglutinins) Auto-antibodies, usually of the IgM type, that cause the erythrocytes agglutination in vitro at temperatures in the range 0–10 °C and hemolysis in 20 °C. In vivo temperature activation is in peripheral cutaneous vessels areas. Erythrocytes bind cold agglutinins, agglutinating in the periphery and binding onto the complement (RBC-IgM-C3b complement) and hemolyzing after the transfer into warmer areas. The most frequent specifity is anti-l, less frequent anti-i, anti-Pr, anti-Gd.
Test Purpose. 1) to help confirm primary atypical pneumonia, 2) to provide additional diagnostic cold agglutinin disease evidence associated with viral infections or lymphoreticular malignancies, 3) to help in problems with blood grouping, compatibility testing, 4) to investigate positive direct antiglobulin test, possible autoimmune hemolysis.

Increased Values
anemia – (atypical hemolytic a., hemolytic a., acquired idiopathic autoimmune hemolytic a. – AIHA), **liver cirrhosis,** pulmonary embolism, **acute/chronic disease from cool agglutinins,** peripheral vascular disease, influenza, bronchopulmonary infection caused by Mycoplasma pneumoniae** (primary atypical pneumonia), cytomegalovirus infection, **viral infections, infectious mononucleosis, malaria,** mumps, measles, tumors – (lymphatic leucemia, lymphoproliferative t., lymphoreticular t., **plasmocytoma** – incl. multiple myeloma, **lymphoma,** reticular sarcoma, **thymic t.**), paroxysmal hemoglobinuria, pneumonia, psittacosis, rheumatic fever, **scleroderma, staphylococcemia, congenital syphilis,** syndrome – (Raynaud's sy, secondary sy from cool agglutinins), **scarlatina,** pregnancy, **trypanosomiasis**

Colony-Stimulating Factors

(CSF) Belong to the cytokines – soluble proteins secreted by monocytes, lymphocytes, macrophages, mastocytes, neutrophils, eosinophils, epithelial cells, endothelial cells, fibroblasts regulating the inflammatory or immune response magnitude. GM-CSF is glycated protein; monomer located on the 5th chromosome near the IL-3, 4, 5 genes. CSFs production is boosted by endotoxin and antigen; they are required continuously to stimulate cellular division. GM-CSF and G-CSF have synergistic influence on neutrophil granulocyte maturation. These factors are absolutely required for the proliferation of hematopoietic progenitor cells. Chronic overproduction leads to tissue destruction. GM-CSF substitution is an important therapeutic agent used after chemotherapy and bone marrow transplantation, in HIV induced neutropenia, aplastic anemia, and hematologic malignant diseases. The secreted factors have an extremely high specific biological activity and are active at very low concentrations.

Function and Effects. **GM-CSF** (granulocyte-macrophage CSF): myeloid stem cell hematopoietic factor, growth of granulocyte and erythroid progenitors, their proliferation and differentiation, macrophage activation; increases eosinophil leukotriene production; increases monocyte tumoricidal activity. It stimulates the proliferation and differentiation of neutrophilic, eosinophilic and monocytic lineages. Enhances cytotoxic and phagocytic neutrophils activity against bacteria, fungi and antibody-coated tumor cells. Inhibits neutrophilic mobility. In granulocytes GM-CSF stimulates the release of arachidonic acid metabolites and the increased generation of reactive oxygen species. Phagocytotic activities of neutrophil granulocytes and the cytotoxicity of eosinophils is also enhanced considerably by GM-CSF. It can be employed for the physiological reconstitution of hematopoiesis in all diseases characterized either by an aberrant maturation of blood cells or by a reduced production of leukocytes. The main and most important clinical application of GM-CSF is probably the treatment of life-threatening neutropenia following chemo- and/or radiotherapy, which is markedly reduced under GM-CSF treatment. **G-CSF** (granulocyte CSF): granulocyte growth, stimulates leukocytosis, enhances neutrophil migration. **M-CSF** (macrophage CSF): monocyte and macrophage growth, increases macrophage antitumor activity.

Complement

Complements are components of humoral immune system. Serum complements comprises a group of glycoproteins that facilitate immunological and inflammatory responses. The so-called complement cascade involves series of enzymatic reactions that take place in the blood and tissue fluids. Complements bind to aggregated IgG, undergo proteolysis, trigger inflammatory response (chemoattractants), solubilize immune complexes to aid in clearance. Complements are markers for intrinsic/extrinsic pathway functions. There are 9 major components labeled C1 through C9. The cascade can be initiated by various means, especially antigen-antibody complexes. The end-product of the activation cascade is the so-called membrane attack unit – MAC (also called terminal complement component), that produces transmembrane channels in the membranes of attacking microorganisms (e. g. gram negative bacteria), thereby causing lysis and death of the cells. CH50 or CH100 are 50% or 100% of „whole" complement activity. There are also a number of side products of the complement cascade that can label other organisms and attract white blood cells and increase the efficiency to engulf bacteria for removal by phagocytic white blood cells. Two different pathways that respond to different factors are available to initiate activation (known as „fixation" for historical reasons). The evolutionarily oldest arm, the alternative pathway, is activated by cell wall components of gram negative bacteria or fungi. The other method of fixing complement is known as the classical pathway. This pathway is activated by antibody bound to a target. The two pathways are considered to be common after C3 since both the substrate and the products are the same. When many microorganisms are exposed to fresh serum, complement is activated by an alternative pathway, that does not require the presence of specific antibodies to the microorganism. These organisms are able to bind C3 directly. Bound C3 (or some modified form of C3b) is able to associate with factor B, held together by Mg ions. This complex is the substrate for an enzyme, factor D that splits B into Ba and Bb. Another component, properdin (or Factor P), binds to the complex and stabilizes it. A stable unit is capable of continuing the complement cascade and is identical to the classical pathway. Alternative pathway differs in that it is initiated by endotoxin (lipopolysaccharide), a component of the cell walls of gram negative bacteria. It may also be initiated by zymosan, a component of yeast cell walls, or by aggregated IgA.

Increased Values – hypercomplementemia
inflammatory conditions that increase acute-phase reactants

Decreased Values – hypocomplementemia
systemic lupus erythematosus, mixed connective tissue disease, **cryoglobulinemia, vasculitis**, short bowel disease, rheumatoid vasculitis, recurrent infectious diseases, septic shock, glomerulonephritis – (acute poststreptococcal g., membranoproliferative g.), subacute bacterial endocarditis, X-linked hypogammaglobulinemia, hereditary angioedema, familial Mediterranean fever, severe combined immunodeficiency, liver failure, severe malnutrition, pancreatitis, prodromal HBV hepatitis, Wegener's granulomatosis, severe burns, Sjögren's syndrome, serum sickness, **atheromatous embolization**

Analyte	Age/Gender	Reference Range	SI Units	Note
Complement				
classical pathway				
components				
– C1r		0.025–0.038	g/l	
– C1s		0.025–0.038	g/l	
– C2	Umbilical blood	0.016–0.028	g/l	
	1 m	0.019–0.039	g/l	
	6 m	0.024–0.036	g/l	
	Adults	0.016–0.040	g/l	
– C3	Umbilical blood	0.570–1.160	g/l	
	1–3 m	0.530–1.310	g/l	
	3 m – 1 y	0.620–1.800	g/l	
	1–10 y	0.770–1.950	g/l	
	Adults	0.830–1.770	g/l	
– C4	Umbilical blood	0.070–0.230	g/l	
	1–3 m	0.070–0.270	g/l	
	3 m – 10 y	0.070–0.400	g/l	
	Adults	0.150–0.450	g/l	
– C5	Umbilical blood	0.034–0.062	g/l	
	1 m	0.023–0.063	g/l	
	6 m	0.024–0.064	g/l	
	Adults	0.038–0.090	g/l	
– C6	Umbilical blood	0.010–0.042	g/l	
	1 m	0.022–0.052	g/l	
	6 m	0.037–0.071	g/l	
	Adults	0.040–0.072	g/l	
– C7		0.049–0.070	g/l	
– C8		0.043–0.063	g/l	
– C9		0.047–0.069	g/l	
– CH50 (total hemolytic activity)		75–160	IU/ml	

Ba, Bb Complement

Ba, Bb complements belong to the complement components (split products). Factor B is cleaved by factor D during alternative pathway activation, generating the two fragments Ba and Bb.

Increased Values
rheumatoid arthritis, congenital deficiency of factor H or I, systemic lupus erythematosus, burns, gram-negative bacterial sepsis, trauma

C1 Complement

The first component of the classical complement pathway. Most of the circulating C1 complement is produced by intestinal epithelial cells. C1 complement biological activity: virus neutralization. C1 binding to antigen bound IgG and IgM initiates the classical pathway.

Increased Values
acute phase response

Decreased Values
acquired angioedema, autoimmune diseases, cryoglobulinemia, lymphopenia, severe malnutrition, circulating immune complexes increase

C1q Complement

Belongs to the classical complement pathway components. C1q complement binds to immunoglobulin in immune complexes. C1q complement is produced by epithelial cells (mainly in intestine, lungs).

Increased Values
kala-azar (Leishmania donovani infection)

Decreased Values
inherited C1q complement deficiency, **X-linked hypogammaglobulinemia**, autoimmune diseases, **systemic lupus erythematosus**, infancy, cryoglobulinemia, lymphopenia, acquired angioedema, severe combined immunodeficiency, increase in circulating immune complexes

C1r Complement

Belongs to the classical complement pathway components.

Decreased Values
rheumatoid arthritis, diseases – (autoimmune d., immune-complex d., renal d.), infectious diseases – (bacterial i. d., recurrent i. d., viral i. d.), **systemic lupus erythematosus**, severe burns, severe trauma

C1s Complement

(syn: C1-esterase) Belongs to the classical complement pathway components. Serum C1s complement is synthesized by intestine and bladder epithelial cells, fibroblasts, monocytes and macrophages.

Decreased Values
rheumatoid arthritis, **C1s complement deficiency**, diseases – (autoimmune d., immune-complex d., renal d.), infectious diseases – (bacterial i. d., recurrent i. d., viral i. d.), systemic lupus erythematosus, severe burns, severe trauma

C2 Complement

Belongs to the classical complement pathway components. C2 complement is synthesized by hepatocytes, monocytes and macrophages.

Increased Values
acute phase response

Decreased Values
hereditary/acquired **angioedema**, rheumatoid arthritis, bacteremia, **C2 complement deficiency**, diseases – (autoimmune d., **immune-complex d.**, renal d.), recurrent infections, lupus nephritis, systemic lupus erythematosus, severe malnutrition, severe burns, severe trauma, viremia
   Interfering Factors: infancy

C3 Complement

Production. C3 is synthesized in liver, macrophages, fibroblasts, lymphoid cells and skin.
Function. Complement is activated by IgG or IgM in the classic pathway. In the alternate pathway by toxins (including endotoxin) and by aggregated IgA. C3 component is a central whole complement system protein. A part of complement system – the body's defense mechanism against infections (defends against gram-negative bacteria). Complement creates a serie of more than 20 plasma proteins (glycoproteins) that bind to antigen-antibody complexes in a specific sequence (cascade) and contribute to humoral immunity via opsonization, phagocytosis, and complement fixation. Complement system activation results in cell lysis, histamine release from mast cells and platelets. Supports phagocytosis, increases vascular permeability, increases smooth muscle contraction, increases leukocytes chemotaxis, increases antibody to antigen immune adherence, plays a role in autoimmune disease → these processes are vitally important in the inflammatory response.
Test Purpose. 1) to help detect immunomediated disease and genetic complement deficiency, 2) to monitor therapy effectiveness, 3) to detect complement activation in SLE, glomerulonephritis and other immune complex diseases.

Increased Values – hypercomplementemia
amyloidosis, **rheumatoid arthritis**, **diabetes mellitus**, gout, viral hepatitis, **rheumatic fever**, diseases – (inflammatory bowel d., inflammatory d., bacterial infectious d., rheumatic d.),

obstructive jaundice, myocardial infarction, ulcerative colitis, tumors, pneumococcal pneumonia, acute phase reaction, sarcoidosis, syndrome – (nephrotic sy, Reiter's sy, pregnancy, typhoid fever, **thyroiditis**

Interfering Factors: medicaments – (corticosteroids)

Decreased Values – hypocomplementemia induced by immunocomplexes production
AIDS, **autoimmune hemolytic anemia**, arteritis temporalis, **rheumatoid arthritis**, babesiosis, liver cirrhosis, gram-negative/positive bacteremia, dermatomyositis, bacterial endocarditis, endotoxemia, glomerulonephritis – (**acute g.**, **membranoproliferative g.**, poststreptococcal g.), hereditary angioedema, Wegener's granulomatosis, paroxysmal nocturnal hemoglobinuria, hepatitis – (h. B, chronic active h.), hypogammaglobulinemia, malignant tumours chemotherapy – (lymphoma), disease – (**immune-complex d.**, acute serum d.), diseases – (**infectious d.**, pyogenic infectious d., parasitic d., inflammatory d.), severe recurrent bacterial infections caused by the homozygote C3 deficiency, systemic candidiasis, **increased complement catabolism**, **disseminated intravascular coagulation**, essential cryoglobulinemia, **hepatic cells lesion**, **partial lipodystrophy**, lupus erythematosus – (discoid l. e., **systemic l. e.**), **malaria**, **malnutrition**, bacterial meningitis, **lupus nephritis**, weakened immune defence, measles, parasitemia, plasmocytoma (incl. multiple myeloma), polyarteritis nodosa, polymyalgia rheumatica, bacterial pneumonia, severe burns, medicamentous hypersensitivity – (cyclophosphamide, chlorpropamide, kalium iodatum, sulfasalazine), purpura – (anaphylactoid p., Henoch–Schönlein p.), **renal transplant rejection**, bacterial sepsis, septicemia, tissue necrosis/injury, scleroderma, ankylosing spondylosis, **Sjögren's sy**, insufficient complement synthesis, trypanosomiasis, thyroiditis, trauma, uremia, **vasculitis**, viremia

Interfering Factors: infancy

Decreased Values – hypocomplementemia without immunocomplexes production
hepatic cirrhosis, embolization, pancreatitis acuta, porphyria, severe nutrition disorders, hereditary causes, thrombocytic–thrombocytopenic purpura, hemolytic–uremic sy, hepatic failure

---

C3a Complement

C3a complement belongs to the complement components (split product). It is a basic peptide. It represents about 6% of the C3 protein mass. C3a complement is one of the anaphylatoxin activity complement fragments. It induces vascular permeability increase, smooth muscle contraction, histamine, serotonin and other mediator release from tissue mast cells and other inflammatory cells. C3a complement is rapidly inactivated by the anaphylatoxin inactivator.

Increased Values
factor H or I congenital deficiency, systemic lupus erythematosus, extracorporeal blood circulation, patients on hemodialysis, patients with the autoantibodies against C3-nephritic factor, burns, sepsis, trauma

---

C4 Complement

Production. A glycoprotein synthesized in the lungs and bone.

Function. Supports phagocytosis. Increases vascular permeability. It is involved in virus neutralization. See also C3 complement.

Test Purpose. To detect complement activation in SLE, glomerulonephritis and other immune complex diseases.

Increased Values
rheumatoid arthritis, **bacterial infections**, **tumors**, acute phase reactions, inflammatory diseases, ulcerative colitis

Decreased Values
autoimmune hemolytic anemia, **rheumatoid arthritis**, deficiency – (alpha-1-antitrypsin d., **inborn C4 complement d.**), bacterial infectious diseases, liver cirrhosis, hepatitis, juvenile dermatomyositis, **hereditary angioneurotic edema**, **bacterial endocarditis**, **glomerulonephritis**, hypergammaglobulinemia, disease – (**immune–complex d.**, serum d.), liver diseases, **cryoglobulinemia**, **systemic lupus erythematosus**, **malaria**, meningitis – (bacterial m., viral m.), **lupus nephritis**, malnutrition, renal transplant rejection, pneumonia, hepatic cells lesion, **anaphylactoid purpura**, sepsis – (staphylococcal s., streptococcal s.), adult respiratory distress sy, autoimmune thyroiditis, vasculitis

   Interfering Factors: infancy, medicaments – (oral contraceptives)

C4a Complement

C4a complement belongs to the complement components (split product). It is a basic peptide that split from C4 complement during classical pathway complement activation. C4a complement has activity similar to C3a but less potent.

Increased Values
congenital/acquired C1-esterase inhibitor deficiency, autoimmune processes involving immune complexes, sepsis

---

C4d Complement

C4d complement belongs to the complement components (split product). It is generated from C4b through further cleavage by factor I. C4d complement represents an end-stage breakdown C4 activation product and can be used as a marker specific for classical pathway activation.

Increased Values
rheumatoid arthritis, congenital C1-esterase inhibitor deficiency, hepatic dysfunction, systemic lupus erythematosus, chronic urticaria with hypocomplementemia

---

C5 Complement

C5 complement belongs to the complement components (terminal pathway component). It is a beta-1-globulin, similar in structure to C3 and C4 complements.

Decreased Values
congenital C5 complement deficiency, immune-complex disease, diseases – (bacterial infectious d., liver d.), systemic lupus erythematosus, burns, trauma, uremia
    Interfering Factors: medicaments – (steroids)

C5a Complement

C5a complement belongs to the complement components (split product). It is released from C5 complement by C5-convertase or by many other enzymes including neutrophil elastase, kallikrein and activated Hageman's factor. C5a is a potent chemotactic factor, anaphylatoxin, and is rapidly inactivated in serum by the anaphylatoxin inactivator.

Increased Values
inherited factor H or I deficiency, hemodialysis, extracorporeal blood circulation, burns, sepsis, trauma

C6 Complement

C6 complement belongs to the complement components (terminal pathway component). It is a glycoprotein, that is synthesized primarily in the liver. It participates in the membrane attack complex of both classical and alternative pathways. Involved in membrane damage, cell lysis.

Decreased Values
congenital C6 complement deficiency, immune-complex disease, diseases – (bacterial infectious d., liver d.), burns, trauma, uremia
    Interfering Factors: medicaments – (steroids)

C7 Complement

C7 complement belongs to the complement components (terminal pathway component). It is a glycoprotein synthesized primarily in the liver. It plays a role in the membrane attack complex formation of both classical and the alternative complement activation pathways. Involved in membrane damage, cell lysis.

Decreased Values
congenital C7 complement deficiency, immune-complex disease, diseases – (bacterial infectious d., liver d.), burns, trauma, uremia
    Interfering Factors: medicaments – (steroids)

C8 Complement

C8 complement belongs to the complement components (terminal pathway component). It is a protein. The liver is the major site of its synthesis. Involved in membrane damage, cell lysis.

Decreased Values
congenital C8 complement deficiency, immune-complex disease, diseases – (bacterial infectious d., liver d.), burns, trauma, uremia
   Interfering Factors: medicaments – (steroids)

C9 Complement

C9 complement belongs to the complement components (terminal pathway component). It is a single protein, the final membrane attack complex constituent. C8 complement initiates the polymerization of at least six C9 molecules in the cell membrane forming the membrane attack complex, which destroys the osmotic integrity of the target cell membrane. C9 is involved in membrane damage and cell lysis. C9 has a long tail that extends through the membrane. When C8 induces the polymerization of C9, it forms a transmembrane channel. The channel lets fluid from the extracellular space rush in due to osmotic pressure, and the cell swells up and eventually ruptures. The C9 tail is soluble only in lipid membranes, so the complete membrane attack complex forms only in gram negative bacteria and animal cells. Gram positive bacteria and fungi are resistant to lysis, but the chemotactic, anaphylatoxic, and opsonic split products are important in eliminating many of these potential pathogens.

Increased Values
rheumatoid arthritis, degenerative joint diseases, systemic lupus erythematosus, acute phase response

Decreased Values
congenital C9 complement deficiency, immune-complex disease, diseases – (bacterial infectious d., liver d.), burns, trauma

CH50 Complement

Functional complement activity determination by the classical method, complex information about all classical complement activation cycle compounds (C1 through C9).
Test Purpose. 1) to evaluate and follow-up systemic lupus erythematosus patient's response to therapy, 2) to screen for complement component deficiency, evaluate complement activity in immune-complex disease, glomerulonephritis, rheumatoid arthritis, and cryoglobulinemia.

Increased Values
acute inflammatory diseases, **acute phase reaction,** trauma

Decreased Values
rheumatoid arthritis, congenital complement components deficiency, membranoproliferative glomerulonephritis, immune-complex disease, diseases – (autoimmune d., infectious d., liver d.), **complement consumption caused by coagulation,** cryoglobulinemia, tumors, severe burns, **insufficient complement compounds production, trauma**

Connective Tissue Growth Factor

(CTGF) Factor is produced by human umbilical vein endothelial cells. CTGF is produced by skin fibroblasts after activation with TGF-beta. It may play a role in the development and progression of atherosclerosis since mRNA and protein are expressed in human arteries in vivo at high levels specifically in advanced lesions. The factor has been shown to induce the proliferation, migration and tube formation of vascular endothelial cells in vitro, and angiogenesis in vivo.

Copper

(Cu, cuprum) Trace metal element, essential micronutrient.

Function. Enzyme component and co-factor (cytochrome oxidase, superoxide dismutase, tyrosinase, dopamine, betahydroxylase, lysyl oxidase, ceruloplasmin, factor V). These enzymes have catalytic roles in melanin synthesis, collagen and elastin cross-linking, iron metabolism, neuronal metabolism, catecholamine conversions. Involved in hemopoiesis, bone production. Copper is bound to proteins. From 40–60% of ingested copper is absorbed by the gut → transported to the liver → complexed to albumin and selected amino acids → stored in hepatocytes, primarily as a cuproprotein. Copper is released into the blood by the liver → incorporated mainly into the blue copper protein ceruloplasmin, the serum ferrooxidase that oxidizes iron prior to plasma transferrin binding. Ceruloplasmin binds about 65% of copper in peripheral blood. Absorbed copper is primarily excreted through the biliary tract (enterohepatic circulation) and gastrointestinal secretions. The renal tubules efficiently reabsorb most of the filtered copper making urinary excretion low. Inorganic copper is very reactive and therefore a cellular toxin. Zinc, cadmium, molybdenum and iron inhibit copper absorption. Highest values are after meals, day-to-day variation is 5%, lowest are in AM, highest in midafternoon. Recommended specimens: serum, cerebrospinal fluid, tissue, urine.

Test Purpose. 1) to screen Wilson's disease along with serum ceruloplasmin and urine copper, 2) to monitor the nutritional adequacy of parenteral or enteral nutrition (gastrointestinal losses), 3) to aid in copper toxicity diagnosis, 4) Menkes' sy diagnosis.

Increased Values – hypercupremia
anemia – (pernicious a., aplastic a., iron-deficiency a., megaloblastic a. of pregnancy), **rheumatoid arthritis, biliary cirrhosis,** hepatolenticular degeneration (Wilson's disease), **smoking,** glomerulonephritis, **hemochromatosis,** hepatitis, **rheumatic fever, hyperthyroidism, hypopituitarism, hypothyroidism, intrahepatic cholestasis,** diseases – (**infectious d., biliary tract d., acute/chronic inflammatory d.**), obstructive icterus, **acute/chronic copper toxicity,** infarction – (brain i., myocardial i.), collagenoses, complications of – (renal dialysis, neonatal transfusion), lactation, **systemic lupus erythematosus,** Addison's disease, tumors – (bone t., cervix t., **leukemia, lymphomas, Hodgkin's disease,** lung t., breast t., hematopoietic system t., gastrointestinal tract t.), pellagra, ankylosing spondylitis, **pregnancy** (3rd trimester), thalassemia minor/major, tuberculosis, typhoid fever, trauma

> **Interfering Factors: elder age,** medicaments – (carbamazepine, estrogens, oral contraceptives, phenobarbital, phenytoin, progesterone, testosterone)

Decreased Values – hypocupremia
anemia, coeliac disease, hepatic cirrhosis, heavy exercise, **hepatolenticular degeneration** (Wilson's disease), diet – (**prolonged total milk d. in infants,** vegetarian d.), **dysproteinemia,** cystic fibrosis, hemochromatosis, persistent infantile diarrhea, chronic diarrhea, long-term

hyperalimentation in adults and infants, **hereditary hypocupremia** (Menkes' kinky hair disease), chronic ischemic heart disease, small bowel diseases, hemolytic jaundice, **kwashiorkor**, **zinc therapy for sickle cell disease**, Bechterew's disease, acute leukemia in remission, **malabsorption**, **malnutrition**, **marasmus**, nephrosis, **premature newborn**, burns, **sprue**, **nephrotic sy**, total parenteral nutrition

   Interfering Factors: medicaments – (penicillamine, zinc salts)

Analyte	Age/Gender	Reference Range	SI Units	Note
Copper	Neonates			
	– premature	2.7–7.7	μmol/l	
	– mature	8.3–11.2	μmol/l	
	Children	10.3–21.4	μmol/l	
	Adults F	12.4–20.6	μmol/l	
	Adults M	11.6–19.2	μmol/l	

Corticosteroid-Binding Globulin

(CBG, syn: cortisol-binding globulin, transcortin) CBG is a glycoprotein primarily synthesized in the liver, binding/transporting cortisol, corticosterone, progesterone, 17-alpha-hydroxy-progesterone and testosterone (to a lesser degree). Its molecular weight is similar to albumin m. w.

Test Purpose. Suspicion of inborn CBG defect.

Increased Values
chronic active hepatitis, ovarian hyperfunction, pregnancy

   Interfering Factors: medicaments – (anticonvulsants, estrogens, lynestrenol, oral contraceptives)

Decreased Values
familial CBG deficiency, hyperthyroidism, ovarian hypofunction, diseases – (chronic liver d., inflammatory d.), nephrosis, fetal death, protein-losing conditions, septic shock, complicated pregnancy

   Interfering Factors: medicaments – (testosterone)

Analyte	Age/Gender	Reference Range	SI Units	Note
Corticosteroid Binding Globulin		28–52	mg/l	

Corticosterone

Increased Values
adrenal adenomas, congenital 18-hydroxylation defect with salt-losing sy, adrenogenital sy with 17-hydroxylase deficiency

Cortisol

(syn: hydrocortisone, serum cortisol, total cortisol).

Production. Main suprarenal cortex glucocorticoid (21-C-corticosteroid), adrenal steroid hormone in plasma bound to cortisol-binding globulin – CBG (about 80%) and albumin (about 10%), 3–10% is in free form. Cortisol is synthesized from cholesterol and secreted by the adrenal cortex in response to corticotropin (ACTH).

Function. 1) carbohydrates metabolism: increases glycogen content in the liver, glucose production, hepatic gluconeogenesis, enhances glucose synthesis from amino acids and fatty acids, decreases peripheral glucose utilization, stimulates the glycolysis. 2) lipid metabolism: increases lipolysis and fatty acids level, decreases glycerol production. 3) protein metabolism: proteolysis, catabolic effects, antianabolic effects by inhibiting amino acid entry into muscles. Normal response to stress. Cortisol has anti-inflammatory effects, inhibits immunologic responses (immunosuppression). Inhibits prostaglandin synthesis, leukotriene synthesis, histamine, bradykinin and SRS-A (slow reacting substance of anaphylaxis) effects. Elicits lymphocytopenia, monocytopenia, eosinopenia. Free cortisol fraction reflexes its determination in saliva. Inhibits fibroblasts activity in skin (healing wound impairment). Inhibits insulin effect – antagonizes insulin (increases cellular resistance to insulin, which leads to decreased glucose entry into cells). Positive inotropic effect on heart, permissive effect on catecholamine action.

Hypophyseous hormone. ACTH. The 17-hydroxysteroids (17-OHCS) are the main cortisol metabolites excreted in urine. Cortisol levels exhibit circadian rhythm (maximum levels are between the rising time and 9 AM, minimum are around midnight to 4 AM). Day-to-day level variation is 15%.

Test Purpose. To aid in Cushing's disease, Cushing's sy, Addison's disease and secondary adrenal insufficiency diagnosis. It is recommended to measure cortisol daily profile with sampling at 7–8 AM, 12 AM, 4–6 PM, 12 PM, or as a functional tests part (ACTH, CRH, dexamethasone).

Increased Values – hypercortisolemia

adrenal adenoma, acute adrenal crisis, heavy smokers, **hyperthyroidism**, chronic active hepatitis, diseases – (generalized d., severe infectious d.), **Cushing's disease** (basophilic pituitary gland adenoma), tumors, **ectopic ACTH-producing tumors, obesity**, operation, small-cell lung cancer, multiple endocrine neoplasia I (MEN I), acute psychosis, stress – (emotional s., physical s.), **Cushing's sy**, chronic renal failure

> **Interfering Factors:** postprandial, **pregnancy** (3rd trimester), medicaments – (ACTH, amphetamines, carbamazepine, estrogens, ethanol, ether, hydrocortisone, interferon gamma, mepacrine, methoxamine, metoclopramide, metoprolol, naloxone, oral contraceptives, prednisolone, prednisone, spironolactone, tricyclic antidepressants, vasopressin)

Decreased Values – hypocortisolemia

suprarenal apoplexy, congenital cortisol-binding globulin deficiency, congenital adrenal hyperplasia, **central hypocorticism, hypopituitarism, hypothyroidism**, diseases – (autoimmune d., **liver d.**), **primary adrenal insufficiency** (Addison's disease), secondary suprarenal insufficiency – (chromophobe adenoma, hypophysectomy, craniopharyngioma, pituitary necrosis, postpartum), **hemorrhage**, malnutrition, tumors, syndrome – (adrenogenital sy, nephrotic sy), **tuberculosis**, renal failure

> **Interfering Factors:** medicaments – (aminoglutethimide, androgens, barbiturates, beclomethasone, betamethasone, danazol, dexamethasone, dextrose, etomidate, levodopa, lithium, methylprednisolone, metyrapone, morphine, oxazepam, phenytoin, prednisone – long-term, prednisolone – long-term, propranolol)

Analyte	Age/Gender	Reference Range	SI Units	Note
Cortisol	7–8 AM	0.14–0.60	µmol/l	
	4–7 PM	0.08–0.46	µmol/l	
	Midnight	0.03–0.11	µmol/l	
	Children – AM	0.14–0.40	µmol/l	

Creatine

An amino acid formed by guanidinoacetic acid methylation. Protein metabolism product in muscle (endogenous creatine) + food intake (exogenous creatine).

Production. Kidney, liver, pancreas → transported in the blood to muscles and nervous tissue.

Function. Creatine is the substrate from which the high-energy phosphate compound creatine phosphate is synthesized by enzyme creatine kinase action. Creatine + ATP ← creatine kinase → creatine phosphate + ADP.

Increased Values – hypercreatinemia
rheumatoid arthritis, cardiac decompensation, progressive muscular dystrophy, **hyperthyroidism**, generalized muscular diseases, renal insufficiency, myasthenia gravis, nephritis, high dietary intake, intestinal obstruction, poliomyelitis, **severe muscular trauma**

   Interfering Factors: medicaments – (testosterone)

Decreased Values – hypocreatinemia
diabetic ketoacidosis (false)

   Interfering Factors: medicaments – (cefoxitin, cimetidine)

Analyte	Age/Gender	Reference Range	SI Units	Note
Creatine	1–14 w	16.8–95.4	µmol/l	
	Adults	12.2–30.5	µmol/l	

Creatine Kinase

(CK, syn: total creatine kinase, creatine phosphokinase – CPK, CP) Creatine kinase production is regulated by 3 different genes, the gene products are named CK-B, CK-M and CK-Mi. Serum activity is realized by cytoplasmic dimers CK-MM, CK-MB and CK-BB. In healthy people the total activity is determined mainly by CK-MM, other isoenzymes and variants are only traces. Variants are relatively frequent, they are divided according to molecular weight.

Function. Enzyme that catalyzes the phosphate group transfer from creatine-phosphate in ADP to yield creatine and ATP – the main usable energy source.

Occurrence. Cytoplasm, mitochondria, skeletal muscle, brain tissue, colon smooth muscle, small intestine, uterus, prostate, lungs and kidneys.

Isoenzymes. 1) **Muscular** MM (CK-3, MM-3, MM-2, MM-1) – major component of all serum samples (94–96%): skeletal muscle (99% of all creatine kinases), cardiac muscle (77%), lungs (26%), spleen (74%), salivary gland (44%), liver (99%), pancreas (14%); 2) **myocardial** MB (CK-2, MB-2, MB-1) – (4–6% of all serum components): myocardium (22%), diaphragm; 3) **cerebral** BB (CK-1, MM-1): brain (100%), nervous tissue, thyroid gland (85%), prostate (93%), kidneys (92%), pancreas (85%), lungs (73%), stomach (95%), uterus (96%), intestine (96%), colon (95%), bladder (92%). Two other CK variants have been described: a) macro-

CK-1 – a CK-BB-IgG or CK-BB-IgA complex, b) macro-CK-2 – a mitochondrial CK. Differential diagnosis of variants is considered relatively often and can be done in regular laboratories. Enzyme tumour marker (CK-BB).

Test Purpose. 1) to detect and diagnose acute MI and reinfarction, 2) to evaluate possible chest pain causes and to monitor the myocardial ischemia severity after cardiac surgery, cardiac catheterization or cardioversion, 3) to detect skeletal muscle disorders that are not neurogenic in origin, such as Duchenne muscular dystrophy and early dermatomyositis, 4) to monitor tricyclic antidepressants cardiotoxic effects, 5) to assess neurological diseases with disordered hematoencephalic barrier – surgery, trauma, hemorrhage, 6) to assess hematological diseases, tumor diseases, upper gastrointestinal tract diseases.

Isoenzymes. 1) to detect or provide early myocardial infarction confirmation, 2) to evaluate reperfusion therapy, 3) newborn screening for muscular dystrophy, 4) testing of carriers, 5) neonatal asphyxia, 6) hypothyroidism, 7) therapy check-up of some oncological diseases.

Increased Values

drug abuse – (phencyclidine, cocaine, lysergide), chronic alcoholism, angina pectoris, **percutaneous transluminal angioplasty, cardiac defibrillation, delirium tremens, acute aortic dissection, dermatomyositis,** dysrhythmia, **pulmonary edema,** electrocardioversion, **electromyography, pulmonary embolism, encephalitis, malignant hyperpyrexia,** hypophosphatemia, **hypokalemia, hypothermia, hypothyroidism,** diseases – (degenerative d., acute cerebrovascular d.), muscular diseases/myopathies – (**progressive muscular dystrophy, myotonic dystrophy, myositis, polymyositis**), prolonged immobilization, infarction – (intestine i., **cerebrum i., lung i.**), **myocardial infarction** (increase 3–12 hrs, maximum at 12–48 hrs, decrease 2–4 d), central nervous system infections, poisoning by – (hypnotics, benzene, xylene, carbon dioxide, carbon monoxide), **central nervous system ischemia, alcoholic cardiomyopathy,** cardiac catheterization, ketoacidosis, coronarography, **subarachnoid hemorrhage, McArdle's disease, meningitis, myocarditis, myxedema,** tumours – (CNS t., colon t., lymphomas, uterus t., bladder t., lung t., prostate t., breast t., testes t.), gastrointestinal tract t.), surgery – (neurosurgery, prostate s., heart s., gastrointestinal tract s.), **pericarditis,** cerebral disorders, cerebrovascular accidents, **muscular polytrauma, burns, psychosis, rhabdomyolysis,** sectio Cesarea (Caesarean section), **sepsis, amyotrophic lateral sclerosis, status epilepticus,** conditions – (**c. following seizures, shock c.,** hemolytic c.), syndrome – (eosinophilia–myalgia sy, diabetic nephrotic sy, **Reye's sy**), **tachycardia, pregnancy,** tetanus, trauma – (central nervous system t., **electric current t.,** thermal t., thorax t., cranium t., **heart t.**), failure – (**renal f.,** congenital heart f.), crush injury, **vigorous physical exercise,** myoglobinuria, familial hypokalemic periodic paralysis

> **Interfering Factors:** intramuscular injections, persons with large muscle mass, athletes, medicaments – (acetylsalicylic acid, aminocaproic acid, amphotericin B, ampicillin, anesthetics, anticoagulants, barbiturates, captopril, carbenoxolone, chlorpromazine, chlortalidone, cimetidine, clindamycin, clofibrate, clonidine, clopamide, colchicine, dexamethasone, diazepam, digoxin, ethanol, etretinate, furosemide, gemfibrozil, haloperidol, halothane, isotretinoin, labetalol, lidocaine, lithium, morphine, penicillamine, perphenazine, phenytoin, pindolol, prochlorperazine, propranolol, quinidine, salicylates, secobarbital, streptokinase, tricyclic antidepressants)

Increased Values – isoencymes

MM (CK-3, MM-3, MM-2, MM-1) – alcoholism, delirium tremens, dermatomyositis, muscular dystrophy, electromyography, pulmonary embolism, acute psychotic episode, hemophilia, malignant hyperpyrexia, hypokalemia, prolonged hypothermia, hypothyroidism, myocardial infarction (high sensitivity and specificity of test), intramuscular injections, poisoning with coma, **electroconvulsive therapy, myocarditis, myositis,** tumours – (colon t., rectum t., lymphoma, bladder t., liver t., lung t., prostate t., breast t., sarcoma, ovary t., stomach t.), pericarditis, **polymyositis, rhabdomyolysis,** conditions – (**convulsion c., c. after surgery,** shock c.), Reye's sy, direct-current countershock, **tachycardia, tetanus,** injury – (head i., brain i., **muscular i., crush i.**), extreme exercise, congestive heart failure

MB (CK-2, MB-2, MB-1) – acromegaly, **unstable angina pectoris,** abuse – (drug a., alcohol a.), bacterial infectious diseases caused by – (Staphylococcus, Streptococcus, Clostridium, Borrelia), coronary angiography, **percutaneous transluminal angioplasty, cardiac defibrillation,** cardiomyopathy – (hypothyroid c., alcohol c.), diabetic ketoacidosis, **protracted dysrhythmia,** dystrophy – (**muscular d., Duchenne's muscular d.**), **hyperthermia, malignant hyperthermia,** hypoparathyroidism, **hypothermia,** hypothyroidism, hyperthyroidism, acute exacerbation of obstructive lung disease, acute cholecystitis, diseases – (infectious d., fungal infectious d., collagen vascular d.), **myocardial infarct** (increase 3–12 hrs, peaking at 12–24 hrs, decrease 72 hrs), poisoning – (carbon monoxide p.), myositis, **myocardial ischemia, subarachnoid hemorrhage,** systemic lupus erythematosus, myoglobinuria, **myocarditis,** parasitic infectious diseases – (trichinosis, toxoplasmosis, schistosomiasis, cysticercosis), tumours – (colon t., rectum t., lymphoma, bladder t., liver t., lung t., **prostate t., breast t.,** sarcoma, ovary t., stomach t.), surgery, open heart surgery, **polymyositis, rhabdomyolysis, Reye's sy, circulatory/cardiogenic shock,** cardio-pulmo-cerebral resuscitation, collagen diseases involving myocardium, prolonged tachycardia, **skeletal muscle trauma, extreme exercise,** failure – (**circulatory f., chronic renal f.**), Rocky Mountain spotted fever, electrical injuries, familial hypokalemic periodic paralysis, burns, viral infectious diseases – (HIV, Epstein–Barr virus, influenza, picornaviruses, coxsackie virus, echoviruses, adenoviruses)

   Interfering Factors: medicaments – (acetylsalicylic acid, halothane, ipecacuanha, tranquilizers)

BB (CK-1) – **anoxia, biliary atresia, aortocoronary bypass, pulmonary embolism,** chronic hemodialysis, **malignant hyperthermia, hypothermia,** infarction – (**pulmonary i.,** mesenterial tract i., brain i.), necrosis of intestine, intestinal ischemia, **subarachnoid hemorrhage, electroconvulsive therapy,** tumors – (**adenocarcinoma, gut t.,** gastrointestinal tract, cervix t., uterus t., bladder t., **brain t.,** liver t., **lung t., prostate t., breast t.,** colon t., lymphomas, testes t., **ovary t.**), **newborn,** surgery – (neurosurgery, prostatic s., gastrointestinal tract s.), **critical care patient,** acute pancreatitis, **cerebrovascular accident** (stroke), syndrome – (**Reye's sy, severe shock sy**), pregnancy, injury – (**head i., brain i.**), **chronic renal failure,** seizure conditions, uremia.

Decreased Values

prolonged bedrest, sedentary lifestyle, alcoholism, pregnancy (1st trimester), metastatic tumors, intensive care unit patients with severe infection/septicemia, hyperthyroidism (untreated), Cushing's disease, alcoholic liver disease, multiple organ failure, malnutrition, rheumatoid arthritis, connective tissue disease, toxins, poisoning by – (insecticides)

   Interfering Factors: elder people, medicaments – (estrogens, ethanol, oral contraceptives, phenothiazines, prednisone, steroids, tamoxifen)

Analyte	Age/Gender	Reference Range	SI Units	Note
Creatine Kinase, Total	1 d	<11.9	μkat/l	
	2–5 d	<10.9	μkat/l	
	6 d–6 m	<4.92	μkat/l	
	7–12 m	<3.38	μkat/l	
	1–3 y	<3.80	μkat/l	
	4–6 y	<2.48	μkat/l	

Analyte	Age/Gender	Reference Range	SI Units	Note
	7–12 y F	<2.57	µkat/l	
	7–12 y M	<4.12	µkat/l	
	13–17 y F	<2.05	µkat/l	
	13–17 y M	<4.50	µkat/l	
	Adults F	<2.78	µkat/l	
	Adults M	<3.17	µkat/l	
Creatine Kinase MB Mass (CK-MB)		<5	µg/l	
Creatine Kinase MB (CK-MB)		<0.40	µkat/l	
Creatine Kinase				
isoenzymes CK-MM		0.97–1.00	µkat/l	
isoenzymes MB		<0.03	µkat/l	
isoenzymes BB		0		
Creatine Kinase				
isoforms MB$_2$/MB$_1$		≤1.5		
isoforms MM$_3$/MM$_1$		≤0.7		
isoform MB$_2$		<2.0	U/l	

Creatinine

Degradation muscle energy metabolism product excreted entirely by the kidney (glomerular filtration), not reabsorbed in the tubules. Creatine-phosphate change end product (creatine catabolism in skeletal muscle). Creatinine concentrations in the serum and urine are governed predominantly by the lean body mass (skeletal muscles) and are slightly affected by diet changes or other factors. The kidneys excrete creatinine very efficiently. Blood flow and urine production levels affect creatinine excretion much less than they affect urea excretion, because temporary alterations in blood flow and glomerular activity are compensated by increased tubular creatinine secretion in urine. The properties have made creatinine the most popular analyte for glomerular filtration determination (renal excretory function). Highest values are in the evening and at night, day-to-day variation is 15–20%.

Test Purpose. 1) to assess renal glomerular filtration in suspected renal function injury in a pathologically changed urine finding in acute or chronic renal disease, hypertension, extrarenal diseases which are secondary influencing the renal function, 2) to screen renal damage, 3) to assess metabolic diseases like hyperuricemic sy, diabetes mellitus, 4) to assess the condition with increased proteosynthesis (plasmocytoma), 5) to assess potential nephrotoxic medicaments indication and dosage, 6) screening and preoperative examination, 7) intensive and postoperative cares monitoring, 8) extrarenal diseases with fluid loss (diarrhea, vomiting), 9) patients on dialysis, 10) pregnancy, especially with complications, 11) malignant tumors monitoring, 12) drug addicts examination, 13) urogenital (genitourinary) system diseases evaluation.

Increased Values – hypercreatininemia
acromegaly, atherosclerosis, salt depletion, **severe dehydration, diabetes mellitus, dialysis program,** thyroid dysfunction, **gigantism, glomerulonephritis, hyperthyroidism,** adrenal hypofunction, diseases – (febrile d., **chronic renal d.**), obstructive icterus, ileus, insufficiency – (**acute/chronic renal i.**, cardiac i.), acetone intoxication, catabolism, coma, leukemia, myasthenia gravis, **myodystrophy, nephritis,** nephropathy, **acute tubular necrosis,** obstruc-

tion – (**urinary ways o.**, intestine o.), decreased renal perfusion, **burns**, functional renal disorders, **pyelonephritis, rhabdomyolysis, shock**, pregnancy, **acute muscular injury**, failure – (**acute/chronic renal f., congestive heart f.**), obstructive uropathy

Interfering Factors: high meat diet, uric acid, medicaments – (acebutolol, acetylsalicylic acid, aciclovir, allopurinol, amikacin, amiloride, aminoglycosides, aminohippuric acid, amoxicillin, amphotericin B, ampicillin, arginine, ascorbic acid, azapropazone, benzyl-penicillin, capreomycin, captopril, carbutamide, cefaclor, cefaloridine, cefamandole, cefazolin, ceforanide, cefoxitin, ceftazimide, cefuroxime, cephalosporins, cephalotin, chlor-propamide, chlortalidone, cimetidine, cisplatin, clindamycin, clometacin, colistin, cotrimoxazole, cyclosporine, diltiazem, diuretics, enalapril, enflurane, fenclofenac, feno-fibrate, fenoprofen, flucytosine, fructose, furosemide, gentamicin, glucose, gold salts, halothane, hydantoin, hydralazine, ibuprofen, indomethacin, levodopa, lidocaine, lith-ium, methoxyflurane, methyldopa, meticillin, mezlocillin, mitomycin, naproxen, neph-rotoxic medicaments, netilmicin, nifedipine, nitrofurantoin, oral contraceptives, oxacil-lin, oxyphenbutazone, paracetamol, paramethadione, paromomycin, penicillamine, penicillin, pentamidine, phenacemide, phenacetin, phenylbutazone, phenytoin, pipera-cillin, piroxicam, polymyxin B, quinine, ramipril, ranitidine, rifampicin, streptokinase, sulfamethoxazole, sulfinpyrazone, sulindac, suprofen, tobramycin, trimethoprim, van-comycin, vasopressin, zimeldine)

Decreased Values – hypocreatininemia
anemia, **muscular dystrophy, myasthenia gravis, pregnancy** ($1^{st}/2^{nd}$ trimester), decreased muscle mass, **ageing**

Interfering Factors: hyperbilirubinemia, hemoglobin, lipemia, medicaments – (ACTH, cephalotin, ibuprofen, N-acetylcysteine, nifedipine)

Analyte	Age/Gender	Reference Range	SI Units	Note
Creatinine	Neonates	<106	µmol/l	
	<6 m	<80	µmol/l	
	>7 m	<88	µmol/l	
	Adults F	<80	µmol/l	
	Adults M	<97	µmol/l	
	Neonates	<115	µmol/l	See ref. ranges note
	<1 w	<88	µmol/l	
	2–4 w	<44	µmol/l	
	Adults F	<97	µmol/l	
	<50 y M	<115	µmol/l	
	>50 y M	<124	µmol/l	

Cryoglobulins

Cryoglobulins are abnormal serum protein complexes (a result of immunoglobulins polym-erization), that undergo reversible precipitation at low temperatures (4 °C) and redissolve when rewarmed (37 °C). These cryoglobulins can precipitate within the finger blood ves-sels when exposed to cold temperatures. This precipitation causes red blood cell sludging within those blood vessels → Raynaud's phenomenon. Cryoglobulins can be divided into 3 groups: type I – no specificity (monoclonal immunoglobulin, IgM-k, IgG, IgA) in plasmo-cytoma, Waldenström's disease, chronic lymphatic leukemia; type II – anti-IgG specificity (mixed type, mono/biclonal immunoglobulin, IgM-k, IgG, IgA) in autoimmune diseases, lymphoproliferative diseases; type III – IgG specificity (mixed type, polyclonal immunoglobulin, IgM) in systemic lupus erythematosus, Sjögren's sy, lymphoproliferative diseases. From cryoglobulins must be separated cryofibrinogen (it appears in stomach, prostate and ovary tumors) and other proteins, like heparin-precipitable fibrinogen complexes, CRP with albumin, or lipoprotein complex with immunoglobulin. Additionally, cryoglobulins can de-monstrate cryoprecipitability as well as rheumatoid activity and binding with cool agglutinins.

Test Purpose. 1) to detect cryoglobulinemia in patients with Raynaud-like vascular symptoms, 2) differential diagnosis of peripheral neuropathies, 3) vasculitides differential diagnosis, 4) cutaneous hemorrhage differential diagnosis.

Increased Values – positive, hypercryoglobulinemia
hemolytic anemia, **rheumatoid arthritis, liver cirrhosis,** endocarditis – (**infective e.,** suba-cute e.), **post-streptococcal glomerulonephritis,** hepatitis – (**chronic active h., viral h.), cytomegalovirus disease, autoimmune diseases,** kala-azar, ulcerative colitis, **essential cryo-globulinemia, leprosy, chronic lymphocytic leukemia, systemic lupus erythematosus, lym-phoma,** lymphosarcoma, **Waldenström's macroglobulinemia, infectious mononucleosis, tumors, plasmocytoma** (incl. multiple myeloma), **polyarteritis nodosa,** sarcoidosis, syphi-lis, syndrome – (nephrotic sy, tropical splenomegaly sy, **Sjögren's sy**), collagen–vascular dis-ease, m. Hodgkin
   Interfering Factors: elder people

Analyte	Age/Gender	Reference Range	SI Units	Note
Cryoglobulins		<80	mg/l	

Cryptococcal Antigen

A negative result does not exclude infection. Antigen levels decrease with effective therapy.
Test Purpose. 1) to help in cryptococcal infection diagnosis, 2) to monitor response to therapy.

Increased Values – positive
Cryptococcosis, cryptococcal meningitis

3, 5-Cyclic Adenosine Monophosphate

(3,5-AMP, syn: adenosine 3,5-cyclic monophosphate – cAMP) cAMP is a neurotransmitter.
Function. Belongs to the 2nd messenger system → carries the hormonal message from the cell membrane to the nucleus. Enzyme adenylate-cyclase converts adenosine triphosphate (ATP) to → cAMP, which activates specific phosphorylating enzymes or protein kinases to produce → the physiological response, cAMP mobilizes resources. Insulin reduces cAMP levels. Epinephrine, norepinephrine and glucose raise cAMP levels. Highest levels appear at noon and the lowest at night, lower in an upright position, highest in spring, lowest in winter.

Increased Values
calcium malabsorption, calcium urolithiasis, exercise, high-protein diet, hypercalcemia in malignancy, manic disorders, obesity, osteomalacia due to vitamin D deficiency, primary hyperthyroidism, pseudohypoparathyroidism
   Interfering Factors: childhood, medicaments – (ACTH, ADH, epinephrine, glucagon, parathormone, phenothiazines, prostaglandins, theophylline, thyrotropin, xanthines)

Decreased Values

depression, ethanol, hypoparathyroidism

    Interfering Factors: medicaments – (probenecid)

Analyte	Age/Gender	Reference Range	SI Units	Note
Cyclic Adenosine Monophosphate	M	17–33	nmol/l	
	F	11–27	nmol/l	

Cyclic Guanosine Monophosphate

(cGMP) Present in plasma as a result of natriuretic peptides (ANP, BNP, CNP) action. Measurement of cGMP helps to evaluate the status of cardiac natriuretic system (ANP, BNP) and vascular natriuretic system (CNP). cGMP evaluation is used also during exercise testing in cardiac patients.

Function. Belongs to the 2nd messenger system of natriuretic peptides.

Test Purpose. 1) to confirm congestive heart failure, 2) to identify asymptomatic cardiac volume overload, 3) to evaluate chronic dialysis program and hydratation status, 4) to evaluate water balance disorders.

Increased Values

cardiovascular diseases with elevated cardiac filling pressure, atrial pacing, **asymptomatic cardiac volume overload**, paroxysmal atrial tachycardia, failure – (renal f., **congestive heart f.**)

Cyclosporine

For bone marrow transplant, the therapeutic intervals vary with the type of transplant (ie. allogeneic, unrelated, syngeneic). The role of therapeutic monitoring is less well established in autoimmune diseases. Monitoring is indicated only if high doses of cyclosporine are used. An elevated result provides an early indication of the toxicity possibility.

Test Purpose. 1) to help in maintenance of therapeutic levels of cyclosporine in patients receiving immunosuppressives, usually to avoid rejection of organ transplants, 2) to detect toxic levels.

Increased Values

cyclosporine overdose

Cystatine C

Cystatine C is a small protein, which does not contain saccharide constituent. It belongs to the particular group of proteins which create amyloid (prealbumin, apolipoprotein A-I, beta-2-microglobulin). Synthesis is not changed in inflammation. It is a low molecular weight protein, its stable level of production is used in GFR measurement and is a better indicator of GFR than creatinine.

Increased Values

diseases – (autoimmune systemic d., renal d.), diseases connected with a very high bilirubin levels

Analyte	Age/Gender	Reference Range	SI Units	Note
Cystatine C	0–50 y	0.63–1.33	ng/l	
	>50 y	0.94–1.55	ng/l	

Cysteine

(Cys) Cysteine is a sulfur-containing nonessential amino acid that is synthesized from methionine. Produced by the digestion or acid hydrolysis of proteins, in the presence of oxygen, two molecules of cysteine are oxidized to form cystine (Cys-Cys, 3,3-dithiobis (2-aminopropionic acid)). Cysteine is the chief sulfurcontaining compound of the protein molecule.

Enzyme defect: defective lysosomal membrane protein.

Increased Values – hypercysteinemia
cystinosis, **sepsis**, chronic renal failure

Decreased Values – hypocysteinemia
protein malnutrition, **after abdominal surgery** (1–2 days)

Cytokine Inhibitors

Cytokine inhibitors are cytokine-specific substances that inhibit the biological activities of specific cytokines in a number of different ways. These proteins probably function to buffer or limit the effects of cytokines as part of a regulatory network. In principle such a specific inhibitor could be an antagonist binding to the same receptor and competing for receptor binding with the genuine cytokine. Another class of cytokine inhibitors of cytokine action are non-specific binding proteins that do not interfere with binding of the cytokines to their respective receptors. One protein capable of binding unspecifically to several cytokines is alpha-2-macroglobulin.

Cytokine Receptor Families

Type-1 cytokine receptor family (IL-2, IL-3, IL-4, IL-5, IL-6, IL-7, IL-9, IL-11, IL-12, GM-CSF, G-CSF, Epo, receptors for thrombopoietin, growth hormone and prolactin). Type-2 cytokine receptor family (IFN-alpha, IFN-beta, IFN-gamma, IL-10 and tissue factor). Forms of the cytokine receptors: membrane-bound and soluble forms. The soluble receptor forms may arise by proteolytic cleavage of transmembrane receptors or by utilizing alternatively spliced receptor mRNAs. They may act as inhibitors of cytokine activities or in a retrocrine fashion.

Cytokines

Cytokine is a generic term for nonantibody proteins released by one cell population on contact with specific antigens acting as intercellular mediators as in immune response generation; they are involved in inflammatory response, amplitude regulation and response duration of these effects. Cytokines belong to low-molecular weight glycoproteins; they are present in lymphatic tissue, peripheral blood cells, monocyte line cells, keratinocytes, fibroblasts, endothelial cells and thymic epithelial cells. The cytokines are a diverse group of proteins, but they share a number of properties. They are produced by lymphoid cells in response to non-specific mitogenic stimulants and specific antigenic stimulants. Once synthesized, the cytokines are rapidly secreted, but their presence is short-lived. Cytokines are non-specific and antigen-independent in activity mode. Their action is autocrine (binding to the same cytokine secreting cell) or paracrine (binding to a adjacent cell). Cytokines posses a great biological potency at low concentrations. They also may have multiple different effects on the same target cell. They react with many different target cell types directly (pleiotropism) through high-affinity cell surface receptors specific for each cytokine/group. Many receptors have two polypeptide chains – a cytokine-specific alpha-chain and a signal-transducing beta-chain. Inflammatory cells (neutrophils, macrophages and lymphocytes) and non-inflammatory cells (endothelial cells, fibroblasts and osteoclasts) belong to target cells. Cytokines co-operate through a network by interconnected induction, transmodulating cytokine cell surface receptors, synergic/antagonistic/additive interaction on cell functions.

Tumor necrosing factors. TNF-alpha, TNF-beta.

Colony stimulating factors. G-CSF (granulocytes colony-stimulating factor), GM-CSF (granulocytes macrophages colony-stimulating factor), M-CSF (macrophages colony-stimulating factor), multi-CSF (IL-3).

Chemokines. IL-8, MCP-1, 2, 3 (monocyte chemoattractant protein, monocyte chemotactic protein, monocyte chemotactic protein and activating factor), MIP-1 (macrophage inflammatory protein), MIP-2, NAP-2 (neutrophil activating protein), PF-4 (platelet factor), beta-TG (beta-thromboglobulin), GCP-2 (granulocyte chemotactic protein), SDF-1-alpha/beta (stromal cell-derived factors), lymphotactin, PBP (platelet basic protein), CTAP-III (connetive tissue-activating protein-3), eotaxin (eosinophil-active chemokine), ENA-78 (epithelial-derived neutrophil attractant 78), MGSA/GRO (melanoma growth-stimulating activity/growth-related oncogen alpha), IP-10 (gamma interferon-inducible protein 10), MIG (monokine induced by interferon gamma), RANTES (regulated on activation, normal T-cell expressed and secreted).

Chemokines involved in hemopoiesis. MIP-1-alpha, MIP-1-beta, MIP-2-alpha, IL-8, IL-10, PF-4.

Interferons (antiviral cytokines). IFN-alpha, IFN-beta, IFN-gamma, IFN-omega, IFN-theta.

Interleukins. IL-1 to IL-18.

Lymphokines. HRFs (histamine releasing factors), LMF (lymphocytic mitogen factor), LMIF (leukocyte migration inhibiting factor), MAF (macrophages activating factor), MCF (macrophage chemotactic factor), MMIF (macrophage migration inhibiting factor), TF (transfer factor), TFN (T-cell fibronectin).

Polypeptide growth factors. ECGF (endothelial cells growth factor), EGF (epidermal growth factor), FGF (fibroblast growth factor), NGF (nerve growth factor), PDGF (platelet-derived growth factor), PD-ECGF (platelet-derived endothelial cell growth factor, gliostatin), SCF (stem cell growth factor, mast cell growth factor, steel factor), VEGF (vascular endothelial growth factor, vasculotropin, vascular permeability factor).

Stress proteins. GRPs (glucose regulated proteins), heme oxidase, HSP 10 (heat shock proteins), HSP 27, HSP 47, HSP 60, HSP 70, HSP 90, HSP 110, SOD (superoxide dismutase), ubiquitine.

Cytokines involved in cellular immunity (Th-1 type). IL-2, IFN-gamma, GM-CSF, TNF.

Cytokines involved in humoral immunity (Th-2 type). IL-4, IL-5, IL-9, IL-10, IL-13.

Other. Lymph nodes permeability factor, suppressor factors, angiogenin, erythropoietin, MGSA (melanoma growth stimulating activity), HGF (hepatocyte growth factor, scatter factor, hematopoietin A), ILGF-I, II (syn. MSA – multiplication stimulation activity), IP-10, LIF (leukemia inhibitory factor, differentiating stimulating factor, DSF), LMW-BCGF (low molecular weight B-cell growth factor), OSM (oncostatin M).

Proinflammatory cytokines of 1st phase activation. Alarm cytokines (IL-1, TNF-alpha), endogenous pyrogens (IL-1, IL-6, TNF-alpha, MIP), inflammatory reaction stimulation (IL-1, IL-6, TNF-alpha, IFN-alpha, IFN-beta, chemokines), stimulation of acute phase protein production (IL-1, IL-6, IL-11, TNF-alpha, IFN-gamma, TGF-beta, LIF, CNTF, OSM).

Proinflammatory cytokines of 2nd phase activation (chemotactic). IL-2, 4, 5, 6, 8, PF4, PBP, NAP-2, beta-TG, MIP-1-alpha, MIP-1-beta, MCP-1, MCP-2, MCP-3, lymphotactin, G-CSF, GM-CSF, M-CSF, IL-1, IL-3, IL-12.

Cytokines supporting growth of hemopoietic cells. IL-3, GM-CSF, M-CSF, G-CSF, erythropoietin, thymic hormones, LIF (leukemia inhibiting factor), SCF (stem cell growth factor), TPO (thrombopoietin).

Cytokines involved in hemopoiesis inhibition. Lactoferrin, TNF-alpha, TNF-beta, IFN-alpha, IFN-beta, inhibin, oncostatin M, LIF, TGF-beta.

Cytokines – interleukins which potentiate hemopoietic factor effects. IL- (1, 2, 4, 6, 7, 9, 11, 12, 13).

Regulatory cytokines. IL – (2, 4, 10), IFN.

Anti-inflammatory cytokines. Proinflammatory cytokine production inhibition IL- (4, 10, 13).

Defensins

Defensins are small basic unglycosylated proteins which are found mainly in segmented neutrophilic granulocytes. They constitute approximately 30–50 percent of all proteins of azurophilic granules. Defensins are released from granules by transport into vacuoles generated after ingestion of microorganisms. They destroy these microorganisms in an oxygen-independent manner by permeabilization of the outer and inner membrane. Defensins also possess a nonspecific cytotoxic activity against a wide range of normal and malignant cells, including cells that are resistant to TNF-alpha and natural killer cytotoxic factor. They kill cells by inserting themselves into the cell membrane, permeabilizing the membranes by the creation of voltage-regulated channels. The family of defensins is diverse and is not restricted to expression in leukocytes. Human defensin 5 is expressed highly in Paneth cells of the small intestine. The existence of enteric defensins suggests that these peptides contribute to the antimicrobial barrier function of the small bowel mucosa, protecting the small intestine from bacterial overgrowth by autochthonous flora and from invasion by potential pathogens that cause infection via the peroral route, such as Salmonella species. Defensins are specific potent chemoattractants for monocytes. HNP-1, the most abundant representative of human defensins, has been found to form very stable complexes with alpha-2-macroglobulin which may function as a scavenger of defensins in inflamed tissues and may constitute an important mechanism for the regulation and containment of inflammation.

Dehydroepiandrosterone

(syn: unconjugated DHEA, dehydroisoandrosterone) Main androgen steroid, adrenal cortex hormone, in peripheral tissues changes into effective androgen testosterone. It is the major androgen precursor in females and the major androgen precursor in postmenopausal women. DHEA does not circulate bound to SHBG and is only weakly androgenic. Day-to-day variation is 30%, highest levels are in AM and lowest in PM.

Increased Values
endurance runners, **bilateral hyperplasia of adrenal cortex, hirsutism, Cushing's disease, ectopic ACTH-producing tumors, adrenal tumours**, neonates, oligomenorrhea, syndrome – (**adrenogenital sy, Cushing's sy, polycystic ovary sy**), virilism

Interfering Factors: medicaments – (clomiphene, corticotropin)

Decreased Values
hyperlipidemia, adrenal hypoplasia, hypogonadism, **adrenal cortex insufficiency**, malnutrition, psoriasis, psychosis, Cushing's sy, pregnancy
   Interfering Factors: elderly people, medicaments – (androgens, carbamazepine, danazol, glucocorticoids, ketoconazole, phenytoin, testosterone)

Analyte	Age/Gender	Reference Range	SI Units	Note
Dehydroepi-androsterone	M			
	<9.8 y	1.07–11.96	nmol/l	
	9.8–14.5 y	3.81–17.16	nmol/l	
	10.7–15.4 y	5.89–20.28	nmol/l	
	11.8–16.2 y	5.55–22.19	nmol/l	
	12.8–17.3 y	8.67–31.21	nmol/l	
	Adults	5.55–27.74	nmol/l	
	F			
	<9.2 y	1.07–11.96	nmol/l	
	9.2–13.7 y	5.20–19.76	nmol/l	
	10.0–14.4 y	6.93–20.80	nmol/l	
	10.7–15.6 y	6.93–24.27	nmol/l	
	11.8–18.6 y	7.45–29.47	nmol/l	
	Adults	5.55–27.74	nmol/l	

Dehydroepiandrosterone Sulfate

(DHEA-S) This test is used to evaluate the function of the adrenal glands (index of adrenal androgen secretion). Highest levels are in AM and lowest in PM.
Test Purpose. 1) measurement of a fertility work-up, 2) to evaluate children with precocious puberty, 3) to screen for rare genetic diseases resulting from deficient steroid-synthetic enzymes.

Increased Values
hirsutism, **congenital adrenal hyperplasia**, Cushing's disease, ectopic ACTH-producing tumors, adrenal cortex tumors, polycystic ovary sy
   Interfering Factors: exercise, smoking, fasting, medicaments – (ACTH, clomiphene, danazol)

Decreased Values
dieting, ethanol, acute illnesses, adrenal insufficiency – (primary a. i., secondary a. i.), malnutrition, **pregnancy**
   Interfering Factors: medicaments – (carbamazepine, dexamethasone, glucocorticoids, ketoconazole, oral contraceptives, phenytoin, prednisone, testosterone)

Analyte	Age/Gender	Reference Range	SI Units	Note
Dehydroepi-androsterone Sulphate	M			
	<9.8 y	0.34–2.16	μmol/l	

Analyte	Age/Gender	Reference Range	SI Units	Note
	9.8–14.5 y	1.09–2.83	µmol/l	
	10.7–15.4 y	1.25–5.20	µmol/l	
	11.8–16.2 y	2.65–10.01	µmol/l	
	12.8–17.3 y	3.12–9.62	µmol/l	
	Adults	4.68–11.70	µmol/l	
	F			
	<9.2 y	0.49–2.96	µmol/l	
	9.2–13.7 y	0.88–3.35	µmol/l	
	10.0–14.4 y	0.83–8.48	µmol/l	
	10.7–15.6 y	1.51–6.76	µmol/l	
	11.8–18.6 y	1.14–6.45	µmol/l	
	Adults	1.56–7.7	µmol/l	

11-Deoxycorticosterone

(DOC) A mineralocorticoid produced in small quantities by the adrenal cortex. DOC increases to maximum value in pregnancy from the 23rd week to term. Highest levels are in AM and lowest in PM.

Increased Values
adrenogenital syndromes due to 17- and 11-hydroxylase deficiencies, **pregnancy**
    Interfering Factors: medicaments – (metyrapone, spironolactone)

Decreased Values
preeclampsia

11-Deoxycortisol

(syn: compound S) An intermediate formed in cholesterol conversion to cortisol in steroidogenesis. Day-to-day level variation is 20–30%.

Increased Values
adrenocortical hyperplasia due to 11-beta-hydroxylase defect, adrenal tumors, pregnancy
    Interfering Factors: medicaments – (metyrapone)

Decreased Values
    Interfering Factors: medicaments – (glucocorticoids, megestrol, phenytoin)

Digoxin

Digoxin half-life is 20–50 hours, prolonged with renal impairment. The therapeutic interval is approximate, toxicity can occur at lower levels, especially if there is associated hypokalemia.
Test Purpose. To assess suspected digoxin toxicity or inadequate response.

Increased Values
digoxin toxicity

Analyte	Age/Gender	Reference Range	SI Units	Note
Digoxin		1.0–2.6	nmol/l	

Dopamine

Belongs to catecholamine.

Function. CNS neurotransmitter, inhibitory transmitter in the carotid body and the sympathetic ganglia. Dopamine elicits many responses not attributable to the stimulation of classic adrenergic receptors: it relaxes the lower esophageal sphincter, delays gastric emptying, causes vasodilation in renal and mesenteric arterial circulations, suppresses aldosterone secretion, directly stimulates renal sodium excretion, suppresses norepinephrine release in sympathetic nerve terminals by a presynaptic inhibitory mechanism.

Increased Values – hyperdopaminemia
ganglioneuroma, neuroblastoma
   Interfering Factors: medicaments – (dopamine)

Decreased Values – hypodopaminemia
Parkinson's disease

Analyte	Age/Gender	Reference Range	SI Units	Note
Dopamine		196–553	pmol/l	

Drug Allergies Detection

Penicillins: benzylpenicillin, phenoxymethylpenicillin, ampicillin, amoxicillin, cloxacillin, flucloxacillin, ticarcillin
Cephalosporins: cephalotin, cefaclor, cephalexin
Other antibacterials: trimethoprim, sulfamethoxazole, cinoxacin
Anesthetic agents: alcuronium, atracurium, succinylcholine, vecuronium, rocuronium, thiopentone
Narcotics: morphine, codeine
Local anesthetics: procaine, lignocaine
Analgesics: paracetamol
Other: latex

Drug Monitoring

Acetaminophen, alcohol, aminophylline, amiodarone, amitriptyline, benzodiazepines, bromide, butabarbital, butalbital, caffeine, carbamazepine, carotene, chlordiazepoxide, clonazepam, cyclosporine, desipramine, diazepam, dicumarol, digitoxin, digoxin, disopyramide, doxepin, ethchlorvynol, ethosuximide, flecainide, flunitrazepam, folate, fluoride, glutethimide, gold, imipramine, isopropanol, lidocaine, lithium, mephobarbital, meprobamate, methaqualone, methotrexate, methsuximide, methyprylon, mexiletine, nitroprusside, nordiazepam, nortriptyline, paracetamol, pentobarbital, phenobarbital, phenytoin, primidone, procainamide, propoxyphene, propranolol, quinidine, salicylates, secobarbital, theophylline, thiocyanate, thioridazine, tocainide, trazodone, trifluoperazine, valproic acid

Antibiotics: amikacin, chloramphenicol, flucytosine, gentamicin, kanamycin, netilmicin, streptomycin, sulfadiazine, sulfamethoxazole, sulfapyridine, sulfisoxazole, tobramycin, vancomycin

Elastase

Functionally belonging to the alpha-1-antitrypsin complex, elastase is an endopeptidase, found in leukocytes, endothelium, pancreatic juice and minimally in serum. Secreted by the pancreas as the proenzyme proelastase and activated in the duodenum via trypsin cleavage, it is involved in protein digestion. It catalyzes the peptide bond cleavage, preferentially on the carboxyl side of leucine, methionine and phenylalanine residues. Unlike other endopeptidases, elastase rapidly hydrolyzes elastin, the yellow elastic connective tissue scleroprotein. Protein of acute phase. PMN-elastase of granulocytes is an important restenoses development indicator after PTCA (2nd – 6th week). PMN-elastase is a neutral lysosomal proteinase. Due to a low substrate specifity and high levels, PMN-elastase has a removal role. After the release into serum it bonds to the alpha-1-proteinase inhibitor (alpha-1-antitrypsin) for the body protection. Only this complex can be measured in the plasma. Elastase II-I is produced in the pancreas; present in young individuals, its activity decreases with age (involved in milk protein digestion). Elastase II-I is secreted with four other proteases, mainly with chymotrypsin. Duodenal and fecal elastase-1 is a sensitive non-invasive test in chronic pancreatitis detection (sensitivity is higher than fecal chymotrypsin sensitivity). Elastase-1 is released in cycles (1 cycle per 150 minutes). In chronic pancreatitis cycle amplitude decreases, not cycle frequency. Sensitivity in moderate and mild conditions is better than with chymotrypsin. Elastase levels are not influenced by substitution therapy (when compared to fecal chymotrypsin).

Test Purpose. 1) septic shock conditions, 2) surgical trauma, polytrauma, 3) joint inflammatory diseases (sensitivity is higher than ESR and other inflammation indicators), 4) intrauterine amniotic infections, 5) cystic fibrosis, pancreatitides, 6) meningitides, 7) artificial material biocompatibility (extracorporal circulation device, dialysis machine), 8) male adnexes infections, 9) adult respiratory distress syndrome diagnosis, 10) diagnosis of Crohn's disease, ulcerative colitis, and non-specific intestinal inflammation (remission/worsening indicator; sensitivity is higher than ESR and other inflammation indicators, except CRP).

Increased Values – hyperelastasemia
rheumatoid arthritis, embolism, rheumatic fever, chorioamnionitis, diseases – (**rheumatic d., inflammatory d.**), **cardiac infarction,** infectious diseases – (**bacterial i. d., neonatal i. d., respiratory system i. d., viral i. d.**), systemic lupus erythematosus, non-specific marker of pulmonary tumours, tumours – (bronchi t., Burkitt's lymphoma, leukemia, t. of pancreas), obstruction of biliary ways, severe surgeries and after surgery, acute/chronic pancreatitis, **inflamed pneumopathy, polytrauma, pyelonephritis, transplant rejection,** sepsis, stress, syndrome – (**adult respiratory distress sy – ARDS,** nephrotic sy), **vasculitis**

Analyte	Age/Gender	Reference Range	SI Units	Note
Elastase	Neonates			
	1–2 d	<75	μg/l	
	3–28 d	<50	μg/l	
	Adults	29–86	μg/l	
Elastase II-1, Pancreatic		<3.5	ng/ml	

Beta-Endorphins

(beta-END) Polypeptides (31-amino acid opioid peptide derived from proopiomelanocortin – POMC) and central neurons neurotransmitter (hypothalamus, amygdala, thalamus, locus coeruleus). After release and interaction with peptidergic (opioid) receptors → hydrolysis by peptidases to smaller inactive peptides and amino acids. Plasma levels show a circadian pattern that is synchronous with that of ACTH. In addition to being an analgesic, beta-endorphins are known to modulate secretion and release of many hormones. Stimulate lymphocytes proliferation. Highest values are in AM and lowest in PM.

Increased Values
electroconvulsive therapy, newborns (during first 24 h of life), obesity, surgery, labor, emotional/physical stress, pregnancy, **physical exercise**, renal failure
  Interfering Factors: ethanol, caffeine, fasting, postprandial

Decreased Values
body weight loss, pregnancy
  Interfering Factors: medicaments – (glucocorticoids, oral contraceptives)

Endothelins

Endothelins belong to cytokines creating in endothelial cells and epithelial cells. The synthesis of endothelins by vascular endothelial cells is increased by bacterial endotoxins, bombesin, thrombin, IL-1, TGF-beta, PDGF, angiotensin and vasopressin. The known endothelin receptors are strongly glycosylated glycoproteins which show a high degree of sequence homology.

Function. Endothelins are mainly known for their pharmacological activities. They are the most potent vasoconstrictors known. They are potent positively inotropic and chronotropic agents for the myocardium. They are involved in vasoconstriction, vasodilation, cellular population proliferation stimulation (mainly smooth muscle cells). Endothelins increase the plasma levels of a number of vasoactive hormones. They increase the secretion of ANP, aldosterone and catecholamines. They reduce renal blood flow and glomerular filtration. The production of endothelins by epithelia, smooth muscle and fibroblasts of the urinary bladder suggests that they may act as an autocrine hormone in the regulation of the bladder wall structure and smooth muscle tone. In addition to their vasoconstrictor actions, endothelins have effects on the central nervous system and on neuronal excitability. They induce the depolarization of spinal neurons, the release of vasopressin and oxytocin, and may be involved in the response of glial cells to tissue injuries. Endothelins act as paracrine modulators of smooth muscle cells and connective tissue cell functions. In human mammary carcinomas endothelins are paracrine growth modulators for mammary stromal cells. They stimulate the proliferation of smooth muscle cells, fibroblasts, mesangial cells, established glioma cells lines and primary astroglial cells. Endothelins are autocrine growth modulators for several human tumor cells lines. Endothelin-1 secreted from human keratinocyes is a mitogen for human melanocytes and may play an essential role in the UV hyperpigmentation in the epidermis. They are also involved in atherosclerosis, pulmonary hypertension, and Raynaud's syndrome pathogenesis. The detection of endothelins in the lung tissues of asthmatic patients suggests that these factors may play an important pathophysiological role as bronchoconstrictors.

Increased Values

hypertension, atherosclerosis, myocardial infarction, cardiogenic shock, Raynaud' syndrome, Crohn's disease

Analyte	Age/Gender	Reference Range	SI Units	Note
Endothelin-1	M	0.38–0.44	pg/ml	
	F	0.36–0.39	pg/ml	
	> 60 y	0.41–0.43	pg/ml	

Enkephalins

(syn: methionine-enkephalin – MEK, leucine-enkephalin – LEK) The enkephalins function as neurotransmitters/neuromodulators in many brain locations, central neurones – globus pallidus, thalamus and the spinal cord; they play a part in pain perception, movement, mood, behavior and neuroendocrine regulation. They are also found in nerve plexuses and in the exocrine glands of the gastrointestinal tract, protecting vessels against damage by granulocytes products. They stimulate antibody production and NK-cells activity and are involved in T-lymphocytes suppression. After releasing and interaction with peptidergic (opioid) receptors, the enkephalins are hydrolyzed by peptidases into smaller inactive peptides and amino acids. Highest levels appear in late afternoon and lowest in AM.

Increased Values
exercise, renal failure

Decreased Values
ethanol, pregnancy

Enolase

Enolase is a dimer of 3 peptides (alpha, beta, gamma). Beta-beta/alpha-beta exist mainly in heart and skeletal muscle, while gamma-gamma and alpha-alpha are located in nerve tissue.

Increased Values – hyperenolasemia
hepatitis, muscle diseases, myocardial infarct

Eosinophil Chemotactic Factor of Anaphylaxis

(ECF-A) Allergic reactions mediator.
Function. Eosinophils chemotactic attraction and deactivation.

Epidermal Growth Factor

(EGF)
Occurrence. Present in most body fluids and sweat gland secretory cells. Cells in various organs, including brain, kidney, salivary gland and stomach produce this factor. The production of EGF has been shown to be stimulated by testosterone and to be inhibited by estrogens. EGF receptors are expressed in almost all types of tissues.

Function. Promotes proliferation/differentiation of mesenchymal and epithelial cells (effective mitogen). Induces epithelial development, promotes angiogenesis, and inhibits gastric secretion. It is a strong chemoattractant for fibroblasts and epithelial cells. EGF alone and also in combination with other cytokines is an important factor mediating wound healing processes. EGF does not influence hemopoietic cells. It strongly influences the synthesis and turn-over of proteins of the extracellular matrix, including fibronectin, collagens, laminin and glycosaminoglycans. EGF increases the release of calcium from bone tissue and promotes bone resorption. It also modulates the synthesis of a number of hormones, including the secretion of prolactin from pituitary tumors and of chorion gonadotropin from chorion carcinoma cells. It is a strong mitogen for many cells of ectodermal, mesodermal and endodermal origin. EGF receptors are in many carcinoma cells (mainly uterine cervix, oral cavity, lung and facies carcinomas); they are coded by c-erb B oncogene. EGF may be a trophic substance for the gastrointestinal mucosa and may play a gastroprotective role due to its ability to stimulate the proliferation of mucosa cells.

Epinephrine

(syn: adrenaline) Epinephrine is a catecholamine hormone.
Production. Secreted by the adrenal medulla and some neurons and stored in the chromaffin granules. Adrenaline is released in response to hypoglycemia, stress and other stimuli.
Function. Neurotransmitter in the central nervous system, a potent stimulator of the sympathetic nervous system (adrenergic receptors, predominantly alpha-receptors). Epinephrine increases: the heart rate and cardiac output, blood pressure, splanchnic and skeletal musculature blood flow (lower levels), platelet aggregation and blood glucose level. Epinephrine enhances release of glucose from glycogen and fatty acids from adipocytes. Epinephrine decreases: peripheral vascular resistance, skin, mucosal and renal blood flow (higher levels). It relaxes bronchial smooth musculature and has antiallergic effects.

Increased Values

electroconvulsion, prolonged exposure to cold, **pheochromocytoma**, ganglioblastoma, ganglioneuroma, anger, hypoglycemia, hypothyroidism, kidney diseases, acute myocardial infarction, diabetic ketoacidosis, adrenal medullary tumors, **physical exertion, neuroblastoma**, paraganglioma, **postoperative states**, fear, severe stress, shock, thyrotoxicosis

   Interfering Factors: medicaments – (alpha-methyldopa, caffeine, dopamine, insulin, isoproterenol, metoprolol, quinidine)

Analyte	Age/Gender	Reference Range	SI Units	Note
Epinephrine		165–468	pmol/l	

C1-Esterase Inhibitor

(C1-INH, syn: C1-esterase inactivator, C1 inhibiting factor) Belongs to the regulatory complement components which checks C1 complement activation. It is a glycoprotein in the enzyme inhibitors family which is capable of binding/inhibiting the plasma enzymes activity, including kallikrein, plasmin, activated factors XI, XII and C1r, and C1s complements. It is synthesized in the liver. With C1 esterase inhibitor defects, there can be a deficiency, mutation in molecule, that means ineffectivity and autoantibody presence. A hereditary and acquired angioedema clinical picture, including death, is an escape of complement activation from the control → production of kinines and anaphylatoxins.

Test Purpose. 1) hereditary angioedema diagnostics due to C1 inhibitor deficiency, acquired C1 inhibitor deficiency in malignancy and SLE, 2) to monitor severity of a disease or determine efficiency of treatment.

Increased Values
congenital hereditary angioedema, **tumors, ulcerative colitis**, acute phase response, pregnancy
> **Interfering Factors:** medicaments – (androgen steroids, danazol)

Decreased Values
angioedema – (**hereditary a.**, acquired a.), **congenital C1-INH deficiency**, diseases – (lymphoproliferative d., d. with B-lymphocyte disorders, bacterial infectious d.), **systemic lupus erythematosus**, lymphoma, **liver cirrhosis, glomerulonephritis, hepatitis**, lupus nephritis, malnutrition, renal transplant rejection

Analyte	Age/Gender	Reference Range	SI Units	Note
C1-Esterase Inhibitor		0.15–0.35	g/l	

Estradiol

(syn: unconjugated estriol)

Production. The major most potent female sex hormone produced mainly by the ovary binds in plasma to the sex hormone-binding globulin (SHBG). Small amounts of estrogens are synthesized also by the adrenal cortex, testes and fetoplacental unit in pregnancy.

Function. Belongs to the estrogens – steroid hormones that control female sexual development, promoting the growth and function of the female sex organs and female secondary sexual characteristics; influences gonadotropins secretion by the anterior pituitary and is involved in bone homeostasis. Marked diurnal variation (50%), highest in late afternoon, lowest around midnight; 25% day-to-day variation of levels. In menstruating women, rises during the follicular phase sharply peak 2–3 d. before ovulation and later rise in the midluteal phase.

Test Purpose. 1) to help in diagnosis of precocious puberty, 2) to monitor estrogen therapy, 3) to monitor ovulation induction in in vitro fertilisation, 4) to assess of women with suspected hypothalamic or pituitary disease.

Increased Values
hepatic cirrhosis, feminization – (f. in children, **testicular f.**), gynecomastia, **hyperthyroidism**, tumors, **estrogen producing tumors**, male sterility, pregnancy
> **Interfering Factors:** smoking, medicaments – (anabolic steroids, androgens, clomiphene, diazepam, digoxin, estrogens, tamoxifen)

Decreased Values
acromegaly, amenorrhea due to – (exercise, weight loss), anorexia mentalis, anovulatory cycles, **gonadal dysgenesis**, congenital adrenal enzymopathies, **hyperprolactinemia, primary/secondary hypogonadism**, hypothyroidism, acute illnesses, primary ovarian insufficiency, malnutrition, **menopause**, corpus luteum insufficiency, syndrome – (Klinefelter's sy, Sheehan's sy), pituitary failure
> **Interfering Factors:** medicaments – (androgens, cimetidine, interferon, ketoconazole, megestrol, oral contraceptives)

Analyte	Age/Gender	Reference Range	SI Units	Note
Estradiol	<10 y	22–140	pmol/l	
	F			
	Follicular phase	37–550	pmol/l	
	Pre-ovulation	400–1400	pmol/l	
	Luteal phase	300–910	pmol/l	
	Post-menopause	40–170	pmol/l	
	Oral contra-ceptives	15–120	pmol/l	
	Pregnancy			
	1st trimester	400–5000	pmol/l	
	2nd trimester	2500–62500	pmol/l	
	3rd trimester	8800–99700	pmol/l	
	M	35–150	pmol/l	

Estriol

(syn: total estriol) Estriol belongs to estrogens as the principal estrogen of pregnancy. In the non-pregnant woman estriol is a major estradiol metabolite; whereas in pregnancy, almost all maternal estriol originates from 16-alpha-OH dehydroepiandrosterone sulfate (DHEA-S) synthesized in the fetal adrenal, which is subsequently converted to estriol by the placenta. Almost all estriol is conjugated with either sulfate or glucuronide and then excreted by the kidneys. Approximately 9% is unconjugated (free) and it is this fraction that is measured.

Function. Stimulates the tissue development involved in reproduction. Estriol has high diurnal variation (50%). In non-pregnant women, parallels changes in the estradiol.

Increased Values
renal insufficiency, pregnancy – (**diabetic p.**, **multiple p.**), tumors – (adrenal t., testicular t., ovarian t.)
   Interfering Factors: medicaments – (ACTH in pregnancy, spironolactone in men)

Decreased Values
anemia, **anencephalic fetus**, **placental sulfatase deficiency**, diabetes mellitus, hemoglobinopathies, **hypoplasia of fetal adrenals**, diseases – (intestinal d., congenital heart d.), **placental insufficiency**, malnutrition, **intrauterine fetal death**, preeclampsia, **postmaturity**, pyelonephritis, Rh isoimmunization, **intrauterine fetal growth-retardation**, high-risk pregnancy – (diabetes mellitus), syndrome – (adrenogenital sy, **Down sy**, Stein–Leventhal sy, Turner's sy), congenital anomalies, failing pregnancy, fetal dysmaturity, fetal distress, hypopituitarism, menopause
   Interfering Factors: high altitude, medicaments – (acetylsalicylic acid, albuterol, ampicillin, penicillin, probenecid, salbutamol, steroids, thyroxine)

Analyte	Age/Gender	Reference Range	SI Units	Note
Estriol, total	pregnancy (week)			
	24–28	104–590	nmol/l	
	28–32	140–760	nmol/l	
	32–36	208–970	nmol/l	
	36–40	280–1210	nmol/l	
	Adult M and non-pregnant F	<7.0	nmol/l	

Estriol, Free

(syn: unconjugated estriol)

Increased Values
imminent delivery

Decreased Values
fetal distress, postmaturity, congenital heart diseases, major malformations of fetal CNS,
fetal Down sy
  Interfering Factors: medicaments – (ampicillin, penicillin)

Analyte	Age/Gender	Reference Range	SI Units	Note
Estriol, free	pregnancy (week)			
	25	12.1–34.7	nmol/l	
	28	13.9–43.4	nmol/l	
	30	15.6–48.6	nmol/l	
	32	17.4–55.5	nmol/l	
	34	19.1–64.2	nmol/l	
	36	24.3–86.8	nmol/l	
	37	27.8–97.2	nmol/l	
	38	31.2–111.0	nmol/l	
	39	34.7–118.0	nmol/l	
	40–41	36.4–86.8	nmol/l	

Estrogens

(syn: total estrogens) Estrogens are female sex hormones that are responsible for female sex
organ development and maintenance and female secondary sex characteristics. In conjunction with progesterone they also participate in menstrual cycle regulation and in pregnancy
maintenance.
Production. By the ovarian follicles, the corpus luteum, and during pregnancy by the placenta. The most potent natural estrogen is estradiol.
Function. Estrogens increase SHBG levels, corticosterone-binding globulin and thyroxine-
binding globulin. They decrease bone reabsorption, in prepubertal girls accelerating linear
bone growth and epiphyseal closure. In the kidney, estradiol enhances sodium reabsorption,
an effect antagonized by progesterone. Estrogens in the uterus stimulate endometrial gland
proliferation, myometrial excitability and increase endometrial cell numbers. In the cervix
they stimulate production of large thin watery mucus amounts. In the breast: stimulate stromal breast development and mammary gland duct growth. In the hypothalamus-pituitary
they sensitize gonadotropins to gonadotropin-releasing hormone and suppress gonadotropin release in pharmacological doses (oral contraceptives). Other functions: follicle growth,
stimulate fat deposition, libido, and hepatic synthesis of transport proteins. In women, increase from nadir at menses peaks in late follicular and luteal phases, similar to estradiol.
Test Purpose. 1) to determine sexual maturation and fertility, 2) to aid diagnosis of gonadal
dysfunction: precocious/delayed puberty, menstrual disorders, or infertility, 3) to determine
fetal well-being, 4) to aid tumors diagnosis known to secrete estrogens.

Increased Values

hepatic cirrhosis, congenital adrenal hyperplasia, hyperthyroidism, diseases – (alcoholic liver d., severe hepatic d.), tumors – (hepatoma, **chorionepithelioma, testicular t., ovarian t. producing estrogens,** granulosa cells and theca cells t.), obesity, precocious puberty, primary testicular failure

> **Interfering Factors:** medicaments – (chlorpromazine, clomiphene, digoxin, estrogens, oral contraceptives, tamoxifen)

Decreased Values

ovarian agenesis, anorexia nervosa, **adrenal cortex hypofunction,** primary/secondary hypogonadism, **hypopituitarism, primary ovarian malfunction, menopause,** psychogenic stress, Turner's sy, ovarian failure

> **Interfering Factors:** prolonged bed rest, medicaments – (cimetidine, ketoconazole, megestrol)

Analyte	Age/Gender	Reference Range	SI Units	Note
Estrogens, total	Children	<30	ng/l	
	M	40–115	ng/l	
	F – cycle day			
	1–10 d	61–394	ng/l	
	11–20 d	122–437	ng/l	
	21–30 d	156–350	ng/l	
	before puberty	<40	ng/l	

Estrone

An oxidation product of estradiol found in pregnancy urine, male urine, plasma and placenta, which is metabolically convertible to estradiol. It is secreted by the ovary but circulating estrone is for the most part derived from peripheral estradiol metabolism, especially androstenedione. 10% day-to-day level variation. In women, increases from nadir at menses peaks at ovulation.

Increased Values
obesity
> **Interfering Factors:** smoking, puberty, pregnancy, medicaments – (digoxin)

Decreased Values
acute illnesses

Factor B

(syn: complement C3 activator, alternate pathway factor B, C3 activator, C3 proactivator, properdin factor B). Factor B belongs to the complement components (alternative pathway component) and is involved in complement activation. Assay of factor B helps distinguish activation of the alternate from the classical complement pathway. It is a protein synthesized by hepatocytes, monocytes and macrophages in other tissues. Decreased values are seen when alternate pathway pathway is activated. Complement proteins are acute phase reactants and have very short half-lives. Their serum levels are a balance of synthesis and catabolism. Thus, serial measurements may be more informative than single values.

Increased Values
acute phase response

Decreased Values
sickle-cell anemia, bacteremia with shock, bacterial endocarditis, glomerulonephritis –
(**hypocomplementemic chronic g.,** membranoproliferative g., post-streptococcal g.), **paroxysmal nocturnal hemoglobinuria,** disseminated intravascular coagulation, systemic lupus
erythematosus, anaphylactic subacute reaction to dextran or radiocontrast media, gram-
negative bacterial sepsis

Factor D

Factor D belongs to the complement components (alternative pathway component). A serine esterase with specificity for factor B, it is the only complement enzyme that circulates
in its active state. It is essential for triggering the alternative pathway activation.

Increased Values
rheumatoid arthritis with secondary amyloidosis, polycystic kidney disease, end-stage kidney disease, systemic lupus erythematosus with renal disease

Factor H

Factor H belongs to the complement components (regulatory component). It is required for
efficient control of the alternative complement pathway.

Decreased Values
congenital factor H deficiency

Factor I

Factor I belongs to the complement components (regulatory component). It is a highly specific serine esterase that acts rapidly to inactivate C3b and C4b. Patients lacking factor I
develop profound hypocomplementemia, primarily due to uncontrolled alternative pathway
activation.

Decreased Values
congenital factor I deficiency

Febrile Agglutinins

(syn: warm agglutinins) Febrile agglutinins are antibodies that cause RBCs aggregation at
high temperatures. Serial dilutions are performed to detect the dilution at which agglutination occurs.
Test Purpose. 1) to identify sera agglutinins in patients thought to have infectious bacterial
diseases characterized by persistent fever, 2) to support clinical findings of diseases caused
by salmonella, Francisella tularensis or brucela, 3) to help to identify cause of fevers of unknown origin.

Increased Values
brucellosis, infections – (rickettsial i., salmonellosis), tularemia, Rocky Mountain spotted fever, typhus, liver diseases, proteus infection
>   **Interfering Factors:** cocaine, hallucinogens, marijuana, narcotics, medicaments – (antibiotics)

Ferritin

(iron hydroxide + protein part → apoferritin). Ferritin is an alpha-1-globulin, tumor marker, and acute phase reactant. Ferritin is the major, water-soluble iron storage protein.
Production. Reticuloendothelial system (liver, spleen, bone marrow, kidney). Ferritin, which is circulating in blood, is a serum ferritin (glycated ferritin, considered as normal secretory cells product) and tissue ferritin mixture, which is released from damaged cells. Ferritin creates complexes with other proteins in blood, e. g. alpha-2-macroglobulin.
Occurrence. Primary protein iron deposits are liver, spleen, bone marrow, and intestinal mucous membrane. Serum ferritin is a protein devoid of iron, and is in a low concentration relative to tissue ferritin. Since it is in equilibrium with tissue ferritin, its concentration correlates well with total body iron stores. Intraindividual level variability is 5–18%, interindividual variability 12–18%.
Test Purpose. 1) to screen and monitor for iron deficiency and iron overload, 2) to measure iron storage, 3) to distinguish between iron deficiency (low iron storage condition) and chronic inflammation (normal storage condition), 4) to help in hemochromatosis diagnosis, 5) stored iron estimation in bone marrow in hemodialyzed patients, 6) to determine response to iron therapy or compliance with treatment, 7) to study population iron levels and response to iron supplement.

Increased Values – hyperferritinemia
chronic alcoholism, anemia – (**hemolytic a.**, **megaloblastic a.**, sideroblastic a., thalassemia, spherocytosis), rheumatoid arthritis, **ineffective erythropoiesis**, hemodialysis, **hemochromatosis**, **hemosiderosis**, **hepatitis**, **hyperthyroidism**, Gaucher's disease, diseases – (**acute/chronic infectious d.**, chronic renal d., **acute/chronic liver d.**, pulmonary infectious d., hepatobiliary tract d., chronic infectious urinary tract d., **acute/chronic inflammatory d.**), obstructive icterus, myocardial infarction, inanition, systemic lupus erythematosus, tumours – (pancreas t., **Hodgkin's/non-Hodgkin's disease**, **leukemia**, renal t., liver t., lung t., **breast t.**, neuroblastoma, testes t.), fasting, osteomyelitis, **plasmocytoma**, burns, porphyria cutanea tarda, **iron intake excess** (iron overload)
>   **Interfering Factors:** hemolytic disorders, recent high iron containing meal ingestion, recent blood transfusions, medicaments – (ethanol, iron preparations, oral contraceptives)

Decreased Values – hypoferritinemia
iron deficiency anemia, **hemodialysis**, **acute severe hemorrhage** (after 2 weeks), malabsorption, **iron intake deficiency**, **protein loss/deficiency**, **polycythemia vera**, nephrotic sy, **pregnancy**
>   **Interfering Factors:** erythropoietin, menstruation

Analyte	Age/Gender	Reference Range	SI Units	Note
Ferritin	1 d–1 w	145–458	µg/l	
	Infants	52–421	µg/l	
	3 m–10 y	9.3–65	µg/l	

Analyte	Age/Gender	Reference Range	SI Units	Note
	11–16 y	12–150	µg/l	
	Adults <50 y F	8–156	µg/l	
	Adults M	8–140	µg/l	
	Adults >50 y F	20–400	µg/l	See ref.
	6 w–18 y	15–120	µg/l	ranges note
	Adults			
	<50 y F	10–160	µg/l	
	>50 y F	30–300	µg/l	
	M	30–300	µg/l	

Alpha-1-Fetoprotein

(AFP, syn: alpha-1-fetoglobulin) Glycoprotein, oncofetal protein (albumin).

Production. Physiologically – fetal hepatocytes, fetal gastrointestinal system, yolk sac. Maximum serum concentration is reached at approximately 10 to 15 weeks' gestation and decreases to an undetectable concentration at about 5 weeks after birth.

Test Purpose. 1) to monitor therapy effectiveness in malignant conditions such as hepatomas, choriocarcinoma, teratocarcinoma and germ cell tumors, and in certain non-malignant conditions such as ataxia-teleangiectasia, 2) to screen a pregnant woman in antenatal neural tube defects diagnosis, Down disease, anencephaly and other congenital anomalies 3) to monitor liver regenerative procedures, 4) a postoperative control of AFP positive patients, 5) differential diagnosis of neonatal hepatitis versus biliary atresia in newborns, 6) to monitor therapy with antineoplastic drugs.

Increased Values

anencephaly, renal aplasia/agenesis, aplasia cutis, **ataxia-teleangiectasia**, atresia of – (**esophagus, duodenum**), **hepatic cirrhosis**, **encephalocele**, **gastroschisis**, partial hepatectomy, **hepatitis, hydrocephalus**, fetal hydrops, cystic hygroma, fetal hypotrophy, disease – (**inflammatory bowel d., alcoholic liver d.**), Rh isoimmunization, **fetal blood contamination**, fetal-maternal hemorrhage, microcephaly, **myelomeningocele**, tumors – (colon t., lymphoma, **Hodgkin's disease, kidney t., pancreas t., liver t.**, lung t., **testes t., sacrococcygeal teratoma, thyroid t.**, biliary tract t., **stomach t.**), embryonic tumours – (choriocarcinoma, **t. of testes, t. of ovary, teratocarcinoma**), nephrosis, hepatic necrosis – (fetal h. n., massive h. n.), oligohydramnios, polycystic kidneys, **omphalocele**, abortion – (impending a., spontaneous a.), secondary to viral infections, **spina bifida**, stenosis of gastrointestinal tract, recovery from hepatitis, syndrome – (Meckel's sy, Wiskott-Aldrich sy, nephrotic congenital sy, **Turner's sy**), **pregnancy** (peak between weeks 16 and 18), **multiple pregnancy**, trisomy 13 (Patau's sy), **tyrosinemia, intrauterine fetal death, tetralogy of Fallot**, underestimated gestational age.

Decreased Values

insulin-dependent diabetes mellitus of mother, hydatidiform mole (molar pregnancy), **choriocarcinoma**, pseudopregnancy, obesity, spontaneous abortion, syndrome – (**Down sy of fetus**, Edwards' sy), pregnancy, fetal demise, overestimated gestational age

Analyte	Age/Gender	Reference Range	SI Units	Note
Alpha-1-Fetoprotein	1–30 d F	18700	µg/l	
	1–30 d M	<16400	µg/l	
	1 m–1 y F	<77	µg/l	
	1 m–1 y M	<28	µg/l	

Analyte	Age/Gender	Reference Range	SI Units	Note
	2–3 y F	<11	µg/l	
	2–3 y M	<7.9	µg/l	
	4–6 y F	<4.2	µg/l	
	4–6 y M	<5.6	µg/l	
	7–12 y F	<5.6	µg/l	
	7–12 y M	<3.7	µg/l	
	13–18 y F	<4.2	µg/l	
	13–18 y M	<3.9	µg/l	
	Adults F	0.8–9.1	µg/l	
	Adults M	0.8–9.5	µg/l	
	Pregnancy			
	4–8 w	<8.4	µg/l	
	15 w	<34.0	µg/l	
	16 w	<38.0	µg/l	
	17 w	<44.0	µg/l	
	18 w	<49.0	µg/l	
	19 w	<56.5	µg/l	
	20 w	<66.0	µg/l	

Fibroblast Growth Factors

(FGF, FGFs) FGF belong to cytokines which are involved in fibroblast proliferation/differentiation, angiogenesis, wound healing, and metastatic processes. They are strong mitogens for mesenchymal/neuroectodermal cells; stimulate endothelial cells to invasion through basal membrane; activate collagenases and plasminogen activators.

Fibroblast growth factor – acidic
(FGF acidic, heparin binding growth factor-1 – HBGF-1, beta-endothelial cell growth factor)
Occurrence. Brain, retina, bone marrow, osteosarcomas.
Function. Mitogenic for mesenchymal and neuroectodermal cells, chemotactic for endothelial cells, it is involved in angiogenesis.

Fibroblast growth factor – basic
(b-FGF, FGF basic, heparin binding growth factor-2 – HBGF-2, astroglial growth factor-2, eye-derived growth factor-1, pituitary growth factor, chondrocytoma growth factor, hepatoma growth factor)
Occurrence. Mesodermal origin tissue, neural tissue, pituitary, adrenal cortex, corpus luteum, placenta, endothelial cells. It is released after tissue injuries and during inflammatory processes and also during the proliferation of tumor cells.
Function. Mitogenic for mesodermal and neuroectodermal cells. Induces differentiation, survival and regeneration of neurons, stimulates astrocyte migration, it is involved in angiogenesis (by controlling the proliferation and migration of vascular endothelial cells). The expression of plasminogen activator and collagenase activity by these cells is enhanced by b-FGF. B-FGF and/or closely related factors may be engaged also in tumor angiogenesis, facilitating the invasive growth and metastasis of tumors by inducing the synthesis of proteases. Stimulates the growth of fibroblasts, myoblasts, osteoblasts, endothelial cells, keratinocytes, chondrocytes. In capillary endothelial cells b-FGF acts in an autocrine manner. Transferrin and HDL-C also support the activity of b-FGF on endothelial cells. For some

cholinergic, dopaminergic and GABA-ergic neuronal cells b-FGF acts as a differentiation factor promoting outgrowth of neurites and promoting survival. In pituitary b-FGF regulates the secretion of thyrotropin and prolactin. It also acts as an ovarian hormone and differentially regulates the expression of steroids. b-FGF modulates the proliferation and differentiation of granulosa cells and inhibits induction of receptors for luteinizing hormone mediated by FSH. It stimulates the synthesis of progesterone. b-FGF and also related factors may be useful to support regeneration of tissues after brain, spinal cord and peripheral nerve injuries. Together with other factors b-FGF can play a role also in neurodegenerative disorders such as Alzheimer's disease, Parkinson's disease and Huntington's disease. Factor is produced in most gliomas and is involved in tumorigenesis and malignant progression, functioning in an autocrine manner. It may play an important role also in tumor neovascularization as a mediator acting in a paracrine manner. Beta-FGF has been shown to improve cardiac systolic function, to reduce infarct size and to increase the number of arterioles and capillaries in the infarct area.

Fibroblast growth factor-3
(syn: heparin binding growth factor-3 – HBGF-3)
Occurrence. Expressed by mammary tumors epithelial cells, various sites and times during embryonic development.
Function. Mitogenic for mesodermal and neuroectodermal cells.

Fibroblast growth factor-4
(syn: heparin binding growth factor-4 – HBGF-4)
Occurrence. Expressed by certain tumor cells and/or by various tissues during embryonic development.
Function. Mitogenic for fibroblasts and endothelial cells, it is involved in angiogenesis.

Fibroblast growth factor-5
(syn: heparin binding growth factor-5 – HBGF-5)
Occurrence. Normal fibroblasts, tumor cells, retinal pigment, epithelium and various tissues during embryonic development.
Function. Mitogenic for fibroblasts and endothelial cells, it is probably involved in angiogenesis.

Fibroblast growth factor-6
(syn: heparin binding growth factor-6 – HBGF-6)
Occurrence. Expressed in tissues during embryonic development and in AIDS Kaposi's sarcoma tissue.
Function. Mitogenic for fibroblasts, it has transforming activity on fibroblasts.

Fibroblast growth factor-7
(syn: heparin binding growth factor-7 – HBGF-7, keratinocyte growth factor – KGF)
Occurrence. Epithelial tissue stromal cells.
Function. Mitogenic for epithelial cells.

Fibronectin

(FN, syn: cold-insoluble globulin, cell surface protein, opsonic alpha-2-surface binding protein) Fibronectins are large adhesive glycoproteins (fibronectin is a dimer) that are integral parts of cell surfaces, extracellular matrices and also occur in intra/extravascular fluids. As adhesive molecules they electrophoretically move in the area of alpha-2-globulins. Fibronectin is in soluble plasma form and insoluble form bound to connective tissue (adhesive function). Fibronectin has three forms: a) plasmatic (soluble dimer form) – in blood and other body fluids, b) cell-surface, c) matrix. VLA-3 molecules (very large antigens) that belong to integrins are the natural fibronectin ligand. The proteins are synthesized by a variety of cells, including endothelium, macrophages, synoviacytes and especially hepatocytes. Fibronectin is also released from alveolar and peritoneal macrophages. Antigen or other mitogen activated T-lymphocytes produce T-lymphocyte fibronectin, which influences monocyte and macrophage functional activities.

Function. In plasma they activate macrophages and act as non-specific opsonins binding bacteria. In tissue: 1) they are involved in fibronectin domain molecular interactions with collagen surface, fibrinogen, DNA, glycosaminoglycans, polyamines, 2) fibronectins on cell surfaces promote cell-cell, cell-matrix and cell-substrate interactions (adhesive protein), 3) they are involved in morphogenesis and oncogenesis (differentiation processes), 4) they are involved in endothelial cells growth inhibition, 5) they also play a role in clot retraction and platelet aggregation, factor XIIIa activation and wound healing. Fibronectins are important in the connective tissue where they cross-link to collagen. Fibronectins are important to collagen fibril restoration and they have pathophysiological importance in biliary concrement creation; they are involved in delayed hypersensitivity reactions. Malignant cells have less fibronectin (→ loss of adhesiveness → metastases).

Test Purpose. 1) osteoporosis diagnosis, 2) delayed hypersensitivity reaction diagnosis, 3) recurrent streptococcal infection diagnosis, 4) prenatal infection and neonatal/infant sepsis diagnosis, 5) to assess protein nutritional state, especially in patients with an acute phase response.

Increased Values
hepatitis – (chronic active h., acute h.), hyperthyroidism, tumors

Decreased Values
burns, biliary cirrhosis, severe infections, DIC, coagulopathies, vascular collapse, malnutrition, tumors, pancreatitis, peritonitis, genetic disorders, splenomegaly, conditions – (septic c., shock c.), protein loss, trauma, liver failure

Analyte	Age/Gender	Reference Range	SI Units	Note
Fibronectin		0.25–0.40	g/l	

Fluorine

(F) Inorganic fluorine is readily absorbed in the small intestine and distributed almost entirely to bone and teeth. Fluorine replaces hydroxyl groups in apatite. Renal excretion is most important in body fluorine content regulation.

Increased Values – hyperfluorinemia
fluorosis, dental enamel, renal failure
> **Interfering Factors:** fluorine-containing toothpaste, medicaments – (flecainide, halothane, methoxyflurane)

Decreased Values – hypofluorinemia
caries (dental decay), osteoporosis

Follicle-Stimulating Hormone

(FSH, syn: follitropin)
Production. Anterior pituitary (adenohypophysis) hormone, gonadotropin, glycoprotein.
Function. Stimulates ovarian follicular cells and the Sertoli cells in the testes. Promotes follicular growth and prepares the follicle for the ovulation-inducing action of luteinizing hormone. Secretion is stimulated by norepinephrine, acetylcholine, gamma-aminobutyric acid, and inhibited by serotonin, dopamine, endorphins. Pulsatile release during day shows a 50% variation, spiking at midcycle in menstruating women. Day-to-day level variation is 40%. Hormone release is governed by: 1) gonadotropin-releasing hormone (GRH) = gonadoliberin → increases gonadotropins release, 2) dopamine → inhibits FSH, LH release.
Test Purpose. 1) to aid in infertility diagnosis and menstruation disorders, 2) to aid in the diagnosis of precocious puberty in girls (before age 9), and boys (before age 10), 3) to aid in a hypogonadism differential diagnosis, 4) to aid in the diagnosis of pituitary tumor.

Increased Values
ovarian/testicular agenesis, acromegaly (early stage), **alcoholism**, climacterium praecox, testes destruction – (x-ray exposure, mumps orchitis) gonadal dysgenesis, hypogonadism – (peripheral h., **primary h.**), primary ovarian insufficiency, **castration, menopause, gonadotropin-secreting pituitary tumors, orchitis, precocious puberty**, seminoma, states after cytostatic therapy, syndrome – (male climacteric sy, **Klinefelter's sy**, Stein-Leventhal sy, **Turner's sy**), **gonadal failure**, postmenopausal women
> **Interfering Factors:** medicaments – (chlorambucil, cimetidine, clomiphene, cyclophosphamide, digitalis, ethanol, ketoconazole, levodopa, naloxone)

Decreased Values
acromegalia, sickle-cell anemia, **anorexia nervosa** (mentalis), aspermatogenesis, **hemochromatosis**, hyperprolactinemia, **anterior pituitary hypofunction, central hypogonadism**, selective hypopituitarism, **several illnesses**, female infertility, **secondary ovarian insufficiency**, malnutrition, obesity, **panhypopituitarism**, pituitary/hypothalamic lesions by – (tumours, trauma), **polycystic ovary sy, pregnancy**
> **Interfering Factors:** medicaments – (anabolic steroids, androgens, corticosteroids, estrogens, megestrol, oral contraceptives, phenobarbital, phenothiazines, stanozolol)

Analyte	Age/Gender	Reference Range	SI Units	Note
Follicle Stimulating Hormone	< 10 y	0.5–2	IU/l	
	F			
	Follicular phase	2–12	IU/l	
	Mid-cycle	10–20	IU/l	
	Luteal phase	2–10	IU/l	
	Postmenopause	>20	IU/l	
	M	<11	IU/l	

Free Fatty Acids

(FFA) Nonesterified fatty acids bound to protein. Free fatty acids are formed by lipoproteins and triacylglycerols breakdown. Free fatty acid and triacylglycerol amounts depend on the dietary sources, fat deposits and body synthesis. In fasting individuals, lowest during sleep. Marked within-day difference (3-fold between highest and lowest).

Increased Values

alcoholism, **uncontrolled diabetes mellitus, hepatic encephalopathy, pheochromocytoma**, prolonged starvation, **hyperthyroidism,** Huntington's chorea, **acute myocardial infarction, von Gierke's disease, obesity, stress, Reye's sy,** excessive lipoactive hormones releasing – (ACTH, adrenaline, glucagon, noradrenaline, thyrotropin)

> **Interfering Factors:** anxiety, smoking, lowered body temperature, postprandial, physical exercise, medicaments – (amphetamine, aminophylline, caffeine, carbutamide, catecholamines, chlorpromazine, desipramine, diazoxide, glucose, growth hormone, heparin, isoproterenol, levodopa, lysergide, nicotine, oral contraceptives, phenformin, prazosin, reserpine, theophylline, thyroxine, tolbutamide, valproic acid)

Decreased Values

cystic fibrosis

> **Interfering Factors:** decreased food intake, medicaments – (acebutolol, acetylsalicylic acid, asparaginase, atenolol, beta-blockers, clofibrate, glucose, insulin, metoprolol, neomycin, niacin, oxprenolol, phenformin, propranolol, salicylates, streptozocin)

Analyte	Age/Gender	Reference Range	SI Units	Note
Fatty Acids, free	Neonates	694–1034	mg/l	
	Infants	1450–2018	mg/l	
	1 y	1433–2075	mg/l	
	2–5 y	2268–3006	mg/l	
	6–10 y	2018–3018	mg/l	
	11–15 y	2200–2800	mg/l	
	Adults	2879–3253	mg/l	
		0.15–0.71	mmol/l	
	F – lactation	5315–6245	mg/l	

Free Oxygen Radicals

Free oxygen radicals are reactive oxygen forms also produced in small amounts in a healthy organism (neutrophils) that belong to the natural protective mechanisms (e. g. phagocytosis process). Chemically, a result of incomplete O_2 reduction through so-called univalent pathway that produces superoxide anion ($\cdot O\downarrow_2$) and very reactive hydroxyl radical ($\cdot OH$). These products react very quickly/effectively with many low/high-molecular agents → their physical, chemical and biological properties are changed. The cells have effective protective systems that are able to eliminate some reactive O_2 forms. The antioxidative enzymes group consists of: superoxide dismutase, glutathione reductase and catalase. Increased free O_2 radicals production (oxidative stress) exceeds the cellular antioxidative system capacity; this starts the intense hydroxyl radical production in iron ions presence and attacks higher unsaturated carboxylic acids preferably → hydroxyperoxides, aldehydes, epoxides are produced. Functionally important substance properties are changing (structural membrane components, enzymes, nucleic acids) → accentuated cell function disorders arise. When investigating polyunsaturated carboxylic acids oxidative products, malone dialdehyde (MDA) determination is considered a dominant lipoperoxide metabolism product. Also a singlet oxygen ($^1O_2$) belongs to reactive oxygen form. All these intermediates have direct cytotoxic effects; they are involved in adhesion molecule expression induction on the endothelial cell surface, in neutrophil margination and diapedesis and in pathogenesis of many pathological conditions (rheumatoid arthritis, pulmonary emphysema, ARDS, silicosis).

Free Thyroxine Index

(FTI, syn: FT4 index) FTI measures the amount of free thyroxine (T4), which is only a fraction of total T4. This index is the calculated product of T3 resin uptake and serum total thyroxine. Free T4 is the unbound T4 entering the cell which is metabolically active. FTI measuring, which is not affected by thyroid-binding globulin abnormalities, correlates more closely with true hormonal status, than total T4 or triiodothyronine (T3) determinations. Index serves as a corrector of misleading results of T3 and T4 determinations caused by conditions that alter the T4-binding protein concentration.

Increased Values
hyperthyroidism

Decreased Values
hypothyroidism

Fructosamine

(syn: serum glycoproteins, glycated/glycosylated serum proteins, ketoamines) Duration and the glycemia level influence plasmatic proteins through non-enzymatically glycation and then irreversible change to ketoamines or fructosamine. Fructosamine reflects the mean glucose blood concentration over a 2–3 week period (in comparison to glycated Hb over 4–10 weeks). The fructosamine levels correlate with HbA_{1c}, serum protein and albumin. The fructosamine assay shows great promise in short-term glycemic control assessment diabetic patients, especially in newborns and in non-pregnant women. Day-to-day concentrations variation is 8%.
Test Purpose. To monitor diabetes mellitus.

Increased Values – hyperfructosaminemia
diabetes mellitus, hyperglycemia, hypothyroidism, **pregnancy** (3rd trimester), uremia, renal failure
> **Interfering Factors:** bilirubin, triacylglycerols

Decreased Values – hypofructosaminemia
early childhood, hypoalbuminemia, obesity, hypoproteinemic states, **pregnancy** (1st trimester), thyrotoxicosis
> **Interfering Factors:** ceruloplasmin, hemoglobin levels, medicaments – (ascorbic acid, pyridoxine)

Analyte	Age/Gender	Reference Range	SI Units	Note
Fructosamine	0–3 y	1.56–2.27	mmol/l	
	3–6 y	1.73–2.34	mmol/l	
	6–9 y	1.82–2.56	mmol/l	
	9–15 y	2.02–2.63	mmol/l	
	Adults	1.6–2.6	mmol/l	

Fructose

(syn: levulose, D-fructose, fructopyranose, fruit sugar) Fructose is a reducing sugar, keto-hexose, occurring in honey, sweet fruits, and as a component of di-/polysaccharides. It can influence glucose metabolism. For analysis a fresh specimen should be obtained, since fructose can undergo conversion to glucose in an alkaline medium.

Increased Values – fructosemia
essential fructosuria, hereditary fructose intolerance

Analyte	Age/Gender	Reference Range	SI Units	Note
Fructose		0.56	mmol/l	
		19–47	µmol/l	

Galactose

Galactose is a reducing sugar, aldohexose. It is a component of lactose and other oligo-saccharides, cerebrosides, gangliosides, and various glycolipids. Galactose creates a substantial part of glycoproteins.

Increased Values – galactosemia
galactose-deficient galactosemia, galactose-1-phosphate uridyl transferase-deficient galactosemia

Analyte	Age/Gender	Reference Range	SI Units	Note
Galactose	Children	0–0.46	mmol/l	
	Adults	0–0.24	mmol/l	
	Umbilical blood	0.417–0.787		See ref.
	0–1 y	0.491–0.779		ranges note

Galactose-1-Phosphate Uridyl Transferase

(GPUT) Enzyme involved in the galactose conversion during lactose metabolism.
Test Purpose. 1) to screen infants for galactosemia, 2) to detect heterozygous galactosemia carriers, 3) to investigate a neonate with a reducing substance in urine that is not glucose, 4) to screen for galactosemia in newborns if one or both parents is a carrier.

Decreased Values
galactose-1-phosphate uridyl transferase deficiency, galactosemia

GALOP Syndrome Antibodies

Patients with GALOP sy (gait disorder, autoantibody, late-age onset, polyneuropathy) have a disorder that appears to be immune mediated and is associated with a high titer of IgM binding to specific CNS myelin lipids (CMA).

Gastric Inhibitory Polypeptide

(GIP) Regulatory GIT peptide with endocrinous effect.
Production. Small intestine K-cells (duodenum, jejunum).
Function. Increases glucose stimulated insulin secretion in hyperglycemia. Inhibits gastric acid juice, gastrin, and pepsin secretions. Reduces gastric and intestinal motility. Increases fluid and electrolyte secretion from small intestine.

Increased Values
diabetes mellitus, prolonged fasting (starvation), hyperlipoproteinemia (type IV), dumping sy, surgical procedures, renal failure

Decreased Values
celiac disease, exocrine insufficiency of pancreas, malabsorption

Analyte	Age/Gender	Reference Range	SI Units	Note
Gastric Inhibitory Polypeptide		8–10	pmol/l	

Gastrin

Production. Polypeptidic hormone produced in the mucous membrane of stomach antral (G-cells) and pyloric regions, duodenum and small intestine (IG and G-cells) pancreatic Langerhans' islets D-cells and from peptidergic vagus nerve fibers.
Function. Secretion is stimulated by food (digestion of amino acids, vagal and adrenergic input, alcohol). Action mechanism is endocrine and partially neuroendocrine. Gastrin is absorbed into the blood and transported to its target organs → 1) in stomach – stimulates the gastric acid juice secretion (HCl secretion) and pepsinogen release, 2) small intestine – releases secretin, 3) pancreas – stimulates bicarbonate (weakly) and pancreatic enzymes production. Gastrin stimulates the mucosa growth that influences RNA, DNA synthesis → creation of colon cells, gastric mucose blood flow, secretion of intrinsic factor, secretin, hepatic bile. Increases lower esophageal sphincter tone, gastric motility (promoting circular stomach muscle contraction), promotes stomach emptying, increases intestinal motility, and relaxes ileocecal the sphincter. Gastrin secretion is inhibited by secretin and by hydrochloric acid (pH <1.5). Three active forms of gastrin exist naturally, with 34 amino acids (G-34, big gastrin), 17 amino acids (G-17, little gastrin) and 14 amino acids (G-14, mini gastrin). Biological half-time of G-34 and G-14 is only 5 minutes. Normal gastrin forms ratio G-13: G-17: G-34 is 8: 2: 1. Lowest levels are in early AM and highest during day, there is 90% fall in values during night. Increased gastrin values should always be interpreted together with gastric secretion levels and the clinical picture.
Test Purpose. 1) to confirm gastrinoma diagnosis, the gastrin-secreting tumor in Zollinger-Ellison sy, 2) to aid differential diagnosis of gastric/duodenal ulcers and pernicious anemia (gastrin estimation has limited value in patients with duodenal ulcer, 3) to help in differential diagnosis of unexplained chronic diarrhea or steatorrhea with or without peptic ul-

cer, 4) to help in diagnosis in peptic ulcer disease with associated endocrine conditions, 5) to test all patients with recurrent ulceration after surgery for duodenal ulcer, 6) to test patient with duodenal ulcer for whom elective gastric surgery is planned.

Increased Values – hypergastrinemia

achlorhydria, **pernicious anemia, rheumatoid arthritis,** hepatic cirrhosis, diabetes mellitus, **pheochromocytoma, gastrinoma,** gastritis, **chronic atrophic gastritis,** hypercalcemia, **hyperparathyroidism, antral G-cell hyperplasia,** hyperthyroidism, **duodenal/gastric ulcer disease,** renal diseases (end-stage), renal insufficiency, gastroduodenal hemorrhage, **stomach tumors, pylorostenosis,** relapse of gastroduodenal ulcer disease (recurrent/resistant ulcers together with diarrhea), resection – (small intestine r., **gastric r.**), **Zollinger-Ellison sy, postvagotomy,** incomplete vagotomy, short-bowel syndrome, recurrent ulcuses after gastroduodenal surgery, **chronic renal failure,** retained gastric antrum, pyloric obstruction, vitiligo

> Interfering Factors: **diabetics taking insulin,** gastroscopy, elderly people, nonfasting patient (postprandial), medicaments – (amino acids, antacids, H2-blocking agents, caffeine, calcium carbonate, calcium chloride, catecholamines, cimetidine, hydrogen pump inhibitors, insulin, omeprazole, ranitidine)

Decreased Values – hypogastrinemia
antrectomy with vagotomy, hypothyroidism

> Interfering Factors: medicaments – (anticholinergics, atropine, lithium, octreotide, phenformin, streptozocin, tricyclic antidepressants)

Analyte	Age/Gender	Reference Range	SI Units	Note
Gastrin	fasting	<48	pmol/l	
	postprandial	46–100	pmol/l	
		40–210	pg/ml	

GC-Globulin

(syn: group-specific component, vitamin D-binding protein – VDBP) Gc-globulin is an inter-alpha-globulin with overlap into alpha-2-globulins and one sterol binding site per molecule.

Production. Gc-globulin is synthesized by the liver.

Function. It binds/transports vitamin D and its metabolites, and also binds monomeric actin. Gc-globulin has three main genetic polymorphisms similar to haptoglobin (Gc 1–1, 2–1, 2–2), that are used only in forensic and paternity diagnosis.

Increased Values
estrogen excess, pregnancy (3rd trimester)

> Interfering Factors: medicaments – (oral contraceptives)

Decreased Values
severe hepatocellular diseases

Analyte	Age/Gender	Reference Range	SI Units	Note
Gc-Globulin		350–450	mg/l	

Globulins

Globulins are the class of proteins characterized by being insoluble in water, but soluble in saline solutions (euglobulins), or water soluble proteins (pseudoglobulins) whose other physical properties closely resemble true globulins.

Production. Gamma globulins – B-lymphocytes, alpha and beta globulins – hepatocytes.

- **alpha-1-globulins:** alpha-1-lipoprotein (HDL-C), alpha-1-antitrypsin, alpha-1-glycoprotein, thyroxine-binding globulin
- **alpha-2-globulins:** alpha-2-macroglobulin, ceruloplasmin, haptoglobin, cholinesterase, prothrombin
- **beta globulins:** beta-lipoproteins, fibrinogen, hemopexin, complement, plasminogen, pre-beta-lipoprotein, transferrin
- **gamma globulins:** immunoglobulin G, A, M, D, E

Increased Values – hyperglobulinemia

AIDS (HIV infection), primary amyloidosis, **rheumatoid arthritis**, hepatic cirrhosis, diabetes mellitus, endocarditis – (**subacute bacterial e.**, infectious e.), monoclonal gammopathy, Wegener's granulomatosis, hepatitis – (chronic active h., autoimmune h.), diseases – (cold agglutinin d., light chain d., heavy chain d.), chronic invasive fungal infections – (histoplasmosis), kala-azar, **collagenoses**, cryoglobulinemia, leprosy, lichen myxedematosus, **systemic lupus erythematosus**, lymphogranuloma venereum, Crohn's disease, Waldenström's macroglobulinemia, tumors – (chronic lymphocytic leukemia, lymphocytic lymphoma, **Hodgkin's disease**, **plasmocytoma**), pyoderma gangrenosum, sarcoidosis, Sjögren's sy, chronic syphilis, trypanosomiasis, **tuberculosis**, immune vasculitis

Decreased Values – hypoglobulinemia
hepatic dysfunction, renal diseases, tumors

Alpha-1-Globulins

Alpha-1-globulins mainly include: alpha-1-antitrypsin, alpha-1-lipoprotein, thyroxine-binding globulin, alpha-1-acid glycoprotein.

Test Purpose. To aid in the diagnosis of hepatic diseases, protein deficiency, renal disorders, gastrointestinal and neoplastic diseases, and to screen for alpha-1-antitrypsin deficiency.

Increased Values
cystitis, endocarditis, phlegmon, monoclonal/oligoclonal gammopathies, rheumatic fever, **febrile conditions**, emphysema, alpha-1-antitrypsin deficiency, cholecystitis, diseases – (**acute/chronic infective d.**, **inflammatory d.**), obstructive icterus, **myocardial infarction**, cachexia, collagenoses, **tumours**, **nephrosis**, tissue necrosis, biliary pathways obstruction, plasmocytoma (incl. multiple myeloma), pneumonia, acute polyarthritis, **burns**, pyelonephritis, acute phase reactions, sarcoidosis, conditions – (after surgery c., septic c.), **nephrotic sy**, pregnancy, tuberculosis, x-ray irradiation

Decreased Values
alpha-plasmocytoma, **hereditary alpha-1-antitrypsin deficiency**, dysproteinemia, **juvenile pulmonary emphysema**, **acute viral hepatitis**, **hypoproteinemia**, chronic diseases of the liver, nephrosis, Tangier disease, **Wilson's disease**, severe liver parenchymatous lesions

Alpha-2-Globulins

Alpha-2-globulins mainly include: serum haptoglobin, alpha-2-macroglobulin, ceruloplasmin, prothrombin and cholinesterase, lipoproteins.
Test Purpose. To aid in the diagnosis of hepatic diseases, protein deficiency, renal disorders, gastrointestinal and neoplastic diseases, acute inflammation.

Increased Values
arteritis, biliary cirrhosis, **rheumatic fever**, cholecystitis, diseases – (**acute infective d., acute/ chronic inflammatory d.**), **tumours**, plasmocytoma (incl. multiple myeloma), acute polyarthritis, **burns**, obstructive jaundice, pyelonephritis, acute phase reactions, **sarcoma, nephrotic sy**

Decreased Values
acute hemolytic anemia, diabetes mellitus, **hemolysis**, pancreatitis, **hepatocellular damage**, transfusions, trauma

Beta Globulins

Beta-1-globulins, as an electrophoretic class, include lipoproteins, transferrin, plasminogen, complement proteins, hemopexin, part of the immunoglobulins. Beta-2-globulin includes fibrinogen.
Test Purpose. To aid in the diagnosis of hepatic diseases, protein deficiency, renal disorders, gastrointestinal and neoplastic diseases.

Increased Values
amyloidosis, biliary cirrhosis, diabetes mellitus, **monoclonal gammopathies**, infectious hepatitis, starvation, **hyperlipoproteinemia**, PIH (pregnancy induced hypertension), **hypothyroidism**, liver diseases, **obstructive icterus**, cachexia, lymphadenosis, Bekhterev's disease, macroglobulinemia, tumours – (beta plasmocytoma, reticulosarcoma), nephrosis, **paraproteinemia, polyarteritis nodosa**, toxic hepatic lesions, **septicemia, nephrotic sy, pregnancy**, tuberculosis, fractures

Decreased Values
abetaglobulinemia, hypocholesterolemia, dysproteinemia, chronic hepatic diseases, malnutrition, hypoprotein disorders, nephrosis

Gamma Globulins

Serum globulins having the slowest electrophoretic migration.
Production. B-lymphocytes. Globulin gamma-fraction mainly contains immunoglobulins G, A, D, E, M. It is necessary to evaluate gamma globulins together with other fractions.
Test Purpose. To aid in the diagnosis of hepatic diseases, protein deficiency, renal disorders, gastrointestinal and neoplastic diseases.

Increased Values – hypergammaglobulinemia
AIDS, amyloidosis, **rheumatoid arthritis, cirrhosis hepatis,** cystitis, endocarditis, oligo and polyclonal gammopathy, hepatitis – (infectious h., **acute viral h.**), starvation, cholecystitis, icterus – (hemolytic i., **obstructive i.**), diseases – (autoimmune d., collagen vascular d., in-

fectious d., chronic d. of liver, pleural d., rheumatic d., **inflammatory d.**), collagenoses, systemic lupus erythematosus, **macroglobulinemia**, tumours – (**chronic lymphocytic leukemia**, lymphoma, **plasmocytoma** incl. multiple myeloma, reticulosarcoma), hepatic tissue necrosis, progressive paralysis, **paraproteinemia**, acute polyarthritis, toxic hepatic lesions, pyelonephritis, sarcoidosis, tuberculosis

Decreased Values – hypogammaglobulinemia
hereditary agammaglobulinemia, **amyloidosis, exudative enteropathy**, hypogammaglobulinemia, intoxication by benzene, radiation therapy, bone metastases, tumours – (**t. of lymphatic system**, lymphogranuloma, lymphomas), nephrosis, undernutrition, **sepsis**, syndrome – (Cushing's sy, **nephrotic sy**)
   Interfering Factors: medicaments – (ACTH, corticosteroids, immunosuppressives)

Glucagon

(syn: hyperglycemic-glycogenolytic factor – HGF) Polypeptide (29 amino acids) with intermediate products pre-proglucagon (180 amino acids) and proglucagon (69 amino acids). Gastrointestinal hormone.
Production. "A" cells (alpha-cells) of the pancreatic Langerhans' islets.
Function. The most potent gluconeogenic peptide hormone effects in the liver; in general, the glucagon action opposes that of insulin. Glucagon causes the rapid mobilization of potential energy sources to glucose by stimulating liver glycogenolysis, gluconeogenesis increase by increased amino acids uptake in the liver as well as into fatty acids by stimulating lipolysis. It inhibits stomach and intestines motility, HCl secretion, gastrin and exogenous pancreatic secretion (enzymes and bicarbonates), and it favourably influences liver cells recovery. The main impulses for glucagon secretion are: protein intake, acetylcholine, epinephrine, physical exertion, stress, blood glucose decrease, growth hormone, pancreatic sympathetic nerves stimulation. Glucose inhibits glucagon secretion; other inhibitors are insulin, serotonin and somatostatin. Glucagon inhibits secretion by feed-back. Released in episodic spikes during day with amplitude up to 35%.
Test Purpose. To help in diagnosis of functional glucagonoma and diabetes mellitus.

Increased Values – hyperglucagonemia
acromegaly, **liver cirrhosis, diabetes mellitus, pheochromocytoma, glucagonoma, familial hyperglucagonemia**, hyperlipoproteinemia, acute hypoglycemia, **infectious diseases**, diabetic ketoacidosis, obesity, surgery, **acute pancreatitis**, burns, Cushing's sy, uremia, trauma, **chronic renal failure**
   Interfering Factors: prolonged fasting, after meal (delay in rise), **severe stress**, moderate to severe exercise, medicaments – (amino acids, atropine, caffeine, calcium gluconate, cimetidine, danazol, epinephrine, gastrin, glucocorticoids, insulin, nifedipine, pancreozymin-cholecystokinin, sympathomimetic amines)

Decreased Values – hypoglucagonemia
idiopathic glucagon deficiency, **cystic fibrosis**, inflammatory disease with a loss of pancreatic tissue, tumors of pancreas, **chronic pancreatitis**, syndrome – (**postpancreatectomy sy**, somatostatin sy)
   Interfering Factors: immediately after meal, medicaments – (atenolol, pindolol, propranolol, secretin)

Analyte	Age/Gender	Reference Range	SI Units	Note
Glucagon		25–250	ng/l	

Glucose

(syn: blood glucose, blood sugar, fasting glucose test, fasting blood sugar – FBS) An aldohexose also known as dextrose, occurring as the D-form is found as a free monosaccharide in fruits and other plants as well as combined in di/oligo/polysaccharides.

Production. It is the end product of carbohydrate metabolism; glucose is formed from carbohydrates digestion (resorbed from jejunum) and glycogen conversion by the liver.

Function. Glucose is the principal fast body fuel. Utilized in the liver, and in muscular, fatty, brain tissues. Excessive glucose uptake → liver glycogen synthesis (glycogenesis) and fat synthesis; in low glucose supply → glycogen converts to glucose (glycogenolysis) in the liver + from amino acids glucose synthesis + from the fat breakdown glycerol (gluconeogenesis). The blood glucose level is regulated by: 1) insulin, epinephrine (2-phase effect) → blood glucose decrease, 2) thyroxine, epinephrine, glucagon, ACTH, corticosteroids, growth hormone, somatostatin → blood glucose increase. Factors affecting glucose control: stress, anxiety, illness, trauma, diet, exercise.

Test Purpose. 1) to screen for diabetes mellitus, 2) to monitor drug or dietary therapy in diabetes mellitus patients, 3) hypoglycemia suspicion, 4) to monitor energy and nutrition mainly with intensively treated patients.

Glycide metabolism. Oral glucose-tolerance test (oGTT): 3 day diet of 250 g carbohydrates per day → after overnight fasting, basal glycemia (blood glucose) is taken → then diluted glucose (75 g) is taken in 250–350 ml of water/tea → blood samples are taken after 30, 60, 90 and 120 minutes.

Factors that affect glucose tolerance: 1) before the test: previous food intake time, GIT surgery and malabsorption, medicaments, age, inactivity, weight, stress, diseases, 2) during the test: posture, nausea, anxiety, caffeine, cigarette smoking, time of day, activity, amount of glucose ingested. Diagnostic criteria in pregnancy screening are different.

Increased Values – hyperglycemia

acidosis, abscess – (perinephric a, pancreatic a.), optic nerve atrophy, **diabetic ketoacidosis**, adenoma of – (**pituitary, pancreas**), **acromegaly**, severe angina pectoris, anoxia, arteriosclerosis, Friedreich's ataxia, hepatic cirrhosis, cutaneous candidiasis, deficiency – (potassium d., growth hormone d.), diabetes mellitus – (**low dose of insulin**, non-insulin dependent d. m., **insulin dependent d. m., d. m. with obesity**, **secondary d. m.**, lipoatrophic diabetes mellitus), myotonic dystrophy, fat embolism, encephalitis, **Wernicke's encephalopathy, non-ketotic hyperosmolar coma**, exposure to extreme cold/heat, cystic fibrosis of pancreas, **pheochromocytoma**, diabetic gangrene, **gigantism**, glucagonoma, **hemochromatosis**, hyperaldosteronism, hyperlipoproteinemia (type III, V), hyperparathyroidism, prostate hyperplasia, essential hypertension, malignant hyperthermia, **hyperthyroidism**, hypothermia, diseases – (adrenal d., chronic d., CNS d., infectious d., pituitary d., renal d., liver d., acute inflammatory d., thyroid d.), prolonged physical inactivity, **myocardial infarction**, renal insufficiency, intoxication by – (CO, phenytoin, fluorine, thallium, isopropyl alcohol, **theophylline),** disease – (Graves' d., **Cushing's d.**), insulin lipodystrophy, infantile malnutrition, mucormycosis, multiplex mononeuritis, tumours, nephritis, diabetic neuropathy, diabetic ophthalmoplegia, obesity, intestinal obstruction, surgeries, pancreatectomy, pancreatitis – (**acute p.**, chronic p., p. due to mumps, acute necrotizing p.), **cerebrovascular accident**, burns, increased glucose intake – (dietary mistake, infusion carbohydrate therapy), hereditary coproporphyria, pseudohypoparathyroidism, diabetic retinopathy, **somatostatinoma**, conditions – (severe pain c., **stress c.**, febrile c., emotional c., **shock c.**, convulsion c.), syndrome – (Alström's sy, ataxia–teleangiectasia sy, **Cushing's sy**, Herrmann's sy, Mauriac sy, Stein-

Leventhal sy, Laurence-Moon-Biedl sy, Prader-Willi sy, Refsum's sy, Schmidt's sy, Werner's sy), cerebral thrombosis, thyrotoxicosis, injuries, uremia, anesthesia, mycotic vulvovaginitis, hemorrhage – (subarachnoid h., cerebellar h.), inborn error of amino acid metabolism **Interfering Factors:** anesthesia, smoking, pregnancy, medicaments – (abacavir, acetazolamide, ACTH, adrenaline, albuterol, aminosalicylic acid, amiodarone, ammonium chloride, amphotericin, amprenavir, analgesics, anesthetics, antineoplastics, antipyretics, ascorbic acid, asparaginase, atenolol, atovaquone, betamethasone, betaxolol, bexarotene, bisoprolol, bumetanide, caffeine, calcitonin, captopril, carteolol, carvedilol, chlorothiazide, chlorpromazine, chlorprothixene, chlortalidone, cimetidine, clobetasol, clonidine, clozapine, corticosteroids, corticotropin, cortisone, cyclosporine, daclizumab, desonide, dexamethasone, dextran, diazoxide, diphenylhydantoin, diclofenac, diuretics, dopamine, encainide, ephedrine, estradiol, estrogens, ethacrynic acid, ethanol, ether, fluoxetine, fluoxymesterone, flurandrenolide, fosinopril, fructose, furosemide, gatifloxacin, gemtuzumab, glucagon, glucocorticoids, human growth hormone, hydrochlorothiazide, hydrocortisone, indapamide, indinavir, indomethacin, interferon, irinotecan, isoniazid, isoprenaline, isoproterenol, isotretinoin, labetalol, levodopa, levonorgestrel, lithium, medroxyprogesterone, megestrol, methylprednisolone, metolazone, metoprolol, modafinil, moexipril, morphine, moxifloxacin, mycophenolate, nadolol, nalidixic acid, nelfinavir, niacin, nicotinic acid, nifedipine, nilutamide, noradrenaline, norethindrone, norgestrel, nystatin, octreotide, oral contraceptives, pantoprazole, pentamidine, pethidine, phenazone, phenothiazines, phenytoin, pioglitazone, pipecuronium, polythiazide, prazosin, prednisolone, prednisone, progesterone, propranolol, psychoactive agents, quinine, reserpine, rifampicin, rimiterol, ritodrine, ritonavir, rosiglitazone, salbutamol, salmeterol, saquinavir, somatropin, somatostatin, sotalol, steroids, streptozocin, sulfonamides, tacrolimus, terbutaline, theophylline, thiazide diuretics, thyroid hormones, torsemide, tranquilizers, triamcinolone, triamterene, trimetaphan, trimethoprim, thyroxine, valproic acid, vitamin A)

Decreased Values – hypoglycemia

hepatic cirrhosis, lactic acidosis, alcoholism, **anorexia nervosa,** acyl-coenzyme A dehydrogenase defects, deficiency of – (ACTH, epinephrine, fructose-1,6-diphosphatase, **glucagon,** carnitine, glucose-6-phosphatase, glycogen synthetase), diabetes mellitus (early stage), **galactosemia,** gastroenterostomy, **glycogenosis, hepatitis, starvation,** diarrhea, **hyperinsulinism, Langerhans' islets hyperplasia, leucine hypersensitivity, hypoadrenalism,** autoimmune hypoglycemia in non-diabetics, hypothalamic lesions, neonatal transient hypoglycemia – (infants of diabetic mothers, infants with erythroblastosis, infants of toxemic mother, small for gestational age, ketotic hypoglycemia, severe respiratory distress, smaller of twins, prematurity), **hypopituitarism, hypothyroidism, maple syrup urine disease,** diseases – (renal d., liver d., congenital heart d.), **dietary mistake,** insufficiency – (adrenal i., chronic renal i.), **inborn fructose intolerance,** poisoning by – (**alcohol,** arsenic, phosphorus, chloroform, Ammanita phalloides, strychnine, tetrachlormethane), **insulinoma** (pancreatic beta-cells tumour), cachexia, disease – (**Addison's d., von Gierke's d.**), **malabsorption, malnutrition,** methylmalonic acidemia, glutaric acidemia, tumours – (diffuse carcinomatosis, carcinoid, **leukemia, fibrosarcoma,** mesenchymal t., **adrenal gland t., liver t.,** gastrointestinal tract t., Wilms' t., **stomach t.**), **excessive physical exertion,** obesity, pancreatitis, **panhypopituitarism,** polycythemia, burns, anti-diabetics overdosage – (**oral antidiabetics, insulin**), decreased intake of glucose, antiinsulin antibodies, antiinsulin receptor antibodies, **bacterial sepsis,** conditions – (febrile c., postsurgery c., post-hyperglycemic c.), syndrome – (**post-gastrectomy sy, Reye's sy, septic shock sy,** Zettersstrom's sy), endotoxic shock, pregnancy (3rd trimester), failure – (**renal f., heart f.**)

Interfering Factors: medicaments – (acebutolol, acetaminophen, acetohexamide, acetyl-salicylic acid – toxic doses, ACTH, amphotericin B, anabolics, androgens, antihistamines, ascorbic acid, atenolol, atropine, beta-blockers, betaxolol, bisoprolol, caffeine, captopril, carbutamide, carteolol, carvedilol, chlorpropamide, chromium, cimetidine, clarithromycin, clofibrate, cyproterone, cysteine, dalfopristin, disopyramide, estrogens, ethanol, fluoxetine, gatifloxacin, ginseng, glimepiride, glipizide, glutathione, glyburide, guanethidine, guanfacine, indomethacin, insulin, interferon beta-1b, levodopa, levofloxacin, MAO inhibitors, marijuana, megestrol, metformin, metoprolol, nadolol, nifedipine, octreotide, oral contraceptives, oxyphenbutazone, oxymetholone, pentamidine, phenformin, phenylbutazone, pindolol, pioglitazone, pivampicillin, potassium chloride, promethazine, propantheline, propranolol, protionamide, quinine, repaglinide, reserpine, ritodrine, rosiglitazone, salicylates, somatotropin, sotalol, spironolactone, streptozocin, sulfadiazine, sulfonamides, sulfonylurea, timolol, tolazamide, tolbutamide, trometamol, valproic acid)

Analyte	Age/Gender	Reference Range	SI Units	Note
Glucose				
capillary blood	Neonates 6 hrs	0.33–3.3	mmol/l	
	> 5 d	0.72–4.2	mmol/l	
	1–2 y	1.8–6.2	mmol/l	
	3–4 y	2.9–5.4	mmol/l	
	5–6 y	3.8–5.5	mmol/l	
	Adults	3.3–5.5	mmol/l	
Glucose				
venous plasma	Adults	3.5–6.4	mmol/l	
Oral Glucose				
Tolerance Test				
capillary blood	fasting – H	<5.6	mmol/l	
	PGT	<7.0	mmol/l	
	DM	>7.0	mmol/l	
	after 1 hour – H	<8.9	mmol/l	
	PGT	>11.0	mmol/l	
	DM	>11.1	mmol/l	
	after 2 hrs – H	<6.7	mmol/l	
	PGT	8.0–11.0	mmol/l	
	DM	>11.0	mmol/l	
venous blood	fasting – H	<6.7	mmol/l	
	PGT	<7.0	mmol/l	
	DM	>7.0	mmol/l	
	after 1 hour – H	<10.0	mmol/l	
	PGT	>10.0	mmol/l	
	DM	>11.1	mmol/l	
	after 2 hrs	<7.0	mmol/l	
	PGT	7,0–10.0	mmol/l	
	DM	>10.0	mmol/l	
venous plasma,				
serum	fasting – H	>7.0	mmol/l	
	PGT	<8.0	mmol/l	
	DM	>8.0	mmol/l	
	after 1 hour – H	<11.0	mmol/l	

Analyte	Age/Gender	Reference Range	SI Units	Note
	PGT	>11.0	mmol/l	
	DM	>11.0	mmol/l	
	after 2 hrs – H	<8.0	mmol/l	
	PGT	8.0–11.0	mmol/l	
	DM	11.1	mmol/l	

Glucose-6-Phosphate Dehydrogenase

(G6PD, G-6-PD) An enzyme found in most body cells which is involved in metabolizing glucose. Enzyme G-6-PD catalyzes the first step in the hexose monophosphate shunt pathway in RBC ($Fe^{2+}Hb \rightarrow Fe^{3+}metHb$) resulting in NADP to NADPH reduction (a co-factor for glutathione reduction) important to protect RBCs from oxidative damage. In the RBCs, a G-6-PD deficiency causes hemoglobin precipitation and cellular membrane changes, that may result in hemolysis of variable severity. Because the G-6-PD gene is located (recessive trait carried) on the X chromosome (sex-linked), full deficiency expression is found in the male hemizygote. Affected males inherit this abnormal gene from their mothers, who are usually asymptomatic. G-6-PD deficiency is the most prevalent congenital RBC enzyme defect.

Test Purpose. 1) to detect hemolytic anemia caused by G-6-PD deficiency, 2) to aid in the hemolytic anemia differential diagnosis, 3) differential diagnosis of recurrent infections in children.

Increased Values
anemia – (**megaloblastic a., pernicious a.**), **hyperthyroidism, myocardial infarction, hepatic coma, chronic blood loss**
> **Interfering Factors:** medicaments – (acetylsalicylic acid, antipyretics, ascorbic acid, nitrofurantoin, phenacetin, primaquine, quinidine, salicylates, sulfonamides, thiazide diuretics, tolbutamide, vitamin K)

Decreased Values
diabetic acidosis, hemolytic anemia caused by G-6-PD deficiency, infections, septicemia, ingestion of fava beans
> **Interfering Factors:** medicaments – (antimalarials, nalidixic acid, nitrofurantoin, phenacetin)

Analyte	Age/Gender	Reference Range	SI Units	Note
Glucose-6-Phosphate Dehydrogenase (RBC)		8–40	µkat/l	

Beta-Glucosidase

Function. Beta-glucosidase is a lysosomal enzyme that is required for glucocerebroside hydrolysis.
Occurrence. Body tissue, fibroblasts, white blood cells. The sample is obtained from skin biopsy.

Decreased Values
Gaucher's disease

Beta-Glucuronidase

Beta-glucuronidase is a lysosomal hydrolase that catalyzes terminal glucuronic acid residues cleavage from a variety of beta-glucuronides. It is important in the degradation of many glycosaminoglycans, including dermatan sulfate, heparan sulfate and the chondroitin sulfates. Present in fibroblasts.

Increased Values
liver cirrhosis, diabetes mellitus, **viral/toxic hepatitis**, hypertension, acute lymphocytic leukemia, tumors of – (colon, cervix, pancreas, liver, breast, stomach), **liver necrosis**, pregnancy (3rd trimester)
> **Interfering Factors:** medicaments – (anabolic steroids, androgens, chlorpromazine, estrogens, ethanol, oral contraceptives, rifampicin)

Decreased Values
mucopolysaccharidosis VII, Marfan's sy, **liver failure**

Glutamate Dehydrogenase

(GD, GMD, GLD, GLDH) GMD is a specific liver zinc containing enzyme.
Function. Mitochondrial enzyme of oxide-reduction, which catalyzes hydrogen cleavage reaction (oxidative deamination) from L-glutamate → alpha-ketoglutarate, using NAD$^+$ or NADP$^+$ as an electron acceptor. The reversible reaction has a major function in both glutamic acid synthesis and degradation. Catalyzes ammonia change arising from amino acids oxidative deamination → prevents the ammonia accumulation in body.
Occurrence. GMD is highly concentrated in the liver (the central liver lobule), erythrocytes, heart muscle, kidneys, brain, skeletal muscles, WBC. Its half-time is 18 hrs.
Test Purpose. To help in hepatopathy diagnosis.

Increased Values
hepatic cirrhosis, acute hepatic dystrophy, hepatitis – (chronic h., viral h.), diseases – (hepatic d., biliary tract d.), intoxication by halothane, **hepatic necrosis**, extra/intrahepatic obstruction
> **Interfering Factors:** medicaments – (ethanol, oral contraceptives, streptokinase)

Analyte	Age/Gender	Reference Range	SI Units	Note
Glutamate Dehydrogenase				
	1–30 d	<163	nkat/l	
	1–6 m	<107	nkat/l	
	13–24 m	<87	nkat/l	
	2–3 y	<63	nkat/l	
	13–15 y	<80	nkat/l	
	Adults F	<88	nkat/l	
	Adults M	<123	nkat/l	

Glutamic Acid

(Glu) A non-essential (glucoplastic) amino acid occurring in proteins. It is important for gluconeogenesis. Intracellular glutamic acid content is high. Glutamic acid determinations clinical importance is mainly with the hereditary metabolic disorder – glutamic aminoacidemia. It also serves as a stimulating neurotransmitter in CNS. Glutathione is the major glutamic acid product in the body. This ubiquitous tripeptide is synthesized and degraded through a complex gamma-glutamyl cycle. Glutathione protects sulfhydrylcontaining compounds from oxidation. It is also involved in peroxide detoxification and keeping the cell content reduced. Plasma glutamic acid is total and free.

Increased Values
glutamic acidemia, rheumatoid arthritis, gout, pancreas tumors
   Interfering Factors: medicaments – (testosterone)

Decreased Values
histidinemia, after abdominal surgery, chronic renal failure
   Interfering Factors: medicaments – (oral contraceptives)

Analyte	Age/Gender	Reference Range	SI Units	Note
Glutamic Acid				
Free	Neonates	0–900	µmol/l	
	1–3 y	<180	µmol/l	
	Adults	25–115	µmol/l	
Total	Adults	517–720	µmol/l	

Glutamic Acid Decarboxylase Antibodies

(anti-GAD, GADA) Glutamic acid decarboxylase (GAD) is the GABA-synthesizing enzyme. Autoimmune processes (caused by the destruction of insulin-secreting pancreatic beta cells) can be confirmed in some patients during latent clinically premanifest diabetes mellitus type I period: islet cell autoantibodies (ICA) as well as insulin autoantibodies (IAA). The clinical onset of the disease is preceded by chronic inflammation of the pancreatic islet cells and the eventual loss of insulin-secreting beta cells. Clinical DM type I occurs only after destruction of 80–90% of these cells. IAA determination has low sensitivity and specificity. ICA determination is limited by vague antigen identification till now. Protein (glutamic acid decarboxylase, GAD) was isolated from Langerhans' islet cell surface; antibodies against this protein are detectable in IDDM. Two isoforms of GADA (GADA65, GADA67) have been identified. GADA65 is the predominant form associated with type I DM. GADA appear prior to clinical symptoms of the disease (can be used to predict who will develop IDDM). GADA are found in about 70% of type I diabetes patients at the time of diagnosis. If GADA appear in NIDDM patients, it can be useful to predict which patients may later require insulin therapy. Other antibodies include antibodies against fragment of tyrosine phosphatase (IA-2) and membrane glycoprotein (glima 38).

Test Purpose. 1) IDDM preclinical stage diagnosis, 2) diagnosis in first-step relatives, mainly in children and adolescents, 3) gestation diabetes differential diagnosis (90% sensitivity, 100% negative specificity, i. e. IDDM exclusion), 4) differential diagnosis of some diabetes mellitus type I and II forms.

Increased Values
insulin-dependent diabetes mellitus, prediabetic phase of diabetes mellitus, **stiff man syndrome**

Analyte	Age/Gender	Reference Range	SI Units	Note
Glutamic Acid Decarboxylase Ab		1–2	U/ml	

Glutamine

(Gln) Glutamine is the most abundant free amino acid in plasma.
Production. Muscle, liver, nervous system.
Function. In ammonia nontoxic storage and transport. A NH_2-groups donor in many substances biosynthesis, it serves also as a main ammonia reserve. Glutamine formation is the major mechanism for the ammonia removal from the brain. Ammonia secreted by the kidney is derived from plasma glutamine.
Test Purpose. To investigate patients with suspected hyperammonemia.

Increased Values – hyperglutaminemia
glutamine aminoacidemia, citrullinemia, hyperammonemia, hyperlysinemia, hyperornithinemia, **hepatic coma**, cerebral hemorrhage, meningitis, **Reye's sy**, total parenteral nutrition
   Interfering Factors: medicaments – (phenobarbital, phenytoin)

Decreased Values – hypoglutaminemia
rheumatoid arthritis
   Interfering Factors: medicaments – (asparaginase)

Analyte	Age/Gender	Reference Range	SI Units	Note
Glutamine	Neonates	20–120	μmol/l	
	Infants	<300	μmol/l	
	Adults	<50	μmol/l	

Gamma-Glutamyltransferase

(GMT, GGT, syn: gamma-glutamyltranspeptidase – GGTP, gamma-GTP) Enzyme – transferase.
Function. Catalyzes gamma-glutamyl group transport from gamma-glutamyl peptides to other peptides, L-amino acids, or water. A key enzyme of gamma-glutamyl cycle which governs transcellular transport of amino acids and peptides.
Occurrence. In tissue cell membranes which have high secretory or absorption capacity as liver, kidney, pancreas, epithelial cells, erythrocytes, intestine, prostate, brain, plasma, bile, cerebrospinal fluid = liquor, leucocytes, spleen, spermatic fluid. Because of the highest enzyme amount in liver (the highest specific activity is in kidney), changes in blood are determined by liver activity (membrane bound hepatic cell marker). In serum it is in heterogenous form, bound mainly onto HDL and LDL. The fraction bound to HDL (biologic half-time 20 hrs) is increased in non-icteric liver disorders forms, in cholestatic disorders the fraction bound onto LDL is increased. Water soluble form (up to 20 %) is increasing in other disorders (biologic half-time 9 hrs). If activity is increased more than twice, or as a com-

bined increase with other enzymes one should also consider parenchymatous damage. Synthesis is stimulated by chronic alcohol abuse and other therapeutic dose medicaments. The GMT level increases in escape from hepatocytes and biliary ways epithelium. Generally parallels changes in serum ALP, LAP and 5-nucleotidase. The most sensitive indicator and a good screening test for alcoholism.

Test Purpose. 1) to provide information about hepatobiliary diseases, to assess liver function and to detect alcohol ingestion, 2) to distinguish between skeletal diseases and hepatic diseases when the serum alkaline phosphatase is elevated.

Increased Values

alcoholism, biliary atresia, rheumatoid arthritis, **cirrhosis hepatis,** primary biliary cirrhosis, diabetes mellitus, myotonic dystrophy, hepatitis – (**chronic alcoholic h., acute/chronic reactive h.,** chronic active h. B, acute h. A, acute h. B, chronic h. C, acute h. D, acute h. E, autoimmune h., cholestatic h.,), **hyperlipidemia, hyperthyroidism,** cholecystitis, cholestasis, **cholelithiasis, intra/extrahepatic cholestasis,** diseases – (**renal d., exocrine pancreatic d., liver d.,** pulmonary d., heart d.), **obstructive icterus, cardiac infarction** (from 2nd–4th day), cardiac insufficiency, poisoning by – (aflatoxin, alcohol, antimony, arsenic, phosphorus, herbicides, mushrooms, chromates, copper, naphthalene, nitrobenzene, lead, solvents, trichlorethylene, iron), **hepatic ischemia,** systemic lupus erythematosus, tumors – (**pancreas t., liver t., prostate t., hypernephroma,** breast t., kidney t., lung t., melanoma), **tumor metastases, infectious mononucleosis,** lipoid nephrosis, **hepatic necrosis, obesity, pancreatitis,** myocardial injury, toxic hepatic lesion caused by – (alcohol, medicaments, poisons), **hepatic steatosis,** syndrome – (nephrotic sy, eosinophilia-myalgia sy), after surgery, primary biliary cirrhosis, septic conditions, pregnancy, renal transplant, **congestive heart failure**

Interfering Factors: medicaments – (abacavir, acarbose, acetaminophen, aciclovir, ajmaline, aldesleukin, allopurinol, alosetron, aminoglutethimide, amiodarone, amlodipine, amoxicillin, amphotericin B, ampicillin, anagrelide, analgesics, antidepressants, antiepileptics, antihemophilic factor, antihyperlipidemics, anticoagulants, anticonvulsants, antirheumatics, ardeparin, argatroban, asparaginase, atenolol, atorvastatin, atovaquone, azapropazone, azathioprine, aztreonam, barbiturates, BCG, benazepril, bexarotene, bicalutamide, bisoprolol, bromfenac, busulfan, candesartan, capecitabine, captopril, carbamazepine, carbenicillin, carbidopa, carbimazole, carboplatin, carmustine, cefepime, cefoperazone, ceftizoxime, celecoxib, cephalosporins, cephradine, cerivastatin, chenodiol, chloramphenicol, chlorzoxazone, cimetidine, cisplatin, clarithromycin, clofazimine, clometacin, clomiphene, coumarin, cyclosporine, cytarabine, cytostatics, dactinomycin, danazol, dantrolene, dapsone, delavirdine, demeclocycline, desmopressin, dexmedetomidine, diazepam, diclofenac, dicloxacillin, dicoumarol, didanosine, diethylstilbestrol, diflunisal, diltiazem, disulfiram, disopyramide, docetaxel, dofetilide, dolasetron, doxycycline, efavirenz, enalapril, eprosartan, erythromycin, estradiol, estrogens, ethambutol, ethanol, ethinyl estradiol, etodolac, etretinate, felbamate, fenofibrate, floxuridine, fluconazole, flucytosine, flurbiprofen, flutamide, fluvastatin, fluvoxamine, fomivirsen, fosinopril, fosphenytoin, gemcitabine, gemtuzumab, granisetron, griseofulvin, haloperidol, halothane, heparin, hydralazine, hydrochlorothiazide, hydrocodone, ibuprofen, idarubicin, imipramine, inamrinone, infliximab, interferon, interleukin 2, irinotecan, isocarboxazid, isoflurane, isoniazid, isotretinoin, itraconazole, ketoconazole, ketoprofen, ketorolac, lamivudine, lansoprazole, leflunomide, levodopa, levonorgestrel, linezolid, loracarbef, losartan, lovastatin, meclofenamate, medroxyprogesterone, mefloquine, megestrol, meloxicam, menotropins, meropenem, mesalamine, mestranol, metaxalone, methimazole, methotrexate, methyldopa, methyltestosterone, metolazone, metoprolol, mexiletine, mezlocillin, minocycline, mirtazapine, mitoxantrone, modafinil, moexipril, moricizine, moxifloxacin, nabumetone, nafcillin, naltrexone, nandrolone, naproxen, narcotics, nefazodone, nevirapine, niacin, nilutamide, nisoldipine, nitrofurantoin, nizatidine, nomifensine, norethindrone, norgestrel, olanzapine, olsalazine, omeprazole, ondasetron, oral contraceptives, oxacillin, oxaprozin, oxyphenbutazone, paclitaxel, palivizumab, pantoprazole, papaverine, pemoline, penicillamine, penicillin G, pentosan, pentostatin, perindopril, phenazone, phenazopyridine, phenelzine, phenobarbital, phenothiazines, phenytoin, pindolol, piperacillin, piroxicam, plicamycin, prasterone, pravastatin, primidone, probucol, progesterone, promazine, propoxyphene, propylthiouracil, pyrazinamide, quetiapine, quinacrine, quinidine, rabeprazole, ranitidine, rifabutin, rifampicin, rifapentine, riluzole, ritodrine, ritonavir, rofecoxib, sedatives, sertraline, sibutramine, simvastatin, sotalol, stavudine, steroids, streptokinase, streptozocin, sulfamethoxazole, sulfasalazine, sulindac, suloctidil, tacrine, tamoxifen, terbinafine, testosterone, tetracycline, thiabendazole, thiamazole, thiazide diuretics, thiopental, thyrostatics, ticarcillin, ticlodipine, timolol, tizanidine, tolcapone, tolmetin, toremifene, trandolapril, tranylcypromine, tretinoin, tricyclic antidepressants, trimethoprim, trimetrexate, troglitazone, trovafloxacin, tuberculostatics, valerian, valproic acid, valsartan, verapamil, verteporfin, warfarin, zafirlukast, zalcitabine, zidovudine, zileuton, zimeldine, zonisamide)

Decreased Values
hypothyroidism, pregnancy (3rd trimester)
> **Interfering Factors:** medicaments – (ascorbic acid, clofibrate, estrogens, fenofibrate, oral contraceptives)

Analyte	Age/Gender	Reference Range	SI Units	Note
Gamma-Glutamyl-Transferase 37 °C	1 d	<2.52	µkat/l	
	2–5 d	<3.08	µkat/l	
	6 d–6 m	<3.40	µkat/l	
	7–12 m	<0.57	µkat/l	
	1–3 y	<0.30	µkat/l	
	4–6 y	<3.38	µkat/l	
	7–12 y	<0.28	µkat/l	
	13–17 F	<0.55	µkat/l	
	13–17 M	<0.75	µkat/l	
	Adults F	<0.53	µkat/l	
	Adults M	<0.82	µkat/l	
	Adults F	<0.75	µkat/l	See ref.
	Adults M	<1.07	µkat/l	ranges note

Glutathione Peroxidase

Antioxidative oxidoreductase class enzyme.
Function. Removes hydrogen peroxide (reactive O_2 form) and organic peroxides with reduced glutathione (detoxifying reduction) via glutathione oxidation. The enzyme requires selenium at the active site. Most enzyme is found in the liver, myocard, lung and brain.

Increased Values
Parkinson's disease

Decreased Values
newborn hemolytic disease, chronic cerebrovascular diseases, acute myocardial infarction
(decrease up to 48 h)

Glutathione S-Transferase

(GST) Elevation of the appropriate GST isoenzyme provides an early, sensitive indicator of
organ damage, particularly rejection of a transplanted organ. p-GST isoenzyme is an indicator of biliary tract damage, especially with rejection of transplanted liver.

Increased Values
renal-transplant rejection, hepatic parenchymal damage, biliary tract damage (p-GST)

Glycerol

(syn: free glycerol) Glycerol is a major component of many lipids and an important intermediate in carbohydrate and lipid metabolism.

Increased Values – hyperglycerolemia
liver cirrhosis, diabetes mellitus, starvation, hyperthyroidism, liver diseases, congenital
absence of glycerol kinase, bacterial contamination of serum, obesity, stress, chronic renal
failure
  Interfering Factors: total parenteral nutrition, medicaments – (adrenaline, ethanol, glucagon, growth hormone, heparin, mannitol, nitroglycerin, thyroxine)

Decreased Values – hypoglycerolemia
  Interfering Factors: medicaments – (amino acids, sulfonylurea, tolbutamide)

Analyte	Age/Gender	Reference Range	SI Units	Note
Glycerol, free	Children	10–110	μmol/l	
	Adults	60–180	μmol/l	

Glycine

(Gly) Glycine a main amino acid in all body fluids is synthesized mainly from serine and
threonine. Participating in many synthetic reactions such as purine formation, it is an inhibitory neurotransmitter in the central nervous system. Glycine concentrations in plasma
depend on nutrition status and fasting duration. Enzyme defect: glycine cleavage enzyme
system.

Increased Values – hyperglycinemia
acidemia – (isovaleric a., methylmalonic a., propionic a.), **glycinemia**, starvation, **hyperammonemia**, hypoglycemia, chronic renal diseases, iminoglycinemia, kwashiorkor, severe
burns, septicemia, chronic renal failure
  Interfering Factors: medicaments – (histidine)

Decreased Values – hypoglycinemia
diabetes mellitus, gout, after abdominal surgery

Analyte	Age/Gender	Reference Range	SI Units	Note
Glycine	Neonates	240–480	μmol/l	
	Infants	100–300	μmol/l	
	Children	170–370	μmol/l	
	Adults	170–260	μmol/l	

Glycol

Test Purpose. To help in diagnosis in suspected ingestion of ethylene glycol, or other glycols.

Increased Values
ethylene glycol ingestion

Beta-2-Glycoprotein I

(Beta2 GpI, syn: apolipoprotein H) Belongs to the electrophoretically divided glycoprotein fraction.

Increased Values
systemic lupus erythematosus

Decreased Values
rheumatoid arthritis, **hereditary deficiency of beta-2-glycoprotein I**

Glycosylated Albumin

(syn: glycated albumin)

Increased Values
renal failure
  Interfering Factors: hemoconcentration

Decreased Values
pregnancy

Growth Hormone

(GH, syn: human growth hormone – hGH, HGH, somatotrophin, somatotropin hormone – STH, SH)
Production. Anterior pituitary (adenohypophysis) hormone.
Function. Insulin antagonist increasing the blood glucose level. Stimulates RNA production, mobilizes fatty acids from fat deposits (increasing the fatty acids breakdown in adipose tissue). STH has a proteoanabolic effect. Essential for postnatal body growth via somatomedins (SM-A, SM-C, IGF-I, IGF-II, MSA) – bone growth prolongation (modulating growth

from birth until the puberty's end) and normal carbohydrate, lipid, nitrogen, and mineral metabolism. In peripheral tissues it supports active peptides production (somatomedin C = insulin-like growth factor). Stimulates thymocyte proliferation, antibody production, cutaneous-graft rejection, NK-cells, and production of IL-1, IL-2, TNF-alpha and thymuline. It is stimuli released: physical exercise, deep sleep, hypoglycemia, proteins ingestion, starvation, injury, overheating, dopamine, epinephrine, norepinephrine. Random GH measurements are not adequate GH deficiency determinants, because hormone secretion is episodic. hGH receptors are localized in many organs, receptor disorder must be eliminated in constitutional low stature and in Laron nanism. hGH, chorion-somatomammotropin, and prolactin are very similar one-chain proteohormones with 90–95% genetic homology.

Hypothalamic Hormones. 1) growth hormone-releasing hormone (GH-RH) = somatoliberin, somatocrinin → increases hGH release, 2) growth hormone-releasing inhibiting hormone (GH-RIH) = somatostatin → inhibits hGH release. Highest levels are just after sleep and in fall, but lowest in spring.

Test Purpose. 1) to aid dwarfism differential diagnosis resulting from hypopituitarism, hypothalamic disorders or thyroid disorders, 2) to confirm acromegaly and gigantism diagnoses, 3) to aid diagnosis of pituitary or hypothalamic tumors, 4) to help in evaluating hGH therapy.

Increased Values

acromegaly, **anorexia nervosa**, hepatic cirrhosis, **long-term endurance exercise**, **diabetes mellitus** (uncontrolled), exposure to heat/cold, **gigantism**, **starvation**, hyperaminoacidemia, selective hyperpituitarism, **hypoglycemia**, **liver diseases**, **malnutrition**, tumors – (pituitary gland t., kidney t., lung t.), **Laron dwarfism** (defective GH receptors), **newborns**, **major surgery**, **excessive protein ingestion**, ectopic GH secretion by tumor – (lung t., stomach t.), stress – **(physical s., psychologic s.)**, **renal failure**

> **Interfering Factors:** fasting, **deep sleep**, medicaments – (ACTH, amphetamines, anabolic steroids, androgens, antiepileptics, apomorphine, arginine, atenolol, baclofen, beta-blockers, clomipramine, clonidine, desipramine, dopamine, estrogens, ethinylestradiol, glucagon, glucocorticoids – short term, histamine, indomethacin, insulin, L-dopa, metoclopramide, metoprolol, methyldopa, metyrapone, nalorphine, nicotinic acid, oral contraceptives, oxprenolol, phenytoin, propranolol, vasopressin)

Decreased Values

growth hormone deficiency, **hemochromatosis**, **adrenocortical hyperfunction**, **hyperglycemia**, hyperthyroidism, **selective hypopituitarism**, **hypothyroidism**, pituitary infarction, **pituitary insufficiency**, elevated free fatty acids, **metastases of malignant tumors**, **tumors**, **nanism** (pituitary dwarfism), **panhypopituitarism**

> **Interfering Factors: obesity**, medicaments – (alpha-blockers, carbamazepine, corticosteroids, glucocorticoids – long term, glucose, growth hormone, isoproterenol, octreotide, phenothiazines, phentolamin, probucol, progesterone, somatostatin)

Growth Hormone-Releasing Hormone

(GH-RH, syn: somatoliberin, somatocrinin) GH-RH is produced by the hypothalamus and stimulates growth hormone release from the anterior pituitary.

Increased Values

acromegaly due to GH-RH secretion by neoplasm – (bronchial carcinoid, thymic carcinoid, pancreatic islet tumors, neuroendocrine tumors)

Guanine Deaminase

(syn: guanase) A hydrolase class enzyme that catalyzes guanine deamination to form xanthine. The reaction is a step in the guanine degradation to uric acid. The enzyme is found in the liver, kidney, spleen and other tissues.

Increased Values
viral hepatitis, heavy metal hepatic toxicity, extrahepatic obstructive jaundice, hepatic metastases

Heat Shock Proteins

(HSP, syn: stress proteins) Heat shock proteins are produced in cells immediately after increased temperature exposure or without the stressor influence. HSP production is caused by environmental stress conditions (higher temperature, ionizing radiation, heavy metals, anoxia, amino acids analogues, hypoglycemia, energetic metabolism inhibitors, infectious/inflammatory diseases, febrile conditions, surgical trauma, malignant tumors and genetic disorders). Immunological production factors are phagocytosis, oxygen/nitrogen reactive, and free-radical forms, T-lymphocytes activation, IFN-gamma, cytokines, tissue transplantation, cell cycle, embryonic development, cell differentiation, and hormonal stimulation. GRPs (glucose regulated proteins) belong to the stress proteins. Synthesis is induced by glucose lack, higher temperature and amino acid analogues. Some of stress proteins are involved in correct protein conformation maintenance, repairing incorrect conformations.

- **GRPs** (glucose regulated proteins)
- **HSP** (heat shock protein) **10:** is present in mitochondria, chloroplasts and bacteria
- **HSP 27:** is present in cytoplasm and nucleus. It is involved in protection against the heat.
- **HSP 47:** is present in endoplasmic reticulum. It is involved in collagen binding.
- **HSP 60:** is present in mitochondria and chloroplasts. Autoantigen.
- **HSP 70:** is present in cytoplasm and nucleus. It is involved in protein transport regulation, molecule marking for lysosome degradation, protection against the heat, protection against TNF-alpha caused cytotoxicity. It has a high afinity for ATP.
- **HSP 90:** is present in cytoplasm and nucleus. It is involved in steroid receptor regulation, binding with protein kinases, actin and tubulin.
- **HSP 110:** is present in nucleolus and nucleus. It is involved in transcriptional process regulation, protection against heat.
- **Heme oxidase:** is present in microsome fraction. It is involved in heme catabolism.
- **SOD** (superoxide dismutase): is present in mitochondria.
- **Ubiquitin:** is present in cytoplasm and lysosomes. It is involved in protein degradation.

Hepatitis Associated Antigens and Antibodies (Markers of Hepatitis)

Hepatitis A (serology)

(syn: HAV, hepatitis A virus serology, HAV serology) Hepatitis A belongs to the most simply, fastest, and most reliably diagnosed viral infections. Hepatitis A antigen examination in the stool and liver is used for diagnosis and monitoring. Antibodies against hepatitis A virus (**anti-HAV**) are evaluated in the serum.

Test Purpose. 1) differential diagnosis of icterus, to rule out current hepatitis A, 2) evidence of immunity. Antibody against hepatitis A IgM (**anti-HAV-IgM**) can be found 2–6 months after disease onset. A negative finding in acute phase rules out hepatitis A.
Test Purpose. Diagnosis or rule out of current hepatitis A.

Positivity	Indicates
anti-HAV-IgM	acute hepatitis
HAV-RNA	infectivity
anti-HAV	immunity to HAV (screen)

Hepatitis B (serology)

(syn: HBV, hepatitis B virus serology, HBV serology) Hepatitis B virus (HBV) is commonly known as serum hepatitis. HBV is made up of an inner core surrounded by an outer capsule. 1) The outer capsule contains the hepatitis B surface antigen (s-antigen) (**HBsAg**), formerly called Australian antigen. The protein-containing surface material manufactured in the infected hepatocytes cytoplasm. 2) The inner core contains HBV core antigen (c-antigen) (**HBcAg**) naturally demonstrable only in the infected hepatocyte nucleus. „Healthy" HBsAg carriers are HBcAg negative. High HBcAg positivity is observed in immunodeficient HBsAg carriers (e. g. dialysis). The hepatitis B e-antigen (**HBeAg**) is also found within core. Antibodies to these antigens are called **anti-HBs, anti-HBc, anti-HBe.** HBsAg generally indicates active infection by HBV (often positive weeks before clinical manifestation and before biochemical abnormalities, earliest indicator of HBV infection). It can be demonstrated 1–4 months from disease onset. It is the most reliable serologic marker of HBV infection. HBsAg is negative in about 5% of patients with hepatitis B. Persistence over 6 months defines carrier state. Hepatitis B vaccination does not cause a positive HBsAg. Titers are not of clinical value. **Anti-HBs** has some but not total protective immunity and this signifies the end of the acute infection phase, indicates absence of infectivity. These antibodies can be demonstrated 4–6 months from disease onset. Indicates recovery from HBV infection. Anti-HBs decline over several years. **Anti-HBc** (total) are positive shortly after HBV inoculation, therefore, a negative finding in clinical onset rules out acute hepatitis B. Occurs at same time as clinical illness, persists for years or for lifetime. Anti-HBc is also present in chronic hepatitis patients (persists for months/years). The anti-HBc level is elevated in the time lag between the HBsAg disappearance and the appearance of anti-HBs. This interval is called the core window, anti-HBc is the only detectable marker of recent hepatitis infection here. Anti-HBc detects virtually all persons who have been previously infected with HBV. **Anti-HBc-IgM** evidence is the method of choice in a negative HBsAg differential diagnosis. Is the earliest specific antibody, usually occurs two weeks after HBsAg. It is the only test unique to recent infection, it can differentiate acute from chronic HBV. **HBeAg** presence correlates with early/active disease, as well as with high infectivity in acute HBV infection. Appears within one week after HBsAg. Occurs early in disease before biochemical changes and disappears after serum ALT peak. It is a marker of active HBV replication in liver. It is useful to determine resolution of infection. Persistent presence of HBeAg in the blood predicts chronic carrier state and chronic HBV infection development. **Anti-HBe** indicates that an acute HBV infection is over and that infection chances are greatly reduced. Appears after HBeAg disappears and remains detectable for years. Suggests good prognosis for resolution of acute infection. Anti-HBe positive patients are often non-infectious, even if they are HBsAg positive. In this case **HBV-DNA** examination is suggested. It is the most sensitive and specific assay for early evaluation of HBV, and may be detected when all other markers are negative. Measures HBV replication even when HBeAg is not detectable. Positive **DNA polymerase** is an evidence of infectiosity. Negative finding, however, does not rule out it (relative low sensitivity and high pretension of method, which incorporates labeled ^{3}H-thymidine into the HBV genome). **HBV-DNA hybridization test** positivity is more sensitive and reliable than the HBeAg evidence. The evidence of **HBV-DNA by PCR** in optimal test conditions can demonstrate the presence of the only virion in the sample. Because of high sensitivity and relatively frequent false positive results (serum contamination), the test is used only in special departments and indications.

Test Purpose. 1) **HBsAg** – to screen blood donors for hepatitis B, 2) to screen high risk hepatitis B contact, such as hemodialysis nurses, 3) to aid in a differential diagnosis of viral hepatitis, 4) **anti-HBc** – to aid in a differential diagnosis of hepatitis syndromes and to assess hepatitis B infection staging, with demonstration of HBsAg and anti-HBs positive findings, 5) **anti-HBe** – to aid in a differential diagnosis, staging and prognosis of hepatitis B infection. Anti-HBe and anti-HBc together confirm the hepatitis B convalescent stage after the HB surface antigen disappearance, 6) **HBeAg** – to aid in a differential diagnosis and prognosis of hepatitis B infection, the evidence of serum infectiosity, monitoring of the chronic hepatitis course and antiviral therapy effect monitoring, 7) **anti-HBs** – evaluates possible immunity in individuals who are at increased risk of further exposure to hepatitis B, evaluates need for hepatitis B immune globulin after needlestick injury, evaluates need for hepatitis B vaccine, evaluates efficacy of hepatitis B vaccine, 8) **HBsAg** – to screen blood donors, to aid differential diagnosis of hepatitis, to evaluate risk in needlestick injuries in health care facilities, to guide use of hepatitis B immunoglobulin, chronic hepatopathies differential diagnosis and chronic hepatitides classification, 9) **HBsAg subtypes** (adw, adr, ayw, ayr) – to demonstrate the epidemiological coherence in frequent focal hepatitides (dialysis, dormitories) and recurrent hepatitis B, 10) **HBsAg** – classification of chronic hepatitis B, bioptic immunohistological evidence in liver tissue, 11) **anti-HBc (IgM)** – diagnosis of acute HBV infection, chronic hepatitis B monitoring, 12) **DNA polymerase** – evidence of serum infectiosity, 13) **HBV-DNA hybridization** – evidence of serum infectiosity, 14) **HBV-DNA by PCR** – evidence of serum infectiosity and blood products negativity.

Increased Values – positive
hepatitis – (**h. A, h. B, chronic h. B, non A non B h.**), **chronic hepatitis B carrier condition**

Increased Values – positive HBsAg
hemophilia, **hepatitis B**, leukemia, Hodgkin's disease

Hepatitis markers

Positivity	Indicates
HBsAg	early acute HBV infection, acute HBV infection, infectivity, HBV carrier status, chronic hepatitis
anti-HBs	recovery, immunity to HBV (screen)
anti-HBc	acute HBV infection, recent hepatitis infection, chronic hepatitis, immunity to HBV (screen), convalescence, recovery, serologic gap
anti-HBc-IgM	acute HBV infection, recent infection, convalescence, serologic gap
anti-HBc-IgG	past infection, HBV carrier status
HBeAg	early acute HBV infection, acute HBV infection, greater infectivity, its persistence indicates an increased risk of chronic liver disease
anti-HBe	convalescence, recovery, better prognosis, less infectivity
DNA polymerase	evidence of infectivity
HBV-DNA	infectivity

Hepatitis C (serology)

(syn: HCV, hepatitis C virus serology, HCV serology) Most cases of post-transfusion non A non B viral hepatitis are caused by HCV. In chronic HCV infection development, anti-HCV testing is positive (80%). Antibodies are positive until the active chronic hepatitis is present. The test has a high false positivity. The test may take up to 6 months from the time of infection to become positive, so the significance of indeterminate results can only be determined by retesting after 3–6 months. Positive HCV RNA is a predictor of worse prognosis and greater infectivity.

Test Purpose. Anti-HCV 1) to aid in a differential diagnosis of acute/chronic hepatitis, cirrhosis, hepatocellular carcinoma, 2) to screen blood units for transfusion safety, to test patients who have received blood or blood products, 3) to test infectivity after needle stick injury, 4) to test infectivity in blood or tissue transplant donors, 5) to investigate patients with mixed essential cryoglobulinemia, 6) anti-HCV – to aid in diagnosis of acute and chronic HCV infection. The demonstration of **HCV-RNA (by PCR)** 1) evidence of HCV positivity and quantity, 2) evidence of blood products infectiosity, 3) evidence of anti-HCV positive findings, therapy monitoring (e. g. with interferon).

Increased Values – positive
hepatitis C (acute non A non B viral hepatitis)

Positivity	Indicates
anti-HCV	acute HCV infection, chronic hepatitis, infectivity
HCV-RNA	infectivity

Hepatitis D (serology)

(syn: HDV, delta antigen serology, hepatitis delta virus, delta hepatitis serology) Parameters evaluated: hepatitis D antigen (HDAg), antibody against hepatitis D virus (anti-HDV), anti-HDV-IgM and HDV-RNA. Hepatitis D is due to a transmissible virus that depends on HBV for expression and replication. It may be found for 7–14 days in the serum during acute infection. The diagnosis of delta hepatitis is dependent on the detection of HBsAg and anti-HDV. Rising titres of anti-HDV suggest acute infection and continuing high titres are consistent with chronic infection. The course depends on the presence of HBV infection. Over 70% of patients with HDV superinfection develop chronic hepatitis. Chronic HDV infection is more severe and has higher mortality than other types of viral hepatitis. IgM anti-HDV persists in chronic delta hepatitis.

Test Purpose. To aid in a differential diagnosis of chronic/recurrent/acute viral hepatitis.

Increased Values – positive
hepatitis D

Positivity	Indicates
HDAg	acute HDV infection, carrier state
anti-HDV	chronic hepatitis, infectivity, carrier state
HDV-RNA	infectivity

Hepatitis E (serology)

(syn: HEV, hepatitis E virus antibodies) Antibody against hepatitis E virus (anti-HEV) develop early in the course of the illness.

Increased Values – positive
hepatitis E

Positivity	Indicates
anti-HEV	acute HEV infection, immunity to HEV (screen)
HEV-RNA	infectivity

Hepatitis G (serology)

(syn: HGV, hepatitis G virus serology, HGV serology) Test is used in acute/chronic hepatitis not attributable to hepatitis A, B, C, D or E virus infection. Infection tends to persist for many years. Detected RT-PCR.

Increased Values – positive
hepatitis G, multiply transfused persons, drug addiction

Hepatocyte Growth Factor

(HGF, syn: scatter factor, hematopoietin A)
Occurrence. Platelets, macrophages, endothelial cells, smooth muscle cells.
Function. Stimulates cellular growth including hepatocytes, epithelial cells, keratinocytes, melanocytes and hematopoietic progenitor cells. Increases motility/invasiveness of various epithelial and endothelial cells. HGF induces plasminogen activator expression. HGF receptors are oncogene c-met product.

Hexosaminidase

(syn: total hexosaminidase) Lysosomal enzyme. Three predominant hexosaminidase isoenzymes have been identified in serum, hexosaminidase A, B and S. It is a group of enzymes necessary for gangliosides metabolism; water-soluble glycolipids are found primarily in brain tissue.
Test Purpose. 1) to confirm/rule out Tay-Sachs disease in neonates, 2) to screen for Tay-Sachs disease carriers, 3) to establish prenatal hexosaminidase A deficiency diagnosis.

Increased Values
hepatic cirrhosis, myocardial infarct, vascular complications of diabetes mellitus, tumors – (myeloma, stomach t.), hydatidiform mole, hepatic necrosis, biliary obstruction, symptomatic porphyria, **pregnancy**
    Interfering Factors: medicaments – (EDTA, ethanol, heparin, isoniazid, oral contraceptives, rifampicin)

Decreased Values
Sandoff's disease, ectopic pregnancy, pregnancy (very early), **Tay-Sachs disease**

Hexosaminidase A

Hexosaminidase isoenzyme.

Increased Values
diabetes mellitus, **pregnancy**
    Interfering Factors: medicaments – (oral contraceptives)

Decreased Values
Sandoff's disease, **Tay-Sachs disease**

Hexosaminidase B

Hexosaminidase isoenzyme.

Increased Values
Tay-Sachs disease

Decreased Values
Sandoff's disease

Histamine

Histamine is a beta-imidazolylethylamine and intercellular mediator with strong effects on many target organs and tissues. A decarboxylation histidine product found in all body tissues, particularly in the mast cells and related blood basophils, the highest concentration is found in the lungs; released by specific allergens or non-specific release agents, e. g. anti-IgE. Histamine effects at the receptors: 1) H_1-receptor: postcapillary venules permeability increase, smooth muscle contraction, pulmonary vasoconstriction, cGMP increase in cells, mucus secretion increase, leukocyte chemotaxis, prostaglandins production in lungs, suppression of cardiac atrioventricular node, bronchoconstriction, 2) H_2-receptor: increase of gastric acid secretion, increase of mucus secretion, increase of cAMP in cells, leukocyte chemotaxis, suppressor T-lymphocytes activation, bronchodilation, induction of idioventricular responses, inhibition of basophilic mediator release, 3) H_1- and H_2-receptors: pruritus, increased vascular permeability, 4) H_3-receptor: histamine release inhibition, histamine synthesis inhibition. It is also a mediator of immediate hypersensitivity, and a neurotransmitter in the CNS. Marked diurnal variation, which is highest in late morning and lowest in afternoon.
Test Purpose. 1) type I immunopathologic reaction suspicion (immediate allergic reaction, anaphylaxis), allergen examination/identification by exposure testing with in vitro/in vivo histamine concentration determination in basophils, plasma, urine, and bronchoalveolar lavage fluid, 2) non-commercial antigens testing, 3) histamine pharmacologic effect determination in gastrointestinal tract, CNS and periphery in research indications.

Increased Values – hyperhistaminemia
ethanol, renal failure, systemic mastocytosis, myeloproliferative disorders, carcinoid syndrome, insulinoma, medullary thyroid carcinoma, pheochromocytoma, vipoma, glucagonoma
    Interfering Factors: radiographic contrast agents, postprandial

Decreased Values – hypohistaminemia
 Interfering Factors: medicaments – (ascorbic acid, erythropoietin, glucocorticoids)

Analyte	Age/Gender	Reference Range	SI Units	Note
Histamine				
plasma		<10	nmol/l	
		<1	ng/ml	
whole blood		200–2000	nmol/l	
		20–200	ng/ml	
cellular		0.10–1.0		
spontaneous release		<0.05		

Histidine

(His) Histidine is an essential amino acid only during infancy; synthetic pathway in older children and adults is poorly understood. Degraded through the urocanic acid pathway to glutamic acid, histidine decarboxylation results in histamine formation. Enzyme defect: L-histidine ammonium lyasis.

Increased Values – hyperhistidinemia
hemolysis, **histidinemia**, transient newborn histidinemia, pregnancy
 Interfering Factors: medicaments – (arginine, asparagine, cystine, histamine, tyrosine)

Decreased Values – hypohistidinemia
rheumatoid arthritis, **after abdominal surgery** (1–16 days)

Analyte	Age/Gender	Reference Range	SI Units	Note
Histidine	Neonates	70–120	μmol/l	
	Infants	50–120	μmol/l	
	Children	50–120	μmol/l	
	Adults	60–100	μmol/l	

HIV-1 RNA

HIV-1 RNA is amplified by PCR. The test measures viral load and provides a predictor of disease course and prognosis, independent of CD4 counts. High viral load is associated with a poor prognosis if detected early in the course of disease. Decreased viral load in response to therapy is associated with an improved long term outcome.

Test Purpose. 1) to monitor the course of HIV infection, including prognosis and response to treatment, 2) in neonates, to assess whether HIV antibody is maternally derived or indicates infection.

Increased Values – positive
HIV infection

Homocysteine

(Hcys) Most homocysteine, an intermediate methionine compound degradation, is normally remethylated to methionine. This methionine-sparing reaction is catalyzed by the enzyme methionine synthase, which requires a folic acid metabolite as a substrate and a vitamin B_{12} metabolite as a co-factor. Homocysteine is a severe ischemic heart disease risk factor.

Test Purpose. 1) to help in diagnosis of homocystinuria and treatment monitoring, 2) to investigate risk factors for early onset cerebral and coronary atherosclerosis.

Increased Values – hyperhomocysteinemia
generalized aminoaciduria, **homocystinuria**, **renal failure**, ischemic heart disease, myocardial infarction, **hypothyroidism**, folate deficiency, **vitamin B_6 deficiency**, smoking

  Interfering Factors: medicaments – (carbamazepine, methotrexate, phenytoin, theophylline)

Analyte	Age/Gender	Reference Range	SI Units	Note
Homocysteine	M			
	<30 y	6–14	μmol/l	
	30–59 y	6–16	μmol/l	
	>60 y	6–17	μmol/l	
	F			
	<30 y	6–14	μmol/l	
	30–59 y	5–13	μmol/l	
	>60 y	7–14	μmol/l	

Hormones and Hormone-Like Substances

	Abbr	Hormone	Site of action
Hypothalamus	TRH	thyrotropin-releasing hormone	anterior pituitary lobe
	GnRH	gonadotropin-releasing hormone, gonadoliberin	anterior pituitary lobe
	CRH	corticotropin-releasing hormone	anterior pituitary lobe
	GH-RH	growth hormone-releasing hormone	anterior pituitary lobe
	GH-RIH	growth hormone-release inhibiting hormone, somatostatin	anterior pituitary lobe
	PRF	prolactin-releasing factor	
	PIF	prolactin-inhibiting factor	
Anterior Pituitary Lobe	TSH	thyroid-stimulating hormone, thyrotropin	thyroid gland
	FSH	follicle-stimulatig hormone, follitropin	ovary, testes
	LH	luteinizing hormone, lutropin	ovary, testes
	PRL	prolactin	mammary gland
	GH	growth hormone, somatotropin, STH	body as a whole
	ACTH	adrenocorticotropic hormone, corticotropin	adrenal cortex

	Abbr	Hormone	Site of action
	beta-LP	beta-lipotropin	?
	beta-END	beta-endorphin	brain
	alpha-MSH	melanocyte-stimulating hormone, melanotropin	skin
	LEK + MEK	leu-enkephalin + met-enkephalin	brain
Posterior Pituitary Lobe	ADH	antidiuretic hormone, adiuretin, vasopressin	arterioles, renal tubules
		oxytocin	smooth muscle of uterus, mammary gland
Pineal Gland		serotonin, 5-hydroxy-tryptamin (5-HT)	cardiovascular/respiratory/gastrointestinal system, brain
		melatonin	hypothalamus
Brain	CCK-PZ	cholecystokinin-pancreozymin	gallbladder, pancreas
	VIP	vasoactive inhibiting polypeptide	GIT
		bombesin	GIT
		neurotensin	GIT, hypothalamus
		substance P	GIT, brain
	LEK + MEK	leu-enkephalin + met-enkephalin	brain
Thyroid Gland	T3, T4	triiodothyronine, thyroxine	general body tissue
		calcitonin, thyrocalcitonin	skeleton
Parathyroid Gland	PTH	parathormone	skeleton, kidney, gastrointestinal tract
Adrenal Cortex		cortisol	general body tissue
		aldosterone	kidney
Adrenal Medulla		epinephrine, norepinephrine	sympathetic receptors
		epinephrine	liver, muscle, adipose tissue
Ovary		estrogens	female accessory sex organs
		progesterone	female accessory reproductive structures
		relaxin	uterus
		inhibin	hypothalamus
Testis		testosterone	male accessory sex organs
		inhibin	hypothalamus
		progesterone	female accessory reproductive structures
		relaxin	uterus
	hCG	choriongonadotropin, human choriongonadotropin	ovary
	hPL	human placental lactogen, somatomammotropin	mammary gland

	Abbr	Hormone	Site of action
Pancreas		insulin	most cells
		glucagon	liver
	PP	pancreatic polypeptide	GIT
Gastrointes-tinal Tract		gastrin	stomach
		secretin	pancreas
	CCK-PZ	cholecystokinin-pancreozymin	gallbladder, pancreas
		motilin	GIT
	VIP	vasoactive inhibiting polypeptide	GIT
	GIP	gastric inhibiting polypeptide	GIT
		bombesin	GIT
		neurotensin	GIT, hypothalamus
		substance P	GIT, brain
	LEK + MEK	leu-enkephalin + met-enkephalin	brain
Kidney		vitamin D	intestine, bone, kidney
	EPO	erythropoietin	bone marrow
Liver	ILGF-I	insulin-like growth factor I, somatomedin C	most cells
	ILGF-II	insulin-like growth factor II	most cells
Thymus		thymosin + thymopoietin	lymphocytes
Heart	ANP	atrial natriuretic peptide, atriopeptin, atrial natriuretic factor, atrial natriuretic hormone	vascular, renal, adrenal tissue
Multiple Cell Types	PTH-RP	parathyroid hormone-related peptide	kidney, bone
		growth factors (e.g. epidermal, fibroblast, transforming, platelet-derived, nerve)	cellular growth stimulation
Monocytes, Lymphocytes, Macrophages		cytokines (e.g. interleukins, tumour necrosing factor, inter-ferons)	

Hormones and Hormone-Like Substances Reported to be Produced by Cancers (Paraneoplastic Secretion)

eosinophilopoietin, erythropoietin, epidermal growth factor, hypophosphatemia-producing factor, insulin-like growth factor, gastrin, glucagon, antidiuretic hormone, growth hormone, follicle-stimulating hormone, melanocyte-stimulating hormone, corticotropin-releasing hormone, growth hormone-releasing hormone, human chorionic gonadotropin, calcitonin, corticotropin, parathyrin, vasoactive intestinal peptide, gastrin-releasing peptide, renin, secretin, somatostatin

Human Chorionic Gonadotropin

(hCG, syn: beta-hCG, beta-human chorionic gonadotropin, human choriongonadotropin)
Placental glycoprotein hormone.

Production. Syncytiotrophoblast placenta cells.

Function. Physiologically supports the corpus luteum until the placenta produces progesterone amounts sufficient to support the pregnancy. Promotes steroidogenesis in the fetoplacental unit and stimulating fetal testicular testosterone secretion.

Test Purpose. 1) to detect early eutopic and mainly ectopic pregnancy, 2) to determine hormonal production adequacy in high-risk pregnancies, 3) to aid in the diagnosis of trophoblastic tumors, such as hydatidiform moles or choriocarcinoma, and discovery of tumors that ectopically secrete hCG, 4) to monitor patients after testicular tumor therapy, who are at high risk for contralateral tumor.

Increased Values
hepatic cirrhosis, ovarian cyst, erythroblastosis fetalis, endometriosis, enteritis regionalis, ulcer disease – (**duodenal u. d.**, gastric u. d.), ulcerative colitis, tumors – (colon t., embryonic t., **pancreas t.**, **liver t.**, **lung t.**, mammary gland t., **seminoma**, thyroid t., **ovarian/testicular teratoma**, **ovary t.**, **stomach t.**), placental tumours – (**chorionepithelioma**, mola hydatidosa – **hydatidiform mole**, non/trophoblastic choriocarcinoma), pregnancy – (**ectopic p.**, **physiological 1st trimester p.**, **multiple p.**), marijuana use, inflammatory bowel disease, missed abortion, fetal death

  Interfering Factors: medicaments – (naloxone)

Decreased Values
abortus imminens (threatened abortion), extrauterine gravidity (ectopic pregnancy)

Analyte	Age/Gender	Reference Range	SI Units	Note
Human Chorionic				
Gonadotropin	M + F	<5	U/l	
	F-postmenopause	<10	U/l	
	Pregnancy			
	after conception	>5	U/l	
	7–10 d	>100	U/l	
	30 d	>2000	U/l	
	40 d	50000–100000	U/l	
	10 w	1000–2000	U/l	
	trophoblast diseases	>100000	U/l	

Human Immunodeficiency Virus Antibodies

Human immunodeficiency virus (HIV) is the virus, that causes acquired immunodeficiency syndrome (AIDS). Viral origin (retrovirus) of immunity acquired impairment, preferably cell-mediated immunity (T-cells). HIV/LAV (lymphadenopathy-associated virus). HIV/HTLV–III virus (human T-lymphotrophic virus, type III).

Test Purpose. 1) document exposure to HIV-1 and HIV-2, 2) to screen blood and blood products for transfusion, 3) to screen organ transplant donors, 4) to study patients in high risk groups (homosexual/bisexual behavior, intravenous drug abusers, male and female prostitutes, hemophiliacs exposed to large amounts of non-heat processed factor VIII).

  HIV1/HIV2 antibodies positive: 8 or more weeks after infection

Human Leukocyte Antigen Antibodies

Increased Values
multitransfused patients, multiparous women

Human Leukocyte Antigen System

(HLA system, syn: major histocompatibility system, leukocyte antigens, histocompatibility antigens, HLA typing) The most histocompatible antigens belong to the HLA system; produced under genetic control and are on all nucleated cells, they are most easily detected on lymphocytes. HLA complex is located in the chromosome number six short arm. Controls many important immune functions. The test is done to determine leukocyte antigens present on the human cell surfaces – histocompatibility level between donor and recipient is identified to determine the possible transplant survival and to forestall rejection episodes. Class I antigens (HLA-A, HLA-B, HLA-C) are derived from T-lymphocytes and class II antigens (HLA-D, DR, DQ, DP) are derived from B-lymphocytes. HLA class I are present in all cells, offering manufactured antigen fragments to the T-cells, CD8. They determine viral infection cell cytolysis, mediated by cells. HLA class II are present on immunocompetent cells, mainly B-cells and macrophages, offering manufactured antigen fragments to the T-cells, CD4. They are required for efficient interaction between immunocompetent cells. Near perfect matching is necessary for bone marrow transplantation. A greater degree of mismatch is acceptable for renal and other organ transplantation.

Test Purpose. 1) to provide histocompatibility tissue recipient typing (transplantation candidate matching) and donors, 2) to aid in family studies for selection of appropriate related bone marrow donors, 3) to assess a risk for family members of an individual with proven hemochromatosis, 4) to aid in genetic counselling, 5) to aid in paternity testing and forensic diagnosis, 6) to aid in autoimmune disease diagnosis.

HLA antigens. Aplastic anemia: DPw3, pernicious anemia: DR2, DR5, psoriatic arthritis: B27, Bw38, Bw39, rheumatoid arthritis: B27, DR4, juvenile rheumatoid arthritis: DR5, barrier to tissue transplantates: A, B, C, D, celiac disease: **B8, DR3**, DR7, DQ2, DQW2, cirrhosis hepatis: DR3, IgA deficiency: DR3, dermatitis herpetiformis: B8, DR3, Dw5, juvenile dermatomyositis: DR3, juvenile diabetes mellitus: DR3, DR4, idiopathic membranous glomerulonephritis: B8, DR3, hemochromatosis: A3, B14, autoimmune chronic active hepatitis: **B8**, DR3, congenital adrenal hyperplasia: BW47, insulin-dependent diabetes mellitus: Bw15, B8, **DR3**, DR4, keratoma: B5, colitis ulcerosa: B5, DR2, tuberculoid leprosy: B8, chronic lymphocytic leukemia: DR5, systemic lupus erythematosus: B8, DR3, Dw3, Burkit's lymphoma: DR7, Addison's disease: B8, **DR3**, Graves' disease: **B8**, B27, **DR3**, Dw3, Hodgkin's disease: A1, myasthenia gravis: **B8**, DR3, nasopharyngeal tumors: B46, narcolepsy: DR2, idiopathic IgA nephropathy: DR4, **DR3**, Dw3, neuritis n. optici: DR2, polycystic kidneys: B5, pemphigus vulgaris: DR4, vulgar psoriasis: Cw6, psoriasis: A13 + B17, B27, Kaposi's sarcoma: DR5, sclerosis multiplex: B27 + Dw2 + A3 + B18, DR2, DR3, schizophrenia: A28, ankylosing spondylitis (Bekhterev's disease): B27, psoriatic spondylitis: B27, Behcet's sy: B5, Goodpasture's sy: **DR2**, Guillain-Barré sy: DR3, nephrotic syndrome in children: DR7, Reiter's sy: B27, Sjögren's sy: B8, DR3, Dw3, Hashimoto's thyroiditis: B37, **DR5**, subacute thyroiditis: B35, acute anterior uveitis: B27, vitiligo: DR7.

Human Placental Lactogen

(hPL, HPL, HCS, syn: human chorionic somatomammotropin).

Production. Polypeptide hormone produced by trophoblast is used to evaluate placental function. Normally, maternal serum hPL increases throughout pregnancy (maximum in 35th week). Maternal serum hPL concentration increase with advancing gestational age is directly correlated with increasing placental tissue mass and functional syncytiotrophoblast.

Function. Lactogenic, metabolic, somatotropic, luteotropic, erythropoietic and aldosterone stimulating effects. The hormone, either directly or in prolactin synergism, has a significant role preparing mammary glands for lactation. Metabolic activities: involved in protein-anabolic body status, glucose uptake inhibition, enhanced lipolysis leading to increased free fatty acids mobilization and nitrogen retention enhancement.

Test Purpose. 1) to assess placental function, fetal well-being, fetal risk level, and to determine the optimal labor term, 2) to aid in hydatidiform mole and choriocarcinoma diagnosis, 3) to aid in the diagnosis and monitor nontrophoblastic tumors treatment that ectopically secrete hPL.

Increased Values
maternal sickle cell anemia, hydrops fetalis, maternal liver diseases, tumors – (pheochromocytoma, lymphoma, breast t., t. of liver, t. of lungs, trophoblastic t.), **large placentas in diabetic women, Rh sensitization, multiple pregnancy**

Decreased Values
fetal anomalies, **fetal distress**, PIH, severely hypertensive women, **choriocarcinoma**, placental insufficiency, vaginal bleeding during pregnancy, hydatidiform mole, **threatened abortion, fetal postmaturity, intrauterine growth retardation**

Analyte	Age/Gender	Reference Range	SI Units	Note
Human Placental Lactogen	Pregnancy >6 w	25–100	μg/l	
	36 w	4–11	mg/l	

Human Soluble Endothelial Cell Leukocyte Adhesion Molecule-1

(h-sELAM-1, syn: E-selectin) h-sELAM-1 is inducible adhesion molecule for neutrophils. It can play a key role in neutrophil extravasation in the acute inflammation sites. ELAM-1 is on the endothelial cell surface after activation by cytokines (IL-1, TNF). Maximum concentration is reached 2–4 hrs after activation which shows ELAM-1 presence in a very early leukocyte adhesion phase to endothelium. ELAM-1 can be detected in healthy people serum as well as in patients with inflammatory diseases.

Increased Values
demyelinization, IDDM, chronic renal insufficiency, dialysis patients, polyneuropathies, Guillain-Barré sy, septic shock, active tuberculosis

Analyte	Age/Gender	Reference Range	SI Units	Note
Human Soluble Endo- thelial Cell Leukocyte Adhesion Molecule-1		0.13–2.8	ng/ml	

Human Soluble Intercellular Adhesion Molecule-1

(h-sICAM-1) Intercellular adhesion molecule natural ligands (ICAM CD54) are LFA-1 (CD11a) (leukocyte function antigen) and Mac (CD11b) which belong to beta-2 integrins. ICAM-1 can be detected on the macrophages, T-/B-cells, fibroblasts, endothelial/epithelial cells. In vivo ICAM-1 expression in healthy tissue is low; it rapidly increases in inflamed tissue. In vitro fibroblast/endothelial cell activation by proinflammatory cytokines (IL-1, TNF, IFN-gamma) leads to rapid ICAM-1 increase on the cell surface.

Increased Values
rheumatoid arthritis, bronchial asthma, atherosclerosis, diabetes mellitus, diseases – (auto-immune d., systemic connective tissue d.), viral diseases – (herpes simplex, HIV), systemic lupus erythematosus, Hodgkin's disease, tumors – (t. of colorectum, melanoma, t. of pan-creas, t. of stomach), tumors with liver metastases, patients with leukocyte adhesion defi-ciency, psoriasis, multiple sclerosis, early type of hypersensitivity, vasculitides

Analyte	Age/Gender	Reference Range	SI Units	Note
Human Soluble Intercellular Adhesive Molecule-1		100–400	ng/ml	

Human Soluble Vascular Cell Adhesion Molecule-1

(h-sVCAM-1) Belongs to immunoglobulin supergene family and has seven extracellular domains which are very similar to immunoglobulin domains, isolated transmembrane do-main and short cytoplasmic chain. VCAM consists of one glycoprotein chain on cell surface with molecular weight 90–110 kD in glycosylation level dependence. Very late activation antigen-4 (VLA-4) is a natural ligand. VCAM belongs to alpha-4 beta-1 integrin. It is expri-mated on lymphocytes, monocytes, basophils, eosinophils, some tumor cells, dendritic cells, bone marrow stroma cells, and endothelial cells. VLA-4 and VCAM-1 induction mediates lymphocyte adhesion to endothelium in the inflammation place.

Increased Values
rheumatoid arthritis, infectious diseases – (cytomegalovirus), diseases – (systemic d., inflammatory d.), systemic lupus erythematosus, tumors, organ transplantation rejection, vasculitides

Analyte	Age/Gender	Reference Range	SI Units	Note
Human Soluble Vascular Cell Adhesion Molecule-1		400–500	ng/ml	

Human T-Cell Lymphotrophic Virus I/II Antibodies

(syn: HTLV I/II antibodies) Human retrovirus (HTLV – human T-cell lymphotrophic virus) HTLV-I is associated with adult T-cell leukemia, HTLV-II is associated with adult hairy-cell leukemia. Positive serum antibody values are not necessarily associated with disease. HTLV I/II infection is not associated with AIDS. HTLV transmission is similar to HIV transmission.

Test Purpose. 1) to screen blood/blood products for transfusion, 2) to aid in the spastic myelopathy differential diagnosis for HTLV-I and chronic neuromuscular diseases (HTLV-II), 3) to aid in the diagnosis of adult T-cell acute lymphoblastic leukemia, 4) to aid in the diagnosis of spastic paraparesis.

Increased Values – positive
neuromuscular diseases, **acute HTLV infection**, **adult T-cell acute lymphoblastic leukemia**, hairy cell leukemia, **tropical spastic paraparesis**

Hydatid Antibodies

Test indicates past or present infection, test remains positive even when cysts are non-viable.
Test Purpose. To confirm diagnosis of hydatid cysts (Echinococcus granulosus, Echinococcus multilocularis).

Increased Values – positive
hydatid cysts

Beta-Hydroxybutyric Acid

(BHBA, BOHB, syn: beta-hydroxybutyrate) BHBA is the predominant ketone body produced by liver. Ketone body accumulation in the blood is referred to as ketosis.

Test Purpose. 1) to diagnose carbohydrate deprivation, which may result from starvation, digestive disturbances, dietary imbalance or frequent vomiting, 2) to aid in disordered carbohydrate utilization diagnosis, 3) to aid in glycogen storage disease diagnosis (glycogenoses), especially von Gierke's disease, 4) to monitor insulin therapy effects during diabetic ketoacidosis treatment, 5) to monitor patient status during emergency hypoglycemia management, acidosis, excessive alcohol ingestion or an unexplained anion gap increase, 6) hereditary metabolic disorders diagnosis (oxoacetyl-CoA-transferase deficiency and alpha-methyl acetoacetic aciduria), 7) monitoring in acetonemic vomiting.

Increased Values
acidosis – (lactic a., metabolic a.), diabetes mellitus, fasting, starvation, diseases – (infectious d., liver d.), catabolism, alcoholic ketoacidosis, obesity, decreased tissue perfusion, shock, renal failure
   Interfering Factors: medicaments – (phenformin, salicylates)

Analyte	Age/Gender	Reference Range	SI Units	Note
Hydroxybutyrate		30–120	µmol/l	
Beta-Hydroxy-butyric Acid	Adults	55–164	µmol/l	

Hydroxybutyric Dehydrogenase

(HBD, syn: alpha-hydroxybutyrate dehydrogenase, a-HBDH) After other enzymes have dropped to normal, HBD remains elevated in myocardial infarction.

Test Purpose. 1) to help in diagnosis of myocardial infarction, 2) to monitor cardiac-iso-enzyme activity after LD has been proved to be elevated, 3) to help to differentiate between heart and liver damage.

Increased Values
myocardial infarction, hemolytic anemia, megaloblastic anemia, muscular dystrophy, liver-cell damage, acute hepatitis, extensive surgery, cardioversion

Analyte	Age/Gender	Reference Range	SI Units	Note
Alpha-Hydroxy-butyrate Dehydrogenase		<3.03	µkat/l	

18-Hydroxydeoxycorticosterone

(18-OH DOC)
Increased Values
primary aldosteronism, 17-α-hydroxylase deficiency, essential hypertension, Cushing's sy

17-Hydroxyprogesterone

(17-OHP) 17-OHP is an intermediate formed in the cholesterol conversion → cortisol, androgens and estrogens. 17-OHP has a marked circadian secretion variation, highest value are in morning, and lowest in afternoon/evening. Day-to-day level variation is 10% in men, and 20% in women. Luteal phase elevation indicates corpus luteum activity.

Test Purpose. 1) to help in diagnosis and management of congenital adrenal hyperplasia, 2) to monitor treatment in patients with congenital adrenal hyperplasia due to 21-hydroxylase deficiency.

Increased Values
congenital adrenal hyperplasia due to 21-hydroxylase deficiency, acute illness of neonates, tumors of – (adrenals, ovary), pregnancy (3rd trimester)
    Interfering Factors: medicaments – (ACTH, ketoconazole)

Decreased Values
Addison's disease, male pseudohermaphrodites, after menopause
    Interfering Factors: medicaments – (anabolic steroids, oral contraceptives)

Analyte	Age/Gender	Reference Range	SI Units	Note
17-Hydroxy-progesterone	M	0.82–6.03	nmol/l	
	F Prolifer. phase	0.66–1.98	nmol/l	
	Secretory phase	3.90–8.90	nmol/l	
	Pregnancy			
	5–20 w	9.5–16.5	µmol/l	
	6–30 w	9.6–35	µmol/l	
	31–40 w	16.1–75	µmol/l	

Hydroxyproline

(Hyp) Enzyme defect: hydroxyproline oxidase. Less than 5% of the total hydroxyproline is free. Peptidebound hydroxyproline is an important measure of total collagen turnover. More than 50% of collagen is placed in bones. Proline as pre-step is used for the collagen synthesis. During the synthesis there is a change of proline to hydroxyproline by posttranslation hydroxylation. Up to 90% of the released hydroxyproline is metabolically changed in the liver to CO_2 and urea, 10% of total hydroxyproline is excreted by urine during collagen breakdown. Excretion of hydroxyproline in the urine is a partial reflection of collagen turnover. Hydroxyproline in the plasma is in 3 forms: free, bound to peptides and bound to proteins. Free and total hydroxyproline in serum can be determined. Day-to-day level variation is 20%, highest values are in spring and fall, they are lower in winter.

Test Purpose. 1) diagnosis and monitoring of primary hyperparathyroidism therapeutic course, 2) to evaluate bone metabolism in dialyzed patients and osteomalacia, 3) examination panel part in osteoporosis diagnosis and therapy monitoring, 4) acromegaly and Paget's disease course and therapy, 5) diagnosis and metabolic activity of bone metastases.

Increased Values – hyperhydroxyprolinemia
acromegaly, rheumatoid arthritis, hepatic cirrhosis, dermatomyositis, diabetes mellitus, **hydroxyprolinemia, hyperthyroidism**, Bekhterev's disease, Hodgkin's disease, **bone metastases, osteitis deformans, osteomalacia, renal osteopathy, osteoporosis**, plasmocytoma, psoriasis, scleroderma, Marfan's sy, bone tuberculosis, uremia

Decreased Values – hypohydroxyprolinemia
hypoparathyroidism, hypothyroidism, nanism, rickets

Analyte	Age/Gender	Reference Range	SI Units	Note
Hydroxyproline				
Total	F	<105.3	µmol/l	
	M	<108.3	µmol/l	
Free	Neonates	4.4–14	µmol/l	
	Boys	11–37	µmol/l	
	Girls	8–32	µmol/l	
	F	7–25	µmol/l	
	M	9–31	µmol/l	

IgA, IgG Antibodies Against Epstein-Barr Virus Viral Capsid Antigen

(anti-EBV-VCA IgG) Infectious mononucleosis diagnosis can be determined via specific EBV protein antigen antibody detection (VCA – viral capsid antigen, EA-D – early antigens-diffuse, EA-R – early antigens-restricted, EBNA – Epstein-Barr nuclear antigen). One to six weeks from infection onset can be EBV-IgM antibodies detected which are specific for infectious mononucleosis diagnosis. EBV-IgG are also early detectable, but they persist for ever. Disease evidence can be performed via other antibody detection, e. g. EA-D, EBNA-IgM, EBNA-IgG. ELISA results in immunodefficient patients should be interpreted carefully; it is needed to repeat them or to do an alternate test method. Specific IgG can compete with IgM (false negativity); in the contrary, rheumatoid factor in positive specific IgG can result in false positive values. Heterotypic (false positive) EBV-IgM can appear in patients who suffer from cytomegalo virus/varicella–zoster infections. **Acute EBV infection phase** (peaking in 3rd week): VCA IgG and IgM, EA-D IgG are present routinely and are increasing during this phase, EBNA-1 IgG are very low to zero level. **Intermediate phase:** VCA IgG persist, VCA IgM are decreasing, EBNA-1 are increasing, EA-D IgG persist. **Convalescence phase:** VCA IgM are decreasing to zero level, VCA IgG, EBNA-1 persist for whole life as overcame infection evidence, EA-D IgG can be temporary/permanently positive. Most of primary infections are transmitted via saliva, are manifesting during childhood and mostly are subclinical. In 50% of children until five year and in 80% of 18 and older are positive antibodies in western civilization. Heterophil antibodies determination is the most frequent method used in acute infection diagnosis (Paul–Bunnell test), but in 20% of acute infectious mononucleosis cases have not positive antibodies, false positive results are in 10%.

Increased Values – positive
EBV infection, false positive values – (cytomegalovirus infection, varicella-zoster virus infection, positive antinuclear antibodies)

Decreased Values
false negative values – (HIV infection, immunodeficient patients)

Immediate Hypersensitivity Mediators

Preformed mediators	Biological effects
histamine	smooth-muscle contraction, vascular permeability increase
serotonin	vascular permeability increase
arylsulfatase	SRS-A inactivation
chymase	Chymotrypsin
heparin	Anticoagulant
HMW-NCF	neutrophil chemotaxia
ECF-A	eosinophil chemotaxia
IMW-ECF	eosinophil chemotaxia
Newly formed mediators	
prostaglandins	bronchial muscle contraction/relaxation, vasodilation, platelet aggregation
leukotrienes C4, D4, E4 (SRS-A)	smooth-muscle contraction, vascular permeability increase
platelet-activating factor (PAF)	platelet aggregation, vasoamine release

Immunoglobulin A

(IgA) Belongs to the antibody, which creates 15–20% of total immunoglobulins. Serum IgA is similar in structure to IgG. It has two subclasses, IgA1 and IgA2. As the main immunoglobulin in body fluids and secretions (sweat, saliva, tears, respiratory, genitourinary, gastrointestinal, colostrum), it provides early antibacterial and antiviral defense. It is largely present in blood and tissue fluid as a monomer (90%), in smaller part as a dimer in secretions (IgA1, IgA2) that is joined with J-chain. Since it is a dimer, it is very effective in aggregating targets which hampers their penetration of the body surface. IgA molecule in mucose cells also have a secretory component (glycoprotein) – secretory immunoglobulin.

Production. B-lymphocytes → plasmocytes → immunoglobulin → humoral immune response.

Function. 1) Secretory immunoglobulin with a protective function in the respiratory, genitourinary, lacrimal, salivary and gastrointestinal systems mucous membranes through the complement activation/fixation via alternative pathway and by preventing microorganisms adherence at mucosal surfaces. Component of serum gamma globulin fraction. Antibodies: antinuclear, anti-insulin, antibacterial agglutinins. 2) Serum IgA protects against brucellae, diphtheria and poliovirus. Subclasses: IgA1 (in circulation and secretions) → against bacterial and food antigens, IgA2 (in large bowel) → against lipopolysaccharides (endotoxins). All immunoglobulin classes and subclasses are taken into account during a clinical evaluation. IgA levels after birth are about 1%, at age 1 about 25%, and at age 3 years about 50% of adult levels. Its half-life is about 6 days.

Test Purpose. 1) to diagnose paraproteinemias, such as plasmocytoma (multiple myeloma) and Waldenström's macroglobulinemia, 2) to detect hypogammaglobulinemia, hypergammaglobulinemia, and non-immunologic diseases such as cirrhosis and hepatitis, 3) to assess the chemotherapy or radiation therapy effectiveness.

Increased Values

AIDS, actinomycosis, **alcoholism**, **rheumatoid arthritis**, **hepatic cirrhosis**, dysgammaglobulinemia, cystic fibrosis, acute/chronic hepatitis, **rheumatic fever**, diseases – (autoaggressive d., autoimmune d., inflammatory bowel d., **infectious d.**, **chronic liver d.**), obstructive jaundice, **systemic lupus erythematosus**, infectious mononucleosis, Crohn's disease, tumors – (monocytic leukemia, Hodgkin's disease, **IgA plasmocytoma**, plasmocytoma incl. multiple myeloma, **t. of gastrointestinal tract**, **t. of hepatobiliary tract**), biliary obstruction, toxic liver lesions – (alcohol t.l. l., medicamentous t.l. l.), mucous membranes lesions, chronic pyelonephritis, sarcoidosis, immunodeficiency conditions, Henoch-Schönlein purpura, syndrome – (Sjögren's sy, **Wiskott-Aldrich sy**), tuberculosis, Hashimoto's thyroiditis, physical exercise, Berger's disease (IgA nephropathy)

   Interfering Factors: medicaments – (ajmaline, ethanol)

Decreased Values

idiopathic agammaglobulinemia, **primary selective IgA deficiency**, subacute bacterial endocarditis, liver cirrhosis, **hereditary thymic aplasia**, exposure to benzene, **protein-losing gastroenteropathies**, **dysgammaglobulinemia** (type I, II, III), chronic sinorespiratory disease, Still's disease, malabsorption, systemic lupus erythematosus, **macroglobulinemia**, tumours – (IgG, IgM monoclonal gammopathy, H-chain disease, L-chain disease, **acute/chronic lymphatic leukemia**, chronic myelogenous leukemia, Hodgkin's disease, non-IgA plasmocytoma), **IgA hypogammaglobulinemia**, recurrent otitis media, acute burns, **immunologic deficiency states**, syndrome – (**ataxia-teleangiectasia sy, hyper-IgM sy, nephrotic sy**), pregnancy (3rd trimester), thyrotoxicosis

   Interfering Factors: healthy persons, medicaments – (carbamazepine, cytostatics, dextran, estrogens, gold salts, immunosuppressives, oral contraceptives, penicillamine, phenytoin, steroids, valproic acid)

Immunoglobulin D

(IgD) An antibody, immunoglobulin D is found with IgM on the cell membranes of circulating B-lymphocytes. Although the H chain of IgD can undergo alternative splicing to a secretory form, IgD serum antibodies in man are uncommon. Involved in lymphocyte differentiation. In children the IgD concentration reaches the adult levels about age 2–4 years.

Component of serum gamma globulin fraction. All immunoglobulin classes and subclasses are taken into account during a clinical evaluation. IgD include antibodies, like ANA, anti-insulin antibodies, antibodies against some medicaments.

Test Purpose. 1) to diagnose paraproteinemias such as plasmocytoma (incl. multiple myeloma) and Waldenström's macroglobulinemia, 2) to detect hypogammaglobulinemia, hypergammaglobulinemia, and non-immunologic diseases such as cirrhosis and hepatitis, 3) to assess the chemotherapy or radiation therapy effectiveness.

Increased Values
diseases – (**infectious d., autoimmune d., liver d., connective tissue d.**), **IgD plasmocytoma**

Decreased Values
non-IgD myeloma, infancy – early childhood, melanoma, preeclampsia, **hereditary/acquired immunodeficiency syndromes**
    Interfering Factors: medicaments – (phenytoin)

Immunoglobulin E

(IgE, syn: reagins, reaginic Ab, skin antibody, skin-sensitising Ab, anaphylactic Ab) Belongs to antibodies with selective distribution like IgA. Serum levels do not represent an effective IgE amount because part of IgE is bond to mastocytes, and part is bound regionally in respiratory and gastrointestinal tracts or in the lymph nodes.

Function. Early-type reaction is allergic type I. reaction – anaphylactic. Polyvalent antigens include pollen, home dust, hair, mites. Defences mainly against parasitic infections.

Production. Mucose membrane B-cells in cooperation with T-CD4+ lymphocytes (regulatory) stimulate creation of specific IgE, which binds to tissue mastocytes and serum basophilic granulocytes by Fc-fragment. The cells degranulate and release the contact antigen mediators (vasoactive compounds – the most important are histamine and slow reactive substance of anaphylaxis) with sensitized mastocytes. B-lymphocytes → plasmocytes → immunoglobulin → humoral immune response in hypersensitivity reactions. Component of serum gamma globulin fraction.

Occurrence. Plasmocytes, skin, mucous membranes, respiratory/gastrointestinal tract, lymphatic nodes, tonsillae, spleen. All immunoglobulin classes and subclasses in complex are clinically evaluated.

Test Purpose. 1) to diagnose paraproteinemias such as plasmocytoma (incl. multiple myeloma) and Waldenström's macroglobulinemia, 2) to detect hypogammaglobulinemia, hypergammaglobulinemia, and non-immunologic diseases, such as cirrhosis and hepatitis, 3) to assess the chemotherapy or radiation therapy effectiveness, 4) to state hyper-IgE syndrome, 5) to monitor allergic bronchopulmonary aspergillosis, 6) to detect bullous skin diseases, intercellular cement pemphigus, basement membrane pemphigoid.

Increased Values
atopic dermatitis, atopic rhinitis, rheumatoid arthritis, inhalant allergy, **basement membrane pemphigoid**, intercellular cement pemphigus, **pulmonary aspergillosis**, **allergic bronchial asthma**, **atopy**, IgA deficiency, **dermatitis**, **eczema**, erythema nodosum, cystic fibrosis, primary pulmonary hemosiderosis, diseases – (infectious d., liver d.), parasitic diseases – (amebiasis, hookworm disease, ascariasis, echinococcosis, fascioliasis, filariasis, capillariasis, onchocerciasis, paragonimiasis, schistosomiasis, strongyloidiasis, toxocarosis, trichinosis, visceral larva migrans), cytomegalovirus infection, candidiasis, coccidioidomycosis, leprosy, hyper-IgE recurrent pyoderma, Hodgkin's disease (far advanced), **Kawasaki's disease**,

infectious mononucleosis, interstitial nephritis, **plasmocytoma**, **bullous pemphigoid**, hypersensitivity pneumonitis, polyarteritis nodosa, burns, **allergic rhinitis** (pollinosis, hay fever), immunodeficiency states, syndrome – (Buckley's sy, DiGeorge sy, hypereosinophilic sy, Guillain-Barré sy, hyperimmunoglobulinemia E sy, **Wiskott-Aldrich sy**), **anaphylactic shock**, sinusitis, urticaria, drug allergy, food allergy

 Interfering Factors: medicaments – (aminophenazone, anticonvulsants, asparaginase, hydralazine, oral contraceptives, phenylbutazone, phenytoin)

Decreased Values

agammaglobulinemia – (**idiopathic a.**, **congenital a.**), hypogammaglobulinemia – (acquired h., congenital h., sex-linked h.), **IgE deficiency**, hereditary/acquired immunodeficiency, **non-IgE myeloma**, radiation therapy, advanced neoplasms, cellular immunity disorders, **syndrome ataxia-teleangiectasia**, pregnancy

 Interfering Factors: medicaments – (methotrexate, phenytoin)

Immunoglobulin G

(IgG) Belongs to the antibodies, creates 70–75% of total immunoglobulins and 10–20% of total serum proteins; it is spreaded in intra/extravascullar space equally. In humans, there are four subclasses of IgG numbered 1–4. IgG is a bilaterally symmetrical tetramer composed of two identical heavy chains and two identical light chains. The chains are held together by disulfide bonds and by hydrophobic interactions.

Production and Function. B-lymphocytes → plasmocytes → immunoglobulin → humoral immune reactions against viruses, some bacteria, fungi, toxins. Antinuclear, antitoxin and antiinsulin antibodies, Rh antibodies, activates complement, and enhances phagocytosis. IgG is the major Ig produced after reimmunization (the memory immune response = secondary immune response) that occurs as a secondary response after IgM response. IgG can fix complements, it is the only immunoglobulin (IgG1, IgG3, IgG4) that crosses the placenta, so it provides the major protection against infection for the first 2–3 months of a baby's life. It is able to do this, because it has a half-life in serum of about 23 days. It is the only immunoglobulin humoral antiinfectious defense in individual who is not breast feeded. It is a component of serum gamma globulin fraction in plasma and extravascular spaces. Many clinically important autoantibodies are in the IgG 3 class (antinuclear, anti-basement membrane, anti-RBC antibodies). IgG subclasses synthesis depend on the nature and amount of antigen, the entry place and exposure duration. IgG subclasses: IgG1 and 3 → against bacterial proteins and viruses. IgG1 and 3 are the immunoglobulins which are most reponsible for labeling targets for removal by the phagocytic system (opsonins), their production depends on T-helper lymphocytes. IgG1 and 3 are most frequently elicited by viral antigens, IgG2 by carbohydrates. IgG2 → creates polysaccharide antigens action answer (e. g. against capsuled bacteria); production is independent of T-helper lymphocytes. After provocation by complex antigen structures (parasites, food components, snake venom) IgG4 is created. IgG4 binds to surface receptors of tissue mastocytes. IgG1 and IgG2 circulating in blood are placed in the B-lymphocytes cytoplasm. IgG1 and IgG3 are placed in tonsil B-lymphocytes. All subclasses except IgG4 can activate complement via the classical pathway, thereby causing the lysis of gram negative bacteria and animal cells. All immunoglobulin classes and subclasses are taken into account during the clinical evaluation.

Test Purpose. 1) to diagnose paraproteinemias such as plasmocytoma (multiple myeloma) and Waldenström's macroglobulinemia, 2) to detect hypo-/hypergammaglobulinemia, as well as non-immunologic diseases such as cirrhosis and hepatitis, 3) to assess chemotherapy or radiation therapy effectiveness, 4) IgG subclasses testing – to reveal immunodeficiency, mainly in recurrent respiratory infections, selective IgG 2 deficiency is typical, 5) therapeutic strategy in selective IgG 4 deficiency.

Increased Values

AIDS, actinomycosis, rheumatoid arthritis, hepatic cirrhosis – (**alcoholic h.c., chronic active h.c., chronic posthepatitic h.c.**), gout, dysgammaglobulinemias, dysproteinemia, subacute bacterial endocarditis, cystic fibrosis, hepatitis – (**chronic active h., acute viral h.**), **rheumatic fever, hyperimmunization,** cholangitis, diseases – (**autoimmune d.**, dermatologic d., **chronic infectious d., parasitic d., chronic liver d.**, inflammatory d.), chronic granulomatous infection, obstructive icterus, **cryoglobulinemia, systemic lupus erythematosus,** Graves-Basedow disease, Waldenström's macroglobulinemia, **malnutrition,** infectious mononucleosis, tumors – (leukemia, lymphoma, Hodgkin's diseases, **plasmocytoma** – IgG type), **paraproteinemia,** chronic pyelonephritis, **sarcoidosis,** scleroderma, Sjögren's sy, pregnancy (1st trimester), intrauterine contraceptive devices (IUD), **tuberculosis**
  Interfering Factors: medicaments – (asparaginase, heparin, methadone, methyldopa, nitrofurantoin, phenytoin, propylthiouracil, valproic acid)

Decreased Values

agammaglobulinemia, AIDS, **amyloidosis, lymphoid aplasia,** cirrhosis hepatis, **congenital IgG deficiency,** dysgammaglobulinemia (type I), muscular dystrophy, **protein-losing enteropathies,** monoclonal gammopathies (non-IgG), **non-IgG macroglobulinemia,** Waldenström's macroglobulinemia, tumours – (**chronic lymphocytic leukemia,** Hodgkin's disease, H-chain disease, **IgA myeloma, non-IgG myeloma**), pemphigus, **burns, preeclampsia,** Bence Jones proteinemia, antiimmunoglobulin antibodies, **immunodeficiency conditions,** syndrome – (**hyper-IgM sy, nephrotic sy,** Wiskott-Aldrich sy), **pregnancy (3rd trimester)**
  Interfering Factors: medicaments – (carbamazepine, cytostatics, dextran, gold salts, immunosuppressives, methylprednisolone, phenytoin)

Immunoglobulin M

(IgM) Antibody forming about 10% of immunoglobulins. IgM in serum is composed of a pentamer of the basic four chain structure held together by inter H chain disulfide bonds. After polymerization the resulting pentamer is further stabilized by another molecule, the joining chain (J-chain).
Production and Function. IgM is the primary immune response immunoglobulin and membrane antigen receptor on non-activated B-lymphocytes. Pentamer IgM molecule have 10 places for antigen bonding, but sterical reasons allow only 5 to be used. IgM also has a sectretory component like IgG. B-lymphocytes → plasmocytes → immunoglobulin → humoral immune reaction against gram-negative microorganisms and rheumatoid factors. First antibody to appear after antigens enter the body (primary antibody answer). It is the most effective Ig at fixing complement and in aggregating targets; IgM serves as agglutinator to assisting the phagocytic system to eliminate many kinds of microorganisms. Forms the natural antibodies of IgM isotype: ABO blood group system (ABO isoagglutinins), cold agglutinins, Wassermann's antibodies, antithyroglobulin antibodies, and rheumatoid factors. IgM can fix complements; a fetus can produce IgM as an intrauterine infection response already from 20th gestational week. Concentrations at the end of 4th month are about 50%

of adult levels, at age 8–14 adult levels are measured. Component of serum gamma globulin fraction. All immunoglobulin classes/subclasses are taken into account during a clinical evaluation.

Test Purpose. 1) recurrent, chronic or severe infections, 2) intrauterine infections screening, 3) monoclonal proteins evaluation, 4) monitoring the progression or therapeutic response of macroglobulinemia patients, 5) to help in diagnosis of hereditary and acquired IgM immunodeficiencies.

Increased Values

AIDS, actinomycosis, rheumatoid arthritis, brucellosis, liver cirrhosis – (alcoholic l. c., primary biliary l. c., posthepatitic l. c.), dysgammaglobulinemia (IgM), subacute bacterial endocarditis, cystic fibrosis, hepatitis – (chronic active h., acute viral h.), cold agglutinin hemolytic disease, diseases – (autoimmune d., chronic hepatocellular d., acute/chronic infectious d., viral infectious d., collagen vascular d., fungal d.), systemic lupus erythematosus, Graves-Basedow disease, Waldenström's macroglobulinemia, malaria, infectious mononucleosis, tumors – (monocytic leukemia, lymphosarcoma, lymphoma, Hodgkin's disease, plasmocytoma), acute/chronic pyelonephritis, reticulosis, sarcoidosis, scleroderma, syndrome – (hyper-IgM sy, nephrotic sy, Sjögren's sy), trypanosomiasis, toxoplasmosis, tuberculosis, Hashimoto's thyroiditis
   Interfering Factors: medicaments – (chlorpromazine)

Decreased Values

idiopathic agammaglobulinemia, amyloidosis, lymphoid aplasia, dysgammaglobulinemia (type II), protein-losing enteropathies, monoclonal gammopathies (non-IgM), chronic hepatitis, H-chain disease, L-chain disease, lymphoproliferative diseases, cryoglobulinemia, tumours – (chronic lymphatic leucemia, Hodgkin's disease, hepatoma, plasmocytoma IgA, IgG, non-IgM myeloma), severe burns, anti-immunoglobulin antibodies, immunodeficiency conditions, nephrotic syndrome, infancy – early childhood
   Interfering Factors: medicaments – (azathioprine, chlorambucil, cytostatics, dextran, gold salts, immunosuppressives, carbamazepine, phenytoin)

Immunoglobulins

Antibodies belong to the class of roughly spherical proteins called globulins. Since they are involved in immunity, they were given the class name immunoglobulin. Immunoglobulins can be subdivided on the basis of physical and fucnctional properties into five classes (G, M, A, D, E). Immunoglobulin protective activities are expressed through antibody action that may act to eliminate antigens by five different mechanisms: neutralization – directly inhibiting binding sites of viruses or various enzymes and toxins produced by bacteria; aggregation; opsonization – which facilitates removal by fagocytes; inducing complement mediated lysis of susceptible organisms, or inducing inflammation.

Analyte	Age/Gender	Reference Range	SI Units	Note
Immunoglobulins				
IgA	1–3 m	0.013–0.53	g/l	
	4–6 m	0.044–0.84	g/l	
	7–12 m	0.11–1.06	g/l	
	2–5 y	0.14–1.59	g/l	

Analyte	Age/Gender	Reference Range	SI Units	Note
	6–10 y	0.33–2.36	g/l	
	Adults	0.70–3.12	g/l	
IgD	Neonates	0	g/l	
	Other	0–0.08	g/l	
IgE	Neonates	<1.5	IU/ml	
	7–12 m	<25	IU/ml	
	6 y	<126	IU/ml	
	11 y	<210	IU/ml	
	Adults	<200	IU/ml	
IgG	1 m	2.51–9.06	g/l	
	2–4 m	1.76–6.01	g/l	
	5–12 m	1.72–10.69	g/l	
	1–5 y	3.45–12.36	g/l	
	6–10 y	6.08–15.72	g/l	
	Adults	6.39–15.49	g/l	
subclasses IgG1		4.0–13.0	g/l	
IgG2		1.2–8.0	g/l	
IgG3		0.4–1.3	g/l	
IgG4		0.01–3.0	g/l	
IgM	1–4 m	0.17–1.05	g/l	
	5–9 m	0.3–1.26	g/l	
	10–12 m	0.41–1.73	g/l	
	2–8 y	0.43–2.07	g/l	
	9–10 y	0.52–2.42	g/l	
	Adults	0.56–2.3		
Immunoglobulin				
kappa chain		1.7–3.7	g/l	
lambda chain		1.1–2.4	g/l	

Immunoreactive Insulin

(IRI)

Increased Values
acromegaly, **diabetes mellitus** (NIDDM), dystrophia myotonica, **liver diseases**, familial fructose/galactose intolerance, **insulinoma** (pancreatic islet cell tumor), obesity, Cushing's sy
    Interfering Factors: medicaments – (albuterol, amino acids, calcium gluconate, chlorpropamide, danazol, fructose, glucagon, glucose, growth hormone, levodopa, niacin, oral contraceptives, pancreozymin, phentolamine, prednisolone, quinine, secretin, spironolactone, terbutaline, tolazolamide, tolbutamide)

Decreased Values
diabetes mellitus (IDDM), hypopituitarism
    Interfering Factors: medicaments – (asparaginase, beta-adrenergic blockers, calcitonin, chlorpropamide, cimetidine, clofibrate, diazoxide, doxazosin, ethacrynic acid, ethanol, ether, furosemide, metformin, nifedipine, phenformin, phenobarbital, phenytoin, propranolol, thiazide diuretics, tolbutamide)

Immunoreactive Proinsulin

Increased Values
hepatic cirrhosis, islet B-cell secretory defects, familial hyperproinsulinemia, hypothyroidism, pancreatic B-cell tumors (insulinoma), chronic renal failure

Immunoreactive Trypsin

(syn: cationic trypsin)

Increased Values
liver diseases, gallstones, acute malnutrition, neonates with cystic fibrosis, acute pancreatitis, peptic gastric ulcer, chronic renal failure

Decreased Values
diabetes mellitus, chronic malnutrition, pancreatic tumors, chronic pancreatitis

Immunosuppressive Acidic Protein

(IAP) IAP is an alpha-1-acid glycoprotein that is produced mainly by macrophages. It exhibits various types of immunosuppressive activities. It lacks disease specificity but it has been shown to increase in the serum of patients with inflammatory neurological diseases and has been described as a tumor associated marker in some solid tumors and hemato-logical diseases.

Inhibins

Inhibins have been shown to regulate the proliferation of multipotential and erythroid progenitor cells in human bone marrow cultures and to modulate hemoglobin accumulation in purified human erythroid progenitor cells. Tumor marker. The test should not be used to screen for the presence of mentioned tumors. Levels must be interpreted with reference to gender and to the stage of the menstrual cycle or menopausal state. Inhibins may have clinical significance as a factors with growth inhibitory and erythroid differentiation activities in the treatment of erythroleukemia and as a general myeloprotective agent.
Test Purpose. 1) to help in diagnosis of granulosa cell tumors and mucinous ovarian tumors, 2) to monitor levels after surgery to detect recurrence.

Increased Values – positive
granulose cell tumors, mucinous ovarian tumors

Inositol

(syn: free inositol, myoinositol) Inositol is a hydroxylated derivative of cyclohexan; a vitamin B-complex member which can be obtained from vegetables, citrus fruits, cereal grains.

Insulin

Production. Biphasic synthesis course, Langerhans' islets pancreatic beta-cells hormone = proinsulin (a biochemically inert peptide fragment known as connecting peptide = C-peptide, breaks off from proinsulin) → equimolar quantities of C-peptide and insulin are released into the circulation → insulin enters the portal circulation → is carried to the liver, the prime target organ. Biological half-time is 30 minutes.

Function. Involved in membrane transport, glucose utilization/metabolism. **Anabolic effect:** 1) liver – synthesis of glycogen and fatty acids (triacylglycerols, LDL, VLDL), 2) fatty tissue – uptake, synthesis and esterification of fatty acids, 3) muscular tissue – amino acids uptake, promotes proteins synthesis (increases amino acid transport, stimulates ribosomal protein synthesis), promotes glycogen synthesis (increases glucose transport, enhances glycogen synthetase activity, inhibits glycogen phosphorylase activity). **Anticatabolic effect:** 1) liver – inhibition of glycogenolysis (glycogen breakdown), gluconeogenesis, ketogenesis, 2) fatty tissue – lipolysis, 3) muscular tissue – proteolysis, amino acids release. In muscle and adipose tissue insulin increases the cellular membranes uptake/permeability to glucose by the cell membrane glucose transporters increase → binding to the insulin receptors → causing channels to open and allowing glucose to pass into cells. Lipid metabolism: insulin causes marked reduction in fatty acids release: 1) decreases in triacylglycerol degradation; insulin decreases circulating fatty acid levels by inhibiting the hormone sensitive lipase activity in adipose tissue, 2) increases triacylglycerol synthesis; insulin increases the glucose transport and metabolism in adipocytes, which provides the substrate glycerol 3-phosphate for triacylglycerol synthesis. Insulin increases lipoprotein lipase adipose tissue activity providing fatty acids for esterification. Brain, liver and RBCs take up glucose independently of the insulin; insulin inhibits glucagon release by pancreatic alpha-cells. Insulin secretion is increased by GIP (gastric inhibitory peptide). Antagonistic action opposing insulin: adrenaline, glucagon, cortisol, growth hormone = counter-regulatory hormones. Insulin is broken down in the liver and by the kidney. Pulsatile secretion with values up to 70% from mean values. Day-to-day variation is 15%.

Test Purpose. 1) to aid in the diagnosis of hyperinsulinemia/hypoglycemia resulting from pancreatic islet cells tumor or hyperplasia, glucocorticoid deficiency, or severe hepatic disease, 2) a part of the functional tests (starvation test, tolbutamide test, glucagon test, oral glucose-tolerance test), 3) to help in the diagnosis of diabetes mellitus and insulin-resistance – metabolic Reaven's sy, 4) glucose/insulin and insulin/glucagon ratios determination, 5) risk factor of early atheromatosis (hyperinsulinemia is an angiotoxic factor).

Increased Values – hyperinsulinemia

acromegaly, endogenous hyperinsulinemia, **insulinoma**, factitious hypoglycemia, insulin overdose, reactive hypoglycemia after glucose ingestion, stress, syndrome – (**Cushing's sy**, insulin resistance sy, insulin autoimmune sy), pregnancy, renal failure

    Interfering Factors: obesity, food, medicaments – (albuterol, amino acids, beclomethasone, calcium gluconate, chlorpropamide, cyclosporine, danazol, fructose, glucagon, glucose, growth hormone, levodopa, niacin, oral antibiotics, oral contraceptives, pancreozymin, phentolamine, prednisolone, quinine, quinidine, salbutamol, secretin, spironolactone, terbutaline, tolazolamide, tolbutamide)

Decreased Values – hypoinsulinemia
exercise, diabetes mellitus (type I)
   Interfering Factors: fasting, medicaments – (asparaginase, beta-adrenergic blockers, calcitonin, calcium channel blockers, chlorpromazine, chlorpropamide, cimetidine, clofibrate, diazoxide, doxazosin, ethacrynic acid, ethanol, ether, furosemide, metformin, nifedipine, pegaspargase, pentamidine, phenobarbital, phenformin, phenytoin, propranolol, streptozocine, thiazide diuretics)

Analyte	Age/Gender	Reference Range	SI Units	Note
Insulin (IRI)	Neonates	3.8–13.6	µIU/ml	
	Children	6.96–26.6	mU/l	
	Adults	8.0–34.5	mU/l	
		58–172	mU/l	
		0.34–1.0	pmol/l	
specific insulin		2–25	µg/l	
Insulin in oGTT	Basal	7–24	µIU/ml	
	30'	25–231	µIU/ml	
	60'	18–276	µIU/ml	
	120'	16–166	µIU/ml	
	180'	4–38	µIU/ml	

Insulin-Like Growth Factor I

(IGF-I, ILGF-I, Sm-C, syn: growth factor, somatomedin C, insulin-like growth hormone, sulfation factor) A biologically active peptide (polypeptide hormone) which monitors the growth of children. Somatomedin quantity provides an indirect measure of present growth hormone quantity.

Production. Liver, cartilage, kidney, heart, lung, fat tissues, glandular tissues and hypophysis – influenced by somatotropin. IGF-I is produced also by chondroblasts, fibroblasts and osteoclasts.

Function. Most growth-producing actions are mediated by ILGF-I; stimulating DNA and RNA synthesis and collagen formation. ILGF-I also shows insulin-like activity in some tissues. The activity is ascribed in part to the similarity of the insulin and ILGF structures. Binding of IGF-I to carrier proteins prevents the establishment of a permanent hypoglycemia in spite of high serum IGF concentrations. These carrier proteins also increase plasma half lives of IGF and prevent the release of IGF from the blood stream into interstitial spaces. ILGF-I inhibits lipolysis, increases glucose oxidation in adipose tissue, and stimulates glucose and amino acid transport to the diaphragm and heart muscle. Synthesis of collagen and proteoglycans is enhanced by ILGF-I, which also has positive effects on Ca, Mg and K homeostasis. The growth hormone stimulates the liver and other body tissues, producing somatomedin, and inducing growth. Because somatomedin peptides are tightly bound to plasma proteins and half-time lasts hours, random measurement provides an accurate reflection of mean plasma concentrations. IGF-I is an autocrine growth modulator for astrocytes and differentiation factor for oligodendrocytes and neurons. It influences the cellular differentiation of ovary granulosa cells. In the ovary IGF-I enhances the activities of estrogens and androgens and upregulates the expression of receptors for luteinizing hormone. IGF-I induces skeletal growth and also differentiation of myoblasts during fetal development. ILGF-I shows about 15 % within-day variation, 30 % decrease at sleep onset with rise to highest values early in the morning.

Test Purpose. 1) to aid acromegaly diagnosis, 2) to evaluate hypopituitarism and hypothalamic lesions in children (dwarfism diagnosis and therapy response), 3) to screen the growth disorders, 4) to assess nutritional status, 5) to monitor the nutritional repletion.

Increased Values

adolescence, **acromegaly**, exercise, **gigantism** (pituitary), thyroid hormones, **hyperpituitarism**, prolactin-secreting tumours, **obesity**, **precocious puberty**, physiological growth of organism, diabetic retinopathy, **pregnancy** (3rd trimester), renal failure
   Interfering Factors: medicaments – (androgens, dexamethasone)

Decreased Values

anorexia nervosa, **liver cirrhosis**, deficiency – (nutrition d., **growth hormone d.**), **children to age 5–6 years**, **diabetes mellitus**, **starvation**, **inactive growth hormone**, hypopituitarism, **hypothyroidism**, diseases – (**acute**/chronic d., liver d.), **kwashiorkor**, malnutrition, tumors of – (pituitary, liver), **nanism** (Laron dwarfism), **delayed puberty**, syndrome – (Down sy, emotional deprivation sy), failure – (chronic renal f., **hepatic f.**)
   Interfering Factors: **elder people**, fasting, medicaments – (estrogens, tamoxifen)

Analyte	Age/Gender	Reference Range	SI Units	Note
Insulin-Like Growth Factor I	M			
	1–2 y	4.05–21.96	nmol/l	
	3–4 y	5.88–30.07	nmol/l	
	5–6 y	6.67–37.65	nmol/l	
	7–8 y	20.66–50.33	nmol/l	
	9–10 y	17.78–40.27	nmol/l	
	11–12 y	23.53–57.52	nmol/l	
	13–14 y	28.76–80.53	nmol/l	
	15–16 y	26.15–109.30	nmol/l	
	17–18 y	37.39–81.97	nmol/l	
	19–20 y	44.32–54.65	nmol/l	
	21– 25 y	26.4–56.61	nmol/l	
	Adults	17.6–58.7	nmol/l	
	F			
	1–2 y	1.43–26.93	nmol/l	
	3–4 y	9.81–41.84	nmol/l	
	5–6 y	9.15–37.65	nmol/l	
	7–8 y	16.34–51.77	nmol/l	
	9–10 y	16.08–43.14	nmol/l	
	11–12 y	24.97–60.40	nmol/l	
	13–14 y	37.39–87.33	nmol/l	
	15–16 y	31.64–87.33	nmol/l	
	17–18 y	31.38–66.15	nmol/l	
	19–20 y	31.64–71.90	nmol/l	
	21–25 y	30.19–59.21	nmol	

Insulin-Like Growth Factor II

(IGF-II, ILGF-II) Unlike ILGF-I (somatomedin C), ILGF-II does not increase in acromegaly but does increase in tumor-related hypoglycemia.

Increased Values
exercise, hepatoma, hypoglycemia associated with non-islet cell tumors, Wilms' tumor

Decreased Values
growth hormone deficiency, severe illnesses

Analyte	Age/Gender	Reference Range	SI Units	Note
Insulin-Like Growth Factor II	Children			
	pre-puberty	44.5–85.6	nmol/l	
	puberty	32.7–98.2	nmol/l	
	Adults	38.4–98.1	nmol/l	

Insulin-Like Growth Factor Binding Protein–1

(IGFBP-1) One of six proteins which binds IGF-I and IGF-II specifically; consists of 234 amino acids. It is synthesized mainly in fetal liver, elder-people liver, and in decidual endometrium. IGFBP is found in various body fluids such as blood serum, amniotic fluid and liquor. Some IGFBP/IGF complexes may contain additional complexed proteins. The formation of these complexes may be inhibited by glycosaminoglycans. Both types of IGF can be released from these complexes by treatment with acids, heparin, proteases and plasmin. IGFBPs modulate IGF activities by increasing their plasma half lives and by inhibiting or promoting the interactions of IGF with receptors on certain target cells. Serum concentration exhibits diurnal variation similar to cortisol. Levels are highest in newborns with subsequent decrease until puberty; next increase starts in 7th decenium. There is an inversion relation between BMI and fasting IGFBP-1 concentration as well as between insulin and fasting concentration; during oGTT 50% decrease is observed. Amniotic fluid concentrations are 10^2–10^3 higher than serum. Fetal membrane rupture leads to vaginal secretion IGFBP-1 concentration increase.
Test Purpose. 1) diabetes mellitus type I differential diagnosis, 2) fetal membrane rupture diagnosis.

Increased Levels
secondary hypoinsulinism, IDDM, fetal membrane rupture, pregnancy, Laron-type dwarfism, growth hormone deficiency

Decreased Levels
acromegaly, NIDDM, obesity, syndrome – (Cushing's sy, polycystic ovary sy)

Analyte	Age/Gender	Reference Range	SI Units	Note
Insulin-Like Growth Factor Binding Protein 1 (ILGFBP-1)		0.6–14.4	ng/ml	
sensitivity		0.2	ng/ml	

Insulin-Like Growth Factor Binding Protein–2

(IGFBP-2) Factor is observed mainly in brain and cerebrospinal fluid.

Increased Levels
prostate tumors

Insulin-Like Growth Factor Binding Protein–3

(IGFBP-3) Factor is the major IGFBP present in serum of humans. Present in serum in two polypeptide forms; binds IGF-I and IGF-II. About 90% of blood IGFBP-3 is in terciary complex con sisting of alpha/beta-subunits and IGF-I/IGF-II; this bound prolongs IGF-I biological half time and serves as metabolic reservoir and regulates IGF access to receptors. If GH and IGF-I concentrations are increased (acromegaly) circulating IGFBP-3 concentration is increasing; alpha subunit is in blood. If IGF-II is not increasing, IGF binding places excess is occupied by IGF-I. On the contrary, if GH/IGF are decreasing (GH deficiency) also IGFBP-3 and alpha subunits are decreasing. Inhibits follicle stimulating hormone. Because of IGFBP-3 exhibits balanced circadian concentration only 1–2 measurements are needed (in comparison to GH).
Test Purpose. The best GH deficiency indicator during the first 5 years of age.

Increased Values
acromegaly, renal failure

Decreased Values
biliary cirrhosis, chronic aggressive hepatitis, severe hepatopathies, growth hormone deficiency, Laron-type dwarfism

Insulin-Like Growth Factor Binding Protein–4

(IGFBP-4) Factor is the predominant IGF binding protein expressed by human osteoblast-like cells.

Insulin-Like Growth Factor Binding Protein–5

(IGFBP-5) Factor is expressed highly in the kidney but is found also in other tissues.

Insulin-Like Growth Factor Binding Protein–6

(IGFBP-6) Factor is abundant in cerebrospinal fluid. Levels of IGFBP-6 have been found to be increased in human breast cancer cells treated with estradiol and IGF-1 and may thus contribute to mitogenesis.

Integrins

Integrins belong to adhesive molecules. These are membrane glycoproteins that consist of alpha- and beta-chains.

- **Beta-1 integrins** (VLA – very late antigens previously): placed on the leukocyte, endothelial cells, fibroblasts, and thrombocytes surface), binding to extracellular matrix proteins (collagen, laminin, fibronectin). They are involved in platelet adhesion to subendothelial matrix and leukocyte concentration at inflammation site.
- **Beta-2 integrins**: placed on leukocyte surface. Involved in circulating leukocytes bound to endothelial cells; it is a condition to their following migration.
- **Beta-3 integrins**: placed (exprimated) on platelets, granulocytes, monocytes, and endothelial cells; they bound fibrinogen and von Willebrand's factor and mediate platelet aggregation.

Inter-Alpha-Trypsin Inhibitor

(I-alpha-TI) It is a labile glycoprotein from proteinase group inhibitors synthesized in the liver (serine protease inhibitor). Substrates of ITI include trypsin, chymotrypsin and a neutrophil elastase. Belongs to acute phase proteins.

Decreased Values
inflammatory diseases, tumors

Interferons

(IFN-alpha, IFN-beta, IFN-gamma) Belong to the cytokines (interleukins) = soluble proteins secreted by fibroblasts, T-cells, and in principle by all nuclear cells, that regulate the magnitude of an inflammatory or immune response (mainly in viral antigens). IFN activates macrophages → increasing their phagocytic and bactericidal ability and NK-cell activity. Interferons are proteins, that place uninfected cells in an antiviral state. Interferons induce the production of a 2nd protein that inhibits viral protein synthesis by degrading viral mRNA (not host mRNA). Production of interferon can be stimulated by viral infection, especially by doublestranded RNA, by intracellular parasites (chlamydiae, rickettsiae), by protozoa (Toxoplasma) and by bacteria (streptococci, staphylococci), by bacterial products (endotoxins). Interferons also have immunoregulatory functions (inhibition of B-cell activation and T-cell antibody production enhancement, NK-cell cytotoxic activity enhancement) and they can inhibit the growth of nonviral intracellular parasites. IFN-gamma is basic glycoprotein (143 amino acids) with two glycosylation places; exists in three monomeric forms in dependence on glycosylation group. N-terminal end is functionally connected with IFN-gamma to receptor bound. Dimer creation is important for biologic activity.

Functions and effects of interferons

- **IFN-alpha**: inhibits viral replication and tumor cell growth, increases antiviral resistance, increases class I (HLA A, HLA B, HLA C) and class II (HLA D, HLA DR, HLA DQ) major histocompatibility complex expression, increases natural killer activity, modulates antibody response (immunomodulatory effects), inhibits antibody production and layed hypersensitivity reactions. IFN-alpha shows antiparasitic and antiproliferative activities. Interferon inhibits cell proliferation, cause increased synthesis of beta-2-

microglobulin, neopterin and matrix metalloproteinases. Stimulates production of interferons, macrophage activity → increase of phagocytic and bactericidal abilities → antigen modulation and transport by T-lymphocytes, Fc-receptor expression, PGE2 production. IFN-alpha inhibits the expression of a number of cytokines in hematopoietic progenitor cells. IFN-alpha has been approved for the treatment of chronic hepatitis C and chronic hepatitis B infections, as well as for the treatment of various neoplasms such as hairy cell leukemia, metastasizing renal carcinoma and Kaposi sarcoma. It is also active against a number of other tumors and viral infections. At least 23 different variants of IFN-alpha are known.

Production. Leukocytes (IFN-alpha), fibroblasts, epithelial cells (IFN-beta), T-helpers, monocytes, macrophages, NK-cells and a number of different cell types following induction by viruses, nucleic acids, glucocorticoid hormones and low-molecular weight substances.

■ **IFN-beta:** In contrast to IFN-alpha IFN-beta is strictly species-specific. Interferon is involved in the regulation of unspecific humoral immune responses and immune responses against viral infections. It increases the expression of HLA class I antigens and blocks the expression of HLA class II antigens stimulated by IFN-gamma. IFN-beta stimulates the activity of NK-cells and hence also antibody-dependent cytotoxicity. IFN-beta has been shown to increase suppressor cell function in multiple sclerosis patients and inhibit the production of IFN-gamma. Interferon beta can be used for topic treatment of condylomata acuminata. Head and neck squamous carcinomas, mammary and cervical carcinomas, and also malignant melanomas respond well to treatment with IFN-beta. It also appears to be very promising for the adjuvant therapy of malignant melanomas with a high potential for metastasis.

Production. Fibroblasts, epithelial cells (IFN-beta). The synthesis of IFN-beta can be induced by common inducers of interferons, including viruses, double-stranded RNA and microorganisms. It is induced also by some cytokines, such as TNF and IL-1.

■ **IFN-gamma:** stimulates expression and increases class I and class II major histocompatibility complex activity (immunomodulatory effects) and macrophage activity, increases natural killer activity, increases IgE and IgG secretion, co-stimulates T- and B-cell growth and differentiation, inhibits viral replication and tumor cells growth (antiproliferative effect); it has antiparasitic effects, activates neutrophils, NK-cells. IFN-gamma inhibits the proliferation of smooth muscle cells of the arterial intima in vitro and in vivo and therefore probably functions as an endogenous inhibitor for vascular overreactions such as stenosis following injuries of arteries. Interferon inhibits the proliferation of endothelial cells and the synthesis of collagens by myofibroblasts. It thus functions as an inhibitor of capillary growth mediated by myofibroblasts and fibroblast growth factors. IFN-gamma induces synthesis of the enzymes that mediate the respiratory burst, allowing macrophages to kill phagocytosed microbes. IFN-gamma plays key role in immune system function regulation. IFN-gamma synergises with TNF-alpha and TNF-beta in inhibiting the proliferation of various cell types. However, the main biological activity of IFN-gamma appears to be immunomodulatory in contrast to the other interferons which are mainly antiviral. IFN-gamma is the main macrophage-activating factor derived from T-cells. It can be used as an antiviral and antiparasitic agent. IFN-gamma has been shown to be effective in the treatment of chronic polyarthritis.

Production. T-cells (CD4+, CD8+), natural killers activated by antigens, mitogens or alloantigens. The synthesis of IFN-gamma is induced by IL-2, EGF. The synthesis is inhibited by 1-alpha, 25-dihydroxy vitamin D3, dexamethasone, cyclosporin A.

■ **IFN-tau:** (syn: TP-1, pregnancy recognition hormone, trophoblast interferon) IFN-tau has been shown to potentiate clonogenic growth of hematopoietic progenitor cells obtained from human fetal liver and neonatal cord blood. IFN-tau behaves like an immunomodulatory cytokine. It appears to interact with several steps of HIV replication cycle and has been shown to inhibit HIV-1 replication in primary peripheral blood lymphocytes, monocyte-derived macrophages and in peripheral blood mononuclear cells. IFN-tau may have therapeutic potential as an antitumor agent without the toxic effects generally associated with IFN.

Gamma Interferon-Inducible Protein 10

(IP-10) Belongs to cytokines.
Occurrence. Monocytes, endothelial cells, fibroblasts, keratinocytes.
Function. Chemoattracts monocytes and T-cells, supports T-cell adhesion to endothelial cells.

Interleukins

(IL) Belong to cytokines (immunoregulative mediators), soluble proteins secreted by monocytes/lymphocytes that regulate the magnitude of an inflammatory or immune response. Interleukins are involved in process of cell activation, cell differentiation, proliferation and cell-to-cell interactions. The same interleukins can be produced by many different cell types and an individual interleukin may act on different cell types, eliciting different biological responses, depending on the particular type of cell. The expression of interleukins is usually strictly regulated, i. e. the factors are often not secreted constitutively. They are synthesized after cell activation as a consequence of a physiological or non-physiological stimulus.

Function and effects

■ **IL-1-alpha, IL-1-beta:** is a major inflammatory mediator that has effects on all bodily systems. Endogenous pyrogen (IL-1-beta mediates fever in response to several inducers), proinflammatory cytokines, involved in acute phase response (acute phase proteins), hypotension, inducing neutrophils, fibroblasts, osteoblasts, epithelial and endothelial cells to grow, differentiate or synthesize specific products. At the brain level – mediate fever, increasing prostaglandins, decreasing REM sleep, anorexia, cause hypoalgesia, increase ACTH. Involved in inflammation or releasing tissue factors, lymphocyte activation, increasing lymphokines production (interferon, IL-2, IL-4, IL-5), T-lymphocytes release stimulation, differentiation B-lymphocytes stimulation, natural killer (NK) cells activation, IL-6 and colony-stimulating factor production. IL-1 protect against lethal effects of radiation, are chemotactic for monocytes and neutrophils, augment B-cell responses, induce collagenase and prostaglandins in synovial cells, increase lipolysis, lipoprotein lipase in adipocytes. At the chondrocytes level – PG, collagenase, plasminogen activator, and cartilage metabolism increase. At the osteoklasts level – collagenase, alkaline phosphatase, and bone resorption decrease. At the synovial cells level – proliferation. At the endothelial cells and smooth muscle cells level – induce proliferation, increase prostaglandins, procoagulation activity, leukocyte adhesion, granulocytic and macrophages colony stimulating factor secretion. At the cardiovascular system level, they are involved in hypotension, increased leukocyte adherence, PGE synthesis, decrease of systemic vascular resistance, and the heart minute volume and heart rate increase. At the adrenals level – increase glucocorticoids production.

Production. Monocytes, macrophages, chondrocytes, keratinocytes, fibroblasts, lymphocytes, endothelial cells, antigen-presenting cells (APC). IL-1 is synthesized as precursor firstly (pro-IL-1). Pro-IL-1-alpha is protein from which an IL-1-alpha is created, both substances are biologically active. Pro-IL-1-beta is biologically inactive protein. This precursor is changed to IL-1-beta by specific ICE (IL-1-beta converting enzyme). Biological properties of IL-1-alpha and IL-1-beta are probably identical; they act as IL-1R I and IL-1R II agonists. IL-1-receptor antagonist (IL-1Ra) is specific IL-1-alpha and IL-1-beta antagonist, but does not trigger any biological signal. Receptors IL-1R I and IL-1R II belong to immunoglobulin superfamily. IL-1R I is biologically active, IL-1R II acts in uptake. Stimuli for IL-1 production: tumor-necrosis factor, IL-2, ultra-violet light, antigen presentation, activated T-cells, immune complexes, C5a, interferon gamma, gram-positive/negative bacteria, yeast, viruses. IL-1 system is created by three ligand molecule types alpha, beta and Ra (receptor antagonist) and by two receptor types IL-1R I and IL-1R II.

■ **IL-2** (T-cell growth factor): T-cell growth/stimulation, co-stimulates B-cell growth and differentiation, thymocyte growth factor, augments natural killers, increases NK-cell cytotoxicity and augments lymphokine-activated killers, increases cytotoxic T-lymphocytes, induces proliferation of mature/immature thymocytes, modulates HLA antigen expression, induces interferon-alpha secretion and other lymphokines, immunoglobulins production. IL-2 is involved in T_H1 and T_H2-lymphocyte balance maintenance via T_H0 to T_H1-lymphocytes differentiation modulation. IL-2 functions in an autocrine fashion as well as a paracrine fashion. IL-2 displays significant anti-tumor activity for a variety of tumor cell types since it supports the proliferation and clonal expansion of T-cells that specifically attack certain tumor types. IL-2 is increasingly used to treat patients with cancers refractory to conventional treatment.

Production. T-helper cells (CD4+, CD8+). These cells react to IL-2 stimulation by IL-2 receptor induction (autocrine loop). IL-2 receptor (IL-2R) is trimeric complex composed of three different polypeptide chains alpha, beta and gamma. IL-2 bounds to alpha- and beta-chain, but not to gamma-chain. IL-2 bounds to trimeric complex or to alpha- and beta-chains differ in affinity. IL-2 is monomer glycosylated protein. Stimulation for production: antigen presentation, IL-1, T-helper cells. Immunostimulatory IL-2 effect is used in tumour immunotherapy.

■ **IL-3:** B-cell stimulatory factor-1, mast cell growth, pluripotential hematopoietic cell growth, granulocytes stimulation, eosinophils, NK-cells, erythrocytes, megakaryocytes and macrophages precursors proliferation, monocytes and macrophages activation; supports growth and differentiation of bone marrow stem cells. IL-3 receptors are expressed on macrophages, mast cells, eosinophils, megakaryocytes, basophils, bone marrow progenitor cells and various myeloid leukemia cells. IL-3 also induces the increased expression of receptors for colony stimulating factors. In LPS-stimulated macrophages IL-3 significantly enhances the secretion of other cytokines including IL-1, IL-6 and TNF. IL-3 alone or in combination with other CSFs or Epo is probably useful in the reconstitution of bone marrow and in stimulating erythropoiesis.

Production. T-cells, mastocytes, keratinocytes, NK-cells, endothelial cells and monocytes. Stimulation for production: antigen and mitogen presentation.

■ **IL-4:** T-cell growth, cytotoxic T-lymphocyte generation, co-stimulates B-cell growth/proliferation/differentiation, synergizes with IL-3 in mast cell growth, induces/increases IgE and IgG production by B-cells, macrophage proliferation, natural-killer cells and T-cells, increases class II major histocompatibility complex in B-cells (HLA D, HLA DR, HLA DQ). IL-4 and IL-10 are involved in T_H0-lymphocytes to T_H2-lymphocytes differentiation. Induces thymocytes proliferation, inhibits thymic epithelial cells growth. Cytokine responsible for arising atopic reactions, an early hypersensitivity reaction. IL-4 acts after binding to specific membrane receptor consisted of alpha- and gamma-chains; it is degraded by various mechanism after binding. IL-4 may be of clinical importance in the treatment of inflammatory diseases and autoimmune diseases since it inhibits the production of inflammatory cytokines such as IL-1, IL-6 and TNF-alpha by monocytes. IL-4 may be useful also in the treatment of solid tumors, of hematopoietic systemic diseases and of immune defects. It also inhibits the growth of colon and mammary carcinomas. IL-4 may play an essential role in the pathogenesis of chronic lymphocytic leukemia disease, which is characterized by the accumulation of slow-dividing and long-lived monoclonal B-cells arrested at the intermediate stage of their differentiation by preventing both the death and the proliferation of the malignant B-cells.

Production. T-helper cells and mastocytes. IL-4 is globular monomer glycoprotein. Many cell types have an IL-4R expression ability; this explains IL-4 pleiotropy. Production stimulation is antigen presentation.

■ **IL-5:** B-cell growth factor, eosinophil production, differentiation, growth and activation (eosinophil differentiation factor), activation of eosinophils to kill helminths. High affinity and low affinity receptors for IL-5 are expressed in all hematopoietic and lymphoid cells. Promotes/increases IgA/IgM production, T- and B-cells differentiation and proliferation. IL-5 is heterogenous glycosylated protein. Active molecule domain needs two monomers. IL-5 is bound to receptor consisting from alpha- and beta-chains. Beta-chain is common receptor for IL-3 and GM-CSF.

Production. T-helper cells (CD4+), mastocytes, eosinophils. Alpha-chain is a specificity carrier, beta-chain is a signal transmitter. Production stimulation is antigen presentation.

■ **IL-6:** B-cell stimulatory factor-2, pyrogen, induces plasmocytes growth, neutrophils stimulation, macrophages and megakaryocytes precursors, enhances Ig production by B-cells, increase class I major histocompatibility complex in fibroblasts (HLA A, HLA B, HLA C), synergizes with IL-2 producing acute phase proteins by hepatocytes, synergizes with IL-3 in hematopoietic cell growth, induces cytotoxic T-lymphocyte differentiation, keratinocyte growth/proliferation. Decreases albumin and prealbumin synthesis. IL-6 effects are mediated via bound to receptor which is composed of two polypeptide chains p80 and gp130. Protein p80 is able to bound IL-6; this complex is bound to gp130 which transfers biological signal. p80 receptor is in soluble form in blood and urine. The determination of IL-6 serum levels may be useful to monitor the activity of myelomas and to calculate tumor cell masses. The deregulated expression of IL-6 is probably one of the major factor involved in the pathogenesis of a number of diseases. It has been suggested that IL-6, due to its effects on hematopoietic cells, may be suitable for the treatment of certain types of anemia and thrombocytopenia.

Production. Macrophages, fibroblasts, endothelial cells, monocytes, activated T-cells, keratinocytes, mastocytes, tumour cells. IL-6 is synthesized as a precursor (240 amino acids) then the peptid is created (212 amino acids) by posttranslation modulation (glycosylation and phosphorylation). Production stimulation is IL-1 and tumor necrosis factor alpha with IL-3, GM-CSF, IFN-gamma.

■ **viral IL-6:** human herpesvirus 8 (HHV-8) or Kaposi sarcoma-associated herpesvirus (KSHV) is a human herpesvirus that have been identified with high frequency in all epidemiological forms of Kaposi's sarcoma. The genome of HHV-8 encodes a structural homolog of IL-6, termed viral IL-6.

■ **IL-7:** proliferation of pro/pre-B-cells, T-cells, T-lymphocytes, and immature thymocytes. In human peripheral monocytes IL-7 induces the synthesis of some inflammatory mediators such as IL-1, IL-6, macrophage inflammatory protein. The human IL-7 receptor is an integral strongly glycosylated membrane protein expressed on activated T-cells. IL-7 receptors are expressed also on B-cells, bone marrow macrophages. It has been suggested that IL-7 alone or in combination with IL-2, may be used as a consolidative immunotherapy for malignancies in patients after autologous bone marrow transplantation.

Production. Bone marrow cells.

■ **IL-8:** neutrophil chemotaxis and activation, lysosomal enzymes release, T-cell activation. IL-8 is chemotactic for monocytes, polymorphonuclears and T-lymphocytes. IL-8 plays key role in local inflammation origin, development and progression; induces basophil histamine and leukotriene release. It inhibits the adherence of neutrophils to vascular endothelium. At relatively high concentrations, IL-8 increases the expression of adhesion proteins on neutrophils. IL-8 is involved also in mediating pain, directly affects B-cells, is chemotactic for all known types of migratory immune cells. It inhibits the adhesion of leukocytes to activated endothelial cells and therefore possesses anti-inflammatory activities. It is a mitogen for epidermal cells, in vivo IL-8 strongly binds to erythrocytes. Macrophage-derived IL-8 supports angiogenesis and may play a role in angiogenesis-dependent disorders as rheumatoid arthritis, tumor growth and wound healing.

Production. Monocytes, macrophages, fibroblasts, endothelial cells, lymphocytes, hepatocytes, keratinocytes, chondrocytes, melanocytes, tumour cells. Stimulation for production: IL-1, IL-3, tumor necrosis factor alpha, phytohemagglutinins, concanavalin A, viruses, bacterial lipopolysaccharides. Inhibition of synthesis: glucocorticoids, IL-4, TGF-beta, inhibitors of 5' lipoxygenase, vitamin D3. There are two IL-8 receptor types IL-8R I and II (G-type receptor protein group); they have similar IL-8 binding afinity, but are different in specificity. Receptors are on neutrophils, basophils and T-lymphocytes.

■ **IL-9:** T-lymphocytes proliferation and growth stimulation in absence of antigen and antigen-presenting cells. Erythroid progenitors stimulation. In the presence of IL-3 IL-9 enhances the proliferation of bone marrow mast cells. It also stimulates erythroid progenitors in normal human bone marrow in the absence of serum. It stimulates the proliferation of fetal thymocytes and promotes the proliferation of some leukemia cell lines. IL-9 is expressed by Reed-Sternberg cells and Hodgkin's lymphoma cells and some large anaplastic lymphoma cells. It may play a role, therefore, in the pathogenesis of Hodgkin's disease and large cell anaplastic lymphoma and has been shown to function as an autocrine growth modulator for Hodgkin's cell lines.

Production. T-cells.

■ **IL-10:** cytokines synthesis inhibition by T_H1-lymphocytes, activated monocytes, and NK-cells incl. itself inhibition, macrophage activity and their bactericidal activity inhibition, augments B-cell proliferation and induces activated B-lymphocytes differentiation to plasma cells, stimulates activated T-cells, and co-stimulates immature/mature thymocyte proliferation/maturation. Inhibits cytotoxic reactions and inflammation; involved in IgA synthesis management. It inhibits the synthesis of a number of cytokines such as IFN-gamma, IL-2 and TNF-beta in Th1 subpopulations of T-cells. IL-10 indirectly suppresses tumor growth of certain tumors by inhibiting infiltration of macrophages which may provide tumor growth promoting activity. IL-10 levels appear to correlate with a poor survival in patients with intermediate or high-grade non-Hodgkin's lymphoma.

Production. T-cells (CD4+), activated mastocytes, keratinocytes and some activated B-cells. IL-10 is composed of T_H0 and T2 CD4+ cell subsets. A strong homology in nucleic acid and amino acid sequences between IL-10 and EBV BCRF-1 protein exists.

Test Purpose. 1) decreased IgA synthesis conditions, 2) chronic EBV infection and lymphoma. In IL-10 determination is needed to examine anti-EBV or EBV because of cross-reactivity.

■ **IL-11:** B-cell development and hematopoiesis stimulation, as well as supporting macrophage growth. It promotes primary and secondary immune responses in vitro and in vivo and modulates antigen-specific antibody reactions. IL-11 inhibits the differentiation of preadipocytes. It induces they synthesis of some acute phase proteins by hepatocytes.
Production. Bone marrow stromal cells and mesenchymal cells.

■ **IL-12:** facilitates proliferation of activated T- and NK-cells, enhances the lytic activity of NK-cells; it is the most potent inducer of IFN-gamma production by resting or activated T- and NK-cells. It selectively induces the differentiation of T_H0 into T_H1-lymphocytes, but suppresses T_H2-dependent functions (e. g. IL-4, IL-10 and IgE antibodies production). Induces GM-CSF, TNF, IL-6, IL-2 production. It synergizes with IL-2 in promoting cytotoxic T-cell responses. IL-12 stimulates the proliferation of human lymphoblasts activated by phytohemagglutinin. It also acts as a co-mitogen and potentiates the proliferation of resting peripheral cells induced by IL-2. IL-12 is involved probably also in the selection of immunoglobulin isotypes. IL-12 is of potential clinical interest since it allows to reduce doses of IL-2 required for the generation of lymphokine-activated killer cells. IL-12 has been shown to augment natural killer-cell mediated cytotoxicity in a number of conditions, including patients with hairy cell leukemia. IL-12 has been shown to inhibit the growth of a variety of experimental tumors in vivo and to have antiangiogenic effects in vivo, which are, at least in part, mediated by IFN-gamma. IL-12 therefore seems to be a potential candidate also for the treatment of angiogenesis-dependent malignancies.
Production. B-cells, macrophages. The most powerful inducers of IL-12 are bacteria, bacterial products and parasites.

■ **IL-13:** induces B- and T-lym growth and differentiation, but inhibits inflammatory cytokine production (IL-1, IL-6, IL-8, IL-10, IL-12) by monocytes and macrophages, induces T_H0 to T_H2 subtypes differentiation and monocyte to dendritic cells differentiation in tissue cultures. IL-13 also decreases the production of nitric oxide by activated macrophages, leading to a decrease in parasiticidal activity. IL-13 is expressed in activated T_H0 cells, T_H1-like cells, T_H2-like cells and T-cells expressing CD8. It is not expressed in heart, brain, placenta, lung, liver and skeletal muscle tissues.
Production. T-cells.

■ **IL-14:** (high-molecular weight B-cell growth factor) induces activated B-cell proliferation and inhibits immunoglobulin mitogen-stimulated B-cells secretion. IL-14 receptors are found only in B-cell line cells. IL-14 is mitogenic for activated B-cells but inhibits antibody production – participates mainly in secondary humoral immune responses.
Production. T-cells, follicular dendritic cells.

■ **IL-15:** stimulates mastocytes, T-lymphocyte growth factor; in antigen stimulus absence IL-15 maintains T-lymphocytes store probably; induces T-cell proliferation. It functions as a signal from nonlymphoid cells for generating T-cell-dependent immune responses. It is widely expressed in placenta, skeletal muscle, kidney, lung, liver, heart, bone marrow stroma. Receptors for IL-15 have been observed on fresh human venous endothelial cells, on stromal cells from bone marrow, fetal liver and thymic epithelium. IL-15 appears to function as a specific maturation factor for NK-cells.

■ **Production.** Non-lymphoid cells (epithelial cells, monocytes). IL-15 has been shown to be produced by human fetal astrocytes and microglia in response to IL-1-beta, IFN-gamma or TNF-alpha and may thus play a role in T-cell mediated immune responses in the human central nervous system.

■ **IL-16**: (lymphocyte chemoattractant factor – LCF) auxiliary factor in HIV virus replication inhibition, growth/chemotactic CD4+ lymphocytes factor. IL-16 is produced in response to histamine stimulation and it induces the directional migration of CD4+ T-cells, eosinophils and monocytes.
Production. T-lymphocytes CD8+.

■ **IL-17**: glycoprotein – soluble co-activating molecule form from CTLA group. Stimulates epithelial/endothelial cells and fibroblasts to IL-6, IL-8, PGE2, GM-CSF production. IL-17 is involved in the early inflammatory reaction induction; mediates immune system – hemopoiesis co-operation. IL-17 enhances expression of the intercellular adhesion molecule-1 in human fibroblasts.
Production. T-lymphocytes CD4+.

■ **IL-18**: (IFN-gamma inducing factor) polypeptide, stimulates T_H1-lymphocytes to IFN-gamma, IL-2 a GM-CSF production. IL-18 induces T_C-lymphocyte and NK-cells activity; inhibits IL-10 production. mRNA for IL-18 is expressed in Kupffer cells and activated macrophages. It is synthesized as a biologically inactive precursor. It has been shown that caspase-1 is responsible for processing pro-IL-18 to the biologically active form. IL-18 may be involved also in mechanisms of tissue injury in inflammatory reactions.
Production. Activated monocytes and macrophages.

Increased IL-2 Values
Hodgkin's disease, graft-versus-host reaction, multiple sclerosis, rheumatoid arthritis, systemic lupus erythematosus, type-1 diabetes mellitus, lepromatous leprosy, AIDS, immunodeficiency sy, severe burns, allogenic bone marrow transplantation

Increased IL-6 Values
rheumatoid arthritis, alcoholic liver cirrhosis, **idiopathic thrombocytemia**, mesangio-capillary proliferative glomerulonephritis, diseases – (autoimmune d., acute systemic inflammatory d.), cardiac myxoma, chronic polyarthritis, plasma cell leukemia, lymphomas, Castleman's disease, myxedema, renal tumors, plasmocytoma, psoriasis, Kaposi's sarcoma, Kawasaki's syndrome

Increased IL-8 Values
rheumatoid arthritis, cystic fibrosis, alcoholic hepatitis, infectious diseases – (meningococcal i. d.), ulcerative colitis, psoriasis, septic shock, tumors

Increased IL-10 Values
non-Hodgkin's lymphoma

Analyte	Age/Gender	Reference Range	SI Units	Note
Interleukin				
Alpha		0–5	pg/ml	
Beta		1–10	ng/ml	
Interleukin 2		<5	pg/ml	
s-Interleukin 2				
Receptor (sIL-2)		25–105	pmol/l	
sensitivity		5	pmol/l	
Interleukin 5		<10	pg/ml	
Interleukin 6		<10	pg/ml	
s-Interleukin 6				
Membrane Receptor				

Analyte	Age/Gender	Reference Range	SI Units	Note
(sIL-6)		10–90	ng/l	
Interleukin 8		<10	ng/l	
Interleukin 10		<5	pg/ml	

Iodine

(I) Basic element of thyroid hormones synthesis. Iodine is transported in iodide form. Each iodide anion is oxidized on I_2 (iodation) after entering thyroid and is bound to thyroxine (iodization). Monoiodothyronine, diiodothyronines, triiodothyronines and thyroxine are created. Unused or released iodine, enters into iodine circulation again, the rest is excreted by the kidney. Stored in thyroid as thyroglobulin form (precursor of triiodothyronine – T3, tetraiodothyronine, thyroxine – T4). These hormones participate in energy mechanism control.

Increased Values
hyperthyroidism, thyroid tumours, stress, struma (goiter), thyrotoxicosis
   Interfering Factors: medicaments – (bismuth salts, bromides, contraceptives, diethyl-stilbestrol, medicaments with iodine)

Decreased Values
hypothyroidism, cretinism, myxedema, struma (goiter), chronic thyroiditis (Hashimoto's)
   Interfering Factors: medicaments – (acetazolamide, aminobenzoic acid, aminosalicylic acid, anabolics, carbimazole, corticosteroids, diphenylhydantoin, phenylbutazone, sulfonamides, sulphonylurea, vitamin A)

Analyte	Age/Gender	Reference Range	SI Units	Note
Iodine				
inorganic		0.78–23.6	nmol/l	
butanol-extractable	Neonates	567–1040	nmol/l	
	Children	335–575	nmol/l	
	Adults	232–504	nmol/l	
bounded to protein	1–2 d	760–1135	nmol/l	
	4–5 w	440–725	nmol/l	
	12 w	400–686	nmol/l	
	52 w	417–575	nmol/l	
	Adults	315–521	nmol/l	

Iron

(Fe, syn: ferrum) Amount absorbed from the diet depends on amount/type of iron ingested, gastric acidity, bone marrow activity, and body iron stores. Although the entire small intestine has the capacity to absorb iron (mainly in a ferrous state), maximal absorption occurs in the duodenum and upper jejunum, owing optimum pH conditions. In severe iron deficiency, the body can increase absorption up to 30% of the dietary intake, to compensate for the depletion. Elementary iron is biologically active in the ferrous (Fe^{2+}) and ferric (Fe^{3+}) forms. In general, an acidic/lower pH, favors the ferrous state and iron absorption; whereas a neutral/alkaline pH favors the ferric state and decreases iron absorption. Iron is transported from the intestine and duodenum mucosal cells to the blood as $Fe(OH)_2 \rightarrow Fe(OH)_3$ bound to protein apoferritin to ferritin $\rightarrow Fe^{2+}$ release $\rightarrow$ apoferritin $\rightarrow$ plasma transport $\rightarrow$ after oxidation to $Fe^{3+} \rightarrow$ bound to a specific iron transport protein free transferrin $\rightarrow$ transferrin (beta-1-globulin, siderophillin) attaches to the developing erythrocyte membrane receptors and releases free iron into erythrocyte for incorporation into heme within the mitochondria. Liver and spleen realize similar reactions to duodenal epithelium ($Fe^{2+} \leftarrow \rightarrow Fe^{3+}$ + apoferritin $\leftarrow \rightarrow$ ferritin). Approximately 10–20% of the total body iron is stored as ferritin. If iron is absorbed in the ferritin storage excess $\rightarrow$ iron is deposited in lysosomal membranes as a pseudocrystalline complex, termed hemosiderin. About 65% (60 mg/kg males, 50 mg/kg females) of the body's iron is bound to heme. 20–25 mg/day are needed for erythropoiesis. 95% of this required iron is recycled iron salvaged from normal RBC turnover and hemoglobin catabolism. Only 1 mg/day (representing 5% of the iron turnover) is newly absorbed to balance minimal iron loss incurred by fecal/urinary secretion.

Function. Essential component in body oxygen transfer and enzyme component.

Occurrence. Hemoglobin, myoglobin, enzymes, ferritin, hemosiderin, plasma, cytochrome, peroxidases, and catalases.

Iron-Storage. Liver, spleen, and bone marrow. Storage iron exists in hemosiderin or ferritin forms. Iron is absorbed from meat, liver (25–30% of iron), eggs, vegetables (5% of iron), best absorbed is inorganic Fe^{2+} and iron coming from hemoglobin. Marked diurnal level variation, up to 40% variation within day, 25% day-to-day. Highest levels are in AM, and lowest are at night.

Test Purpose. 1) to help in malnutrition and Plummer-Vinson sy diagnosis, 2) to help in hemochromatosis diagnosis, 3) suspicion of latent or manifest iron deficiency, iron overdose, iron processing disorders, 4) prolonged parenteral nutrition, 5) to monitor an overload in renal dialysis patients or patients with transfusion dependent anemias.

Increased Values – hypersideremia

portocaval anastomosis, anemia – (**aplastic a.**, **hemolytic a.**, **hypoplastic a.**, sickle cell a., **pernicious a.**, **sideroblastic a.**, sideroachrestic a., **thalassemia**), congenital atransferrinemia, **hepatic cirrhosis**, deficiency of – (folate, pyruvate kinase, vitamin B_6, **vitamin B_{12}**), decreased/ineffective erythropoiesis, hemolysis, hepatitis – (**acute h., viral h.**), **primary hemochromatosis**, **hemosiderosis**, **hemolytic icterus**, insufficiency – (chronic renal i., pancreatic i.), intoxication by – (**lead, iron**), acute leukemia, nephritis, **hepatic necrosis**, porphyria, **increased iron intake, frequent transfusions**, renal dialysis patients

   Interfering Factors: medicaments – (chloramphenicol, cisplatin, dextran, estrogens, ethanol, iron preparations, methotrexate, methyldopa, oral contraceptives, salicylates)

Decreased Values – hyposideremia

inadequate iron absorption, achlorhydria, anemia – (**sideroblastic a.**, **sideropenic a.**), avitaminosis C, **celiac disease, premature infants, prolonged total milk diet in infants, diverticulitis**, duodenitis, enteritis regionalis, **increased erythropoiesis**, gastrectomy, **atrophic gastritis, helminthiasis, hematuria**, hemodialysis, paroxysmal nocturnal hemoglobinuria, hemoglobinuria, **prolonged hemoptysis, hemorrhoids**, hiatal hernia, chronic diarrhea, hypothyroidism, diseases – (**acute/chronic infectious d.**, inflammatory renal d., chronic hepatic d., **chronic inflammatory d.**), myocardial infarction, **chronic renal insufficiency, ulcerative colitis**, hemorrhage – (**acute h., chronic h., gastrointestinal h., menstruating h.**), kwashiorkor, lactation, vitamin B_{12} deficiency treatment (shortly after), **malabsorption, malnutrition, tumours**, nephrosis, blood sampling – (diagnostic, blood donors), **extensive surgery**, polyps, **decreased intake in conjunction with gut infestation with hookworm, negative iron balance during the growth spurts**, chronic gastrointestinal blood loss, syndrome – (**Good-**

pasture's sy, **malabsorption sy**, **nephrotic sy**), steatorrhea, **pregnancy** (3rd trimester), small intestine teleangiectasis, urolithiasis, **trauma**, **esophageal varices**, volvulus, **peptic ulcers**, recovery from pernicious anemia

   Interfering Factors: adolescence, infancy, medicaments – (acetylsalicylic acid – large doses, ACTH, allopurinol, anabolic steroids, chloramphenicol, cholestyramine, colchicine, cortisone, deferoxamine, metformin, methicillin, oxymetholone, testosterone)

Analyte	Age/Gender	Reference Range	SI Units	Note
Iron	2 w	11–36	µmol/l	
	6 m	5–24	µmol/l	
	12 m	6–28	µmol/l	
	<12 y	4–24	µmol/l	
	F <25 y	6.6–29.5	µmol/l	
	40–60 y	4.1–24	µmol/l	
	>60 y	7.0–26.7	µmol/l	
	Pregnancy			
	0–12 w	7.6–31.6	µmol/l	
	36–40 w	4.5–24.5	µmol/l	
	6 w post-labor	2.9–26.9	µmol/l	
	M <25 y	7.2–27.7	µmol/l	
	40–60 y	6.3–30.1	µmol/l	
	>60 y	7.2–21.5	µmol/l	

Isocitrate Dehydrogenase

(ICD, ICDH) Exists in 2 isoenzyme forms (mitochondrial, cytoplasmic). Enzyme ICD NAD$^+$ (or NADP$^+$) catalyzes isocitrate oxidative decarboxylation to alpha-ketoglutarate using NAD$^+$ (or NADP$^+$) as an electron acceptor. Enzymes require Mg^{2+} and Mn^{2+}, they are activated by ADP, citrate, Ca^{2+}, and inhibited by NADH, NADPH and ATP. Increased ICD activity is a sensitive indicator of parenchymal liver disease.

Test Purpose. 1) to detect early viral hepatitis and infectious mononucleosis, 2) to distinguish between liver disease and myocardial infarction, when AST is elevated, 3) to assess presence and extent of liver damage.

Increased Values

ethanol abuse, megaloblastic anemia, neonatal biliary duct atresia, **hepatic cirrhosis**, hepatitis – (**chronic toxic h.**, infectious h., **viral h.**), pregnancy induced hypertension, hepatic hypoxia due to hemodynamic causes, **acute biliary tract inflammatory diseases**, icterus – (hepatotoxic i., obstructive i.), severe pulmonary infarct, kwashiorkor, **infectious mononucleosis**, tumours – (myeloid leukemia, **metastatic t. to liver, liver t.**), hepatic obstruction, necrotizing processes of liver, pregnancy

   Interfering Factors: medicaments – (allopurinol, aminosalicylic acid, amphotericin B, anabolic steroids, androgens, anesthetics, chlorpromazine, clindamycin, ethanol, isoniazid, methotrexate, phenylbutazone)

Decreased Values

heavy metals intoxication

   Interfering Factors: medicaments – (EDTA, fluoride, isocitrate, natrium chloride, oxalate)

Analyte	Age/Gender	Reference Range	SI Units	Note
Isocitrate-Dehydro-genase	Neonates	33–146	nkat/l	
	Children	0–85.5	nkat/l	
	Adults	13.3–73	nkat/l	

Isoenzyme BB of Glycogenphosphorylase B

(GP-BB) It is a dominant isoform of glycogenphosphorylase in the myocard. As a cytosol enzyme, it escapes cardiomyocyte early after ischemic injury. More sensitive early marker for acute myocardial infarction and unstable angina than is CK-MB, troponin T and myoglobin. Sensitive marker of perioperative myocardial damage in coronary artery bypass surgery.

Test Purpose. 1) acute myocardial infarction diagnosis, 2) thrombolytic therapy success control.

Increased Values
myocardial infarction (increase after 2 hrs, decrease 24–36 hrs), unstable pectoral angina

Isoleucine

(Ile) Amino acid produced by fibrin and other proteins hydrolysis, essential for optimal growth in infants and for nitrogen equilibrium in adults. Enzyme defect: O-acetyl-coenzyme thiolase.

Increased Values – hyperisoleucinemia
acidemia – (methylmalonic a., propionine a.), accumulation of alpha-methylacetate, carboxylase deficiency, viral hepatitis, starvation, methylmalonic homocystinuria, maple syrup urine disease (branched-chain ketoaciduria), obesity

Decreased Values – hypoisoleucinemia
hepatic encephalopathy, acute hunger, hyperinsulinism, Huntington's chorea, carcinoid, kwashiorkor, severe burns, conditions after abdominal surgery
    Interfering Factors: medicaments – (alanine, glucose, histidine, oral contraceptives)

Analyte	Age/Gender	Reference Range	SI Units	Note
Isoleucine	Neonates	<50	µmol/l	
	Children	20–80	µmol/l	
	Adults	30–60	µmol/l	

Isopropanol – Methanol

Test Purpose. To confirm cause and extent of intoxication caused by methanol or isopropanol suspected from patient history and clinical examination.

Increased Values
intoxication – (isopropanol i., methanol i.)

Ketobodies

Ketobodies (ketones) include acetone, acetoacetic acid, beta-hydroxybutyric acid. They are produced in liver by fatty acid oxidation. Ketogenesis is quite a complicated process, which is controlled actively and regulated by the fatty acid beta-oxidation rate. Free fatty acids are activated by bonding with CoA, they are esterified onto triacylglycerol, or they react with carnitine (a very important enzyme carnitine acyltransferase, inhibited by malonyl-CoA) and enter mitochondria. Ketobody concentration is increased in acetyl-CoA overproduction (as a fatty acids beta-oxidation result) by glucose lack. Insulin shortage stimulates carnitine acyltransferase and leads to malonyl-CoA decrease and finally blocks glucose utilization on the periphery (musculature). Insulin shortage (absolute and relative) causes: 1) lipolysis stimulation, 2) accelerates and promotes beta-oxidation, 3) decreases ketobody utilization on the periphery.

Increased Values
acetonemic vomiting in children, acidosis – (lactic a., metabolic a.), **alcohol intoxication,** active acromegaly, **alcoholism, anorexia nervosa, branched-chain ketonuria,** bulimia, **catabolism, catecholamines excess,** conditions – (**febrile c.,** septic c., shock c., **post-anesthesia c.**), decreased tissue perfusion, diseases – (infectious d., liver d.), **exercise in untrained subjects, glycogen storage diseases, hyperglycemia,** hypoglycemic encephalopathy, **hyperinsulinism, increased fat intake,** infantile organic acidemias, **intestinal diseases,** ketoacidosis – (**diabetic k.,** alcoholic k., fasting k.), **methylmalonic aciduria,** obesity, **persistent vomiting,** pregnancy, **prolonged fasting** (most common in children 1 to 6 years old), **prolonged excessive insulin administration in diabetics, severe carbohydrate intake restriction, severe thyrotoxicosis, starvation, stress, weight-reducing diets,** renal failure

> **Interfering Factors:** medicaments – (amprenavir, asparaginase, diazoxide, indinavir, nelfinavir, ritonavir, saquinavir)

Analyte	Age/Gender	Reference Range	SI Units	Note
Ketobodies, total	Neonates	40–180	µmol/l	
	0–1 w	90–1900	µmol/l	
	Infants	30–890	µmol/l	
	1–6 y	30–1100	µmol/l	
	Adults	5–280	µmol/l	

Lactic Acid

(LA, syn: lactate, L-lactate) Glucose metabolism end product in oxygen absence (anaerobic glycolysis), which provides energy anaerobically in skeletal muscles during heavy exercise; it can be oxidized aerobically (Krebs' cycle) in the heart for energy production or converted back to glucose (gluconeogenesis, Cori's cycle). Marker of tissue hypoperfusion. Main source: skin, erythrocytes, brain, skeletal muscles, intestine, leukocytes. Lactic acid and pyruvate together form a reversible reaction that is regulated by the oxygen supply. When O_2 levels are deficient → pyruvate converts to lactic acid, when O_2 levels are adequate → lactic acid converts to pyruvate. Lactate concentration depends on pH, NADH/NAD+ ratio (it determines so-called redox cells condition), metabolization rate and → pyruvate concentration. Day-to-day value variation is 25%.

Test Purpose. 1) to assess tissue oxidation in metabolic and shock conditions and circulation failures, 2) tissue hypoxia diagnosis in low pO_2 levels, 3) to help determine the lactic acidosis and metabolic acidosis causes, 4) to help in differential diagnosis of myopathies (glycogenoses), 5) differential diagnosis of inborn enzymopathies, 6) differential diagnosis of comatose conditions and intoxications, 7) diagnosis of mesenteric vessels thrombosis and embolia, 8) perinatal asphyxia, 9) 2nd type diabetes mellitus and incorrect biguanids indication, 10) hereditary metabolic disorders (some metabolic organic acidurias and differential diagnosis of glycogenoses in function tests). Diagnostic importance has only a parallel acid base balance status evaluation.

Increased Values – hyperlactacidemia

acidosis – (**lactate a.**, nonketotic a., **metabolic a.**), **alcoholism**, **anemias**, narcosis, arteriosclerosis, chronic bronchitis, hepatic cirrhosis, dehydration, deficiency – (fructose-1,6-diphosphatase d., thiamine d.), **diabetes mellitus**, **subacute bacterial endocarditis**, **pulmonary embolism**, impaired renal/hepatic function, **glycogenoses** (glycogen storage disease), pregnancy induced hypertension, **hyperventilation**, hypotension, diseases – (severe vascular d., **infectious d.**, **hepatic d.**, severe pulmonary d., inflammatory d., cyanotic heart d.), decompensated inborn heart disorders, **myocardial infarction**, ketoacidosis, hepatic insufficiency, intoxication – (**ethanol i.**, ethylene glycol i., propylene glycol i., salicylate i.), acute hemorrhage, leukemia – (**acute l., chronic myeloid l.**), lymphomas, **von Gierke's disease**, tumour metastases, myopathies, **tumors**, extracorporeal circulation, **insufficient tissue oxygenation/ perfusion**, pneumonia, poliomyelitis, **pyelonephritis**, **septicemia**, conditions – (postictal c.), shock – (hypoglycemic s., s. **after surgery**, traumatic s.), pregnancy (3rd trimester), tuberculosis (advanced), uremia, tissue hypoperfusion, hypoxia, cardiac arrest, **physical exertion**, failure – (liver f., renal f., pulmonary f., **cardiac f.**), defective biotin metabolism
    Interfering Factors: medicaments – (acetaminophen, acetylsalicylic acid, albuterol, beclomethasone, biguanides, carbamazepine, catecholamines, disopyramide, epinephrine, ethanol, fructose, glucagon, glucose, insulin, isoniazid, metformin, methanol, methylprednisolone, nalidixic acid, oral contraceptives, phenformin, phenobarbital, salicylates, sodium bicarbonate, sorbitol, terbutaline, valproic acid)

Decreased Values – hypolactacidemia

anemia, weight loss
    Interfering Factors: medicaments – (morphine)

Analyte	Age/Gender	Reference Range	SI Units	Note
Lactate (Lactic acid)	Neonates	<2.9	mmol/l	
	Adults	<2.4	mmol/l	
		<1.8	mmol/l	See ref.
Capillary blood		1.0–1.8	mmol/l	ranges note
Venous blood		<1.8	mmol/l	
Arterial blood		<1.5	mmol/l	
Venous plasma		<2.2	mmol/l	
Arterial plasma		<1.8	mmol/l	
Umbilical blood		<3.3	mmol/l	

Lactic Acid Dehydrogenase

(LD, LDH, syn: lactate dehydrogenase, lactic dehydrogenase) Enzyme, oxidoreductase, a tetramer containing M (muscle) and H (heart) subunits. Subunits also determine elimination rate. Multiorgan cytosol enzyme activity is determined by 5 isoenzymes. LD 1 isoenzyme has a special position, because of higher hydroxybutyrate (HBDH) substrate afinity; other enzymes have afinity to 2-oxobutyrate. LD increase indicates cellular death.

Function. Enzyme – catalyzes L-lactate interconversion (reversible reaction) → pyruvate under aerobic/anaerobic conditions with $NADH/NADH_2$. The reaction is the glycolysis final step (white muscle fibers). The reversible reaction is the first lactate combustion step (heart, red muscle fibers) or its conversion to glucose (liver).

Occurrence. Myocardium, brain, muscle, liver, kidneys, lungs and erythrocytes cytoplasm.

Isoenzymes: 1) LD 1, H4 type (HBDH – hydroxybutyrate dehydrogenase) – cardiac: kidneys (60% of all isoenzymes), pancreas, heart, fetal skeletal muscle, brain, RBC, lungs, serum (25%), 2) LD 2, H3M type (HBDH – hydroxybutyrate dehydrogenase) – cardiac: kidneys (30%), spleen, lymph nodes, brain, RBC, lungs, thyroid, heart, uterus, serum (35%), 3) LD 3, H2M2 type: spleen, lymph nodes (31%), brain (19%), RBC (13%), lungs (28%), uterus (50%), serum (20%), thyroid, adrenals, 4) LD 4, HM3 type – hepatic: hepar, skeletal muscle, spleen, lymph nodes, adrenals, brain (31%), lungs, uterus, serum (10%), 5) LD 5, M4 type – hepatic: hepar (94%), skeletal muscle (76%), spleen, lymph nodes (18%), lungs (21%), uterus, serum (10%), granulocytes. Enzyme tumour marker. LD isoenzyme patterns cannot be interpreted without the clinical history.

Test Purpose. 1) to aid in MI, pulmonary infarction (late diagnosis), embolism, anemias, jaundice and hepatic disease differential diagnosis, 2) when CK-MB samples are drawn too late to support CK isoenzyme tests for diagnosing myocardial infarction, 3) to monitor patient chemotherapy response, 4) to help in skeletal muscles diseases diagnosis, 5) to help in suspected intravascular hemolysis, 6) to help in malignant tumors diagnosis – tumor marker, 7) patient monitoring after invasive cardiosurgery procedures.

Increased Values

anemia – (**hemolytic a.**, sickle cell a., **megaloblastic a.**, **pernicious a.**), **anoxia**, hepatic cirrhosis, **acute cardiac decompensation, delirium tremens, skeletal muscle dystrophy, pulmonary embolism, fractures, hemolysis**, hepatitis – (**acute h.**, viral h.), **hypotension**, hypothyroidism, **hypoxia**, prosthetic heart valve, cholangitis, diseases – (skin d., renal d., **liver d.**, cardiopulmonary d., collagen vascular d.), **obstructive jaundice**, infarction – (**intestinal i., myocardial i.** – increase at 6–24 hrs, peaking at 24–72 hrs, decrease 7–14 d., **renal i., pulmonary i.**), **intestinal ischemia**, carcinomatosis, **collagenoses**, meningitis, **tumor metastases, infectious mononucleosis, myocarditis, myopathies**, myxedema, tumours – (t. of colorectum, **acute leukemia**, myeloid leucemia, **lymphomas**, Hodgkin's disease, myeloproliferative t., t. of lung, t. of testes, liver t., seminoma, Ewing's sarcoma), necrosis – (**skeletal muscle n., hepatic n.**, tissue n., tubular n.), intestinal obstruction, pancytopenia, **pancreatitis, cerebrovascular accidents**, polycythemia, injury of – (erythrocytes, **skeletal muscle**, skin, brain, kidney, liver, lungs, heart), pyelonephritis, sprue, nephrotic sy, transfusions, **shock, heat stroke**, trauma, **congestive heart failure**, Epstein-Barr virus infection

Interfering Factors: strenuous exercise in children, erythrocytes hemolysis – blood sample freezing/healing/shaking, skin diseases, seasonal variations, medicaments – (acebutolol, acetylsalicylic acid, ajmaline, alcohol, amiodarone, amphotericin B, anabolic steroids, anesthetics, azlocillin, captopril, cephalosporins, ceftizoxime, chloramphenicol, chlorpropamide, cimetidine, clofibrate, dicumarol, disopyramide, erythromycin, etretinate, fluorides, fluorouracil, flucloxacillin, heparin, imipramine, interferons, isoniazid, isotretinoin, ketoconazole, ketoprofen, labetalol, metoprolol, methotrexate, mithramycin, morphine, narcotics, nitrofurantoin, nomifensine, oxacillin, penicillamine, phenothiazines, phenytoin, piperacillin, plicamycin, procainamide, propoxyphene, quinidine, streptokinase, sulfonamides, sulindac, tetracyclines, thiamazole, thiopental, ticarcillin, tretinate, triamterene, trimethoprim, valproic acid, verapamil)

Increased Isoenzymes

■ **LD 1:** anemia – (**hemolytic a.**, **acute sickle cell a.**, megaloblastic a., **pernicious a.**), hemolytic hyperbilirubinemia, **acute myocardial infarction** (increase at 6–24 h, peaking at 24–72 h, decrease at 4th d), **renal infarction**, germ cell tumors – (**dysgerminoma of ovary**, **seminoma of testis, teratoma**), acute renal cortical necrosis, skeletal muscle injury

■ **LD 1, 2:** anemia – (**hemolytic a.**, **acute sickle cell a.**, megaloblastic a., **pernicious a.**), hemolytic hyperbilirubinemia, **myocardial infarction**, **renal infarction**, acute renal cortical necrosis

■ **LD 1, 2, 3:** progressive muscular dystrophy

■ **LD 2:** malignant lymphoma

■ **LD 2, 3, 4:** massive platelet destruction, pulmonary embolism, lymphocytic leukemia, lymphomas, infectious mononucleosis, tumors, skeletal muscle injury, extensive blood transfusion, collagenoses, pulmonary infarction, congestive heart failure, viral infectious diseases

■ **LD 3:** pernicious anemia, pulmonary embolism, pulmonary infarction, infectious mononucleosis, extensive pneumonia, idiopathic sprue, malignant lymphoma, active chronic granulocytic leukemia, systemic lupus erythematosus

■ **LD 4:** malignant lymphoma, systemic lupus erythematosus, strenuous exercise

■ **LD 5: hepatic cirrhosis**, progressive muscular dystrophy, **liver diseases**, degenerative/inflammatory skeletal muscle diseases, passive liver congestion, tumors, skeletal muscle injury, trauma, burns – (electrical b., thermal b.), hepatitis (early), dermatomyositis, strenuous exercise, prostate carcinoma, CNS tumors

Decreased Values

positive response to cancer therapy

Interfering Factors: medicaments – (ascorbic acid, clofibrate, fluoride, ketoprofen, metronidazole, oxalate, urea)

Analyte	Age/Gender	Reference Range	SI Units	Note
Lactate				
Dehydrogenase 37 °C	1 d	<22.1	μkat/l	
	2–5 d	<28.9	μkat/l	
	6 d – 6 m	<16.3	μkat/l	
	6–12 m	<18.3	μkat/l	
	1–3 y	<14.2	μkat/l	
	4–6 y	<10.3	μkat/l	
	7–12 y F	<9.67	μkat/l	
	7–12 M	<12.7	μkat/l	
	13–17 y F	<7.27	μkat/l	
	13–17 M	<11.4	μkat/l	
	Adults	<7.5	μkat/l	See ref.
		<6.3	μkat/l	ranges note
Lactate Dehydro-				
genase – isoenzymes	Adults I (heart)	0.175–0.36		
	II	0.304–0.50		
	III	0.192–0.25		
	IV	0.096–0.10		
	V (liver)	0.055–0.13		

Lactoferrin

Lactoferrin is an iron-binding protein found in specific neutrophil granules where it exerts antimicrobial activity by withholding iron from ingested bacteria and fungi. It is involved in granulocytopoiesis, hydroxyl radicals bonding, showing bacteriostatic effects. It also occurs in many secretions (milk, tears, mucus, saliva, bile) and exudates.

Increased Values
bacterial infectious diseases mainly in children, meningitis, pneumonia, sepsis

Analyte	Age/Gender	Reference Range	SI Units	Note
Lactoferrin		170–440	µg/l	

LDL-Receptors

LDL-receptor "Apo BE receptor" – recognizes Apo BE particles (i. e. Apo B-100, or Apo E). It recognizes and takes up LDL particles, widely distributed throughout different tissues. The delivery of the cholesterol to the cell inhibits this receptor. That is, the product of the endocytosis gives a negative feedback. Functions as a regulator of LDL levels in blood; in redistribution and utilization of cholesterol.

Remnant receptor Apo E – it is found only in the liver. It recognizes chylomicron remnants and Apo E rich HDL receptors. Remnants are the leftovers of the chylomicron particles, after they have already dumped off their fatty acids. Chylomicrons remnants still have lots of cholesterol in them. It functions in uptake of cholesterol-loaded remnants and delivery of cholesterol to the liver.

Scavenger receptor – uptake of oxidized or chemically modified LDL-particles by monocytes in circulation or macrophages in tissues. It functions in degradation and uptake of modified (damaged) lipoproteins and uptake of bacteria to protect us from endotoxic shock.

LE Cells

(syn: lupus erythematosus cells, systemic lupus erythematosus cells) LE factor has the characteristics of an antinuclear antibody. LE cells are neutrophils, the cytoplasm contains large masses of depolymerized DNA from the polymorphonuclear leukocytes nuclei. Examination of LE cells is successively replaced by determination of antinuclear antibodies.

Increased Values – positive
rheumatoid arthritis, hepatitis, chronic active hepatitis, diseases – (rheumatic d., connective tissue d.), **systemic lupus erythematosus, scleroderma**
    Interfering Factors: medicaments – (acebutolol, acetazolamide, aminosalicylic acid, chlorothiazide, chlorpromazine, chlorprothixene, griseofulvin, hydralazine, isoniazid, labetalol, methyldopa, nitrofurantoin, oral contraceptives, penicillamine, penicillin, phenylbutazone, phenytoin, pindolol, practolol, primidone, procainamide, quinidine, streptomycin, sulfonamides, tetracyclines)

Decreased Values
    Interfering Factors: false negative results – (steroids)

Lead

(Pb) An ubiquitous constituent of the environment, lead has been, and to a lesser degree still is, used as a component of paints and petrol additive. Other settings that may result in exposure are lead mining and smelting, storage battery manufacturing and recycling, brass foundries, glass industries and plastics industries. General exposure to lead is elated to airborne fume emitted from motor vehicles and industrial emissions. Airborne lead eventually drops-out to contaminate soil, dust, sediments and waterways. Human exposure is almost always associated with inhalation or ingestion. Lead accumulates in bone and teeth where it displays a half-life of years. A much smaller proportion of the body burden is distributed to the soft tissues including red blood cells. The half-life of this compartment is 1 month. 95% of lead in whole blood is associated with the RBC's. Lead is mainly eliminated from the body in the urine by glomerular filtration and tubular secretion. Altered heme synthesis is found early after lead exposure and is due to inhibition of delta-aminolevulic acid dehydratase. Lead is also a neurotoxin. Whole blood lead is the sample of choice for the investigation of lead exposure. It is a short-term marker of exposure and also reflects redistribution of lead from the skeleton. Guidelines for evaluation of occupational exposure represent biological levels of chemicals that correspond to workers with inhalation exposure equivalent to the threshold limit value (TLV) of the chemicals. TLVs refer to maximal airborne concentrations that workers may be repeatedly exposed to without adverse effects.

Test Purpose. 1) to reveal lead exposure, 2) monitoring of people working with lead semi/products, 3) in patients, when the symptomatology can show lead intoxication. Lead levels and the clinical picture are assessed in chronic intoxications together with other parameters (e. g. DALA).

Increased Values
ethanol, **industrial exposure**, smoking, **lead poisoning**, ingestion of – (Pb-containing paint, ceramic glazes)

Analyte	Age/Gender	Reference Range	SI Units	Note
Lead	Neonates	<0.48	µmol/l	
Whole blood	Adults F	0.15–0.41	µmol/l	
	M	0.14–0.48	µmol/l	

Lecithin-Cholesterol Acyltransferase

(LCAT) LCAT activity represents the endogenic cholesterol esterification rate, which depends on functionally active enzyme and also on enzyme substrates, co-factors and other plasma constituents. It is involved in HDL3 → HDL2 → HDL1 conversion.

Increased Values
hypertriacylglycerolemia

Decreased Values
mild hemolytic anemia, early atherosclerosis, familial LCAT deficiency, hyperlipidemia, fish eye disease, hepatocellular diseases, corneal opacitates, renal failure

> **Interfering Factors:** medicaments – (oral contraceptives)

Analyte	Age/Gender	Reference Range	SI Units	Note
Lecithin–Cholesterol Acyltransferase		18.3–23.7	*	*nmol ³H.CE/ substr/hrs

Leptin

Leptin is a fatty tissue polypeptide hormone (167 amino acids) known as so-called ob gene product (e. g. obesity gene). It functions as a signal for food intake ending; it shows a circadian secretion rhythm.

Increased Values
glucocorticoids, **obesity**, metabolic syndrome with parallel insulin/leptin resistance

Decreased Values
type I diabetes mellitus, starvation, hypogonadism, sterility

Analyte	Age/Gender	Reference Range	SI Units	Note
Leptin	normosthenic	0.1–15	ng/ml	
	obese	5–50	ng/ml	

Leucine

(Leu) An amino acid essential for optimal infant growth and for adult nitrogen equilibrium maintenance. It is obtained by digestion or hydrolytic protein cleavage. Enzyme defect: branched ketonic acids decarboxylase.

Increased Values – hyperleucinemia
isovaleric acidemia, beta-hydroxy-isovaleric aciduria, viral hepatitis, starvation, **maple syrup urine disease** (branched-chain ketoaciduria), obesity

Decreased Values – hypoleucinemia
hepatic encephalopathy, acute hunger, hyperinsulinism, Huntington's chorea, kwashiorkor, severe burns, conditions after abdominal surgery

Interfering Factors: medicaments – (alanine, glucose, histidine, oral contraceptives)

Analyte	Age/Gender	Reference Range	SI Units	Note
Leucine	Neonates	46–109	µmol/l	
	Infants	40–150	µmol/l	
	Children	50–200	µmol/l	
	Adults	80–150	µmol/l	

Leucine Aminopeptidase and Leucine Aryl-Amidase

(LAP, LAA syn: aryl-amidase, naphthylamidase) LAP is a collective name for a exopeptidases group which occurs in high concentrations and activities in many organs.

Production. By the liver.
Function. Catalyzes protein and peptide breakdown by slow amino acids breakdown.
Occurrence. Biliary system, pancreas, small intestinal mucosa. LAP levels tend to parallel ALP levels in hepatic disease.
Test Purpose. 1) to help in hepatobiliary system diseases diagnosis and cholestasis differential diagnosis, 2) to help to differentiate between liver disease and diseases of bones and joints, 3) to detect difference between inherited blockage of bile ducts and hepatitis in newborns.

Increased Values
chronic alcohol abuse, **hepatic cirrhosis,** hepatitis – (**acute h., chronic active h.**), gallstones, **cholestasis, obstructive hepatobiliary diseases,** acute alcohol intoxication, hepatic ischemia, tumors of – (**pancreas, liver**), pancreatitis, severe preeclampsia
    Interfering Factors: pregnancy (3rd trimester), medicaments – (chlorpromazine, estrogens, hepatotoxic drugs, morphine, oral contraceptives, progesterone)

Analyte	Age/Gender	Reference Range	SI Units	Note
Leucine-Aminopeptidase	Neonates		10–50	U/l
	Adults F	10–32	U/l	
	Adults M	20–35	U/l	

Leukemia Inhibitory Factor

(LIF, syn: differentiating stimulating factor – DSF, differentiation inducing factor – DIF, differentiation inhibitory activity – DIA)
Occurrence. Stromal cells of bone marrow, fibroblasts, T-cells, monocytes, macrophages, astrocytes, endometrial cells, tumorous cells.
Function. Maintaining the pluripotent phenotype of embryonic stem cells. Promotes the IL-3 dependent hematopoietic progenitors proliferation.

Leukotrienes

Leukotrienes (LTB4, LTC4, LTD4, LTE4) are specialized fatty acids within eicosanoids, the lipooxygenase pathway end products (formed from arachidonic acid by enzyme 5-lipoxygenase initial action). Leukotrienes have histamine-like actions (vascular permeability enhancement, bronchospasm induction, mediator activities for leukocytes). LTC4, LTD4, LTE4 combined have been identified as slow-reacting substance of anaphylaxis (SRS-A). Leukotriene A4 (syn. LTA4): produced in leukocytes, monocytes, macrophages, lymphocytes, platelets, mast cells, heart and lung vascular tissue → 1) LTB4 (major source – neutrophils): increases polymorphonuclear leukocyte chemotaxis, releases lysosomal enzymes, promotes white blood cells adhesion, inhibits immunoglobulin synthesis, enhances NK-cell activity and monocyte cytokine production, 2) LTC4 → LTD4 → LTE4 (major source – mastocytes, basophils, eosinophils): smooth muscle contraction, bronchoconstriction, vasoconstriction, coronary blood flow and cardiac contractility decrease, vascular permeability increase – plasma exudation, slow-reacting substance of anaphylaxis components (SRS-A), mitogen-induced lymphocyte proliferation inhibition.

Light Chains

(syn: free light chains, L-chains) All five immunoglobulin classes contain light chains as an integral portion of the whole molecule, but there are only two L-chain types, kappa and lambda. The amino terminal portion of the heavy chains and the light chain form the antigen binding site with its enormously diverse specificity. Constant part determines division type into subclasses kappa and lambda. Light and heavy chains are synthesized in B-lymphocytes separately. Single B-cell (its clone resp.) produces one light chain type. In malignant clone turn an excessive L-chains synthesis is present, they are not connecting to H-chains → excreted as Bence Jones protein. Molecules exist as monomers/dimers produced as such by immunocytes or they exist in conjunction with intact immunoglobulins. L-chains are cleared and destroyed by the kidney.

Increased Values
amyloidosis, Waldenström's macroglobulinemia, plasmocytoma (incl. multiple myeloma)

Lipase

(LPS, syn: triacylglycerol acylhydrolase) Glycoprotein with hydrolytic activity on TAG (long-chain fatty acids cleavage).
Production. Secreted in pancreas (pancreatic acinar cells) 99% through apical pole into ductus pancreaticus and duodenum along with other pancreatic digestive enzymes. 1 % is excreted in the opposite direction through lymph into capillaries (blood to duodenal fluid concentration ratio is 1: 800). Biological half-time is 7–14 hrs.
Function. Pancreatic enzyme, splits (hydrolyzes) triacylglycerols (long chain fatty acids) to glycerol and unesterified fatty acids.
Occurrence. Pancreas, small intestine (intestinal mucosa), gastric mucosa, lingual glands, leukocytes, pulmonary mucosa, breast, vascular intima, adipose tissue adipocytes. Lipase secretion is stimulated by: glucagon, norepinephrine, epinephrine, adrenal steroids, vasopressin, thyrotropin, ACTH, luteotropin, somatotropin. Inhibited by: insulin.
Test Purpose. 1) to aid in acute pancreatitis diagnosis, 2) suspicion on pancreatic carcinoma, 3) pancreas cystic fibrosis, 4) to help find sudden abdominal accident cause, 5) to help in diagnosis of peritonitis, strangulated/infarcted bowel.

Increased Values
alcoholism, liver cirrhosis, pancreatic cyst/pseudocyst, diabetes mellitus (severe), cystic fibrosis of pancreas (mucoviscidosis), **endoscopic retrograde choledochopancreatography** (ERCP), **acute/chronic cholecystitis, gastric ulcer disease,** diseases – (biliary ways d., acute/chronic renal d.), **mesenterial infarction, renal insufficiency,** diabetic ketoacidosis, gallstone colic, intracranial bleeding, tumors – (**pancreas t.,** lymphoma, lung t.), **high intestinal obstruction,** pancreatic duct obstruction by – (**calculus, tumors**), **acute pancreatitis** (usually rise 24 to 48 hrs after the onset, remain elevated up to 14 days), chronic pancreatitis, **parotitis with pancreatic lesion, intestine perforation,** peritonitis, adipose tissue polytrauma, rachitis, transplant rejection – (kidney t. r., liver t. r., heart t. r.), ruptured tubal pregnancy, conditions after abdominal surgery, strangulated bowel, mesenterial thrombosis, tuberculosis (early), **duodenal ulcus perforating into pancreas, acute turn of chronic pancreatitis, perforated peptic ulcer,** hyperlipidemias (types I, IV), post-cholecystectomy, **acute/chronic renal failure,** bone fracture, crush injury, fat embolism

Interfering Factors: medicaments – (bethanechol, cholinergics, codeine, heparin, indomethacin, meperidine, methacholine, methylprednisolone, morphine, narcotics, secretin, sulindac)

Decreased Values
atherosclerosis, pancreatic parenchyma atrophy, diabetes mellitus, cystic fibrosis, essential hyperlipidemia, chronic intrahepatic cholestasis, insufficiency of pancreas, cachexia
Interfering Factors: medicaments – (calcium ions, EDTA, protamine, quinine)

Analyte	Age/Gender	Reference Range	SI Units	Note
Lipase		<3.17	µkat/l	
		<2.67	µkat/l	See ref.
		7.7–56	U/l	ranges note

Lipid Associated Sialic Acid

(LASA) Lipid-associated sialic acid is considered a tumor marker that lacks the specificity and sensitivity needed for routine cancer detection and diagnosis. Sialic acid is a name for a group of compounds derived from or related to N-acetylneuraminic acid. Sialic acids are found in glycoproteins, gangliosides and glycolipids. Sialic acids on cell membranes facilitate the binding of biologically active molecules and mediate a number of cellular interactions (antigenicity, adhesion, recognition). LASA is a complex marker that measures the amount of sialic acid including sialic acid from gangliosides that are bound to serum proteins and sialic acid contained in circulating glycoproteins (e. g. acute phase reactants). Malignant cells often exhibit aberrant sialylation, which has been implicated in the loss of contact inhibition and the metastatic potential of these cells. Increased levels of sialic acid reflect the release and accumulation of sialyl compounds from malignant cells.
Test Purpose. 1) in conjunction with other tumor markers LASA may be useful in managing selected cancer patients, 2) monitoring tumor therapy in connection with other tumor markers.

Increased Values
tumors – (breast t., **melanoma**, **colorectum t.**, gastrointestinal tract t., **ovarian t.**, **pulmonary t.**, **leukemia**, **Hodgkin's lymphoma**, **lymphoma**, **sarcoma**), diseases – (inflammatory d.), tissue necrosis

Lipids

(syn: total lipids) Lipids are heterogenous fat and fatlike water-insoluble substance compounds. The body stored lipids serve as a fuel source, are an important cell structure constituent, and serve other biological functions. Lipids include fatty acids, neutral fats, waxes and steroids. Compound lipids are glycolipids, lipoproteins and phospholipids.

Increased Values – hyperlipidemia
amyloidosis, alcoholism, anesthesia, anemia, liver cirrhosis, **diabetes mellitus**, chronic glomerulonephritis, hemodialysis, acute hepatitis, **essential hyperlipidemia**, **hypothyroidism**, **obstructive icterus**, poisoning by – (phosphorus, chloroform, cobalt, tetrachlormeth-

ane), leukemia, **lipoidosis**, nephritis, nephrosclerosis, nephrosis, nephrotic sy, pancreatic ducts obstruction, food fat intake, pregnancy (gravidity), renal transplantation, tuberculosis (severe), uremia

  Interfering Factors: coffee, medicaments – (amprenavir, beta-blockers, bexarotene, cyclosporine, diuretics, enoxaparin, estrogens, goserelin, indinavir, levobetaxolol, miconazole, moxifloxacin, nelfinavir, ritonavir, saquinavir, sirolimus, steroids, tamoxifen)

Decreased Values – hypolipidemia
coeliac disease, lipoprotein synthesis defect, pancreatic cystic fibrosis, **hyperthyroidism**, autoimmune diseases, catabolism, malabsorption, niacin

---

Lipoprotein (a)

(Lp [a]) Lipoprotein related to LDL class. Lp(a) is a protein attached to Apo B-100 by disulfide bond, also bound to Apo A. Lp(a) synthesis occurs in the liver, where it appears attached to Apo B. Lp(a) is strongly associated with the atherosclerotic process (independent risk factor for coronary artery disease and cerebral infarction). Plasma concentrations are genetically determined. Race dependent differences in Lp(a) concentrations are known.
Test Purpose. 1) early atherosclerotic risk recognition, 2) early ischemic heart disease symptoms without hypercholesterolemia, 3) differential diagnosis of high HDL-C levels, 4) isolated extracranial a. carotis sclerosis in young people (mainly in non-smokers), 5) genetic family examination.

Increased Values
atherosclerosis, ischemic heart disease

Analyte	Age/Gender	Reference Range	SI Units	Note
Lipoprotein (a) [Lp (a)]		<0.28	g/l	

Lipoprotein X

(LP-X) Lipoprotein X differs physicochemically/immunologically from other lipoproteins. Electrophoretically migrates with beta-fraction (LDL). Abnormal LDL lipoprotein in cholestasis patients. It differs from LDL, because it does not react to statins administration. Increased GMT activity is always connected with LP-X. Composition: 65% phospholipids, 20% free cholesterol, 7% proteins (apolipoprotein X).
Test Purpose. 1) to help in the diagnosis/differential diagnosis of jaundice, 2) to assess cholestasis (without differentiating intra/extrahepatic cholestases).

Increased Values
cirrhosis – (primary biliary c., hepatic c.), LCAT deficiency, hepatitis – (acute h., chronic h., h. with cholestasis), pregnancy cholestasis, obstruction – (extrahepatic o., intrahepatic o.)

Analyte	Age/Gender	Reference Range	SI Units	Note
Lipoprotein X		<30	mg/l	

Lipoprotein Lipase

(LP lipase) Hydrolase class enzyme that catalyzes hydrolytic fatty acyl group cleavage from triacyl-glycerols in chylomicrons, VLDL lipoproteins and LDL lipoproteins. It occurs on capillary endothelial surfaces, especially in mammary, muscle and adipose tissue, requires apolipoprotein C-II as a co-factor.

Increased Values
hemolysis, diets high in carbohydrates and polyunsaturated fats
   Interfering Factors: medicaments – (clofibrate, nicotinic acid)

Decreased Values
alcoholism, untreated diabetes mellitus, primary hyperchylomicronemia (type I lipoproteinemia), endogenic hypertriacylglycerolemia associated with obesity, hypothyroidism, pancreatitis, renal failure
   Interfering Factors: medicaments – (steroids)

Lithium

(Li) Lithium half-life is 8–20 hours, may be prolonged in renal failure.
Test Purpose. To monitor lithium therapy.

Increased Values
lithium therapy overdose, sodium depletion
   Interfering Factors: medicaments – (diuretics)

Analyte	Age/Gender	Reference Range	SI Units	Note
Lithium		0.3–1.3	mmol/l	

Long-Acting Thyroid Stimulator

(LATS, syn: 7S gamma globulin, thyroid stimulatory immunoglobulin – TSI, thyroid-stimulating immunoglobulin, thyroid stimulatory antibodies – TSA)
Production. Polyclonal autoantibodies, created in thyroid lymphocytes and directed against the thyroid-cell plasma membrane.
Function. LATS mimics thyroid-stimulating hormone action having more prolonged effects. LATS stimulates the thyroid gland to produce and secrete excess thyroid hormones. This factor inhibits TSH secretion through the normal negative feedback mechanism.
Test Purpose. 1) to confirm Graves' disease diagnosis, 2) to aid in suspected thyroid disease evaluation, 3) to aid in suspected thyrotoxicosis diagnosis, especially in patients with exophthalmos, 4) to monitor thyrotoxicosis treatment.

Increased Values
exophthalmos, Graves' disease, relapse of hyperthyroidism, thyroiditis acuta, thyrotoxicosis

Low-Molecular Weight B-Cell Growth Factor

(LMW-BCGF)
Occurrence. T-cells.
Function. Stimulates growth of activated B-cells and B-cell lines.

Lupus Inhibitor

(syn: lupus anticoagulant, circulating anticoagulant – CAC) Belongs to antiphospholipid auto-antibody. The lupus inhibitor is an immunoglobulin (IgA, IgG, IgM) which can interfere with phospholipid-dependent coagulation reactions without inhibiting the activity of any specific coagulation factor. It is a circulating anticoagulant that inhibits prothrombin to thrombin conversion.
Test Purpose. 1) to investigate prolonged APTT not corrected by normal plasma, 2) to aid in diagnosis of systemic lupus erythematosus, 3) to investigate unexplained recurrent fetal loss, 4) to aid in diagnosis of vascular thrombosis.

Increased Values – positive
rheumatoid arthritis, dysproteinemias, diseases – (autoimmune d., gynecologic d., neurologic d., viral infectious d.), ulcerative colitis, postpartum complications, **systemic lupus erythematosus,** healthy people, tumors, fetal loss, multiple transfused patients, plasmocytoma (incl. multiple myeloma), drug reactions
   Interfering Factors: medicaments – (chlorpromazine)

Luteinizing Hormone

(LH, syn: lutropin, interstitial cells stimulating hormone – ICSH, gonadotropin-2) The hormone consists of an alpha chain that is identical with FSH, thyrotropin or chorionic gonadotropin, and a beta chain that is hormone-specific.
Production. Anterior pituitary (adenohypophysis) hormone, gonadotropin, glycoprotein.
Function. Stimulates the progesterone production by corpus luteum cells, testosterone by the Leydig's cells, ovulation, and corpus luteum formation. Induces estrogen release. Secretion is stimulated by norepinephrine, acetylcholine, gamma-aminobutyric acid and inhibited by serotonin, dopamine, and endorphins. Apart from its documented physiological role LH appears to be involved also in immune functions thus establishing it as one component of the neuroimmune network. LH has been shown to be produced also by lymphocytes. LH is secreted by human thymocytes and appears to act as a co-mitogen in lymphoproliferation in an autocrine fashion. Released in episodic spikes during day, there is 30 % variation day to day. Values are highest in early sleep, lowest in late afternoon, highest in summer, and lowest in winter. In women sharp spike appears before ovulation.
Hypothalamic Hormone. 1) gonadotrophin-releasing hormone (GRH) = gonadoliberin and luteinizing hormone-releasing hormone (LH-RH) → increases LH release, 2) follistatin and dopamine → inhibit FSH, LH release.
Test Purpose. 1) to detect ovulation, 2) to assess male or female infertility, 3) to evaluate amenorrhea, 4) to monitor therapy designed to induce ovulation, 5) hypogonadism differential diagnosis mainly in male, 6) differential diagnosis of pubertas tarda and hypogonadotropic eunuchoidism, 7) in so-called global test with hypophyseous hormones, to assess presence of hypopituritarism, 8) to evaluate the normalcy of hypothalamic-pituitary-gonadal axis.

Increased Values

pituitary adenoma, acromegaly (early stage), anorchia, destruction of testes, **primary gonadal dysfunction,** hyperthyroidism, **hypogonadism,** liver diseases, **menopause,** obesity, orchiectomy, **precocious puberty,** psychic stress, syndrome – (**Klinefelter's sy, Stein-Leventhal sy,** complete testicular feminization sy, Turner's sy), failure – (**gonadal f.,** renal f.)

    Interfering Factors: medicaments – (antiepileptics, clomiphene, cyclophosphamide, ethanol, ketoconazole, naloxone, propranolol in men)

Decreased Values

amenorrhea, anorexia nervosa, isolated LH deficiency, diabetes mellitus, secondary gonadal dysfunction (male), eosinophilic granuloma, hemochromatosis, starvation, hypogonadotropism, severe illnesses, pituitary infarction, radiation therapy, malnutrition, metastases of malignant tumors, tumors – (germinoma, gliomas, hamartroma, craniopharyngioma, meningioma, pinealoma), obesity, sarcoidosis, severe stress, syphilis, shock, tuberculosis, trauma, failure – (**pituitary f., hypothalamic f.**)

    Interfering Factors: heavy exercise, high altitude, medicaments – (anabolic steroids, androgens, digitalis, digoxin, estrogens, oral contraceptives, phenobarbital, phenothiazines, progesterone, propranolol, stanozolol, testosterone)

Analyte	Age/Gender	Reference Range	SI Units	Note
Luteinizing Hormone (LH)	< 10 y	0.5–1.0	IU/l	
	F			
	Follicular phase	0.5–18	IU/l	
	Mid-cycle	15–80	IU/l	
	Luteal phase	0.5–18	IU/l	
	Postmenopause	18–64	IU/l	
	M	0.5–10	IU/l	

Lymphocytotoxic Antibodies

(LCA, LCAb) Component of the cross match procedure in organ transplantation.

Increased Values

rejection of renal transplant

Lysine

(Lys) Lysine is an essential dibasic amino acid needed for optimal infant growth (growth and differentiation) and for adult nitrogen equilibrium maintenance. Highest lysine need is after birth and during puberty. Lysine degradation goes through saccharopine, which is quickly degraded. Enzyme defect: lysine ketoglutarate reductase and pipekolate oxidase.

Test Purpose. 1) mental retardation differential diagnosis, 2) neuromuscular disorders differential diagnosis.

Increased Values – hyperlysinemia

hyperlysinemia type I (specific enzyme defect), hyperlysinemia type II (transport disorder), congenital lysine intolerance, saccharopinuria

Decreased Values – hypolysinemia
conditions after abdominal surgery, carcinoid sy

Analyte	Age/Gender	Reference Range	SI Units	Note
Lysine		100–250	µmol/l	

Lysozyme

(syn: muramidase) Highly basic, carbohydrate free, low-molecular-weight protein with enzyme effect.
Production. Synthesized by macrophages, neutrophils, monocytes.
Occurrence. Lysosomes, serum, urine, saliva, sputum, tears, lung, kidney (tubular cells), blood cells.
Function. Catalyses cell wall destruction (by disrupting N-acetylglucosamine) of certain bacteria = bacteriolysis. External secretions, containing very high lysozyme levels, which act as a first defense line against bacterial pathogens. Proximal renal tubulus impairment indicator.
Test Purpose. 1) tubular dysfunction indicator, 2) graft-rejection reaction, 3) leukemia diagnosis and monitoring, 4) differential diagnosis of bacterial and viral meningitides, 5) neonatal sepsis, 6) intrauterine infections.

Increased Values
diseases – (chronic infectious d., kidney d.), heavy metals intoxication, leukemia – (**monocyte l.**, chronic myeloid l., **myelomonocyte l.**), polycythemia vera, pyelonephritis, renal graft rejection, sarcoidosis, tuberculosis
   Interfering Factors: medicaments – (nephrotoxic antibiotics – aminoglycozides)

Decreased Values
heparin, bone marrow hypoplasia, immunosuppressive therapy after transplant rejection, leukemia – (granulocytic l., lymphocytic l.)

Analyte	Age/Gender	Reference Range	SI Units	Note
Lysozyme		2–9	mg/l	

Alpha-2-Macroglobulin

(Alpha-2 M, A2MG)
Function. Glycoprotein binding hormones. Represents about 1/3 of alpha-2-globulin fraction. Plasmin/protease inhibitor. It is a broad-spectrum, stoichiometric inhibitor of nearly all enzymes that split proteins internally (endoproteases). In 22 % influences ESR. Irreversibly inactivates trypsin, plasmin, kallikrein, chymotrypsin, pepsin, granulocyte elastase, collagenase, cathepsin, thrombin, factor Xa, thrombin. Alpha-2-macroglobulin appears to be important physiologically in clotting control, clot lysis, complement cascades, as well as in collagenase control from leukocytes, lysosomal cathepsin, pancreatic trypsin and chymotrypsin. It combines rapidly with activated proteases, acting initially as a substrate, then sterically "enfolding" them and blocking further proteolytic activity toward proteins and other large peptides. A2M-protease complexes are then rapidly removed from circulation by the liver Kupffer's cells. Alveolar macrophages have destroy similar complexes. The interactions between A2MG and cytokines are thought to modulate the expression of acute phase proteins in liver hepatocytes. A2MG inhibits the growth of several tumors in vitro.

Test Purpose. Increased protease release condition diagnosis.

Increased Values

rheumatoid arthritis, liver cirrhosis, exercise, alpha-1-antitrypsin deficiency, **diabetes mellitus, emphysema,** chronic hepatitis, acute inflammatory diseases, cerebral infarction, lupus erythematosus systemicus, tumors, nephrosis, **plasmocytoma** (incl. multiple myeloma), **hepatic parenchyma lesions,** syndrome – (Down sy, **nephrotic sy**), **pregnancy** (gravidity, graviditas).

   Interfering Factors: medicaments – (estrogens, mestranol, oral contraceptives).

Decreased Values

arthritis – (rheumatoid a., juvenile rheumatoid a.), fibrinolysis, gastroenteritis, peptic ulcer disease, disseminated intravascular coagulation (DIC), extracorporeal circulation, **acute pancreatitis,** plasmocytoma, preeclampsia, sepsis, terminal stages of critically ill liver failure patients.

   Interfering Factors: 30 to 50-year old males, medicaments – (dextran, fibrinolytics, streptokinase).

Analyte	Age/Gender	Reference Range	SI Units	Note
Alpha-2-Macroglobulin	F	1.30–3.0	g/l	
	M	1.10–2.5	g/l	

Macrophage Inflammatory Protein

(MIP-1-alfa, MIP-1-beta)
- **Macrophage inflammatory protein 1-alpha.**
  Occurrence. T-cells, B-cells, monocytes, mastocytes, fibroblasts.
  Function. Chemoattracts monocytes, T-cells and eosinophils. Inhibits early hematopoietic stem cell proliferation.
- **Macrophage inflammatory protein 1-beta.**
  Occurrence. T-cells, B-cells, monocytes, mastocytes, fibroblasts.
  Function. Chemoattracts monocytes and T-cells. Induces T-cells adhesion via beta-1 integrins to endothelial cells.

Magnesium

(Mg) Primary intracellular electrolyte. In serum, one-third is protein bound, about 20% is complexed to phosphate (ATP), citrate/other compounds, and the remainder is free. This electrolyte is critical in nearly all metabolic processes. The kidney is the major organ that controlls Mg concentration in serum.
Function. In extracellular space, affects neuromuscular irritability, response, permeability characteristics. Co-factor for carbohydrate metabolism enzymes (glycolysis), protein/nucleic acid synthesis (cell replication, nucleotide metabolism), oxidative phosphorylation, cell respiration. Mg is involved in cation transport i. e. Ca, Na. Mg^{2+} inhibits neurotransmitter release (competes with Ca^{2+}), stabilizes nerve axons. Mg maintains a low resting intracellular Ca ions concentration, it competes with Ca^{2+} for membrane binding sites, and stimulates Ca sequestration by the sarcoplasmic reticulum, a necessary prerequisite for the calcium "trigger function" in several cellular processes. Magnesium stabilizes cellular membranes by producing lipid complexes. Influences cardiovascular system function by cardiomyocyte ion transport system regulation as well as vascular smooth musculature tonus and reactivity.

Important for adenosine triphosphate (ATP) use as energy source and in clotting mechanisms (Ca^{2+} antagonist). Mg has intimate relationship to Ca and K; therefore, reduction in ion creates a comparable reduction in the others. About 50–60% of body Mg is in bones, skeletal muscles (20%), other cells (19%), extracellular fluid (1%). Highest values are in winter, lowest are in summer. In women decreased with menses. Changes inversely with plasma glucose. Day-to-day values variation is 5%.

Test Purpose. 1) to evaluate electrolyte status, 2) to assess neuromuscular or renal function, 3) cardiac dysrhythmias, 4) differential diagnosis of ECG changes (QT interval prolongation), 5) acute myocardial infarction diagnosis and monitoring, 6) prolonged diuretic therapy and potential nephrotoxic medicament monitoring, 7) alcoholism assessment, 8) renal diseases assessment, 9) parenteral nutrition monitoring. Magnesium value increases with intracellular determination.

Increased Values – hypermagnesemia

acidosis, adrenalectomy, **diabetic acidosis before treatment, dehydration,** diabetes mellitus (in elder), accidental ingestion of large amount of sea water, dialysis, eclampsia, hyperpituitarism, hypokalemia, **hypothyroidism, renal insufficiency,** lithium intoxication, catabolism, diabetic coma, systemic lupus erythematosus, **Addison's disease,** menstruation, necrosis – (extensive cellular n., acute tissue n.), **oliguria, plasmocytoma, muscular polytrauma,** toxic cellular injury, increased magnesium intake – **(parenteral, oral),** rhabdomyolysis, **uremia,** failure – **(renal f.,** acute hepatic f.).

> **Interfering Factors:** hemolysis, enemas containing magnesium, medicaments – (acetylsalicylic acid – prolonged therapy, aminoglycoside antibiotics, antacids with magnesium, calcium-containing medications, diuretics, estrogens, ethacrynic acid, laxatives, lithium, magnesium salts, progesterone, salicylate, thiazides, thyroid medications, triamterene).

Decreased Values – hypomagnesemia

acidosis – **(diabetic a.,** metabolic a., **renal tubular a.), chronic alcoholism,** atherosclerosis, jejuno-ilial bypass, **hepatic cirrhosis,** phosphate depletion, disease – (celiac d., **Crohn's d.,** Paget's d.), decreased absorption, neonatal gut immaturity, diabetes mellitus, osmotic diuresis, postobstructive diuresis, postoperative drains, postoperative electrolyte dysbalance, epilepsy, **gastrointestinal fistulas, glomerulonephritis,** hemodialysis, chronic hepatitis, **starvation, acute/chronic diarrhea,** osteolytic processes healing, **hyperaldosteronism,** hyperglycemia, **hypercalcemia, primary hyperparathyroidism, pregnancy induced hypertension, hyperthyroidism,** primary neonatal hypomagnesemia, **hypoparathyroidism, chronic renal diseases,** insufficiency – (renal i., hepatic i.), cardiomyopathies, **ulcerative colitis, kwashiorkor, excessive lactation, prolonged parenteral therapy, malnutrition, tumors,** newborns – (physiologically, n. of diabetic mothers, exchange transfusion in n.), interstitial nephritis, postobstructive nephropathy, **acute tubular necrosis** (diuretic phase), **prolonged nasogas-tric suction** (gastric probes), **acute/chronic pancreatitis, plasmocytoma** (incl. multiple myeloma), porphyria, **burns, decreased magnesium intake,** excessive sweating, puncture of – (ascites, hydrothorax), **chronic pyelonephritis, extensive small gut resection,** celiac sprue, postrenal transplantation conditions, loss – (excessive renal l. of magnesium, l. of enteric fluids), idiopathic renal wasting, multiple transfusions with citrated blood, syndrome – **(malabsorption sy,** SIADH), cardiosurgery procedures, **renal failure,** abdominal irradiation, villous adenoma, acute alcoholism, hypothermia, septic conditions.

> **Interfering Factors:** extreme physical exertion, pregnancy, medicaments – (aldesleukin, aminoglycosides, amphotericin B, antibiotics, atenolol, benazepril, bisoprolol, calcium gluconate, calcium salts, capreomycin, captopril, carbenicillin, carboplatin, chlor-

talidone, cimetidine, cisplatin, cyclosporine, digitalis, digoxin, diuretics, enalapril, ethacrynic acid, ethanol, fosinopril, furosemide, gemtuzumab, gentamicin, glucagon, glucose, hydrochlorothiazide, insulin, irbesartan, laxatives, mannitol, mercurial diuretics, metolazone, neomycin, oral contraceptives, pamidronate, pentamidine, phenytoin, plicamycin, rimiterol, salbutamol, thiazides, ticarcillin, tobramycin, triamterene, urea).

Analyte	Age/Gender	Reference Range	SI Units	Note
Magnesium	Neonates	0.83–1.11	mmol/l	
	Children	0.87–1.07	mmol/l	
	Adults	0.79–1.09	mmol/l	

Malate Dehydrogenase

(MDH, MD) MD (NAD$^+$) is an oxidoreductase class enzyme catalyzing L-malate to oxaloacetate oxidation, reducing NAD$^+$. Enzyme occurs both in the mitochondria/cytosol. The reaction is important in the tricarboxylic acid cycle and malate-aspartate electron shift. MD (NADP$^+$) is an oxidoreductase class enzyme that catalyzes oxidative L-malate decarboxylation to form pyruvate, reducing NADP$^+$. Cytosolic and mitochondrial forms are isozymes. The cytosolic enzyme is a major NADPH source for fatty acid synthesis.

Increased Values
anemia – (sickle cell a., megaloblastic a.), diseases – (acute hepatic d., skeletal muscle d.), myocardial infarct, tumors, hemolytic conditions, trauma

Analyte	Age/Gender	Reference Range	SI Units	Note
Malate Dehydrogenase	Neonates	1.6–4.0	µkat/l	
	Children	1.0–2.32	µkat/l	
	Adults	0.83–1.73	µkat/l	

Malone Dialdehyde

(MDA) One of dominant lipoperoxid metabolism products (polyunsaturated carboxylic acids oxidative product) in increased free oxygen radicals production.

Increased Values
diabetes mellitus, chronic cerebrovascular diseases, acute myocardial infarction (increase 24–48 hrs, decrease up to 12 d), leukemia – (acute lymphocytic l., acute myeloid l.), Parkinson's disease, acute pancreatitis, preeclampsia, **stress**, pregnancy, uremia, procedures – (revascularization p., cardiosurgery p.).

Decreased Values
hemodialysis patients

Analyte	Age/Gender	Reference Range	SI Units	Note
Malone Dialdehyde		<6.5	µmol/l	

Mammary-Derived Growth Inhibitor

(MDGI) MDGI is a polypeptide isolated from mammary gland epithelial cells belonging to cytokines and involved in cell proliferation inhibition during lactation. It has an inhibitory effect to malignant breast carcinoma cells.

Manganese

(Mn) An ubiquitous element with eleven oxidation states. Manganese's major use is in the production steels. It is also used in the production of non-ferrous alloys, dry cell batteries, fertilisers, dyes, catalysts, wood preservatives, glass and ceramics, chemical industry, lead-free gasoline. Organic manganese containing compounds are used as an anti-knock petrol additives and fungicides. Workplace exposure to manganese fume and dusts may occur during mining and processing of the ore. Exposure of the general population to manganese from air, water and food sources is very low. Mn is trace essential metal element bound to protein. Absorbed manganese entering the portal blood may be rapidly bound to alpha-2-macroglobulin or remains free before rapid transport (bound to transferrin) to the liver → where it is almost completely removed to bile. There is extensive enterohepatic circulation of manganese. The liver therefore has relatively high manganese content.

Function. Mn is enzyme co-factor (glycosyl transferases, alkaline phosphatase, arginase, cholesterol biosynthesis enzymes, hydrolases, kininases, superoxide dismutase). Manganese is associated mainly with connective and bony tissue formation, growth and reproductive functions, carbohydrates and lipid metabolism. Manganese toxicity may result from manganese dust or fume inhalation (steel and dry cell battery industries), or from contaminated water ingestion. Chronic manganese poisoning has occurred in miners, foundry workers, welders, workers manufacturing drugs, ceramic, glass, varnish and food additives.

Occurrence. Mitochondria of bone, liver, pancreas.

Test Purpose. 1) manganese intoxication suspicion, 2) to follow manganese concentrations in parenteral nutrition, 3) to detect manganese deficiency (e. g. increased nutritional requirements, pregnancy, alcohol abuse, chronic severe diseases).

Increased Values – hypermanganesemia
rheumatoid arthritis, phenylketonuria, **acute hepatitis**, maple syrup urine disease, hepatobiliary diseases, **myocardial infarction**, **chronic manganese poisoning** (professional, occupational – industrial exposure), mineral supplements, pregnancy.
   Interfering Factors: water

Decreased Values – hypomanganesemia
dialysis, epilepsy, phenylketonuria, sexual function disorders, seizure states, increased nutritional requirements, pregnancy, breast feeding, alcohol abuse, drugs abuse, chronic severe diseases, excessive stress conditions, postsurgery conditions, gastrectomy, severe burns, severe injuries.
   Interfering Factors: medicaments – (estrogens, oral contraceptives)

Analyte	Age/Gender	Reference Range	SI Units	Note
Manganese				
whole blood		115–119	nmol/l	
serum		8–14	nmol/l	

Matrix Metalloproteinases

(MMPs) Enzymes, known collectivelly also as matrixins, are zinc-dependent endopeptidases that function extracellularly at neutral pH and mediate the degradation of extracellular matrix components. For full activity these enzymes also require extrinsic calcium ions. These proteases constitute a large and growing family of proteins which are highly related in terms of structure and enzymatic properties (MMP-1, MMP-2, MMP-3, MMP-7, MMP-8, MMP-9, MMP-10, MMP-11, MMP-12, MMP-13, MMP-14, MMP-15, MMP-16, MMP-17, MMP-18, MMP-19, MMP-20, MMP-21, MMP-22, MMP-23). Some MMPs have been found to exist also as membrane-bound proteins (MMP-14, MMP-15, MMP-16, MMP-17). Their location at the surface of cells implies that these enzymes could play a role in the modulation of cell-matrix interactions. MMPs are usually not expressed constitutively. The expression of MMP genes can be modified by a variety of physiological and pharmacological signals, including cytokines and growth factors, bacterial endotoxins and hormones. All MMPs are synthesized as fairly large preproenzymes. Most of them are secreted from the cells as proenzymes (promatrixins). They require activation before becoming fully active and this involves regulated proteolysis causing the loss of the propeptide. The regulatory propeptide sequence contains a free cysteine residue which has the ability of binding to zinc. This interaction maintains latency of the enzymes, which become active once the propeptide is removed from the catalytic domain of the protein. MMP activation can be achieved by autoactivation and by a variety of other proteases, including furin, urokinase, plasmin, and various other members of the MMP family. The activation of these proenzymes is one of the critical steps that leads to extracellular matrix breakdown. MMPs have been linked with a wide array of biological activities and play important roles during organ development and pathological processes. Collectively MMPs are key enzymes for the metabolism of extracellular matrix proteins, including fibrillar and non-fibrillar collagens, fibronectin, laminin and basement membrane or interstitial stroma glycoproteins. Due to their activities these enzymes are considered to be important therapeutic targets for the treatment of various diseases where tissue degradation is part of the pathology, such as cancer and arthritis. Under physiological conditions MMPs are involved in extracellular degradation and breakdown of matrix proteins during normal tissue remodelling processes such as wound healing, pregnancy and angiogenesis. MMPs are believed to facilitate cellular migration across basement membranes. The release of these enzymes by various cell types has been implicated in the pathogenesis of many dis-eases and diverse invasive processes, including tissue destruction during inflammatory reactions, and diseases such as arthritis, periodontitis, glomerulonephritis, atherosclerosis, tissue ulceration, cancer and multiple sclerosis. Cytokines, growth factors and hormones have been found to regulate expression of MMPs and their inhibitors.

- **matrix metalloproteinase-1 (MMP-1, previously collagenase-1, interstitial collagenase)** initiates cleavage of interstitial type I, type II and type III collagens. Also cleaves collagens of types VII and X. Requires calcium and zinc as cofactors for activity. Can be activated without removal of the activation peptide. Belongs to peptidase family M10a, also known as matrixin subfamily.

- **matrix metalloproteinase-2 (MMP-2, previously type IV collagenase, gelatinase A, TBE-1)** cleaves type IV collagen, the main structural component of basal membrane. It cleaves also collagen types V, VII, X. Requires calcium and zinc as cofactors for activity. MMP-2 is produced by normal skin fibroblasts.

- **matrix metalloproteinase-3 (MMP-3, previously stromelysin-1, transin-1, SL-1)** has the wide substrate specificity. It degrades proteoglycans, laminin, fibronectin and gelatins of type I, III, IV, V, collagens type III, IV, X, IX, cartilage proteoglycans. Activates procollagenase. Requires calcium and zinc as cofactors for activity. MMP-3 is secreted by connective tissue cells.

- **matrix metalloproteinase-7 (MMP-7, previously matrilysin, uterine metalloproteinase, matrin)** degrades casein, gelatins of type I, III, IV, V, fibronectin. Activates procollagenase. Requires calcium and zinc as cofactors for activity. Released from stores – secretory epithelial cells of skin, gastrointestinal and respiratory systems.

- **matrix metalloproteinase-8 (MMP-8, previously neutrophil collagenase)** can degrade fibrillar type I, II, III collagens. It cleaves interstitial collagens in the triple helical domain. Requires calcium and zinc as cofactors for activity. Cannot be activated without removal of the activation peptide. It is stored in intracellular granules (neutrophils, eosinophils). Tissue specificity – neutrophils.

- **matrix metalloproteinase-9 (MMP-9, previously gelatinase B, gelB)** could play a role in bone osteoclastic resorption. It cleaves gelatin type I, V and collagen type IV and V. Requires calcium and zinc as cofactors for activity. It is stored in intracellular granules (neutrophils, eosinophils). Tissue specificity – produced by normal alveolar macrophages and granulocytes.

- **matrix metalloproteinase-10 (MMP-10, previously stromelysin-2, transin-2, SL-2)** can degrade fibronectin, gelatins of type I, III, IV and V, weakly collagens III, IV and V. Activates procollagenase. Catalytic activity is similar to stromelysin 1, but action on collagen type III, IV, V is weak. Requires calcium and zinc as cofactors for activity.

- **matrix metalloproteinase-11 (MMP-11, previously stromelysin-3, ST3, SL-3)** may play an important role role in the progression of epithelial malignancies. Requires calcium and zinc as cofactors for activity. Tissue specificity – specifically expressed in stromal cells of breast carcinomas.

- **matrix metalloproteinase-12 (MMP-12, previously macrophage metalloelastase)** may be involved in tissue injury and remodelling. MMP-12 has significant elastolytic activity and catalytic activity (hydrolysis of soluble and insoluble elastin). Requires calcium and zinc as cofactors for activity. Tissue specificity – fond in alveolar macrophages but not in peripheral blood monocytes. MMP-12 is induced by exposure to lipopolysaccharide, inhibited by dexamethasone.

- **matrix metalloproteinase-13 (MMP-13, previously collagenase-3)**, has wide substrate specificity, degrading collagen type-1, type-2, type-3 and type-4. MMP-13 also cleaves gelatin and cartilage aggrecan. MMP-13 is inhibited by the tissue inhibitors of metalloproteinases (TIMP-1, TIMP-2, TIMP-3). MMP-13 is expressed by stromal cells in breast carcinomas and produced at significant levels during fetal ossification and in arthritic processes. Expression of MMP-13 in osteoarthritic cartilage and its activity against type II collagen indicates that enzyme plays a significant role in cartilage collagen degradation. MMP-13 is expressed selectively in rheumatoid arthritis synovial fluid.

- **matrix metalloproteinase-14 (MMP-14)**, exists in a membrane-bound rather than a secreted form. MMP-14 seems to specifically activate of pro-gelatinase A. May thus trigger invasion by tumor cells by activating pro-gelatinase A on the tumor cell surface. Requires calcium and zinc as cofactors for activity. MMP-14 is expressed on fibroblasts activated by concanavalin A and also in osteoclasts. MMP-14 is expressed in trophoblastic cells in the decidual membrane and may have general importance in the tissue organization of the early human placenta. Also has been found to be expressed on cancer cell membranes and probably plays an important role in tumor invasion and angiogenesis. It is most often overexpressed in malignant tumor tissues, including lung and stomach carcinomas. TIMP-2 is a naturally occurring inhibitor of MMP-14. Tissue specificity – stromal cells of colon, breast, head and neck.

- **matrix metalloproteinase-15 (MMP-15, membrane-type matrix metalloproteinase 2, MT-MMP-2, SMCP-2)** has been shown to activate the zymogen of another endoproteinase, MMP-2. MMP-15 is an endopeptidase that degrades various components of the extracellular matrix. May activate pro-gelatinase A. Requires calcium and zinc as cofactors for activity. Tissue specificity – appeared to be synthesized preferentially in liver, placenta, colon and intestine. Substantial amounts are also detected in pancreas, lung, heart and skeletal muscle. Also has been shown to play a key role in tumor invasion and metastasis by being predominantly responsible for activation of the inactive zymogen pro-form of MMP-2. MMP-13 is expressed selectively in rheumatoid arthritis synovial fluid.

- **matrix metalloproteinase-16 (MMP-16, membrane-type matrix metalloproteinase 3, MT-MMP-3, MMP-X2)** is an endopeptidase that degrades various components of the extracellular matrix, such as collagen type III and fibronectin. Activates pro-gelatinase A. Involved in the matrix remodeling of blood vessels. The short isoform cleaves fibronectin and also collagen type III, but at lower rate. Requires calcium and zinc as cofactors for activity. Tissue specifictiy – MMP-16 is expressed in human brain tissues (microglial cells), heart, placenta, ovary and small intestine. The short isoform is found in the ovary. Present also in fetal tissues, especially in brain. Expression seems to decline with advanced development.

- **matrix metalloproteinase-17 (MMP-17)** is expressed mainly in human brain, leukocytes, the colon, the ovary and the testis. It has been found to be expressed in all breast carcinomas.

- **matrix metalloproteinase-18 (MMP-18)**. Its mRNA is expressed in a wide variety of normal human tissues, including mammary gland, placenta, lung, pancreas, ovary, small intestine, spleen, thymus, prostate, testis, colon and heart.

- **matrix metalloproteinase-19 (MMP-19)** has been detected on the surface of activated peripheral blood mononuclear cells, Th-1 lymphocytes. Expression was detected in placenta, lung, pancreas, ovary, small intestine, spleen, thymus and prostate. Autoantibodies directed against MMP-19 have been found in patients with rheumatoid arthritis and in patients with systemic lupus erythematosus.

- **matrix metalloproteinase-20 (MMP-20 previously enamelysin)** is expressed in the ameloblasts of the enamel organ and the odontoblasts of the dental papilla. The formation of dental enamel involves the cleavage and removal of most of the protein components of the extracellular enamel matrix, on which amelogenin is the major protein. These proteins are replaced by mineral ions, calcium and phosphorus, leading to a fully mineralized mature tissue. MMP-20 can play a central role in tooth enamel formation.

- **matrix metalloproteinase-21 (MMP-21)** does not contain a highly conserved cysteine residue in the proenzyme domain, shown to be involved in the autocatalytic activation of many metalloproteinases.

- **matrix metalloproteinase-22 (MMP-22)** does not contain a highly conserved cysteine residue in the proenzyme domain, shown to be involved in the autocatalytic activation of many metalloproteinases.

- **matrix metalloproteinase-23A and B (MMP-23A, MMP-23B)** is expressed predominantly in ovary, testis, heart, pancreas and prostate.

- **matrix metalloproteinase-24 (MMP-24, MT5-MMP)** is expressed in a variety of brain tumors (astrocytomas, glioblastomas, mixed gliomas, oligodendrogliomas, ependymomas, meningiomas).

- **matrix metalloproteinase-26 (MMP-26)** is expressed in placenta, uterus, malignant tumors from different sources as well as in diverse tumor cell lines. It was suggested MMP-26 may play a role in some of the tissue remodeling events associated with tumor progression.

Mediators of Inflammation

- **Vasoactive mediators and smooth muscle constriction mediators:** stored (histamine), serotonin, bradykinin, produced after cell activation (arachidonic acid metabolites – PGD2, PGE2, LTB4, LTC4, LTD4, platelet activating factor – PAF, adenosine), TXA2, C3a, C5a, fibrinopeptides, HMWK

- **Chemotactic mediators:** with effect on eosinophils (eosinophilic chemotactic factor of anaphylaxis – ECF-A, PAF), with effect on neutrophils (high-molecular chemotactic factor of neutrophils – HMW-NCF, LTB4, PAF), endothelial cells adhesion increase (IL-1, TNF-alpha, MCP-1, LTB4, LPS)
- **Enzymes:** neutral proteases (tryptase, chymase), lysosomal hydrolases (arylsulfatase, beta-glucuronidase, beta-hexosaminidase), other enzymes (superoxide dismutase, peroxidase)

Melanocyte Stimulating Hormone

(MSH, syn: melatonin) Hormone synthesized by the pineal gland. Secretion increases by light exposure. It influences hormone production, implicated in sleep regulation, mood, puberty and ovarian cycles. MSH is antiinflammatory mediator, inhibiting IL-1 inflammatory activity. Highest concentrations are at 4 AM and falls gradually to nadir at 8 PM.

Increased Values
exercise, pregnancy (3rd trimester), renal failure
> **Interfering Factors:** medicaments – (progesterone)

Decreased Values
ethanol, smoking, fasting
> **Interfering Factors:** medicaments – (beta-blockers)

Analyte	Age/Gender	Reference Range	SI Units	Note
Melanocyte Stimulating Hormone	Adults			
	7–8 AM	0.8–18.3	µg/l	
	12 AM	0–33	µg/l	
	12 PM	0–200	µg/l	

Melanoma Growth Stimulating Activity

(MGSA)
Occurrence. Fibroblasts, chondrocytes, epithelial cells, monocytes, macrophages, neutrophils, platelets.
Function. Chemoattraction and activation of neutrophils and stimulation of melanoma cell proliferation.

Mercury

(Hg) Mercury and its organic and inorganic compounds have been used in medicine for centuries as cathartics, desiccants, antiseptics, vermicides and diuretics. Mercury is a component of some materials used in dentistry. Hg compounds are found in some medications, fungicides and industrial processes. Mercury in the natural environment arises from outgassing of mercury vapour from the earth's surface and burning of fossil fuels. Microorganisms that live in marine and freshwater sediments methylate mercury. Methyl mercury is concentrated up the food chain and can be present in high concentrations in top predators. Elevated concentrations of mercury have been found in freshwater fish species living in areas subject to acid rain. Occupational exposures occur during the mining and processing of mercury ores, the manufacture, use and disposal of scientific instruments, batteries and fungicides. The major component of exposure to organic mercurials is seafood. Metallic mercury is readily absorbed by inhalation, whereas little is absorbed after ingestion. Inorganic mercury compounds are also poorly absorbed from the gut. Organic Hg compounds are very well absorbed from either the lungs or the gut. Inorganic Hg-compounds are lipid soluble. Once the compounds are absorbed, the divalent oxidation state is favored and the compounds concentrate in the CNS (except the brain) and the kidney. Over 90% of whole blood Hg is associated with erythrocytes (binds to hemoglobin). Inorganic mercury is excreted in the urine. Methyl mercury is secreted into the bile and mostly reabsorbed from the gut. Recommended specimens: whole blood, erythrocytes, urine and hair.

Increased Values – hypermercuremia
industrial exposure, mercury poisoning, excessive therapeutic intake
> Interfering Factors: newborn, medicaments – (penicillin)

Decreased Values – hypomercuremia
> Interfering Factors: platinum, gold

Analyte	Age/Gender	Reference Range	SI Units	Note
Mercury	Children	6.2–7.0	nmol/l	
	Adults	9.5–23.5	nmol/l	

Methionine

(Met) Essential glucoplastic amino acid important in sulphur metabolism. Methionine catabolism pathway produces S-adenosylmethionine, which serves as a methyl group donor for body compounds methylation. After adenosine transmethylation and cleavage, L-homocysteine is produced → L-cysteine. Methionine to homocysteine change is connected with methyltetrahydrofolate, vitamin B_{12} and B_6. Because of hereditary metabolic anomaly importance, sulphur amino acids are examined/evaluated together, frequently in load tests (L-methionine, vitamin B_6). Neonatal screening has insufficient sensitivity, it reveals only high methionine values. Methionine is a main methyl group source (choline, creatinine, epinephrine, and N-methyl-nicotinamide synthesis).
Enzyme defect. Cystathionine synthase and cystathionase.

Increased Values – hypermethioninemia
acidemia – (methylmalonic a., propionine a.), cystathioninemia, methionine adenosyltransferase deficiency, homocystinemia, homocystinuria, hypermethioninemia, severe liver diseases, septicemia, carcinoid sy, tyrosinemia

Decreased Values – hypomethioninemia
protein malnutrition

Analyte	Age/Gender	Reference Range	SI Units	Note
Methionine		10–40	µmol/l	

Beta-2-Microglobulin

(B2M) Lymphatic system non-glycated polypeptide. Renal tubular dysfunction indicator. Found on nucleated cells surfaces (cell membrane-associated amino acid peptide) associated with HLA beta-chain (human leukocyte antigen subunit). As beta-2-microglobulin has been demonstrated on the surface membranes of both T- and B-lymphocytes, it is also a histocompatibility Y-chromosome antigen subunit as well as tumour-associated and transplantation antigens.

Test Purpose. 1) to evaluate renal disease, chronic lymphocytic leukemia activity, AIDS activity, 2) to evaluate prognosis and progression in multiple myeloma, 3) prediction of prognosis in HIV infection, 4) to detect dialysis amyloidosis, 5) to monitor glomerular filtration in renal disease.

Increased Values

AIDS, amyloidosis, renal dialysis, hepatitis, hyperthyroidism, diseases – (viral infectious d., renal d., lymphatic system d., inflammatory d.), lymphogranuloma, Crohn's disease, tumours – (adenocarcinoma of the colon, chronic lymphocytic leukemia, lymphomas, melanoma, liver t., plasmocytoma including multiple myeloma, breast t., ovary t., t. from beta-cells), renal grafting rejection, renal injury, sarcoidosis, Felty's sy, vasculitis, renal failure, Wilson's disease, non-cancer specific increase – (hepato-biliary tract diseases, heavy metal intoxication, immunodeficiency conditions)

> **Interfering Factors:** healthy persons, medicaments – (nephrotoxic antibiotics – aminoglycozides)

Analyte	Age/Gender	Reference Range	SI Units	Note
Beta-2- Micro-globulin	Adults <60 y	0.80–2.4	mg/l	
	Adults >60 y	1.00–3.00	mg/l	

Mitochondrial Aspartate Aminotransferase

(mAST) Isoenzymes of AST are cAST (cytosolic form) and mAST (mitochondrial form). In the human liver and most other organs, mAST represents 80% of the total, but, in the serum it is less 12% for both healthy and diseased condition. Serum levels slightly increase as a sign of severe cellular damage.

Increased Values

chronic alcohol abuse, hepatitis – (alcoholic h., fulminant viral h.), acute liver diseases, myocardial infarction, liver injury, organ damage, severe heart failure

Molybdenum

(Mo) Trace metal element.
Occurrence. In trace amounts in nearly all biological materials, the highest molybdenum amounts are retained in the liver, skeleton, kidney. Oxidation-reduction active metal element occurring in three human metalloenzymes: xanthine oxidase, aldehyde oxidase, sulfite oxidase. Molybdenum is absorbed mainly in the stomach and small intestine. After absorption, most molybdenum is rapidly turned over and eliminated via the urine and excreted in the bile.

Test Purpose. Suspect industrial intoxication.

Increased Values
industrial exposure

Decreased Values
inborn molybdenum metabolism error

Analyte	Age/Gender	Reference Range	SI Units	Note
Molybdenum		8–60.3	nmol/kg	

Monoclonal Proteins

Increased – positive
amyloidosis, pernicious anemia, rheumatoid arthritis, benign monoclonal gammopathy, chronic liver diseases, leukemia, chronic lymphocytic leukemia, systemic lupus erythematosus, lymphomas, Waldenström's macroglobulinemia, tumours, plasmocytoma (incl. multiple myeloma), polyarteritis nodosa, syndrome – (systemic capillary leak sy, Sjögren's sy), thyroiditis

Monocyte Chemotactic Protein–1

(MCP-1, syn: monocyte chemotactic and activating factor – MCAF).
Occurrence. Monocytes, macrophages, fibroblasts, B-cells, epithelial cells, smooth muscle cells and glioblastoma cells.
Function. Chemoattracts monocytes, regulates adhesion molecule expression and cytokine production in monocytes.

Motilin

Motilin is an acid peptide, widely distributed in the gastrointestinal tract, from the esophagus to the colon (small intestine M-cells), including the gallbladder, biliary tract, pineal, and pituitary glands.
Function. It is a strong stimulant for upper gastrointestinal tract smooth muscle contraction, increases fundus/antrum/duodenum motility, as well as lower esophageal sphincter contractions. Action mechanism is endocrine. Fat ingestion stimulates motilin release, release is inhibited by somatostatin and oral glucose. Motilin is unique because actions are generally restricted to fasting condition.

Increased Values
acute diarrhea, acute intestinal infection, ulcerative colitis, Crohn's disease, tropical sprue, irritable bowel sy

Analyte	Age/Gender	Reference Range	SI Units	Note
Motilin	Neonates	28–36	pmol/l	
	1 m	100–147	pmol/l	
	Adults	16–28	pmol/l	

Mucoproteins

Glycoprotein, seromucoid and plasmatic protein globulin fraction; term "mucoproteins" is used for glycoproteins (protein group name, which contain saccharide component) having more than 4% hexosamine and which pass into filtrate after deproteinization by sulfosalicylic acid, and perchloric acid. Also sialic acid (N-acetyl neuramine acid) belongs to saccharide components. To the mucoproteins belong: orosomucoid (acid alpha-1-glycoprotein), haptoglobin, alpha-2-macroglobulin, ceruloplasmin, thyroxine-binding globulin, group specific components Gc, beta-2-microglobulin, transcortin.

Test Purpose. 1) acute and chronic inflammations diagnosis, 2) postsurgery conditions assessment, 3) myocardial infarction monitoring, 4) malignant tumors diagnosis, 5) systemic and rheumatic diseases diagnosis and monitoring, 6) liver injury, 7) perinatal infections diagnosis.

Increased Values
rheumatoid arthritis, bacterial endocarditis, diseases – (infectious d., rheumatic d., **inflammatory d.**), systemic lupus erythematosus, Hodgkin's disease, tumours, nephritis, osteomyelitis, pneumonia, poliomyelitis, chronic progressive polyarthritis, postoperative states, tuberculosis, **ankylosing spondylitis**.

Decreased Values
hepatic cirrhosis, infectious hepatitis, adrenal insufficiency, lipoid nephrosis, hepatic parenchyma injury, Marfan's sy

Analyte	Age/Gender	Reference Range	SI Units	Note
Mucoproteins		<386	µmol/l	

Müllerian Inhibiting Substance

(MIS, syn: anti-Müllerian hormone) MIS is expressed during the development of mammalian embryos. It is secreted by Sertoli cells in undifferentiated gonads and also by granulosa cells of the ovaries. It causes the regression of the Müllerian duct in male embryos which develops into tubes, uterus and upper vagina of female embryos. MIS has been implicated also in fetal lung development. It has been reported that MIS also inhibits the meiosis in oocytes and the growth of tumor cell lines.

Increased Values
ovarian sexcord tumor

Decreased Values
Hirschprung's disease

Myoglobin

(Mb) Myoglobin is an oxygen-binding iron containing protein not present in smooth musculature. Skeletal muscle and myocardium hemoprotein (found in the cytosolic fraciton). In comparison to hemoglobin, myoglobin binds only one oxygen mol. Myoglobin measurement is a myocardium damage index. Because of its small size and relatively high tissue concentration, very rapid and pronounced increases are seen after skeletal and/or cardiac damage. Increases in myoglobin can be measured in many cases within 1 hour of the cardiac event (the occlusion of a coronary artery). Thus, myoglobin is an early marker of cardiac injury but lacks the specificity of an ideal marker. The protein is excreted in the urine and clears rapidly from the blood.

Function. Normally transports an oxygen in mammalian muscles; red muscle tissue oxygen stores; with oxygen deprivation, this O_2 is released by muscle mitochondria to generate energy through glucose combustion to carbon dioxide and water.

Test Purpose. 1) myocardial infarction diagnosis (focus size estimation) and reperfusion therapy efficiency monitoring, 2) rhabdomyolysis evidence, 3) crush sy, blast sy and thermic damage diagnosis and monitoring, 4) medicamentous intoxication diagnosis (hypnotics, hypolipemics), 5) endocrinopathies differential diagnosis (hypothyroidism, Conn's sy, diabetes mellitus), 6) hereditary metabolic muscular phosphorylase disorders (McArdle's disease), fructokinase, carnitine palmityltransferase, 7) malignant hyperthermia assessment, 8) renal damage evidence, 9) sport traumatology diagnosis, 10) systemic diseases diagnosis and monitoring.

Increased Values – hypermyoglobinemia

muscle enzyme deficiencies, **muscular dystrophy**, **dermatomyositis**, glycogenoses, **malignant hyperthermia**, hypoglycemia, hypokalemia, hypothyroidism, viral infectious diseases, **cardiac infarction** (increase at 2–6 hrs, peaking at 6–12 hrs, decrease at 12–24 h.), intoxication by – (carbon dioxide, water), **skeletal muscle ischemia**, cardioversion, **postinfectious myoglobinuria**, myopathies, narcotics, **polymyositis**, systemic lupus erythematosus, inborn disorders of muscular metabolism – (phosphofructokinase, phosphorylase, carnitine palmitoyltransferase), **muscle injury, overload of skeletal muscle during physical exertion, rhabdomyolysis**, syndrome – (Conn's sy, crush sy), tetanus, typhoid fever, skeletal muscle trauma, **skeletal muscle inflammation**, shock conditions, recent pectoral angina attack, renal failure.

Interfering Factors: intramuscular injections, medicaments – (suxamethonium)

Decreased Values – hypomyoglobinemia

rheumatoid arthritis, myasthenia gravis, circulating antibodies to myoglobin.

Analyte	Age/Gender	Reference Range	SI Units	Note
Myoglobin	F	17.0–65.5	µg/l	
	M	16.5–76	µg/l	

Myosin

(syn: myosin light chain – MLC) Myosin is found in the thick muscle myofibrilar sarcomere filament. Following myocardial cell necrosis, myosin is released into serum as myosin light/heavy-chain fragments (L – light chains are specific for heart). These chains are detectable from 2 to 10 days after myocardial infarction onset (retrospective myocardial cell damage detection). Cytosol MLC is in blood after 6–14 hrs, structure bounded MLC is released after 22 hrs (2-phase releasing). MLC washing is performed independently from related myocardial area perfusion, it is necrotic changes range expression in the affected cardiomyocytes. MLC is considered to be a very good marker for infarcted area range determination (better than Mb or CK-MB).

Test Purpose. 1) myocardial infarction diagnosis (focus size estimation) and reperfusion therapy efficiency, 2) rhabdomyolysis evidence, 3) crush sy, blast sy and thermic damage diagnosis and monitoring, 4) medicamentous intoxication diagnosis (hypnotics, hypolipemics), 5) endocrinopathies differential diagnosis (hypothyroidism, Conn's sy, diabetes mellitus), 6) hereditary metabolic muscular phosphorylase disorders (McArdle's disease), fructokinase, carnitine palmityltransferase diagnosis, 7) malignant hyperthermia assessment, 8) renal damage evidence, 9) sport traumatology diagnosis, 10) systemic diseases diagnosis and monitoring, 11) to state unstable angina pectoris prognosis.

Increased Values
acute myocardial infarction (increase 6–14 hrs, decrease at 14th d.), acute/chronic myocarditis, cardiac surgery, cardiac trauma.

Decreased Values
cardiac atrophy due to – (AIDS, cachexia, severe malnutrition, tumors)

Natrium

(Na, syn: sodium) Principal extracellular cation.

Function. Extracellular fluid volume control, acid-base balance maintenance and electrical potential maintenance in the neuromuscular system, and osmotic pressure maintenance. Mechanisms for maintaining plasma and extracellular fluid Na levels are renal blood flow, carbonic anhydrase activity, natriuretic factors, aldosterone, renin and ADH. The average diet provides between 8–15 g of NaCl per day; the body requires between 1–2% of the intake. Excess is excreted in the urine. Between 60–70% of the filtered load is reabsorbed in the proximal tubules with bicarbonate and water. A further 25–30% is reabsorbed in Henle's ascending loop, thus only a small original filter load fraction is presented to the dis-tal tubule. However, in the distal tubule, most important Na regulation aspect occurs under ACTH and aldosterone influence. Coupled with potassium exchange and/or H^+ determines the sodium amount excreted in the urine. Highest values are in summer and lowest in winter.

Test Purpose. To evaluate fluid-electrolyte, acid-base balance, and related neuromuscular/renal/adrenal functions.

Increased Values – hypernatremia
diabetic acidosis, liver cirrhosis, **dehydration**, cardiac decompensation, diabetes insipidus – (**central d. i., nephrogenic d. i.**), **osmotic diuresis**, encephalitis, **febrile conditions, hemodialysis,** diarrhea, primary hyperaldosteronism, idiopathic hypernatremia, prolonged hyperpnea, diseases – (pituitary d., hypothalamic d.), insufficiency – (renal i., cardiac i.), dia-betic coma, Cushing's disease, tumours, nephritis, cystic kidney, severe burns, disorders – (**endocrine d.,** water metabolism d.), excessive sweating, increased intake of natrium – (in-fusion, hyperosmolar solutions, salt water, parenteral alimentation), comatous conditions, **predominant loss of water,** nephrotic sy, decreased total body water, increased temperature of environment, tracheobronchitis, trauma, vomiting, **decreased natrium excretion.**

> **Interfering Factors:** old people, medicaments – (ACTH, anabolic steroids, androgens, antibiotics, betamethasone, captopril, carbenicillin, carbenoxolone, cholestyramine, clonidine, corticosteroids, cortisone, dexamethasone, diazoxide, diuretics, enoxolone, estrogens, ethanol, glucose, guanethidine, hydrocortisone, lactulose, mannitol, methoxyflurane, methyldopa, methylprednisolone, oral contraceptives, Na penicillin, prednisone, prednisolone, oxyphenbutazone, phenylbutazone, phosphorus salts, reserpine, sodium bicarbonate, sodium lactate, triamcinolone, triamterene, urea)

Decreased Values – hyponatremia

acidosis – (metabolic a., renal tubular a.), bronchial asthma, **hepatic cirrhosis**, diabetes mellitus, diuresis – (**osmotic d.,** postobstructive d.), encephalopathy, gastroenteritis, gastrointestinal fistulas, diarrhea, **hypersecretion of ADH** (SIADH), hyperglycemia, hyperlipidemia, hyperosmolality, **hypopituitarism, hypothyroidism,** polycystic renal disease, diseases – (renal d. with polyuria, primary chronic tubular renal d., **liver d.**), **ileus**, insufficiency – (primary/secondary adrenocortical i., **renal i., cardiac i.**), intoxication – (alcohol i., ethylene glycol i., methanol i., water i.), ketonuria, hemorrhage, infusion therapy, **Addison's disease**, tumours – (bronchogenic t., mediastinal t., cerebral t.), nausea, interstitial nephritis, **acute tubular necrosis**, pyloric obstruction, small bowel suction, surgery, panhypopituitarism, **pancreatitis**, peritonitis, pleural effusion, pneumonia, **polydipsia**, burns, porphyrias, **increased sweating, insufficient natrium intake,** repeated ascitic/pleural transudate puncture, chronic pyelonephritis, transurethral prostate resection, conditions – (**painful c., edematous c.**), loss of – (**increased l. of natrium, gastrointestinal fluid**), emotional stress, syndrome – (malabsorption sy, **nephrotic sy**), tuberculosis, trauma, **vomiting**, parenteral alimentation, extreme physical exertion, failure – (acute renal f., **hepatic f., congestive cardiac f.**).

Interfering Factors: medicaments – (ACE inhibitors, acetazolamide, acetohexamide, aldesleukin, amiloride, aminoglycosides, amitriptyline, ammonium chloride, amphotericin B, atovaquone, bexarotene, bicarbonate, bumetanide, captopril, carbamazepine, carboplatin, chlorpropamide, chlortalidone, cholestyramine, cisplatin, citalopram, clofibrate, clonidine, codeine, cyclophenthiazide, cyclophosphamide, dalfopristin, desmopressin, dextran, dextrose, diuretics, ethacrynic acid, fentanyl, fluoxetine, fluvoxamine, furosemide, gentamicin, glimepiride, glucose, glyburide, haloperidol, heparin, hydrochlorothiazide, hydrocodone, hydromorphone, imipramine, indapamide, indomethacin, ketoconazole, lactulose, lithium, lorcainide, losartan, mannitol, meperidine, mercurial diuretics, methadone, metolazone, miconazole, morphine, nonsteroidal antiinflammatory agents, oxcarbazepine, oxycodone, oxytocin, paroxetine, phenothiazines, polymyxin, polythiazide, propafenone, saluretics, sertraline, spironolactone, thiazides, ticlopidine, tolazamide, tolbutamide, triamterene, tricyclic antidepressants, trimethoprim, trimetrexate, urea, vasopressin, vinblastine, vincristine, vinorelbine).

Analyte	Age/Gender	Reference Range	SI Units	Note
Natrium (Sodium)	1 d–4 w	132–147	mmol/l	
	2–12 m	129–143	mmol/l	
	>1 y	132–145	mmol/l	
	Adults	135–145	mmol/l	

Neopterin

Neopterin is a pteridine derivative, a pyrazinopyrinidine compound. It is produced by macrophages after induction by interferon gamma and serves as a marker of cellular immune system activation. Neopterin levels can be used as prognostic predictors for certain types of malignancies. It is eliminated primarily in the urine, so evaluation of urinary neopterin levels may be useful in assessing activation of the cellular immunity system even in the absence of typical clinical symptoms.

Increased Values – positive

HIV infection, rheumatoid arthritis, systemic lupus erythematosus, viral infectious diseases, **tumors,** tetrahydrobiopterin biosynthesis disorders, graft rejection, viral infection in transplant patients, conditions with impaired – (cellular immunity, renal function), autoimmune diseases.

C-3 Nephritic Factor

(C3 NeF) C-3 nephritic factor is an autoantibody belonging to the complement components (regulatory component). It is a potent alternative pathway activator due to its bonding and stabilizing abilities C3 convertase to prevent its dissociation by factors H and I. Levels of C3 and C4 should be determined before this test is requested.

Test Purpose. Distinguishing types of mesangiocapillary glomerulonephritis.

Increased Values

glomerulonephritis – (membranoproliferative g., **mesangiocapillary g.,** post-streptococcal g.), **partial lipodystrophy,** systemic lupus erythematosus.

Nerve Growth Factor

(NGF) NGF belongs to neurotrophins and cytokines, it is a protein complex of three subunits (alpha-2, beta, gamma-2). Beta-subunit is a 7S subunit component responding for biological activity; it is a dimer consisting of two identical subunits. NGF is involved in Alzheimer's disease pathogenesis, in autoimmune/sensoric neuropathy development.

Occurrence. Smooth muscle cells, fibroblasts, activated macrophages, epithelial cells, neurons, astrocytes, Schwann's cells.

Function. Stimulates growth and differentiation of B-cells. Plays a critical role in the development of sympathetic and some sensory neurons. NGF is involved in vitality development/maintenance of embryonic neurons. Enhances histamine release from mast cells.

Test Purpose. 1) dementia differential diagnosis, 2) peripheral neuropathy diagnosis from etiopathogenesis point of view.

Analyte	Age/Gender	Reference Range	SI Units	Note
Nerve Growth Factor Beta		5–10	pg/ml	

Neuron-Specific Enolase

(NSE) Neuron-specific enolase is one of the five isozymes of the glycolytic enzyme, enolase. This enzyme is released into the CSF when neural tissue is injured. Neoplasms derived from neural or neuroendocrine tissue may release NSE into the blood. The test may have value in predicting response to therapy. NSE is a useful adjunct in the monitoring of patients with small cell lung cancer. There is evidence that the level of serum NSE correlates with tumor burden. NSE is a tumor marker.

Test Purpose. To monitor a progress of neural crest tumors, including small cell carcinoma of lung.

hemolysis, lung diseases, pneumonia, septic shock, cranial trauma, tumors – (pheochromo-cytoma, gastrinoma, carcinoid, **bronchogenic small-cell carcinoma**, medulloblastoma, mela-noma, **neuroblastoma**, retinoblastoma, seminoma, t. of pancreas, t. of kidney, t. of thyroid, Wilm's tumor), uremia on dialysis.

Analyte	Age/Gender	Reference Range	SI Units	Note
Neuron-Specific Enolase		0–12	ng/ml	

Neurotensin

Gastrointestinal hormone with neuroendocrine and partial paracrine action mechanism. Neurotensin is an amino acid peptide, that is produced by endocrine ileal mucosa and large intestine N-cells and then released by mixed meal and long-chain fatty acids.
Function. Inhibits gastric acid and gastric emptying, decreases pancreatic bicarbonate juice, intestinal secretions, esophageal/intestinal sphincter tonus, increases intestinal motor ac-tivity, induces vasodilation and hypotension. Neurotensin serves as neurotransmitter in the brain. Gastrocolic reflex is probably a neurotensin function.

Increased Values
after meals, renal failure

Decreased Values
    Interfering Factors: medicaments – (morphine)

Neutrophil Chemotactic Factor

(syn: high-molecular weight neutrophil chemotactic factor – HMW-NCF)
Function. Neutrophils chemotactic attraction, deactivation, and allergic reaction mediator.

Nickel

(Ni) Serum and urine levels are useful indices of chronic environmental exposure and expo-sure to ink, magnets, spark plugs, paints, stainless steel, enamels, ceramics, batteries, electro-nics, glass and alloys manufactures. Exposure most often occurs in the industrial environ-ment either through the inhalation of nickel dust or dermal contact with nickel compounds.

Increased Values
ethanol, **industrial exposure**, **acute myocardial infarction**, tissue necrosis, dialysis patients, burns, **acute stroke**, trauma, renal failure

Decreased Values
diseases – (renal d., hepatic d.)

Analyte	Age/Gender	Reference Range	SI Units	Note
Nickel		0.13–0.76	µmol/l	

Non-protein Nitrogen

(NPN) The nitrogenous blood constituents exclusive of the protein bodies consists of the nitrogen of urea, uric acid, creatine, creatinine, amino acids, polypeptides and an undetermined part known as a rest nitrogen. These compounds are by-products of proteins or nucleic acids.

Increased Values
prerenal azotemia, high-protein diet, renal diseases, urinary tract obstruction, pregnancy (3rd trimester)

Decreased Values
severe hepatic insufficiency, hepatic necrosis

Norepinephrine

(syn: noradrenaline, levarterenol) One of the naturally occurring catecholamine, neurohormone.
Production. Adrenal gland (by the medulla in response to splanchnic stimulation; stored in the chromaffin granules), peripheral nerve endings (postganglionic adrenergic nerves) and some brain neurons. Tyramine provokes release. Major urine metabolite source.
Function. It is a major neurotransmitter that acts on alpha- and beta-1 adrenergic receptors, increases blood pressure, peripheral vascular resistance and blood glucose level (slightly), decreases heart rate, skin and renal blood flow, and splanchnic blood flow. Predominantly released in response to hypotension and stress.

Increased Values
progressive muscular dystrophy, pheochromocytoma, **ganglioblastoma**, **ganglioneuroma**, hypoglycemia, hypothyroidism, diseases – (kidney d., thyroid d.), acute myocardial infarction, diabetic ketoacidosis, myasthenia gravis, neuroblastoma, **paraganglioma**, burns, postoperatively, severe stress, shock, thyrotoxicosis, anxiety, **extreme exercise**.
    Interfering Factors: medicaments – (alpha-methyldopa, desipramine, dopamine, ethanol, felodipine, fenoterol, furosemide, hydralazine, insulin, isoproterenol, metoprolol, prazosin, quinidine, salbutamol)

Decreased Values
anorexia nervosa, autonomous nervous system dysfunction, orthostatic hypotension
    Interfering Factors: medicaments – (nifedipine)

5-Nucleotidase

(5-NT, syn: nucleotidase) Enzyme specific to the liver, phosphatase that acts only on nucleoside-5 phosphates (such as AMP) releasing inorganic phosphate. The enzyme is widely distributed throughout body tissues and it is principally localized in the cell cytoplasmic membrane (mainly in hepatobiliary tract). 5-NT levels measurement helps determine whether ALP elevation originates from skeletal or hepatic diseases. 5-NT remains normal in skeletal disease and pregnancy, thus more specific for assessing hepatic dysfunction than ALP or leukocytic ALP. 5-NT parallels the increases of alkaline phosphatase and leucine aminopeptidase in hepatobiliary diseases. It is a relatively good intrahepatic lesion indicator.

Test Purpose. 1) to distinguish between hepatobiliary and skeletal disease, when elevated ALP level source is uncertain, 2) to help differentiate biliary obstruction from acute hepatocellular damage, 3) to detect hepatic metastasis in jaundice absence, 4) primary biliary cirrhosis diagnosis, 5) to aid in differential diagnosis of hepatobiliary disease during pregnancy.

Increased Values
hepatic cirrhosis, hepatitis, cholelithiasis, cholestasis, graft vs. host disease, diseases – (hepatobiliary d., bone d.), hepatic ischemia, hepatic tumors, liver metastases, hepatic necrosis, extra/intrahepatic biliary obstruction, acute lymphoblastic leukemia, pregnancy (3rd trimester)

> **Interfering Factors:** children, elderly people, medicaments – (acetaminophen, acetylsalicylic acid, androgens, anticonvulsants, asparaginase, chloramphenicol, chlorpromazine, estradiol, hepatotoxic agents, indomethacin, meperidine, methyltestosterone, morphine, nandrolone, penicillamine, penicillin, phenothiazines, tolazamide, tolbutamide)

Analyte	Age/Gender	Reference Range	SI Units	Note
5-Nucleotidase		33–250	nkat/l	

Oncostatin M

(OSM) OSM belongs to glycoprotein-character cytokine.
Occurrence. T-cells, monocytes, macrophages.
Function. Inhibits proliferation of certain melanomas and other solid tumors, endothelium and embryonic stem cell proliferation; stimulates normal fibroblasts and AIDS-Kaposi's sarcoma-derived cell growth. The antiproliferative activity of OSM for some cells lines is synergised by TGF-beta and IFN-gamma. It promotes the growth of human fibroblasts, vascular smooth muscle cells and some normal cell lines. Oncostatin M is involved in acute phase protein and vasoactive peptide synthesis; induces leukemic cell, fibroblasts and neuronal cell differentiation.

Ornithine

(Orn) Non-essential amino acid, belongs to so-called ornithine cycle amino acid group (ornithine, citrulline, arginine, argininosuccinic acid). Ornithine is one urea cycle intermediate metabolite that is not incorporated into natural proteins. Rather, it is arginine generated in the cytosol and must be transported into the mitochondria where it is used as a enzyme OTC substrate (ornithine transcarbamoylase) to form citrulline.
Enzyme defect. Ornithine keto-acid-transaminase.

Increased Values
hemolysis, hyperornithinemia, severe burns

Decreased Values
conditions after abdominal surgery, carcinoid sy, chronic renal failure

Analyte	Age/Gender	Reference Range	SI Units	Note
Ornithine	Neonates	120–220	µmol/l	
	Children	50–200	µmol/l	
	Adults	50–120	µmol/l	

Ornithine Carbamoyltransferase

(OCT, syn: ornithine transcarbamoylase)

Function. OCT catalyzes the second enzymatic urea cycle reaction and the ornithine carbamoyl phosphate carbamoylation to form citrulline. The enzyme is located almost exclusively in the liver mitochondria, the intestinal mucosa, and leucocytes. OCT is a sensitive indicator of hepatocellular damage.

Test Purpose. 1) infant hyperammonemias differential diagnosis, 2) to detect minimal liver-cell damage in various disorders.

Increased Values

hepatic cirrhosis, drug toxicity, alcoholism, enteritis, **acute viral hepatitis**, myocardial infarction, liver diseases – (infective l. d., parasitic l. d.), collagen vascular diseases, **obstructive jaundice, metastatic liver tumors, liver cancer, liver necrosis, congestive heart failure**

> **Interfering Factors:** alcoholism, dietary changes, medicaments – (acetaminophen, amiodarone, anabolic steroids, androgens, anti-thyroid agents, azlocillin, carbamazepine, carmustine, dantrolene, daunorubicin, disulfiram, doxorubicin, erythromycin, estrogens, etrenitate, gold compounds, halothane, isoniazid, ketoconazole, mercaptopurine, methotrexate, methyldopa, mezlocillin, naltrexone, nitrofurantoin, oral contraceptives, phenothiazines, phenytoin, piperacillin, plicamycin, rifampin, sulfonamides, tetracyclines, valproic acid)

Decreased Values

inborn metabolic defect of OCT, congenital hyperammonemia

> **Interfering Factors:** mercuric salts

Orosomucoid

(syn: alpha-1-acid glycoprotein – AGP) Early acute phase reactant, high-weight molecular protein belonging to the main serum glycoproteins. Orosomucoid saccharides proportion weight is up to 45%, giving properties of solubility and thermostability. It has a great genetic polymorphism (saccharide proportion and protein component), looks like CEA with amino acid homology and partially immunologically, bonds progesterone, is bound to cyanocobalamin, and involved in hemocoagulation and immunological processes. Biological half-time is 5 days. Orosomucoid is used as an early glomerular filtration decrease indicator. Examination sensitivity is lower in chronic inflammatory diseases.

Test Purpose. 1) it is mainly used to monitor acute phase reactions, 2) malignancy monitoring, 3) renal diseases diagnosis.

Increased Values

rheumatoid arthritis, alcoholic liver cirrhosis, glomerulonephritis, acute hepatitis, diseases – (autoimmune d., **severe infectious d., severe inflammatory d.**), myocardial infarction, systemic lupus erythematosus, Crohn's ileitis, **tumors**, surgery, pneumonia, burns, **acute phase reactions**, trauma

> **Interfering Factors:** medicaments – (corticosteroids, oxymetholone)

Decreased Values

hepatic cirrhosis, pulmonary embolism, malnutrition, severe hepatic damage, severe protein losing, nephrotic sy, pregnancy (1st trimester)

Interfering Factors: early childhood, medicaments – (estrogens, oral contraceptives, tamoxifen)

Analyte	Age/Gender	Reference Range	SI Units	Note
Orosomucoid	F	0.40–1.20	g/l	
	M	0.50–1.30	g/l	

Osmolal Gap

Difference between measured and calculated values.

Increased Values
acidosis – (lactate a., diabetic a.), ethanol ingestion, hyperlipidemia, hyperproteinemia, intoxication by – (acetone, ethylene glycol, paraldehyde, methanol, isopropyl alcohol), shock conditions, renal failure.

Osmolality

(syn: serum osmolality) Osmolality measures the concentration of all dissolved osmotically active particles in a solution. It is the most important parameter for internal water balance assessment. For interpretation it is necessary to consider water regulatory mechanisms, electrolyte, and acid-base balance. Osmolality can be calculated according to the formula: Osm (mosmol/kg) = 2 x Na + glucose + urea. If the measured osmolality exceeds the calculated osmolality by more than 5 mosmol/kg → osmotic gap arises. This gap arises mainly in osmotic active agents intoxication; with unclear origin comatose conditions the gap more than 15 mosmol/kg, suggests intoxication, or endogenous osmotic active agent accumulation, lactate is the most frequent. Hyperosmolality → antidiuretic hormone secretion stimulation → ↑ water reabsorption in renal tubules → more concentrated urine and less concentrated serum. A low serum osmolality leads to ADH release → results in ↓ water reabsorption and large dilute urine amount. Water deficiency – dehydration – hyperosmolality. Water excess – hyperhydration – hypoosmolality. The same conditions that reduce/increase serum sodium affect osmolality.
Test Purpose. 1) to evaluate electrolyte and water balance, 2) to evaluate hyperosmolar status and hydration status, 3) to evaluate dehydration and acid-base balance, 4) to evaluate seizures, 5) to evaluate clue to alcoholism, methanol toxicity, ethylene glycol ingestion, 6) to evaluate antidiuretic hormone function, liver disease, hyperosmolar coma, hypernatremia.

Increased Values – hyperosmolality
azotemia, alcoholism, relative water deficiency in solutes excess – (glucose, mannitol, NaCl, urea), **hypertonic dehydration**, **diabetes insipidus**, **diabetes mellitus**, gastrointestinal fistulas, **diarrhea**, **hyperglycemia**, **hypertonic hyperhydration**, **hypercalcemia**, **hypernatremia**, hyperventilation, hypokalemia, chronic renal diseases, sickle cell disease, renal insufficiency, poisoning by – (**ethanol, ethylene glycol, methanol**), acute catabolism, **diabetic ketoacidosis**, **ketosis**, **diabetic coma**, cerebral lesions, Addison's disease, **renal tubular necrosis**, burns, sweating, insufficient water intake – (parenterally, orally), **severe pyelonephritis**, sepsis, water loss, **shock**, **uremia**, **vomiting**, incorrect parenteral alimentation, febrile conditions
Interfering Factors: medicaments – (corticosteroids, diuretics, ethanol, insulin, inulin, mannitol, methoxyflurane, urea)

Decreased Values – hypoosmolality

liver cirrhosis, natrium deficiency, **hypotonic dehydration, osmotic diuresis**, diarrhea, starvation, **hypotonic hyperhydration, hypoproteinemia + hyponatremia**, hypothyroidism, insufficiency – (renal i., cardiac i.), chronic catabolism, Addison's disease, **water excess**, relative water excess in electrolyte deficiency, replacement of isotonic fluid loss with water, nephritis, panhypopituitarism, burns, pancreatitis, peritonitis, excessive endogenous/exogenous water intake, conditions – (painful c., postoperative c.), stress, syndrome – (adrenogenital sy, **sy of inappropriate ADH secretion, paraneoplastic sy associated with lung carcinoma**, nephrotic sy), decreased water excretion, proximal renal tubular acidosis, salt-losing nephropathy, genito-urinary tract obstruction, vomiting, pyelonephritis, polycystic kidney disease, congestive heart failure

> **Interfering Factors:** medicaments – (carbamazepine, chlortalidone, cisplatin, citalopram, cyclophosphamide, diuretics, fluoxetine, fluvoxamine, hydrochlorothiazide, lorcainide, polythiazide, terbutaline, thiazides)

Analyte	Age/Gender	Reference Range	SI Units	Note
Osmolality	Neonates	265–275	mmol/kg	
	Adults <60 y	275–295	mmol/kg	
	Adults >60 y	280–300	mmol/kg	

Osteocalcin

(syn: bone Gla protein – BGP) Vitamin K-dependent, calcium-binding bone protein; the most abundant/best determined non-collagen protein (49 amino acids) in bone.

Production. Osteocalcin is synthesized in the skeleton by osteoblasts, the cells responsible for bone formation, and under the vitamin D3 control ↓ incorporation into extracellular bone matrix. Osteocalcin creates 1–2% of the bone proteins. Increased total osteocalcin in serum reflects new osteoblastic synthesis, not bone resorption. N-terminal fragment is a main osteocalcin fragment. Gamma-glutamic acid fragment gamma-carboxylation level can be problematic during examination (gamma-carboxylation changes immunoreactivity, low-molecular osteocalcin increases with ageing and changes with vitamin intake). Incompletely carboxylated osteocalcin concentration is a prospective femur collum fracture risk indicator.

Function. Osteocalcin appears to be a sensitive non-invasive bone metabolism marker (osteoformation). Its physiological importance is not clear; it seems to inhibit Ca and P deposition into bones and prevent excessive mineralization. It bounds hydroxyapatite with high affinity during osteoclastic resorption; bone matrix osteocalcin is released into circulation as nonimmune fragments. These fragments are cleared by the kidney and appear in the urine as gamma-carboxyglutamic acid metabolites (Gla). The serum osteocalcin levels parallel alkaline phosphatase activity. Osteocalcin is excreted via the kidney; concentration rises intensely in glomerular filtration decrease. Highest values are at night and early in the morning, falls to nadir in early afternoon, increases later afternoon, with women higher concentrations are in luteal phase. Within-day level variation is 50–100%. Day-to-day variation is 50%.

Test Purpose. 1) osteoporosis diagnosis and bone turn-over differential diagnosis, 2) diagnosis and monitoring of malignant tumors with bone metastases, 3) primary hyperparathyroidism diagnosis, 4) renal osteopathies diagnosis, 5) to help in patogenetically unclear ALP activity increase, 6) to help in renal failure diagnosis.

Increased Values – hyperosteocalcinemia
adolescent growth spurt, **acromegaly**, exercise, menstruation cycle, hypercalcemia of malignancy, hyperparathyroidism, **primary/secondary hyperthyroidism**, lactation, **Paget's disease**, tumors, metastatic skeletal tumors, obesity, **renal osteodystrophy**, osteogenesis imperfecta, osteoarthritis, osteoporosis, recent fractures, **chronic renal failure**
  Interfering Factors: female gender, race, diurnal rhythms, seasonal variation, age over 50 years, medicaments – (anticonvulsants, calcitrol, fluorides, growth hormone, omeprazole, thyroid hormones, vitamin D3)

Decreased Values – hypoosteocalcinemia
anorexia nervosa, primary biliary cirrhosis, menstruation cycle, **growth hormone deficiency**, ethanol, hypercalcemia of malignancy, hypoparathyroidism, hypothyroidism, diseases – (acute d., liver d.), metastases of malignant tumors, osteoarthritis, osteomalacia, postmenopausal osteoporosis, plasmocytoma (incl. multiple myeloma), **pregnancy** (1st trimester)
  Interfering Factors: race, diurnal rhythms, seasonal variation, medicaments – (calcitonin, corticosteroids, coumarine anticoagulants, estrogens, glucocorticoids, oral contraceptives, tamoxifen, thiazides, warfarin)

Analyte	Age/Gender	Reference Range	SI Units	Note
Osteocalcin		3.0–5.4	µg/l	

Oxalate

Normal oxalate is derived from dietary oxalic acid (about 10%), from food, ascorbic acid metabolism (35–50%) and glycine (40%). Oxalic acid and its salts are used as cleaning and bleaching agents.

Increased Values
hereditary primary hyperoxaluria, oxalate poisoning
  Interfering Factors: medicaments – (methoxyflurane)

Oxytocin

Production. Posterior pituitary hormone (neurohypophysis).
Release. Nipple irritation during breast feeding (suckling). Stretch receptors in the uterus and possibly in the vaginal mucosa may also initiate oxytocin release. Emotional stress inhibits lactation. Placental enzyme oxytocinase breaks oxytocin during pregnancy.
Function. Uterine contraction during labour (uterokinetic effect), breast milk flow stimulation by myoepithelial muscle fibre contractions in the milk ducts → milk ejection. In women the levels increase to peak near ovulation time, nadir in late luteal phase.

Increased Values – hyperoxytocinemia
hemoconcentration, pregnancy (3rd trimester)
  Interfering Factors: medicaments – (oral contraceptives)

Decreased Values – hypooxytocinemia
psychic factors, stress

Pancreatic Polypeptide

(PP) Gastrointestinal hormone with endocrine and paracrine mechanism action.

Production. Pancreatic and duodenal PP-cells. All ingested nutrients stimulate PP release, e. g. triacylglycerols and glucose; protein is the most potent. PP release is mediated by vagal stimulation and insulin-induced hypoglycemia.

Function. PP has a biphasic effect, initially increasing → then inhibiting pancreatic enzymes, water and electrolytes secretion. PP thus opposes secretin and CCK stimulatory effects. PP also increases gut motility and gastric emptying, as well as pyloric, ileocecal sphincters, colon and gallbladder relaxation. Marked episodic level fluctuations, average 200% within-day variation.

Test Purpose. 1) suspect endocrinous active gastrointestinal tract tumor, 2) secretory diarrhea diagnosis/monitoring.

Increased Values
diabetes mellitus, duodenal ulcer disease, pancreatic insufficiency, carcinoid, advancing age, metastases of islet tumors, tumors – (adenocarcinoma of pancreas, t. of colon, **gastrinoma**, **glucagonoma**, **insulinoma**, t. of rectum, t. of thyroid, **VIPoma**, t. of stomach), multiple endocrine neoplasia (MEN), **renal failure**
    Interfering Factors: postprandial condition, stress

Decreased Values
chronic pancreatitis with exocrine insufficiency
    Interfering Factors: medicaments – (anticholinergics, morphine)

Analyte	Age/Gender	Reference Range	SI Units	Note
Pancreatic Polypeptide		<150	pmol/l	

Pantothenic Acid

Beta-alanine and pantoic acid amide. Vitamin B-complex component (vitamin B_5). Pantothenic acid is widely spreaded naturally in coenzyme A form. Pantothenic acid eaten with food is hydrolyzed on pantein in the intestine and together with pantothenate is absorbed. Human intestine flora synthesizes a sufficient amount of acid.

Test Purpose. Deficiency evidence.

Decreased Values
anorexia nervosa, conditions – (immunodeficiency c., septic c.), malabsorption sy, prolonged parenteral nutrition

Analyte	Age/Gender	Reference Range	SI Units	Note
Vitamin B_5 (pantothenic acid)		4.7–8.4	µmol/l	

Paraproteins

Monoclonal immunoglobulin forms come from one plasmocyte or cell clone. To the monoclonal immunoglobulins belong complete immunoglobulin molecules, Bence Jones protein, and free immunoglobulin H-chains.

Test Purpose. 1) to help in diagnosis of myeloma, Waldenström's disease, heavy chain disease, Bence Jones myeloma, 2) to help in diagnosis of anemias, blood clotting disorders, hyperproteinemias, Bence Jones proteinuria, and unexplained ESR acceleration.

Increased Values – paraproteinemia

gammapathy – (benign monoclonal g., polyclonal g.), heavy chain disease (Franklin disease), Bence Jones myeloma, myelomatosis, **Waldenström's macroglobulinemia**, malignant lymphoproliferative diseases, cryoglobulinemia.

Parathyroid Hormone

(PTH, syn: parathormone, parathyrin)

Production. Polypeptide hormone (a molecule of 84 amino acids) synthesized and secreted from parathyroid chief epithelial cells. There are 2 pre-steps (pre-PTH and pro-PTH) in intact PTH synthesis. It is metabolized in circulation on 2 main fragments, the N-terminal (biologically active, half-time few minutes) and the C-terminal fragment. Mid-regional fragment (antibody against synthetic fragment 44–68, biologically inactive, half-life about 3 – 5 hours) also exists. This first generation of PTH assays measure many blood borne fragments of PTH along with PTH. The second generation PTH assays are called "intact" PTH assays and they measure a large fragment of PTH (likely PTH 7-84) along with PTH. This PTH 7-84 fragment is a biological inhibitor of PTH. The third generation of PTH assays (most sensitive) measure only PTH 1-84.

Function. Calcium/phosphate homeostasis regulating hormone through its combined actions on the bone, intestine and kidney. Parathormone increases the extracellular calcium fluid level by the osteolysis stimulation which effects the osteoclasts. Increases Ca^{2+} and Mg^{2+} renal tubular reabsorption, decreases phosphate and bicarbonate renal tubular reabsorption. PTH also increases lactate and ALP production. PTH causes the intestine to increase calcium and phosphorus absorption. Parathormone is involved in calcium resorption from small intestine by vitamin D3. PTH stimulates the $1,25(OH)_2D3$ production via 25-hydroxy-cholecalciferol hydroxylation $\rightarrow$ which stimulates calcium and phosphorus intestinal absorption. A substantial part of the PTH effect can be focused on the calcitriol effect. In dialysis patients good laboratory medicine is to identify which dialysis patients have adynamic low bone turnover disease in order to avoid soft tissue and vascular calcification from mistreatment with vitamin D. A large bone histology study revealed that neither the 1st or 2nd or 3rd generation of PTH assays could satisfactorily identify which dialysis patients who had never received vitamin D therapy had adynamic low bone turnover disease. However, when a ratio of 3rd generation PTH/PTH 7-84 was calculated that then those patients with adynamic low bone turnover disease could be identified as they all had a ratio value of less than one. The PTH 7-84 is calculated by subtracting the 3rd generation PTH test value from a 2nd generation PTH test value (when that 2nd generation PTH test has 100% cross reactivity with PTH 7-84). Then the ratio is determined by dividing the 3rd generation PTH test value by the calculated PTH 7-84 value. A ratio of less than 1. 0 indicates adynamic low bone turnover.

Release. Mainly by calcium level decrease, magnesium level decrease, phosphorus level increase. Release inhibition is mediated by increased calcium levels. Metabolism: in the liver and kidney. Highest values are at 4 PM, it gradually decreases to nadir at 8 AM. Within-day variation is 30%. Values are higher in summer than in winter; in women gradual increase peaks at midcycle.

Test Purpose. 1) to aid differential diagnosis of parathyroid disorders, 2) C-terminal PTH – secondary and terciary hypoparathyroidism assessment, 3) N-terminal PTH – diagnosis of primary hypoparathyroidism, 4) mid-regional PTH is the most potent parameter because of the great indication range and possibility of parathyroidism assessment, 5) to monitor patients undergoing renal dialysis, 6) to help in the diagnosis of tumors and hyperplasia of the parathyroid gland as well as in localizing hyperfunctioning parathyroid tissue by assay of samples obtained via venous catheterization.

Increased Values

vitamin D deficiency, fluorosis, primary hyperparathyroidism – (adenocarcinoma, **parathyroid hyperplasia**), **secondary hyperparathyroidism**, familial hypocalciuric hypercalcemia, hyperthyroidism, **hypocalcemia**, transient neonatal hypocalcemia, hypomagnesemia, diseases – (**chronic renal d.**, liver d.), renal insufficiency, tumors of – (kidney, pancreas, lung, ovary, pituitary gland, liver, breast), ectopic PTH-producing tumors, nephrolithiasis, obesity, **osteomalacia**, **pseudohypoparathyroidism**, pseudogout, **rickets**, syndrome – (DiGeorge sy, malabsorption sy, paraneoplastic sy, Zollinger-Ellison sy), pregnancy (1st trimester), spinal cord trauma, urolithiasis, renal failure

> **Interfering Factors:** lactation, postprandial, medicaments – (antiepileptics, anticonvulsants, corticosteroids, estrogens, furosemide, glucocorticoids, isoniazid, lithium, octreotide, omeprazole, phenytoin, rifampicin)

Decreased Values

hemochromatosis, **hypercalcemia**, hyperthyroidism, transient neonatal hypocalcemia, **hypomagnesemia**, **hypoparathyroidism**, thymic hypoplasia, diseases – (**autoimmune d.**, hereditary d.), intoxication by – (aluminium, vitamin A and D), **Graves' disease**, Wilson's disease, **metastatic bone tumors**, hematopoietic malignancies, following I 131 therapy, **sarcoidosis**, postoperative states, syndrome – (**DiGeorge sy, milk alkali sy**), pregnancy (3rd trimester)

> **Interfering Factors:** exercise, high-protein diet, milk ingestion, medicaments – (cimetidine, calcium gluconate, pindolol, propranolol, ranitidine, thiazides)

Analyte	Age/Gender	Reference Range	SI Units	Note
Parathormone	Children	55–195	ng/l	
	Adults M	67–135	ng/l	
	Adults F	50–88	ng/l	
		1.5–6.5	pmol/l	
	pregnancy	80–230	ng/l	

Parathyroid Hormone-Related Protein

(PTHrP) The test is of value as a tumor marker in some malignancies to monitor progress.

Increased Values

tumors, lymphedema, renal insufficiency, non-malignant pheochromocytoma, mammary hypertrophy, normal lactation

Analyte	Age/Gender	Reference Range	SI Units	Note
Parathyroid Hormone-Related Protein	Antibodies 1–34		<2.5	pmol/l
	Antibodies 53–84		<21	pmol/l

Pemphigoid Antibodies

Test Purpose. To help in diagnosis of bullous skin diseases.

Increased Values – positive
bullous pemphigoid

Pemphigus Antibodies

Intercelullar cement substance antibody is specific for pemphigus.
Test Purpose. To help in diagnosis of bullous skin diseases, 2) to help in differentiation between pemphigus and pemhigoid.

Increased Values – positive
pemphigus, burns, drug reactions, extensive skin damage

Pepsin

Production. Main gastric cells, mucous neck cells. It is in serum as an inactive precursor (pepsinogen), which activates to pepsin by acidifying. Pepsin begins proteolysis, stimulated by cholinergic (vagal) input and local gastric acid.

Analyte	Age/Gender	Reference Range	SI Units	Note
Pepsin	Neonates	10–138	nkat/l	
	Children	17–51	nkat/l	
	Adults	13–43	nkat/l	

Pepsinogen

(PSG) Pepsinogen is an inactive pepsin precursor.
Production. Most pepsinogen (99%) is synthesized and stored as zymogen granules and secreted by gastric mucose glands main cells → enters the stomach where it is activated to pepsin. Seven pepsinogen blood fractions have been identified; 5 of them are called group I (PSG I, pepsinogen A) and are found only in fundus main and mucous neck cells, two are called group II (PSG II, pepsinogen C) and are found in other stomach and duodenum glands. Pepsinogen I is present in serum and urine (higher levels). Pepsinogen II is present in serum and seminal fluid. Pepsinogen A is a marker of mucous membrane atrophy and a subclinical marker of duodenal ulcer disease in genetic studies. Pepsinogen is a marker of gastric mucous membrane state and a marker of Helicobacter pylori infection eradication. Secretion stomach lumen pepsinogen level is related to the main cell mass and controlled by gastrin. Pepsinogen secretion is stimulated by the vagus nerve and gastrointestinal hormones (gastrin, secretin, cholecystokinin). Secretion is inhibited by gastric inhibitory polypeptide, anticholinergics, histamine H_2-receptor antagonists and vagotomy. Blood group "A" carriers have lower PSG levels in comparison to "O" group carriers.
Test Purpose. 1) gastric secretion assessment, 2) monitoring in gastric neoplasia, 3) to help in gastric ulcer and gastric cancer differential diagnosis, 4) monitoring of Helicobacter pylori infection eradication.

Increased Values – hyperpepsinogenemia
gastrinoma, acute/chronic gastritis, hypergastrinemia, ulcer disease – (**duodenal u. d., gastric u. d.** – PSG I), **Zollinger-Ellison sy, increased gastric acid output**

Decreased Values – hypopepsinogenemia
achlorhydria, histamine-resistant achlorhydria, **pernicious anemia, atrophic gastritis,** hypogastrinemia, hypopituitarism, gastric ulcer disease, **Addison's disease, myxedema, gastric neoplasia,** gastric resection

C-Peptide

The presence of C-peptide distinguishes endogenous insulin secretion from exogenous insulin administration. C-peptide is formed during insulin creation by proinsulin proteolytic splitting to insulin in the pancreas Langerhans' islands beta-cells. Normally a strong correlation exists between insulin levels and C-peptide. C-peptide is an endogenous insulin synthesis by-product and endogenous insulin production marker. Insulin and C-peptide are secreted simultaneously by equimolar quantities into the portal blood. During the first-pass circulation, a considerable variable insulin proportion is extracted by the liver, but almost all C-peptide enters the systemic circulation intact. Most C-peptide is degraded in the kidney, a small intact peptide amount is excreted in the urine unchanged. Day-to-day variation is 10%.

Test Purpose. 1) to assess serum insulin concentrations, 2) to help in insulinoma suspicion diagnosis and differential diagnosis, 3) to assess post-pancreatitis and post-pancreatectomy conditions, 4) to assess beta-cell function in diabetes, 5) to evaluate a hypoglycemia.

Increased Values
decreased renal function, hyperinsulinism, **insulinoma, non-insulin dependent diabetes mellitus** (NIDDM, type II), insulin-secreting neoplasms, obesity, **pancreas/beta-cells transplants, renal failure**
> **Interfering Factors:** medicaments – (chloroquine, danazol, ethinylestradiol, oral hypoglycemic agents, oral contraceptives)

Decreased Values
starvation, **factitious hypoglycemia,** hypoinsulinism – (NIDDM, **IDDM**), Addison's disease, **radical pancreatectomy**
> **Interfering Factors:** medicaments – (insulin)

Analyte	Age/Gender	Reference Range	SI Units	Note
C-Peptide		1.1–3.6	ng/ml	
		206–934	pmol/l	

Phenothiazines

Test Purpose. 1) to check for suspected phenothiazine toxicity from patient history or clinical examination, 2) to monitor compliance with therapy, 3) to detect phenothiazines for medical-legal purposes.

Increased Values
phenothiazines overdose

Phenylalanine

(Phe, syn: phenylalanine screening, phenylketonuria test, PKU test, Guthrie screening test)
Phenylalanine is an essential amino acid necessary for growth; however, any excess must be converted to tyrosine. Enzyme defect: phenylalanine hydroxylase, converting phenylalanine to tyrosine. An infant with phenylalanine hydroxylase deficiency lacks the ability to make this necessary conversion; thus, phenylalanine accumulates and spills over into the urine.
Test Purpose. To screen infants for possible phenylketonuria.

Increased Values – hyperphenylalaninemia
low-birth-weight infants, hepatic encephalopathy, false positive values – (premature infants), **phenylketonuria,** galactosemia, viral hepatitis, severe burns, sepsis, transient tyrosinemia in newborns
    Interfering Factors: medicaments – (ampicillin, aspartame, cotrimoxazole)

Decreased Values – hypophenylalaninemia
false negative values – (infants tested before 24 hours of age, feeding problems)
    Interfering Factors: medicaments – (ascorbic acid, glucose, histidine, progesterone – high doses)

Phenytoin

This drug exhibits Michaelis–Menten kinetics, i. e. as serum levels rise, a stage is reached when a small increase in dose causes a large increase in serum levels.
Test Purpose. To monitor therapy.

Increased Values
phenytoin overdose

Analyte	Age/Gender	Reference Range	SI Units	Note
Phenytoin	Premature infants	24–56	µmol/l	
	Adults	20–80	µmol/l	

Phospholipase A2

(syn: human soluble phospholipase A2 – h-sPLA2) Lipolytic enzyme which hydrolyzes phospholipids in position 2 creating equivalent FFA and lysophospholipid amounts. Enzyme is widely spreaded in nature; present in leukocytes, macrophages, erythrocytes, thrombocytes, vascular smooth muscle cells, and chondrocytes. It is released from cells into inflammatory exudation in pathological conditions. The highest organ activity is in pancreas, stomach, intestine, heart, lung, and ejaculate with two isotypes 14 kD (type 1–3) and 85 kD (type 4). High activity can be determined in synovial fluid and inflammatory exudates (isoform 2). Cytokines stimulate their production/secretion. PLA2 presence in atherosclerotic plaque and its development is discussed.

Increased Values
rheumatoid arthritis, diseases – (autoimmune d., intestine inflammatory d., cardiovascular d., inflammatory d.), myocardial infarction, ulcerative colitis, acute pancreatitis, bacterial pneumonia, psoriasis, bacterial sepsis, septic shock, vasculitides.

Analyte	Age/Gender	Reference Range	SI Units	Note
Phospholipase		<1	ng/ml	
	sensitivity	1.25	ng/ml	

Phospholipids

(PL) Phospholipids are involved in cell membrane composition and permeability, as well as controlling enzyme activity within the membrane. They are involved in fatty acids and lipids transport across the intestinal barrier, from the liver and other fat depots to other body tissues. They are essential for pulmonary gas exchange, as a component of lung surfactant, and participate in signal transmission across membranes. There are two phospholipids classes, those that have glycerol as a backbone (phosphoglycerides) and those that contain sphingosine (sphingolipids, sphingomyelin). Phospholipids are synthesized in the smooth endoplasmic reticulum. Lung surfactant is dipalmitoyl phosphatidyl choline secreted by pneumocytes. Although phospholipids create the 2nd biggest part of lipids (30%), the clinical importance/applications are inferior.

Test Purpose. 1) to aid in the fat metabolism evaluation, 2) to aid in the diagnosis of hypothyroidism, diabetes mellitus, nephrotic sy, chronic pancreatitis, obstructive jaundice and hypolipoproteinemia.

Increased Values – hyperphospholipidemia
alcoholism, hepatic cirrhosis – (alcoholic h. c., primary biliary h. c.), **diabetes mellitus**, viral hepatitis, hyperlipoproteinemia IIa, IIb, hypothyroidism, cholestasis, **obstructive jaundice**, myocardial infarction, von Gierke's disease, **chronic pancreatitis**, **nephrotic sy**, pregnancy

   Interfering Factors: medications – (adrenaline, chlorpromazine, estrogens, oral contraceptives)

Decreased Values – hypophospholipidemia
abetalipoproteinemia, anemia – (sickle-cell a., pernicious a., hereditary spherocytosis), severe viral hepatitis, hyperthyroidism, **hypolipoproteinemia**, **Tangier disease**, sclerosis multiplex, neonatal respiratory distress sy, LCAT deficiency

   Interfering Factors: medications – (acetylsalicylic acid, asparaginase, cholestyramine, clofibrate, niacin, thyroxine)

Analyte	Age/Gender	Reference Range	SI Units	Note
Phospholipids, Total	Neonates	0.75–1.70	g/l	
	Infants	1.00–2.75	g/l	
	Children	1.80–2.95	g/l	
	Adults	1.25–2.75	g/l	

Phosphorus

(P, syn: inorganic phosphorus, inorganic phosphate, phosphate, phosphates, PO_4) Most of the blood phosphorus exists as phosphates or esters.

Function. Phosphorus is required for bony tissue generation (85%), teeth, in the metabolism of glucose and lipids, in acid-base balance maintenance, in energy storage/transfer. Component of DNA, RNA, vitamins – thiamine, niacin, riboflavin, pyridoxine. Phosphorus levels are always evaluated in relation to ALP activity, serum calcium levels, urine calcium and phosphorus levels respectively; there is an inverse relationship between the two. Phosphorus entering the cell with glucose is lowered following carbohydrate ingestion. Phosphorus levels are determined by calcium metabolism, parathormone (PTH) and to a lesser degree by intestinal absorption. Phosphate PTH regulation is such that PTH tends to decrease phosphate reabsorption in the kidney. Dietary phosphorus is absorbed in the small bowel. There are marked differences in patterns from person to person. Overall day-to-day concentrations variation is 5 – 10%; highest are in summer and lowest in winter. In women, lower during menstruation.

Test Purpose. 1) to aid renal disorders and acid-base imbalance diagnosis, 2) to detect endocrine, skeletal and calcium disorders.

Increased Values – hyperphosphatemia

acidosis – (diabetic a., **lactate a.,** respiratory a.), **acromegaly,** anemia – (**sickle cell a.,** thalassemia), acute yellow hepatic atrophy, dehydration, dysproteinemia, ethylism, **hemolysis,** hyperbilirubinemia, **familial intermittent hyperphosphatemia,** hyperlipidemia, **secondary hyperparathyroidism, hypervitaminosis D, malignant hyperthermia, hyperthyroidism,** juvenile hypogonadism, **hypocalcemia, hypomagnesemia, hypoparathyroidism,** diseases – **(liver d., bone d.), vitamin D intoxication, acute/chronic renal insufficiency,** tissue ischemia, **tumoral calcinosis, catabolism,** diabetic coma, chemotherapy, lysis – (cell l., **acute tumour l.), Addison's disease,** Paget's disease, **bone metastases,** tumours – (t. of bone, **leucemia,** lymphoma, plasmocytoma – incl. multiple myeloma), intestinal obstruction, burns, increased intake of phosphates intravenously/orally – (**phosphorus,** alkaline agents), ectopic production of parathormone, **pseudohypoparathyroidism, rhabdomyolysis, sarcoidosis, transfusion of stored blood, milk-alkali syndrome, fractures in the healing stage, renal failure**

> **Interfering Factors:** children, phosphate enemas, menopause, prolonged sample cooling, medicaments – (anabolics, androgens, asparaginase, calcifediol, calcitriol, clonidine, contraceptives, cytostatics, dihydrotachysterol, doxercalciferol, ergocalciferol, etidronate, growth hormone, laxatives, methicillin, nephrotoxic medicaments, paricalcitol, phosphorus salts, vitamin D)

Decreased Values – hypophosphatemia

alcohol abuse, acidosis – (lactic a., renal tubular a.), alkalosis – (metabolic a., **respiratory a.),** anorexia nervosa, **renal tubular defects, vitamin D deficiency, gout, diabetes mellitus, chro-nic ethylism,** glycosuria, **hemodialysis, starvation, diarrhea, hyperalimentation, hyper-insulinism, hypercalcemia,** idiopathic hypercalciuria, hypercorticism, **primary**/secondary **hyperparathyroidism,** hyperventilation, **hypokalemia, hypomagnesemia,** hypoparathyroidism, **primary hypophosphatemia,** hypothyroidism, hepatic diseases, **chronic renal insufficiency,** fructose intolerance, salicylate poisoning, cardiomyopathy, **diabetic ketoacidosis,** ketoacidosis treatment, **malabsorption, malnutrition,** menstruation, tumours, nasogastric suction, metabolic causes, **osteomalacia,** osteoporosis, pseudohypoparathyroidism, severe burns, disorders – (neuromuscular d., renal d., **severe nutritional d.),** hepatocellular impairment, increased carbohydrate intake, **vitamin D resistant rachitis** (rickets), **sepsis,** prolonged hypothermia, postrenal transplantation conditions, total parenteral nutrition, syndrome – (**Fanconi's sy,** Cushing's sy), urolithiasis, pregnancy, tetany, recovery from starvation, **vomiting**

> **Interfering Factors:** medicaments – (acetazolamide, ACTH, adrenaline, aldesleukin, alendronate, aluminium hydroxide, anabolic steroids, androgens, antacids, bumetanide, calcitonin, calcium carbonate, carboplatin, catecholamines, cisplatin, continuous administration of iv. glucose, contraceptives, corticosteroids, diuretics, estradiol, estrogens, fructose, glucagon, indapamide, insulin, lithium, mannitol, mithramycin, mycophenolate, niacin, pamidronate, phenothiazines, phenytoin, plicamycin, risedronate, salicylates, steroids, streptozocin, sucralfate, thiazide diuretics, total parenteral nutrition)

Analyte	Age/Gender	Reference Range	SI Units	Note
Inorganic Phosphate	Neonates	1.6–3.1	mmol/l	
	2–12 m	1.6–3.5	mmol/l	
	> 1 y	1.1–2.0	mmol/l	
	Adults	0.87–1.45	mmol/l	

Phytanate

Test Purpose. To help in diagnosis of Refsum's disease and some other peroxisomal diseases.

Increased Values
Refsum's disease, Zellweger disease, large intake of dairy foods

Plasma Volume

Increased Values
acidosis, anemia, hepatic cirrhosis, emphysema, overhydration, renal insufficiency, macro-globulinemia, plasmocytoma, recumbency, polycythemia, splenomegaly, pregnancy (3rd trimester), thyrotoxicosis, vasodilation, cardiac failure
  Interfering Factors: carbon dioxide, chloroform, medicaments – (anesthetics, halothane, morphine, thiopental, vasodilators)

Decreased Values
dehydration due to salt loss, diabetes mellitus, smoking, arterio-venous fistula, diarrhea, tissue hypoxia, chronic infectious diseases, acute hemorrhage, older people, upright position, preeclampsia, radiation, vomiting
  Interfering Factors: medicaments – (vasoconstrictors)

Platelet Derived Endothelial Cell Growth Factor

(PD-ECGF)
Occurrence. Platelets, stromal cells of placenta, fibroblasts, vascular smooth muscle cells, some tumor cells.
Function. Stimulates angiogenesis, inhibits astrocyte and glial cell growth. Promotes survival, differentiation and regeneration of CNS neurons.

Platelet Derived Growth Factor

(PDGF) PDGF is a cytokine dimer composed from two polypeptide chains. Platelets synthesize a mixture of isomorphs AA, AB, BB. PDGF is synthesized mainly by megakaryocytes.
Occurrence. Platelet alpha granulations, endothelial cells, monocytes, macrophages, smooth muscle cells, fibroblasts, cytotrophoblasts, myoblasts, glial cells, neurons. PDGF receptors are expressed at a density of 40.000–300.000 copies per cell in fibroblasts, osteoblasts, chondroblasts, smooth muscle cells, glial cells and endothelial cells.
Function. Potent mitogen for dermal fibroblasts, glial cells, smooth muscle cells, epithelial and endothelial cells (angiogenic factor). Chemotactic for fibroblasts, smooth muscle cells, neutrophils and mononuclear cells. Inhibits NK-cells activity. PDGF is probably involved in myelofibrosis, atherosclerosis, rheumatoid arthritis and some glomerulonephritides patho-

genesis; also involved in tumor growth acceleration (melanoma, sarcoma, thyroid tumors). Stimulates granule release by neutrophils and monocytes. Stimulates collagen synthesis. PDGF binds to several plasma proteins and also to proteins of the extracellular matrix which facilitates local concentration of the factor. The factor functions as a local autocrine and paracrine growth factor. In the adult organism PDGF is involved in wound healing processes.

Increased Values
obliterative bronchiolits

Polyspecific Antibodies

IgM and IgG antibodies that are polyspecific bind to a wide range of glycolipids. They occur in many disorders and do not predict a specific neurologic disorder or clinical syndrome. They probably reflect the presence of an ongoing immune phenomenon with analogy to an elevated sedimentation rate or a moderately positive ANA.

Porphyrins

Production. From porphin. Porphyrins or heme synthesis disorders lead to accumulation and increased excretion of some porphyrin metabolism components. Porphyrins metabolism is always evaluated totally, serum and RBC porphyrins, and total urine porphobilinogen excretion determination, with distinguishing coproporphyrin I and III, uroporphyrin resp. and intermediary urine porphyrins, and delta-aminolevulic acid excretion.

Function. Porphyrins form chelates, which are hemoglobin, myoglobin, cytochrome biosynthesis constituents. Proteins used in the hemoglobin heme synthesis. The majority of blood porphyrins are found in the erythrocytes. Coproporphyrins, uroporphyrins and protoporphyrins belong to porphyrins. Enzyme activities in porphyrin biosynthesis: delta-aminolevulic dehydratase (porphobilinogen synthase), uroporphyrinogen-I synthase (URO-S, porphobilinogen deaminase), uroporphyrinogen decarboxylase (URO-D).

Test Purpose. 1) to help in diagnosis of congenital erythropoietic porphyria, erythropoietic protoporphyria, 2) diagnosis of chronic hepatic porphyrias, incl. porphyria cutanea tarda, acute hepatic porphyrias, acute intermittent porphyria and variegate porphyria, 3) lead and heavy metals intoxication, 4) iron metabolism disorders diagnosis, 5) bone marrow tumours monitoring. Sometimes it is necessary to determine porphyrins in stools, bone marrow or in liver biopsy samples as a part of the differential diagnosis. Delta-aminolevulinic dehydratase – diagnosis of: 1) lead intoxication, 2) chronic alcoholism, 3) alcohol-liver-porphyrin syndrome, 4) hereditary synthesis defect. Uroporphyrinogen-I-synthase – diagnosis of: 1) genetically determined enzymopathies, 2) acute intermittent porphyria, 3) differential diagnosis of variegate porphyria and hereditary coproporphyria. Uroporphyrinogen decarboxylase – diagnosis of: 1) chronic hepatic porphyria, 2) porphyria cutanea tarda, 3) hepatoerythropoietic porphyria.

Increased Values
anemia – (hemolytic a., iron deficiency a.), chronic renal insufficiency, **lead intoxication**, iron deficiency, porphyria – (**acute p.,** erythropoietic p., **chronic p.**), porphyria cutanea tarda, increased protoporphyrin production

Decreased Values
acute intermittent porphyria (URO-S), alcoholism, low-carbohydrate diet, bleeding disorders, liver diseases

Potassium

(K, syn: kalium, kalium cation)

Function. Principal intracellular cation and primary intracellular buffer. Together with sodium it helps to maintain the nervous system electrical potential and muscle excitability, acid-base balance and osmotic pressure. It is essential for nerve and muscle functioning. Potassium is filtered at the glomerulus → approximately 90% is reabsorbed in the proximal tubule and the ascending Henle's loop and about 10% of the filtered load reaches the distal tubule where the body potassium regulation occurs through secretion in exchange for sodium under the aldosterone influence. Serum potassium concentration depends on: 1) aldosterone – increases potassium renal loses, 2) sodium reabsorption – as sodium is reabsorbed, potassium is lost, 3) acid-base balance – alkalotic states tend to lower serum potassium levels by causing potassium shift into the cell. Acidotic states tend to raise serum potassium levels by reversing that shift. Highest values are at 8 AM, decreasing during day, within-day variation is 20%.

Test Purpose. 1) to evaluate clinical signs of potassium excess/depletion with special interest on intensively treated patients, 2) to monitor renal functions, 3) to monitor acid-base balance and glucose metabolism, 4) to evaluate neuromuscular disorders, 5) to evaluate endocrine disorders, 6) to detect arrhythmia origins, 7) to monitor diuretic therapy, 8) to monitor hypertension, 9) intestinal secretion loss monitoring, 10) mineral disorders monitoring.

Increased Values – hyperkalemia

acidosis – (**metabolic a.,**respiratory a.), anemia – (sickle-cell a., hemolytic a.), renal tubular acidosis, **amyloidosis**, anorexia nervosa, anuria, **insulin deficiency**, **dehydration**, diabetes mellitus, dialysis, coronary bypass, **hemolysis**, blood hemolysis during venipuncture, **acute starvation**, congenital adrenal hyperplasia, **malignant hyperpyrexia**, **hypoaldosteronism**, **chemotherapy**, diseases – (**infectious d., renal d.**), interstitial nephritis, prostaglandin synthesis inhibition, insufficiency – (**acute/chronic renal i.**, adrenal i.), **digitalis intoxication**, **catabolism**, diabetic coma, **internal hemorrhage, leucocytosis, systemic lupus erythematosus, tumorlysis**, Addison's disease, **tissue necrosis**, sickle cell nephrosis, familial **hyperkalemic periodic paralysis, burns, crush injuries, plasmocytoma** (incl. multiple myeloma), renal tubular disorders, **prolonged tourniquet use during blood sampling**, increased potassium intake – (**infusion, peroral, old blood transfusion**, exchange transfusion in neonates), pseu-dohypoaldosteronism, factitious hyperkalemia, **rhabdomyolysis**, syndrome – (Liddle's sy, Bartter's sy), status epilepticus, **postoperative states**, shock, **renal transplantation, severe thrombocytosis**, severe trauma, **obstructive uropathy**, medium physical exertion, failure – (**acute/chronic renal f.**, heart f.), transfusion reaction, ureteral implants into jejunum, cephalohematoma in newborns, intracranial hemorrhage in newborns

Interfering Factors: medicaments – (ACE inhibitors, ACTH, adrenaline – initial effect, aldesleukin, amiloride, aminocaproic acid, amlodipine, amphotericin B, arginine, benazepril, beta-blockers, bromfenac, candesartan, captopril, ce-phalosporins, cyclophosphamide, cyclosporine, cytostatics, dextrose, digitalis, digitoxin, digoxin, diltiazem, disopyramide, enalapril, epoietin, eprosartan, ethanol, fosinopril, glycosides, heparin, histamine, hydrochlorothiazide, hydrocodone, ibuprofen, indomethacin, interferon, irbesartan, isoniazid, lisinopril, lithium, losartan, mannitol, menotropins, methicillin, moexipril, mycophenolate, naproxen, nonsteroid anti-inflammatory agents, penicillins, pentamidine, perindopril, phenformin, phosphorus salts, pindolol, pipecuronium piroxicam, potassium sparing diuretics, potassium supplements, propranolol, quinapril, ramipril, spirapril, spironolactone, succinylcholine, sulfamethoxazole, suxamethonium, tacrolimus, telmisartan, tetracyclines, timolol, trandolapril, triamterene, trimetaphan, trimethoprim, valsartan, vincristine)

Decreased Values – hypokalemia

renal tubular acidosis, vilous rectum adenoma, alkalosis – (**metabolic a., respiratory a.**), **anorexia nervosa, anuria, bulimia,** delirium tremens, **magnesium depletion, osmotic diuresis,** ileostomy drainage, ectopic ACTH production, delirium tremens, pheochromocytoma, **intestinal/biliary fistulas, chronic starvation, diarrhea, primary/secondary hyperaldosteronism, primary adrenal hyperplasia,** dexamethasone suppression, hypertension – (**malignant h.,** renovascular h.), hyperthyroidism, **hypomagnesemia,** diseases – (endocrine d., infectious d., liver d. with ascites, **renal d.**), **acute/chronic renal insufficiency, diabetic ketoacidosis, acute leukemia,** infusion therapy, Cushing's disease, **malabsorption, malnutrition, mineralocorticoid excess, renin producing tumors,** pancreatic VIPoma, **acute/chronic nephritis, nephrosclerosis, pyloric obstruction, gastrointestinal suctioning, hypokalemic periodic paralysis, severe burns, sweating, insufficient potassium intake, pyelonephritis,** conditions – (anabolic c., chronic febrile c., **post-surgical c.**), **excessive potassium depletion,** gastrointestinal loss, stress, syndrome – (**Bartter's sy,** Conn's sy, **Cushing's sy,** Liddle's sy, **Fanconi's sy,** Zollinger-Ellison sy), tobacco chewing, toluene intoxication, thyrotoxicosis, **ureterosigmoidostomy,** vasculitis, vomiting, radiation, cystic fibrosis, draining wounds, treatment of severe megaloblastic anemia with vitamin B_{12} or folic acid, neonatal asphyxia

   Interfering Factors: highly trained athletes, medicaments – (acetazolamide, ACTH, beta-adrenergic agonists, albuterol, aldesleukin, alprostadil, aminoglycosides, aminophylline, aminosalicylic acid, ammonium chloride, amphotericin B, ampicillin, asparaginase, atenolol, azlocillin, barbiturates, benzylpenicillin, betamethasone, bisacodyl, bisoprolol, bumetadine, calcitonin, capreomycin, captopril, carbamazepine, carbenicillin, carbenoxolone, carboplatin, chlorothiazide, chlortalidone, cholestyramine, cisplatin, clindamycin, clopamide, corticosteroids, cortisone, cyanocobalamin, dexamethasone, dextrose, diclofenamide, digitoxin, digoxin, disopyramide, diuretics – initial effect, dobutamine, enoloxone, epinephrine, ergocalciferol, estrogens, ethacrynic acid, fenoldopam, fenoterol, fluconazole, fludrocortisone, fluorides, foscarnet, fosinopril, furosemide, gastrin, gemtuzumab, gentamicin, glucagon, glucocorticoids, glucose, hydrochlorothiazide, hydrocortisone, indapamide, insulin, irbesartan, isoniazid, itraconazole, lactulose, laxatives, levodopa, magnesium salts, mannitol, methicillin, methylprednisolone, metolazone, mezlocillin, mifepristone, mineralcorticoids, mycophenolate, nafcillin, nifedipine, oprelvekin, pamidronate, penicillin G, phenothiazines, phenytoin, phosphates, piperacillin, plicamycin, polymyxin B, polythiazide, prednisolone, prednisone, rimiterol, ritodrine, salbutamol, salicylates, salmeterol, sirolimus, sodium bicarbonate, sodium chloride, sodium polystyrene sulfonate, steroids, terbutaline, tetracyclines, theophylline, thiazides, ticarcillin, torsemide, triamcinolone, urea, vitamin B_{12})

Analyte	Age/Gender	Reference Range	SI Units	Note
Potassium (Kalium)	1 d–4 w	3.6–6.1	mmol/l	
	2–12 m	3.6–5.8	mmol/l	
	>1 y	3.1–5.1	mmol/l	
	Adults	3.6–4.8	mmol/l	

Prealbumin

(PA, syn: tryptophan-rich prealbumin, transthyretin – TTR, thyroxine-binding prealbumin – TBPA).

Production. Prealbumin is synthesized by the liver.

Function. Transport protein for T3, T4 (TBPA) and retinol-binding protein – RBP, up to 50% of circulating prealbumin is bounded to this protein. Binds about 10–25% of T4 and less than 10% of T3. It has a low affinity, therefore it plays a greater role in delivering iodothyronines to the tissue. TTR probably functions by inhibiting processing of newly synthesized peptides for secretion. TTR thus may act as an endogenous antiinflammatory mediator. Transthyretin is a very sensitive negative acute phase protein.

Test Purpose. 1) liver diseases diagnosis, 2) protein synthesis assessment in parenteral nutrition, 3) nutrition status assessment.

Increased Values
adrenal hyperfunction, hypothyroidism, Hodgkin's disease
  Interfering Factors: medicaments – (anabolic steroids, androgens, corticosteroids, estrogens, non-steroid antiinflammatory agents, prednisolone)

Decreased Values
hepatic cirrhosis, zinc deficiency, cystic fibrosis, hyperthyroidism, diseases – (chronic d., inflammatory d.), **malnutrition**, tumours
  Interfering Factors: medicaments – (amiodarone, androgens, estrogens, oral contraceptives)

Analyte	Age/Gender	Reference Range	SI Units	Note
Prealbumin		0.1–0.4	g/l	

Alpha-2-Pregnancy-Associated Glycoprotein

(alpha-2-PAG, SP3, syn: pregnancy zone protein – PZP) This protein is a major pregnancy associated serum protein; this large globulin is synthesized in the liver. Tissue localization has identified the protein in the syncytiotrophoblast and on B-lymphocytes and monocytes surface.

Increased Values
tumors, pregnancy
  Interfering Factors: medicaments – (estrogens, oral contraceptives)

Pregnancy-Associated Plasma Protein A

(PAPP-A)

Increased Values
eclampsia, tumors
  Interfering Factors: medicaments – (oral contraceptives)

Pregnenolone

Intermediate in steroid hormones synthesis which is formed by cholesterol side chain cleavage.

Increased Values
hirsutism, adrenal tumors, ectopic ACTH secreting tumors, Cushing's sy
  Interfering Factors: medicaments – (ACTH, metoclopramide)

Prenatal Infectious Disease Antibodies

Test detects TORCH antibodies (toxoplasma, rubella, cytomegalovirus, herpes). Test includes: cytomegalovirus antibodies (IgM), herpes simplex I antibodies (IgM), herpes simplex II antibodies (IgM), rubella antibodies (IgM), Toxoplasma gondii antibodies (IgM). Demonstration of IgM antibody or rising titers of IgG antibody can confirm a diagnosis of specific infection. The availability of IgM specific assays also determines whether antibody in cord blood represents passive transfer from the mother (IgG antibody) or signifies congenital infection (IgM antibody).

Increased Values – positive
infectious diseases – (toxoplasmosis, rubella, cytomegalovirus infection, herpervirus infection)

Primidone

Phenobarbitone is an active metabolite of primidone. Steady state level of primidone is reached after 48 hours. Mean half-life is 10 hours (3–20 hours).
Test Purpose. To monitor drug therapy.

Increased Values
primidone overdose

Analyte	Age/Gender	Reference Range	SI Units	Note
Primidone		23–69	µmol/l	

Procainamide

Both procainamide and its major metabolite N-acetyl procainamide are active pharmacologically and should be measured, as the relative levels differ in slow or fast acetylators. Procainamide half-life is about 3 hours, whereas N-acetyl procainamide has a half-life of about 6–9 hours.
Test Purpose. To monitor drug therapy.

Increased Values
procainamide overdose

Analyte	Age/Gender	Reference Range	SI Units	Note
Procainamide		15–42	µmol/l	

Procalcitonin

(PCT) Precursor of calcitonin synthesized from pre-procalcitonin. Cleavaged into N-terminal end of calcitonin and katacalcin (PDN 21), which is known as other peptide placed on procalcitonin C-terminal end. PCT has a higher diagnostic validity in evaluation, monitoring and prognosis of severe infectious and septic conditions in comparison to other inflammatory parameters. PCT concentration increases during first 2–3 hours after infection beginning.

Test Purpose. 1) to help in early diagnosis of system infectious complications, 2) to monitor and follow therapeutic effect of bacterial, parasitic and mycotic infectious diseases treatment, 3) to help in differential diagnosis of febrile conditions of unclear etiology, 4) to monitor critically ill patients, 5) to help in prognostic evaluation of septic and shock conditions, multiorgan failure and acute pancreatitis.

Increased Values

severe infectious diseases – (**bacterial i. d., parasitic i. d., mycotic i. d.**), conditions – (**febrile c., shock c., septic c.**), multiorgan failure, acute pancreatitis, surgery, trauma of – (abdomen, thorax).

Analyte	Age/Gender	Reference Range	SI Units	Note
Procalcitonin		<0.5	µg/l	

Progesterone

The most important female sex hormone, gestagen.

Production. Ovarian corpus luteum, placental, adrenal cortex and testicular steroid hormone. In non-pregnant women, progesterone is secreted mainly by the corpus luteum; corpus luteum is a main progesterone production source until 8th pregnancy week. During pregnancy, the placenta becomes the major source of this hormone.

Function. Responsible for endometrium preparation during pregnancy, pregnancy maintenance, and prevents additional egg release from the ovary; involved in lactic gland development. Especially important in preparing the uterus for blastocyst implantation. Progesterone stimulates endometrial glandular secretion, decreases myometrial excitability and thick cervical mucus production, increases body temperature, inhibits gonadotropins (LH, FSH). Progesterone metabolites are pregnanolones, pregnanediones and pregnanediols. Plasma progesterone levels start to rise with the luteinizing hormone surge, continuing rise for approximately 6 to 10 days, and then falling. Released in episodic spikes during day in women. 20% day-to-day levels variation, highest levels are at bedtime and lowest are at 8 AM.

Test Purpose. 1) to assess corpus luteum function in infertility study algorithms, 2) to evaluate corpus luteum function and later placental function during pregnancy, 3) to aid in confirming ovulation; test results support basal body temperature readings, 4) to assess placental function during pregnancy and ovarian function.

Increased Values – hyperprogesteronemia

ovarian cysts, deficiency – (21-hydroxylase d., 17-alpha-hydroxylase d., **11-beta-hydroxylase d.**), **congenital adrenal hyperplasia,** tumors – (**chorionepithelioma of ovary, luteinizing t.,** adrenal t., ovary t.), **ovulation, pregnancy,** molar pregnancy

> **Interfering Factors:** medicaments – (clomiphene, corticosterone, 11-deoxycortisol, dihydroprogesterone, estrogens, ketoconazole, pregnanedione, progesterone)

Decreased Values – hypoprogesteronemia

amenorrhea, bulimia, exercise, **gonadal dysfunction, pregnancy induced hypertension, primary/secondary hypogonadism, panhypopituitarism, threatened abortion, galactorrhea, amenorrhea sy, fetal death,** short luteal phase syndrome

Interfering Factors: postprandial, medicaments – (ampicillin, cyclophosphamide, dana-zol, ethinylestradiol, interferon, oral contraceptives)

Analyte	Age/Gender	Reference Range	SI Units	Note
Progesterone	F			
	Follicular phase	0.95–3.5	nmol/l	
	Luteal phase	5.7–67	nmol/l	
	>60 y	<3.2	nmol/l	
	1st trimester	29–121	nmol/l	
	2nd trimester	60–413	nmol/l	
	3rd trimester	165–776	nmol/l	
	M	<0.95	nmol/l	

Proinsulin

Insulin precursor. Proinsulin is formed within the pancreatic beta-cells, with approximately 95% cleaved to insulin and C-peptide and 5% is directly secreted into the circulation.

Increased Values – hyperproinsulinemia
diabetes mellitus (type II), familial hyperproinsulinemia, hyperthyroidism, **insulinoma**, insulin-producing tumours, after meals, impaired glucose tolerance, factitious hypoglyc-emia (sulfonylurea).
    Interfering Factors: medicaments – (glucocorticoids, growth hormone, sulfonylurea)

Analyte	Age/Gender	Reference Range	SI Units	Note
Proinsulin		<25	ng/l	See ref.
		<3	pmol/l	ranges note.
		<25	ng/l	
		<3	pmol/l	
		77–102	ng/l	
		8.5–11.3	pmol/l	

Prolactin

(PRL, syn: luteotrophic hormone, lactogenic hormone, lactotropin, mammotropin, luteotro-pin)
Production. Anterior pituitary (adenohypophysis) hormone. Target organ is mammary gland. PRL production is stimulated by breast irritation, hypoglycemia, pregnancy, nursing, stress, exercise, norepinephrine, and endorphins; production is inhibited by dopamine.
Function. Involved in the female breast development and differentiation, in lactation initia-tion and maintenance, fetoplacental unit osmoregulation maintenance. Once milk produc-tion is established, lactation can continue without supranormal prolactin levels. Stimulates the corpus luteum progesterone production. Prolactin levels rise late in pregnancy, peaks with the lactation initiation and will surge each time lactating woman suckles the baby. Pro-lactin is a physiological infertility central regulator during lactation. Prolactin increases male prostate testosterone binding, it has a regulative effect on spermatozoa metabolism and sur-vival rate. Stimulates thymocyte proliferation, antibody production, cutaneous-graft rejec-tion, NK-cells, production of IL-1, IL-2, TNF-alpha and thymuline. Prolactin has been shown

also to have cytokine-like activities and to have important immunoregulatory activities. A prolactin-like molecule is synthesized and secreted by concanavalin A stimulated human peripheral blood mononuclear cells and functions in an autocrine manner as a growth factor for lymphoproliferation. Prolactin has been reported to activate cellular proliferation in nonreproductive tissue, such as liver, spleen and thymus. It induces significant proliferation in aortic smooth muscle cells. PRL also appears to be directly mitogenic for pancreatic beta cells. Growth hormone augments superoxide anion secretion of human neutrophils by binding to the prolactin receptor.

Hypothalamic Hormone. 1) both gonadotrophin-releasing hormone (GRH) and thyrotropin-releasing hormone (TRH) → increase prolactin production, 2) both prolactin-release inhibiting hormone (PRIH) and dopamine → inhibit prolactin release. Prolactin is very sensitive to stress stimuli before sampling. Released in episodic spikes during the day, 2–3 times higher values are at night, lowest are in early afternoon. Day-to-day level variation is 5–10% in men, 40% in women.

Test Purpose. 1) to facilitate pituitary dysfunction diagnosis, possibly due to pituitary adenoma, 2) to aid in hypothalamic dysfunction diagnosis regardless of cause. **Females:** 3) to evaluate secondary amenorrhea, oligomenorrhea and galactorrhea, menorrhagia and anovulatory cycles, 4) to help in ovarian hypofunction differential diagnosis, 5) to help in diagnosis of fertility disorders, libido disorders, gynecomastia and mastopathy, 6) corpus luteum disorders diagnosis, 7) virilism diagnosis, 8) lactation psychosis and postdelivery psychosyndromes diagnosis, 9) prolactinoma suspicion. **Males:** 10) potency or libido disorders diagnosis, 11) gynecomastia and galactorrhea, 12) hypogonadism diagnosis.

Increased Values – hyperprolactinemia

acromegaly, **amenorrhea**, **anorexia nervosa**, **anovulation**, hepatic cirrhosis, smoking in men, **galactorrhea**, chronic cocaine abuse, gigantism, eosinophilic granuloma, gynecomastia, **herpes zoster**, histiocytosis X, **selective hyperpituitarism**, benign prostate hyperplasia, **idiopathic hyperprolactinemia**, **hypoglycemia**, hypogonadism, **hypothyroidism**, liver diseases, insufficiency – (**adrenal i.**, acute renal i.), Cushing's disease, spinal cord lesions, tumours – (t. of pituitary gland, t. of hypothalamus, acute myeloid leukemia, lymphomas, **prolactinoma**, **renal t., lung t.,** craniopharyngioma, ovarian teratomas), spinal cord lesion, ectopic prolactin production of malignant tumours – (hypernephroma, bronchogenic carcinoma), irradiation, bilateral oophorectomy, **sarcoidosis**, corpus luteum insufficiency, seizure conditions, **stress during operation**, **stress**, syndrome – (Forbes-Albright sy, MEN sy, acute cardiac allograft rejection, **empty sella sy**, **polycystic ovary sy**), **tuberculosis**, precocious puberty, head/chest injury, uremia, failure – (liver f., **renal f.**)

> **Interfering Factors: nursing, postpartum lactation, newborns, food intake, sleep, nipple stimulation, pregnancy**, high altitude, **physical exercise**, medicaments – (amitriptyline, amoxapine, amphetamines, antidepressants, antiemetics, antihistamines, antihypertonics, antipsychotics, arginine, benserazide, butyrophenones, carbamazepine, chlorpromazine, cimetidine, clomipramine, cyclosporine, desipramine, domperidone, enflurane, estrogens, fentanyl, flunarizine, fluphenazine, furosemide, haloperidol, imipramine, insulin, isoniazid, labetalol, MAO inhibitors, methadone, methyldopa, metoclopramide, morphine, neuroleptics, olanzapine, opiates, oral contraceptives, perphenazine, phenothiazines, phenytoin, pimozide, prochlorperazine, promazine, promethazine, ranitidine, reserpine, risperidone, sulpiride, thiethylperazine, thioridazine, thiothixene, thioxanthines, TRH, tricyclic antidepressants, tricyclic antidepressants, trifluoperazine, tryptophan, verapamil, zimeldine)

Decreased Values – hypoprolactinemia

bulimia, **pituitary destruction from tumor**, ethanol, smoking in women, selective hypopituitarism, idiopathic hypogonadotropic hypogonadism, acute illnesses, malnutrition, panhypopituitarism, pseudohypoparathyroidism, syndrome – (galactorrhea/amenorrhea sy, empty sella sy, **Sheehan's sy** – pituitary apoplexy sy), lactation failure in lactating mother

   Interfering Factors: fasting, medicaments – (apomorphine, bromocriptine, calcitonin, clonidine, dopamine, lergotrile, levodopa, lisuride, propranolol, rifampicin, tamoxifen, valproic acid)

Analyte	Age/Gender	Reference Range	SI Units	Note
Prolactin	1–30 d F	8–2620	U/l	
	1–30 d M	102–2 240	U/l	
	<1 y F	6–825	U/l	
	<1 y M	8–800	U/l	
	2–3 y F	28–470	U/l	
	2–3 y M	63–365	U/l	
	4–6 y F	44–360	U/l	
	4–6 y M	22–465	U/l	
	7–9 y F	8–355	U/l	
	7–9 y M	52–320	U/l	
	10–12 y F	52–265	U/l	
	10–12 y M	25–355	U/l	
	13–15 y F	83–400	U/l	
	13–15 y M	44–460	U/l	
	16–18 y F	58–510	U/l	
	16–18 y M	75–420	U/l	
	Adults F	3.8–23.2	µg/l	
	Adults M	3.0–14.7	µg/l	
	F	91–557	mU/l	
	M	72–353	mU/l	

Proline

(Pro) Imino acid. Proline is synthesized from glutamic acid. Proline and hydroxyproline are found highly concentrated in collagen.

Enzyme defect. Proline oxidase and pyroline-5-carboxyl dehydrogenase.

Increased Values – hyperprolinemia

protein malnutrition in infants, severe burns (1 day after), prolinemia

Decreased Values – hypoprolinemia

Huntington's chorea, severe burns (4 days after), conditions after abdominal surgery

Analyte	Age/Gender	Reference Range	SI Units	Note
Proline	Neonates	130–350	µmol/l	
	Infants	100–300	µmol/l	
	Children	60–300	µmol/l	
	Adults	120–240	µmol/l	

Properdin

Properdin belongs to the complement components (alternative pathway component). It [is]
a polypeptide, synthesized in the blood by monocytes. The alternative pathway role is to st[a]-
bilize C3-convertase, so that factor H and I cannot dissociate and inactivate it. Properd[in]
deficiency is the only X-linked complement deficiency.

Test Purpose. 1) to help in diagnosis of complement abnormalities, 2) to help in defini[ng]
the cause of glomerulonephritis.

Decreased Values
properdin deficiency (X-linked), activated alternative complement pathway

Analyte	Age/Gender	Reference Range	SI Units	Note
Properdin	Umbilicus	190–320	µmol/l	
	< 3 m	285–545	µmol/l	
	< 1 y	600–838	µmol/l	
	Adults	527–1167	µmol/l	

Prostaglandins

(PG, PGs) PGs belong to eicosanoids that are derived from 20-carbon unsaturated fa[tty]
acids (primarily arachidonic acid) via the cyclooxygenase pathway. Prostaglandin gro[up]
consists of prostaglandins, thromboxanes, and leukotrienes.

Function. Extremely potent mediators of diverse physiological processes. Prostaglandins a[re]
in synthesized and surrounding cells; actions and effects vary with the concentration, h[or]-
monal environment and cell type. Function in arterial smooth muscle – blood press[ure]
alterations; in uterine muscle – induce labor, therapeutic abortion; in lower gastrointestin[al]
tract – increase motility; in smooth muscle – induce bronchospasm; in platelets – decrea[se]
coagulability; in stomach – increase gastric acid secretion; in capillaries – increase perm[e]-
ability with flushing; in adipose tissue – inhibit triacylglycerol lipolysis. PG increase [to]
renal blood flow and natrium secretion. Total peripheral vascular resistance, renal vasc[u]-
lar resistance, cardiac output, baroreceptor activity and plasma volume are optimal. Indu[ce]
luteolysis, decrease progesterone secretion, stimulate pregnant uterus contraction. PG a[re]
hormone and cyclic nucleotides modulators, gastric secretion and thrombocyte aggregati[on]
inhibitors. At the hypothalamo-pituitary level they act as LH releasing factor mediators [in]
LH secretion.

- **PGA2:** potent vasodilator in kidney (antihypertensive function). Stimulates renin pr[o]-
  duction.
- **PGD2:** the major prostaglandin produced by mast cells and platelets; an immediate h[y]-
  persensitivity mediator synthesized and released in response to mast cell receptors [Ig]
  binding. Its effects include nonvascular smooth muscle vasodilation and contractio[n],
  bronchoconstriction, skin vasodilation, granulocyte chemokinesis, chronotropic effe[ct]
  on the heart, increase in vascular permeability, sneezing, rhinorrhea.
- **PGE1:** the analogue of PGE2. Many of its effects, including vasodilation, are similar [to]
  PGE2 but unlike PGE2, it inhibits platelet aggregation. Used as a neonate vasodilat[or]
  with congenital heart disease treatment.
- **PGE2:** an important PG having many effects. It is synthesized by platelets, produced [in]
  the renal medulla, gastrointestinal mucosa and other tissues, causes renal vasodilati[on]
  (antihypertensive function) and renal tubular sodium resorption inhibition, gast[ric]

secretion inhibition and may cause smooth muscle contraction/relaxation depending on the tissue. It is also released by macrophages, modulating several inflammatory responses. It increases vascular permeability, and pain sensitivity; it is pyrogenic and suppressing lymphocyte transformation, and mediators release from mast cells and cell-mediated cytotoxicity. Other effects include bronchodilatation (relaxes smooth muscle), vasodilatation. PGE2 produced by some tumors causes osteoclasts bone resorption stimulation hypercalcemia. It is a potent endogenous lipolysis regulator (inhibits lipolysis – antilipolytic substance). It is an important induction factor in a normal delivery.

■ **PGF2-alpha:** a stable prostaglandin formed from PGH2 or PGE2; it stimulates uterine and bronchial smooth muscle contractions and produces vasoconstriction in some vessels (microvasculature and pulmonary vasculature). Decreases luteal body blood flow, inhibits progesterone synthesis. Produced by most tissues. It is an important induction factor in a normal delivery.

■ **PGG2:** a prostaglandin cyclic endoperoxide formed from arachidonic acid by incorporation of two oxygen molecules; it is an unstable intermediate that converts rapidly and spontaneously to PGH2.

■ **PGH2:** a prostaglandin cyclic endoperoxide formed from PGG2; as an unstable intermediate it converts to several important prostaglandins and thromboxanes.

■ **PGI2 (syn: prostacyclin):** derived from arachidonic acid in the vascular endothelium. Effects – smooth muscle relaxation, bronchodilation, pulmonary vasodilation, coronary artery vasodilation. Inhibits platelet aggregation, increases cAMP formation. It is synthesized by adipose tissue, it is a potent endogenous lipolysis regulator.

Renal prostaglandin production stimuli
■ **Peptide hormones:** vasopressin, bradykinin, angiotensin II, endothelin 1
■ **Miscellaneous stimuli:** calcium, intravenous loop diuretics, alpha-adrenergic catecholamines, adenosine triphosphate, dietary supplementation with arachidonic acid precursors, interleukin 1-alpha, tumor necrosis factor alpha, serotonin, endotoxin, estradiol
■ **Diseases:** glomerulonephritis, cirrhosis, congestive heart failure, Bartter's sy, renal ischemia, ureteral obstruction

Prostate Specific Antigen

(PSA) Organ-specific (prostate-tissue specific) glycoprotein enzyme (serine protease) is found in the cytoplasm, localized in prostate ductal epithelial cells and within the prostatic ducts lumina. PSA is excreted in urine and seminal plasma. In the seminal fluid, PSA cleaves a seminal vesicle-specific protein into several low-molecular-weight proteins as part of the seminal coagulum liquefaction process. PSA possesses chymotrypsin-like and trypsin like activity. Serum PSA (89%) is bound onto alpha-2-macroglobulin and alpha-1-antichymotrypsin, the rest of the PSA is in a free form. In healthy males this is present in low serum levels. Increased levels appear in children (first months of life, then after 10 years). Specific prostate tissue enzyme tumour marker. PSA is released into blood via injured tissue. Repetitive measurements are extremely valuable for treatment evaluating response to prostatic cancer. Determination of free PSA fractions is of great value when decisions must be made in borderline levels. PSA levels may precede clinically detectable metastasis development by as much as 6–12 months. Day-to-day variation is 15–20%.
Test Purpose. 1) to monitor the prostate cancer course, 2) to aid in evaluation of treatment, 3) to check for recurrence after treatment has finished.

Increased Values

prostatic needle biopsy, cystoscopy, **benign prostate hyperplasia**, **inflammatory prostate diseases**, acute myocardial infarction, **prostatic infarction**, **prostate ischemia**, permanent bladder catheter, benign prostate tumors, tumors – (bone metastases, sweat glands t., colorectal t., salivary glands t., kidney t., lung t., **prostate t.,** breast t., gastrointestinal tract t., ovary t., genitourinary tract t.), **prostate palpation/massage**, **prostatitis**, growth of children, digital rectal examination, radiation therapy, **transurethral resection of prostate**, **acute urinary retention**, transrectal ultrasonography, vigorous bicycle exercise, full term placenta, treadmill stress test, **acute renal failure**.

    Interfering Factors: medicaments – (testosterone)

Decreased Values

prolonged supine position, radical prostatectomy, sedentary patient, ejaculation (within 24–48 hrs), castration, radiation therapy

    Interfering Factors: medicaments – (estrogen, antiandrogens, finasteride)

Analyte	Age/Gender	Reference Range	SI Units	Note
Prostate Specific Antigen		<4.0	ng/ml	

Prostate Specific Antigen, Free

(free PSA) It is a specific prostate tissue product in prostate/seminal fluid, healthy/hyperplastic prostate and malignant prostate tumor/metastases. There are three free PSA forms in serum: a) free, b) bound to alpha-2-macroglobulin (imunulogically inactive), c) bound to alpha-1-antitrypsin. Free PSA to total PSA ratio is decreased in the malignant prostate tumor compared to benign prostate hyperplasia. Paralel free/total PSA determination has a differential diagnostic value.

Test Purpose. 1) differential diagnosis between benign prostate hyperplasia and malignant prostate tumor, 2) examination in the case of total PSA increase.

Analyte	Age/Gender	Reference Range	SI Units	Note
Prostate Specific Antigen, Free		2.4–3.5	ng/ml	

Prostatic Acid Phosphatase

(PAP) Acid phosphatase is a lysosomal enzyme, glycoprotein. The prostatic enzyme is found in prostate epithelium lysosomes and normally is present only in small amounts in the blood. Prostatic acid phosphatase is an enzyme tumour marker.

Test Purpose. 1) diagnosis of prostate tumors, 2) differential diagnosis of bone metastases, 3) to check malignant tumor therapy effectivity.

Increased Values

benign prostatic hyperplasia (BPH), hyperparathyroidism, hepatitis, **prostate infarction**, disease – (**Gaucher's d.,** Niemann–Pick d., Paget's d., sickle-cell d.), bone diseases, obstructive jaundice, acute renal insufficiency, **prostatic tumors**, **prostatic surgery/biopsy** (1–2 d after), prostatitis, following prostatic manipulation/massage/catheterization, leukemia, non-Hodgkin's lymphoma, osteoporosis, liver cirrhosis, pulmonary embolism, hyperparathy-

roidism, hemolytic conditions, leukemic reticuloendotheliosis, metastatic carcinoma of bone, plasmocytoma (incl. multiple myeloma), partial translocation trisomy 21, excessive platelet destruction, **thromboembolism**, idiopathic thrombocytopenic purpura
  Interfering Factors: medicaments – (alglucerase, androgens, buserelin, clofibrate)

Decreased Values
  Interfering Factors: medicaments – (fluoride, heparin, ketoconazole, oxalate)

Protein S-100

Proteins S-100 are acid, related calcium binding proteins found in nervous tissue, melanocytes, adipocytes, chondrocytes, epidermal Langerhans' cells, myoepithelial cells of the salivary and mammary glands. Its dimer molecule consist of alpha- and beta- subunits. Dimer beta-beta is present in glial and Schwann cells, dimer alpha-alpha is present in skeletal muscle, myocard and kidney. Protein S-100 seems to be a prognostic marker in malignant melanoma (staging and therapeutic effectivity information). Protein S-100 is a prognostic marker in brain injuries. S-100 also inhibits the activities of some tyrosine-specific protein kinases involved in receptor-mediated processes of intracellular signal transduction.
Test Purpose. 1) to evaluate the extent of brain damage (injury, surgery, tumors), 2) to monitor staging and therapy in malignant melanoma.

Increased Values
brain injury, brain surgery, extracorporeal surgeries, tumors – (glioma, melanoma, **Schwannoma**, differentiated neuroblastoma, granular cell tumors, **neurofibroma**)

Analyte	Age/Gender	Reference Range	SI Units	Note
Intracellular Protein S-100		<0.20	µg/l	

Proteins

(T. P., syn: total proteins)
Function. Proteins and nucleic acids as the structural components of a cell, serve as biocatalysts – enzymes; hormone metabolism regulators; the conjugated proteins – lipoproteins, glycoproteins, metal binding proteins; components of genetic makeup – chromosomes. Support colloid-osmotic plasma pressure that maintains equilibrium in the capillaries. They are involved in the transport of lipids, amino acids, hormones, bilirubin, anions, cations, medicaments, acting in an acid-base balance, nutrition, immunity and energy source.
Test Purpose. 1) to aid in edema, polyuria, hemorrhage diagnosis, 2) to aid in chronic disease diagnosis (kidney, diarrhea, liver, connective tissue), 3) to help in bone ache diagnosis, 4) to aid in lymphoproliferative disease and infectious disease diagnosis.

Increased Values – hyperproteinemia
rheumatoid arthritis, bronchiectasis, **hepatic cirrhosis** (compensated, early stage), **dehydration**, diabetes insipidus, **exsicosis**, phlegmon, impaired renal function, **hemoconcentration**, hypergammaglobulinemia, **diarrhea**, diseases – (**severe infectious d.,** acute hepatic d., **inflammatory d.**), diabetic ketoacidosis, **collagenosis**, systemic lupus erythematosus, Addison's disease, **Waldenström's macroglobulinemia**, myxedema, tumors – (bronchial t.,

monocytic leukemia, lymphogranuloma, **plasmocytoma** incl. multiple myeloma), **parapro**tein-emia, polyuria, burns (early stages), inadequate fluid intake, **sarcoidosis**, sepsi strumec-tomy, lung tuberculosis, **vomiting**, collagen vascular disease

Interfering Factors: medicaments – (ACTH, anabolics, androgens, clofibrate, corticost roids, dextran, digitoxin, epinephrine, growth hormone, insulin, oral contraceptive phenazopyridine, progesterone, propranolol, sulfasalazine, thyroid preparations)

Decreased Values – hypoproteinemia

agammaglobulinemia, **amyloidosis**, posthemorrhagic anemia, **ascites**, bronchiectasi **hepatic cirrhosis**, potassium deficit, dermatitis, diabetes mellitus (uncontrolled), **hepat dysfunction**, **exudative enteropathy**, eczema, cystic fibrosis, **glomerulonephritis**, **starvatio diarrhea**, **overhydration**, **essential hypertension**, **hyperthyroidism**, hypoalimentation, di eases – (**acute/chronic infectious d., chronic hepatic d.**, infective pulmonary d., inflamm tory d.), obstructive icterus, mechanic ileus, insufficiency – (pancreatic i., hepatic i., **cardia i.**), intoxication by – (benzene, carbon tetrachloride), **collagenoses**, **colitis ulcerosa**, massi hemorrhage – (hemorrhagic diathesis, gastrointestinal tumours/ulcers, injuries), **kwas iorkor**, **systemic lupus erythematosus**, disease – (**Crohn's d., Hodgkin's d., Whipple's d. malnutrition**, marasmus, **tumours**, **nephrosis**, **hepatocellular necrosis**, **chronic pancrea tis**, **pemphigus vulgaris**, peritonitis, plasmapheresis, pleuritis exudativa (pleural effusior **severe burns** (late stage), toxic hepatic impairment, decreased intake/resorption of protein **water/minerals retention**, **decreased protein consumption**, **sprue**, conditions – (**cachect c.**, febrile c., postoperative c.), shock states – (**surgery, trauma**), **idiopathic steatorrhe increased protein loss**, syndrome – (**malabsorption sy**, SIADH sy, **nephrotic sy**), **pregnanc** (3rd trimester), tuberculosis, failure – (**acute/chronic renal f.**, congenital heart f.), wat intoxication

Interfering Factors: medicaments – (allopurinol, contraceptives, estrogens, hepatotox drugs, rifampicin)

Analyte	Age/Gender	Reference Range	SI Units	Note
Proteins, Total	Premature			
	infants, 1 d	34–50	g/l	
	1 d–4 w	46–68	g/l	
	2–12 m	48–76	g/l	
	>1 y	60–80	g/l	
	Adults	66–87	g/l	
Electrophoresis	Adults			
Albumin		0.55–0.69		
		55.3–68.9	%	
alpha-1-globulins		0.02–0.06		
		1.6–5.8	%	
alpha-2-globulins		0.06–0.11		
		5.9–11.1	%	
beta globulins		0.08–0.14		
		7.9–13.9	%	
gamma globulins		0.11–0.18		
		11.4–18.2	%	
Albumin	Neonates	32.7–45.3	g/l	
	<1 y	35.7–51.3	g/l	
	1–5 y	33.1–52.2	g/l	
	6–15 y	40–52.2	g/l	
	Adults	35.2–50.4	g/l	

Analyte	Age/Gender	Reference Range	SI Units	Note
alpha-1-globulins	Neonates	1.1–2.5	g/l	
	<1 y	1.3–2.5	g/l	
	1–5 y	0.9–2.9	g/l	
	6–15 y	1.2–2.5	g/l	
	Adults	1.3–3.9	g/l	
alpha-2-globulins	Neonates	2.6–5.7	g/l	
	<1 y	3.8–10.8	g/l	
	1–5 y	4.3–9.5	g/l	
	6–15 y	4.3–8.6	g/l	
	Adults	5.4–9.3	g/l	
beta globulins	Neonates	2.5–5.6	g/l	
	<1 y	3.5–7.1	g/l	
	1–5 y	3.5–7.6	g/l	
	6–15 y	4.1–7.9	g/l	
	Adults	5.9–11.4	g/l	
gamma globulins	Neonates	3.9–11	g/l	
	<1 y	2.9–11	g/l	
	1–5 y	4.5–12.1	g/l	
	6–15 y	5.9–13.7	g/l	
	Adults	5.8–15.2	g/l	

Psoriasin

Psoriasin is a calcium binding protein, belonging to the S-100 family of proteins. Significant levels of psoriasin are found in ear, skin and tongue tissues. It is a potent and selective chemotactic inflammatory protein for CD4 T-lymphocytes and neutrophils. Psoriasin may thus be a factor that plays an important role in inflammatory skin disorders such as psoriasis. Psoriasin has been shown to be externalitzed to the urine of bladder squamous cell carcinoma.

Pyroglobulins

Abnormal proteins (monoclonal immunoglobulins) that irreversibly precipitate/gel when blood serum is heated to 56 °C.

Increased Values – positive
systemic lupus erythematosus, lymphoma, myeloma, polycythemia vera

Pyruvic Acid

(syn: pyruvate) Embden–Meyerhof glucose metabolism pathway end product. It is also produced by several amino acid catabolism. Pyruvate can be converted to acetyl coenzyme A, which enters the tricarboxylic acid cycle for aerobic energy production or to be used for fatty acid synthesis. Pyruvate can also be converted to oxaloacetate, the first step in gluconeogenesis. The relation between lactate and pyruvate is determined with the equation: lactate + $NAD^+ \leftarrow \rightarrow$ pyruvate + NADH + H^+, reaction is bilaterally catalyzed with LD. Amino acids that form pyruvate: alanine, serine, glycine, cystine, threonine.

Test Purpose. 1) to assess tissue oxidation, 2) to help determine lactic acidosis causes, 3) differential diagnosis of hereditary organic acidurias disorders (pyruvate dehydrogenase deficiency), 4) to provide an index of the severity of circulatory failure.

Increased Values
acute advanced beriberi, thiamine deficiency, diabetes mellitus, hepatolenticular degeneration, malignant hyperthermia, advanced liver diseases, heavy metal poisoning by – (antimony, arsenic, mercury, gold), muscular dystrophy, tumors, diabetic ketoacidosis, von Gierke's disease, Reye's sy, uremia, severe cardiac failure

Analyte	Age/Gender	Reference Range	SI Units	Note
Pyruvate	Children	11–86	mmol/l	
	Adults F	41–67	mmol/l	
	Adults M	34–102	mmol/l	

Quinidine

Mean half-life is about 7 hours (4–12 hours).
Test Purpose. To monitor drug therapy.

Increased Values
quinidine overdose

Analyte	Age/Gender	Reference Range	SI Units	Note
Quinidine		6–15	μmol/l	

RANTES

(Regulated upon activation, normal T-cell expressed, and presumably secreted) RANTES is produced by circulating T-cells. The expression of RANTES is inhibited following stimulation of T-lymphocytes. It is chemotactic for T-cells, human eosinophils and basophils and plays an active role in recruiting leukocytes into inflammatory sites. Activates eosinophils to release, for example, eosinophilic cationic protein. Increases the adherence of monocytes of endothelial cells. It selectively supports the migration of monocytes and T-lymphocytes expressing the cell surface markers CD4. RANTES is expressed by human synovial fibroblasts and may participate in the ongoing inflammatory process in rheumatoid arthritis. It has been observed that antibodies to RANTES can dramatically inhibit the cellular infiltration associated with experimental mesangioproliferative nephritis. RANTES appears to be expressed highly in human renal allografts undergoing cellular rejection.

C-Reactive Protein

(CRP) CRP is a protein with electrophoretical mobility in the gamma globulin area; functionally it is analogous to immunoglobulin G but it is not antigen specific.
Production. An abnormal protein synthesized primarily by the hepatocytes during an acute inflammatory processes. CRP synthesis is initiated by cytokines, antigens, immune complexes, bacteria, fungi and trauma (as early as 4–6 hrs after injury). CRP rises more than 6 hours after triggering stimulus, peaks within 48–72 hours, rapidly declines after condition resolves.

Occurrence. Serum, inflammatory fluids and exudates.

Function. Acute phase protein, polysaccharide transport protein that increases phagocytosis, initiates opsonization, lyses foreign cells and acts as a detoxification agent. Non-specific inflammatory reaction, infectious and tissue destruction/necrosis index. CRP is able to interact with complement system. The determination has its specific advantages when compared to ESR, WBC count and body temperature measurement. CRP shows an earlier, more intense increase rise than ESR; with recovery, disappearance of CRP precedes the return to normal of ESR. CRP generally parallels ESR but is not influenced by anemia, polycythemia, spherocytosis, macrocytosis, congestive heart failure and hypergammaglobulinemia. After surgery the failure of CRP to fall is more sensitive indicator of complications than WBC, ESR, temperature and pulse rate.

Test Purpose. 1) inflammatory/infective disorders screening, detection, monitoring, 2) quick determination of inflammatory processes in intensively treated patients, in neonatology, in patients with antineoplasm therapy and transplantation, 3) antibiotic therapy response control, 4) differential diagnosis between viral and bacterial inflammation, 5) false low ESR during acute phase and unexplained high ESR, 6) rheumatic activity follow-up, 7) to aid in diagnosis of neoplastic conditions (tumor marker).

Increased Values

rheumatoid arthritis, unstable angina, tissue ischemia, hepatic cirrhosis, **gouty arthritis, embolism**, viral hepatitis, **rheumatic fever, chorioamnionitis**, diseases – (**inflammatory bowel d., rheumatic d., inflammatory d.**), infarction – (**cardiac i.** – appears within 24–48 hrs, peaks at 72 hrs, becomes negative after 7 days, **pulmonary i.**), infections – (**bacterial i.**, intrauterine i., **neonatal i., respiratory system i., viral i.**), leprosy, **systemic lupus erythematosus, Crohn's disease, non-specific marker of pulmonary malignant tumours**, bacterial meningitis, tumours – (t. of bronchi, **leukemia, Burkitt's lymphoma, t. of lung**, breast t., gastrointestinal tract t., t. of pancreas), nephritis, **tissue necrosis**, obstruction of biliary ways, **severe surgeries and after surgery**, pericarditis, peritonitis, **pneumonia, inflamed pneumopathy, severe burns**, pyelitis, **pyelonephritis**, transplant rejection – (**renal t. r.**, marrow t. r.), multiple sclerosis, neonatal septicemia and meningitis, stress, syndrome – (Guillain-Barré sy, nephrotic sy, **Reiter's sy**), **scarlet fever, tuberculosis, trauma, varicella, vasculitis**.

> **Interfering Factors:** intrauterine device, pregnancy (3rd trimester), medicaments – (oral contraceptives)

Decreased Values

> **Interfering Factors:** medicaments – (atenolol, nonsteroidal antiinflammatories, oral contraceptives, salicylates, steroids)

Analyte	Age/Gender	Reference Range	SI Units	Note
C-Reactive Protein		0.07–8.2	mg/l	

Renin

(syn: plasmatic renin activity, plasma renin activity – PRA, plasma renin concentration) Enzyme, proteinase, endopeptidase.

Production. Renin is a hydrolytic enzyme that is synthesized and stored in the juxtaglomerular apparatus epitheloid cells. Released into renal veins in response to stress, sodium depletion, hypovolemia, baroreceptor/macula densa stimulation, beta-adrenergic system, prostacyclines. Renin release decrease is caused by: kalium, calcium, vasopressin, and angiotensin II.

Function. The enzyme is a renin-angiotensin-aldosterone system component that regulate blood pressure, plasma volume, and electrolyte balance. Renin converts angiotensinoge produced by the liver to angiotensin I → that is converted in the lung to angiotensin II, th most potent vasopressor agent responsible for renal origin hypertension and aldosteror release from the adrenal cortex. Angiotensin II and aldosterone increase blood pressure. R nin level increases when there is decreased renal perfusion pressure, decreased sodium an water delivery to the glomerulus vascular pole, decreased plasma volume and blood pre sure, and as a neural stimulation response. Highest values are at 4 AM, lowest are at 4–6 PM in women, increases during menses. Most of plasma renin is enzymatically inactive. On the active form has diagnostic value. Its performance is assessed only by functional tes (basal secretion and stimulated with saluretics and/or orthostasis). Examination shoul follow when aldosterone concentrations are known.

Test Purpose. 1) to screen for renal hypertension origin, 2) to help in essential hypertensic plan treatment, 3) to help identify unilateral renovascular disease hypertension by renal vei catheterization, 4) to help identify primary aldosteronism resulting from aldosterone-secre ting adrenal adenoma, 5) to confirm primary aldosteronism, 6) to help in Addison's diseas diagnosis, 7) to help in differential diagnosis of hypertension and edematous states, 8) dia nosis of tumors producing renin (reninomas), 9) functional diagnosis in sonographic an CT findings on adrenals, 10) Bartter's sy diagnosis.

Increased Values – hyperreninemia

hepatic cirrhosis, edema – (hepatic e., renal e., cardiac e.), **pheochromocytoma**, hepatiti hypertension – (**essential h., renovascular h., malignant h.**), hypoaldosteronism – (primar h., **secondary h.**), **secondary hyperaldosteronism, hypokalemia**, hypovolemia, diseases (gastrointestinal tract d., renal/liver parenchymal d.), **hemorrhage, Addison's disease**, adre nal tumours, **renin-secreting tumors, salt-losing nephropathy, nephrosis, transplant reje tion**, syndrome – (**Bartter's sy**, Cushing's sy), failure – (**chronic renal f., congestive heart f.**

Interfering Factors: **low salt diet, upright body position, pregnancy, early in the morr ing**, last half of menstrual cycle, medicaments – (ACE inhibitors, amiloride, antihype tensives, calcium antagonists, captopril, chlorpropamide, chlortalidone, diazoxide, diu retics, dobutamine, enalapril, estrogens, felodipine, furosemide, glucocorticoids, gua nethidine, heparin, hydralazine, hydrochlorothiazide, lisinopril, minoxidil, nifedipin nitroprusside, oral contraceptives, prazosin, salbutamol, saralasin, spironolactone, th azide diuretics, triamterene, vasodilating agents)

Decreased Values – hyporeninemia

adrenal cortex adenoma, diabetes mellitus, aldosteronism – (idiopathic a., **primary a.**), hy perkalemia, adrenal cortex hyperplasia, essential hypertension, benign hypertension, hype tension due to unilateral renal artery stenosis, hypertension due to unilateral renal parer chymal disease, hypervolemia, secondary hypoaldosteronism, hypotension – (essential l with low renin levels, postural h.), renal parenchymal diseases, pituitary insufficiency, ac renal tumors with mineralocorticoid excess, bilateral/unilateral nephrectomy, renal injur increased fluid intake, pseudohyperaldosteronism (Liddle's sy), **high-sodium diet**, syr drome – (**Conn's sy**, Cushing's sy)

Interfering Factors: healthy people, ageing, medicaments – (acetylsalicylic acid, ang otensin, beta-adrenergic blocking agents, antidiuretic hormone, carbenoxolone, cis platin, clonidine, deoxycorticosterone, digoxin, guanethidine, indomethacin, methyl dopa, oral contraceptives, oxprenolol, pindolol, potassium preparations, prazosin, prc pranolol, reserpine, steroids, timolol)

Analyte	Age/Gender	Reference Range	SI Units	Note
Renin	rest	0.5–1.9	ng/ml/h	
	exertion	1.9–6.0	ng/ml/h	

Respiratory Syncytial Virus Antigen

Test Purpose. To investigate severe respiratory illness in infants (bronchiolitis, pneumonia, croup).

Increased Values – positive
respiratory syncytial virus infectious diseases

Retinol-Binding Protein

(RBP) RBP is one of two proteins responsible for transporting vitamin A in the blood. Retinol is binding with RBP (ratio 1:1) → bound to prealbumin. It is synthesized/secreted by the liver parenchymal cells and circulates in serum as a protein-protein complex with prealbumin. The kidneys play a major role in RBP catabolism. Clinical importance is similar to prealbumin, when used as a nutrition status indicator and in parenteral nutrition. Probably one of the most sensitive hepatocyte function and protein synthesis indicator found to date.

Increased Values
alcohol hepatitis, **chronic renal diseases**, fatty liver
  Interfering Factors: medicaments – (estrogens, oral contraceptives, phenobarbital, phenytoin)

Decreased Values
hepatic cirrhosis – (alcoholic h. c., cryptogenic h. c., primary biliary h. c.), zinc deficiency, **cystic fibrosis**, hepatitis – (chronic active h., acute viral h.), hyperparathyroidism, hyperthyroidism, diseases – (**hepatocellular d.,** infectious d.), **kwashiorkor**, proteinuria

Analyte	Age/Gender	Reference Range	SI Units	Note
Retinol-Binding	0–5 d	8–45	mg/l	
Protein	1–9 y	10–78	mg/l	
	10–13 y	13–99	mg/l	
	14–19 y	30–92	mg/l	

Reverse Triiodothyronine

(rT3, syn: reverse T3) rT3 represents an alternate T4 deiodination pathway. Reverse T3 is a biologically inactive thyroxine metabolite. It is created via type III deiodase action.

Increased Values
starvation, diseases – (hepatic d., severe systemic d.), treatment of obesity by starvation, acute surgical stress, hyperthyroidism, syndrome of low triiodothyronine
  Interfering Factors: advancing age, postpartum women, medicaments – (amiodarone, glucocorticoids, methylthiouracil, oral cholecystographic agents, propranolol, propylthiouracil, salicylates)

Decreased Values
hypothyroidism

Analyte	Age/Gender	Reference Range	SI Units	Note
Triiodothyronine, Reverse	1–5 y	0.23–1.1	nmol/l	
	5–10 y	0.26–1.2	nmol/l	
	10–15 y	0.29–1.36	nmol/l	

Rheumatoid Factor

(RF) Macroglobulin serum autoantibodies that bind a many antigenic determinants in the Fc portion of IgG, usually the IgM (IgG, IgA) class, which are directed against human IgG forming immune complexes. Incidence of rheumatoid arthritis increases with duration of disease (33% at 3 months, 45% at 6 months, 75% at 12 months, 90% at 18 months). Prognosis is worse with high titre at onset.

Test Purpose. 1) to confirm rheumatoid arthritis, especially when clinical diagnosis is doubtful, 2) diagnosis of connective tissue disease.

Increased Values
ankylosing spondylitis, **cryptogenic fibrosing alveolitis**, brucellosis, **hepatic cirrhosis, dermatomyositis**, endocarditis – **(subacute bacterial e., infective e.)**, filariasis, **autoimmune chronic active hepatitis**, gout, **chondrocalcinosis**, arthritis – (suppurative a., psoriatic a., **rheumatoid a.,** enteropathic a.), **mixed connective tissue disease**, diseases – **(viral infectious d., kidney d., liver d., lung d.)**, influenza, **cryoglobulinemia, leprosy, leukemia, systemic lupus erythematosus**, lymphomas, **Waldenström's macroglobulinemia, malaria, infectious mononucleosis**, tumors, osteoarthritis, osteomyelitis, plasmocytoma (incl. multiple myeloma), polymyalgia rheumatica, postvaccination infections, **polymyositis**, cryoglobulinemic purpura, **sarcoidosis**, schistosomiasis, **scleroderma, syphilis**, syndrome – (CREST sy, **Felty's sy**, Reiter's sy, **Sjögren's sy, Still's sy**), allografts – (skin a., kidney a.), trypanosomiasis, **tuberculosis**

 Interfering Factors: circulating immune complexes, cryoglobulins, lipemia, elderly people, relatives of patients with rheumatoid arthritis, medicaments – (chemotherapeutics, methyldopa)

Analyte	Age/Gender	Reference Range	SI Units	Note
Rheumatoid Factor		<14	kU/l *	See ref.
		<79	U/l	ranges note
		<40	kU/l	

Salicylates

Test Purpose. 1) to confirm suspected toxicity from patient history or clinical examination, 2) to monitor therapeutic levels of blood salicylate.

Increased Values
salicylates overdose

Decreased Values
low therapeutic levels

Secretin

Gastrointestinal tract (small intestine S-cells, mucosal granular cells) regulative polypeptide (27 amino acids) with endocrine effect. Secretin is a duodenal mucosa hormone.
Production. Duodenum, jejunum, CNS.
Function. Stimulates pancreatic bicarbonate secretion (after administration it can be used in functional pancreas testing, pancreatic secretion sampling, gastrinoma diagnosis). Natural antacid. Duodenal pH less 4.5 is a stimulus for secretin release in response to gastric acid, digestive products and proteins entering the duodenum. Involved in pyloric sphincter contraction and slows stomach emptying, increases bile secretion, augments cholecystokinin-induced pancreatic digestive enzymes secretion, and reduces acid secretion in the stomach.

Increased Values – hypersecretinemia
exercise, diabetes mellitus, **gastrinoma**, starvation, **gastric acid hypersecretion**, duodenal ulcer disease, **chronic pancreatitis**, severe physical stress, Zollinger-Ellison sy, chronic renal failure
    Interfering Factors: postprandial, stress

Decreased Values – hyposecretinemia
achlorhydria, pernicious anemia, celiac disease (gluten-sensitive enteropathy)
    Interfering Factors: medicaments – (cimetidine, somatostatin)

Selectin

(syn: selectin P, E, L, cell adhesion molecule) Selectins are surface glycoproteins, they play a role in leukocyte endothelial adhesion during transition into extracellular space. P-selectin (platelet) is placed on platelets, megakaryocytes, and after thrombin/histamine activation appears also in endothelial cell membranes. E-selectin (endothelial) is a molecule, which exprimates on the endothelial cell surface after activation by cytokines IL-1, TNF-alpha and lipopolysaccharide. There are selectin E receptors which are placed on the granulocyte, monocyte and T-lymphocyte surfaces. Adhesion among endothelial cells and leukocytes is fast; it leads to rapid leukocyte aggregation and facilitates their diapedesis through the vessel into inflammation focus. L-selectin (leukocyte) occurs constitutively in T- and B-lymphocyte membranes, monocytes, NK-cells, neutrophils and eosinophils. L-selectin is an adhesion receptor group member, its receptor is highly glycosylated molecule. It consists of three extracelluar domains (lectin, epidermal growth-like factor, complement-regulatory protein), the most important is lectin domain. It is responsible for specific lymphocyte migration into lymphatic nodes.

Increased Values
diabetes mellitus, smoking, ischemic heart disease, peripheral vascular diseases

Analyte	Age/Gender	Reference Range	SI Units	Note
P-Selectin		19–521	ng/ml	

Selenium

(Se, selen) Trace element. A widely, but unevenly distributed essential micronutrient that can also be toxic in excess. Selenium is used in photoelectric cells, glass, ceramics, cosmetics, pigments and sheep dips. Occupational hazards result from exposure to dust or fume. The selenium content of foodstuffs varies markedly in proportion to the selenium content of the soils in which the animal feed or cereals and vegetables have grown. Seafood provides a stable and relatively abundant source of selenium. Selenium is absorbed after inhalation of aerosol (small respirable particles), non-respired selenium is cleared to the gut. Organoselenium compounds found in cereals (mainly seleno-methionine) are well absorbed. Once absorbed organo-selenium coumpounds are rapidly transferred to plasma and RB cells. Circulating selenium is primarily partitioned to brain, kidney and liver, but body stores are not large relative to metabolic demand. Body balance of selenium is maintained through regulation of excretion of trimethyl-selenonium to urine. Plasma selenium levels respond rapidly to either stress or selenium uptake.

Function. Glutathione peroxidase compound (antioxidant, detoxified lipid hydroxyperoxide), is closely related to vitamin E. Glutathione peroxidase protective properties help prevent Heinz bodies formation in RBC, hemolytic anemia, oxidative compounds hepatic damage, in phagocytic cells protecting the cell from auto-oxidation, deiodases component in thyroid hormone metabolism.

Test Purpose. 1) to monitor selenium nutritional condition in long-term parenteral nutrition, 2) to monitor exposure/intoxication to selenium, 3) to detect selenium deficiency in dietary deficiency.

Increased Values

industrial intoxication – (electro-industry, glass-industry), **reticuloendothelial tumors**, renal failure

> **Interfering Factors:** medicaments – (glucocorticoids, oral contraceptives, selen containing preparations)

Decreased Values

AIDS, rheumatoid arthritis, hepatic cirrhosis, smoking, phenylketonuria, cystic fibrosis, **hemodialysis**, hepatitis, diseases – (acute d., skin d.), **cardiomyopathies**, catabolism, **protein-caloric malnutrition**, tumors, **gastrointestinal tumors**, **decreased selenium dietary intake**, muscle pain conditions, **stress conditions**, premature neonates, **pregnancy**, **long-term parenteral nutrition**, renal failure

> **Interfering Factors:** medicaments – (valproic acid)

Analyte	Age/Gender	Reference Range	SI Units	Note
Selenium		3–6.2	µmol/l	

Serine

(Ser) A naturally occurring, non-essential amino acid, it may be synthesized from glycine and used as a dietary supplement.

Increased Values

lysinuric protein intolerance, oral intake of glycine/histidine

Decreased Values
gout

Analyte	Age/Gender	Reference Range	SI Units	Note
Serine	Infants	23–172	µmol/l	
	Adults	76–164	µmol/l	

Serotonin

(5-HT, syn: 5-OH tryptamine) Biogenic amine and tissue hormone. Tryptophan metabolite.
Function. Potent vasoconstrictor, increases blood pressure, smooth muscle contraction, peristalsis stimulator. Neurotransmitter especially in the sleep process. Involved in body temperature regulation, pain perception, social behavior, and mental depression.
Occurrence. Platelets, gastric, small and large intestinal wall enterochromaffin cells, central nervous system serotoninergic neurons. It is transported in the blood by the platelets. Free to bound serotonin concentration ratio change can be present in migraine attacks. Serotonin oxidative deamination by the enzyme monoamine oxidase leads to 5-hydroxyindole-acetic acid formation (the most significant serotonin metabolite). Highest levels are at noon, lowest are at night. In women are lowest levels during menses. Highest concentrations are in summer, lower in fall and winter.

Increased Values – hyperserotoninemia
anxiety, autism, benign cystic dermoids, cystic fibrosis, hepatitis, inflammatory diseases, postoperative ileus, acute myocardial infarction, **carcinoid**, colitis ulcerosa, acute intestinal obstruction, food – (pineapple, bananas, walnuts, tomatoes), enterochromaffin cell proliferation, schizophrenia, nontropical sprue, dumping sy, benign cystic teratomas, oat cell carcinoma of lung, islet tumors of pancreas, medullary carcinoma of the thyroid, multiple endocrine neoplasia (types I and II)
  Interfering Factors: medicaments – (estrogens, MAO inhibitors, mephenazine, methocarbamol)

Decreased Values – hyposerotoninemia
AIDS, migraine headaches, severe depression, untreated phenylketonuria, Parkinson's disease, syndrome – (Down sy, Kleine-Levin sy), renal failure, degenerative changes in serotonin-ergic system
  Interfering Factors: medicaments – (ranitidine, reserpine)

Analyte	Age/Gender	Reference Range	SI Units	Note
Serotonin	F	500–900	nmol/l	
	M	300–700	nmol/l	
	platelet plasma	1000–2500	nmol/l	
	deplateled plasma	4–15	nmol/l	

Serum Amyloid A

(SAA, syn: amyloid A protein, serum amyloid A protein) SAA is a normal serum protein closely related to the fibrotic tissue protein, it is a prompt and vigorous acute phase protein.

Increased Values

secondary amyloidosis, rheumatoid arthritis, inflammatory diseases, myocardial infarction, tumors, problems during pregnancy

Analyte	Age/Gender	Reference Range	SI Units	Note
Serum Amyloid A		0.17–10	mg/l	

Serum Factors Suppressing Lymphocyte Activity

- **Serum proteins:** albumin (high concentration), specific antibodies against stimulating antigens, immunoregulatory globulin, acid alpha-1-glycoprotein, CRP, serum alpha globulin of amyloid, alpha globulins in tumors, chronic infections, inflammatory diseases, AFP, LDL, complexes antigen-antibody, antibodies against HLA antigens, antibodies against T-lymphocytes
- **Hormones:** glucocorticoids, progesterone, estrogens, androgens, prostaglandins
- **Medicaments:** acetylosalicylic acid, chloroquine, ouabaine
- **Other:** interferon, cyclic nucleotides

Sex Hormone-Binding Globulin

(SHBG, syn: testosterone-binding globulin, sex steroid-binding globulin) Beta globulin. SHBG levels are under the positive control of estrogens and thyroid hormones, and are suppressed by androgens. These influences dynamically control the liver synthesis of this carrier protein.

Production. SHBG is synthesized in the liver and testes Sertoli's cells.

Function. Plasmatic carrier of testosterone and estradiol. Day-to-day level variation is 10%, highest levels are in early afternoon, and lowest around midnight.

Increased Values

anorexia nervosa, **hepatic cirrhosis**, androgens deficiency, smoking, hepatitis, **hyperthyroidism**, male hypogonadism, pregnancy, thyrotoxicosis, testicular feminization, prepubertal children

> **Interfering Factors:** fasting, ageing, medicaments – (androgens, antiepileptics, anticonvulsants, carbamazepine, contraceptives, diphenylhydantoin, estrogens, rifampicin, tamoxifen, thyroid hormones)

Decreased Values

acromegaly, **hirsutism**, hyperinsulinism, **hypercortisolism**, hyperprolactinemia, **hypothyroidism**, **obesity**, puberty, syndrome – (nephrotic sy, polycystic ovary sy), virilization, obese postmenopausal women, women with diffuse hair loss

> **Interfering Factors:** exercise, medicaments – (androgens, danazol, lynestrenol, norgestrel, stanozolol, testosterone)

Silver

(Ag, syn: argentum) Silver alloys and compounds are extensively used in electronics, electrical circuits and batteries. Alloys of silver are utilized in the production of tableware and jewelry. Approximately 30% of the silver consumption in industry is associated with photography.

Test Purpose. To monitor an exposure to silver through dermal contact and inhalation.

Increased Values
silver exposure

Soluble CD4

CD4 expression is mainly on cortical thymus cells, microglia, dendritic cells, and main peripheral T-lymphocyte subclasses. CD4+ T-cells are mature immunocompetent lymphocytes which include T-helper population involved in immunoregulatory functions. CD4+ T-cells recognize peptide antigen only in connection with syngenic proteins of MHC II (main histocompatibility complex) membrane complex. These antigen presenting cells (APC) are able to present CD4+ T-cells antigen peptides in connection with MHC II. APC to T-cell interaction is partially mediated by T-cell receptor (TCR) and CD4.

Test Purpose. Complex cellular immunity assessment and signs of immune system activation.

Increased Values
autoimmune diseases, HIV infections

Analyte	Age/Gender	Reference Range	SI Units	Note
Soluble CD4		0–20	ng/ml	
	sensitivity	<0.25	ng/ml	

Soluble Fas-Ligand

(syn: soluble Fas-L) Fas ligand is named also death factor; binds to Fas receptor and plays an important role in early apoptose phase. Ligand is changed to soluble form and its serum and cell culture concentrations are measurable.

Test Purpose. 1) lymphoproliferative disease therapeutic effect evaluation, 2) resistance/therapy assessment.

Increased Values
LGL leukemia, NK-type lymphomas

Analyte	Age/Gender	Reference Range	SI Units	Note
Soluble Fas Ligand		<0.11	ng/ml	

Soluble Granulocyte Macrophage Colony Stimulating Factor Receptor

(sGM-CSFR) Membrane GM-CSF receptor is composed of two membrane glycoproteins, specific GM-CSFR-alpha (CDw116) and GM-CSFR-beta (KF97) which are essential for biological signal creation. As in many hematopoietic receptors also soluble alpha-chain form exists which has similar afinity like membrane receptor. Soluble receptor task is not completely explained; they are probably important in cytokine activity regulation; they act as cytokine reservoir and transport protein, as antagonist or receptor agonist in dependence on cytokine concentration.

Analyte	Age/Gender	Reference Range	SI Units	Note
Soluble GM-CSF				
Receptor		16–50	pmol/L	
sensitivity		5	pmol	

Soluble Interleukin 2 Receptor

(sIL-2R) IL-2 is bound to receptor (IL-2R) with high afinity which has three different sub-units alpha, beta and gamma. Beta-subunit is stable lymphocyte membrane part, alpha-subunit is inducable IL-2 bound, this subunit corresponds with low afinity IL-2 receptor; increased number testifies cell activation → subunit part is released as protein from membrane → creates soluble IL-2 receptor → circulating cell activation marker.

Test Purpose. 1) diagnosis and monitoring of T-lymphocyte activation in organ transplantation, 2) AIDS and secondary immunodeficiency diagnosis, 3) lymphoproliferative disease diagnosis (hairy cell leukemia especially), 4) autoimmune disease diagnosis.

Increased Values
AIDS, autoimmune diseases, leukemia – (lymphocytic l., hairy-cell l.)

Soluble Interleukin 6 Receptor

(sIL-6R) Membrane IL-6 receptor consists of two glycoprotein chains IL-6-alpha-R and IL-6-beta-R. Membrane IL-6-alpha-R receptor is splitted → soluble protein is created which circulates in blood stream → into urine; this protein is named sIL-6R. IL-6 is binding to IL-6R (IL-6-alpha-R and sIL-6R) and creates binary complex → which bounds with two IL-6-beta-R molecules. Homodimer IL-6-beta-R subunit is responsible for signal transfer; the subunit is activated by LIF, CNTF, oncostatin M, IL-11, and cardiolipin 1. sIL-6R mediates acute phase protein synthesis stimulation and acute/chronic liver inflammations are involved in its modulation.

Increased Values
HIV infection, B-lymphocyte leukemia, plasmocytoma (incl. multiple myeloma)

Somatostatin

(syn: somatotropin release inhibiting hormone, SIH) Gastrointestinal tract regulative polypeptide (it exists in more forms, 14 and 28 amino acids) with neurocrine (neurotransmitter), endocrine/paracrine effects.

Production. Stomach D-cells (mainly antrum), duodenum, pancreas Langerhans' islets, large intestine. Somatostatin is released after food intake and by gastric acid in lumen. Release of somatostatin from the hypothalamus has been shown to be inhibited by VIP, enhanced by IGF-1, IL-1 beta.

Function. Inhibits gastrin, secretin, cholecystokinin, gastrointestinal polypeptide, insulin, glucagon, substance P, enteroglucagon, motilin, VIP, pancreatic polypeptide, ACTH, TSH and GH secretion, motility and splanchnic hyperemia, portal pressure, liver hyperemia. It is one of the most potent endocrine secretion inhibitor known. Decreases aldosterone, catecholamines, T3, T4, and calcitonin. Inhibits acid gastric juice production, pancreatic exocrine secretion (pepsinogen), gallbladder contraction/emptying, small intestinal fluid secretion, and bile secretion. Inhibits T-lymphocyte activation, tumoricidal macrophage activity induced by IFN-gamma, and early hypersensitivity. Also inhibits immune responses, including IFN-gamma secretion, leukocytosis induced by endotoxins and release of colony stimulating factors.

Occurrence. Hypothalamus, central and peripheral nervous system, stomach antrum, upper small intestine, pancreas. Somatostatin has been detected also in platelets, mononuclear leukocytes, mastocytes, and polymorphonuclear leukocytes. Somatostatin is rapidly degraded in the blood and has a very short half-time (1–4 min), one of the most quickly acting polypeptides. 20% diurnal variation, increases during evening to peak at midnight, gradually decreases to low at 8 AM.

Increased Values – hypersomatostatinemia
anemia (normocytic, normochromic), pheochromocytoma, cholelithiasis, disease – (alcoholic liver d., duodenal ulcer d.), active ulcerative colitis, medullary thyroid tumors, tumour from D-cells of pancreatic Langerhans' islets, **somatostatinoma**, steatorrhea, irritable bowel sy, pregnancy, renal failure
> **Interfering Factors:** after meals

Decreased Values – hyposomatostatinemia
conditions following vagotomy
> **Interfering Factors:** medicaments – (oral contraceptives, theophylline)

Analyte	Age/Gender	Reference Range	SI Units	Note
Somatostatin		0–20	ng/l	

Sorbitol Dehydrogenase

(SD, SDH, syn: iditol dehydrogenase) Enzyme, which catalyzes sorbitol to fructose change. It is localized in hepatic cell cytoplasma, its value in liver diseases diagnosis is similar to aldolase and isocitrate dehydrogenase. Its NIDDM diagnosis importance is in complication development monitoring. Measurable activity appearance indicates parenchymal cell damage.

Increased Values
hepatic cirrhosis, hepatitis – (acute infectious h., toxic h.), primary/secondary liver tumors, hypoxic liver damage

Decreased Values
> **Interfering Factors:** medicaments – (cysteine, EDTA, glutathione, phenothiazines)

Stem Cell Factor

(SCF)
Occurrence. Stromal cells of bone marrow, endothelial cells, fibroblasts, and Sertoli's cells.
Function. With various growth factors synergizes/stimulates myeloid, erythroid and lymphoid progenitors. Stimulates the mast cell proliferation and maturation.

Substance P

Peptide composed of 11 amino acids, within nerve cells scattered throughout the body and in special gut endocrine cells. GIT hormone with GIT and brain function. It increases gastrointestinal smooth muscle contractions and causes vasodilatation; it is one of the most potent vasoactive substances known. It seems to be a sensory neurotransmitter mediating pain (analgesic factor), touch and temperature. It increases salivation and histamine release, stimulates early hypersensitivity, mastocyte mediators release, macrophage superoxide production and tumoricid macrophage activity. Substance P may prove to be a better tumor marker for carcinoid tumor than serotonin or 5-HIAA.

Increased Values
tumors – (**carcinoid**, chronic leukemia, medullary t. of the thyroid)

Superoxide Dismutase

(SOD) Antioxidative oxidoreductase class enzyme that protects cells against dangerous superoxide levels. The key enzyme catalyzing high-reactive oxygen removal reaction (free-oxygen radicals, superoxide) → hydrogenperoxide. Enzyme contains the metal elements (Cu-SOD and Zn-SOD) in cytosol and Mn-SOD in mitochondria.
Occurrence. Liver, kidney, lungs, erythrocytes.

Increased Values
diabetes mellitus, cytomegalovirus hepatitis, Parkinson's disease, uremia, revascularization procedures (early reperfusion)

Decrease Values
hemodialysis, hepatitis – (chronic active h., chronic persistent h.), chronic cerebrovascular diseases, acute myocardial infarction (decrease 24–48 hrs, increase 2 w), cardiosurgery procedures

Syphilis Antibodies

Test Purpose. To detect syphilis (Treponema pallidum). Tests used for detection of Treponema pallidum antibody include: Venereal Disease Research Laboratory – VDRL, Rapid Plasma Reagin – RPR, Automated Reagin Test – ART, Standard Test for Syphilis – STS. Tests used for detection of Treponema antigen precipitating antibody include: Fluorescent Treponemal Antibody – Absorption Test – FTA, Microhemagglutination – Treponema pallidum – MHA-TP.

Positive Values	False Positive Values
syphilis	atypical pneumonia, brucellosis, infectious hepatitis, infectious mononucleosis, leprosy, malaria, miliary tuberculosis, post-vaccination state, pregnancy, related Treponemal infection – (yaws, pinta, bejel), systemic lupus erythematosus, typhus

Taurine

(Tau) Belongs to non-essential amino acids, which are involved in sulphur metabolism. It is cysteine metabolism end-product. Taurine is an oxidized, sulfur-containing amine conjugated in the bile, usually with cholic acid to form cholyltaurine (taurocholate), or with chenodeoxycholic acid to form chenodeoxycholyltaurine. Found also in platelets and skeletal musculature; taurine is thought to be a central nervous system neurotransmitter or neuromodulator. Taurine passes to urine after breakdown.

Increased Values – hypertaurinemia
sulfite oxidase deficiency, liver insufficiency, leukemia, tissue necrosis, increased protein intake, sepsis
   Interfering Factors: medicaments – (histidine)

Decreased Values – hypotaurinemia
depressive neurosis, manic depressive disorder, conditions following abdominal surgery (day 4)

Analyte	Age/Gender	Reference Range	SI Units	Note
Taurine	Neonates	70–240	μmol/l	
	Infants	70–180	μmol/l	
	Adults	40–140	μmol/l	

Telopeptides

Bone collagen type I molecules contain two chains which create a helix structure with short non-helix parts (telopeptide) on both sides of the molecule. Telopeptides are important points of stabilizing the cross inter-/intramolecular link creation. Intermolecular cross-links of pyridinoline type are created at the molecular ends. Bone resorption is mediated by osteoclasts, which dissolve the mineral compartment and degrade the organic matrix. This process leads to Ca, P, enzyme and matrix degradation product washout, which have variable bone specificity and are used to bone resorption level measurement. These are mainly the products of collagen (hydroxyproline, hydroxylysine glycosides, pyridine derivatives, and so-called cross-link type I C-terminal telopeptides – ICTP or CTx) and type I N-terminal telopeptides (INTP or NTx). a) The ICTP fragment comes from cross-linked C-terminal telopeptides of a type I collagen alpha-1-chain with alpha-1 or the alpha-2-chain helix area of other collagen molecules. It is released during bone resorption. This fragment is probably specific only for bone. ICTP concentration values in rheumatoid arthritis correlate with disease activity; in plasmocytoma they are prognostic indicators of therapy response and survival prediction. Serum concentration shows a circadian rhythm with maximum after midnight. The concentration differences can be about 25%. b) CTx – antibodies against octapeptide epitope (synthetic) overlapping cross-link area in type I collagen chain are used. CTx is used mainly in urine determination (so-called cross-labs). This part of the telopeptide alpha-1-chain region can be isomeric (alpha and beta isomers) in the aspartate remnant. Isomeric forms can/cannot correlate in different diseases; this can be a disadvantage. Antibodies (cross-labs ELISA) are directed against beta isomers. c) INTP – different pyridinoline and deoxypyridinoline production in bone collagen is based upon N-terminal telopeptide linkage with the helix area of other collagen molecules. Pyridinoline and deoxy-pyridinoline concentration in collagen tissue is very low; the highest ratio is in bone tissue (3.5 : 1), so deoxypyridinoline is thought to be a more specific bone resorption marker than pyridinoline. These fragments are similar to the collagen type from which they split. INTP is used in urine determination. The increased specificity results form the non-reacting peptides, which have a collagen II origin (rheumatoid arthritis, osteoarthritis, Paget's disease), collagen III (synovia), and II (cartilage). Collagen degradation products belong to post-translational collagen modifications; they are not reutilized. The metabolic end is different; specificity is based upon difference between the post-translational modification of type I bone collagen and type I soft tissue collagen. These very sensitive determinations need method standardization to be comparable.

Test Purpose. ICTP – 1) diagnosis of osteoporosis, rheumatoid arthritis, Paget's disease, secondary metabolic osteopathy, 2) plasmocytoma diagnosis (incl. multiple myeloma), 3) hyperparathyroidism diagnosis.

Increased Values – ICTP
rheumatoid arthritis, plasmocytoma (incl. multiple myeloma)

Increased Values – NTx
primary hyperparathyroidism, hyperthyroidism, m. Paget, postmenopause

Analyte	Age/Gender	Reference Range	SI Units	Note
Telopeptide		1.8–5.0	mg/l	

N-Terminal Atrial Natriuretic Peptide

(NT-pro-ANP) Precursor pro-ANP, produced in cardiomyocytes, is splitted into C-terminal polypeptide ANP (half-life about 2 minutes) and N-terminal pro-ANP (half-life about 2 hours, more stabile). High correlation exists between NYHA classification and NT-pro-ANP levels.

Function. Involved in water balance homeostasis, blood pressure regulation. Functions through natriuresis stimulation, vasodilation, RAA system inhibition. Its secretion is stimulated by atrial preload.

Test Purpose. 1) to help in diagnosis, follow-up, therapy and prognosis estimation of chronic heart failure, 2) to help in long-term prognosis evaluation after acute myocardial infarction, to evaluate the left ventricle dysfunction and mortality, 3) to help in evaluation of dilation cardiomyopathy.

Increased Values
cardiovascular diseases with elevated cardiac filling pressure, atrial pacing, **asymptomatic cardiac volume overload**, **dilation cardiomyopathy**, kidney insufficiency, liver cirrhosis, paroxysmal atrial tachycardia, diseases – (renal d., liver d.), failure – (renal f., **congestive heart f.**)

    Interfering Factors: exercise

Analyte	Age/Gender	Reference Range	SI Units	Note
N-Terminal Atrial Natriuretic Peptide		0.11–0.60	nmol/l	

C-Terminal Propeptide Procollagen Type I

(PICP) Type I collagen is a main bone collagen form (97%). Procollagen type I is a collagen precursor which contains two indentical alpha-1 chains and one alpha-2 chain which create helix through non-helix parts on both molecule sides. They are synthesized independently and are modified posttranslationally (hydroxylation and glycosylation). One C-terminal propeptide is released into collagen fibril from each collagen molecule through complicated processes with important space setting. Procollagen has also the N-terminal end (aminoterminal propeptide – PINP). PICP is released as unstable subunit. Good correlation between total ALPI (alkaline phosphatase isoenzyme) plasmatic acitivity and serum PICP concentration exists as well as between serum PICP and bone production.

Increased Values
Paget's disease, metabolically active osteoporosis (values decrease after 50–60 weeks of therapy)

Decreased Values
liver diseases, thyrotoxicosis

Testosterone

(syn: total testosterone) Main male sexual steroid hormone, plasma androgen is bound (about 30%) strongly to sex hormone-binding globulin (SHBG, TeBG – testosterone-binding globulin) and to albumin loosely (about 68%). In males only 1–3% of testosterone remains unbound (0.5–1.3% in female). 5-alpha-dihydrotestosterone (biologically active) is created in target organs and bound to specific cytoplasmic receptors. Steroid complex travels to the cell nucleus and affects gene transcription. Factors that may increase SHBG production are estrogens and thyroid hormones. Testosterone and androstenedione are the main precursors of estradiol and estrone. Blood levels reflect LH secretion and Leydig's cell function.

Production. 1) male: testes – Leydig's cells (90%), 2) female: ovary (15%), liver, adrenal cortex (25%), peripheral conversion from other androgens.

Function. Involved in sexual differentiation, spermatogenesis, secondary sexual organs and sex characteristic development (genital tract masculinization), anabolic metabolism, gene regulation, and male patterned behavior. Testosterone contributes to muscle bulk, bone mass, sex drive, sexual performance and ovulation. Testosterone is metabolized via two pathways to: 1) estradiol (stronger hypophyseous gonadotropic activity inhibitor) and 2) dihydrotestosterone. Released in episodic spikes during day with highest spikes in early AM. In women peaking at ovulation. 10–20% day-to-day level variation.

Test Purpose. 1) to facilitate differential diagnosis of male sexual precocity in boys under age 10, 2) to aid in differential diagnosis of hypogonadism, primary hypogonadism must be distinguished from secondary hypogonadism, 3) to evaluate male infertility or other sexual dysfunction and impotence, 4) to evaluate anovulation, amenorrhea, hirsutism and virilization in women, 5) to evaluate hypopituitarism and Klinefelter's sy, 6) to help in the masculinizing ovary tumors diagnosis, adrenal cortex tumors and congenital adrenal hyperplasia.

Increased Values – hypertestosteronemia
testicular feminization, **hirsutism**, adrenal hyperplasia, congenital adrenal hyperplasia – (21-hydroxylase deficiency, **11-beta-hydroxylase deficiency**), **hyperthyroidism**, male infertility, tumors – (**arrhenoblastoma**, virilizing luteoma, virilizing ovarian t.), testosterone producing tumours – (**adrenal glands t.,** liver t., testes t., ovary t.), **precocious puberty in boys**, syndrome – (adrenogenital sy, Cushing's sy, **polycystic ovary sy – Stein-Leventhal sy**), virilism, short intensive physical exertion
    Interfering Factors: medicaments – (antiepileptics, anticonvulsants, barbiturates, cimetidine, clomiphene, estrogens, gonadotropin – males, oral contraceptives, phenytoin, rifampicin)

Decreased Values – hypotestosteronemia
drug abuse, acromegaly, narcosis, **liver cirrhosis**, myotonic dystrophy, hyperprolactinemia, **primary/secondary hypogonadism**, hypothyroidism, severe diseases, immobilization, **hepatic insufficiency, cryptorchidism**, tumors of – (prostate, testes), obesity, **orchidectomy**, delayed male puberty, stress, syndrome – (**Down sy, Klinefelter's sy**), **uremia**, prolonged intensive physical exertion
    Interfering Factors: medicaments – (anabolic steroids, androgens, antiepileptics, carbamazepine, corticosteroids, cyproterone, danazol, dexamethasone, diethylstilbestrol, digitalis, digoxin, estrogens, ethanol, glucocorticoids, glucose, gonadotropin-releasing hormone, halothane, ketoconazole, methadone, metoprolol, metyrapone, oral contraceptives, phenothiazines, spironolactone, stanozolol, steroids, tetracycline)

Analyte	Age/Gender	Reference Range	SI Units	Note
Testosterone	F	<2.98	nmol/l	
	Oral contracept.	<0.35	nmol/l	
	M	7.0–29.5	nmol/l	

Testosterone, Free

Free (non-protein-bound) testosterone is independent of concentrations changes in the principal testosterone transport protein sex hormone-binding globulin (SHBG).

Increased Values
hirsutism/virilism in females, androgen resistance, polycystic ovary sy
    Interfering Factors: medicaments – (danazol)

Decreased Values
hypogonadism, luteotropin hormone-dependent hyperandrogenism

Thallium

(Tl) Trace element, tissue poison. After intake, thallium is excreted by bile → kidney, a part is stored in tissues (kidney, hair, nails).
Test Purpose. 1) suspicion of intoxication after poison intake, 2) industrial intoxication (metal foundry, cement factory, coke factory, glass foundry, chemical industry, cosmetic industry).

Increased Values
industrial exposure, poisoning

Analyte	Age/Gender	Reference Range	SI Units	Note
Thalium		<25	nmol/l	

Threonine

(Thr) Natural amino acid essential for optimal growth in infants and nitrogen equilibrium in adults. Enzyme defect: carboxylase of propionyl coenzyme A.

Increased Values – hyperthreoninemia
acidemia – (methylmalonic a., propionic a.), carboxylase propionyl coenzyme A deficiency

Thymic Hormones

thymulin serum thymic factor, FTS, thymomodulin, thymopoietin, thymopentin, thymostimulin, thymosins) The thymic epithelium is involved in the differentiation of T-cells through several mechanisms, involving the direct contact with stem cells and the secretion of a variety of biochemically characterized proteins, called thymic hormones. The intrathymic environment is characterized by a complex network of paracrine, autocrine and endocrine signals, involving both cytokines and thymic peptides. The endocrine influences of thymic hormones decline with age and are associatted with "thymic menopause" and cellular immune senescence, contributing to the development of diseases in the aged. The exact physiological roles of thymic hormones are largely unknown. These biologically active proteins and peptides are present in various thymus fractions and participate in the regulation, differentiation and function of thymus-derived lymphocytes. They may act directly or indirectly also on other cells and may have more general functions than those in cellular immunity and differentiation of lymphoid cells. Thymulin needs a zinc ion to express its immunoregulatory properties. Production is stimulated by IL-1, prolactin and growth hormone. Thymulin influences a variety of T-cell differentiation markers and functions in vivo and enhances several functions of the various T-cell subsets.

Thyroglobulin

(Tg) Thyroglobulin is composed of high-molecular weight glycoprotein produced by thyroid gland follicular cells → excreted into follicular lumen where it is iodinated → thyroglobulin iodinated tyrosyl moieties form iodothyronines (thyroxine, triiodothyronine). Thyroglobulins are taken up by endocytosis into follicular cells, where the iodothyronines are liberated by proteolysis → released into extracellular fluid and hence into the blood stream.
Function. Matrix for thyroid hormones synthesis and hormone thyroid gland store forms. Present also in the blood in small amounts. After thyroid gland elimination, Tg is an important tumor marker with a high diagnostic specificity and sensitivity. Day-to-day level variation is 5%. Tg determination must be performed with all antithyroid antibodies determination because antibodies can interfere with thyroglobulin determination.
Test Purpose. 1) to aid in thyroid disorders (goiter, thyroid hyperfunction, inflammation and thyroid physical injury) diagnosis, 2) to aid in differentiated thyroid tumors diagnosis, 3) monitoring after strumectomia (surgical and isotopic) in differentiated thyroid carcinomas, concentration must be unmeasurable, 4) to assess thyroid dystrophy, 5) to aid in subacute/autoimmune thyroiditis diagnosis.

Increased Values – hyperthyroglobulinemia
benign thyroid adenoma, hyperthyroidism, tumors of the thyroid, toxic/non-toxic goiter, liver failure, posttraumatic conditions, pregnancy (3rd trimester), thyroiditis – (Hashimoto's t., subacute t.), thyrotoxicosis

Decreased Values – hypothyroglobulinemia
thyroid agenesis in newborn, thyroidectomy
> **Interfering Factors:** medicaments – (neomycin, thyroid hormones)

Analyte	Age/Gender	Reference Range	SI Units	Note
Thyroglobulin		0–50	µg/l	

Thyroid-Stimulating Hormone

(TSH, syn: thyrotropin, thyreotropic hormone) Glycoprotein which consists of 2 polypeptide chains; alpha-chain has the same homology as have LH, FSH and hCG alpha-chains.
Production. Anterior pituitary (adenohypophysis) hormone. TSH secretion is physiologically mainly regulated by T3 and secondarily by T4 (negative feedback inhibition).
Function. Stimulates thyroid gland vascularity and follicular cells proliferation. Stimulates the thyroid function to produce thyroid hormones (T3, T4) effecting follicular cells via cAMP system activation, including iodine uptake and organic binding. Stimulates antibody production and proliferation of B- and T-lymphocytes.
Hypothalamic Hormones. 1) thyrotropin-releasing hormone (TRH, thyroliberin) → augments TSH release. Low triiodothyronine and thyroxine levels are underlying stimuli for TRH and TSH. 2) growth hormone-release inhibiting hormone (GH-RIH, somatostatin) → inhibits TSH release. Released in episodic spikes, the highest concentrations appear at midnight, falls are to nadir at 4 PM. Day-to-day level variation is 20%. Highest levels are in winter, and lowest are in summer.
Test Purpose. 1) to confirm or rule out primary hypothyroidism and distinguish it from secondary hypothyroidism (pituitary, hypothalamic), 2) to monitor drug therapy in patients with primary hypothyroidism, 3) hyperthyroidism diagnosis (borderline thyroiditides forms), 4) thyroliberin test segment (borderline thyrotoxicosis and thyrotropic reserve evidence, differential diagnosis of pituitary and hypothalamic hypothyroidism, and prolactin secretion pituitary reserve).

Increased Values
surgical/radioactive thyroid ablation, **TSH antibodies,** thyroid agenesis, smoking, **secondary hyperthyroidism, primary hypothyroidism,** congenital cretinism, euthyroid patient with thyroid tumors, euthyroid sick syndrome (recovery), ectopic TSH secretion – (tumors of lung, breast t.), **psychological stress,** endemic goiter, post-subtotal thyroidectomy, pregnancy, thyroiditis – (**Hashimoto's t.,** subacute t. – recovery phase), renal failure
> **Interfering Factors:** TSH autoantibodies, oral radiographic dyes, medicaments – (amiodarone, antiarrhytmics, benserazide, carbamazepine, chlorpromazine, cimetidine, clomiphene, domperidone, growth hormone, haloperidol, interleukin 2, iodine, iopanoic acid, ipodate, ketoconazole, lithium, methimazole, metoclopramide, morphine, phenothiazines, phenytoin, potassium iodide, prednisone, propylthiouracil, sulfapyridine, thyrotropin-releasing hormone, TSH injection)

Decreased Values

TSH autoantibodies, primary hyperthyroidism (except of TSH-producing tumors), subclinical hyperthyroidism, **selective hypopituitarism**, hypothyroidism – (central h., **secondary h.** – pituitary dysfunction), **severe dehydration**, hyponatremia, tertiary hypothyroidism (hypothalamic), **acute illnesses**, pituitary infarction, **malnutrition**, pituitary tumors, thyroid adenoma (autonomous), Graves' disease (treated), euthyroid sick syndrome, acute psychiatric disease, panhypopituitarism, autonomous thyroid hormone secretion, **toxic multinodular goiter, thyroiditis**, pituitary trauma

Interfering Factors: medicaments – (acetylsalicylic acid, amiodarone, anabolic steroids, androgens, apomorphine, benziodarone, bromocriptine, carbamazepine, clofibrate, clomifene, corticosteroids, cotrimoxazole, danazol, dexamethasone, dopamine, glucocorticoids, heparin, iodine, levodopa, lithium, methysergide, opiates, phentolamine, propylthiouracil, pyridoxine, salicylamide, salicylates, somatostatin, steroids, sulfonamides, thiamazole, triiodothyronine)

Analyte	Age/Gender	Reference Range	SI Units	Note
Thyroid Stimulating Hormone	Neonates	<20	mU/l	
	Adults	0.23–4.0	mU/l	

Thyroxine

(T4, TT4, syn: tetraiodothyronine, total thyroxine) About 75% of thyroxine is bound to thyroxine-binding globulin (TBG), about 15% to thyroxine-binding prealbumin (TBPA) – transthyretin (TTR), and about 9% to albumin in plasma. T4 is converted in some peripheral tissues (liver, kidney, muscle) to the more active T3. Free/unbounded thyroxine (FT4, about 0.03–0.5%) is available to the tissues and is metabolically active hormone form. The half-life of T4 in the circulation is 6 to 7 days and for T3 is 24 to 36 hours.

Function. Important for normal metabolic processes (carbohydrates, lipids, proteins), enhances glucose release from glycogen, sugar absorption from intestine; important for mental and physical development, normal respiratory center reactivity, increases the adrenergic receptors number, increases O_2 utilization, bone metabolic turnover, and muscle relaxation rate. T4 is involved in heat production and thermoregulation. T4 has chronotropic and inotropic effects on the heart.

Hypophyseous Hormone. Thyrotropic hormone – thyroid-stimulating hormone (TSH) → stimulates the thyroid function.

Hypothalamic Hormone. 1) thyrotropin-releasing hormone (TRH, thyroliberin) → causes pituitary TSH secretion, 2) growth hormone-release inhibiting hormone (GH-RIH, somatostatin) → inhibits pituitary TSH secretion. 15% day-to-day level variation, highest are in winter, and lowest are in summer. Within-day variation is 50%.

Test Purpose. 1) to evaluate thyroid function, 2) to aid in hyperthyroidism and hypothyroidism diagnosis, 3) to monitor response to antithyroid medication in hyperthyroidism or thyroid replacement therapy in hypothyroidism.

Increased Values – hyperthyroxinemia

autonomic thyroid gland adenoma, acromegaly, **autoantibodies to thyroxine**, cirrhosis – (primary biliary c., liver c.), hepatitis – (chronic active h., viral h.), **hyperemesis gravidarum, hyperthyroidism, acute psychiatric illnesses**, Basedow's disease (Graves' disease), **mola hydatidosa, **pituitary tumors**, thyroid cancer, narcotic addiction, obesity, **acute intermittent porphyria**, euthyroid sick syndrome, **thyroid hormone overdose**, thyroiditis – (**chronic Hashimoto's t.** – early stage, **Quervain's t.** – early stage), **thyrotoxicosis T4**, familial increase of – (thyroxine-binding globulin, thyroxine-binding prealbumin), toxic multinodular goiter, transport proteins increase – (albumin, hepatic diseases, prealbumin in pregnancy, **thyroxine-binding globulin**)

Interfering Factors: oral cholecystographic agents, newborns, after x-ray iodinated contrast studies, pregnancy (1st trimester), medicaments – (albumin, amiodarone, amphetamines, clofibrate, estradiol, estrogens, ether, ethinylestradiol, fluorouracil, heroin, levarterenol, levodopa, lithium, mestranol, methadone, opiates, oral contraceptives, perphenazine, phenothiazines, propranolol, propylthiouracil, thyroid preparations, thyrotropin)

Decreased Values – hypothyroxinemia

acromegaly, **liver cirrhosis**, strenuous physical exercise, **iodine deficiency, hypoproteinemia, primary/secondary hypothyroidism, chronic liver diseases, pituitary insufficiency, malnutrition, myxedema**, hypothalamic disease, **nephrosis**, panhypopituitarism, familial decrease in thyroxine-binding globulin, **antithyroid antibodies**, pseudohypoparathyroidism, **iodine radiotherapy**, thyroid resection, **nephrotic sy**, Hashimoto's thyroiditis (far advanced), subacute thyroiditis, thyrotoxicosis T3, uremia, previous treatment of hyperthyroidism, failure – (renal f., hepatic f.), **decreased transport proteins/thyroxine-binding proteins**

Interfering Factors: adolescents, medicaments – (acetylsalicylic acid, ACTH, aminoglutethimide, aminosalicylic acid, amiodarone, anabolic steroids, androgens, anticonvulsants, antiepileptics, antithyroid drugs, asparaginase, barbiturates, carbamazepine, chlorpromazine, chlorpropamide, cholestyramine, colestipol, corticoids, danazol, diazepam, diphenylhydantoin, dopamine, ethionamide, fenclofenac, fluorouracil, furosemide, glucocorticoids, heparin, interferon, interleukin 2, iodides, isotretinoin, lithium, penicillin, phenobarbital, phenothiazines, phenylbutazone, phenytoin, propranolol, propylthiouracil, reserpine, retinol, rifampicin, salicylates, somatotropin, stanozolol, steroids, sulfonamides, sulfonylurea, testosterone, thiourea, tolbutamide, triiodothyronine, trimethoprim, valproic acid)

Analyte	Age/Gender	Reference Range	SI Units	Note
Thyroxine, Total	1–2 d	138–332	nmol/l	
(T4)	3–30 d	100–253	nmol/l	
	2–12 m	69.5–178	nmol/l	
	1–7 y	68.2–158	nmol/l	
	8–13 y	77.2–143	nmol/l	
	14–18 y	63.1–138	nmol/l	
	Adults	60–155	nmol/l	

Thyroxine, Free

(FT4, syn: free tetraiodothyronine) FT4 is a very small metabolically active total thyroxine fraction (0.04%). 15% day-to-day level variation, highest are in winter, and lowest are in summer.

Test Purpose. 1) to measure the metabolically active thyroid hormones, 2) to aid in the diagnosis of hyperthyroidism or hypothyroidism when TBG levels are abnormal.

Increased Values

hyperthyroidism, Graves' disease, dysalbuminemic hyperthyroxinemia, **hypothyroidism treated with thyroxine,** toxic adenoma, subacute thyroiditis, Hashimoto's thyroiditis, thyroid cancer, toxic multinodular goiter, choriocarcinoma, hydatidiform mole, **euthyroid sick syndrome,** postoperative conditions, pregnancy (1st trimester)

> **Interfering Factors:** medicaments – (acetylsalicylic acid, amiodarone, danazol, furosemide, heparin, lithium, propranolol, valproic acid)

Decreased Values

hemodialysis, **primary/secondary hypothyroidism, hypothyroidism treated with triiodothyronine,** pregnancy (3rd trimester), **sick euthyroid syndrome,** Hashimoto's thyroiditis, idiopathic myxedema, previous treatment of hyperthyroidism, subacute thyroiditis, pituitary dysfunction, hypothalamic disease

> **Interfering Factors:** medicaments – (acetylsalicylic acid, amiodarone, anabolic steroids, androgens, antiepileptics, anticonvulsants, carbamazepine, colestipol, fenclofenac, fenoprofen, heparin, interferon, levothyroxine, lithium, methadone, nitroprusside, para-aminosalicylic acid, phenylbutazone, phenytoin, rifampicin, sulfonamides, thiourea, valproic acid)

Analyte	Age/Gender	Reference Range	SI Units	Note
Thyroxine, Free (FT4)	1–2 d	21–49	pmol/l	
	3–30 d	19–39	pmol/l	
	2–12 m	14–23	pmol/l	
	1–13 y	12–22	pmol/l	
	14–18 y	12–23	pmol/l	
	Adults	12–25	pmol/l	

Thyroxine Autoantibodies

Increased Values – positive

primary hypothyroidism, Graves' disease, thyroid tumors, diffuse/nodular goiter, **Hashimoto's thyroiditis**

Thyroxine-Binding Globulin

(TBG, syn: thyroid-binding globulin)

Function. Principal protein-carrier for T4 and T3 in the plasma. Binds about 70–75% of T4 and 70–80% of T3 because of its relatively high binding affinity and slower dissociation (in comparison with transthyretin) providing a stable hormone plasma reservoir. Hormone balance is carried out by transthyretin (prealbumin). In some conditions it is needed to assess thyroid status by TBG determination (e. g. when dysproteinemia is present). Increased TBG reduces total T4 and T3 measurements and vice versa. The index TT4/TBG is considered as a diagnostic criterion.

Test Purpose. 1) to evaluate abnormal thyrometabolic states not correlating with thyroid hormone values, 2) to identify TBG abnormalities.

Increased Values

cirrhosis – (hepatic c., biliary c.), infectious diseases, hepatitis – (**chronic active h., infectious h., acute viral h.**), **hypothyroidism**, heroin, genetic/idiopathic hepatic diseases, **hereditary TBG excess, estrogen-producing tumors**, familial hyperthyroxinemia, **acute intermittent porphyria, newborns**, subacute thyroiditis, acute liver damage, **pregnancy**

> **Interfering Factors:** medicaments – (acetylsalicylic acid, carbamazepine, clofibrate, estrogens, ethinylestradiol, fluorouracil, heroin, methadone, oral contraceptives, perphenazine, phenothiazines, progesterone, stilbol, tamoxifen)

Decreased Values

uncompensated acidosis, active acromegaly, hepatic cirrhosis, estrogen deficiency, **protein-losing enteropathy, hyperthyroidism**, ovarian hypofunction, **hypoproteinemia**, diseases – (**generalized d. connected with cachexia**, genetic/**chronic**/idiopathic hepatic d., severe d.), malabsorption, **malnutrition**, corticosteroid excess, testosterone producing tumors, hereditary TBG deficiency, **nephrosis, surgical stress**, syndrome – (**Cushing's sy, nephrotic sy**), thyrotoxicosis, liver failure, obstructive jaundice

> **Interfering Factors:** medicaments – (ACTH, anabolic steroids, androgens, asparaginase, carbamazepine, colestipol, corticosteroids, danazol, diazepam, glucocorticoids, lithium, metandienone, neomycin, oxymetholone, perphenazine, phenylbutazone, phenytoin, prednisone, propranolol, salicylates, stanozolol, steroids, testosterone, thyrostatics, valproic acid)

Analyte	Age/Gender	Reference Range	SI Units	Note
Thyroxine Binding Globulin	1 d–1 y F	18–34	mg/l	
	1 d–1 y M	18–32	mg/l	
	2–3 y F	19–34	mg/l	
	2–3 y M	17–32	mg/l	
	4–6 y F	18–31	mg/l	
	4–6 y M	17–30	mg/l	
	7–12 y F	15–30	mg/l	
	7–12 y M	17–29	mg/l	
	13–18 y F	14–29	mg/l	
	13–18 y M	14–26	mg/l	
	Adults F	14–26	mg/l	
	Adults M	9.6–18.5	mg/l	
Thyroxine Uptake (Free thyroxine-binding capacity, T4-uptake)	M	0.29–0.40		

Tissue Polypeptide Antigen

(TPA) Component of the cytoskeleton, tumour marker, a so-called proliferative-kinetic antigen produced in epithelial cells with a high proliferative activity (in S-phase), with the tendency to produce homologous aggregates. Determination specifity is lower because it is positive also in benign disorders of the liver, pancreas and lung. TPA exists in about 90% of all carcinomas, unfortunately it passes into the blood only after cell disintegration or in extreme proliferation.

Test Purpose. To monitor a malignant tumors course and therapy.

diabetes mellitus, hepatitis, infectious diseases, tumors – (colorectum t., uterus t., urinary bladder t., pancreas t., liver t., lung t., prostate t., mammary gland t., testes t., ovary t., thyroid gland t.), pneumonia, dialysis program, conditions after surgery

Analyte	Age/Gender	Reference Range	SI Units	Note
Tissue Polypeptide Antigen Specific Tissue		<80	U/l	
Polypeptide Antigen (TPSA)		<95	U/l	

Total Iron-Binding Capacity

(TIBC) Transport metal-binding globulin. Total amount of iron bound to transferrin/siderophilin. TIBC correlates with serum transferrin levels. Interpretation may be complicated by the presence of an acute phase response, which is associated with decreased iron and iron binding capacity with increased ferritin. High plasma capacity to bound the iron is present in iron deficiency. Highest values are at 4–8 PM and lowest are at 8 AM.

Test Purpose. 1) to estimate total iron storage, 2) to aid in hemochromatosis diagnosis, 3) to help distinguish iron deficiency anemia from chronic disease anemia, 4) to help evaluate nutrition status.

Increased Values

anemia – (hemolytic a., **hypochromic a., sideropenic a.**), exercise, dietary iron deficiency in – **(children, infants), acute hepatitis,** icterus – (mechanical i., obstructive i.), hemorrhage, **hepatic necrosis, polycythemia vera,** conditions post subtotal gastrectomy, **acute/chronic blood loss, pregnancy** (3rd trimester)

Interfering Factors: medicaments – (estrogens, fluorides, oral contraceptives, parenteral iron preparations)

Decreased Values

anemia – (**hemolytic a.,** hyperchromic a., **sickle cell a.,** chronic a. following numerous transfusions, **pernicious a.,** a. in infectious diseases, sideroblastic a., **thalassemia major**), rheumatoid arthritis, atransferrinemia – (**acquired a. from nephrotic sy, congenital a.**), **hepatic cirrhosis, hemochromatosis,** hemosiderosis, hepatopathy, starvation, hyperthyroidism, **hypoproteinemia,** diseases – (chronic infectious d., liver d., renal d., **inflammatory d.**), **chronic renal insufficiency, kwashiorkor, malnutrition, tumours, nephrosis,** acute/chronic liver lesion, **protein loss states,** nephrotic sy

Interfering Factors: medicaments – (ACTH, asparaginase, chloramphenicol, cortisone, glucocorticoids, testosterone)

Analyte	Age/Gender	Reference Range	SI Units	Note
Iron-Binding	1 d	24–57	µmol/l	
Capacity, Total	1 w	34–58	µmol/l	
(TIBC)	1 w–2 m	27–61	µmol/l	
	3–12 m	52–78	µmol/l	
	1–3 y	49–85	µmol/l	
	4–10 y	47–89	µmol/l	
	11–16 y	52–79	µmol/l	
	Adults F	49–89	µmol/l	
	Adults M	52–77	µmol/l	

Tranquilizers and Hypnotics

Test Purpose. To detect suspected toxicity from patient history or clinical observations of central nervous system depression.

Increased Values
tranquilizers overdose, hypnotics overdose

Transcobalamin II

(TC II) Transcobalamin II (glycoprotein) binds and transports plasma vitamin B_{12} to the tissues, predominantly the liver, where the complex is absorbed by the cells via receptor mediated endocytosis.

Increased Values
myeloproliferative diseases

Decreased Values
TC deficiency II – (functional d., congenital d.), infants with severe megaloblastic anemia

Transferrin

(Tf, syn: siderophilin) Beta-1-globulin exists in many genetic polymorphisms.
Production. In the liver, and in small extent in reticuloendothelial system, testes, and ovaries.
Function. Reversibly binds iron, copper, zinc and calcium. Transferrin carries 2 iron atoms per molecule. It is responsible for 50–70% of the iron binding capacity of serum. Mucous membrane intestinal cells iron is transferred on transferrin-glycoprotein blood iron carrier (shuttles iron to liver and to bone marrow). Transferrin carries the iron from macrophages where iron is released after old RBCs breakdown or from the intestines where iron is absorbed. In the bone marrow, transferrin-iron complex attaches to a transferrin receptor on the developing RBC surface. When this complex enters the cell by endocytosis, the iron is released and transferrin is returned to the plasma. Transferrin regulates iron absorption; iron binding capacity reflects the transferrin serum content. Transferrin is measured by the iron amount with which it can bind (total iron-binding capacity – TIBC). In iron deficiency the transferrin level is increased (high plasma capacity to bind iron), in excess levels are decreased. It is an index of nutritional status. Normally about 30% of transferrin is saturated with iron. The second iron store form is hemosiderin. Transferrin is responsible for circadian variation in serum iron due to variable activity of the reticuloendothelial system.
Occurrence. Hepar, bone marrow, lien, lymphatic nodes.
Test Purpose. To aid in the diagnosis of anemias, liver lesions, hemochromatoses, and protein-energetic malnutrition.

Increased Values – hypertransferrinemia
anemia – (aplastic a., posthemorrhagic a., sideropenic a.), hepatitis – (acute h., viral h.), polycythemia, inadequate iron intake
> Interfering Factors: children 2 to 10 years of age, **pregnancy** (3rd trimester), medicaments – (estrogens, ethanol, oral contraceptives)

Decreased Values – hypotransferrinemia

anemia – (sickle-cell a., pernicious a., **thalassemia**), rheumatoid arthritis, **congenital atransferrinemia**, hepatic cirrhosis, **hemochromatosis**, chronic hepatitis, diseases – **(acute/chronic infectious d., renal d., liver d., inflammatory d.)**, **iron poisoning**, **kwashiorkor**, **malnutrition**, **tumors**, **nephrosis**, plasmocytoma (incl. multiple myeloma), septic conditions, **protein loss**, **nephrotic sy**, uremia, **systemic lupus erythematosus**

> **Interfering Factors:** medicaments – (ACTH, asparaginase, chloramphenicol, corticosteroids, dextran, testosterone)

Analyte	Age/Gender	Reference Range	SI Units	Note
Transferrin	1–3 y	2.18–3.47	g/l	
	4–9 y	2.08–3.78	g/l	
	10–19 y +	2.24–4.44	g/l	
	Adults			

Transferrin Receptor

(sTfR, syn: soluble transferrin receptor) Transferrin receptor is a transmembrane, disulfide-linked dimer of two identical polypeptide subunits that binds and internalizes diferric transferrin, thereby delivering iron to the cell cytosol. Each monomer consists of extracellular, membrane and intracellular domain. When a cell needs iron, TfR expression is increased to facilitate iron uptake. Since the major use of iron is for hemoglobin synthesis, about 80% of total TfR is on erythroid progenitor cells. The TfR number in erythropoietic tissue cells is regulated by iron need and intracellular iron levels. Soluble transferrin receptor arises from proteolysis of the intact protein on the cell surface, leading to monomers that can be measured in plasma and serum. Thus, the concentration of soluble TfR in plasma or serum is an indirect measure of total TfR. The serum level of sTfR reflects either the cellular need for iron or the rate of erythropoiesis. The concentration of sTfR in plasma or serum is correlated with erythron transferrin uptake, a ferrokinetic measure of erythropoietic activity. Used for the detection of true iron deficiency and differentiate it from the anemia of chronic disease. An increase in transferrin receptor provides a sensitive measure of iron deficiency, as it reflects the total body mass of tissue receptor. Transferrin receptor is the major mediator of iron uptake by cells.

Test Purpose. 1) to detect the iron deficiency anemia, 2) to help in differential diagnosis of sideropenias and anemias, 3) to monitor an iron utilization (e. g. in patients on dialysis), 4) to evaluate the iron storage status (pregnancy, children, growth spurt, active athletes, conditions after transplantation, chronic inflammatory diseases, cancers).

Increased Values

anemia – (**iron deficiency a., hemolytic a.,** megaloblastic a., beta-thalassemia), polycythemia, **hyperplastic erythropoiesis**, myelodysplastic sy, persons living at high altitude, erythropoietin therapy

Decreased Values

hypoplastic erythropoiesis, chronic renal failure, anemia – (aplastic a., post-transplant a.), iron overload

Analyte	Age/Gender	Reference Range	SI Units	Note
Soluble Transferrin Receptor (sTfR)		10–30	nmol/l	
Transferrin Receptor		1.2–2.8	mg/l	

Transferrin Saturation

(syn: iron saturation, percent transferrin saturation) Percent transferrin saturation is a better iron metabolism index than serum iron is alone.

Increased Values
anemia – (aplastic a., hemolytic a., chronic a. following numerous transfusions, untreated pernicious a., sideroblastic a., thalassemia major), atransferrinemia – (acquired a. in nephrotic sy, congenital a.), vitamin B_6 deficiency, **hemochromatosis, hemosiderosis**, acute iron poisoning, excessive iron intake
  Interfering Factors: medicaments – (parenteral iron preparation)

Decreased Values
anemia – (hemolytic a., **hypochromic a.,** pernicious a. – early treatment), rheumatoid arthritis, hepatic cirrhosis, dietary iron deficiency (infants and children), **acute/chronic infectious diseases**, inflammatory diseases, myocardial infarction, tumors of – (small intestine, stomach), polycythemia vera, conditions post-subtotal gastrectomy, acute/chronic blood loss, pregnancy
  Interfering Factors: diurnal rhythm – (evening)

Analyte	Age/Gender	Reference Range	SI Units	Note
Transferrin Saturation	2 w	30–99	%	
	6 m	10–93	%	
	12 m	10–47	%	
	1–15 y	7–46	%	
	M	16–45	%	
	F	16–45	%	
	Pregnan. 12–16 w	18–50	%	
	3rd trimester	2–30	%	
	1–2 m post-labor	9–49	%	

Transforming Growth Factor

(TGF) Belongs to the cytokines – soluble proteins secreted by solid tumors, monocytes, platelets, keratinocytes, placenta, kidney, bone, T- and B-cells that regulate the magnitude of an inflammatory/immune response and cell growth. It is considered to be an autocrine mitogene of some tumors.

Function and effects

■ **TGF-alpha:** angiogenesis, keratinocyte proliferation, pathological bone resorption, tumor growth, DNA synthesis stimulation. TGF-alpha is produced by a number of human carcinomas and cell lines transformed by viral and cellular oncogene. The factor is found also in urine and plasma. Factor is produced by keratinocytes, macrophages, hepatocytes, platelets. Its synthesis is stimulated by infection with viruses. In mammary tissue its synthesis is induced by estrogens. It is produced also by some non-transformed cells during the development of mammalian embryos. TGF-alpha is probably also involved in the regeneration of liver tissue. Factor may play a role in the vascularisation of tumor tissues since it is produced by tumor cells and macrophages residing in this tissue. Also affects bone formation and remodeling by inhibition of the synthesis of collagen and release of calcium. Factor promotes the generation of osteoblast-like cells in long-term bone marrow cultures. An enhanced production of TGF-alpha has been observed in the development of psoriatic lesions. The factor may be involved, therefore, also in the pathogenesis of psoriasis. The simultaneous expression of TGF-alpha and EGF receptors in primary tumors of advanced gastric cancer appears to correlate significantly with a very poor prognosis.

■ **TGF-beta:** fibroblast proliferation, collagen and fibronectin synthesis, inhibition of cytotoxic T-lymphocyte, natural killers, lymphokine-activated killers, inhibition of T- and B-cell proliferation, wound healing, extracellular matrix stabilization, inhibits protease synthesis, increases their inhibitor production. TGF-beta is involved in immunoglobulin production inhibition (immunosuppression), mitotic endothelial activity inhibition (antiangiogenic effects), connective tissue overproduction pathogenesis (e.g. lung fibrosis, scleroderma); allograft rejection, hematopoiesis, NK-cell activity and T-/B-cell proliferation decrease. It inhibits the synthesis of GM-CSF, IL-3 and the expression of the receptor for G-CSF. TGF-beta also inhibits the growth of immature hematopoietic progenitor cells induced by IL-3, GM-CSF and M-CSF. TGF-beta is a potent chemoattractant for monocytes and fibroblasts; induces the production of other cytokines by monocytes including IL-1-beta, TNF-alpha, platelet-derived growth factor and basic fibroblast growth factor. TGF-beta receptors are at nearly all cell type. Factor is produced in inactive form; it is effective by acidification, alkalization or medicamentous activation. TGF-beta is the most potent known growth inhibitor for normal and transformed epithelial cells, endothelial cells, fibroblasts, neuronal cells, lymphoid cells and other hematopoietic cell types, hepatocytes and keratinocytes. It stimulates the synthesis of the major matrix proteins including collagen, proteoglycans, glycosaminoglycans, fibronectin, integrins, thrombospondin, osteonectin and osteopontin. It also regulates the expression of plasminogen activator and plasminogen activator inhibitor. TGF-beta exists in at least five isoforms (TGF-beta-1, TGF-beta-2, TGF-beta-3, TGF-beta-4, TGF-beta-5). Many of the biological activities of the TGF-beta point to the fact that it may be a potent regulator of wound healing, of bone fracture healing and in the treatment of osteoporosis.

Transketolase

Transferase class enzyme catalyzing specific glycolaldehyde group ketose phosphates transfer to aldose phosphates, a reaction that occurs in the pentose phosphate pathway. The enzyme contains thiamine pyrophosphate and Mg^{2+}. Functional thiamine test.

Increased Values
pernicious anemia

Decreased Values
diabetes mellitus, polyneuritis

Triacylglycerols

(TAG) Triacylglycerols are the major neutral fats found in mammalian tissue; excess is stored in adipose tissue. TAG constitute about 95% of fatty tissue (tissue storage fat).
Production. They are mainly synthesized in the small intestine, liver (from glycerol, fatty acids, and their triesters) and adipose tissue. TAG from intestinal mucosal cells are transported via the thoracic lymph duct to systemic circulation mainly in chylomicron form (triacylglycerols are not soluble in blood) and to a smaller extent as VLDL-C (triacylglycerols

from endogenic source). Chylomicrons contain about 84% TAG, 7% cholesterol, 7% phospholipids and 2% proteins. TAG synthesized in the liver are released to circulation as VLDL-C. Chylomicrons and VLDL-C are further catabolized by lipoprotein lipase to TAG, the chylomicron remnant and LDL-C. HDL-C found in circulation also contains TAG. 30% day-to-day level variation. In women are highest levels at midcycle. Highest levels are in winter, lowest are in fall.

Test Purpose. 1) to screen for hyperlipidemia, 2) to help identify nephrotic sy, 3) to determine the coronary artery disease and atherosclerosis risk, 4) to evaluate nephropathies, thyropathies, 5) to eliminate hypertriacylglycerolemia in hyperuric sy, pancreatitis, diabetes mellitus, alcoholism, 6) genetic screening, 7) to evaluate turbid samples of blood, plasma and serum.

Increased Values – hypertriacylglycerolemia

ethanol abusus (abuse), anorexia nervosa, **atherosclerosis**, cirrhosis – (**hepatic c.,** alcoholic hepatic c.), familial lipase defect, **lipoprotein lipase co-factor deficiency (Apo C-II), familial lipoprotein lipase deficiency, diabetes mellitus,** dialysis program, **gout, familial dysbetalipoproteinemia**, renal dysfunction, **dysproteinemia, glycogenoses,** viral hepatitis, idiopathic hypercalcemia, **familial/essential hyperlipidemia, essential hypertension,** PIH (pregnancy induced hypertension), **familial**/secondary **hypertriacylglycerolemia, hyperuricemia, hypothyroidism,** cholestasis, **chronic ischemic heart disease, liver diseases, obstructive icterus, myocardial infarction,** systemic lupus erythematosus, tumours – (hepatoma), **nephrosis, obesity, biliary obstruction, acute/chronic pancreatitis,** acute intermittent porphyria, excessive caloric intake, increased fat/carbohydrates intake, **high-carbohydrate and fatty diet,** stress, syndrome – (respiratory distress sy, Down sy, **nephrotic sy,** Werner's sy), thalassemia major, impaired glucose tolerance, toxemia, cerebral vessels thrombosis, uremia, **xanthomatosis, chronic renal failure**

> **Interfering Factors:** heavy meals, pregnancy, medicaments – (abacavir, acetylsalicylic acid, amiodarone, amprenavir, androgens, ascorbic acid, asparaginase, atenolol, benazepril, beta-blockers, betaxolol, bexarotene, bisoprolol, captopril, carteolol, carvedilol, catecholamines, chlortalidone, cholestyramine, corticosteroids, cyclosporine, danazol, diazepam, diuretics, enalapril, enoxaparin, estradiol, estrogens, ethanol, ethinylestradiol, etretinate, fosinopril, furosemide, glucocorticoids, hydrochlorothiazide, indapamide, indinavir, interferon, isotretinoin, itraconazole, ketoconazole, losartan, mepindolol, mestranol, methyldopa, metolazone, metoprolol, miconazole, moexipril, nadolol, nelfinavir, oral contraceptives, oxprenolol, phenformin, phenytoin, pindolol, practolol, propranolol, retinol, ritonavir, salicylates, saquinavir, sirolimus, sotalol, spironolactone, tamoxifen, theophylline, thiazides, timolol, torsemide, tretinoin, verapamil)

Decreased Values – hypotriacylglycerolemia

abetalipoproteinemia, severe anemia, **exudative enteropathy,** starvation, hyperparathyroidism, **hyperthyroidism,** hypolipoproteinemia, chronic obstructive lung disease, parenchymal liver disease (end stage), **brain infarction, cachexia,** lactosuria, intestinal lymphangiectasia, **malnutrition,** vigorous exercise, burns, **malabsorption sy**

> **Interfering Factors:** omega-3 fatty acids, fish oil, medicaments – (acetylsalicylic acid, aminosalicylic acid, amiodarone, androgens, ascorbic acid – high doses, asparaginase, celiprolol, chenodeoxycholic acid, cholestyramine, clofibrate, colestipol, doxazosin, estrogens, gemfibrozil, glibenclamide, glucagon, guanfacine, heparin, insulin, metandienone, metformin, metyrapone, neomycin, nicotinic acid, nifedipine, norethisterone, norgestrel, oxymetholone, phenformin, prazosin, probucol, progestins, spironolactone, sulfonylurea, terazosin)

Analyte	Age/Gender	Reference Range	SI Units	Note
Triacylglycerols	Umbilicus	0.10–0.90	mmol/l	
	1–6 y	0.32–0.95	mmol/l	
	6–10 y	0.35–1.14	mmol/l	
	Puberty	0.40–1.33	mmol/l	
	Adults M	0.40–1.60	mmol/l	
	F	0.35–1.40	mmol/l	
		<1.6	mmol/l	

Triiodothyronine

(T3, TT3, syn: total triiodothyronine) Thyroid gland hormone binds to: 1) thyroxine-binding globulin (TBG), 2) thyroxine-binding prealbumin (TBPA; transthyretin – TTR), 3) plasma albumin.

Production. Main part of T3 is created from T4 (prohormone) by deiodinase I in the liver and kidney.

Function. Important for normal metabolic processes, mental and physical development. T3 has greater biological activity than T4 and binds to carriers less tightly than T4.

Hypothalamic-Hypophyseous Relations and Function (see thyroxine). 20% day-to-day value variation, highest levels are in winter, lowest are in summer.

Test Purpose. 1) to aid in T3-toxicosis diagnosis, 2) to aid in hyper/hypothyroidism diagnosis, 3) to monitor clinical response to hypothyroidism therapy.

Increased Values

autonomic thyroid gland adenoma, acromegaly, severe hepatic cirrhosis, **hereditary TBG deficiency, T3 hyperthyroidism, Graves' disease**, increased transport proteins – (albumin, thyroxine-binding globulin, prealbumin), toxic nodular goiter, nephrotic sy, **pregnancy, thyroiditis**

  Interfering Factors: high altitude, medicaments – (amiodarone, clofibrate, dextrothyroxine, estrogens, fenoprofen, fluorouracil, heparin, heroin, insulin, lithium, mestranol, methadone, methimazole, opiates, oral contraceptives, prostaglandin F2-alpha, rifampicin, terbutaline, valproic acid)

Decreased Values

hepatic cirrhosis, uncontrolled diabetes mellitus, smoking, infectious hepatitis, **starvation**, hyperparathyroidism, **hypothyroidism**, severe chronic diseases, systemic diseases, **cachexia, protein-caloric malnutrition, major surgery**, protein loss, acute stress, fasting, decreased transport proteins – (albumin, thyroxine-binding globulin, prealbumin), severe injuries, renal failure, **hereditary increase in TBG**

  Interfering Factors: oral cholecystographic agents, radioopaque contrastagents, elder people, newborns, pregnancy, medicaments – (alprenolol, amiodarone, anabolic steroids, androgens, anticonvulsants, asparaginase, atenolol, benziodarone, carbamazepine, cholestyramine, cimetidine, clomipramine, colestipol, danazol, dexamethasone, ethanol, ethionide, fenclofenac, glucagon, glucocorticoids, growth hormone, heparin, interferon, iodides, isotretinoin, lithium, methylthiouracil, metoprolol, neomycin, penicillin, phenobarbital, phenylbutazone, phenytoin, potassium iodide, prednisone, propranolol, propylthiouracil, reserpine, salicylates – large doses, stanozolol, steroids, sulfonamides, trimethoprim, valproic acid)

Analyte	Age/Gender	Reference Range	SI Units	Note
Triiodothyronine, Total				
	1–2 d	1.2–4.0	nmol/l	
	3–30 d	1.1–3.1	nmol/l	
	2–12 m	1.7–3.5	nmol/l	
	1–7 y	1.8–3.1	nmol/l	
	8–13 y	1.7–3.1	nmol/l	
	14–18 y	1.5–2.8	nmol/l	
	Adults	1.2–2.7	nmol/l	

Triiodothyronine, Free

(FT3) FT3 is the minute T3 portion not bound to TBG and other serum proteins. This unbound hormone is responsible for the thyroid's effects on cellular metabolism. FT3 measurement is the best thyroid function indicator.
Test Purpose. 1) to measure the metabolically active thyroid hormone forms, 2) to aid in the diagnosis of hyperthyroidism or hypothyroidism when TBG levels are abnormal.

Increased Values
hyperthyroidism, T3 toxicosis
    Interfering Factors: high altitude, medicaments – (alprenolol, amiodarone, dextrothyroxine, oral contraceptives, propranolol)

Decreased Values
hypothyroidism, pregnancy (3rd trimester)
    Interfering Factors: cholecystographic agents, medicaments – (amiodarone, atenolol, heparin, metoprolol, phenytoin, propranolol, valproic acid)

Analyte	Age/Gender	Reference Range	SI Units	Note
Triiodothyronine, Free (FT3)				
	1–2 d	5.2–14.3	pmol/l	
	3–30 d	4.3–10.6	pmol/l	
	2–12 m	5.1–10.0	pmol/l	
	1–7 y	5.2–10.0	pmol/l	
	8–13 y	6.1–9.5	pmol/l	
	14–18 y	5.2–8.6	pmol/l	
	Adults	5.4–12.4	pmol/l	

T

Triiodothyronine Resin Uptake

(T3 resin uptake)
Test Purpose. To calculate free thyroxine index.

Increased Values
uncompensated acidosis, **active acromegaly, hepatic cirrhosis,** estrogen deficiency, **protein-losing enteropathy, hyperthyroidism,** ovarian hypofunction, **hypoproteinemia,** diseases – (**generalized d. connected with cachexia,** genetic/**chronic**/idiopathic hepatic d., severe d. systemic d.), malabsorption, **malnutrition,** corticosteroid excess, testosterone producing tumors, X-linked hereditary TBG deficiency, **nephrosis, surgical stress,** syndrome – (**Cushing's sy, nephrotic sy**), thyrotoxicosis, liver failure, obstructive jaundice

Interfering Factors: medicaments – (ACTH, anabolic steroids, androgens, asparaginase, carbamazepine, colestipol, corticosteroids, danazol, diazepam, glucocorticoids, lithium, metandienone, neomycin, oxymetholone, perphenazine, phenylbutazone, phenytoin, prednisone, propranolol, salicylates, stanozolol, steroids, testosterone, thyrostatics, valproic acid)

Decreased Values

cirrhosis – (hepatic c., biliary c.), infectious diseases, hepatitis – (**chronic active h., infectious h., acute viral h.**), **hypothyroidism,** heroin, genetic/idiopathic hepatic diseases, **X-linked hereditary TBG excess, estrogen-producing tumors,** malnutrition, familial hyperthyroxin-emia, **acute intermittent porphyria, newborns,** subacute thyroiditis, acute liver damage, **pregnancy**

Interfering Factors: medicaments – (acetylsalicylic acid, carbamazepine, clofibrate, estrogens, ethinylestradiol, fluorouracil, heroin, methadone, oral contraceptives, perphenazine, phenothiazines, progesterone, stilbol, tamoxifen)

Tropomyosin

Muscle protein of the I-band that inhibits contraction till its position is modified by troponin, enabling the myosin molecule contact with the actin molecules.

Increased Values

alcohol, cocaine, viral/bacterial infectious diseases, **myocardial infarction,** ischemia, **myopathy,** severe muscle damage due to trauma

Troponin I

(cTnI) Cardiac specific troponin I is one of three myofibrilar proteins found in the troponin regulatory complex (troponin C, I, T). Isoforms distribution varies between cardiac muscle and slow- and fast-switch skeletal muscle. Troponin I is present both as a minor cytosolic and a major structural bound protein pool.

Function. Troponin I is the actomyosin-adenosine triphosphatase-inhibiting troponin subunit. Troponin complex mediates the actin interaction and myosin through tropomyosin position alterations in the groove between the two active strands. Troponin I remains increased longer than CK-MB and is more cardiac specific. Principal AMI diagnosis biochemical marker (100% myocardial infarction sensitivity, low specificity).

Test Purpose. 1) to aid in acute myocardial infarction diagnosis, 2) subacute myocardial infarction and microinfarction diagnosis, 3) noninvasive infarction focus size determination, 4) acute myocardial infarction therapy monitoring, 5) after revascularization procedures (PTCA, CABG), 6) myocardial injury in trauma, sport.

Increased Values

chronic ischemic heart disease, unstable angina, **myocardial infarction** (increase 2–8 hrs, peak at 12–24 hrs, decrease 5–10 days after), acute skeletal muscle injury, cardiogenic shock, ventricular dysrhythmia, new complete heart block, intraaortic balloon pumping, **myocardial anoxia, myocardial contusion,** intubation, coronary artery bypass graft, percutaneous transluminal coronary angioplasty

Analyte	Age/Gender	Reference Range	SI Units	Note
Troponin I		<0.1	µg/l	

Troponin T

(cTnT) Cardiac specific troponin T is the tropomyosin-binding subunit of troponin. It is a structural protein, troponin regulatory system segment present in the contractile striated musculature system thin filament. The whole troponin complex is bound to tropomyosin fiber by troponin T. Troponin T is present both as a minor cytosolic and a major structural bound protein pool.

Function. The complex has two other regulatory proteins: troponin I inhibiting actomyosin ATP-ase in conjunction with Ca^{2+} amount, that binds to a third complex component – troponin C that binds Ca and regulates fiber activation process during muscular contraction. A small part of troponin T is free in the cardiomyocyte cytoplasm and probably is a troponin complex synthesis precursor. Principal AMI diagnosis biochemical marker (94% myocardial infarction sensitivity, low specificity). Less specific than troponin I.

Test Purpose. 1) to help in acute myocardial infarction diagnosis, 2) subacute myocardial infarction and microinfarction diagnosis, 3) noninvasive infarction focus size determination, 4) acute myocardial infarction therapy monitoring, 5) after revascularization procedures (PTCA, CABG), 6) trauma/sport myocardial injury.

Increased Values – positive
unstable angina pectoris, false positive values – (chronic muscle disease, acute/**chronic renal failure**), **myocardial infarction** (increase 2–8 hrs, peak at 12–96 hrs, decrease 5 days – 3 months after), perioperative myocardial infarction, myocardial contusion, **myocardial microinfarction** (minor myocardial damage), myocarditis, myocardial damage following percutaneous transluminal coronary angioplasty (PTCA) or coronary artery bypass grafting (CABG).

Analyte	Age/Gender	Reference Range	SI Units	Note
Troponin T		<0.1	µg/l *	See ref. ranges note

Trypsin

A serine protease (201 amino acids).

Production. Trypsin originates from the pancreas (acinar cells). Enzymatically inactive trypsin pancreatic gland precursors are found in two isoforms (trypsinogens I, II) – cationic and anionic, stored in zymogen granules (proenzymes, zymogens) → secreted into the duodenum under vagus nerve or intestinal hormone cholecystokinin-pancreozymin stimulus. Trypsinogens are converted to active enzyme trypsin in the intestinal tract by the intestinal enzyme enterokinase (enteropeptidase) or by preformed trypsin (autocatalysis). Trypsin activity is stimulated by calcium, magnesium, cobalt, and manganese.

Function. When exposed to proteolytic intestine enzymes, cationic and anionic trypsinogens cleave to form cationic and anionic trypsins, which play major roles in dietary protein digestion. Trypsin hydrolyzes peptide bonds formed by lysine or arginine carboxyl groups with other amino acids. Enzymatically active trypsin can activate several coagulation cascade factors, and lead to intravascular clotting. To prevent this occurrence in vivo, active trypsin released into the blood is rapidly inactivated by alpha-1-antitrypsin and alpha-2-macroglobulin. These inhibitors protect plasma and other proteins against trypsin hydrolysis.

Test Purpose. 1) acute and acutely relapsing pancreatitis diagnosis, 2) chronic relapsing pancreatitis diagnosis and monitoring, 3) cystic fibrosis diagnosis, 4) pancreas tumors diagnosis and monitoring.

Increased Values – hypertrypsinemia
gallstones, disease – (Bornholm d., neonatal fibrocystic d.), diseases – (viral infectious d., liver d.), pulmonary infarction, insufficiency – (chronic renal i., cardiac i.), meningitis, mumps, **acute pancreatitis**, relapsed chronic pancreatitis, peptic ulcer
> **Interfering Factors:** after ERCP, after meals, medicaments – (bombesin, cholecystokinin, secretin)

Decreased Values – hypotrypsinemia
diabetes mellitus, pancreatic tumors, chronic pancreatitis

Tryptase

Increased tryptase levels indicate mast cell degranulation with mediator release, thereby demonstrating an allergic basis for the reaction. A negative results does not exclude an allergic basis.
Test Purpose. To identify anaphylaxis as a cause of collapse or death (e.g. during anesthesia, after insect sting, administration of drugs, administration of biological agents).

Increased Values
anaphylactic reactions

Tryptophan

(Trp) Tryptophan is an essential glucoplastic amino acid needed for infant growth and adult nitrogen equilibrium. Trp is a precursor to nicotinic acid, nicotinamide (main pathway), serotonin and indole agents (secondary pathway). Trp majority is used in protein synthesis, minor part in biogenic agents synthesis.

Increased Values – hypertryptophanemia
hepatic encephalopathy, sepsis

Decreased Values – hypotryptophanemia
enteritis regionalis, hypothermia, Hartnup disease, **protein-caloric malnutrition** (kwashiorkor), **pellagra**, conditions after abdominal surgery (1–2 days), carcinoid sy
> **Interfering Factors:** medicaments – (acetylsalicylic acid, glucose, indomethacin)

Analyte	Age/Gender	Reference Range	SI Units	Note
Tryptophan	Infants	45–65	μmol/l	
	Adults	45–75	μmol/l	

TSH Alpha-Subunit

Increased Values
TSH-secreting **pituitary tumours**, post-menopausal women, hypogonadal men

Tumor Markers

(TM) Tumor marker is a substance either in or produced by tumors (or by the body in response to the presence of tumor), that can be used to differentiate the tumor from normal tissue, found in cells, tissues or body fluid. Tests help to determine the characteristics of the tumor (aggressiveness, rate of growth, degree of abnormality). **Potential TM utilization: 1)** screening in general population, 2) diagnosis and differential diagnosis in symptomatic patients, 3) clinical carcinoma staging, 4) estimating tumor volume, 5) prognostic indicator for disease progression, 6) planning and evaluating treatment process and success, 7) detecting carcinoma recurrence, 8) monitoring therapy response, 9) tumor mass radio immunolocalization, 10) determining immunotherapy direction. Measurements of tumor marker levels can be useful when used along with x-rays or other tests, in the detection and diagnosis of some types of cancer. However, measurements of tumor marker levels alone are not sufficient to diagnose cancer for the following reasons: 1) TM levels can be elevated in people with benign conditions, 2) TM levels are not elevated in every person with cancer, especially in the early stages of the disease, 3) many tumor markers are not specific to particular type of cancer, the level of a TM can be raised by more than one type of cancer.

- **Blood group antigen-related cancer markers: CA 19-9** (pancreas, liver, breast, gastrointestinal tract), **CA 19-5** (pancreas, breast, gastrointestinal tract, ovary), **CA 50** (colon, pancreas, liver, gastrointestinal tract), **CA 72-4** (colon, lung, breast, gastrointestinal tract, ovary), **CA 242** (gastrointestinal tract, pancreas)
- **Enzymes: acid phosphatase** (prostate, prostate metastases), **aldolase** (colon, rectum, liver, lungs, stomach, CNS, leukemia, lymphoma, melanoma, pancreas, prostate, breast, gastrointestinal tract, genitourinary tract), **alcohol dehydrogenase** (liver), **ALP** (leukemia, Hodgkin's lymphoma, bone metastases, liver, liver metastases, lung, breast, sarcoma, seminoma, testes, gastrointestinal tract, trophoblast, ovary), **ALP – placental isoenzyme** (ovary, endometrium, lung, breast, seminoma, seminoma metastases, smokers), **ALP - intestinal isoenzyme** (hepatoma, gastrointestinal tract), **AMS** (pancreas), **prostate specific antigen** (prostate), **arylsulfatase B** (colon, breast), **AST** (mammary gland), **beta-glucosidase** (colon), **beta-glucuronidase** (acute lymphocytic leukemia, stomach), **neuron-specific enolase** (NSE) (pheochromocytoma, carcinoid, bronchogenic small-cell carcinoma, melanoma, neuroblastoma, pancreas, Wilm's tumor, thyroid gland, kidney, testes, APUD tumors), **esterase** (breast), **specific acid prostatic phosphatase** in prostatic tumors, **galactosyltransferase** (colon, bladder, gastrointestinal tract), **glycosyltransferase** (ovary), **GMT** (liver, liver metastases), **hexokinase** (liver), **cathepsin, creatine kinase BB** (colon, lymphomas, uterus, bladder, lung, prostate, breast, testes, gastrointestinal tract, ovary), **lactic dehydrogenase** (colorectal tumors, leukemia, lymphomas, non-Hodgkin's lymphoma, liver, seminoma, Ewing's sarcoma), **LD-1** (testes), **L-dopa decarboxylase** (lungs), **leucine aminopeptidase** (pancreas, liver), **myeloperoxidase** (acute myeloblastic leukemia), **5-nucleotidase** (acute lymphoblastic leukemia, liver), **pyruvate kinase** (liver), **ribonuclease** (large bowel, lung, ovary), **sialyltransferase** (colon, lung, breast), **terminal deoxynucleotidyl-transferase** (leukemia), **thymidine kinase** (pulmonary small cell carcinoma, leukemia, lymphomas)
- **Globulins:** monoclonal immunoglobulin in paraproteinemia
- **Hormones: Bombesin** (lung small cell carcinoma), **erythropoietin** (paraneoplastic erythrocytosis), **gastrin** (gastrinoma, stomach, pancreas, parathyroid, pituitary), **antidiuretic hormone** (bladder, duodenum, lung small cell carcinoma, carcinoid, Hodgkin's disease, adrenal cortex, pancreas), **adrenocorticotrophic hormone** (adrenals, lung small cell carcinoma), **human growth hormone** (pituitary adenoma, kidney, lung), **beta-human**

chorionic gonadotropin (choriocarcinoma, embryonal carcinoma, testes), **insulin, calcitonin** (medullar thyroid carcinoma, breast, liver, kidney, lung carcinoid), **human placental lactogen** (gonads, trophoblastic carcinoma, lung, breast), **neurophysins** (lung small cell carcinoma), **parathormone** (pituitary adenoma, kidney, liver, lung, breast), **parathormone-related protein** (lung, ovary, thymoma, carcinoid, islet cell tumor of pancreas, medullary carcinoma of thyroid), **renin** (kidney), **vasoactive intestinal polypeptide** (pheochromocytoma, bronchogenic carcinoma, neuroblastoma, pancreas), **prolactin** (pituitary adenoma, kidney, lung), **thyroglobulin** (thyroid)

■ Proteins: **melanoma associated antigen** (melanoma), **pancreas associated antigen** (pancreas, stomach), **beta-2-microglobulin** (chronic lymphatic leukemia, B-cell lymphoma, Waldenström's macroglobulinemia, multiple myeloma), **C-peptide** (insulinoma), **ferritin** (leukemia, liver, lungs, breast), **immunoglobulins** (lymphomas, multiple myeloma, Waldenström's macroglobulinemia), **chromogranin A** (pheochromocytoma)

■ Others: **estrogen and progesterone receptors** (breast), **hydroxyproline** (urine) (bone metastases, plasmocytoma), **homovanillic acid, 5-hydroxy-indoleacetic acid** (carcinoid), **lipid-bound sialic acid** (LSA) (lymphoma, melanoma, lung, prostate, mammary glands, gastrointestinal tract), **catecholamines metabolites** (vanilmandelic acid, metanephrines in urine) – (pheochromocytoma, neuroblastoma), **polyamines** (cerebrospinal fluid), **tumour necrosis factor** (cachectin + lymphotoxin)

■ Mucin tumor markers: **MCA** (mucin-like carcinoma-associated antigen) – (breast, ovary), **CA 15-3** (colorectum, pancreas, lungs, breast, ovary, uterus, prostate), **CA 125** (endometrium, ovary, peritoneum, pleura, pancreas, liver, lung, breast, gastrointestinal tract, fallopian tube), **CA 549** (lungs, prostate, breast, ovary), **CA 27. 29** (colorectum, pancreas, lungs, breast, ovary), **DU-PAN-2** (pancreas, lung, gastrointestinal tract, ovary)

■ Oncofetal antigens: **carcinoembryonic antigen** (colorectum, pancreas, lung, breast, gastrointestinal tract), **beta-oncofetal antigen** (colon), **pancreatic oncofetal antigen** (pancreas), **squamous cell antigen** (cervix, head, skin, neck, lung), **Tennessee antigen** (colon, bladder, gastrointestinal tract), **tissue polypeptide antigen** (colorectum, bladder, breast, ovary), **alpha-fetoprotein** (germ cells tumor, liver), **tumor associated glycoprotein** (TAG 72)

■ Oncogenic markers: **N-ras-mutation** (acute myelogenic leukemia, neuroblastoma), **c-myc-translocation** (B- an T-cell lymphomas, bronchogenic small-cell carcinoma), **c-erb-B-2-amplification** (breast, gastrointestinal tract, ovary), **c-abl/bcr-translocation** (chronic myelogenous leukemia), **N-myc-amplification** (neuroendocrine tumors)

Tumour Marker BCL-2

Apoptotic and tumour marker (intracellular protein) characteristic for B-cell lymphoma-2. It plays main role in apoptosis regulation, inhibiting apoptosis induced by different factors. BCL-2 determination gives strategic information about prognosis and tumour chemotherapy resistance. It is useful also in HIV infection diagnosis.
Test Purpose. 1) lymphoma diagnosis, 2) AIDS diagnosis.

Tumour Marker BTA

(bladder tumor antigen) Proteins which regulate complement (incl. factor H) are coded with gene cluster in so-called RCA locus of the first chromosome (complement activation regulators). Some cell lines of human malignant tumors synthesize complement related to CFH (complement factor H). BTA is a member of RCA gene group; it has proven factor H biological activity. The best determination is in urine. It has a 20% higher sensitivity than cytological determination in each stage and grade. Healthy individuals and persons with non-genitourinary carcinoma have negative BTA test results by 95% and 93% respectively; in benign prostate hyperplasia by 84% and 78% in prostate carcinoma. Non-specific positive results are found in malignant kidney tumors, lithiasis, nephritides and relatively recent genitourinary tract injury (catheterization microtrauma).

Test Purpose. Bladder carcinoma diagnosis.

Increased Values – positive
kidney tumours, nephritis, nephrolithiasis, gastrointestinal tract injury

Tumour Marker – Cancer Antigen 15-3

(CA 15-3) (BCM – breast cancer mucin) CA 15-3 is a mucin-like high-molecular-weight glycoprotein localized in the alveoli apices and mammary glands ducts. It is a circulating antigen.

Increased Values – positive
tumors – (uterus t., pancreas t., prostate t., **lung t., mammary gland t., ovary t.**), non-cancer specific increase in – (benign breast diseases, hepatobiliary tract diseases, lung diseases, pancreatitis, benign ovarian diseases, endometriosis, pelvic inflammatory disease, hepatitis, pregnancy, lactation)

Analyte	Age/Gender	Reference Range	SI Units	Note
CA 15-3		<28	U/ml	

Tumour Marker – Carbohydrate Antigen 19-9

(CA 19-9) CA 19-9 is a Lewis blood group derivative.

Increased Values – positive
tumors – (**biliary ways t., colorectal t., pancreas t., liver t., lung t.,** ovary t., **stomach t.**), non-cancer specific increase in – (hepatic cirrhosis, cystic fibrosis, **acute cholecystitis, gallstones,** hepatobiliary tract diseases, alcoholic liver disease, lung diseases, ulcerative colitis, inflammatory bowel disease, inflammatory diseases, **acute pancreatitis**, renal failure)

Analyte	Age/Gender	Reference Range	SI Units	Note
CA 19-9		<37	U/ml	

Tumour Marker – Cancer Antigen 27-29

(CA 27-29)

Increased Values – positive
tumors – (biliary ways t., renal t., uterus t., **colorectal t., pancreas t., liver t., lung t., ovary t., stomach t.**), non-cancer specific increase in – (pregnancy – 1st trimester, endometriosis, ovarian cysts, benign breast disease, renal diseases, liver diseases)

Tumour Marker – Cancer Antigen 50

Increased Values – positive
tumors – (colon-rectum t., biliary ducts t., intestine t., kidney t., **pancreas t.,** lung t., prostate t., breast t., ovary t., stomach t.), non-cancer specific increase in – (hepatobiliary tract diseases, inflammatory diseases)

Analyte	Age/Gender	Reference Range	SI Units	Note
CA 50		<25	U/ml	

Tumour Marker – Cancer Antigen 72-4

(CA 72-4, syn: tumor-associated glycoprotein – TAG 72) CA 72-4 is a high-molecular-weight mucin-like, tumor-associated antigen.

Increased Values – positive
tumors – (biliary ducts t., intestine t., pancreas t., lung t., breast t., stomach t.)

Analyte	Age/Gender	Reference Range	SI Units	Note
CA 72-4		<4	U/ml	

Tumour Marker – Cancer Antigen 125

(CA 125) CA 125 is a high-molecular-weight glycoprotein, present in normal endometrial tissue, serous and mucinous uterine fluids; it does not circulate except when natural barriers are destroyed. It is not possible to state the meaning of an abnormally high CA 125 without additional information about the particular patient being evaluated. The reason is that this protein can be increased in many different benign and malignant conditions. The two most frequent situations in which CA 125 is used is to monitor patients with a known malignancy or as one of several tests in the workup of a patient suspected of having a tumor. In the patient who is known to have a malignancy, such as ovarian carcinoma, the CA 125 level can be monitored periodically. A decreasing level indicates effective therapy while an increasing level indicates tumor recurrence.

Increased Values – positive
tumors – (**metastatic peritoneal carcinomatosis,** colorectum t., **endometrium t.,** spinal cord t., **pancreas t., liver t., lung t., breast t., ovarian t., gastrointestinal tract t.,** fallopian tube t., peritoneal t., pleural t.), non-cancer specific increase in – (**hepatic cirrhosis, endometriosis,** gynecological diseases, hepatobiliary tract diseases, **onset of menstrual period, pancreatitis, peritonitis,** pelvic inflammatory disease, **pleuritis, pregnancy** – 1st trimester, ovarian cysts, fibroids, inflammatory bowel disease)

Analyte	Age/Gender	Reference Range	SI Units	Note
CA 125		<35	U/ml	

Tumor Marker CA 242

Belongs to the membrane associated glycoproteins with CA 19-9 and CA 72-4. These markers are also named human pancarcinoma tumor mucines. CA 242 is an independent progression indicator in colorectum carcinoma, high levels mean lymph node metastases. Significant CA 242 decrease or normalization mean longer periods without disease. Its sensitivity is higher than CEA and other markers. Sensitivity and specificity are much higher when compared to Dukes B, C and D stages (marker is positive from stage B). Examination of this parameter does not improve tumor staging. Determination in colon and rectum carcinoma advantages over CEA and CA 19-9 have not been proven; combination with CEA will increase examination sensitivity to 57% and 62% respectively in these tumors.

Test Purpose. 1) colorectum carcinoma diagnosis, 2) pancreas carcinoma differential diagnosis, 3) stomach carcinoma diagnosis.

Increased Values – positive
liver cirrhosis, diseases – (gynecological d., lung d., hepatobiliary d.), tumors of – (esophagus, pancreas, breast, biliary ducts)

Analyte	Age/Gender	Reference Range	SI Units	Note
CA 242		16–20	U/ml	

Tumor Marker CA 549

(syn. cancer-associated antigen) Tumor marker CA 549 is high-molecular acid glycoprotein complex, which is placed mainly in mammary gland membranes, colon, urinary bladder, biliary ducts, pancreas, ovary, prostate, liver and kidney. CA 549 consists of two subunits which bond differently with sialic acid. Two monoclonal antibody types immunochemically distinguish epitops; epitops also differ in mammary gland spread (luminal/membranous and cytoplasmatic).

Test Purpose. To monitor metastasing mammary gland carcinoma when combined with TPS (tissue polypeptide substance), MCA and CEA.

Increased Values – positive
diseases – (liver d., breast d.), tumors of – (bronchi, prostate, **breast**, ovary), non/metastasing mammary gland tumors, metastatic tumors – (colon, endometrium, lungs, prostate, ovary), benign liver tumors, benign breast tumors, non-cancer specific increase in – (liver diseases, pregnancy)

Analyte	Age/Gender	Reference Range	SI Units	Note
CA 549	F	0–11	U/ml	
	M	1.1–6.7	U/ml	

Tumor Marker M2-PK

(M2 isoform of pyruvate kinase) Glycolytic enzyme pyruvate kinase exists in four isoforms (type R, L, M1, M2). Isoforms have tissue-specific distribution. All active isoforms are homotetramers. Pyruvate kinase M2 iso-form is present in tumor cells and has a lower substrate affinity (tumor M2-PK). Tumor marker M2-PK evaluation together with CEA and/or CA 19-9 evaluation lead to higher sensitivity in colorectum and pancreatic cancers diagnosis with small decrease of specificity.

Test Purpose. 1) to help in diagnosis of malignant tumors, 2) to monitor course and therapy of tumors (breast, lung, kidney, stomach, esophagus, colorectum) in combination with other tumor markers.

Increased Values – positive
tumors of – (breast, lung, kidney, stomach, esophagus, colorectum), non-cancer specific increase in – (inflammatory diseases of intestine, ulcerative colitis)

Tumour marker organ specificity:
■ **Good organ specificity**
- **AFP:** tumors – (chorion t., acute lymphocytic leukemia, **liver t.,** mammary gland t., **testes t., ovary t., thyroid t.**), non-cancer specific increase in – (fetal abnormalities, hepatobiliary tract diseases, digestive disorders, **pregnancy**)
- **beta-hCG:** tumors – (**choriocarcinoma, mola hydatidosa, testes t., ovary t., thyroid t.**), non-cancer specific increase in – (ovarian cysts, endometriosis, pregnancy)
- **immunoglobulins:** myeloma, Waldenström's disease
- **insulin:** insulinoma
- **calcitonin:** tumors – (pancreas t., **lung t.,** mammary gland t., **medullary thyroid gland t.**), non-cancer specific increase in – (polyadenomatosis)
- **MCA:** tumors – (**breast t.**), non-cancer specific increase in – (hepatobiliary tract diseases, pregnancy)
- **NSE:** tumors – (**bronchogenic small-cell t.,** pheochromocytoma, gastrinoma, carcinoid, medulloblastoma, brain t., Wilm's t., testes t., **neuroblastoma**, kidney t., retinoblastoma, thyroid t.), non-cancer specific increase in – (hemolysis, lung diseases, pneumonia, septic shock, cranial trauma)
- **prostate specific antigen:** bone metastases, **prostate tumors**, non-cancer specific increase in – (prostatic infarction, bladder catheterisation, benign prostatic tumors, prostatitis)
- **thyroglobulin:** tumors – (**thyroid gland t.**), non-cancer specific increase in – (benign thyroid diseases)

■ **Relatively good organ specificity**
- **ACP:** tumors – (bone metastases of t., prostate t.), non-cancer specific increase in – (prostatic adenoma, hepatobiliary tract diseases, bone diseases, kidney diseases, prostatic infarct, bladder catheterization, rectal examination)
- **SCCA (squamous cell carcinoma antigen):** tumors – (esophagus t., head t., epidermoid t. of uterus cervix, neck t., large-cell epidermoid t. of lung), non-cancer specific increase in – (bronchopneumonia, benign gynecologic diseases, inflammatory diseases of kidney/liver)
- **beta-2-microglobulin:** tumors – (**lymphomas**, melanoma, plasmocytoma, lung t., breast t.), non-cancer specific increase in – (hepatobiliary tract diseases, chronic inflammatory diseases, renal insufficiency, heavy metal intoxication, immunodeficiency states)
- **CA 15-3:** tumors – (uterus t., pancreas t., prostate t., **lung t., mammary gland t., ovary t.**), non-cancer specific increase in – (benign breast diseases, hepatobiliary tract diseases, lung diseases, pancreatitis, benign ovarian diseases, endometriosis, pelvic inflammatory disease, hepatitis, pregnancy, lactation)

- **CA 19-9:** tumors – (**biliary ways t.,** colon t., **pancreas t., liver t., lung t.,** ovary t., stomach t.), non-cancer specific increase in – (hepatic cirrhosis, cystic fibrosis, **acute cholecystitis**, gallstones, hepatobiliary tract diseases, alcoholic liver disease, lung diseases, inflammatory diseases, acute pancreatitis, renal failure)
- **CA 50:** tumors – (colon-rectum t., kidney t., **pancreas t.,** lung t., prostate t., breast t., ovary t., stomach t.), non-cancer specific increase in – (hepatobiliary tract diseases, inflammatory diseases)
- **CA 72-4:** tumors – (biliary ducts t., intestine t., pancreas t., lung t., breast t., stomach t.)
- **CA 125:** tumors – (**metastatic peritoneal carcinomatosis, endometrium t.,** uterus t., spinal cord t., **pancreas t., liver t.,** lung t., breast t., **gastrointestinal tract t., ovary t.,** fallopian tube t., peritoneal t., pleural t.), non-cancer specific increase in – (**hepatic cirrhosis, endometriosis,** gynecological diseases, hepatobiliary tract diseases, **onset of menstrual period, pancreatitis, peritonitis,** pelvic inflammatory disease, **pleuritis, pregnancy** – 1st trimester)
- **CA 195:** tumors – (colorectum t.)
- **CA 549:** tumors – (**breast t.**), metastatic tumors – (colon, endometrium, lungs, prostate, ovary), benign liver tumors, benign breast tumors, non-cancer specific increase in – (liver diseases, pregnancy)
- **CYFRA 21-1:** tumors – (bronchogenic non-small cell t., gynecologic epidermoid t.), non-cancer specific increase in – (gynecological diseases, chronic renal diseases)
- **TAG 72:** tumors – (**colorectum t.**)
- **thymidine-kinase:** tumors – (bronchogenic small-cell carcinoma, leukemia, lymphomas), non-cancer specific increase in – (vitamin B_{12} depletion, viral infections)

- **Relatively small organ specificity**
  - **CEA:** tumors – (chorion t., **colon-rectum t.,** bone t., leukemia, bladder t., neuroblastoma, pancreas t., liver t., lung t., prostate t., mammary gland t., testes t., gastrointestinal tract t., ovary t., stomach t., thyroid t., gallbladder t.), non-cancer specific increase in – (alcoholism, smoking, hepatic and biliary tract diseases, pulmonary inflammatory diseases, digestive disorders)
  - **ferritin:** tumors – (**acute myeloblastic leukemia,** lymphomas, **non-Hodgkin's lymphomas, Hodgkin's disease,** neuroblastoma, pancreas t., liver t., **plasmocytoma** (incl. multiple myeloma), lung t., breast t., testes t.), non-cancer specific increase in – (sideroblastic anemia, hemochromatosis, hemosiderosis, hepatobiliary tract diseases, inflammatory diseases, iron overload)
  - **5-OH indoleacetic acid:** carcinoid
  - **TPA:** tumors – (colorectum t., uterus t., urinary bladder t., pancreas t., **lung t., mammary gland t.,** ovary t., stomach t., thyroid t., bile duct t.), non-cancer specific increase in – (gastrointestinal tract diseases, diseases of breast/lung, inflammatory diseases)

Tumor markers with described relation to organs/systems, pathological and physiological conditions:

Tumorous diseases	Tumor markers
biliary ways	CEA, CA 19-9
large intestine	ACTH, ADH, AFP, aldolase, AMS, Tennessee Ag, arylsulfatase B, beta-glucosidase, beta-lipotropin, beta-oncofetal antigen, CA 15-3, CA 19-9, CA 27.29, CA 50, CA 72-4, CA 195, CA 242, CA 549, CEA, CK-BB, galactosyltransferase, LD, ribonuclease, sialyltransferase, TAG 72, TPA

Tumorous diseases	Tumor markers
small intestine	CA 72-4
adrenal marrow	**chromogranin A, B**
duodenum	ADH
embryo	AFP, hCG
head	SCCA
hypophysis	**PRL** (adenoma), PTH, STH
chorion	AFP, CEA, **hCG, SP-1**
rectum	aldolase, CA 15-3, CA 27.29, CA 50, CA 195, CEA, LD, TAG 72, TPA
bone	ALP, CEA
skin	melanoma-associated Ag, **B2M**, hCG, sialic acid, NSE, **intracellular S-100 protein**, SCCA, thymidine kinase
neck	SCCA
leukemia	AFP, ALP, beta-glucuronidase, B2M, c-abl/bcr-translocation, CEA, **ferritin, chromogranin A, B**, sialic acid, LD, myeloperoxidase, N-ras-mutation, 5-nucleotidase, **glucocorticoid receptors**, terminal deoxytransferase, thymidine kinase
lymphomas	ALP, **BCL-2, B2M, CD 30+**, CK-BB, c-myc-translocation, **ferritin, fibronectin**, immunoglobulins, sialic acid, LD, **thymidine kinase**
uterus + cervix	ACTH, CA 15-3, CA 125, CEA, CK-BB, beta-glucuronidase, hCG, **SCCA, TPA**
bladder	ACTH, Tennessee Ag, beta-lipotropin, **BTA**, CEA, CK-BB, galactosyl-transferase, **TPA**
metastases into bones	ACP, ALP, hydroxyproline (urine), PSA
tumor metastases	CA 549
adrenals	ACTH, ADH, hCG, NSE, VIP
neuroendothelium	**chromogranin A, B**, VIP
kidney	ACTH, AFP, beta-lipotropin, CA 50, NSE, PRL, PSA, PTH, STH
ENT	**CA 50**, CEA, **NSE**, SCCA, **thymidine kinase**, TPA
pancreas	ACTH, ADH, AFP, AMS, pancreas-associated antigen, beta-lipotropin, CA 15-3, CA 19-5, **CA 19-9**, CA 27.29, CA 50, CA 72-4, CA 125, CA 195, **CA 242, CEA**, DU-PAN-2, ferritin, galactosyltransferase, hCG, chromogranin A, B, calcitonin, LAP, NSE, pancreatic oncofetal Ag, SPAN-1, TPA, VIP
pharynx	CEA, **SCCA**, TPA
liver	**AFP**, aldolase, alcohol dehydrogenase, ALP, CA 15-3, **CA 19-9**, CA 125, CEA, feritin, GMT, hCG, hexokinase, LAP, LD, 5-nucleotidase, placental lactogen, PTH, pyruvate kinase, TPA
plasmocytoma (incl. multiple myeloma)	**B2M, ferritin, fibronectin**
lung	ACTH, ADH, AFP, aldolase, ALP, B2M, bombezin, CA 15-3, CA 19-9, CA 27.29, CA 50, CA 72-4, **CA 125** (small-cell, epithelial), CA 549, CEA (**small-cell**, epithelial), CK-BB, c-myc-translocation, CYFRA 21-1, DU-PAN-2, ferritin, hCG, hPL, **chromogranin A, B** (small-cell), calcitonin, sialic acid, L-dopadecarboxylase, MCA, neurophysins, **NSE** (small-cell), PRL, PSA, PTH, ribonuclease, **SCCA** (epithelial), sialyltransferase, SP-1 (small-cell), STH, TPA (small-cell), thymidine kinase (small-cell), VIP
prostate	ACP, ACTH, ALP, CA 50, CA 549, CEA, CK-BB, sialic acid, **PSA**, TPA

Tumorous diseases	Tumor markers
breast	ACTH, AFP, alpha-lactalbumin, ALP, arylsulfatase B, AST, **BCM**, B2M, beta-lipotropin, **CA 15-3**, CA 19-5, CA 27.29, CA 50, CA 72-4, CA 125, CA 242, **CA 549**, **CEA**, c-erb-B-2-amplification, CK-BB, esterase, ferritin, hCG, hPL, calcitonin, sialic acid, **MCA**, PSA, PTH, estrogen/glucocorticoid/progesterone receptors, sialyltransferase, **TPA**
neural system	CA 125, CEA, ferritin, N-myc-amplification, N-ras-mutation, NSE, VIP
testes	ACTH, **AFP**, ALP, CEA, CK-BB, ferritin, **hCG**, hPL, LD, SP-1, TPA
gastrointestinal tract	ALP, Tennessee Ag, CA 19-5, CA 19-9, CA 50, CA 72-4, CA 125, CA 242, CEA, c-erb-B-2-amplification, CK-BB, DU-PAN-2, galacto-syltransferase, sialic acid, PSA, SCCA
ovary	AFP (germinative cells), ALP, CA 15-3 (epithelial cells), CA 19-5, **CA 19-9** (epithelial cells), CA 27.29, CA 50, CA 72-4 (epithelial cells), **CA 125** (epithelial cells), CA 549, CEA, c-erb-B-2-ampli-fication, CK-BB, DU-PAN-2, galactosyltransferase, glycosyltrans-ferase, hCG (germinative cells), hPL, MCA, PRL, ribonuclease, TPA (epithelial cells)
stomach	AFP, aldolase, pancreas-associated Ag, beta-glucuronidase, **CA 19-9**, CA 50, **CA 72-4**, CA 125, CA 195, **CA 242**, **CEA**, hCG, chromogranin A, B, TPA
parathyroid	**PTH**
thyroid	AFP, CEA (follicular, medullar), calcitonin (medullar), NSE, TPA (medullar), thyroglobulin (follicular)

Tumor markers in non-tumor diseases and other conditions:

Non-tumorous diseases	Tumor markers
alcoholism	CEA
smoking	CEA
bone diseases	ACP
blood diseases	ferritin
uterus diseases	CA 125, hCG
renal diseases	ACP, B2M, CYFRA 21-1, SCCA
pancreas diseases	CA 15-3, CA 19-9, CA 125
lung diseases	CA 15-3, CA 19-9, CEA, NSE, SCCA, TPA
prostate diseases	ACP, PSA
breast diseases	CA 15-3, CA 549, TPA
gastrointestinal tract diseases	AFP, TPA
hepatobiliary tract diseases	ACP, AFP, B2M, CA 15-3, CA 19-9, CA 50, CA 125, CA 549, CEA, ferritin, MCA, SCCA
ovary diseases	CA 125, hCG
inflammatory diseases	CA 50, ferritin, TPA
thyroid diseases	thyroglobulin
shock conditions	NSE
pregnancy	AFP, CA 125, CA 549, hCG, MCA
trauma	NSE

Ectopic tumour production of hormones:

Hormones	Tumor production
ACTH (MSH, beta-endorphins)	small-cell bronchial carcinoma, about 15% of Cushing's disease is induced by paraneoplastic process
ADH	tumors – (colorectum t., lymphomas, adrenal t., pancreas t., bronchi and lung t., prostate t., uterus body t., thymomas)
erythropoietin	uterus myomatosis, tumors – (pheochromocytoma, cerebellar hemangioblastomas, hepatomas, renal t. – hypernephroma)
FSH, LH	mola hydatidosa, tumors – (chorionepithelioma, insulinoma, melanomas, pancreas t., breast t.)
gastrin	tumors – (medullary t., mesodermal t., insular pancreatic t., ovary t., stomach t., parathyroid t.)
hCG	mola hydatidosa, tumors – (chorionepithelioma, pancreas t., testes t., ovary t., VIPoma)
calcitonin	tumors – (paranasal sinuses t., urinary bladder t., pancreas t., bronchi t., uterus body t.)
parathormone	tumors – (hypernephroma, uterus cervix t., bronchi t., breast t.)
prolactin	tumors – (hypernephroma, lymphomas, bronchial t.)
renin	tumors – (hemangiopericytoma, hypernephroma, bronchial t., Wilms' tumor)
serotonin	tumors – (carcinoid, insular pancreatic t., bronchi t.)
somatomedin	tumors – (hepatoma, hypernephroma, mesothelioma, adrenal t., stomach t.)
STH	tumors – (bronchi – adenocarcinoma, stomach t.)

Tumor Necrosis Factor

(syn: TNF-alpha – cachectin, TNF-beta – lymphotoxin)

Production. TNF-alpha – activated macrophages, T-cells, NK-cells, monocytes, mastocytes, fibroblasts. Stimulated peripheral neutrophilic granulocytes but also unstimulated cells and also a number of transformed cell lines, astrocytes, microglial, smooth muscle cells and fibroblasts also secrete TNF. TNF-alpha is synthesized as transmembrane precursor (stimulation by lipopolysaccharides, IL-1, IFN-gamma) which is changed to monomer; trimer is an active form. Produced and secreted by macrophages exposed to endotoxin. The production of TNF-alpha is inhibited by IL-6, TGF-beta, vitamin D3, prostaglandin E2, dexamethasone and antagonists of platelet activating factor. TNF-beta – product of T-cells, B-cells, monocytes. TNF exists in isomorphs with a great homology, which functionally competitively bind to the same receptor. TNF-alpha consists of 157 amino acids.

Function. TNF-alpha belongs to the cytokines, soluble proteins that regulate the inflammatory/immune response magnitude (immunomodulatory effects). Other effects: induces interleukin 1, 2, 6, 8 production, increases molecules adhesion, pyrogen, induces CSF (colony-stimulating factors), cytolytic, cytotoxic, cytostatic effects, induces IFN-gamma secretion. TNF-alpha shares many biologic activities of IL-1, except those related to immunostimulation. Selective tumoricidal activity, studies have documented a direct cytostatic and cytotoxic effects of TNF-alpha against subcutaneous human xenografts. Catabolic effects on bone and cartilage, inhibits adipocyte lipoprotein lipase, stimulates neutrophils function, activates endothelial cells (increasing prostaglandins, procoagulation activity, thrombotic process promotion). Plays an important role in pathological processes such as venous thrombosis, arteriosclerosis, vasculitis and disseminated intravascular coagulation. In synovial cells mediates proliferation, increases prostaglandins and collagenase. In brain mediates fever, increases prostaglandins, sleep, and anorexia. In bone tissue increases collagenase and bone resorption. In hepatocytes increases acute phase proteins. In fibroblasts increases IL-1, IL-6, IL-8, prostaglandins, collagenase, and proliferation. In chondrocytes increases prosta-glandins, collagenase, plasminogen activator, and cartilage metabolism, as well as mediates pathophysiology of bacterial sepsis and septic shock. Biological activities of TNF-alpha: cau-ses cachectization by fat metabolism increase (lipoprotein lipase activization), causes fever (endogenous pyrogen), involved in slow-wave sleep, hemodynamic shock, increases hepatic acute phase protein synthesis, decreases albumin synthesis, activates endothelium, priming neutrophils, priming macrophages, decreases iron and zinc plasma levels, increases fibro-blasts proliferation, increases synovial cell collagenase and PGE2 levels. TNF-alpha is invol-ved in muscular glycogenolysis increase. It has angiogenic and antiviral effects. TNF-alpha interacts with two specific membrane receptors p55 (CD120a) and p75 (CD120b). TNF-al-pha appears to be an important autocrine modulator promoting the survival of hairy cell leukemia cells. It may be important, therefore, in the patogenesis of this disease. Soluble receptor form plays probably an important regulatory role; it can be detected in plasma and urine. **Biological activities of TNF-beta:** induces the synthesis of GM-CSF, G-CSF, IL-1, colla-genase and prostaglandin E2 in fibroblasts. It is cytolytic or cytostatic for many tumor cells. In monocytes TNF-beta induces the terminal differentiation and the synthesis of G-CSF. TNF-beta is a mitogen for B-lymphocytes. In neutrophils TNF-beta induces the production of reactive oxygen species. It is also a chemoattractant for these cells, increases phagocytosis and also increases adhesion to the endothelium. It inhibits the growth of osteoclasts and keratinocytes. Administration of TNF-beta induces metabolic acidosis, decreases the par-tial pressure of CO_2, induces synthesis of stress hormones (epinephrine, norepinephrine, glucagon) and also alters glucose metabolism. The clinical application of this factor is in its initial stages. The intrapleural administration of TNF-beta may significantly reduce liquid volumes in some metastasizing tumors. TNF-beta levels in the sera of patients with menin-gococcal septicemia have been shown to correlate with morbidity and mortality. TNF fac-tors compete to bind to common membrane receptors which are placed nearly at all cells except RBCs.

Test Purpose. 1) latent infection demonstration before clinical/laboratory signs manifesta-tion in immunodeficient patients, 2) patients after transplantation, 3) acute leukemias, 4) HIV-positive patients, 5) septic shock monitoring.

Increased Values
rheumatoid arthritis, infectious diseases, tumors, septic shock

Analyte	Age/Gender	Reference Range	SI Units	Note
Tumor Necrosis Factor-2		<5	pg/ml	

Tyrosine

(Tyr) Tyrosine is a non-essential glucoplastic, ketoplastic (in phenylalanine deficiency) amino acid.

Function. Proteins component, key precursor in catecholamines, pigments and thyroid hor-mones synthesis. Hypertyrosinemia is the most frequently encountered metabolic disorder in neonates. Differential diagnosis methods: tyrosinuria determination, ascorbic acid load-ing test, galactose and fructose metabolites, urine succinylacetate, fumarylacetoacetase enzymatic activity. Tyrosine determination derivatives: thyroxine, dopamine, epinephrine, and melanin. Enzyme defect: tyrosine alpha-ketoglutarate aminotransferase and tyrosine aminotransferase.

Increased Values – hypertyrosinemia
hyperthyroidism, sepsis
   Interfering Factors: medicaments – (acetylsalicylic acid, triiodothyronine, tryptophan, tyrosine)

Decreased Values – hypotyrosinemia
rheumatoid arthritis, phenylketonuria, Huntington's chorea, hypothermia, hypothyroidism, myxedema, polycystic kidney disease, carcinoid sy, chronic renal failure
   Interfering Factors: medicaments – (adrenaline, androgens, ascorbic acid, estrogens, glucagon, glucose, hydrocortisone, oral contraceptives, testosterone)

Analyte	Age/Gender	Reference Range	SI Units	Note
Tyrosine	Premat. neonates	<180	µmol/l	
	1 w	90–180	µmol/l	
	Infants	60–140	µmol/l	
	Adults	40–100	µmol/l	

Unsaturated Vitamin B$_{12}$-Binding Capacity

(UBBC) Most UBBC is due to vitamin B$_{12}$ binding to transcobalamin II.
Test Purpose. 1) to aid in polycythemia vera vs. secondary/relative polycythemias differential diagnosis, 2) to evaluate macrocytic/megaloblastic anemias, 3) to diagnose congenital transcobalamin I, II, III absence.

Increased Values
pernicious anemia, folic acid deficiency, tumors – (liver t., lymphoproliferative t., myeloproliferative t.), polycythemia vera, pregnancy
   Interfering Factors: medicaments – (oral contraceptives)

Decreased Values
neonatal megaloblastic anemia, hepatic cirrhosis, infectious hepatitis, recurrent infectious diseases, malabsorption, growth disorders

Urea

Urea x 2. 14 = urea nitrogen in the blood (blood urea nitrogen, BUN, azotemia). The name urea and urea nitrogen are used as synonyms in some of medical communications. Urea nitrogen reflects the ratio between urea production and its clearance.
Production. In the liver from ammonia and CO_2 = urea cycle. Quantitatively it is the most important protein metabolism end-product. During ingestion, protein is broken down into amino acids → amino acids are catabolized in the liver and free ammonia is formed → ammonia is combined to form urea → in the blood and transported to the kidney → concentrated, filtered freely, excreted by the kidney (glomeruli), and reabsorbed slightly by the

tubules. It is excreted also by stools and sweat. Therefore, urea is directly related to the protein content in food, metabolic liver function and excretory kidney function. Urea diffuses freely into both intracellular and extracellular fluids. Urea production is controlled by acid-base balance. Urea is produced almost exclusively in neutral or basic conditions. In acidosis, a higher glutamine amount is produced, instead of urea in musculature and liver, which is transported by the blood to kidneys. NH_3 is released in the kidneys, which bounds $H^+ \rightarrow NH^{4+} \rightarrow$ excreted in urine. Urea concentration in blood is determined by: 1) urine volume during a defined time together with water excreted, 2) urea production level (protein intake and endogenic protein breakdown), 3) glomerular filtration.

Test Purpose. 1) to evaluate renal function and aid in renal disease diagnosis, 2) to aid in hydration assessment, 3) to assess nitrogen balance, 4) dialyzed patient status assessment, 5) comatose conditions differential diagnosis, 6) patients on intensive care.

Increased Values

diabetic acidosis, acromegaly, amyloidosis, anuria, **atherosclerosis, dehydration, diabetes mellitus,** dialysis program, gout, **acute muscular dystrophy,** dementia, dysentery, epilepsy, **glomerulonephritis, starvation, diarrhea,** hyperalimentation, malignant hypertension, **prostatic hyperplasia, hypovolemia,** cholera, diseases – (infectious d., renal d.), ileus, **acute myocardial infarction, acute/chronic renal insufficiency, renal ischemia, catabolism, gastrointestinal bleeding, leukemia, Addison's disease,** tumors – (myeloproliferative t., t. of prostate, t. of genitourinary tract), nephritis – (**interstitial n.,** lupus n.), nephrolithiasis, nephropathy – (acute ischemic n., diabetic n.), **nephrosclerosis,** nephrosis, **acute tubular necrosis, urinary tract obstruction, severe operations,** peritonitis, polytrauma, **severe burns, severe muscular injury, excessive sweating,** increased intake of – (**protein,** lipids), **pyelonephritis, increased protein disintegration,** conditions – (hemolytic c., **febrile c.,** c. after transplantation, septic c., stress c., **shock c.),** blood loss, syndrome – (**hepatorenal sy,** Alport's sy, acute nephritic sy, **Goodpasture's sy,** hemolytic-uremic sy), **typhoid fever, urinary tract stones, vomiting,** failure – (**acute/chronic renal f., congestive heart f.)**

Interfering Factors: pregnancy (3rd trimester), medicaments – (abacavir, aciclovir, aldesleukin, allopurinol, amikacin, amiloride, aminoglycosides, amlodipine, ammonium salts, amphotericin B, anabolics, androgens, bacitracin, benazepril, bisoprolol, bromfenac, bumetanide, candesartan, captopril, carbamazepine, carboplatin, carmustine, ceftizoxime, celecoxib, cephalosporins, cephalotin, cephradine, chloral hydrate, chloramphenicol, chlortalidone, cidofovir, cisplatin, colistin, corticosteroids, cyclosporine, denileukin, diclofenac, diltiazem, enalapril, ethacrynic acid, ethambutol, ethinylestradiol, etidronate, etodolac, flurbiprofen, foscarnet, fosinopril, furosemide, ganciclovir, gentamicin, guanethidine, hydantoins, hydrochlorothiazide, ibuprofen, ifosfamide, indomethacin, interleukin 2, irbesartan, kava kava, ketorolac, lisinopril, lithium, lomustine, losartan, meclofenamate, mefenamic acid, meloxicam, mestranol, methicillin, methotrexate, methyldopa, minocycline, mitomycin, moexipril, nabumetone, naproxen, neomycin, nephrotoxic medicaments, nilutamide, nisoldipine, oxaprozin, penicillamine, pentamidine, perindopril, phenacetin, piroxicam, plicamycin, polymyxin B, quinapril, ramipril, salicylates, sirolimus, sparfloxacin, spirapril, spironolactone, steroids, streptomycin, streptozocin, sulfonamides, sulfonylurea, sulindac, tacrolimus, telmisartan, tetracyclines, thiabendazole, thiazide diuretics, thyroxine, tobramycin, tolmetin, torsemide, trandolapril, triamterene, trimethoprim, valsartan, zonisamide)

Decreased Values

acromegaly, **negative nitrogen balance, celiac disease,** liver cirrhosis decompensation, dehydration, hepatic dystrophy, hepatitis, eclampsia, **anabolic phase of metabolism after catabolism, inherited hyperammonemia, hyperhydration,** isovolemic hypotonic hyponatremia, hypotension, **glomerular diseases**, **liver diseases**, parenchymatous icterus, acute hepatic insufficiency, **malnutrition**, nephritis, urinary obstruction, disorders – (inborn urea cycle metabolism d., hepatic d.), reduced renal blood flow, intake – (**decreased protein i., increased carbohydrate i.,** excessive i. v. fluid i.), imbalanced realimentation and rehydration, syndrome – (**nephrotic sy,** SIADH), **pregnancy** (gravidity, graviditas, 3rd trimester), i. v. feeding only, **acute hepatic failure,** poor nutrition

Interfering Factors: children, **elderly people,** medicaments – (anabolic steroids, chloramphenicol, growth hormone, streptomycin)

Analyte	Age/Gender	Reference Range	SI Units	Note
Urea	Neonates	<7.0	mmol/l	
	<6 m	<7.0	mmol/l	
	>7 m	<8.0	mmol/l	
	Adults F	2.2–6.7	mmol/l	
	Adults M	3.8–7.3	mmol/l	

Urea/Creatinine Ratio

Test Purpose. To differentiate prerenal, postrenal and renal azotemia.

Increased Values – Ratio >20:1

prerenal azotemia, high protein intake, impaired renal function, decreased glomerular filtration, increased tissue breakdown, heart failure, dehydration, ureterocolostomy, Cushing's sy, blood loss, salt depletion, conditions – (catabolic c., febrile c.), urine reabsorption, reduced muscle mass, surgery, burns, cachexia, gastrointestinal bleeding, thyrotoxicosis, obstructive uropathy, infectious diseases

Interfering Factors: medicaments – (glucocorticoids, tetracycline)

Decreased Values – Ratio <10:1

acute tubular necrosis, inherited hyperammonemia, SIADH, starvation, decreased urea secretion, renal failure, low protein diet, severe liver diseases, patients on hemodialysis, pregnancy, rhabdomyolysis

Interfering Factors: medicaments – (phenacemide)

Uric Acid

(syn: urate) An important part of antioxidative systems connected with tocopherols and ascorbic acid concentrations. Important ischemic heart disease risk indicator.

Production. Uric acid is a nitrogenous compound: a) the last purine nucleotide degradation product (adenine, guanine – nucleic acids constituents), b) an important antioxidative agent. It is synthesized primarily in the liver, reaction is catalyzed by the enzyme xanthine oxidase → filtered and excreted in the urine and stools. Renal handling of uric acid is complex and involves four sequential steps: 1) glomerular filtration of virtually all uric acid in the capillary plasma entering the glomerulus, 2) reabsorption in the proximal convoluted tubule, about 98–100% of the filtered uric acid, 3) subsequent uric acid secretion into the lumen of proximal tubule distal portion, 4) further reabsorption in the distal tubule. The net urinary uric acid excretion is 6 to 12% of the amount filtered. 95% of gout cases are induced by selective uric acid excretion disorder. Hyperuricemia leads to sodium urate crystal deposits to renal interstitium → nephropathy and to joint synovial fluid → gout (uratic arthritis, gouty arthritis). Uric acid is poorly soluble in water → urate crystals readily precipitate from urine in low pH to produce urate or urate-oxalate kidney stones. Organ meats, legumes and yeasts are especially high in purines. Highest values are in AM and lowest are in afternoon, day-to-day variation is 10%. Higher levels are in summer, lower are in winter.

Test Purpose. 1) to confirm gout diagnosis, 2) to help detect kidney dysfunction (e. g. gouty nephropathy), fat metabolism disorders, 3) to help in arthritides, urolithiasis diagnosis, 4) to help reveal obesity causes, 5) to help in diagnosis of myeloproliferative diseases, hemoblastoses and malignant tumors, 6) part of ischemic heart disease screening profile, part of oxidative stress evidence.

Increased Values – hyperuricemia

pulmonary abscess, acidosis – (alcoholic a., **diabetic a., lactate a., metabolic a.**), alkaptonuria, alcoholism, amyloidosis, anemia – (**hemolytic a., sickle cell a., pernicious a.**), **arthritis, atherosclerosis, chemotherapy/radiotherapy**, chronic berylliosis, glucose-6-phosphatase deficiency, **dehydration, nephrogenic diabetes insipidus, diabetes mellitus**, diet – (yeast, legumes), **gout** (arthritis urica – uratic arthritis), **eclampsia**, exsiccation, fasting, glomerulonephritis, **glycogenoses**, hemoblastoses, **hemoglobinopathies**, hereditary fructose intolerance, starvation, **hyperlipoproteinemia, hyperparathyroidism, hypertension**, PIH, hypertriacylglycerolemia, prostate hyperplasia, **hypoparathyroidism, hypothyroidism**, hypoxanthineguanine-posphoribosyl transferase deficiency, **tissue hypoxia**, disease – (**polycystic renal d., maple syrup urine d.,** Addison's d., Gaucher's d., **von Gierke's d.**), diseases – (febrile d., **acute infectious d., lymphoproliferative d., myeloproliferative d., chronic renal d.**, inflammatory d.), weight reduction – („zero" diet), hemolytic jaundice, ileus, metabolic myopathy, **myocardial infarction**, renal insufficiency – (**acute r. i., chronic r. i.**, prerenal r. i.), poisoning by – (**beryllium, lead**, methyl alcohol, ammonia, carbon monoxide), **calcinosis**, carcinomatosis, **ketoacidosis, diabetic coma, leucemia, chronic lymphocytic leukemia, malignant tumours treatment, lymphomas**, Waldenström's macroglobulinemia, **metastatic tumours, infectious mononucleosis**, myxedema, **tumours, nephritis, nephrolithiasis, obesity, plasmocytoma** (incl. multiple myeloma), **pneumonia, polycythemia, polycythemia vera**, disorders of – (purine degradation/synthesis, renal function, lipid metabolism, glucose tolerance), **preeclampsia**, pseudohyperparathyroidism, excessive food intake of – (meat, **proteins, purines**), **psoriasis**, pyelonephritis, sarcoidosis, hemolytic conditions, syndrome – (**Bartter's sy, Down sy, Lesch-Nyhan sy**, Reaven's metabolic sy, adult respiratory distress sy), **shock**, tuberculosis, **strenuous exercise**, failure – (**acute/chronic renal f., congestive heart f.**), nephropathy – (acute uric acid n., chronic urate n.)

> **Interfering Factors:** stress, medicaments – (acetaminophen, acetazolamide, acetylsalicylic acid, adrenaline, anabolic steroids, androgens, angiotensin, ascorbic acid – large doses, asparaginase, atenolol, azathioprine, barbiturates, benazepril, beta-blockers, bisoprolol, bromfenac, bumetanide, busulfan, caffeine, capreomycin, captopril, carboplatin, chlorambucil, chlorothiazide, chlortalidone, cimetidine, cisplatin, citrates, clofibrate, cyclophosphamide, cyclosporine, cysteine, cystine, cytarabine, cytostatics, dextran, diazoxide, didanosine, diuretics, edetate disodium, enalapril, ethacrynic acid, ethambutol, ethanol, fludarabine, flurbiprofen, fosinopril, fructose, furosemide, gemtuzumab, glucose, glutathione, halothane, hydrochlorothiazide, hydrocodone, hydroxyurea, ibuprofen, idarubicin, indapamide, indomethacin, interferon alfa-2b, irbesartan, laxatives, levodopa, mechlorethamine, mefruside, melphalan, mercaptopurine, methicillin, methoxyflurane, methyldopa, metolazone, mitomycin, moexipril, nadolol, niacin, nicotinic acid, norepinephrine, phenothiazines, phenylbutazone, phenytoin, polythiazide, prednisone, propranolol, pyrazinamide, salicylates – low dose, spironolactone, theophylline, thiazide diuretics, thioguanine, thiotepa, timolol, torsemide, triamterene, tuberculostatics, vasopressin, vinblastine, vincristine, viomycin, warfarin)

Decreased Values – hypouricemia

alcohol, anemia, acromegaly, **cystinosis, renal-tubular defects,** deficiency – (adenosine deaminase d., **congenital xanthine oxidase d.,** purine-nucleoside phosphorylase d.), **diabetes mellitus, low purine/protein diet, galactosemia,** hemochromatosis, hypophosphatemia, isovolemic hypotonic hyponatremia, **severe liver diseases, obstructive icterus,** hereditary fructose intolerance, hereditary renal hypouricemia, **intoxication by heavy metals, x-ray contrast agents,** Hodgkin's disease, **hepatolenticular degeneration** (Wilson's disease), **tumors,** plasmocytoma (incl. multiple myeloma), **acute intermittent porphyria,** syndrome – (**Fanconi's sy, sy of inadequate ADH secretion** – SIADH, hypereosinophilic sy), **decreased uric acid synthesis,** pregnancy, **xanthinuria,** familial hypouricemia, celiac disease, coronary artery bypass

Interfering Factors: tea, coffee, radiographic contrast agents, medicaments – (acetylsalicylic acid – high doses, ACTH, adipiodone, allopurinol, anticoagulants, antiepileptics, ascorbic acid, azathioprine, azauridine, azlocillin, benziodarone, chlorpromazine, chlorprothixene, citrate, clofibrate, corticoids, cortisone, coumarins, dextrose, dicoumarol, diflunisal, estrogens, ethacrynic acid, ethinylestradiol, expectorants, fenofibrate, furosemide, glucose infusion, glycine, guaifenesin, ibuprofen, indomethacin, mannitol, methotrexate, orotic acid, phenothiazines, phenylbutazone, probenecid, salicylates – high doses, sodium chloride, tetracyclines, vinblastine, vitamin C – high doses, warfarin, zoxazolamine)

Analyte	Age/Gender	Reference Range	SI Units	Note
Uric Acid	1–2 d	<340	µmol/l	
	6 d	<220	µmol/l	
	Infants	<150	µmol/l	
	Children	<390	µmol/l	
	Adults F	180–340	µmol/l	
	Adults M	180–420	µmol/l	

Uroporphyrinogen Carboxylase

Porphyrin biosynthesis enzyme.
Test Purpose. Inborn forms of chronic hepatic porphyria diagnosis.

Decreased Values
porphyria cutanea tarda

Valine

(Val) Essential glucoplastic amino acid, produced in digestion or by protein hydrolysis. Valine, leucine and isoleucine have similar properties. First steps (deamination, aerobic decarboxylation and dehydrogenation) create fatty acid. Needed for optimal infant growth and adult nitrogen equilibrium. Enzyme defect: branched ketoacids decarboxylase.

Increased Values – hypervalinemia
acidemia – (methylmalonic a., propionic a.), methylmalonic homocystinuria, branched-chain ketoaciduria (maple syrup urine disease)

Decreased Values – hypovalinemia

hepatic encephalopathy, acute hunger, Huntington's chorea, hyperinsulinism, protein malnutrition (kwashiorkor), severe burns (day 4), carcinoid sy

Interfering Factors: medicaments – (alanine, glucose, histidine, oral contraceptives, progesterone)

Analyte	Age/Gender	Reference Range	SI Units	Note
Valine	Neonates	100–250	µmol/l	
	Infants	100–300	µmol/l	
	Children	150–300	µmol/l	
	Adults	150–250	µmol/l	

Vascular Endothelial Growth Factor

(VEGF, syn: vascular permeability factor – VPF) VEGF is a highly specific mitogen for vascular endothelial cells.

Occurrence. Aortic smooth muscle cells, tumor cells, epithelial cells, macrophages.

Function. Promotes angiogenesis and vascular permeability. VEGF is involved in wound healing process, embryonic development in physiological conditions; in tumor neovascularization and rheumatoid arthritis in pathological conditions. VEGF inhibition suppresses tumor growth in vivo. In endothelial cells VEGF induces the synthesis of von Willebrand's factor. It is also a potent chemoattractant for monocytes and thus has procoagulatory activities. In microvascular endothelial cells VEGF induces the synthesis of plasminogen activator and plasminogen activator inhibitor type-1. VEGF also induces the synthesis of the metalloproteinase, interstitial collagenase, which degrades interstitial collagen type I-III under normal physiological conditions. VEGF secreted from the stromal cells may be responsible for the endothelial cell proliferation in capillary hemangioblastomas which are composed of abundant microvasculature and primitive angiogenic elements represented by stromal cells. The production and secretion of VEGF by human retinal pigment epithelial cells may be important in the pathogenesis of ocular neovascularization.

Vasoactive Intestinal Polypeptide

(VIP)

Production. Gastrointestinal tract regulative acid polypeptide (24 amino acids) produced by neuroendocrine cells and pancreatic D-cells. VIP is distributed throughout the gut and nervous system, greatest concentration is in the distal small bowel and large bowel.

Occurrence. GIT, heart, lungs, hypophysis, nervous system, epiphysis, kidney, and spleen.

Function. Stimulates lipolysis, glycogenolysis, intestinal and pancreatic juice secretion, bile flow. Action mechanism is paracrine and neuroendocrine. Induces the GIT sphincters, genitourinary system, tracheobronchial tree, and non/vascular smooth muscle relaxation. Cardiovascular system: hypotension, moderate inotropic effect. Respiratory system: augmented ventilation, bronchial secretion stimulation. Stimulates immunoglobulin synthesis; inhibits mitogen-induced T-lymphocytes transformation, mast cell histamine release and platelet aggregation. Stimulates adenylate cyclase activity, glycogenolysis and lipolysis, bone resorption and hyperglycemia. VIP stimulates prolactin, hGH, ACTH, endorphins, insulin, glucagon, somatostatin, renin and steroids secretion; inhibits gastrin, gastric acid secretion and hypothalamic somatostatin secretion. VIP is believed to be a neurotransmitter limited to the peripheral and central nervous system. VIP mediates water transport, stimulates chloride secretion, and inhibits sodium absorption in the intestine.

Test Purpose. 1) differential diagnosis of profuse persistent diarrhea followed by hypokalemia, 2) Verner–Morrison sy and VIPoma diagnosis.

Increased Values
hepatic cirrhosis, exercise, pheochromocytoma, ganglioneuroma, **ganglioneuroblastoma,** **pancreatic islet cell hyperplasia,** pancreatic cholera – (**Verner–Morrison sy,** watery diarrhea-hypokalemia-hypochlorhydria syndrome - WDHH), liver diseases, **tumour from Langerhans' islets, medullary thyroid tumors,** obesity, MEN sy type I (multiple endocrine sy), pancreatic VIP-secreting tumors (VIPomas), chronic renal failure, bronchogenic carcinoma

Analyte	Age/Gender	Reference Range	SI Units	Note
Vasoactive Intestinal Polypeptide		<20	pmol/l	

Vasoactive Mediators

Mediator	Source
Vasoconstriction	
neurogenic	nerves
LTC4, LTD4, LTE4	mast cells, basophils
Vasodilation	
PGI2	endothelial cells
PGE2, PGD2	monocytes, macrophages, mast cells
histamine	mast cells, basophils
serotonin	platelets
bradykinin	contact activation system (plasma)
Increased vascular permeability	
histamine	mast cells, basophils
serotonin	platelets
C3a, C5a	plasma via histamine release
bradykinin	contact activation system (plasma)
LTC4, LTD4, LTE4	eosinophils, mast cells, monocytes
PAF	mast cells, basophils, monocytes, macrophages, neutrophils, eosinophils, plateles, endothelial cells

VDRL

(syn: Venereal Disease Research Laboratory test)
Test Purpose. 1) test is widely used to screen for primary and secondary syphilis, 2) to confirm primary and secondary syphilis when syphilitic lesions appear, 3) to analyze syphilis quantitatively, 4) to monitor response to treatment.

Positive Values
syphilis, related Treponemal infection – (yaws, pinta, bejel)

False Positive Values
alcoholism, AIDS, bacterial endocarditis, brucellosis, connective tissue disease (mixed form, MCTD), chronic liver disease, leprosy, leptospirosis, systemic lupus erythematosus, lymphogranuloma venereum, elder people, malaria, infectious mononucleosis, mycoplasmosis, ad-

vanced tumors, progressive paralysis, plasmocytoma (incl. multiple myeloma), pneumococcal pneumonia, atypical pneumonia, psittacosis, rickettsial disease, relapsing fever, scarlet fever, pregnancy, multiple blood transfusions, trypanosomiasis, typhus, tuberculosis, post-vaccination state, general paresis, nephrotic sy, rheumatoid arthritis

Viscosity

Plasma and whole blood viscosity are distinguished clinically. Blood hyperviscosity may be due to elevated plasma/serum viscosity, elevated cell count, or increased cell resistance to blood vessels shape and accommodation size. Plasma viscosity is remarkably stable and can be evaluated with great precision. Plasma can be considered as Newton's fluid; this is not true in complex fluid (whole blood). In general, ESR and plasmatic viscosity react equally. Indirectly, macromolecules which are responsible for increased viscosity often cause increased RBC aggregation. Larger aggregates settle quickly. Similarly, increased plasmatic viscosity slows down RBC movement and decreases aggregometry findings. Changes are complex in clinical cases, so it is always necessary to assess ESR, plasmatic viscosity and RCA (aggregometry) together, because the changes can be contradicting. Patients suffering from vascular diseases have increased HCT, plasmatic viscosity, and RBC aggregability. RCA and ESR can be normal. Contrarily, therapeutic RBC aggregation improvement, if it is connected with HCT decrease, effects the RCA and ESR increase.

Test Purpose. 1) to evaluate hyperviscosity syndrome associated with monoclocal gammopathy states, 2) to evaluate inflammatory diseases.

Increased Values – hyperviscosity
AIDS, amyloidosis, sickle cell anemia, **rheumatoid arthritis,** hepatic cirrhosis, dyslipoproteinemia, dysproteinemias, **monoclonal gammopathy,** chronic active hepatitis, hyperfibrinogenemia, hypercryofibrinogenemia, lymphoproliferative diseases, **cryoglobulinemia,** leukemia, leukocytosis, **systemic lupus erythematosus, Waldenström's macroglobulinemia, IgA/IgG myeloma, polycythemia,** severe burns, spherocytosis, **splenectomy,** syndrome – (**polyclonal hyperviscosity sy, neonatal hyperviscosis sy,** Sjögren's sy), thrombocytosis

Analyte	Age/Gender	Reference Range	SI Units	Note
Viscosity				
venous plasma		1.09–1.15	mPa.s	
blood in 0.7/s		21.2–25.6	mPa.s	
blood in 95/s		4.3–4.7	mPa.s	

Vitamin A

(syn: retinol) Fat soluble vitamin having two natural forms, retinol (A1) and 3-dehydroretinol (A2), which are absorbed in the small intestine. The provitamin A (beta-carotene), can be cleaved in the intestinal mucosa to retinal, that largely reduces to retinol. Retinol is esterified with long chain fatty acids in the mucosal cells and transported with chylomicrons to the liver. If needed, retinol is released from liver storage, binds to retinol-binding protein (RBP), and then to thyroxine-binding prealbumin (TBPA) as a protective action against loss via the kidney. Retinol in this complex binds on specific receptors.

Occurrence. Retinol (fish oil, liver, egg yolk), provitamin beta-carotene (green leaf and yellow vegetables, yellow fruits).

Storage. Liver.

Function. Retina photoreceptor mechanisms, epithel, lipoprotein membranes and subcellular structure integrity, lysozyme stability; involvement in glycoprotein and steroid synthesis, a key component in reproduction and immunosystem integrity. 25% day-to-day level variation.

Test Purpose. 1) to investigate suspected vitamin A deficiency or toxicity, 2) to aid in visual disturbance diagnosis, especially night blindness and xerophthalmia, 3) to aid in skin disease diagnosis, such as keratocytosis follicularis or ichthyosis, 4) to screen for malabsorption.

Increased Values
diabetes mellitus, hepatomegaly, **hypervitaminosis A**, hypercholesterolemia, idiopathic hypercalcemia in infants, hyperlipidemia, chronic kidney diseases, **vitamin A intoxication, excessive intake of vitamin A**, pregnancy, renal failure
> **Interfering Factors:** alcohol (moderate intake), medicaments – (estrogens, glucocorticoids, oral contraceptives, phenytoin)

Decreased Values
abetalipoproteinemia, celiac disease, deficiency – (**vitamin A d. in food**, zinc d.), **cystic fibrosis of pancreas**, infectious hepatitis, perifollicular hyperkeratosis, hypothyroidism, diseases – (**infectious d.**, pancreatic d., **liver d.**), obstructive jaundice, keratomalacia, kwashiorkor, malabsorption, **protein malnutrition**, chronic nephritis, impaired fat absorption, growth retardation, sprue, **fever conditions**, sterility, carcinoid sy, night blindness, **pregnancy**, teratogenesis, disseminated tuberculosis, **xerophthalmia**, xerosis
> **Interfering Factors:** alcoholism, medicaments – (allopurinol, cholestyramine, colestipol, diethylstilbestrol, neomycin)

Analyte	Age/Gender	Reference Range	SI Units	Note
Vitamin A	Neonates	1.22–2.60	µmol/l	
	Children	1.05–2.80	µmol/l	
	Adults F	0.85–1.75	µmol/l	
	M	1.05–2.27	µmol/l	

Vitamin B$_1$

(syn: thiamine, aneurin, vitamin F, antineuritic vitamin) Water soluble heat labile vitamin, absorbed by active/passive transport in the small intestine → phosphorylated to the active coenzyme – thiamine pyrophosphate (TPP) in the liver. Free vitamin B$_1$ is present in plasma, TPP in musculature, liver, heart and kidney.

Occurrence. Yeasts, grain, cereals, meat, nuts, legumes.

Function. Carbohydrate metabolism (glycolytic and pentose phosphate pathways), co-factor for alpha-keto acids (pyruvate, alpha-ketoglutarate) and transketolase/transaldolase oxidative decarboxylation, involved in central and peripheral nervous system cell function, myocardium function. In the body vitamin B$_1$ concentration assessment is not important, but RBC transketolase activity or a blood lactate/pyruvate ratio after glucose loading is measured.

Increased Values
leukemia, Hodgkin's disease, polycythemia vera

Decreased Values

alcoholism, megaloblastic anemia of unknown origin, **beriberi**, exercise, diabetes mellitu subacute necrotizing encephalopathy, impaired pyruvate carboxylase function, long-term hyperalimentation, hyperthyroidism, diseases – (diarrheal d., **febrile d., chronic d., liver d.** lactation, **elderly people**, tumours, peripheral neuropathy, **insufficient intake** (thiamine-poo diets), demented patients, excessive consumption of tea, excessive consumption of raw fis. dialysis program, **pregnancy**, cardiac failure

   Interfering Factors: medicaments – (barbiturates)

Analyte	Age/Gender	Reference Range	SI Units	Note
Vitamin B$_1$		<75	nmol/l	

Vitamin B$_2$

(syn: riboflavin) Water soluble heat labile vitamin, integral flavoenzymes component – fl vin mononucleotide (FMN), flavin adenine dinucleotide (FAD). In the form of FAD an FMN coenzymes, vitamin B$_2$ is a flavoprotein dehydrogenases and oxidases componen Then it is involved in many redox-processes, e. g. oxidative phosphorylation, synthesis an fatty acids breakdown. Specific enzyme compound (xanthine oxidase, glutathione reduc ase, amino acids oxidase). Dietary flavins are converted to free riboflavin by intestinal en zymes before intestinal absorption, occurs primarily in the proximal small bowel.

Occurrence. Cereals, milk, cheese, liver, and eggs.

Function. Energetic metabolism, protein metabolism, mucous membrane integrity, oxi reduction reactions. Actual body vitamin status is assessed as free vitamin B$_2$ in urine/m creatinine or by RBC glutathione reductase activity determination.

Decreased Values

chronic alcoholism, anorexia nervosa, celiac disease, **seborrhoic dermatitis**, dermatose high carbohydrate low protein diet, infectious enteritis, ethanol, phototherapy of infan with jaundice, atrophic glossitis, hypothyroidism, diseases – (chronic diarrheal d., **liver d.** conjunctivitis, **malabsorption**, tumors, gastrointestinal/biliary tract obstruction, decrease dietary intake of riboflavin, small bowel resection, tropical sprue, **angular stomatitis/cheil tis**, stress, irritable bowel sy, pregnancy

Analyte	Age/Gender	Reference Range	SI Units	Note
Vitamin B$_2$				
blood		361–1770	nmol/l	
serum		133–478	nmol/l	

Vitamin B$_3$

(syn: niacin, nicotinic acid amid, niacinamide, pellagra preventing factor) Water solubl vitamin that can be synthesized in people using tryptophan as a precursor.

Occurrence. Yeasts, fishes, legumes.

Function. Oxide-reduction reactions, carbohydrate metabolism, cellular metabolism, vas dilation, plasma cholesterol reduction. Niacin is in tissues as a coenzyme: nicotinamide a nicotinamide adenine dinucleotide (NAD) and in nicotinamide adenine dinucleotide pho phate (NADP).

Decreased Values

alcoholism, hepatic cirrhosis, dietary deficiency, diarrhea, Hartnup disease, pellagra, excessive dietary intake of leucine, carcinoid sy

    Interfering Factors: medicaments – (isoniazid)

Analyte	Age/Gender	Reference Range	SI Units	Note
Niacin				
serum		2–12	μmol/l	
whole blood		16–73	μmol/l	

Vitamin B$_6$

(PLP, syn: pyridoxine, pyridoxal phosphate) Water soluble heat labile vitamin, resorbed largely from the jejunum. Vitamers are pyridoxine, pyridoxamine, and pyridoxal, they become phosphorylated in the tissues. Vitamin B$_6$ is synthesized by plants and many microorganisms but not in higher animals.

Function. Pyridoxal-5-phosphate is the most important compound; it is the coenzyme form of B$_6$ enzymatic reactions – amino acid and protein metabolism, lipid and carbohydrate metabolism (decarboxylation, transsulfuration, transamination, and deamination), tryptophan conversion → nicotinic acid, heme and sphingosine synthesis. Glycogen phosphorylase requires vitamin B$_6$ as does delta aminolevulinic acid synthetase, and pyridoxal phosphate is required for DNA synthesis. All of the vitamers are urine excreted in small amounts; the main catabolite, 4-pyridoxic acid, is found in high concentrations. With dietary deficiency, conservation of pyridoxal phosphate-dependent enzymes occurs with redistribution of available coenzyme and maintenance of more essential functions, thus rendering some clinical deficiency states difficult to define. Vitamin B$_6$ deficiency impairs immune function by inhibiting interleukin-2 production and lymphocyte proliferation.

Occurrence. Widely available in natural diets, fish, poultry, fruits, vegetables, and germ wheat.

Test Purpose. To detect vitamin B$_6$ deficiency (dermatitis, seborrhea, hyperpigmentation, depression, neuritides).

Decreased Values

chronic alcoholism, asthma bronchiale, gestational diabetes, diabetes mellitus, preeclamptic edema, industrial exposure to hydrazine compounds, smoking, acute myocardial infarction, neonatal seizures, **lactation**, leukemia, **malabsorption**, malnutrition, pellagra, renal dialysis program, carpal tunnel sy, **pregnancy**, uremia, renal failure, inflammatory diseases, sideroblastic anemia

    Interfering Factors: medicaments – (amiodarone, anticonvulsants, carbamazepine, cycloserine, disulfiram, ethanol, hydralazine, isoniazid, L-dopa, oral contraceptives, penicillamine, phenobarbital, phenytoin, primidone, pyrazinoic acid, theophylline, tricyclic antidepressants)

Analyte	Age/Gender	Reference Range	SI Units	Note
Vitamin B$_6$		30–144	nmol/l	

Vitamin B₁₂

(syn: cobalamin, cyanocobalamin, antipernicious factor) Water soluble vitamin, a cyclic tetrapyrol compound with bounded cobalt. Vitamin B_{12} represents a group of substances which contain porphyrin core and cobalt as the central atom. They differ one another according to ligands. The most important cobalamines are: coenzyme B_{12}, methylcobalamin, and hydroxy/aquacobalamin.

Occurrence. Eggs, milk/milk products, liver, and meat.

Function. Antipernicious factor, RBC maturation, nervous function, essential co-factor for DNA synthesis, methionine, and acetate synthesis. Homocysteine methyltransferase prosthetic factor – enabling homocysteine change to methionine in DNA synthesis. Function is closely related to folic acid, it is involved in monocarbon remnants transfer in amino acid and DNA metabolism; there it is indirectly involved in proteosynthesis and body growth. Within methylmalonyl-CoA to succinyl-CoA change it is involved in lipid and porphyrin synthesis. Vitamin B_{12} is synthesized in nature by microorganisms. Humans cannot synthesize vitamin B_{12} in sufficient amounts, so acquire necessary amounts by eating animal tissues. Intestinal flora synthesize vitamin B_{12}, but the amount is inadequate to prevent deficiency; manifesting by megaloblastic anemia and neurological damage. The vitamin requires gastric parietal cell intrinsic factor synthesis for absorption across the ileal mucosa (terminal ileum). In the blood vitamin B_{12} is bounded to: a) storage protein transcobalamin I (TC I – cobalamin transport from the cells to the tissues – a passive reservoir. TC I is primarily derived from granulocytes), b) transport protein transcobalamin II (TC II – cobalamin transport from the intestine to the liver and into the cells, comes predominantly from the liver). TC II is probably an acute-phase reactant. STORAGE: liver, muscular tissue, and kidney. Normal body stores are sufficient to withstand zero vitamin intake for a year or more. Vitamin B_{12} level interpretation is usually considered in conjunction with serum and RBC folate. Schilling's test is ordered for vitamin B_{12} resorption disorders (chronic atrophic gastritis, ileal diseases). Suspicion of decreased vitamin intake when increased urine methylmalonate or homocysteine is excreted. Methylmalonic aciduria can be a hereditary enzymopathies result (e. g. methylmalonyl-CoA-mutase, methylmalonyl-CoA-racemase).

Test Purpose. 1) to aid in megaloblastic anemia differential diagnosis, 2) to aid in central nervous system disorder differential diagnosis that affect peripheral and spinal myelinated nerves, 3) chronic gastric diseases with mucous membrane atrophy, conditions after gastric resection, terminal ileum diseases, 4) intestinal parasitic diseases, 5) diagnosis of conditions connected with prolonged colchicine administration (inhibited resorption), 6) nutritional causes (some vegetarians), 7) chronic liver and renal diseases.

Increased Values

hepatic cirrhosis, diabetes mellitus, **severe hepatic dystrophy**, erythroleukemia, acute/chronic hepatitis, increased levels of transcobalamin, drug induced cholestasis, diseases – **(myeloproliferative d., liver d.)**, hepatic coma, leukemia – (chronic lymphatic l., acute/chronic myelogenic l., myelomonocytic l.), **leukocytosis**, protein malnutrition, **tumours with liver metastases, polycythemia vera**, failure – (chronic renal f., severe congestive heart f.), uremia

Interfering Factors: medicaments – (anticonvulsants, estrogens, vitamin A, vitamin C)

Decreased Values

protein transport abnormalities, achlorhydria, alpha-thalassemia, **chronic alcoholism**, anemia – **(pernicious a., megaloblastic a.,** aplastic a.), **coeliac disease, congenital deficiency of transcobalamin II**, deficiency – (iron d., folate d.), gastric mucous membrane destruction, delirium, dementia, fashionable diets, jejunal diverticula, smoking, cystic fibrosis, **gastrec-**

tomy, **chronic atrophic gastritis**, hemodialysis, **hyperthyroidism**, hypermetabolic state, **primary hypothyroidism**, diseases – (CNS d., intestine d., endocrinous d., kidney d., liver d.), **lack of intrinsic factor**, **regional ileitis**, parasitic infection by – (Diphyllobothrium latum), pancreatic insufficiency, leukemia, **specific vitamin B$_{12}$ malabsorption**, malnutrition, **breast feeding of vegan mother**, tumours of – (intestine, **stomach**), chronic pancreatitis, plasmocytoma (incl. multiple myeloma), **decreased intake of vitamin B$_{12}$**, radiation, **bowel resection, scleroderma, sprue**, syndrome – **(malabsorption sy, blind loop sy, Zollinger-Ellison sy)**, **pregnancy** (3rd trimester), **veganism**

Interfering Factors: children, elder people, medicaments – (acetylsalicylic acid, aminoglycosides, aminosalicylic acid, antibiotics, anticonvulsants, ascorbic acid, cholestyramine, cimetidine, colchicine, metformin, methotrexate, neomycin, nitroprusside, oral contraceptives, pentamidine, phenformin, phenobarbital, phenytoin, primidone, ranitidine, tranquilizers, triamterene)

Analyte	Age/Gender	Reference Range	SI Units	Note
Vitamin B$_{12}$				
Total cobalamins	Adults	244–730	pmol/l	
Vitamin B$_{12}$	Neonates	118–959	pmol/l	
	Adults	162–694	pmol/l	
	Pregnancy	<125	pmol/l	

Vitamin C

(syn: ascorbic acid, antiscorbutic vitamin) Water soluble heat labile vitamin, that is absorbed in the small intestine. Some absorbed ascorbic acid is oxidized to other active vitamer – dehydroascorbic acid (DHAA) → both vitamers are present in plasma.

Occurrence. Citrus, hips, tomatoes, potatoes, and green pepper, green-leafy vegetables.

Function. Important in osteoid tissue production, necessary for proline and lysine hydroxylation during collagen production, vessel function, involved in connective tissue matrix protein synthesis, tissue respiration, wound healing, tyrosine, folic acid, and histamine metabolism, carnitine, norepinephrine, and 5-OH tryptophan synthesis, corticosteroids release, bile acid formation, and iron transfer to ferritin. Vitamin C functions as a donor/acceptor in many hydroxylation reactions (e.g. collagen, catecholamines, and steroids synthesis). Ascorbate is involved via complex reactions in WBC function, immune response, and allergic responses. Ascorbic acid is found in most tissues and body fluids, very high concentrations are found in endocrine tissue. Vitamers are excreted into the urine. Day-to-day level variation is 25%, highest levels are in early AM, falls during day, highest are in summer and lowest are in winter, in women peaking at ovulation time.

Test Purpose. To aid in the diagnosis of scurvy, scurvy-like conditions and metabolic disorders, such as malnutrition and malabsorption syndromes.

Increased Values
increased vitamin C intake

Decreased Values
alcohol abuse, anemia, smoking, hemodialysis, hyperthyroidism, diseases – (**acute/ chronic infectious d.,** rheumatoid d., chronic inflammatory d.), heavy metal poisoning, malabsorption, male sex, tumors, **obesity**, dietary iron overload, **scurvy**, febrile states, steatorrhea, **severe stress, pregnancy**

Interfering Factors: medicaments – (acetylsalicylic acid, aminopyrine, barbiturates, estrogens, nitrosamines, oral contraceptives, paraldehyde)

Analyte	Age/Gender	Reference Range	SI Units	Note
Vitamin C	Adults	34–114	µmol/l	

Vitamin C in WBC

Decreased Values
gastroduodenal disorders, scurvy, postoperative states, peptic ulcer

Vitamin D

(syn: ergocalciferol – vitamin D2, cholecalciferol – vitamin D3, calcitriol, 1,25-(OH)$_2$D3) Fat soluble vitamin.
Occurrence. Fish oil and egg yolk. 95% of vitamin D3 and 5% of vitamin D2 occurs in serum.
Production. In skin by sunbathing (D3) – natural provitamin 7-dehydrocholesterol skin irradiation. Ergocalciferol is manufactured commercially from the plant sterol ergosterol. Vitamin D is readily absorbed in the normal jejunum → carried to the liver by lymphatic system and bound directly to chylomicrons → in the liver hydroxylation occurs producing 25-OH-D2 (vitamin D2), which circulates bound to alpha globulin (vitamin D-binding globulin, DEP). Second hydroxylation by 25-OH vitamin D-1-hydroxylase occurs in the kidney mitochondria to create the active vitamin form → 1-alpha-25-dihydroxy-cholecalciferol (1,25-(OH)$_2$D3, vitamin D3) → the active vitamin is carried in the blood to the target organs by DEP. The final step in active hormone production is regulated closely by a number of factors, including parathyroid hormone, plasma calcium, phosphate, calcitonin, thyroid status, estrogens, growth hormone, prolactin, insulin, glucocorticoids and vitamin D metabolites.
Function. Calcium and phosphorus absorption by the small intestine, calcium bone resorption in concert with parathormone, calcium reabsorption from the distal renal tubules, bone mineralization, and collagenization. The vitamin D effect is an increase of the total/ionized plasma calcium, inorganic phosphate concentrations, and calcium urinary excretion increase. Higher levels are in winter than summer. In women, sharply increases at ovulation. 20% day-to-day level variation.
Test Purpose. 1) to evaluate bone diseases, such as rickets, renal osteodystrophy and osteomalacia, 2) to aid in hypercalcemia diagnosis, 3) to detect vitamin D deficiency or toxicity, 4) to monitor therapy with vitamin D, 5) to aid in the diagnosis of primary hyperparathyroidism, hypoparathyroidism, pseudohypoparathyroidism, 6) to aid in the diagnosis of psoriasis.

Increased Values
anorexia nervosa, excessive exposure to sunlight/ultraviolet light, idiopathic hypercalciuria, **hyperparathyroidism,** tumoral calcinosis, **lactation,** lymphoma, non-Hodgkin's lymphoma, obesity, **excessive intake of vitamin D,** normal growing children, **sarcoidosis, pregnancy,** tuberculosis, renal calculi
Interfering Factors: medicaments – (estrogens, octreotide, prednisone)

Decreased Values

rheumatoid arthritis, **celiac disease**, biliary/portal hepatic cirrhosis, dietary deficiency of vitamin D, insulin-dependent diabetes mellitus (adolescents), cystic fibrosis, familial hypophosphatemia, hypercalcemia of malignancy, hypoparathyroidism, diseases – (inflammatory bowel d., hepatic d., **cholestatic liver d.**), **exposure to sunlight lack**, insufficiency – (**renal i.**, pancreatic i.), **malabsorption**, osteitis fibrosa cystica, renal osteodystrophy, **osteomalacia** (in adults), tumor-induced osteomalacia, osteopetrosis, postmenopausal osteoporosis, pancreatitis, **pseudohypoparathyroidism**, rhachitis – (**vitamin D dependent r. in children, vitamin D resistant r.**), bowel/stomach resection, steatorrhea, syndrome – (infantile hypercalcemia sy, **nephrotic sy**, Williams' sy), thyrotoxicosis, chronic renal failure

    Interfering Factors: medicaments – (carbamazepine, cholestyramine, colestipol, glucocorticoids, isoniazid, isotretinoin, ketoconazole, phenobarbital, phenytoin, primidone, rifampicin)

Analyte	Age/Gender	Reference Range	SI Units	Note
Vitamin D	Children	75–175	pmol/l	
1,25 – (OH)$_2$ D3	Adults	50–200	pmol/l	
25 – OH-D2	summer	50–300	nmol/l	
	winter	25–125	nmol/l	

Vitamin E

(syn: alpha-tocopherol, tocopherol) The name vitamin E should be understand as group mark of naturally occurring tocolens and tocotrienolens. They have biological function like alpha-tocopherol and a 6-chromanol nucleus structure. Tocopherol is a group name for methylated tocols. Alpha-tocopherol from this tocol group was named vitamin E (less realistic). Fat soluble vitamin. The vitamin is absorbed from the small intestine with bile's aid assistance, transported to the systemic circulation via the lymphatic system, and incorporated into chylomicrons and VLDL.

Occurrence. Plant oils, leafy vegetables, egg yolk, grain germs.

Function. a) intracellular antioxidant mainly for polyunsaturated (saturated) membrane phospholipids fatty acids, b) protecting the body from free radicals that could oxidize vitamin A and DNA, c) part of other antioxidative systems connected with uric acid, d) mutagens production inhibiton in GIT. Membrane integrity, normal neurological structure and function maintenance. Protects RBCs from hemolysis. Tocopherol deficiency (also relative) leads to increased lipoperoxide concentrations, subsequently to membrane damage and cellular death (resp. precoccious atheromatosis). Vitamin E is stored in diverse tissues, but especially adipose tissue. 15% day-to-day levels variation.

Test Purpose. 1) to evaluate vitamin E deficiency in premature newborns and infants hemolytic disease, neuromuscular disorders in infants, chronic cholestasis patients, 2) evaluate patients on long-term parenteral nutrition, 3) to evaluate patients with malignancy and malabsorption.

Increased Values

hyperlipidemia, obstructive liver diseases, **excessive vitamin E intake**, pregnancy, renal failure

Decreased Values

abetalipoproteinemia, reflexes absence, hemolytic anemia, cerebellar ataxia, **biliary atresia**, celiac disease, hepatic cirrhosis, premature infants, encephalomalacia, regional enteritis, gluten enteropathy, retrolental fibroplasia, **cystic fibrosis**, hemolysis, chronic cholestasis, lymphangiectasis, **malabsorption**, pancreatic tumors, peripheral neuropathy, chronic pancreatitis, fat absorption disorders, steatorrhea

> **Interfering Factors:** medicaments – (anticonvulsants, cholestyramine, carbamazepine, clofibrate, ethanol, phenobarbital, phenytoin)

Analyte	Age/Gender	Reference Range	SI Units	Note
Vitamin E	0–1 m	8–28	µmol/l	
	1–6 m	10–31	µmol/l	
	6 m–6 y	20–30	µmol/l	
	Adults	11–45	µmol/l	

Vitamin K

(syn: phylloquinone, coagulation vitamin) Fat soluble vitamin. Principal vitamin K vitamers are plant origin phylloquinones (K1 type) and bacterial origin menaquinones (K2 type). It is assumed, that one-half of the body's supply originates from intestinal flora and the other half from the diet. The jejunum and ileum are the predominant absorption sites. Gut bile is required for absorption, as with other fat-soluble vitamins. The absorbed vitamin is transported primarily through the lymphatics bound chylomicrons to the liver and distributed systematically. Excretion is mainly in the bile as metabolites; a small amount is eliminated through the urine.

Occurrence. Leafy vegetables, plant oils.

Function. Vitamin K is essential for the post-translational carboxylation of several gamma-carboxyglutamic acid-containing proteins, including the procoagulation factors: prothrombin (II) and hemocoagulation factors VII, IX, X, the thrombolytic factors, protein C and protein S, and copper-binding proteins modulation.

Decreased Values

cystic fibrosis, diarrhea – (**chronic d.,** d. treated by antibiotics), **hypoprothrombinemia**, hemorrhagic disease of the newborn, diseases – (pancreatic d., hepatic d., gastrointestinal tract d.), **obstructive jaundice, chronic fat malabsorption, breast milk low in vitamin K,** newborn infants, hemorrhagic states

> **Interfering Factors:** medicaments – (antibiotics, anticoagulants, cholestyramine, hydantoin, vitamin K antagonists)

Analyte	Age/Gender	Reference Range	SI Units	Note
Vitamin K	Adults	0.3–2.64	nmol/l	

Xanthine Oxidase

Enzyme, oxidoreductase catalyzes hypoxanthine to xanthine and xanthine to uric acid oxidation; the final step in purine degradation. It is an iron-molybdenum flavoprotein containing FAD.

Increased Values

acute hepatic jaundice

Zinc

(Zn) Trace metal element. Quantitatively the 2nd most important micronutrient.

Function. An enzyme component (metalloenzymes which play a direct role in catalytic enzyme action – carbonic anhydrase, pancreatic carboxypeptidase A, thymidine kinase, alkaline phosphatase, alcohol dehydrogenase, RNA, DNA polymerases) and an insulin component. Involved in skin integrity, wound healing, and organism growth. Zinc is absorbed in the distal small intestine → in plasma bound to albumin (60–70%) and globulin (alpha-2-macroglobulin 30–40%) → excreted primarily into gastrointestinal tract, urine and sweat.

Occurrence. Bones, teeth, hair, skin, liver, muscles, testes, erythrocytes, leucocytes, thrombocytes, breast milk, prostate, semen fluid, kidney, and retina.

Sources. High-protein foods (meat, fish, dairy products). Zinc bioavailability from vegetables and cereal grains is reduced, because phytates, cellulose, hemicellulose and other dietary fibers inhibit zinc absorption. Dietary zinc availability is decreased by high dietary calcium, phosphates, iron and copper. Diets rich in proteins stimulate zinc absorption, whereas low-protein diets have the opposite effect. Highest levels are at 9 AM, lowest at 9 PM. Day-to-day level variation is 15%.

Test Purpose. 1) to detect zinc deficiency or toxicity, 2) to help in dermatitides differential diagnosis, 3) to help in immunity disorders diagnosis, 4) to monitor wound healing disorders, 5) to help in chronic infectious disease diagnosis, 6) to monitor prolonged parenteral nutrition, 7) to monitor zinc exposure, 8) to follow therapy.

Increased Values – hyperzincemia

anemia, arteriosclerosis, exercise, accidental/professional exposure, diabetes mellitus, **familial hyperzincemia**, coronary heart disease, primary osteosarcoma

> **Interfering Factors:** protein and carbohydrates intake, medicaments – (carbonic anhydrase inhibitors, chlortalidone, glucocorticoids, penicillamine)

Decreased Values – hypozincemia

acrodermatitis, **alcoholism**, drugs abuse, alopecia, anemia – (sickle cell a., pernicious a., **thalassemia major**), arthritis, rheumatoid arthritis, intestinal bypass, **hepatic cirrhosis**, tissue destruction, diabetes mellitus, conditions – (postsurgery c., febrile c., **stress c.**, septic c.), gluten-sensitive enteropathy, rapid growth phase of children, gastrectomy, major fractures, viral hepatitis, hypoalbuminemia, **hypogonadism**, diseases – (**acute infectious d., renal d.**, parasitic d., chronic liver d., gastrointestinal tract d., inflammatory d.), ileitis, acute myocardial infarction, **renal insufficiency**, ulcerative colitis, **leukemias**, systemic lupus erythematosus, lymphomas, **Crohn's disease**, **malnutrition**, lactating women (breast-feeding), tumors, **hypogonadal dwarfism, severe burns, growth retardation, sprue**, severe injuries, steatorrhea, **pregnancy**, pulmonary tuberculosis, parenteral nutrition, **chronic renal failure, uremia**

> **Interfering Factors:** medicaments – (anabolics, captopril, chemotherapeutics, cisplatin, corticosteroids, diuretics, estrogens, ethacrynic acid, interferon, metal chelating agents, oral contraceptives, penicillamine, phenytoin, thiazides)

Analyte	Age/Gender	Reference Range	SI Units	Note
Zinc	Neonates			
	premature	6.8–11	μmol/l	
	mature	9.4–13.7	μmol/l	
	Adults F	10.1–16.8	μmol/l	
	Adults M	10.6–17.9	μmol/l	

Zinc Protoporphyrin

(ZPP, Zn-Proto, Zn-PP)

Test Purpose. 1) to help in differential diagnosis of disorders of heme production versus diseases of globin synthesis, 2) to detect lead toxicity or chronic exposure.

Increased Values

anemia – (iron deficiency a., a. of chronic disease, sideroblastic a.), iron deficiency, accelerated erythropoiesis, protoporphyria, inflammatory diseases, **chronic lead poisoning**

Interfering Factors: hemolysis, increased bilirubin, medicaments – (digitalis, riboflavin)

Analyte	Age/Gender	Reference Range	SI Units	Note
Zinc Protoporphyrin		19–38	μmol/mol heme	

Acid-base Balance

D. Mesko, R. Pullmann

The acid-base systems function is to maintain the blood and intracellular pH within a narrow range with normal, increased or decreased metabolic acid production and excretion rates. The usual end point of metabolism is the production of an acid, primarily carbonic acid (H_2CO_3) as well as sulfuric, phosphoric and small amounts of organic acids. The pH is regulated by physiologic buffers, by production of base (primarily bicarbonate) and by control of acid excretion by the lungs and kidneys. The primary volatile acid, H_2CO_3 is excreted as CO_2 by the lungs and as H^+ and ammonium ion (NH^{4+}) by the kidneys. Fixed acids such as sulfuric, phosphoric and the organic acids are excreted by the kidneys. Carbonic acid and bicarbonate amount balance in the blood must be maintained at a constant ratio of 1:20 in order to keep the plasma's hydrogen ion concentration at a constant value (pH 7.4).

- **Cation:** ionized particle with a net positive charge travelling in an electrical field toward the negative pole – cathode.
- **Anion:** ionized particle with a net negative charge travelling in an electrical field toward the positive pole – anode.
- **Acid:** dissociated substance that releases hydrogen ion (H^+) into a solution. An acid is a proton (hydrogen ion) donor. Hydrochloric, sulfuric, phosphoric and carbonic acids are conventional acids, each dissociating to liberate protons. A strong acid is one that is highly dissociated, therefore, presenting a high hydrogen ions concentration. A weak acid: dissociable compound that separates and yields H^+ ions only when few other H^+ ions are present, or at a fairly high pH. Weak acids are poorly dissociated. When excreted through the urine, fixed acid must be in salt form accompanied by a cation. Volatile acids can be excreted as gas without requiring a cation (carbonic acid).
- **Base:** a dissociable substance capable of combining with a hydrogen ion in solution. The base is a hydrogen ion acceptor; thus binding free hydrogen ions and reducing their concentration.
- **Hydroxyl ion:** anion OH^- is capable of combining with H^+ to form uncharged water.
- **Salt:** compound formed by acid and base combination. Acid H^+ is replaced by a cation that does not affect the pH.
- **Buffer pair:** solution containing a weak acid and salt of the same acid. A buffer is defined as a substance that reduces changes in free hydrogen ion concentrations of a solution by the addition of an acid or base. Buffer increases the amount of acid or alkali that must be added to cause a pH change. Addition of a strong acid to any of these buffer systems results in the production of a neutral salt and a weak acid. Undissociated weak acid formation removes free H^+ from the solution and the solution pH changes are relatively small; this action is called "buffering". By generating a poorly dissociated acid, the buffer significantly reduces free hydrogen ion concentration increment, when the reaction is compared to one that is not buffered. Physiologically important buffers are: bicarbonate, hemoglobin, protein and phosphate. The principal buffer found in extracellular fluid is bicarbonate-carbonic acid system, intracellular buffers include various proteins and organic phosphates. In the urine, phosphate in mono/dihydrogen form is the major buffer.

■ **Standard bicarbonate:** defined as the plasma HCO_3^- in blood that has been equilibrated at 37 °C with a gas mixture having a $pCO_2 = 40$ mmHg and pO_2 greater than 100 mmHg.

Characteristics of disorders

	pCO2	pH	SB	compensation
MAC – primary decreased HCO_3^-				
a) non-compensated	=	<	<	
b) fully compensated	<	=	<	hyperventilation
MAL – primary increased HCO_3^-				
a) non-compensated	=	>	>	
b) fully compensated	>	=	>	hypoventilation
RAC – primary increased pCO_2				
a) non-compensated	=	<	=	
b) fully compensated	>	=		acid urine
RAL – primary decreased pCO_2				
a) non-compensated	=	>	=	
b) fully compensated	<	=		alkaline urine

MAC-RAC	<standard bicarbonate	>pCO_2		<pH
MAL-RAL	>standard bicarbonate	<pCO_2		>pH
MAC-RAL	<standard bicarbonate	<pCO_2		< >pH
MAL-RAC	>standard bicarbonate	>pCO_2		< >pH

Acid-base balance disorders

pCO_2	HCO_3^- <21 mmol/l	21–29 mmol/l	>29 mmol/l
>6 kPa	combined MAC-RAC	RAC	combined MAL-RAC
4.5–6 kPa	MAC	NORMAL	MAL
<4.5 kPa	combined MAC-RAL	RAL	combined M-RAL

Acid-base abnormality	Initiating event	Alteration in acid-base balance	Immediate response (lungs)	Delayed response (kindneys)
MAC	↑ acid production ↑ alkali loss	↓ pH secondary to ↓ HCO_3^-	↓ pCO_2 by increasing ventilation	↑ acid excretion ↑ HCO_3^- retention
RAC	↓ gas exchange in lungs	↓ pH secondary to ↑ pCO_2	↓ pCO_2 by increasing ventilation	↑ HCO_3^- retention ↑ acid excretion
MAL	↑ alkali gain ↑ acid loss	↑ pH secondary to ↑ HCO_3^-	↑ pCO2 by decreasing ventilation	↑ HCO_3^- excretion ↓ acid excretion
RAL	↑ gas exchange in lungs due to hyperventi-lation	↑ pH secondary to ↑ HCO_3^-	↑ pCO_2 by decreasing ventilation	↑ HCO_3^- excretion ↓ acid excretion

Acid-base balance (homeostasis) systems

■ **Buffer system:** extracellular fluid – mainly bicarbonates (HCO_3^-)
■ **Respiratory system:** elimination of CO_2
■ **Kidney:** H^+ elimination – mainly ammonium ions (NH^{4+})

Actual Bicarbonates

(AB) Bicarbonate is filtered by the glomerulus and mainly reabsorbed in the proximal and distal renal tubules. Bicarbonate concentrations are readily calculated from the measured values of pH and pCO_2 using the modified Henderson–Hasselbach equation. Bicarbonate levels are controlled by renal reabsorption and production of bicarbonate.

Increased Values
mixed metabolic alkalosis + respiratory acidosis, compensated respiratory acidosis, metabolic alkalosis

Decreased Values
metabolic acidosis, compensated respiratory alkalosis, mixed metabolic acidosis + respiratory alkalosis, severe acute respiratory acidosis

Anion Gap

Increased Values
acidosis – (primary lactic a.), alcoholism, shock – (cardiogenic s., hypovolemic s., septic s.), hepatic coma, epilepsy, **diabetic ketoacidosis**, chronic renal failure, poisoning – (glycol p., carbon monoxide p., methyl alcohol p., salicylate p.), seizure conditions, inborn error of amino acid metabolism

Analyte	Age/Gender	Reference Range	SI Units	Note
Anion Gap (Na + K)– (Cl + HCO_3^-)		14.1–18.1	mmol/l	

Arterial Blood Gases

(ABG, syn: blood gases) Clinical laboratory gas analyzers measure pO_2, pH and pCO_2. Additional acid-base parameters of interest are calculated from these values.

Base Excess

(BE, syn: base excess/deficit, total base excess/deficit) BE is the total buffer anion concentration in whole blood = bicarbonate ions (in plasma and erythrocytes) + hemoglobin + plasma proteins + phosphates (in plasma and red blood cells). BE indicates the metabolic component of the acid-base. It represents increase/decrease in the buffer base needed to achieve the measured acid-base status. A negative value for BE implies decrease in available buffer base caused by increased acid production or increased alkali loss. Positive values for BE imply base excess for the measured acid-base status.

Increased Values

compensated respiratory acidosis, mixed metabolic alkalosis + respiratory acidosis, metabolic alkalosis

> **Interfering Factors:** medicaments – (chlortalidone, ethacrynic acid, polythiazide)

Decreased Values

metabolic acidosis, mixed metabolic acidosis + respiratory alkalosis, severe acute respiratory acidosis, lactic acid accumulation, compensated respiratory alkalosis, ketoacidosis, dietary intake of organic/inorganic acids

Analyte	Age/Gender	Reference Range	SI Units	Note
Base Excess	Neonates	(-10)–(-2)	mmol/l	
	Infants	(-7)–(-1)	mmol/l	
	Children	(-4)–(+2)	mmol/l	
	Adults	(-3)–(+3)	mmol/l	

Bicarbonates

(HCO_3^-, syn: bicarbonate ions) The major extracellular buffer in blood is the bicarbonate/carbonic acid system (HCO_3^-/H_2CO_3). Conventionally it is defined to include plasma bicarbonate, carbonate, and CO_2 bound in plasma carbamino compounds. Bicarbonate (carbonic acid) buffer is one of the most important buffer systems for maintaining body fluids normal pH by the acid-base balance system. Secondary importance lies in electrical neutrality of extracellular/intracellular fluids. Levels of HCO_3^- are regulated by the kidneys. As long as the ratio of plasma HCO_3^- to dissolved CO_2 (H_2CO_3) remains at 20 : 1, the blood pH remains at 7. 4, even if the absolute concentrations of HCO_3^- and H_2CO_3 change. Bicarbonate/bicarbonic acid are renewable, even before the pulmonary and renal mechanisms restore the constituents, the lung alters the ratio of the numerator (HCO_3^-) to the denominator (H_2CO_3) by blowing off CO_2. Through CO_2 excretion rate regulation, the lungs attempt to maintain the ratio at/near 20:1, and pH changes are minimized. Day-to-day level variation is 30 %. Highest levels are in spring and lowest in summer, for women the lowest levels occur during menses.

Increased Values

respiratory acidosis in – (poor diffusion in alveolar membrane disease, **pulmonary emphysema**, heart failure with pulmonary edema/congestion), metabolic alkalosis in – (hypokalemia, ingestion of large quantities of sodium bicarbonate or alkali, severe vomiting in pyloric stenosis), **hyperaldosteronism, gastric suction, shock, protracted vomiting of acid gastric juice accompanying K^+ deficit, renal failure**, ventilatory failure – (narcotics, inadequate artificial respiration), respiratory dysfunction, Cushing's sy

> **Interfering Factors:** medicaments – (aldosterone, barbiturates, bicarbonates, diuretics, flurazepam, glucocorticoids, hydrocortisone, carbenicillin, ethacrynic acid, laxatives, metolazone, morphine, steroids)

Decreased Values

metabolic acidosis – (**diabetic ketoacidosis, lactic m. a., starvation m. a.**), renal tubular acidosis with coexisting hyperchloremia, respiratory alkalosis in – (**hyperventilation**), dehydration, intestinal fistula, **persistent diarrhea**, hypotension, renal insufficiency, intoxication by – (ethylene glycol, methanol, paraldehyde, salicylates), insufficient tissue perfusion, excess ingestion of acidifying salts, ureteral transplant to ileum or colon, renal failure, renal diseases, **Addison's disease**

Interfering Factors: medicaments – (ammonium chloride, acetazolamide, cyclosporine, thiazide diuretics, phenformin, cholestyramine, lithium, methicillin, nitrofurantoin, paraldehyde, spironolactone, tetracyclines, triamterene)

Analyte	Age/Gender	Reference Range	SI Units	Note
Bicarbonates				
arterial blood		21–28	mmol/l	
venous blood		22–29	mmol/l	

Combined Metabolic Acidosis + Respiratory Acidosis

(MAC + RAC) phosphorus depletion, pulmonary edema, chronic obstructive pulmonary disease with hypoxia, intoxication by – (ethylene glycol, hypnotics, colchicine, narcotics, sedatives), diabetic ketoacidosis, hypophosphatemic + hypokalemic myopathy, cardiopulmo-cerebral resuscitation, acute cardiac and respiratory arrest

Combined Metabolic Acidosis + Metabolic Alkalosis

(MAC + MAL) eritis, diarrhea + vomiting, hemorrhagic shock with massive transfusions

Combined Metabolic Acidosis + Respiratory Alkalosis

hepatic cirrhosis – (alcoholic h. c., primary biliary h. c.), assisted respiration, pulmonary edema, glomerulonephritis, Wegener's granulomatosis, hypoxia, diseases – (CNS d., hepatic d.), SLE, polyarteritis nodosa, sepsis, rapid correction of severe metabolic acidosis, pulmonorenal sy, tuberculosis, salicylate intoxication, septicemia due to gram-negative organisms

Combined Metabolic Alkalosis + Respiratory Alkalosis

(MAL + RAL) critical states, pregnancy, blood transfusion, hepatic insufficiency with hyperventilation, severe vomiting

Combined Metabolic Alkalosis + Respiratory Acidosis

(MAL + RAC) pulmonary edema, severe vomiting, chronic obstructive pulmonary disease, myopathies, pneumonia, gram-negative sepsis, chest trauma

Hyperchloremic Metabolic Acidosis

villous adenoma, aldosterone deficiency, gastrointestinal fistula, diarrhea, hyperkalemia, advanced renal insufficiency, chloride containing ascid, ileus, posthypocapnia, uretero-sigmoidostomy

Interfering Factors: medicaments – (cholestyramine, carbonic anhydrase inhibitors)

Hyperkalemic Metabolic Acidosis

distal renal tubular acidosis, renal amyloidosis, sickle-cell hemoglobinopathies, hypoaldosteronism – (hyper-/hypo-/normoreninemic h.), prostaglandin synthesis inhibitors, acute hypersensitivity interstitial nephritis, diabetic nephropathy, pseudohypoaldosteronism, obstructive uropathy

Interfering Factors: medicaments – (amiloride, cyclosporin A, heparin, angiotensin converting enzyme inhibitors, spironolactone, trimethoprim)

Lactate Acidosis

- **with hypoxia:** anemia, hemorrhage, asphyxia, hypotension, marathon running, seizure conditions, cardiopulmonary disorders, shock
- **without hypoxia:** deficiency – (fructose-1,6-diphosphatase d., pyruvate dehydrogenase d., pyruvate carboxylase d.), diabetes mellitus, glycogenosis (type I), diseases – (infectious d., liver d.), renal insufficiency, poisoning by methanol, tumors – (lymphoma, leukemia, sarcoma), seizure conditions, uremia, alkaloses, methylmalonicaciduria, propionicaciduria, short bowel sy

   Interfering Factors: medicaments – (abacavir, biguanids, didanosine, ethanol, ethylene glycol, fructose, lamivudine, metformin, methanol, salicylates, sodium bicarbonate, sorbitol, stavudine, streptozocin, xylitol, zalcitabine, zidovudine)

Metabolic Acidosis

(MAC) Metabolic acidosis occurs when there is increased acid production or increased bicarbonate loss, such that the blood pH decreases below the reference range.

Increased acid supply

anemia, acidosis – (renal tubular a., primary lactic a.), terminal stage of hepatic cirrhosis, primary biliary cirrhosis, strenuous exercise, **diabetes mellitus**, pulmonary edema, epilepsy, **ethylism**, food poisoning – (staphylococcal f. p., Clostridium perfringens f. p., salmonella f. p.), fructose intake, gastroenteritis, **starvation**, hyperkalemia, **primary**/secondary **hyperparathyroidism**, **hypoxemia**, **malignant hyperthermia**, hypervitaminosis D, diarrhea, **hypothermia**, **cholera**, **glycogen storage disease** (type I), Whipple's disease, diseases – (infectious d., hepatic d.), insufficiency – (heart i., mesenteric vascular i., renal i.), intoxication by – (arsenic, CO, **ethylene glycol**, formaldehyde, cyanide, acids, **methylalcohol**, paraldehyde, phenol, salicylate, toluene), **diabetic ketoacidosis**, **hepatic coma**, leukemia, toxic conditions – (acetazolamide, biguanids, phenformin, isoniazid, laxative, paraldehyde, salicylates, sedatives, strychnine, thiazides), melanoma, methemoglobinemia, tumours, chronic lead nephropathy, analgesic neuropathy, sarcoma, conditions – (hypoxic c., convulsion c., hemorrhagic c., septic c., seizure c., **shock c.**), **Fanconi's syndrome**, chronic toxoplasmosis, **acute/chronic renal failure**, inborn error of amino acid metabolism

Increased HCO_3^- loss

renal tubular acidosis (proximal, type II), fistulas – (intestinal f., pancreatic f.), diarrhea, ileostomy, colostomy, uretherosigmoidostomy

Decreased elimination of acids
renal tubular acidosis (distal, type I), hereditary enzymatic defects, hypoaldosteronism, renal insufficiency/failure

Other causes
hyperkalemia, chloride retention – (renotubular acidosis, increased intake of arginine/lysine/NH^4Cl)
> Interfering Factors: medicaments – (acetazolamide, acetylsalicylic acid, aldesleukin, amiloride, biguanids, cidofovir, cyclosporine, dalfopristin, dimercaprol, epinephrine, isoniazid, levobupivacaine, paraldehyde, phenformin, salicylates, sedatives, spironolactone, strychnine, theophylline, thiazides)

Metabolic Alkalosis

(MAL) Metabolic alkalosis occurs when increased intake or alkali production or increased acid loss rate lead to net increase in blood HCO_3^- concentrations.

Increased loss of acids
severe kalium deficiency, diuretics – (furosemide, ethacrynic acid, thiazides), corticosteroids, Conn's disease, Cushing's disease, **prolonged nasogastric suction**, gastric juice loss

Increased HCO_3^- supply
antacids, HCO_3^- metabolization of ketones and lactate, sodium bicarbonate i. v. administration, excessive artificial respiration in chronic hypocapnic patient, milk-alkali sy, blood transfusion, decreased HCO_3^- elimination

Other causes
deficiency – (11-hydroxylase d., 17-hydroxylase d.), diarrhea, **primary hyperaldosteronism**, hypercalcemia, hyperreninism, hypokalemia, hypoproteinemia, insufficient chloride intake, excessive chloride depletion, syndrome – (Bartter's sy, Liddle's sy), **vomiting**
> Interfering Factors: medicaments – (aldesleukin, betamethasone, corticotropin, cortisone, dexamethasone, fludrocortisone, hydrocortisone, indapamide, methylprednisolone, metolazone, prednisolone, prednisone, sodium bicarbonate, sodium lactate, triamcinolone)

Normal Buffer Base

Increased Values
hyperproteinemia, hypohydration, polyglobulia

Decreased Values
anemia, hyperhydration, hypoproteinemia

Osmolal Gap

Increased Values
intoxication by – (**methanol, ethylene glycol**, diuretics, mannitol, **isopropyl alcohol**, ethanol, sorbitol, glycerol, acetone, ether trichloroethane, paraldehyde)

Oxygen Saturation

(O_2 sat.) A significant parameter for the evaluation of O_2 transport, oxygen saturation defined as the ratio of oxyhemoglobin to the total hemoglobin in percent. Represents t[] hemoglobin percentage carrying O_2, the higher the O_2 sat., the larger amount of O_2 bei[] transported by the hemoglobin.

Increased Values
physical exercise, **hyperventilation**, breathing O_2-enriched air, **polycythemia**

Decreased Values
anemia, anesthesia, **asthma bronchiale**, **atelectasis**, bronchiectasis, **cardiac decompensatio[]** suffocation, **dysrhythmia**, **pulmonary edema**, **pulmonary embolism**, **pulmonary emphysem[]** carbon monoxide exposure, **hypoventilation due to neuromuscular diseases**, pulmona[] diseases – (**chronic obstructive p. d.**, **restrictive p. d.**), congenital heart diseases, **pulmona[] infarction**, **circulatory collapse**, mucoviscidosis, tumors, airway obstruction by – (retaine[] secretions, foreign body), phrenic nerve paralysis, **high altitude aircraft pilots**, pneumoc[] niosis, **pneumonia**, **pneumothorax**, acute poliomyelitis, drug overdose, resection/compre[] sion of the lung, sarcoidosis, **shock conditions**, shunts – (extrapulmonary s., intrapulmona[] s., intracardiac s.), syndrome – (sleep apnea sy, **adult respiratory distress sy, respirato[] distress sy in newborns**, Hamman–Rich sy, **pickwickian sy**), tetanus, submersion, cran[] trauma, decreased cardiac output, **pleural effusion**, **high altitude**, **atmospheric pO_2 decrea[]**
   Interfering Factors: medicaments – (barbiturates, diazepam, heroin, meperidine, mid[] zolam, morphine)

Analyte	Age/Gender	Reference Range	SI Units	Note
Oxygen Saturation	Neonates	0.85–0.90		
arterial blood	Others	0.95–0.99		

Partial Carbon Dioxide Pressure

(pCO_2, $PaCO_2$) As a measure of respiratory function, pCO_2 is considered to be directly rel[] ted to ventilation. High ventilation rates lead to low pCO_2 values and low ventilation rat[] lead to high pCO_2 values. An increase in pCO_2 is a bad sign, indicating inadequate capaci[] of the pulmonary system to compensate further.

Increased Values – hypercapnia
respiratory acidosis, metabolic alkalosis, anesthesia, **asthma bronchiale**, bronchitis – (**chr[] nic b.**, **chronic obstructive b.**), pulmonary fibrosis, cardiac defects, **pulmonary emphysem[]** hyperaldosteronism, reduced function of respiratory center in – (tumors, head trauma, dru[] overdose), hypokalemia, **severe hypothyroidism**, **alveolar hypoventilation**, diseases – (ol[] structive lung d., cardiac d., muscular d.), chest wall abnormalities, **compensation of met[] bolic alkalosis**, mucoviscidosis, myopathies, myxedema, **poliomyelitis**, **polymyositis**, acu[] intermittent porphyria, airway obstruction, scoliosis, severe electrolyte disturbances, co[] ditions – (**shock c.**, febrile c., seizure c.), syndrome – (**pickwickian sy**, Cushing's sy, Guillair[] Barré sy), multiple sclerosis, vomiting, foreign body in the airways, **tuberculosis**
   Interfering Factors: medicaments – (antacids, barbiturates, diazepam, midazolam, na[] cotic analgesics, opiates)

respiratory alkalosis, **anxiety**, **diabetic ketoacidosis**, metabolic acidosis, pulmonary embolism, loss of bicarbonate, idiopathic pulmonary fibrosis, severe diarrhea, hyperthermia, **hyperventilation**, **hypoxia**, disease – (**high altitude d.**, legionnaires d.), **compensation of metabolic acidosis**, leptospirosis, nervousness, influenza, pneumonia – (aspiration p., pneumococcal p., Pneumocystis carinii p., staphylococcal p., streptococcal p., viral p.), pneumoconiosis, stress, pregnancy, head injury with damage to respiratory center, overventilation on a mechanical ventilator (mechanical artificial ventilation), chronic renal failure

Interfering Factors: medicaments – (salicylates, trometamol)

Analyte	Age/Gender	Reference Range	SI Units	Note
Carbon Dioxide	M	4.7–6.4	kPa	
Partial Pressure (pCO$_2$)	F	4.3–6.0	kPa	

Partial Oxygen Pressure

(pO$_2$, PaO$_2$) Hypoxemia = decreased blood pO$_2$, hypoxia = inadequate delivery of O$_2$ to the tissues such that anaerobic pathways are activated.

Increased Values

physical exercise, **hyperventilation**, breathing O$_2$-enriched air, **polycythemia**

Interfering Factors: medicaments – (barbiturates, diazepam, heroin, meperidine, midazolam, morphine)

Decreased Values – hypoxemia

anemia, anesthesia, **asthma bronchiale**, **atelectasis**, bronchiectasis, **cardiac decompensation**, suffocation, **dysrhythmia**, **pulmonary edema**, **pulmonary emphysema**, **pulmonary embolism**, carbon monoxide exposure, **hypoventilation due to neuromuscular diseases**, pulmonary diseases – (**chronic obstructive p. d.**, **restrictive p. d.**, interstitial p. d.), congenital heart diseases, **pulmonary infarction**, **circulatory collapse**, tumors, mucoviscidosis, airway obstruction by – (retained secretions, foreign body), phrenic nerve paralysis, **high altitude aircraft pilots**, **pneumonia**, pneumoconiosis, **pneumothorax**, acute poliomyelitis, drug overdose, resection/compression of the lung, **sarcoidosis**, shunts – (extrapulmonary s., intrapulmonary s., intracardiac s.), **shock conditions**, syndrome – (sleep apnea sy, **adult respiratory distress sy**, **respiratory distress sy in newborns**, Hamman–Rich sy, **pickwickian sy**), tetanus, submersion, cranial trauma, decreased cardiac output, **pleural effusion**, **high altitude**, **atmospheric pO$_2$ decrease**

Interfering Factors: medicaments – (amifostine, barbiturates, beractant, calfactant, colfosceril, dalfopristin, dexmedetomidine, diazepam, fludarabine, gemtuzumab, heroin, meperidine, midazolam, morphine, nitrous oxide, poractant alfa, rituximab, sargramostim, trastuzumab, vinorelbine)

Analyte	Age/Gender	Reference Range	SI Units	Note
Partial Oxygen Pressure	Neonates	1.1–3.2	kPa	
arterial PaO$_2$	5–10 min	4.4–10.0	kPa	
	30 min	4.1–11.3	kPa	
	>1 hour	7.3–10.6	kPa	
	1 d	7.2–12.6	kPa	
	Others	11–14.4	kPa	
pO$_2$		8.66–13.3	kPa	

pH

pH is a quantitative measure of the solution acidity/alkalinity with reference to pure water. pH is the negative logarithm of the hydrogen ion concentration in the blood. The sources of H ions are in volatile acids (H_2CO_3) and in non-volatile acids (lactic acid, ketoacids, dietary acids). pH is normally controlled by HCO_3^- and Hb buffer systems; the protein and phosphate buffers account for less than 5% of the blood buffer capacity. Blood pH is controlled by the ratio of HCO_3^- to pCO_2, not the level of the individual components. Only when the ratio of HCO_3^- to H_2CO_3 deviates from the usual value of about 20:1 is the pH abnormal. The HCO_3^- concentration, controlled by the kidneys, is a metabolic component; pCO_2, controlled by the lungs, is a respiratory component of acid-base balance. The primary renal mechanism of acid-base control are interrelated excretion of H^+ and resorption of HCO_3^-.

Increased Values – alkalosis, alkalemia

alkalosis – (**metabolic a.**, respiratory a.), **hyperventilation**, hypokalemia, loss of acids – (enteral l. of a., renal l. of a.)

> **Interfering Factors:** medicaments – (antacids, sodium bicarbonate, bumetanide, citrates, diuretics, mercurial diuretics, phenylbutazone, furosemide, carbenicillin, acetylsalicylic acid – initially RAL, ethacrynic acid, glutamic acid, lactate, laxatives, triamcinolone)

Decreased values – acidosis, acidemia

acidosis – (**lactate a.**, **metabolic a.**, respiratory a.), **diabetes mellitus**, **hypoventilation**, poisoning by – (acetone, ether, ethylene glycol, fluorides, methanol)

> **Interfering Factors:** medicaments – (acetazolamide, ammonium chloride, amphotericin B, arginine, citrates, dimercaprol, ethanol, ether, phenformin, chloramphenicol, cholestyramine, isoniazid, calcium chloride, acetylsalicylic acid – late effect, aminobenzoic acid, aminosalicylic acid, nalidixic acid, methoxyflurane, spironolactone, terbutaline, tetracyclines, trimethadione)

Analyte	Age/Gender	Reference Range	SI Units	Note
pH		7.35–7.45		

Respiratory Acidosis

(RAC) The three major mechanisms of respiratory acidosis are: decreased ventilation (hypoventilation), decreased respiration, and increased production of CO_2.

Central causes

cerebral edema, general anesthesia, **encephalitis**, **primary central hypoventilation**, spinal cord diseases, respiratory center inhibition, **intoxication**, intracranial hemorrhage, meningitis, myxedema, **CNS tumors**, bulbar poliomyelitis, **respiratory center functional disorders**, **CNS disorders**, **comatose states**, CNS trauma

> **Interfering Factors:** medicaments – (anesthetics, hypnotics, narcotics, sedatives)

Thoracic/abdominal causes

cryptogenic fibrosing alveolitis, aortic aneurysm, **ascites, foreign body aspiration, asthma bronchiale**, bronchiolitis, bronchospasm, bronchoscopy-associated hypoventilation/respiratory arrest, muscular dystrophy, **pulmonary edema**, embolism – (thromboembolism, fat e., air e.), pulmonary emphysema, epiglottitis, fibrothorax, cystic fibrosis of lung, hydrothorax, **obstructive pulmonary disease**, pulmonary diseases, kyphoscoliosis, laryngitis, **laryngospasm, myasthenia gravis**, myopathies, myxedema, obstruction – (**upper airway o.**, postintubation laryngeal o.), diaphragmatic paralysis, peritonitis, shock lungs, **severe pneumonia, pneumothorax**, poliomyelitis, polymyositis, disorders – (hypoventilation d., laryngeal d., respiratory mechanics d., pulmonary structural d., chest wall d.), **cardio-pulmo-cerebral resuscitation** (reanimation), scoliosis, ankylosing spondylitis, **status asthmaticus**, tracheal stenosis, **adult respiratory distress sy**, scleroderma, thoracoplasty, misplacement/displacement of airway cannula during anesthesia/mechanical ventilation, trauma, **pleural effusion**, breathing arrest

Peripheral nervous system disorders

botulism, poisoning by – (curare, organophosphates), hypokalemic myopathy, tumors – (cord t., larynx t., thymoma), poliomyelitis, paralysis of vocal cords, sclerosis – (amyotrophic lateral s., multiple s.), myasthenic crisis, status epilepticus, **tetanus**

    Interfering Factors: medicaments – (aminoglycosides, succinylcholine)

Other causes

angioedema, extreme obesity (pickwickian sy), general anesthesia, sleep disorders, febrile conditions, syndrome – (sleep apnea sy, **Guillain–Barré sy**), myopathies

---

Respiratory Alkalosis

(RAL) Respiratory alkalosis is initiated by increased ventilation rate or depth (hyperventilation), lowered pCO_2 and increased pCO_2 to HCO_3^- ratio.

Central causes

psychogenic hyperventilation, hypoxemia, hysteria, carbon monoxide poisoning, **subarachnoid hemorrhage**, meningoencephalitis, **CNS tumors**, exertion, **intracranial surgery, central nervous system disorders**, cerebrovascular accidents, conditions – (painful c., febrile c., anxious c.), **respiratory center stimulation**, stress, **trauma to CNS**, CNS inflammation

Thoracic causes

aspiration, **bronchial asthma**, atelectasis, pulmonary edema, pulmonary embolism, **cystic fibrosis of lung**, hemothorax, pulmonary hypertension, diseases – (interstitial pulmonary d., cyanotic heart d.), myocardial infarction, pneumonia, pneumothorax, **reflex stimulation of respiratory center**, left-right pulmonary shunts, respiratory distress sy, foreign body in respiratory system, acute/chronic heart failure

Other causes

anemia, hepatic cirrhosis, encephalitis, **metabolic encephalopathy**, G-negative endotoxemia, hepatopathy, **hyperthyroidism**, hyperventilation, hypotension, **hepatic insufficiency**, hepatic coma, infectious diseases, laryngospasm, meningitis, tumours, nicotine, hot conditions, conditions – (**septic c.**, shock c.), **pregnancy** (3rd trimester), drowning, trauma, prolonged artificial ventilation, vomiting, high altitude, **hepatic failure**, recovery from MAC

    Interfering Factors: medicaments – (analeptics, angiotensin II, dinitrophenol, doxapram, thyroid hormones, catecholamines, nikethamide, progesterone, salicylates, vasopressors, xanthines)

Shifted Oxygen Saturation Curve

- **Left shift (same O_2 saturation implies lower p_aO_2):** increased pH, decreased temperature, decreased p_aCO_2, decreased 2,3-DPG
- **Right shift (same O_2 saturation implies higher p_aO_2):** increased temperature, increased p_aCO_2, increased 2,3-DPG, decreased pH

Increased Values

vagal hyperfunction, G-cell hyperplasia, **duodenal ulcer disease**, basophilic leukemia, systemic mastocytosis, syndrome – (postresection sy, **Zollinger-Ellison sy**)

Decreased Values

pernicious anemia, gastric tumors

Amniotic Fluid

D. Mesko

Amniotic fluid is produced from amniotic membrane cells (1ˢᵗ trimester); later most is derived from maternal blood (direct filtration), fetal urine, metabolic intestinal tract and fetal respiratory tract products and fetal skin coverage. During pregnancy the amniotic fluid increases in volume as the fetus grows. At full term (40 weeks gestation) there is approximately 1000 ml of amniotic fluid surrounding the baby. This fluid is circulated by the fetus approximately every 3 hours. Amniotic fluid is obtained by aspiration during amniocentesis.

Physiologically amniotic fluid is a clear, slightly yellowish, slightly alkaline, contains albumin, urea, uric acid, creatinine, lecithin, sphingomyelin (phosphatidylglycerol), bilirubin, fat, glucose, fructose, hormones, epithelial cells, leukocytic enzymes and lanugo.

Test Purpose. 1) to detect fetal abnormalities, particularly chromosomal/genetic and neural tube defects, 2) to detect hemolytic disease of newborn, 3) to diagnose metabolic disorders, amino acid disorders and mucopolysaccharidoses, 4) to determine fetal age and maturity, especially pulmonary maturity, 5) to assess fetal health meconium or blood detection, or measuring amniotic levels of estriol and fetal thyroid hormone, 6) to assess intrauterine growth retardation, 7) to assess postdate pregnancies, 8) to identify fetal gender when one or both parents are carriers of a sex-linked disorder, 9) in higher maternal age, 10) when metabolic diseases are suspected, 11) in maternal insulin-dependent diabetes mellitus.

Acetylcholinesterase

Increased Values
exomphalos, **open neural tube**, until about the 11th week of fetal development

Adrenocorticotropic Hormone

Decreased Values
anencephalic fetus

Alanine Aminotransferase

Increased Values
placental infarction

Alkaline Phosphatase

Increased Values
cystic fibrosis, meconium in amniotic fluid

Amino Acid Profile

(syn: fractionated amino acids, quantitative amino acids).
Test Purpose. 1) to aid in prenatal diagnosis of argininosuccinic aciduria, 2) to evaluate recurrent intrahepatic cholestasis, 3) to evaluate Rhesus incompatibility, 4) to evaluate central nervous system malformations.

Aspartate Aminotransferase

Increased Values
placental infarction

Bilirubin

Increased Values
erythroblastosis fetalis (Rh isoimmune disease), hemolysis in the fetus, maternal infectious hepatitis, maternal sickle cell crisis, maternal hyperbilirubinemia, maternal hemolytic anemia, maternal cholestasis, threatened abortion

Blood

Positive Values
contamination with blood, intraamniotic hemorrhage, damage to – (umbilical cord vessels, placenta, fetus)

Catecholamines

Decreased Values
pregnant drug addicts

Color

- ■ **colorless/pale straw:** physiologically
- ■ **yellow:** blood incompatibility, Rh isoimmunization, fetal RBC hemolysis, fetal ascitic fluid, amniotic cysts, maternal urine (accidental)
- ■ **red:** contamination with blood, intraamniotic hemorrhage, trauma, hemolysis, abruptio placentae
- ■ **green:** erythroblastosis, contamination with meconium, fetal distress
- ■ **yellow-brown:** intrauterine fetal death, oxidized Hb from degenerated RBC
- ■ **brown-black:** fetal maceration

Cortisol

Decreased Values
fetal hypotrophy, prematurity, pregnancy with anencephalic fetus

Creatine Kinase

Increased Values
intrauterine fetal death

Creatinine

Production. Creatinine is a by-product of fetal muscle metabolism in amniotic fluid.
Function. Level is a reflection of increased fetal muscle mass and the mature kidney ability
to excrete creatinine into the amniotic fluid. Creatinine progressively increases as pregnancy
advances. An indicator of fetal physical maturity, creatinine correlates with pulmonary maturity.

Increased Values
diabetic mothers, preeclampsia, prematurity, growth-retarded infants of hypertensive
mothers, hypercreatininemia, maternal renal disease

Decreased Values
fetal kidney abnormalities, fetus – (smaller f. than normal, immature f.), gestation less advanced

Dehydroepiandrosterone

Increased Values
sulfatase deficiency in placenta

Decreased Values
congenital fetal adrenal hypoplasia

Dehydroepiandrosterone Sulfate

Increased Values
sulfatase deficiency in plasma

Decreased Values
anencephaly

DNA-Testing

abetalipoproteinemia, acatalasemia, disease – (Canavan's d., Bloom d., Fabry's d., Farber's
d., Gaucher's d., Krabbe's d., maple syrup urine d., Niemann-Pick d., Pompe's d., Wolman's
d., sickle cell d., Tay-Sachs d.), deficiency – (acylcoenzyme A d., alpha-1-antitrypsin d., G6PD
d., multiple sulfatase d.), Duchenne muscular dystrophy, familial dysautonomia, fragile X-
syndrome, gangliosidosis GM1, hemophilia, Huntington's chorea, X-linked adrenoleukodystrophy, metachromatic leukodystrophy, mucolipidosis, phenylketonuria, retinoblastoma,
syndrome – (Hunter's sy, Hurler's sy, Lesch-Nyhan sy, Maroteaux-Lamy sy, Morquio sy, Sanfilippo's sy, Scheie's sy), thallasemia, tyrosinemia (type I)

Estriol

Decreased Values
anencephaly, erythroblastosis fetalis, fetal distress, fetal death, fetal hypotrophy

Analyte	Age/Gender	Reference Range	SI Units	Note
Estriol, Free	Pregnancy			
	16–20 w	3.5–11.1	nmol/l	
	20–24 w	7.3–27.1	nmol/l	
	24–28 w	7.3–27.1	nmol/l	
	28–32 w	13.9–47.2	nmol/l	
	32–36 w	12.5–53.8	nmol/l	
	36–38 w	16.0–62.5	nmol/l	
	38–40 w	18.7–68.7	nmol/l	

Alpha-1-Fetoprotein

(AFP) Fetal glycoprotein synthesized by embryonic liver and gastrointestinal tract.

Increased Values
anencephaly, **esophageal/duodenal atresia**, **neural tube defects**, fetal distress, encephalocele, hydrocephaly, **myelomeningocele**, congenital nephrosis, fetal hepatic necrosis, gastrointestinal tract obstruction, **omphalocele**, missed/**imminent** abortion, preeclampsia, severe Rh isoimmunization, **spina bifida**, syndrome – (Meckel's sy, Turner's sy), Fallot's tetralogy
   Interfering Factors: fetal blood contamination, multiple pregnancy

Decreased Values
PIH (pregnancy induced hypertension), Down sy

Analyte	Age/Gender	Reference Range	SI Units	Note
Alpha-1-Fetoprotein	Pregnancy			
	15 w	10.8–16.92	µg/ml	
	16 w	8.32–15.08	µg/ml	
	17 w	7.27–13.33	µg/ml	
	18 w	6.28–12.72	µg/ml	
	19 w	4.24–9.96	µg/ml	
	20 w	2.55–7.45	µg/ml	

Follicle Stimulating Hormone

Increased Values
alcoholism

Decreased Values
anterior pituitary hypofunction

Glucose

Increased Values
hypertrophy of fetal pancreas (near the term)

Decreased Values
fetal hypoxia

Alpha-Glucosidase

(syn: alpha-D-glucoside glucohydrolase)

Decreased Values
cystic fibrosis, Pompe's disease, necrotizing pancreatitis

Growth Hormone

Decreased Values
anencephalic fetus

Human Chorionic Gonadotropin

Increased Values
severe erythroblastosis fetalis, chorioncarcinoma, hydatidiform mole

Decreased Values
Down sy

17-Hydroxyprogesterone

17-OHP has a marked circadian secretion variation (highest values in the morning). Luteal phase elevation indicates corpus luteum activity. 17-OHP is the substrate for subsequent 21- and 11-hydroxylation in cortisol production.

Increased Values
congenital adrenal hyperplasia due to 21-hydroxylase deficiency

Interleukin 6

Increased Values
intra-amniotic infections

17-Ketosteroids

Increased Values
at term

Lactate Dehydrogenase

Increased Values
chronic fetal hypoxia, placental infarction

Lecithin/Sphingomyelin Ratio

(L/S ratio) Surfactant factor components. Phospholipids in amniotic fluid are predictors of fetal lung maturity. Lecithin is a primary component of the phospholipids that make up the majority of the alveolar lining and accounts for alveolar stability. Phosphatidylglycerol and phos-phatidylinositol serve to stabilize surfactant; surfactant is necessary to keep the air spaces open when the infant is born. The following factors may increase surfactant production: maternal diabetes, toxemia, hypertension, malnutrition, placenta previa, drug addiction, premature rupture of membranes, intrauterine growth retardation, female fetus, hemoglobinopathy. The following factors may decrease surfactant production: anemia, polyhydramnions, hypothyroidism, male fetus, twins, isoimmune disease, liver disease, renal disease, advanced maternal age, syphilis and toxoplasmosis.
Production. Lung.
Function. Lecithin and sphingomyelin stabilize the neonatal alveoli and prevent collapse on expiration and consequential atelectasis. Ratio is used as an index of fetal lung maturity.

Decreased Values
fetal pulmonary immaturity, fetal respiratory distress sy

Analyte	Age/Gender	Reference Range	SI Units	Note
Lecithin/Sphingomyelin		2.0–5.0		

Malate Dehydrogenase

Increased Values
placental infarction

Meconium

Positive Values
fetal distress, fetal hypotension

Phosphatidylglycerol

The presence of phosphatidylglycerol is evidence, that the fetus is whitin 2–6 weeks of full-term.

Test Purpose. 1) to evaluate fetal lung maturity and prevent respiratory distress syndrome from low surfactant in early delivery, 2) indicator to determine optimal time for obstetrical intervention in cases of possible fetal distress (maternal diabetes, toxemia, hemolytic disease of the newborn, postmaturity).

Decreased Values
pulmonary immaturity

Placental Lactogen

Increased Values
severe erythroblastosis, preeclampsia, multiple pregnancy

Prolactin

Increased Values
hydramnios secondary to Rh isoimmunization

Prostaglandin F2-Alpha

Decreases progesterone level, increases uterus sensitivity onto oxytocin.

Increased Values
pregnancy

Reverse Triiodothyronine

Increased Values
diabetes mellitus, anemic fetuses

Uric Acid

Increased Values
pregnancy induced hypertension, chronic maternal nephritis

Volume

Increased Values – polyhydramnion
fetal anemia, agenesis of ears, **anencephaly**, **duodenal/esophageal atresia**, **diabetes mellitus** (maternal), **tracheoesophageal fistula**, diaphragmatic hernia, **hydrocephaly**, hydrops fetalis, diseases – (neuromuscular d., polyuric renal d., congenital heart d., genitourinary tract d.), idiopathic polyhydramnion, cystic adenomatoid lung malformation, microcephaly, mongolism, congenital malformations, lip/palate cleft, deformity of limbs, spina bifida, **severe Rh isoimmune disease**, pyloric stenosis, imperforate anus, fetal heart failure, **multiple pregnancy**

Decreased Values– oligohydramnion

agenesis – (bladder a., renal a.), anomalies – (fetal a., a. of the fetal urinary tract), urethral atresia, preeclampsia, pregnancy induced hypertension, fetal pulmonary hypoplasia, placental insufficiency, **intrauterine fetal growth retardation**, syndrome – (postmaturity sy, donor-twin sy), amniotic fluid leak

    Interfering Factors: medicaments – (indomethacin, ACE inhibitors)

Increased Values

vagal hyperfunction, G-cell hyperplasia, **duodenal ulcer disease**, basophilic leukemia, systemic mastocytosis, syndrome – (postresection sy, **Zollinger-Ellison sy**)

Decreased Values

pernicious anemia, gastric tumors

Bronchoalveolar Lavage Fluid

D. Mesko

Bronchoalveolar lavage fluid (BALF) is sampled by back-aspiration after isotonic NaCl solution application into bronchial stroma.

BALF examinations: biochemical, cytological, cultivation, molecular-biological, microscopic, tissue culture and flow cytometry examination.

Test Purpose. 1) to investigate possible bronchial neoplasia, bacterial, viral and fungal bronchopulmonary infections, alveolar proteinosis, inflammatory and fibrosing lung disorders. Lavage is used in peripheral lesions that cannot be reached by bronchoscope. Lavage has a higher yield for Pneumocystis carinii than does brush or wash. Lavage is contraindicated in suspected tuberculosis.

Bacteriological Picture

Non-specific and specific flora, anaerobic microorganisms and fungi
- **Bacillus Koch (Mycobacterium tuberculosis):** pulmonary tuberculosis
- **non-specific flora:** bronchiectasis, acute/chronic bronchitis, bronchopneumonia, pulmonary empyema, lung tumors, pneumonia

Cellular Constituents

Increased Values
- **eosinophils:** exogenous allergic alveolitis
- **lymphocytes:** exogenous allergic alveolitis, **sarcoidosis**
- **neutrophils: cryptogenic fibrosing alveolitis**, allergic exogenous alveolitis, smokers

Decreased Values
- **alveolar macrophages:** cryptogenic fibrosing alveolitis, allergic exogenous alveolitis, **sarcoidosis**

Color

- **white-yelowish:** pus – (empyema)
- **red** (transparent): exudates in – (tumors, acute pancreatitis, tuberculosis, uremia), pulmonary infarction, perforation of pulmonary and subphrenic abscesses/cysts, pneumothorax
- **red** (non-transparent): blood – (malignant exudate, trauma)
- **white cream:** fatty degenerated malignant cells – (lymphomas), chylothorax, pseudochylothorax
- **straw-yellow** (transparent): transudate or exudate of various etiology

Cytological Picture

The looking for malignant cells on malignant lung tumours suspicion
- **activated macrophages:** fibrosing cryptogenic alveolitis
- **eosinophils:** asbestosis, idiopathic pulmonary fibrosis
- **erythrocytes:** exudates in – (tumors, acute pancreatitis, tuberculosis, uremia), pulmonary infarction, perforation of pulmonary/subphrenic abscesses/cysts, pneumothorax, trauma
- **physiologically:** alveolar macrophages, bronchial epithelial cells, lymphocytes, polymorphonuclear cells
- **lymphocytes:** exogenous allergic alveolitis (CD4+), fibrosing cryptogenic alveolitis, alveolitides, rheumatoid arthritis, asbestosis (CD4+), berylliosis (CD4+), metal exposure (CD4+), systemic connective tissue diseases (CD8+), radiation pneumonitis (CD8+), sarcoidosis (CD4+), silicosis (CD8+), tuberculosis
- **macrophages:** pulmonary hemorrhage, aspergillosis
- **mesothelial cells:** fluidothorax, mesothelioma
- **tumorous cells:** exudates of malignant etiology, carcinomatous lymphangoitis, bronchogenic tumors
- **neutrophils:** fibrosing cryptogenic alveolitis, drug reaction, alveolitides, asbestosis, silicosis, scleroderma, Sharp's sy, bacterial infectious diseases, acute respiratory distress syndrome
- **altered polymorphonuclears:** pulmonary abscess, metal exposure, inflammatory lung diseases, purulent lung processes

D-Dimers

Increased Values
fibrosing pulmonary processes

Fibronectin

Increased Values
fibrosing cryptogenic alveolitis

Flow Cytometry

Immunoregulative index (CD4/CD8, T4/T8)

Increased Values
lymphocytic alveolitis, asbestosis, berylliosis, sarcoidosis

Decreased Values
exogenous allergic alveolitis, fibrosing cryptogenic alveolitis, alveolitides, silicosis

Free Oxygen Radicals

(O_2^-, H_2O_2, $\cdot OH$)

Increased Values
fibrosing cryptogenic alveolitis, inflammatory pulmonary diseases

Gene Probes

DNA-DNA or DNA-RNA hybridization, amplification by speed polymerase chain reaction (PCR).

Positive
tuberculosis

Globulins

Increased Values
inflammatory pulmonary processes

Immunoglobulins

Increased Values
inflammatory activity

Interleukins

(IL-1, 2, 6, 10)

Increased Values
fibrosing cryptogenic alveolitis, inflammatory pulmonary processes

Lactate Dehydrogenase

Decreased Values
pulmonary alveolar proteinosis

Mucin-Like High-Molecular Glycoprotein

Increased Values
fibrosing cryptogenic alveolitis

Proteins

Increased Values
exudate

Short-Term Cultures

- **gene expression of particular cytokines**: fibrosing cryptogenic alveolitis, inflammatory processes
- **surface differentiated molecules expression (CD11, CD18, CD4, CD8)**: fibrosing cryptogenic alveolitis, inflammatory pulmonary processes
- **cytokine production (IL-1, 2, 6, 8, 10, TNF-alpha, TNF-beta), their receptors and free O_2 radicals**: fibrosing cryptogenic alveolitis, inflammatory pulmonary processes

Surface Differentiated Molecules

(CD11, CD18, CD4, CD8)

Increased Values
fibrosing cryptogenic alveolitis, inflammatory pulmonary diseases

Transforming Growth Factor Beta

Increased Values
fibrosing cryptogenic alveolitis

Tumour-Necrosis Factor Alpha

Increased Values
fibrosing cryptogenic alveolitis, inflammatory pulmonary processes

Increased Values
vagal hyperfunction, G-cell hyperplasia, **duodenal ulcer disease**, basophilic leukemia, systemic mastocytosis, syndrome – (postresection sy, **Zollinger-Ellison sy**)

Decreased Values
pernicious anemia, gastric tumors

Cerebrospinal Fluid

D. Mesko, R. Pullmann

Cerebrospinal fluid functions like "protective pillow" for nervous tissue. Cerebrospinal fluid (CSF) is produced in the ventricle plexus choroideus (choroid plexus) by the plasma ultra-filtration, active plexus cell activity, differential absorption, active secretion, and intensive metabolic change through cerebral ventricles ependyma and basal glial membrane. Metabolic change is carried out also among pial vessels and liquor spaces. CSF fills the subarachnoid space within/around the CNS and is absorbed by the dural arachnoid villi sinuses. The subarachnoid space, which lies between the arachnoid membrane externally and the pia mater internally, carries the flow from the cerebral ventricles to its points of absorption. The subarachnoid space extends superficially over the whole surface of the brain and spinal cord. Every blood vessel entering or leaving the nervous system must pass across it. Total CSF volume is about 70–150 ml (10–60 ml in newborn), 500–600 ml is formed daily, and the entire volume is renewed every 5–7 hours. There is also known to be a constant process of dialysis with exchange of various chemical constituents between the CSF and the blood across the ventricular ependyma, the perivascular spaces and the arachnoid membrane at all levels. Some CSF constituants concentrations are regulated within narrow limits: K^+, H^+, Mg^{2+}, Ca^{2+}. Glucose, urea and creatinine diffuse freely but require several hours for equilibration. CSF analytes concentrations should always be compared with those in plasma, because alterations in the latter are reflected in the CSF even when CNS metabolism is normal.

CSF provides fluid medium to enhance brain nutrition, remove metabolic by-products, and protect against mechanical injury. Most CSF constituents appear in equal/lower concentrations than in plasma. Under pathological conditions, elements ordinarily restrained by the socalled blood-brain barrier may enter the spinal fluid and establish higher concentrations. Cerebrospinal fluid is usually obtained by lumbar puncture.

Examination of the liquor: color, appearance, consistency, clots, pressure, cells, biochemical, bacteriological/viral + culture, cytological, and serological analysis, phase contrast microscopy, antigen detection, nucleic acid probes after PCR amplification, specific serological testing, stain for eosinophils.

Physiologically: colorless, crystal-clear fluid, slightly alkaline with a composition similar to blood electrolytes and containing small protein amount.

Most blood plasma changes will also affect the cerebrospinal fluid.

Test Purpose. 1) to measure CSF pressure as an aid in detecting CSF circulation obstruction, 2) to aid in the diagnosis of viral or bacterial meningitis, subarachnoid or intracranial hemorrhage, tumours and brain abscesses, 3) to aid in neurosyphilis and central nervous system infections diagnosis.

Acid Proteinases

Increased Values
central nervous system inflammatory diseases, sclerosis multiplex

Adenylate Kinase

(AK) Is an ATP:AMP phosphotransferase that results in AMP and ATP production employing ADP as a substrate (2ADP = ATP + AMP).

Increased Values
acute cerebrovascular disease, subarachnoid hemorrhage, **bacterial meningitis**, tumors, Guillain–Barré sy, cerebral trauma

Albumin

Albumin in CSF is in a dynamic balance with plasmatic albumin.

Increased Values
cerebrospinal fluid flow blockage, choroid plexus lesions, vascular-central nervous system damage

Analyte	Age/Gender	Reference Range	SI Units	Note
Albumin				
Suboccipital Liquor		61–180	mg/l	
Ventricular L.		110–350	mg/l	
Spinal L.		112–354	mg/l	
Albumin CSF/Serum Ratio		<0.007		

Aldolase

Increased Values
amaurotic familial idiocy, Niemann-Pick disease

Amino Acids

(AA, syn: alpha-amino acids, fractionated amino acids, quantitative amino acids) Amino acid levels are highest in midafternoon and lowest in early morning (30% less).
Test Purpose. 1) diagnosis and evaluation of genetic diseases that lead to amino acid disorders.

Increased Values
conditions with severe liver damage, diabetes mellitus with ketosis, eclampsia, hereditary fructose intolerance, malabsorption, maple sugar urine disease, phenylketonuria, renal failure, Reye's syndrome, urea cycle disease
   Interfering Factors: hemolysis, medicaments – (bismuth salts, glucocorticoids, heparin, levarterenol, 11-oxysteroids, sulfonamide, testosterone)

Decreased Values
adrenocortical hyperfunction, GM2 gangliosidosis, metachromatic leukodystrophy, amyotrophic lateral sclerosis, multiple sclerosis, Hartnup's disease, Huntington's chorea, nephrotic syndrome, phlebotomy fever, rheumatoid arthritis

Interfering Factors: medicaments – (epinephrine, estrogens, glucose, oral contraceptives, progesterone)

Gamma-Aminobutyric Acid

Decreased Values
Huntington's d.

Analyte	Age/Gender	Reference Range	SI Units	Note
Gamma-Aminobutyric Acid		190–280	nmol/l	

Amylase

Increased Values
choledocholithiasis, acute pancreatitis

Angiotensin-I-Converting Enzyme

Increased Values
neurosarcoidosis

Antibodies Against Mumps Virus

Test Purpose. To help in diagnosis of infection with mumps virus (paramyxovirus).

Increased Values – positive
mumps meningitis

Antibodies Against Rabies Virus

Antibodies can be detected in most patients with clinical rabies within two weeks of onset. High CSF antibody titres are seen in clinical rabies, but not after vaccination.
Test Purpose. To support a clinical diagnosis of rabies.

Increased Values – positive
rabies virus infection

Antibodies Against St. Louis Encephalitis Virus

Test is used to support the diagnosis of St. Louis encephalitis virus infection. Demonstration of IgM antibody in CSF rapidly establishes a diagnosis of arboviral encephalitis.

Increased Values – positive
St. Louis encephalitis

Antidiuretic Hormone

Increased Values
pseudotumor

Decreased Values
Alzheimer's disease

Anti-Hu Antibodies

Increased Values – positive
gangliopathy, limbic encephalitis, cerebellar disorders, gastrointestinal dysfunction

Arginine

Increased Values
bacterial meningitis

Decreased Values
multiple sclerosis

Aspartate Aminotransferase

Increased Values
acute anterior poliovirus meningitis, subarachnoid hemorrhage, cortical stroke, cerebral embolism, cerebral infarction, tumors, head injury

Bacterial Antigens

Bacterial antigen detection may be useful for the diagnosis of meningitis which has been partially treated.
Tests are available for: Haemophilus influenzae type b, Neisseria meningitidis, Streptococcus pneumoniae, group B streptococcus.

Basophils

Increased Values
diseases – (inflammatory CNS d., parasitic infectious d.), chronic myelogenous leukemia involving meninges, convulsive states, foreign body reaction

Blood

Increased Values – positive
bleeding – (intracranial b., subarachnoid b.), traumatic tap

Carcinoembryonic Antigen

Increased Values
metastatic meningeal tumors – (breast t., lung t., bowel t.)

Chloride

Increased Values
encephalitis, nephrosis, meningeal infection, hypochloremia

Decreased Values
hypochloremia, meningitis – (bacterial m., purulent m., **tuberculotic m.**), Addison's disease, pneumonia

Cholesterol

Increased Values
cerebral abscess, cerebral hemorrhage, meningitis, CNS tumours, sclerosis multiplex

Cholinesterase

Increased Values
brain abscess, CNS bleeding, brain parenchyma destruction, hydrocephalus, meningitis, brain tumors, multiple sclerosis, Guillain–Barré syndrome

Citrulline

Increased Values
citrullinemia

Color + Turbidity

- ◼ **red:** bleeding – (cerebral b., subarachnoid b.), trauma, primary amebic meningoencephalitis, spinal cord obstruction, traumatic lumbar puncture
- ◼ **physiologically:** crystal clear, colorless, does not coagulate
- ◼ **pus:** purulent meningitis
- ◼ **slightly yellow:** meningitis – (acute pyogenic m., tuberculous m.), acute poliomyelitis, **proteins**
- ◼ **viscous:** tuberculotic meningitis, metastatic mucinous adenocarcinoma, cryptococcal infection, severe meningeal infection, injury to annulus fibrosus
- ◼ **xanthochromic** (xanthochromasia – pale pink to yellow): **bilirubinemia**, immature newborns, **hypercarotenemia**, hyperproteinorrhachia, jaundice, **intracerebral/intra-/ventricular/subarachnoid hemorrhage**, meningeal melanosarcoma, methemoglobinemia, spinal cord/brain tumours, **conditions after bleeding**, toxoplasmosis

- **turbid** (cloudy): **bacteria, proteins, erythrocytes**, contrast media, epidural fat aspiration during lumbar puncture, yeasts, **leukocytes**, meningitis – (purulent m., tuberculous m., viral m.), amebae
- **dark:** metastatic melanoma, jaundice (hyperbilirubinemia)

Copper

Increased Values
brain infarction

Corticotropin Releasing Hormone

Increased Values
depression

Creatine Kinase

Creatine kinase is normally present in CSF, primarily as the CK-BB isoenzyme (97–98% of total CK activity), derived from brain tissue.
Test Purpose. 1) to assess focal cerebral ischemia, 2) acute subarachnoid hemorrhage diagnosis, 3) hydrocephalus diagnosis, 4) brain injuries, 5) coma after cardio-pulmo-cerebral resuscitation assessment.

Increased Values
hydrocephalus, cerebral infarction, cerebral ischemia, coma, subarachnoid hemorrhage, bacterial meningitis, **viral meningoencephalitis, CNS tumors, metastatic tumors involving CNS, demyelinating disorders**, sclerosis multiplex, **following epileptic seizures**, Guillain–Barré sy, increased intracranial pressure, cerebral thrombosis, **cerebral injury** (CK-BB), vasculitis

Cryptococcal Antigen

A negative result does not exclude infection. Antigen levels decrease with effective therapy.
Test Purpose. 1) to help in cryptococcal infection diagnosis, 2) to monitor response to therapy.

Increased Values – positive
cryptococcal meningitis

Cyclic Adenosine Monophosphate

Decreased Values
after intracranial hemorrhage, trauma of CNS

Analyte	Age/Gender	Reference Range	SI Units	Note
Cyclic Adenosine Monophosphate		4–19	nmol/l	

Cytological Examination

The detection of malignant cells indicates meningeal involvement with carcinoma, lymphoma or leukemia.

DNA-Testing

PCR amplification, followed by specific nucleic acid probes, provides a sensitive technique for detection of Mycobacterium tuberculosis, herpes simplex virus, enteroviruses, cytomegalovirus and Toxoplasma gondii.

Endorphins

Increased Values
after local electrical brain stimulation, Nelson's sy

Analyte	Age/Gender	Reference Range	SI Units	Note
Beta-Endorphins		6–15	pmol/l	

Enkephalins

(syn: leu-enkephalin, met-enkephalin)

Increased Values
Leigh's sy, after electroacupuncture

Analyte	Age/Gender	Reference Range	SI Units	Note
Leu-Enkephalin		124–369	pmol/l	
Met-Enkephalin		19–108	pmol/l	

Enolase

Enolase is found in three naturally forms, the brain-specific enolase (alpha-alpha form) is the most acidic. Both liver-specific enolase and the isoenzyme form are non-neuronal enolase enzymes.

Increased Values
astrocytoma, demyelination, lymphoma, Hodgkin's disease, malignant CNS metastases

Eosinophils

Increased Values
allergy, **coccidioidomycosis**, obstructive hydrocephalus, parasitic CNS infections – (Cysticercus, Fasciola hepatica, Hypoderma bovis, Paragonimus westermani, Schistosoma spp., Taenia solium, Toxoplasma, Trichinella), hemorrhage into the CNS, lymphocytic leukemia with spread to CNS, **intrathecal drugs and dyes**, **malignant lymphoma**, Hodgkin's disease,

meningitis – (bacterial m., fungal m., rickettsial m., tuberculous m., viral m.), myelography, subacute sclerosing panencephalitis, periarteritis nodosa, pneumoencephalography, **acute polyneuritis**, sarcoidosis, sclerosis multiplex, intracranial shunt, cerebrospinal syphilis, rabies vaccination, Rocky Mountain spotted fever

Ependymal Cells

Increased Values
hydrocephalus, following pneumoencephalography, intrathecal chemotherapeutic agent administration

Erythrocytes

Increased Values
bleeding – (**cerebral b., subarachnoid b.**), **hemorrhagic central nervous system lesions**, primary amebic meningoencephalitis, **lumbar puncture**, arterio-venous malformation, cerebral aneurysm, delirum tremens, epilepsy, Guillain-Barré sy, hemorrhagic stroke, neurosyphilis, primary lymphoma of the brain, spinal tumors, syphilitic aseptic meningitis, syphilitic myelopathy

Ferritin

Injured cells connected with hemato-liquor barrier disorders are the main ferritin liquor source. The stimulus for local ferritin synthesis are probably free iron/iron compounds in extracellular and subarachnoid spaces.

Increased Values
CNS infectious diseases, cerebral infarction, subarachnoid hemorrhage, circulation disorders in vasculitis, intraparenchymatous cerebrovascular accident

Alpha-1-Fetoprotein

Increased Values – positive
CNS dysgerminomas, meningeal carcinomatosis, embryonal tumors

Fibrinogen

Increased Values
spinal cord channel obstruction

Fibronectin

Fibronectin is a high-molecular weight glycoprotein found in blood and various tissues.

Increased Values
astrocytoma, acute lymphoblastic leukemia, metastatic tumors in CNS

Glial Fibrillary Acidic Protein

Fibrous astrocyte protein as part of the intermediate filaments, which can be extracted from the white matter.

Increased Values
hydrocephalus with normal pressure, Alzheimer's disease, glial tumors

Analyte	Age/Gender	Reference Range	SI Units	Note
Glial Fibrillary Acidic Protein		<9.5	µg/l	

Gamma Globulins

Test Purpose. To aid in diagnosis of multiple sclerosis.

Increased Values
chronic central nervous system infections, **neurosyphilis, subacute sclerosing panencephalitis, sclerosis multiplex** (multiple sclerosis), **Guillain-Barré sy**, general paresis, herpes encephalitis, myxedema, meningeal carcinomatosis, carcinomatous cerebellar degeneration, connective tissue disease, demyelinating disease, liver cirrhosis, plasmocytoma (incl. multiple myeloma), rheumatoid arthritis, sarcoidosis

Glucose

Normally 2/3 to 1/2 of fasting blood glucose levels. Glucose reaches the CSF by facilitated diffusion via a choroid plexus membrane transport system. CSF plasma glucose changes are reflected in about two hours, and normally reach equilibrium in four hours.
Test Purpose. 1) to aid in diagnosis of meninges and brain inflammation, 2) to evaluate comatose states, 3) to evaluate hypoglycemic shock, 4) to help diagnose of bacterial or fungal infections.

Increased Values – hyperglycorrhachia
cerebral abscess, **diabetes mellitus, encephalitis, hyperglycemia**, viral CNS infections, acute cerebral infarction, meningitis, cerebral tumours, poliomyelitis, **CNS syphilis**, CNS trauma

Decreased Values – hypoglycorrhachia
cysticercosis, encephalitis – (mumps e., **bacterial e.**, HSV e.), **hypoglycemia, meningeal carcinomatosis, subarachnoid hemorrhage, meningeal spread leukemia**, meningeal spread lymphomas, melanoma, meningitis – (**amebic m., bacterial m.**, cryptococcal m., parasitic m., **fungal m., purulent m.**, acute pyogenic m., rheumatoid m., acute syphilitic m., trichinotic m., **tuberculotic m.**), Lyme disease, viral meningitis in – (**herpes simplex, herpes zoster, mumps**, lymphocytic choriomeningitis), meningoencephalitis – (**primary amebic m., mumps m.**), **lupus myelopathy, CNS tumors**, metastatic CNS tumors, **neurosyphilis**, antidiabetics overdose, parameningeal processes, **sarcoidosis**, hypoglycemic shock

Analyte	Age/Gender	Reference Range	SI Units	Note
Glucose	Children <16 y	1.8–4.6	mmol/l	
	Adults	2.7–4.2	mmol/l	
blood/liquor coefficient	Adults	1.1–1.6		

Beta-Glucuronidase

Increased Values – positive
meningeal carcinomatosis, metastatic leptomeningeal adenocarcinoma, acute myeloblastic leukemia

Glutamic Acid

Increased Values
meningitis – (bacterial m., carcinomatous m.), Garin–Bujadoux–Bannwarth meningoradiculitis

Glutamine

Glutamine is synthesized in brain tissue from ammoniaic and glutamine acid, glutamine production provides a mechanism for removing ammonia from the central nervous system. This glutamine formation protects the CNS from toxic ammonia effects.

Increased Values
hepatic cirrhosis, **genetic urea cycle enzyme deficiencies**, **hepatic encephalopathy**, encephalopathy – (e. secondary to respiratory failure, septic e.), histidinemia, hypercapnia, **hepatic coma**, meningitis – (**bacterial m.**, **carcinomatous m.**), **Garin–Bujadoux–Bannwarth meningoradiculitis**, neonates, **Reye's syndrome**

Gamma-Glutamyltransferase

Increased Values
cerebral infarction, electroconvulsive shock therapy

Glycine

Increased Values
non-ketotic hyperglycinemia, meningitis – (aseptic m., bacterial m., carcinomatous m.), meningoradiculitis

Alpha-2-Glycoprotein

Glial-cell-specific protein high in neuraminic acid content.

Increased Values
multiple sclerosis

Human Chorionic Gonadotropin

(hCG, syn: beta-hCG, beta-human chorionic gonadotropin, human choriongonadotropin)

Increased Values
CNS dysgerminomas, CNS metastatic choriocarcinoma, meningeal carcinomatosis

Human Soluble Vascular Cell Adhesion Molecule–1

(h-SVCAM-1)

Increased Values
systemic lupus erythematosus, vasculitides

Human T-Cell Lymphotrophic Virus I/II Antibodies

(syn: HTLV I/II antibodies) Human retrovirus (HTLV – human T-cell lymphotrophic virus)
Test Purpose. To aid in the spastic myelopathy diagnosis and differential diagnosis for HTLV-I and chronic neuromuscular diseases (HTLV-II).

Increased Values – positive
neuromuscular diseases, **acute HTLV infection, adult T-cell acute lymphoblastic leukemia,** hairy cell leukemia, tropical spastic paraparesis

5-Hydroxyindoleacetic Acid

(5-HIAA) Metabolite of serotonin.

Decreased Values
diffuse brain dysfunction, encephalopathy

Analyte	Age/Gender	Reference Range	SI Units	Note
5-Hydroxyindole-acetic Acid		145–205	nmol/l	

Hydroxyproline

Increased Values
bacterial meningitis

Immunoglobulin A

Measurement of IgA in CSF and serum can be used to determine the IgA index. The index is a measure of intra-blood-brain-barrier synthesis.

Increased Values
CNS lupus erythematosus, multiple sclerosis, viral meningitis

Analyte	Age/Gender	Reference Range	SI Units	Note
Immunoglobulin A				
Suboccipital liquor		0–1.8	mg/l	
Ventricular l.		0–3.9	mg/l	
Spinal l.		379–4250	mg/l	

Immunoglobulin G

(CSF IgG, CSF gamma G, syn: cerebrospinal fluid IgG, CSF immunoglobulin) All inflammatory CNS processes lead to higher IgG values.
Test Purpose. 1) to evaluate central nervous system involvement through infection, neoplasm or primary neurologic disease, 2) to evaluate the integrity and permeability of the blood-cerebrospinal fluid barrier and IgG synthesis within the CNS.

Increased Values
rubella encephalitis, diseases – (**infectious d.**, connective tissue d.), CNS diseases – (chronic infectious phase, inflammatory CNS d.), CNS hemorrhage, **subacute sclerosing leukoencephalitis,** lupus erythematosus involving CNS, **meningitis,** viral meningoencephalitis, healthy persons, CNS tumours, **neurosyphilis,** sarcoidosis, **sclerosis multiplex** (multiple sclerosis), **Guillain-Barré sy**

Analyte	Age/Gender	Reference Range	SI Units	Note
Immunoglobulin G				
Suboccipital liquor		5.0–23	mg/l	
Ventricular l.		13.9–37.5	mg/l	
Spinal l.		284–860	mg/l	

Immunoglobulin M

Increased Values – positive
bacterial meningitis, tumours of – (meninges, brain), sclerosis multiplex (multiple sclerosis)

Analyte	Age/Gender	Reference Range	SI Units	Note
Immunoglobulin M				
Suboccipital Liquor		<350	µg/l	
Ventricular l.		<450	µg/l	
Spinal l.		2658–24800	µg/l	

Interferon

Increased Values
viral infections

Interleukin 6

Increased Values
meningitis – (**bacterial m.**, **viral m.**)

Isocitrate Dehydrogenase

Increased Values
vascular cerebral lesions, acute bacterial meningitis, cerebrospinal tumor – (metastatic c. t., primary c. t.)

Isoleucine

Increased Values
meningitis – (bacterial m., carcinomatous m.), Garin-Bujadoux-Bannwarth meningoradiculitis

Lactate Dehydrogenase

LD liquor sources: diffusion through the barrier blood-cerebrospinal fluid, the barrier brain-cerebrospinal fluid, leucocytes, bacteria, and tumorous cells.
Test Purpose. 1) cerebrovascular accident diagnosis, 2) cerebral tumors, 3) meningeal and cerebral inflammation, 4) polyradiculoneuritides, 5) lumboischialgic syndrome diagnosis.

Increased Values
brain abscess, lumbar discopathy, encephalitis, hemorrhage – (neonatal intracranial h., **subarachnoid h.** – LD3,4,5), **leukemia** – LD3,4,5, **lymphoma**, lymphosarcoma, meningitis – (**bacterial m.** - LD4,5, viral m. – LD1,2, cryptococcal m., tuberculotic m. – LD1,2,3), **CNS tumours**, **metastatic CNS tumors**, **cerebral ischemic necrosis**, severe cerebral hypoxia, **cerebral apoplexy** (cerebrovascular accident, LD1), CNS inflammation/infection

Lactic Acid

(syn: lactate) CNS anaerobic metabolism is a primary source of liquor lactic acid.
Test Purpose. 1) to help in the diagnosis of purulent meningitis and brain inflammation, 2) cerebral ischemia.

Increased Values
brain abscess, respiratory alkalosis, atherosclerosis, cerebral edema, **hydrocephalus**, **hypocapnia**, **hypotension**, **cerebral infarct** (prognostic factor), **cerebral ischemia**, hemorrhage – (intracranial h., **subarachnoid h.**), leukemia, **lymphoma**, meningitis – (**bacterial m.**, fungal m., serous m., tuberculous m.), **CNS tumors**, cerebral malaria, ischemic necrosis, metastatic CNS tumors, reduced cerebral blood flow, **sclerosis multiplex**, conditions – (**hypoxic c.**, **seizure c.**), increased intracranial pressure, **CNS trauma**

Decreased Values
viral CNS infectious diseases

Analyte	Age/Gender	Reference Range	SI Units	Note
Lactate	6 m–15 y	1.1–1.8	mmol/l	
	16–50 y	1.5–2.1	mmol/l	
	51–75 y	1.7–2.6	mmol/l	

Leucine

Increased Values
generalized aminoaciduria, starvation, maple syrup urine disease, Hartnup disease, meningitis – (aseptic m., bacterial m., carcinomatous m.), Garin–Bujadoux–Bannwarth meningoradiculitis, severe burns, pregnancy (1st trimester), hepatic failure

Leukocytes

Increased Values – pleiocytosis
abscess – (**cerebral a.**, spinal epidural a., retropharyngeal a., epidural a.), spinal anesthesia, **septic emboli due to bacterial endocarditis**, delirium tremens, dementia, cerebral embolism, epilepsy, **subdural empyema**, **amebic encephalomyelitis**, encephalitis – (**AIDS e.**, herpes e., Japanese B e.), postinfectious e., postvaccinal e., St. Louis e.), subacute necrotizing encephalomyelopathy, lead encephalopathy, dural sinuses phlebitis, **cerebral infarct**, intoxication by – (arsenic, mercury), hemorrhage – (central nervous system h., **subarachnoid h.**), leptospirosis, **chronic granulocytic leukemia**, intrathecal medication, cerebral malaria, meningitis – (aseptic m., **bacterial m.**, carcinomatous m., granulomatous m., purulent m., listeria m., **meningococcal m.**, Mollaret's m., mycotic m., fungal m.), rickettsial m., acute luetic m., tuberculous m., viral m.), **meningoencephalitis**, myelography, lymphoma, **CNS tumors**, metastatic CNS tumors, infectious mononucleosis, skull osteomyelitis, otitis/sinusitis, pneumoencephalography, polyneuritis, **repeated lumbar puncture, neonatal sepsis, sclerosis multiplex, meningovascular syphilis**, Behcet's sy, toxoplasmosis, trichinosis, cerebral thrombophlebitis, **intracranial vein thrombosis**, trypanosomiasis, endemic typhus, vasculitis, demyelinating diseases, Rocky Mountain spotted fever
   Interfering Factors: medicaments – (ibuprofen, sulfamethoxazole, sulindac, tolmetin)

Decreased Values
encephalitis, myelitis, CNS tumours

Lymphocytes

Increased Values
chronic alcoholism, brain abscess, granulomatous arteritis, **aseptic/viral encephalitis, drug abuse encephalopathy**, herpes zoster, **choriomeningitis, parasitic CNS diseases**, meningitis – (aseptic m., **bacterial m., leptospiral m., fungal m., tuberculous m., viral m.**), syphilitic meningoencephalitis, **brain tumours**, measles, **subacute sclerosing panencephalitis**, periarteritis involving the CNS, poliomyelitis, polyneuritis, **meningeal sarcoidosis, sclerosis multiplex** (multiple sclerosis), acute disseminated sclerosis (encephalomyelitis), **cerebrospinal syphilis, Guillain-Barré sy**, cerebral thrombosis

Lysine

Increased Values

meningitis – (bacterial m., carcinomatous m.), Garin-Bujadoux-Bannwarth meningora-diculitis

Lysozyme

Present in granulocytes.

Increased Values

meningitis – (bacterial m., fungal m., tuberculous m.), CNS tumors, **leukemia**, CNS system sarcoidosis

Alpha-2-Macroglobulin

Increased Values

inflammatory CNS disease, cerebral/spinal metastases, polyneuropathy

Analyte	Age/Gender	Reference Range	SI Units	Note
Alpha-2-Macroglobulin				
Suboccipital liquor		0–2.2	mg/l	
Ventricular l.		0–3.3	mg/l	
Spinal l.		469–2957	mg/l	

Macrophages

Increased Values

cerebral abscess, ischemic cerebral infarct, **acute intracranial bleeding**, contrast media, meningitis – (mycotic m., tuberculous m.), reaction to – (foreign bodies, erythrocytes, lipids in cerebrospinal fluid), CNS trauma

Magnesium

Decreased Values

ischemic brain disease, meningitis

Malignant Cells

positive

primary malignant and metastatic brain tumors

Methionine

Increased Values
homocystinuria, bacterial meningitis

Beta-2-Microglobulin

Test Purpose. Diagnosis and monitoring of progression of neurological involvement in leukemia, lymphoproliferative disorders and HIV infection.

Increased Values
acute leukemia, **lymphoma with CNS involvement, CNS involvement in acute lymphoblastic leukemia,** multiple sclerosis, CNS disease in HIV infection

Microscopic Examination

- ■ **cells – physiologically:** mononuclear cells – (lymphocytes, monocytes)
- ■ **cells – pathologically:** ependymal, glial, white blood cells, macrophages, malignant cells
- ■ **bacteria:** inflammatory CNS diseases, bacterial meningitis
- ■ **plasmocytes:** sclerosis multiplex

Analyte	Age/Gender	Reference Range	SI Units	Note
Cells	Neonates	<32	WBC/l	
	Adults	0	WBC/l	
Leukocytes – Spinal l.		0–5		
Suboccipit. l.		0–3		
Ventricular l.		0–1		
Lymphocytes – Spinal l.		0.6–0.85		
Suboccipit. l.		0.8–0.95		
Ventricular l.		0.9–1.00		
Granulocytes – Spinal l.		0.15–0.40		
Suboccipit. l.		0.05–0.20		
Ventricular l.		0–0.10		

Monocytes

Increased Values
chronic alcoholism, **aseptic/viral encephalitis,** drug abuse encephalopathy, herpes zoster, parasitic CNS diseases, meningitis – (**aseptic m.,** leptospiral m., **fungal m., tuberculous m., viral m.**), brain tumours, measles, periarteritis involving the CNS, poliomyelitis, polyneuritis, meningeal sarcoidosis, **sclerosis multiplex,** acute disseminated sclerosis, **subacute sclerosing panencephalitis,** cerebrospinal syphilis, Guillain-Barré sy

Myelin Basic Protein

(MBP) CNS myelin contains approximately 70% lipid and 30% protein, produced by the oligodendroglia; two proteins make up 80% of the total protein content. The larger is called proteolipid protein and the smaller is called myelin basic protein because of its solubility in acid solutions. MBP is released into the CSF whenever there is damage to neural tissue; it reflects intact myelin sheath destruction in the course of demyelinating disease of the CNS. MBP comprises 30% of the protein of the myelin sheath.

Test Purpose. 1) to estimate central nervous system demyelinating diseases activity, especially multiple sclerosis, 2) to determine whether active demyelination is occurring in patients being treated by intrathecal chemotherapy or radiation therapy for CNS neoplastic diseases, 3) to diagnose acute brain tissue destruction in children, 4) to assess the efficacy of potential treatments for multiple sclerosis.

Increased Values

diabetes mellitus, Wernicke's encephalopathy, encephalitis – (St. Louis e., herpes e., e. lethargica, Japanese B e.), hydrocephalus – (**h. with normal CSF pressure**, communicating h., obstructive h.), hypoxia, **intrathecal chemotherapy**, disease – (Krabbe's d.), cerebral infarction, HIV infection, leukemia, **leukodystrophies, metachromatic leukodystrophy**, necrotizing leukoencephalopathy, **CNS systemic lupus erythematosus, leptomeningeal metastases**, meningoencephalitis, myelitis, **CNS tumors, peripheral neuropathy**, neurosyphilis, **subacute sclerosing panencephalitis, stroke, sclerosis multiplex**, postneurosurgery, **Guillain-Barré sy, cerebrovascular injury**, head trauma, vasculitis, encephalopathies, CNS hemorrhage, amyotrophic lateral sclerosis, cranial irradiation, chronic renal failure, immune complex diseases, beriberi

Analyte	Age/Gender	Reference Range	SI Units	Note
Myelin Basic Protein		<2.5	µg/l	

Neuron-Specific Enolase

(NSE) Neuron-specific enolase is one of the five isozymes of the glycolytic enzyme, enolase. This enzyme is released into the CSF when neural tissue is injured. Neoplasms derived from neural or neuroendocrine tissue may release NSE into the blood. The test may have value in predicting response to therapy. NSE is a tumor marker.

Increased Values

neural tissue injury, tumors – (pheochromocytoma, gastrinoma, carcinoid, **bronchogenic small-cell carcinoma**, medulloblastoma, melanoma, **neuroblastoma**, retinoblastoma, seminoma, t. of pancreas, t. of kidney, t. of thyroid)

Oligoclonal Bands

(syn: oligoclonal proteins) Qualitative interpretation in diagnosis of bacterial, viral or fungal meningitis, encephalitis, malignant infiltrates (acute leukemia, lymphoma), disorders with local immunoglobulin production in the CNS (e. g. multiple sclerosis), subarachnoid hemorrhage, spinal canal blockage, Guillain-Barré syndrome, crebrovascular accident.

sclerosis multiplex, viral encephalitis, progressive rubella encephalitis, subacute sclerosing panencephalitis, bacterial meningitis, trypanosomiasis, meningeal carcinomatosis, cerebral infarction, neurosyphilis, toxoplasmosis, cryptococcal meningitis, inflammatory neuropathies

Ornithine

Increased Values
bacterial meningitis, Garin-Bujadoux-Bannwarth meningoradiculitis

pH

Test Purpose. 1) acute acid-base balance disorders diagnosis, 2) dialysis patients monitoring, 3) pulmonary ventilation control, 4) consciousness disorders diagnosis in encephalopathies, 5) cerebral circulation disorders, 6) atraumatic cerebral edema diagnosis.

Decreased Values – acid pH
cerebral infarction, subarachnoid hemorrhage, purulent meningitis, head injury

Phenylalanine

Increased Values
meningitis – (aseptic m., bacterial m., carcinomatous m.), hyperphenylalaninemia, meningoradiculitis Garin-Bujadoux-Bannwarth

Phosphorus

Increased Values
meningitis, CNS tumours, degenerative cerebral processes, blood phosphate retention

Plasma Cells

Increased Values
subacute viral encephalitis, CNS diseases – (parasitic CNS d., chronic inflammatory CNS d., subacute inflammatory CNS d.), leukoencephalitis, meningitis – (fungal m., tuberculous m., viral m.), **syphilitic meningoencephalitis**, cerebral tumors, delayed hypersensitivity response, subacute sclerosing panencephalitis, sarcoidosis, **sclerosis multiplex**, Guillain-Barré sy

Prealbumin

Increased Values
obstructive hydrocephalus

Pressure

Cerebrospinal fluid pressure is directly related to pressure in the jugular and vertebral veins. The brain, spinal cord and CSF are enclosed in a rigid container composed of the skull and vertebral column. Normal pressure is maintained by CSF absorption in amounts equal to its production through the arachnoid villi and choroid plexus.

Increased Values
abscess – (**epidural a.**, **brain a.**), arachnoiditis, blockage of liquor outflow – (arachnoid granulations, foramen magnum), encephalitis, **cerebral edema**, subdural empyema, lead encephalopathy, subacute bacterial endocarditis, myelographic dye, hydrocephalus, overproduction of CSF, **hypoosmolality due to hemodialysis**, diseases – (degenerative CNS d., infectious d., bone d., **inflammatory d. of meninges**), intoxication by – (bromide, mushrooms, methanol, lead, thallium, toluene), meningeal carcinomatosis, collagen-vascular disease, **subarachnoid hemorrhage**, leptospirosis, leukemia, Paget's disease, meningitis – (aseptic m., bacterial m., fungal m., purulent m., tuberculous m., viral m.), **amebic meningoencephalitis**, mucolipidosis, mucopolysaccharidosis, tumors of – (**CNS**, bone, **choroid plexus**), pathway obstruction/restriction – (intracranial subarachnoid o. /r., ventricular o. /r., spinal subarachnoid o. /r.), **acute superior vena cava obstruction**, hypertrophic osteoarthritis, osteomyelitis, osteoporosis, vertebral discs disorders, CNS sarcoidosis, ankylosing spondylitis, cervical/thoracic spondylosis, CNS syphilis, toxoplasmosis, thrombophlebitis, **intracranial venous sinus thrombosis**, bacterial ventriculitis, **congestive heart failure**
> **Interfering Factors:** anxious person, knee flexion against the abdomen, hypoxia, involuntarily breath holding or muscle tension, medicaments – (corticosteroids, nalidixic acid, tetracyclines, theophylline, vitamin A)

Decreased Values
cerebral abscess, adhesions, complete spinal subarachnoid block, severe dehydration, fistulae – (surgery f., osteomyelitis f., previous lumbar puncture f., traumatic f.), **vertebral fracture, herniated intervertebral disc, hyperosmolality, circulatory collapse, CNS tumors**, CSF otorrhea – (via the petrous bone), CSF rhinorrhea – (via ethmoid, frontal, sphenoid sinuses or cribriform plate), **spinal fluid leakage**, shock conditions, diabetic coma

Proline

Increased Values
meningitis – (aseptic m., bacterial m., carcinomatous m.), Garin-Bujadoux-Bannwarth meningoradiculitis

Prostaglandins

Prostaglandin D2 and PGF2-alpha are the predominant brain prostaglandins.

Increased Values
meningitis, stroke, cerebral trauma

Proteins

More than 80% CSF protein contents originate from plasma by ultrafiltration through the capillaries walls in the meninges and choroid plexuses, the remainder originates from intrathecal synthesis. As the CSF passes down to the lumbar spine protein concentrations increases. Dysproteinemia leads to liquor disorder, to the hemato-liquor barrier permeability changes for proteins, cerebrogenous proteins hyperproduction. Albumin to globulin proportion is higher in cerebrospinal fluid than in blood plasma since the albumin molecule is significantly smaller and can more easily cross the blood-brain barrier.

Test Purpose. 1) circulation disorders or blood stasis in CNS, 2) CNS cell elements breakdown detection, 3) causal determination of liquor-brain barrier higher permeability.

Increased Values – hyperproteinorrhachia

abscess – (epidural a., **brain a.**), AIDS, anemia – (pernicious a.), giant cell arteritis, cerebral arteriosclerosis, beta plasmocytoma, liver cirrhosis, dehydration, **diabetes mellitus**, cerebral embolism, subdural empyema, encephalitis – (St. Louis e., herpes e., Japanese B e., echo e., e. lethargica, California e.), **encephalomyelitis**, hypertensive encephalopathy, **subacute bacterial endocarditis**, brain ependymoma, epilepsy, myelographic dye, fever – (Rocky Mountain spotted f.), malignant histiocytosis, hyperadrenalism, hematoma – (**cerebral h.**, subdural h.), hypercalcemia, hypercapnia, hypoparathyroidism, hypothyroidism, intoxication by – (arsenic, ethanol, lead), heavy metal intoxication by – (lead, mercury), **meningeal carcinomatosis**, collagenoses, disease – (**Cushing's d.**, Creutzfeldt–Jakob d., Hodgkin's d., Refsum's d.), myxedema coma, hemorrhage – (**subarachnoid h.**, **intracerebral h.**, cerebellar h.), cryptococcosis, leptospirosis, leukemia, listeriosis, progressive multifocal leukoencephalopathy, systemic lupus erythematosus, lymphoma – (Burkitt's l., lymphocytic l.), meningitis – (**aseptic m.**, **bacterial m.**, meningococcal m., listerial m., carcinomatous m., cryptococcal m., granulomatous m., pneumococcal m., leptospiral m., fungal m., **purulent m.**, **tuberculous m.**, Mollaret's m., viral m.), primary amebic meningoencephalitis, infectious mononucleosis, mumps, mycosis fungoides, myeloma, **myxedema**, **CNS tumours**, neuroborreliosis, neuropathy – (**diabetic n.**, alcoholic n.), **neurosyphilis**, **intracranial obstruction**, **subacute sclerosing panencephalitis**, general paresis, periarteritis, **poliomyelitis**, **polyneuritis**, **chronic inflammatory polyneuropathy**, rabies, **CNS sarcoidosis**, **sclerosis multiplex**, sporotrichosis, syphilis, syndrome – (**Guillain-Barré sy**, Behcet's sy, Arnold-Chiari sy), toxoplasmosis, thrombophlebitis, trypanosomiasis, **cerebral thrombosis**, **cerebral trauma**, **uremia**, CNS vasculitis

Interfering Factors: medicaments – (acetylsalicylic acid, chlorpromazine, ibuprofen, imipramine, isopropanol, lidocaine, methicillin, methotrexate, morphine, penicillin, phenacetin, phenytoin, phenothiazines, procaine, streptomycin, sulindac, tyrosine)

Decreased Values – hypoproteinorrhachia

hyperthyroidism, **large liquor volume removal**, **increased intracranial pressure**, cerebrospinal fluid leakage – (CSF otorrhea, CSF rhinorrhea), rapid CSF production

Analyte	Age/Gender	Reference Range	SI Units	Note
Proteins, Total	Premat. infants			
	27–32 w of pregn.	0.68–2.40	g/l	
	33–36 w of pregn.	0.67–2.30	g/l	
	37–40 w of pregn.	0.58–1.50	g/l	
	1 d–1 m	0.25–0.72	g/l	
	2–3 m	0.20–0.72	g/l	
	4–6 m	0.15–0.50	g/l	
	7–12 m	0.10–0.45	g/l	

Analyte	Age/Gender	Reference Range	SI Units	Note
	2 y	0.10–0.40	g/l	
	3–4 y	0.10–0.38	g/l	
	5–8 y	0.10–0.43	g/l	
	Adults	<0.45	g/l	
Electrophoresis				
Prealbumin		0.054–0.090		
Albumin		0.553–0.659		
alpha-1-globulins		0.028–0.056		
alpha-2-globulins		0.028–0.048		
beta globulins		0.099–0.155		
gamma globulins		0.082–0.146		

C-Reactive Protein

Increased Values
false positive values – (subarachnoid hemorrhage, increased intracranial pressure), inflammatory CNS diseases, bacterial meningitis

Somatostatin

Increased Values
CNS damage

Decreased Values
Alzheimer's disease, sclerosis multiplex (multiple sclerosis)

Specific Antibodies

borrelia, cytomegalovirus, herpes, HIV, fungi, yeasts, mycobacteria, parazites, rubeola, toxoplasmosis

Taurine

Increased Values
meningitis – (bacterial m., carcinomatous m.)

Transferrin

Transferrin can be used as a marker for the presence of CSF in patients presenting with discharge of clear fluid.

Tryptophan

Increased Values
hepatic cirrhosis, hepatic encephalopathy, meningitis – (bacterial m., carcinomatous m.)

Tumor Markers

- ◼ **Embryonic proteins**
    - ▪ **alpha-fetoprotein:** pineal germ cell tumors
    - ▪ **human chorionic gonadotropin:** trophoblastic tumors, teratoma
    - ▪ **carcinoembryonic antigen:** metastatic colon cancer into CNS
- ◼ **Peptide hormones**
    - ▪ **ACTH, FSH, LH, GH, TSH:** pituitary tumors
- ◼ **Products of proteolysis**
    - ▪ **fibronectin, laminin, polyamines:** medulloblastoma
- ◼ **Brain specific proteins**
    - ▪ **myelin basic protein, glial fibrillary acidic protein:** glioma
    - ▪ **S-100 protein:** glioma/medulloblastoma
- ◼ **Enzymes**
    - ▪ beta-glucuronidase, enolase
- ◼ **Others**
    - ▪ beta-2-microglobulin, desmosterol, monoclonal antibodies to specific tumor types

Tyrosine

Increased Values
meningitis – (bacterial m., carcinomatous m.)

Urea

Increased Values
uremia

Valine

Increased Values
meningitis – (aseptic m., bacterial m., carcinomatous m.), Garin-Bujadoux-Bannwarth meningoradiculitis

VDRL

Increased Values – positive
neurosyphilis

Vitamin C

Decreased Values
encephalitis, poliomyelitis

Gastric Fluid

D. Mesko

Gastric acid secretion is proportional to parietal cell mass. Its secretion is stimulated by the presence, smell or taste of food → food in the stomach promotes neural (vagus nerve) and hormonal (gastrin) mediated secretion. Gastric acid secretion is not stimulated by fat or glucose. With gastric acid and already activated pepsin → pepsinogen is quickly converted to its active proteolytic form pepsin. Pepsinogen secretion is promoted by neural (vagal) and hormonal (gastrin, secretin, cholecystokinin-pancreozymin) stimulation. Gastric inhibitory peptide, anticholinergics, histamine antagonists and vagotomy oppose pepsinogen secretion.

The stomach itself contains cells/cell groups of many different types: 1) the surface epithelial cells secrete mucus, 2) the parietal cells secrete hydrochloric acid and intrinsic factor, 3) the chief (zymogen, peptic) cells secrete pepsinogens, 4) the neck chief cells (mucus cells) secrete mucus and pepsinogens, 5) enterochromaffin cells secrete serotonin, 6) and a number of different types of endocrine-secreting cells.

Physiological findings show fluid consistency which may be slightly viscous from mucus; it is colorless, sour smelling and contains bile (25% in normals). The blood is negative. Anacidity: pH never falls below 6, even after stimulation.

Acidity

Increased – (Decreased pH)
anemia, coeliac disease, febrile diseases, chronic cough, undernutrition, rhachitis, duodenal regurgitation, **hypertrophic hypersecretory gastropathy**, massive resection of small intestine (early), systemic mastocytosis, ulcer disease – (**duodenal u. d.**, gastric u. d.), **Zollinger-Ellison sy**, tetany
   Interfering Factors: medicaments – (ACTH, corticoids)

Decreased – (Increased pH)
pernicious anemia, **atrophic gastritis**, alopecia areata, **gastric carcinoma**, vitiligo, adenomatous stomach polyps, gastric ulcer, Ménétrier's disease, rheumatoid arthritis, thyrotoxicosis, chronic renal failure, postvagotomy, postantrectomy

BAO

(basal acid output) BAO can either be calculated from an overnight 12-hour or a 60-minute collection in basal condition. BAO represents gastric acid secretion (HCl) in stimulation absence. It follows circadian rhythm and is highest from 2–11 PM.

Increased Values
vagal hyperfunction, G-cell hyperplasia, **duodenal ulcer disease**, basophilic leukemia, systemic mastocytosis, syndrome – (postresection sy, **Zollinger-Ellison sy**)

Decreased Values
pernicious anemia, gastric tumors

Basal Secretion of the Gastric Juice

Increased Volume
gastrinoma, duodenal ulcer disease, **pyloric obstruction**, **regurgitated duodenal content**

Decreased Volume
gastric ulcer disease, healthy people, gastric tumors

Bile

Increased Values – positive
partial gastrectomy, gastroenterostomy, obstructing lesions of the small intestine distal to the ampulla/papilla of Vater, bile regurgitation

Blood

Appearance of blood will vary with the pH of the gastric content; strong acid pH in the stomach causes acid hematin formation which has a brownish appearance and resembles coffee grounds.

Increased Values – positive
interfering factors – (bleeding gums), **severe gastritis**, hemophilia, **gastroduodenal ulcer disease**, leukemia, **stomach tumors**, purpura, scorbutus

Beta-Glucuronidase

Increased Values
stomach cancer

Hydrochloric Acid

(syn: free HCl) Secreted by the parietal cells, the parietal secretion pH is about 0.9. As secretion mixes with other gastric constituents such as mucus, saliva, regurgitated material, and ingested food, the final hydrogen ions concentration decreases and the pH increases to 1.5 to 3.5.

Increased Values – hyperchlorhydria
hypertrophic hypersecretory gastropathy, massive resection of small intestine (early), systemic mastocytosis, ulcer disease – (**duodenal u. d., gastric u. d.**), **Zollinger-Ellison sy**
  Interfering Factors: medicaments – (ethanol, caffeine, corticotropin, pilocarpine, propanidid, rauwolfia, reserpine, calcium salts, thiopental, tolazoline)

Decreased Values – hypochlorhydria
pernicious anemia, alopecia areata, **gastric carcinoma**, vitiligo, **adenomatous stomach polyps**, gastric ulcer, Ménétrier's disease, rheumatoid arthritis, thyrotoxicosis, chronic renal failure, **postvagotomy**, **postantrectomy**
> Interfering Factors: healthy persons, medicaments – (acetazolamide, H2-receptor antagonists, atropine, cimetidine, diazepam, ganglionic blocking agents, glucagon, 5-hydroxytryptamine, insulin, loperamide, propranolol, ranitidine, secretin)

Intrinsic Factor

(syn: vitamin B_{12} intrinsic factor)

Decreased Values
pernicious anemia, atrophic gastritis

Lactic Acid

Increased Values
gastric ulcer disease, **stomach tumors**, **pyloric obstruction/stenosis**

MAO

(maximal acid output) MAO is defined as the average hourly output (HCl) obtained from the four 15-minute collections following pentagastrin.

Increased Values
duodenal ulcer disease, **Zollinger-Ellison sy**

Decreased Values
pernicious anemia, chronic atrophic gastritis, gastric tumors

Mucus

Mucus is produced by the surface epithelial cells and the neck chief cells of the stomach.

Increased Values
mechanical irritation due to passage of a stomach tube, gastritis, gastric tumors

PAO

(peak acid output) PAO is an average of the two fractions with the highest free acid.

Increased Values
duodenal ulcer disease, healthy people, **Zollinger-Ellison sy**

Pepsin

Proteolytic enzyme.

Increased Values
ulcer disease – (duodenal u. d., gastric u. d.)

Decreased Values
histamine resistant achlorhydria, pernicious anemia, gastric ulcer disease, stomach tumors

Potassium

Increased Values
damage to gastric mucosal membrane

Volume

Increased Values
duodenal ulcer disease, stomach tumors, pyloric obstruction, duodenal content regurgitation, increased gastric secretion, Zollinger-Ellison sy, delayed stomach emptying

Decreased Values
    Interfering Factors: medicaments – (atropine, diazepam, ganglionic blocking agents, 5-hydroxytryptamine, insulin)

Hair

D. Mesko

Arsenic

Increased Values
intoxication

Chromium

Decreased Values
diabetes mellitus, **professional exposure**

Manganese

Increased Values
diabetes mellitus, **professional exposure**

Zinc

Decreased Values
celiac disease, diabetes mellitus, protein malnutrition

Hematology

D. Mesko, R. Pullmann

Plasma is the liquid part of fluid blood. Outside the vascular system, blood can be kept fluid by either removing fibrinogen or by adding anticoagulants, most of which prevent coagulation by chelating or removing calcium ions. Citrate, oxalate and EDTA are chelating category anticoagulants. Heparin prevents coagulation via direct thrombin inhibition, and fibrinogen to fibrin conversion by augmenting a natural anticoagulant antithrombin III molecule to neutralize thrombin. Heparin fails to influence the calcium concentration in its anticoagulant effect. Freshly drawn plasma contains all the proteins of circulating blood; in stored plasma, however, factor V and VIII activity gradually declines.

Serum is the fluid which remains after blood coagulates. Coagulation converts all fibrinogen into solid fibrin, consuming factors V, VII and prothrombin in the process. Other coagulation proteins and proteins not related to hemostasis remain in serum as in plasma levels. Normal serum lacks fibrinogen, prothrombin, factors V, VIII, XIII, but contains factors VII, IX, X, XI, XII. If the coagulation process proceeds abnormally, serum may contain residual fibrinogen and fibrinogen cleavage products in unconverted prothrombin.

Acetylcholinesterase in Erythrocytes

(syn: RBC cholinesterase, erythrocytic cholinesterase, red cell cholinesterase, "true" cholinesterase) The enzyme is limited to the outer membrane surface. The red cell enzyme is synthesized during erythropoiesis. Activity is higher in young erythrocytes, decreasing rapidly with age. Red cell cholinesterase is a better chronic organic phosphate poisoning indicator than serum pseudocholinesterase (better measure of acute toxicity). The cholinesterase activity in human red cells is highly but not exclusively specific for acetylcholine. Cholinesterase activity present in the serum/plasma hydrolyses both choline and aliphatic esters, has a broader range of esterolytic activity and is referred to as "pseudo-" or "nonspecific" cholinesterase. It hydrolyses acetylcholine only slowly. Test is used also to detect atypical forms of the enzyme. Cholinesterase is irreversibly inhibited by organophosphate insecticides and reversibly inhibited by carbamate insecticides.

Increased Values
sickle cell anemia, hemolytic conditions, thalassemias, spherocytosis, acquired hemolytic anemias

Decreased Values
paroxysmal nocturnal hemoglobinuria, organophosphate toxicity, pyridostigmine therapy for myasthenia gravis, megaloblastic anemia relapse

Activated Protein C Resistance

(syn: APC resistance) It is an anticoagulatory protein C system action disorder with high thrombotic risk, caused by molecular F V defect (i. e. factor V Leiden is less sensitive to anticoagulative activated protein C influence than normal F Va) with modified activated protein C splitting properties.

Test Purpose. 1) differential diagnosis of thrombophilic conditions (APC resistance is the most frequent genetic thrombosis cause).

Positive Resistance
inborn APC resistance, acquired APC resistance in – (protein C/S deficiency, increased F VIII values, antiphospholipid syndrome)

Adenylate Kinase in Erythrocytes

Decreased Values
autosomal recessive hemolytic anemia

Aminolevulinate Dehydratase in Erythrocytes

Decreased Values
ALAD deficiency, lead poisoning, hereditary tyrosinemia
   Interfering Factors: medicaments – (EDTA)

Alpha-2-Antiplasmin

(alpha-2 AP, syn: alpha-2-plasmin inhibitor) Antiplasmin is a glycoprotein, the primary plasmin inhibitor synthesized in the liver.

Function. Antiplasmin serves as a regulator of fibrinolysis – a) it blocks the enzymatic activity of plasmin, b) inhibits binding of plasminogen to fibrin, c) it binds to fibrin with factor XIII, making the clot more difficult to lyse by plasmin.

Test Purpose. 1) to evaluate serum alpha-2-antiplasmin functional activity, 2) differential diagnosis of bleeding conditions (e.g. accelerated fibrinolysis).

Increased Values
diabetes mellitus

Decreased Values
congenital antiplasmin deficiency, primary fibrinogenolysis with prostate tumors, liver diseases, bleeding diathesis, consumptive coagulopathy, therapy – (fibrinolytic t., **thrombolytic t. with streptokinase**), hereditary bleeding disorders

Analyte	Age/Gender	Reference Range	SI Units	Note
Alpha-2-Antiplasmin		0.8–1.2		
		80–120	%	
		50–70	mg/l	

Antithrombin III

(AT III, syn: functional antithrombin III assay, AT III antigen assay, heparin co-factor, immunologic AT III, A-Th3, serine protease inhibitor) AT III is a plasma protein that inhibits thrombin by binding to its active site.

Function. AT III is the strongest/most important physiological serine coagulation protease inhibitor. The main AT III inhibitory effect goal are factor IIa (activated thrombin), and factor Xa; AT III has smaller inhibitory effect against factor XIa and XIIa, but is the only factor IXa inhibitor. AT III action is catalyzed by heparin. The heparin – antithrombin III complex will rapidly neutralize any thrombin that is generated by coagulation cascade activation. Homeostasis results from a balance between AT III and thrombin. AT III deficiency increases coagulation risk or tendency toward thrombosis. Platelets lysis releases PF 4 → inhibits AT III activity.

Production. Liver, vascular endothelium.

Test Purpose. 1) to evaluate thromboembolic disease conditions, 2) to evaluate hypercoagulable or fibrinogenolytic conditions and response to heparin, 3) to test for hereditary AT III deficiency, 4) thrombophilic conditions differential diagnosis, e.g. congenital or acquired AT III deficiency associated with severe cirrhosis, chronic liver failure, DIC, thrombolytic therapy, pulmonary embolism, nephrotic sy or postsurgical conditions.

Increased Values
vitamin K deficiency, **acute hepatitis**, hyperglobulinemia, **cholestasis**, **inflammatory diseases**, obstructive jaundice, **menstruation**, **kidney transplant** (recent), increased values of
– (CRP, ESR, globulins), post-myocardial infarction
> **Interfering Factors:** medicaments – (anabolic steroids, androgens, coumarins, oral contraceptives – containing progesterone, sodium warfarin)

Decreased Values
liver cirrhosis, **hereditary antithrombin III deficiency**, dialysis, diffuse venoocclusive disease, **pulmonary embolism**, enteropathy, partial hepatectomy, pregnancy induced hypertension, diseases – (**liver d.**, renal d.), **acute myocardial infarction**, **disseminated intravascular coagulopathy**, leukemia, malnutrition, tumours, **surgery**, **CNS surgery/trauma**, plasmapheresis, immature fetus, burns, **polytrauma**, **hepatic parenchyma lesions**, **preeclampsia**, increased AT III consumption, conditions – (**septic c.**, shock c.), severe blood loss, **nephrotic sy**, decreased AT III synthesis, **pregnancy** (3rd trimester), **liver transplant**, **thrombophlebitis**, **deep vein thrombosis**, increased AT III excretion, **chronic liver failure**
> **Interfering Factors:** medicaments – (asparaginase, contraceptives containing estrogens, fibrinolytics, heparin, L-asparaginase)

Analyte	Age/Gender	Reference Range	SI Units	Note
Antithrombin III		0.8–1.2		
		80–120	%	
		180–300	mg/l	

Autohemolysis

Hemolysis: RBC breakdown and hemoglobin outflow from RBC into surrounding environment. Determined by the spontaneous hemolysis amount occurring in blood over 24–48 hour period under special laboratory conditions (ATP, glucose). Autohemolysis: RBC hemolysis caused by RBC antibody production which are bound to RBC membrane as an immune system disorder result. Antibody types: warm, cold, bitermic. Autohemolysis causes are: a) congenital RBC inferiority (inner construction disorder, enzymatic set, or RBC hemoglobin), b) acquired RBC inferiority (RBC damaged by extraerythrocyte causes).

Test Purpose. 1) hemolysis level determination, 2) differential diagnosis of hemolytic anemias (congenital, acquired), paroxysmal nocturnal hemoglobinuria.

Decreased Values
congenital nonspherocytic hemolytic anemia (decreased less markedly), hereditary spherocytosis (decreased markedly)

Analyte	Age/Gender	Reference Range	SI Units	Note
Autohemolysis		2.5–5	% relat.	

Basophils

(bas) Granulocytic developmental stem cells with specific granules.

Function. Phagocytosis, fat metabolism, functionally similar to mastocytes. Contain heparin, histamine, serotonin, release chemotactic factors; involved with mast cells in immediate hypersensitivity reactions, have receptors for the complement C3, C5 components, and high affinity receptors for IgE. Binding of C3a and C5a or cross-linking of membrane bound IgE by allergens induces release 60–80% of the granules of both cell types. Tissue basophils receptors react with allergens and IgE to induce vasoactive mediators release. These factors cause contraction of endothelial cells and vasodilation of capillaries resulting in the redness, warmth and fluid accumulation in tissues characteristic of inflammation. Massive granule content release may evoke sudden death – anaphylactic shock.

Increased Values – basophilia, basophilic leukocytosis
chronic hemolytic anemia, hepatic cirrhosis, **hypothyroidism**, diseases – (**myeloproliferative d.**, chronic inflammatory d.), **ulcerative colitis**, leukemia – (**basophilic l., chronic myelocytic l.**), **mastocytosis, myeloid metaplasia, morbilli, Hodgkin's disease**, myelofibrosis, **myxedema, nephrosis, polycythemia, polycythemia vera**, radiotherapy, recovery from infection, chronic sinusitis, **splenectomy**, allergic conditions – (inhalants, drug, food), **stress**, syndrome – (**myelodysplastic sy, nephrotic sy**), pregnancy, urticaria, **varicella**, variola, foreign protein injection, ionizing radiation
  Interfering Factors: medicaments – (antithyroid preparations, contraceptives)

Decreased Values – basophilic leukopenia, basopenia
hemorrhagic conditions, **hyperthyroidism**, diseases – (**infectious d., inflammatory d.**), myocardial infarction, prolonged steroid therapy, ovulation, reactions – (**acute allergic r., hypersensitive r.**), **stress reactions, Cushing's sy, anaphylactic shock, urticaria**, bleeding peptic ulcer, **pregnancy**
  Interfering Factors: medicaments – (ACTH, adrenaline, corticosteroids, progesterone)

Analyte	Age/Gender	Reference Range	SI Units	Note
Basophilic Granulocytes	Neonates	<3	%	
	Infants	<3	%	
	Adults	0–7	%	
		0–0.07		
		0–0.25	x 10⁹/l	

Bleeding Time (Duke's Method)

(BT, syn: Duke's bleeding time, time of bleeding) Bleeding time is an interval between a standard cut/prick and bleeding stoppage; Duke's method is bleeding time after a 4th finger-tip prick. It is a primary hemostasis phase measure, platelet interaction with the blood vessel wall and hemostatic plug formation. Bleeding time duration depends upon the platelet quantity and quality, von Willebrand's factor, and the blood vessel walls ability to constrict.

Test Purpose. 1) to obtain information about normal or insufficient primary hemostatic plug formation, 2) to assess overall hemostatic function (platelet response to injury and functional vasoconstriction capacity), 3) to detect congenital and acquired platelet function disorders.

Bleeding Time (Ivy's Method)

An in vivo functional test for platelet and capillary function. Bleeding time is measured from standard forearm cut under standard pressure.

Test Purpose. 1) screening used to assess capillary function, platelet count and function, platelet ability to adhere to vessel wall and form a plug, 2) to assess overal platelet response to injury, 3) to assess functional capacity of vasoconstriction, 4) to detect congenital and acquired blood disorders, 5) to evaluate ecchymosis, spontaneous bruising and bleeding, bleeding tendency.

Increased Values – prolonged bleeding time
alcohol, amyloidosis, aplastic anemia, hepatic cirrhosis, coagulation factor defect/deficiency – (I, II, V, VII, VIII, IX, XI), congenital protein C or S deficiency, **capillary fragility, hemophilia, hypersplenism,** disease – (**Cushing's d.,** Henoch-Schönlein d., **hemolytic newborn d., von Willebrand's d.**), diseases – (**collagen vascular d., liver d.,** viral infectious d., myeloproliferative d.), ecchymosis, **primary/metastatic tumor bone marrow infiltration, disseminated intravascular coagulation** (DIC), **leukemia, Hodgkin's disease, Waldenström's macroglobulinemia,** parahemophilia, plasmocytoma (incl. multiple myeloma), disorders – (**platelet function d.,** blood vessel wall d.), preleukemia, **senile purpura,** scurvy, fibrinolytic states, syndrome – (**Bernard-Soulier sy,** Wiskott-Aldrich sy, myelodysplastic sy, Chédiak-Higashi sy, Hermansky-Pudlak sy, Ehlers-Danlos sy), hereditary teleangiectasia, massive transfusions, **Glanzmann's thrombasthenia, thrombocytoasthenia** (thrombasthenia), **thrombocytopathy, thrombocytopenia,** thrombocytosis, **uremia, vasculopathies,** failure – (**bone marrow f.,** renal f.), hemorrhagic conditions, deep intracerebral hemorrhage, hemorrhagic stroke

> **Interfering Factors:** medicaments – (acetylsalicylic acid, allopurinol, aminocaproic acid, aminophylline, amitriptyline, amoxicillin, ampicillin, anticoagulants, antibiotics, antihistamines, antiinflammatory agents, asparaginase, azlocillin, beta-blockers, caffeine, calcium channel blockers, carbenicillin, cefoperazone, ceftizoxime, cephalosporins, chlorpromazine, clarithromycin, corticoids, dextran, dihydralazine, diltiazem, diuretics, ethanol, halothane, heparin, hydroxychloroquine, ibuprofen, imipramine, indomethacin, ketoprofen, lansoprazole, lipid-lowering drugs, meropenem, moxalactam, nafcillin, nandrolone, naproxen, nifedipine, nitrates, nitric oxide, nitrofurantoin, nitroglycerin, nonnarcotic analgesics, non-steroidal antiinflammatory drugs, nortriptyline, panthenol, penicillin, phenylbutazone, piperacillin, piroxicam, plicamycin, promethazine, propra-

nolol, prostacyclin, salicylates, streptodornase, streptokinase, sulfonamides, theophylline, thiazides, ticarcillin, tricyclic antidepressants, trifluoperazine, urokinase, valproic acid, warfarin)

Analyte	Age/Gender	Reference Range	SI Units	Note
Bleeding Time				
Ivy's		4–8	min	
Duke's		2–5	min	

Blood Culture

Test Purpose. 1) to establish the diagnosis in suspected septicemia, endocarditis, bacterial meningitis, pericarditis, septic arthritis, osteomyelitis, pyelonephritis, enteric fever, 2) to identify the causative organisms in severe pneumonia, postpartum fever, pelvic inflammatory disease, cannula sepsis, neonatal epiglottitis and sepsis.

Capillary Fragility Test

(syn: Rumpel–Leede positive pressure test, tourniquet test, negative pressure test) The infotest about primary phase hemostasis components (vascular wall and platelet condition). Test is used to demonstrate capillary fragility defects due to abnormalities in the capillary walls or thrombocytopenia by positive/negative pressure → forearm area petechiae are counted. **Test Purpose.** 1) to assess the capillary wall fragility, 2) to identify platelet deficiency.

Positive

deficiency of – (factor VII, fibrinogen, prothrombin, vitamin K), diabetes mellitus with vascular complications, dysproteinemia, hypertension, chronic renal diseases, influenza, DIC, **von Willebrand's disease**, measles, polycythemia vera, purpura – (**senile p.**, **vascular p.**), scurvy, scarlet fever, **thrombasthenia**, thrombocytopathies, **thrombocytopenia**, vasculopathies

> **Interfering Factors:** healthy persons, before menstruation, women over age 40

Analyte	Age/Gender	Reference Range	SI Units	Note
Capillary Fragility Test (Rumpel–Leede)		<10	*	*petechiae over 16 cm^2

Carboxyhemoglobin

(COHb) Carbon monoxide bound to Hb molecule (e.g. in intoxication) is irreverzible. Hb to CO affinity is 300-times higher when compared to O_2 afinity.
Test Purpose. Investigation of possible carbon monoxide exposure and poisoning. Toxicity relates more to inhibition of mitochondrial cytochrome respiration than to interference with blood oxygen transport.

Increased Values

CO poisoning, intestinal hemorrhage, following exercise, intestinal bacteria reactions, caloric reduction, hemolytic conditions

Interfering Factors: medicaments – (enflurane, halothane, isoflurane)

Analyte	Age/Gender	Reference Range	SI Units	Note
Carboxyhemoglobin	Non-smokers	<0.012		
	Smokers	<0.085		
	Lethal	>0.5		

Catalase in Erythrocytes

Catalase is iron containing hemin bound to protein by porphyrin circle, catalase is necessary for cell peroxide production. This enzyme is in all oxidative procedures performing cells.

Increased Values
beta-thalassemia minor

Decreased Values
acatalasemia, iron deficiency anemia

CD Antigens

(CD – cluster of differentiation) Lymphocytes, in the course of development from precursor cells into functionally mature forms, display a complex pattern of surface antigens, some of which are acquired at certain stages, while others are lost. The CD antigen nomenclature was introduced when it was found out that different monoclonal antibodies from different sources recognized identical antigens. Use of these antibodies also helps to delineate the biologic traits that distinguish normal immune and hematopoietic cells from their malignant counterparts, which is of fundamental importance in understanding hematological malignancies.

Cells of Inflammation

1) **circulating:** neutrophils, eosinophils, basophils, thrombocytes,
2) **tissue:** mastocytes, macrophages, endothelial cells.

Clot Retraction

(syn: clot retraction test, whole-blood clot retraction test) Blood clot investigation incubated in thermostat and the serum amount dislodged from blood clot is measured. In vitro testing is based on the fact that normally clotted whole blood will retract or recede from the container sides, resulting in transparent serum separation and contracted blood clot.

In vivo platelets play a major part in the clot retraction mechanism by active fibrin blood coagulum fibre shrinkage followed by wound edge contraction creating compact mass. It is the final definitive plug creation process. Clot retraction depends upon normal platelet function, contractile proteins in the platelet membrane (thrombostenin), magnesium, ATP and pyruvate kinase. It is also influenced by the hematocrit level, fibrinogen structure, and concentration.

Test Purpose. 1) to help in Glanzmann's thrombasthenia diagnosis, 2) to assess platelet function and fibrin structure in clot retraction induction.

Increased Values
severe anemia, hypofibrinogenemia

Decreased Values
erythrocytosis, hyperfibrinogenemia, **von Willebrand's disease**, **Waldenström's macro-globulinemia, thrombasthenia, Glanzmann's thrombasthenia, thrombocytopenia**

Analyte	Age/Gender	Reference Range	SI Units	Note
Clot Retraction		>0.88		
		>88	%	

Clotting Time (Lee-White)

(CT, ACT, syn: whole blood clotting time, coagulation time, activated coagulation time, activated clotting time, ground glass clotting time) Blood clot formation in 37 °C.
Test Purpose. 1) it gives rough information about plasmatic prothrombin activator production (without thrombocytes), prothrombin to thrombin change, and fibrinogen to fibrin change influenced by this activator, 2) to monitor heparin effect during cardio-pulmonary bypass surgical procedures, 3) screening test for coagulation deficiencies, with special application to heparin effect monitoring, 4) to monitor heparin administration.

Increased Values – prolonged
anemia, coagulative factors deficiency – (II, V, VII, X, XII), **hemophilia A, B,** hypo/**afibrinogenemia,** von Willebrand's disease, **disseminated intravascular coagulation,** biliary ducts obstruction, vitamin K metabolism disorders, hepatic parenchyma injury
  Interfering Factors: medicaments – (anticoagulative agents, coumarin, heparin, tetracyclines)

Analyte	Age/Gender	Reference Range	SI Units	Note
Clotting Time	37 °C	6–10	min	
Lee–White	20 °C	6–12	min	

Coagulation Tests – hemostasis

Vascular function and platelet function – **primary hemostasis**
■ bleeding time, capillary fragility test/Rumpel–Leede test
Platelet function – **primary hemostasis**
■ platelet adhesiveness, platelet aggregation, activated bleeding time, activated recalcification time, bleeding time, clotting time, platelet factor 3, prothrombin consumption, platelet count, recalcification time, clot retraction
Overall clotting ability
■ activated partial thromboplastin time, fibrinogen, PT, TT
Internal coagulation system – **contact phase** (stage I hemostasis)
■ activated clotting time, activated partial thromboplastin time, activated recalcification time, clotting time, prothrombin time, partial thromboplastin time, recalcification time, thromboplastin generation time
External coagulation system (stage II hemostasis)
■ prothrombin time

Common coagulation phase (stage III hemostasis – 3rd coagulation phase)
- ethanol gelation test, fibrin stabilizing factor – (factor XIII), fibrinogen, protamine sulfate, thrombin time

Fibrinolytic process (stage IV hemostasis – fibrinolytic activity)
- euglobulin lysis time, ethanol gelation test, fibrin-degradation products, partial thromboplastin time, plasminogen, protamine sulfate, clot lysis test, thrombin time

Complete Blood Count

(CBC, syn: blood count, blood cell profile)
hemoglobin (Hb), hematocrit (HCT), erythrocytes (red blood cell (corpuscle) count, RBC), leukocytes (white blood cell count, WBC), thrombocytes (platelet count, PLT), differential white cell count, red blood cell indices – Wintrobe blood indices (mean corpuscular volume/MCV, mean corpuscular hemoglobin/MCH, mean corpuscular hemoglobin concentration/MCHC), microscopical stained cellular blood elements examination (film/peripheral blood smear)
Test Purpose. Differential diagnosis of anemias, polyglobulias, leukopenias, leukocytoses, thrombocytopenias, and thrombocytoses.

Cryofibrinogen

A test for one of the cold-precipitating plasma proteins in patients with cold intolerance.
Test Purpose. To evaluate coagulation disorders.

Increased Values – positive
pregnancy phlebitis, inflammatory diseases, neonatal infections, tumors, scleroderma
   Interfering Factors: medicaments – (oral contraceptives)

Analyte	Age/Gender	Reference Range	SI Units	Note
Cryofibrinogen		<60	mg/l	

Differential White Cell Count

(syn: differential, leukogram, blood smear, smear evaluation, white blood cell slide differential, differential WBC count, leukocyte differential, manual differential) Differential gives the WBC category percentage in a particular blood sample obtained microscopically from stained blood smear or from native blood using a blood cell computer.
Test Purpose. 1) to evaluate the body's capacity to resist and overcome infection, 2) to detect and identify various leukemia types, 3) to determine infection degree and severity, 4) to detect allergic reactions, 5) to assess allergic reaction severity.
Leukocytes types
- **basophilic granulocytes** = basophils
- **eosinophilic granulocytes** = eosinophils
- **lymphocytes**
- **monocytes**
- **mononuclear leucocytes** = lymphocytes + monocytes
- **neutrophilic segmented granulocytes** = segmented neutrophils

- **neutrophilic sticks** = band neutrophils
- **plasmocytes**
- **polymorphonuclear leukocytes** = neutrophils + eosinophils + basophils = granulocytes

Analyte	Age/Gender	Reference Range	SI Units	Note
Leukogram				
Granulocytes				
neutrophilic sticks	Adults	3–5	%	
		0.03–0.05		
		0.6–1.2	x 10⁹/l	
neutrophilic g.	Neonates	<65	%	
	Infants	<25	%	
	Adults	47–79	%	
		0.47–0.79		
		2.5–5.6	x 10⁹/l	
eosinophilic g.	Neonates	<3	%	
	Infants	<3	%	
	Adults	1–7	%	
		0,01–0.07		
		0.03–0.25	x 10⁹/l	
basophilic g.	Neonates	<0.75	%	
	Infants	<0.25	%	
	Adults	0–2	%	
		0–0.02		
		0<0.03	x 10⁹/l	
Monocytes	Neonates	<8	%	
	Infants	<10	%	
	Adults	2–11	%	
		0.02–0.11		
		0.15–0.58	x 10⁹/l	
Lymphocytes	Neonates	<22	%	
	Infants	<60	%	
	Adults	12–40	%	
		0.12–0.40		
		1.2–3.1	x 10⁹/l	
Plasmocytes	Neonates	<0.25	%	
	Infants	<0.5	%	

D-Dimers

(syn: fragment D-dimer, fibrin degradation fragment) D-dimers are fibrin derivatives (DD-fragments with preserved cross covalent bonds in the D-domain area; produced in stabilized blood fibrin coagulum creation) produced during fibrinolysis by plasmin effect onto fibrin coagulum. They are a terminal stabilized fibrin degradation product. The fragment D-dimer assesses both thrombin and plasmin activity. This fragment is formed after thrombin converts fibrinogen to fibrin; factor XIIIa stabilizes it to a clot, and plasmin lyses the clot. **Test Purpose.** 1) screening test for deep-vein thrombosis detection, embolism, bleeding conditions, liver diseases, malignant tumors and differential diagnosis, 2) to evaluate acute myocardial infarction, unstable angina pectoris and disseminated intravascular coagulation.

arthritis, unstable pectoral angina, cellulitis, **pulmonary embolism, fibrinolysis primary/ secondary,** false-positive values – (high rheumatoid factors titers), diseases – (inflammatory d., infectious d.), acute myocardial infarction, **disseminated intravascular coagulation, vaso-occlusive sickle cell anemia crisis, thrombolytic/defibrination therapy with tissue plasminogen activator, tumors, surgery** (within 2 days), severe trauma, pneumonia, pregnancy (3rd trimester), **arterial thromboembolism, deep-vein thrombosis,** failure – (renal f., liver f., cardiac f.)

Analyte	Age/Gender	Reference Range	SI Units	Note
D-dimers		0.2–0.4	μg/ml	

2,3-Diphosphoglycerate

(syn: 2,3-DPG in erythrocytes) 2,3-DPG is a RBC enzyme that controls oxygen transport to the tissues. Enzyme deficiency results in RBC oxygen dissociation curve alterations controlling oxygen release to the tissues. An increase in 2,3-DPG decreases the hemoglobin oxygen binding capacity → increased oxygen amount is released and becomes available to tissues at lower oxygen tensions. The oxygen red cells affinity is inversely proportional to 2,3-DPG concentration.
Test Purpose. Enzyme hemolytic anemias differential diagnosis.

Increased Values
anemia, **hepatic cirrhosis,** pyruvate kinase deficiency, **cystic fibrosis with pulmonary involvement, hyperthyroidism, hypoxia, obstructive lung disease,** diseases – **(lung d., heart d., congenital cyanotic heart d.), after vigorous exercise conditions,** thyrotoxicosis, **uremia, high altitudes, chronic renal failure**

Decreased Values
acidosis, inherited genetic defects, deficiency – (phosphofructokinase d., hexokinase d.), **hemoglobin C diseases,** banked blood, polycythemia, respiratory distress sy
   Interfering Factors: medicaments – (acetanilid, adriamycin, amylnitrite, isosorbide dinitrate, nalidixic acid, niridazole, nitrofurantoin, phenazopyridine, primaquine, sulfacetamide, sulfamethoxazole, sulfanilamide, sulfapyridine, sulfasalazine)

Eosinophil Cationic Protein

(ECP) ECP is an eosinophil granule-derived protein which is released during activation of eosinophils. Assay of ECP is claimed to assist in monitoring bronchial inflammation in acute asthma, serving as an index of disease severity and as an adjunct to quantitation of the reponse to bronchial provocation.
Test Purpose. To determine in vivo eosinophil activity.

Increased Values
bronchial asthma

Eosinophils

(eos, eo) Granulocytic developmental stem cells with a two-lobed nucleus and moderately large granules.

Function. Eosinophils are active in later inflammation stages. Active in allergic reactions and parasitic infections (ability to damage certain helminth parasites) via cationic proteins (major basic protein – MBP; eosinophil-derived neurotoxin – EDN; eosinophil cationic protein – ECP; eosinophil peroxidase – EPO). Eosinophils bear receptors for IgG, complement components C3, C5 and low-affinity receptors for IgE. Involved in chemotaxis and antigen–antibody complex engulfment. Eosinophils release enzymes that are able to inactivate biologically active substances (histamine). This is important in type I hypersensitivity reactions. Involved in detoxication processes (against chemical mediators, in hypersensitive reactions, in tissue lesion, in fibrin deposit removal). Eosinophil circulation half-time is about 12–18 hours and 3–10 days in tissues.

Increased Values – eosinophilia, eosinophilic leukocytosis

allergy – (**medicamentous a.**, milk protein a., **food a.**), **amebiasis, pernicious anemia, rheumatoid arthritis, ascariasis, aspergillosis, bronchial asthma, atopy, brucellosis, eosinophilic cellulitis,** hepatic cirrhosis, **excessive exercise,** IgA deficiency, dermatitis – (exfoliative d., **herpetiformis d.**), dermatomyositis, peritoneal dialysis, **eczema, Löffler's endocarditis,** protein losing enteropathy, **erythema multiforme,** eosinophilic fasciitis, **eosinophilic gastroenteritis,** acute hemolysis, cholestatic hepatitis, hay fever (pollinosis), **adrenal hypofunction,** hypopituitarism, serum sickness, diseases – (**allergic d., autoimmune d.,** collagen-vascular d., inflammatory bowel d., gastrointestinal d., **dermatologic d., myeloproliferative d.,** parasitic d., **professional pulmonary d., connective tissue d.,** chronic inflammatory d.), infectious diseases – (bacterial i. d., **fungal i. d.,** viral i. d.), Pneumocystis carinii infection, **eosinophilic pulmonary infiltrate,** colitis ulcerosa, acute hemorrhage, leukemia – (**eosinophilic l., chronic granulocytic l., chronic myeloytic l.**), **systemic lupus erythematosus,** lymphogranulomatosis, **non-Hodgkin's lymphoma, Addison's disease, Hodgkin's disease,** malaria, tumour metastases – (kidney, lungs, gastrointestinal tract), infectious mononucleosis, tumours of – (colon, bone, uterus, melanoma, pancreas, lung, ovary), thymic disorders, interstitial nephritis, tumor necrosis, **graft rejection** (graft-versus-host disease), intestinal parasites, **pemphigus,** pityriasis rubra, pneumonia – (chlamydial p., eosinophilic p.), **polyarteritis nodosa,** polycythemia, **psoriasis, radiotherapy,** tropical eosinophilia, drug hypersensitivity reaction, **hyperimmune reactions, sarcoidosis, scleroderma, splenectomy, scabies,** syndrome – (**angioneurotic sy,** Dressler's sy, **eosinophilia-myalgia sy,** Goodpasture's sy, Wiskott-Aldrich sy, **hypereosinophilic sy**), **scarlet fever, toxocarosis,** toxoplasmosis, **trichinosis,** trichuriasis, tropical eosinophilia, **tuberculosis,** urticaria, vasculitis, ionizing radiation

   Interfering Factors: medicaments – (acarbose, acetylsalicylic acid, ajmaline, aldesleukin, allopurinol, aminosalicylic acid, amoxapine, amoxicillin, amphotericin B, ampicillin, antithymocyte globulin, aztreonam, bacitracin, beclomethasone, captopril, carbamazepine, carbenicillin, carisoprodol, cefalexin, cefalotin, cefamandole, cefazolin, cefoperazone, cefoxitin, cefradine, ceftazidime, ceftizoxime, ceftriaxone, cephalosporins, chloral hydrate, chloramphenicol, chlorpromazine, chlorpropamide, chlorprothixene, chlortetracycline, clindamycin, clofibrate, clometacin, clomipramine, codeine, dacarbazine, dapsone, demeclocycline, desipramine, digitalis, digitoxin, disulfiram, doxepin, doxycycline, enflurane, erythromycin, ethosuximide, etretinate, fenofibrate, flavoxate, fluconazole, flunisolide, fluorides, fluphenazine, flurbiprofen, fluticasone, fomepizole, fosphenytoin, gemfibrozil, glibenclamide, gold salts, halothane, imipramine, indomethacin, interferons, isoniazid, iodides, kanamycin, lamotrigine, levofloxacin, lomefloxacin, loracarbef, mebendazole, mephenytoin, meprobamate, mercaptopurine, meropenem, methotrexate, methyldopa, methysergide, meticillin, mezlocillin, minocycline, modafinil, montelukast, moxifloxacin, nalidixic acid, naproxen, nevirapine, nitrofurantoin, nomifensine, nortriptyline, oxacillin, oxcarbazepine, papaverine, penicillamine, penicillins, perphenazine, phenazopyridine, phenothiazines, phenytoin, piperacillin, potassium iodide, probucol, procainamide, procarbazine, prochlorperazine, promethazine, protriptyline, ranitidine, rifampicin, streptokinase, sulfadoxine, sulfafurazole, sulfamethoxazole, sulfasalazine, sulfonamides, sulindac, tetracyclines, thioridazine, thiothixene, ticlopidine, tocainide, triamterene, trifluoperazine, trifluperidol, verapamil, viomycin)

Decreased Values – eosinopenia, eosinophilic leukopenia
anoxia, aplastic/pernicious anemia, cold environment, hemodialysed patients, Löffler's endocarditis, hypersplenism, diseases – (**severe bacterial infectious d.**, severe viral infectious d., **inflammatory d.**), hormone secreting tumors, Hodgkin's disease, infectious mononucleosis, myocardial infarction, tumours, surgery, **morbilli**, pancytopenia, polyarteritis nodosa, **burns**, sarcoidosis, seizure conditions, splenectomy, states after radiation, **stress**, syndrome – (**Cushing's sy**, Löffler's sy), shock, **typhoid fever, trauma**, congestive heart failure

> **Interfering Factors:** intermenstrual period, medicaments – (ACTH, adrenaline, aminophyllin, amphotericin B, cefuroxime, corticosteroids, cortisone, glucocorticoids, gold salts, histamine, hydrocortisone, nortriptyline, prednisone, thyroxine)

Analyte	Age/Gender	Reference Range	SI Units	Note
Eosinophilic Granulocytes	Neonates	<3	%	
	Infants	<3	%	
	Adults	1–7	%	
		0.01–0.07		
		0.03–0.25	x 10^9/l	

Erythrocyte Sedimentation Rate

(ESR, FW, SR, syn: Fahraeus–Westergren, sed rate test) Complex RBC sedimentation process in unclotted blood sample based on equable blood plasma RBC division which depends on RBC movement and suspension plasma stability. ESR consists of three phases: a) early period (slow RBC decrease, nearly according to Stockes' formula), b) RBC agglomeration (faster RBC conglomerates fall), c) resistance/packing stage, when RBC in close contact decrease slowly. ESR means RBC settling rate in the unclotted blood sample in milimeters which is measured between fluid column top and settled RBC column top in a specific period. Test is based on the fact that inflammatory and necrotic processes cause an alteration in blood proteins and result in red blood cells aggregation, making them heavier and more likely to fall rapidly. A highly non-specific screening test (high sensitivity, low specificity). Normal ESR cannot be used to exclude organic disease. ESR depends on RBCs size/specific concentration, and blood plasma specific concentration/viscosity, as well as earth gravitation acceleration (Stockes' formula). ESR rises >24 hours after inflammation onset and symptoms, gradually returns to normal until 4 weeks after resolution. Factors influencing ESR: 1) plasma factors (fibrinogen concentration, globulin concentration, serum cholesterol), 2) red cell factors (red cell surface area – microcytes sediment more slowly than macrocytes).

Test Purpose. 1) to monitor inflammatory or malignant diseases, 2) to aid detection and diagnosis of occult disease, such as TB, tissue necrosis, or connective tissue diseases, rheumatic conditions, 3) to monitor disease course or activity and treatment, 4) may help grade severity in emergency setting.

Increased Values

- ■ ↑ **100 mm/1st hour:** autoimmune hemolytic anemia, liver cirrhosis, hemolytic-uremic sy, chronic myelogenous leukemia, collagenosis, dermatomyositis, giant-cell arteritis, rheumatoid arthritis, endocarditis, phlegmon, hemoblastosis, rheumatic fever, cholecystitis, systemic lupus erythematosus, malaria, Hodgkin's disease, Waldenström's disease, tumours, nephrosis, osteomyelitis, peritonitis, plasmocytoma (incl. multiple myeloma), polyarthritis, polymyalgia rheumatica, renal diseases, pyelitis, pyelonephritis, sepsis, nephrotic sy, vasculitis, chronic granulomatous disease
- ■ ↑ **50 mm:** severe anemia, liver cirrhosis, glomerulonephritis – (acute g., chronic g.), lupoid hepatitis, infectious hepatitis, hemodilution, hyperfibrinogenemia, hypergammaglobulinemia, hypothyroidism, diseases – (bacterial infectious d., renal d., chronic hepatic d., inflammatory bowel d.), cardiac infarction (increase at 12–48 hrs, peaking at 4th–5th d., decrease at 1–4 months), acute heavy metal poisoning, cachexia (advanced), Henoch–Schönlein purpura, Mediterranean fever, collagenoses, leptospirosis, leukemia, lymphoma, metastatic tumours, pleuritis, pneumonia, polyarteritis nodosa, polymyalgia rheumatica, toxic liver disorders, necrotic states, sarcoidosis, infantile cortical hyperostosis, scleroderma, syphilis, pregnancy, thrombophlebitis, thyroiditis, cat scratch disease, primary atypical pneumonia, systemic fungal infections, acute pancreatitis, burn injury, drug hypersensitivity reaction
- ■ ↓ **50 mm:** anemia, diabetes mellitus, leucemia, menses, undernutrition, postoperative states, pregnancy (2nd, 3rd trimester), tuberculosis
  Interfering Factors: ↓ **50 mm:** acanthocytosis, macrocytosis, hypercholesterolemia, hyperfibrinogenemia, hyperglobulinemia, poikilocytosis, medicaments – (acetylsalicylic acid, allopurinol, clometacin, cyclosporine, dextran, globulin, heparin, hydralazine, methyldopa, methysergide, naproxen, nitrofurantoin, nomifensine, oral contraceptives, penicillamine, phenylbutazone, procainamide, retinol, theophylline, thiabendazole, trifluperidol, vitamin A, zimeldine)

Decreased Values

afibrinogenemia, acanthocytosis, HbC disease, alkalosis, sickle-cell anemia, angina pectoris, disseminated intravascular coagulation, exsicosis, hemoconcentration, hyperalbuminemia, hyperglycemia, severe plasma hyperviscosity, hypofibrinogenemia, obstructive icterus, cachexia, cardiac insufficiency, poisoning by – (CO, phosphorus), cryoproteinemia, leukocytosis, macroglobulinemia, microcytosis, infectious mononucleosis, massive hepatic necrosis, poikilocytosis, polycythemia, polycythemia vera, polyglobulia, defibrination sy, shock – (allergic s., anaphylactic s.), spherocytosis, old blood specimen, congestive heart failure
  Interfering Factors: medicaments – (ACTH, adrenal steroids, amphotericin B, calcium, cardiotonics, cortisone, quinine, salicylates)

Analyte	Age/Gender	Reference Range	SI Units	Note
Erythrocyte Sedimentation Rate				
	3 m–13 y	12–24	mm	
	Adults M	5–10	mm	
	F	10–20	mm	

Erythrocyte Survival

Test Purpose. To confirm decreased RBC survival.

Increased Values
thalassemia minor

Decreased Values
anemia – (idiopathic acquired hemolytic a., sickle cell a., pernicious a., megaloblastic a., congenital nonspherocytic hemolytic a., hereditary spherocytosis), elliptocytosis with hemolysis, HbC disease, paroxysmal nocturnal hemoglobinuria, chronic lymphatic leukemia, pregnancy, uremia

Erythrocytes

(RBC, syn: red blood cells, red blood cell count, red blood corpuscle count) RBC are biconcave disc shape cells without nuclei, characterized by red color caused by hemoglobin. They do only glycolysis, they have no mitochondria.

Function. O_2 transport from the lungs to the body tissues + transfer CO_2 from the tissues to the lungs through the hemoglobin. They also function in acid-base balance. They continually produce lactate, which is continually excreted out of the RBC, in exchange for OH^- coming in.

Production. Formed in the red bone marrow (ribs, sternum, vertebrae, pelvis) = erythropoietin effect erythropoiesis from clone cells. In O_2 decrease a renal hormone erythropoietin stimulates RBC production.

Test Purpose. 1) to provide data for calculating MCV and MCH that reveals RBC size and Hb content, 2) to support other hematological tests for diagnosing anemia or polycythemia.

- ■ **Peripheral blood smear** (syn. stained red cell examination/film, smear evaluation, stained blood film, blood smear, red blood cell morphology, RBC smear): used for evaluation of changes in numbers or morphology of red cells, white cells and platelets. Blood film examination clarifies abnormalities detected by automated hematology instruments and guides further investigation.
- ■ **Physiologic:** normochromic normocytes
- ■ **Acanthocytes → acanthocytosis** (irregularly spiculated surface, spur cells): **abetalipoproteinemia**, alcoholic cirrhosis with hemolysis, hepatic necrosis, asplenia, **pyruvate kinase deficiency**, liver diseases, postsplenectomy sy, irreversibly abnormal membrane lipid content, uremia, infantile pyknocytosis
- ■ **Anisocytes → anisocytosis** (variable size, simultaneous macrocytes and microcytes occurrence): severe anemia, deficiency of – (folic acid, vitamin B_{12}, iron), reticulocytosis, transfusing normal blood into microcytic or macrocytic cell population
- ■ **Anisochromia** (different RBC staining caused by non-equal RBC Hb content)
- ■ **Anulocytes → anulocytosis** (erythrocytes deficient in hemoglobin which is localized in the erythrocyte periphery): anemia – (hypochromic a., severe sideropenic a.)
- ■ **Echinocytes → echinocytosis** (syn. crenated cells, burr cells, regularly spiculated cell surface): anemia, reversible membrane lipid content abnormalities, bile acids abnormalities, pyruvate kinase deficiency, high plasma free fatty acids, gastrointestinal bleeding, hypophosphatemia, hypomagnesemia, medicaments – (barbiturates, salicylates), gastric tumors, uremia, peptic ulcer

■ **Elliptocytes** → **elliptocytosis** (syn: ovalocytes, oval cells, oval/sickle shaped): anemia – (hemolytic a., megaloblastic a., **hereditary ovalocytosis** – **elliptocytosis, sickle cell a.**, refractory normoblastic a., sideropenic a., **thalassemia**), iron deficiency, myelofibrosis

■ **Hyperchromic** (hyperchromasia, more colored): anemia – (macrocytic a., spherocytic a.), concentrated hemoglobin (usually caused by dehydration)

■ **Hypochromic** (enlarged pallor area, RBC are insufficiently hemoglobinised): **iron deficiency, cardiac diseases**, heme synthesis disorder, **thalassemia**

■ **Macrocytes** ($\uparrow$ 8.5 μm) → **macrocytosis**: alcoholism, anemia – (**aplastic a., hemolytic a., macrocyte a., megaloblastic a., pernicious a., postsplenectomic a.**, sideroblastic a.), deficiency of – (folic acid, vitamin B_{12}), smoking, interfering factors – electronic cell sizing artifact – (cold agglutinins, severe hypoglycemia, hyponatremia, stored blood), **hypothyroidism**, diseases – (myeloproliferative d., **chronic hepatic d., chronic lung d.**), obstructive icterus, **leukemia**, medicaments – (alcohol, chemotherapeutics, hydroxyurea, immunosuppressives, zidovudine), myxedema, tumors, **newborn, plasmocytoma** (incl. multiple myeloma), **reticulocytosis secondary to increased erythropoiesis, myelodysplastic sy**, pregnancy, old age

■ **Megalocytes** (10–16 μm) → **megalocytosis**: megaloblastic anemia, folate/vitamin B_{12} deficiency, chemotherapy, myeloproliferative diseases

■ **Microcytes** (<6.5 μm) → **microcytosis**: anemia – (a. of chronic disease, sickle cell a., **spherocytic a., sideropenic a., thalassemia**), **hemoglobinopathies**, tumours, nephritis, increased iron consumption, chronic hemorrhage conditions, polycythemia vera, toxic chronic diseases effects on bone marrow, tuberculosis

■ **Microspherocytes** (small, round): autoimmune hemolytic anemia, hemolysis, hereditary spherocytosis

■ **Normocytes** (biconcave disc): physiologically

■ **Poikilocytes** → **poikilocytosis** (variations in shape, irregular shape): anemia – (sickle cell a., pernicious a., severe a.), extramedullary hematopoiesis, microangiopathic hemolysis, leukemias, post-transfusion reaction, marrow stress of any cause

■ **Polychromasia** (RBC with blue or gray-violet color in the partially basophilic cytoplasm): hemolytic anemia, increased young RBC outflow – (tumor metastases to bone marrow, newborn, polycythemia), increased erythropoiesis, increased reticulocytopoiesis

■ **Pyknocytes** → **pyknocytosis** (distorted/contracted/spiculed): hemolytic anemia, newborn

■ **Schistocytes** → **schistocytosis** (syn. helmet cell, burr cell, fragmented RBC with bizarre shape, triangular or spiral, helmet-shaped): hemolytic anemia, eclampsia, glomerulonephritis, giant hemangioma, hemoglobinuria, hemolytic-uremic sy, **microangiopathic hemolysis, malignant hypertension, artificial/prosthetic heart valves, disseminated intravascular coagulation** (DIC), **metastatic tumors**, normal newborn, severe burns, thalassemia, **thrombotic thrombocytopenic purpura**, renal graft rejection, severe valvular heart diseases, snakebite, increased intravascular mechanical trauma, uremia, **vasculitis**

■ **Sickle cells** (syn. drepanocytes, ERCs that assume a crescent or sickle shape due to some abnormal hemoglobins, half-moon shape): anemia – (hemolytic a., **sickle cell a.**, thalassemia), hemoglobinopathies (HbI, HbC)

■ **Siderocytes** → **siderocytosis**: anemia – (chronic hemolytic a., pernicious a., hereditary spherocytosis, thalassemia), hemochromatosis, lead poisoning, newborn, polycythemia vera, post-splenectomy

■ **Spherocytes** → **spherocytosis** (smaller, round, cells with no central pallor, biconcave shape loss): anemia – (**congenital hemolytic a., acquired immunohemolytic a., hereditary spherocytosis**), accelerated red blood cell destruction by reticuloendothelial system, acute alcoholism, hemoglobin C disease, severe burn injury, hemolytic transfusion reactions, severe hypophosphatemia, acute oxidant injury (hexose monophosphate shunt defect), Clostridium Welchii septicemia, recent blood transfusion

■ **Stomacytes** → **stomatocytosis** (syn. stomatocytes, slit-like central pallor area in erythrocyte): **acute alcoholism**, diseases – (cardiovascular d., hepatobiliary d.), hemolytic anemia, Rh null disease, medicaments – (phenothiazines), liver diseases, tumors, **hereditary stomatocytosis**

■ **Target cells** → **leptocytosis** (syn. leptocytes, codocytes, hypochromic cells, dark peripheral hemoglobin rim and dark central ring, often microcytic): decreased lecithin-cholesterol acyltransferase activity, anemia – (hypochromic a., sickle cell a., sideropenic a., **thalassemia**), severe iron deficiency, hemoglobinopathies – (HbC, HbD, HbE, HbS), **liver diseases**, obstructive icterus (jaundice), hemoglobin C and S presence, lead intoxication, **splenectomy**

■ **Tear-shaped** (dacrocytes, dacryocytes, drop-shaped RBCs, often microcytic): anemia – (myelophthisic a., severe hemolytic a.), erythroleukemia, **extramedullary erythropoiesis**, marrow infiltration with tumor, **myelofibrosis, thalassemia**

■ **RBC intracellular structures:**

  ■ **basophilic stippling** – basophilic RNA – (**hemolytic anemia, megaloblastic anemia, pernicious anemia**, arsenic poisoning, sideroblastic anemia, **lead poisoning, leukemia, reticulocytosis, thalassemia**), unstable hemoglobin, increased erythropoiesis,

  ■ **Heinz bodies** – insoluble oxidatively denatured Hb masses and the end-product of oxidative degradation of Hb – (**hemolytic anemia, G6PD deficiency, hemoglobinopathies**, acute hemolytic crisis, **methemoglobinemia, drug-induced RBC injury, following splenectomy, severe oxidative stress**, excessive globin-chain production, **thalassemia**, intoxication), medicaments – (analgesics, antimalarials, antipyretics, furazolidine, nalidixic acid, nitrofurans, phenazopyridine, phenylhydrazine, primaquine, procarbazine, sulfacetamide, sulfamethoxazole, sulfapyridine, sulfonamides, tolbutamide, large vitamin K doses),

  ■ **Howell–Jolly bodies** (nuclear remnants) – nuclear DNA fragments – (**hemolytic anemia, megaloblastic anemia, intense erythrocyte production, postsplenectomy**, vitamin B_{12} deficiency, hyposplenism, thalassemia, folic acid deficiency),

  ■ **nucleus – nucleated red blood cells**, nucleated RBC – (marrow-occupying neoplasm or fibrotic tissue in: **myeloma, leukemia, erythroleukemia**), (physiologic response to RBC deficiency in: **hemolytic anemias, sickle cell crisis, transfusion reaction, erythroblastosis fetalis**), (physiologic response to hypoxemia in: **congenital heart disease, congestive heart failure**), "**normal" for infants blood**, tumors – (breast t., lung t., prostate t., thyroid t.), disease – (**Niemann-Pick d., Gaucher's d., Hodgkin's d.**), **osteopetrosis, Hand-Schüller-Christian sy**, plasmocytoma (incl. multiple myeloma), **leukemoid reaction, thrombotic thrombocytopenic purpura, miliary tuberculosis**, agnogenic myeloid metaplasia with myelofibrosis

  ■ **parasitized RBCs** – (malarial stippling, Bartonella parasites)

  ■ **siderotic granules** (Pappenheimer bodies) – iron-containing granules – (after splenectomy, iron-overload sy, sideroblastic anemia, thalassemia, lead poisoning, pyridoxine-un-/responsive anemias)

Increased Values – erythrocytosis

cryptogenic fibrosing alveolitis, anaphylaxis (capillary leak syndromes), **cor pulmonale, renal cysts**, deficiency of – (**2,3-DP-glycerate**, salt), **dehydration**, long-term hemodialysis, enteropathy, familial erythrocytosis, CO exposure, **smoking, diarrhea, hydronephrosis**, alveolar hypoventilation, diseases – (neuromuscular d., **hypoxic pulmonary d., cyanotic congenital heart d.**, renal d.), **carboxyhemoglobinemia**, diabetic hyperosmolar coma, methemoglobinemia, tumours – (pheochromocytoma, uterus t., cerebellum t., adrenal t., **kidney**

t., liver t., lung t., ovary t.), **secondary response to hypoxia, polycythemia due to plasma volume contraction, polycythemia vera, polyglobulia,** burns, chronic osmoregulation disorders, **increased erythropoietin production, cardiovascular right-to-left shunt,** low-output cardiac states, **renal artery stenosis,** blood loss due to hemolysis/hemorrhage, **physical/psychic stress,** syndrome – (sleep apnea sy, **Bartter's sy,** Cushing's sy, hypoventilation sy, nephrotic sy, pickwickian sy), **renal transplantation, high altitude,** vomiting, **chronic congestive heart failure**

Interfering Factors: medicaments – (androgens, corticosteroids, diuretics, gentamicin, methyldopa, methyltestosterone, testosterone)

Decreased Values – erythrocytopenia

amyloidosis, anemia – (**hereditary nonspherocytic hemolytic a., sickle cell a., pernicious a., hereditary spherocytosis, thalassemia, a. from dietary deficiency of** – iron, vitamin B_6, B_{12}, folic acid), **subacute endocarditis,** erythropoietin deficiency, erythroleukemia, **hemoglobinopathies, acquired paroxysmal nocturnal hemoglobinuria, hemolysis,** viral hepatitis, **rheumatic fever, hyperhydration,** hypothyroidism, diseases – (bone marrow d., chronic renal d., **rheumatic d., chronic inflammatory d.**), infectious diseases – (fungal i. d., viral i. d.), intoxication by – (arsenic, benzene, copper, lead), **hemorrhage, leukemia,** systemic lupus erythematosus, malnutrition, mastocytosis, myelofibrosis, Addison's disease, Gaucher's disease, **Hodgkin's disease,** infectious mononucleosis, **myelofibrosis, tumors, plasmocytoma** (incl. multiple myeloma), **radiation, sepsis, pregnancy,** transfusion reaction, tuberculosis, failure – (**bone marrow f., renal f.**)

Interfering Factors: medicaments – (antiarthritic preparations, antibiotics, antidepressants, antidiabetics, antiinflammatory drugs, antihistamine preparations, anticonvulsants, antineoplastics, antithyroid preparations, chloramphenicol, diphenylhydantoin, methotrexate, penicillin, phenacetin, quinidine, quinine)

Analyte	Age/Gender	Reference Range	SI Units	Note
Erythrocytes	Neonates	4.5–5.6 *		
	3 m–13 y	3.8–5.0 *		* x 10^{12}/l
	Adults M	4.6–5.5 *		
	Adults F	4.2–5.0 *		

Erythrocytic Folate

Since serum folate values fluctuate significantly with diet, measurement of red cell folate is a better measure of tissue folate stores. Attention to clinical setting is important since a normal red cell folate level can be found in a rapidly developing folic acid deficiency such as the stress of pregnancy. Test is used to detect folate deficiency and monitor therapy with folate.

Erythrocytic Indices

(syn: Wintrobe red cell indices, blood indices) Erythrocytic indices derived from RBC parameters inform about RBC size and blood stain, calculated from hemoglobin, RBC count, and hematocrit values.

- ■ MCV – mean corpuscular volume
- ■ MCH – mean corpuscular hemoglobin
- ■ MCHC – mean corpuscular hemoglobin concentration

Erythrocytic Protoporphyrin

(FEP, syn: free erythrocyte protoporphyrin, RBC protoporphyrin) It is a heme pre-step in biosynthesis created by oxidation from protoporphyrinogen and protoporphyrin oxidase action. Free erythrocyte protoporphyrin expresses the noncomplexed, nonheme protoporphyrin amount in red cells. Increased lead absorption is reported in the presence of iron deficiency.

Test Purpose. 1) to aid in congenital/acquired erythropoietic porphyrias diagnosis, 2) to help confirm diagnosis of disorders affecting red blood cell activity, 3) to screen for lead poisoning, iron deficiency and iron deficiency anemia, 4) to monitor chronic industrial exposure to lead.

Increased Values
anemia – (severe hemolytic a., **a. of chronic disease, sideroblastic a., iron-deficiency a.**), diseases – (infectious d., chronic d.), increased erythropoiesis, **lead poisoning, chronic industrial exposure, lead intoxication porphyria, erythropoietic protoporphyria**

Decreased Values
anemia – (thalasemia minor, pyridoxine-responsive a.)

Erythropoietin

(EPO)

Production. EPO is a glycoprotein hormone produced principally by the kidney (renal cortex peritubular cells). The liver is the major extrarenal production site and accounts for about 10% of EPO in adults. EPO synthesis is governed by mild mechanisms where the peripheral oxygen saturation and hemoglobin concentration play an important feed-back regulatory role; their decrease leads to EPO synthesis increase. It is released in response to renal hypoxia (tissue oxygen delivery reduction).

Function. Major stimuli for erythropoiesis effecting erythroid clone cells (erythroid progenitors proliferation and maturation) and accelerating erythropoiesis in bone marrow. EPO concentrations are relatively low in healthy persons. In some anemias, e.g. aplastic, EPO production regulation is not impaired; it leads to high EPO levels (up 1000 x higher). EPO kinetics in hemorrhage and acute hypoxic conditions is in hours. Basal EPO concentration determination is an important EPO therapy condition. During renal anemias evaluation (the most frequent EPO therapy indication) it is needed to take into consideration: 1) renal tissue decrease during ageing and by synthesis place number diminution, 2) metabolic synthesis influence by toxic, uremic and inhibitory substances, 3) chronic renal insufficiency patients have lowered endogenous EPO marrow answer, 4) less quality synthesis by RBC, 5) possible increased blood loss caused by examination, dialysis, and hemorrhage. Lowest levels are in early afternoon, increase to peak around midnight. Within-day variation is 60%.

Test Purpose. 1) to aid in anemia and polycythemia diagnosis, 2) to aid in malignant tumor diagnosis/therapy, 3) to detect erythropoietin abuse by athletes, 4) to monitor erythropoietin therapy in chronic renal failure.

Increased Values
AIDS, cryptogenic fibrosing alveolitis, anemia – (**aplastic a., hemolytic a.**), exercise, chronic iron deficiency, high-altitude hypoxia, chronic obstructive pulmonary disease, tumors – (testicular t., breast t.), erythropoietin-producing tumors – (**pheochromocytoma, cerebel-**

lar hemangioblastoma, **hepatoma**, hemangiosarcoma, leiomyoma, renal adenocarcinoma, meningioma, **nephroblastoma**), myelodysplasia, **polycystic renal disease, secondary polycythemia, kidney transplant rejection**, following moderate normal individual bleeding, athletes using EPO as doping, **pregnancy**

Interfering Factors: medicaments – (anabolic steroids)

Decreased Values

congenital erythropoietin absence, AIDS, rheumatoid arthritis, chronic disease anemia in – (**malignancy, chronic inflammation**), decreased renal function, **starvation**, hypogonadism, hypocorticism, **hypopituitarism, hypothyroidism, severe renal diseases**, plasmocytoma (incl. multiple myeloma), tumors, **polycythemia vera, renal tissue loss**, bone marrow transplant, autonomic neuropathy, nephrotic sy, **renal failure**

Interfering Factors: high plasma viscosity, medicaments – (ACE inhibitors, amphotericin B, beta-adrenergic blockers, enalapril, estrogens)

Analyte	Age/Gender	Reference Range	SI Units	Note
Erythropoietin		6–20	mU/ml	See ref.
		25–125	mU/ml	ranges note

Ethanol Gelation Test

(syn: ethanol gel) Screening test which identifies abnormal exaggerated intravascular coagulation activation. Test detects fibrin monomers by gelification with ethanol.

Test Purpose. 1) dissolved plasma fibrin monomer amount evaluation, 2) information about abnormal intravascular blood coagulation (e.g. DIC).

Positive Values

pulmonary embolism, phlebothrombosis, disseminated intravascular coagulation

Euglobulin Lysis Time

(syn: whole blood clot lysis, euglobulin clot lysis, euglobulin lysis) Euglobulins are precipitated proteins coming from acidified dilute plasma. The euglobulin plasma fraction contains fibrinogen, plasminogen, and plasminogen plasma activators, but only antiplasmin traces. Thrombin added to the euglobulin solution converts fibrinogen to fibrin and activates plasminogen. Fibrinolytic activity evaluation which measures fibrin coagulum lysis time of clotted plasma endoglobulin fraction (fibrinogen, prothrombin, fibrinolytic enzymes). The fibrinolytic system normally breaks down small fibrin deposits. When this system is abnormally overactive, as in primary fibrinolysis, any fibrin clot formed will be dissolved immediately that results in a bleeding tendency. Usually, fibrin formed in the euglobulin plasma fraction is very rapidly dissolved by plasmin (fibrinolysin). The time measured from clot formation to clot lysis is referred to as the euglobulin lysis time. These tests are generally not practical, since it is difficult to determine whether fibrinolysis has occurred through a primary mechanism specifically activating the fibrinolytic pathway, or through secondary intravascular coagulation with secondary fibrinolytic activation.

Test Purpose. 1) to assess the fibrinolytic system, 2) to detect abnormal fibrinolytic states, 3) to monitor streptokinase/urokinase therapy, 4) to investigate possible acquired bleeding disorders.

Increased Values – (increased, prolonged lysis time, shortened, decreased fibrinolysis) hypoxia, **diabetes mellitus, disseminated intravascular coagulation,** fibrinolytic system insufficiency, **premature infants,** pyrogen reactions, **incompatible blood transfusion**
Interfering Factors: hyperventilation

Decreased Values – (decreased, shortened lysis time, prolonged, increased fibrinolysis) amniotic fluid embolism, primary fibrinolysis, extracorporeal circulation, **liver cirrhosis,** fetal death, **thrombolytic therapy** (streptokinase, urokinase), **obstetric complications, antepartum hemorrhage,** hereditary deficiency of fibrinogen, **leukemia, mola hydatidosa,** plasminogen rich organs surgery – (uterus, pancreas, lungs, prostate, heart), **septic abortion, shock conditions,** trauma – (acute t., **extensive vascular t.**), tumours of – (pancreas, **prostate**), **thrombocytopenic purpura,** first 48 hours after surgery, systemic fibrinolytic states
Interfering Factors: arterial blood, **elder people, physical exercise, normal newborns, obesity, postmenopause,** medicaments – (ACTH, alteplase, anistreplase, asparaginase, dextran, clofibrate, steroids, streptokinase, urokinase)

Analyte	Age/Gender	Reference Range	SI Units	Note
Euglobulin Lysis Time		10–18	hrs	

Ferritin

(see ferritin in blood-plasma-serum parameters chapter) (iron hydroxide + protein part → apoferritin). Ferritin is an alpha-1-globulin, tumor marker, and acute phase reactant. Ferritin is the major, water-soluble iron storage protein.
Production. Reticuloendothelial system (liver, spleen, bone marrow, kidney). Ferritin, which is circulating in blood, is a serum ferritin (glycated ferritin, considered as normal secretory cells product) and tissue ferritin mixture, which is released from damaged cells. Ferritin creates complexes with other proteins in blood, e.g. alpha-2-macroglobulin.

Analyte	Age/Gender	Reference Range	SI Units	Note
Ferritin	M	30–310	ng/ml	
	F	22–180	ng/ml	

Fetal Hemoglobin

(HbF, syn: hemoglobin F, alkali-resistant hemoglobin) Fetal hemoglobin is normal hemoglobin manufactured in the fetal/infant RBCs and composes 50 to 90% of the newborn hemoglobin. This hemoglobin type disappears from circulation during the 1st year. The remaining hemoglobin portion in the newborn is made up of adult type hemoglobin A1 and A2.
Test Purpose. 1) to state HbF percentage, 2) differential diagnosis of hemolytic anemias (sickle-cell, beta thalassemia) and hereditary disorders (elliptocytosis, hereditary HbF persistence).

Increased Values
anemia – (**aplastic a., sickle cell a., pernicious a.,** chronic infection a., blood loss a., megaloblastic a., spherocytic a., sideroblastic a., **heterozygous/homozygous beta-thalassemia**), elliptocytosis, erythroleukemia, benign monoclonal gammopathies, paroxysmal nocturnal

hemoglobinuria, hyperthyroidism, diseases – (hemoglobin H d., myeloproliferative d., chronic renal d.), infants who are small for gestational age, fetomaternal hemorrhage, leukemia – (**acute/chronic l.**, juvenile chronic myeloid l.), **hydatidiform mole**, plasmocytoma (incl. multiple myeloma), cancer with marrow metastases, **hereditary HbF persistence**, erythropoietic porphyria, pregnancy, **trisomy D**, Down sy, chronic renal failure

Decreased Values
hemolytic anemia in the newborn

Analyte	Age/Gender	Reference Range	SI Units	Note
Hemoglobin F	1 d	0.62–0.92		
	5 d	0.65–0.88		
	3 w	0.55–0.85		
	6–9 w	0.31–0.75		
	3–4 m	0.02–0.59		
	6 m	0.02–0.09		
	Adults	<0.02		

Fibrin Degradation Products

(FDP, FDPs, syn: fibrin/fibrinogen split products – FSPs, fibrin breakdown products – FBP, fibrinogen degradation products) Fibrin/fibrinogen split products by plasmin during fibrinolysis. Test is used in consumptive coagulopathy degree determination. When plasma acts to dissolve fibrin blood clots FDPs (X, D, E, Y) are formed. Split products have an anticoagulant action and inhibit clotting when there is an product excess. Tests for FDP are done on serum; since FDPs do not coagulate, they remain in the serum after fibrinogen is removed through clotting. Normal serum contains neither fibrinogen nor FDP → there is nothing present to react with antifibrinogen antibodies.

Test Purpose. 1) to detect fibrin degradation products in the circulation, 2) to help determine presence and approximate hyperfibrinolytic condition severity that may result in primary fibrinogenolysis or hypercoagulability, 3) to help determine the disseminated intravascular coagulation diagnosis, 4) to determine thrombolytic condition in thrombolytic therapy patients.

Increased Values
alcoholic cirrhosis, pulmonary embolism, primary/secondary fibrinolysis, hypoxia, diseases – (infectious d., renal d., liver d., congenital heart d.), myocardial infarction, disseminated intravascular coagulation (DIC), obstetric complications – (abruptio placentae, intrauterine fetal death, preeclampsia), coma due to hypnotics, acute leukemia, fibrinolytic therapy, tumors, surgery of the – (thorax, heart), polycythemia vera, burns, renal injury, transplant rejection, sepsis, portocaval shunt, thromboembolic states, pregnancy (3rd trimester), blood transfusion – (incompatible b. t., massive b. t.), renal transplantation, venous thrombosis, exercise, anxiety, stress conditions, sunstroke, trauma, following Cesarean birth
  Interfering Factors: medicaments – (barbiturates, heparin, streptokinase, tissue plasminogen activator, urokinase)

Analyte	Age/Gender	Reference Range	SI Units	Note
Fibrin Degradation Products		<5	mg/ml	

Analyte	Age/Gender	Reference Range	SI Units	Note
		<10	mg/ml	See ref. ranges note

Fibrinogen

(F I, syn: factor I, fibrinogen level) Factor I in hemocoagulation. Protein fibrin precursor needed for fibrin fibre production and definitive coagulant plug creation. Substrate for thrombin which splits 3-chain fibrinogen molecules to fibrin monomers, they are connecting (polymerization) by hydrogen bonds → this leads to unstable fibrin net creation. Fibrinogen is not present in serum. Activity is destroyed during coagulation process. Protective acute phase protein (reactant) produced by the liver. Fibrinogen is characterized with genetic polymorphism; as an inflammatory protein it increases with 24–48 hrs latency. Synthesis is decreased during liver diseases. It is involved in platelet aggregation processes, determines some blood attributes, and via interaction with vascular wall has a direct relation to thrombosis and atherosclerosis origin. It is assumed, that it plays a key role in ischemic heart disease origin and development.

Test Purpose. 1) to aid in the diagnosis of suspected clotting or bleeding disorders caused by fibrinogen abnormalities (congenital/acquired a/hypo/dysfibrinogenemia) and liver diseases, 2) to identify disseminated intravascular coagulation (DIC) and fibrinolytic activity, 3) to estimate ischemic heart disease and cerebrovascular disorders, peripheral angiopathy risks and prognoses, 4) to aid in the diagnosis of inflammatory disorders and neoplastic conditions, 5) to aid in the diagnosis of unexplained high ESR, 6) to monitor disease activity.

Increased Values – hyperfibrinogenemia

rheumatoid arthritis, **atherosclerosis**, diabetes mellitus, **smoking**, **glomerulonephritis**, hepatitis, rheumatic fever, hypertension, **coronary artery disease**, diseases – (**cerebrovascular d., acute infectious d., acute/chronic inflammatory d.**), **myocardial infarction**, compensated disseminated intravascular coagulation (DIC), collagenosis, leukemia, fibrinolytic treatment, non-specific pulmonary malignant tumours marker, menstruation, bone metastases, tumours – (bronchial t., pancreatic t., **plasmocytoma** (incl. multiple myeloma), nephrosis, **tissue necrosis**, obesity, biliary ways obstruction, paraproteinemia, pleuritis, pneumopathies, pneumonia, polyarthritis, burns, hypercoagulative disorders, septicemia, conditions – (hemorrhagic c., postsurgery c.), **stress**, nephrotic sy, pregnancy (3rd trimester), tuberculosis, trauma, uremia

> **Interfering Factors:** elderly people, medicaments – (acetylsalicylic acid, estrogens, nandrolone, oral contraceptives, oxymetholone)

Decreased Values – hypofibrinogenemia

abruption/ablation of placenta, **afibrinogenemia**, hepatic cirrhosis, **dysfibrinogenemia**, **acute hepatic dystrophy**, eclampsia, amniotic fluid embolism, **primary/secondary fibrinolysis**, **hypofibrinogenemia**, severe infections with septicemia, **acute/chronic hepatic diseases with insufficiency**, acute inflammatory diseases, obstructive icterus, phosphorus poisoning, **cachexia**, **DIC**, leukemia – (acute l., myeloid l.), thrombolytic treatment by – (streptokinase, urokinase), meningococcal meningitis, prostate tumour metastases, tumors of – (**bone marrow, pancreas, lung, prostate**), nephrosis, polycythemia vera, **severe surgery**, spontaneous abortion, defibrination sy, shock, pregnancy, **large blood transfusion**, typhoid fever, **trauma**

> **Interfering Factors:** medicaments – (anabolic steroids, androgens, antiepileptics, asparaginase, dextran, heparin – in high concentrations, oral contraceptives, metformin, phenobarbital, streptokinase, testosterone, valproic acid)

Analyte	Age/Gender	Reference Range	SI Units	Note
Fibrinogen (Factor I)	Neonates	1.25–3.0	g/l	
	Adults	1.5–3.5	g/l	
		4.0–10.0	µmol/l	

Fibrinopeptide A

(FPA) Thrombin fibrinogen to fibrin conversion is associated with peptides (A, B) release. Reflects active intravascular blood clotting as in subclinical disseminated intravascular coagulation. Fibrinogenesis marker.

Increased Values
pulmonary emboli, early leukemia treatment phase, DIC, leukemic patients at time of initial diagnosis or during relapse after remission, **deep-vein thrombosis**

Decreased Values
clinical leukemia remission after chemotherapy

Analyte	Age/Gender	Reference Range	SI Units	Note
Fibrinopeptide A		<3	ng/ml	

Folic Acid

(syn: folate) Active folic acid form = folinic acid. It is a pteridine, para-aminobenzoic acid and glutamic acid derivative. One of water soluble B vitamin group. Food folates are polyglutamates that are broken down by intestinal mucosal conjugase enzymes to a more soluble monoglutamates before absorption. This folate form circulates in the plasma freely or loosely bound to albumin, rapidly entering the tissues. To utilize liver folate stores, it is necessary to excrete into the bile and reabsorb the matter by jejunum – enterohepatic circulation.
Function. Necessary for normal red and white blood cells function, and important for the cellular genes and DNA production. Folic acid is a part of the coenzymes involved in purine and thymine synthesis, pyrimidine DNA methylation reactions, conversion of homocystine to methionine, conversion of serine and glycine, degradation of histidine; it plays a key role in cell growth and reproduction. Tetrahydrofolic acid is an active folic acid form serving as a co-factor in monocarbon radicals metabolism. It transfers activated formic acid and activated formaldehyde. Folate absorption depends on normal intestinal mucosa functioning.
Occurrence. Fresh green vegetables, fruits, beans, nuts, liver, kidney. It is stored in the liver. Highest values are in winter, lower are in summer.
Test Purpose. 1) questionable deficiency in conditions like megaloblastic anemias, undernutrition, malabsorption sy (celiac disease, conditions after intestine resection), alcoholism, neurological diseases, 2) to assess folate stores in pregnancy, 3) long term therapy monitoring with antiepileptics (mainly phenytoin), antibiotics, and cytostatics, 4) dialyzed patient monitoring, 5) dermatological disease diagnosis (e.g. psoriasis).

Increased Values
vitamin B_{12} deficiency, blood transfusion, distal small bowel disease, **inadequate folate intake**, blind loop sy, **vegetarianism**
  Interfering Factors: medicaments – (metformin, phenformin)

Decreased Values

amyloidosis, alcoholism, anemia – (**hemolytic a.,** macrocytic a., megaloblastic a., **pernicious a., sideroblastic a.,** hereditary spherocytic a., thalassemia), nutritional megaloblastic anemia in – (infants, **infectious diseases**), **anorexia nervosa, coeliac disease,** hepatic cirrhosis, vitamin B_{12}/C deficiency, **dermatitis herpetiformis,** exfoliative dermatitis, diabetes mellitus, diabetic enteropathy, smoking, **partial gastrectomy, hemodialysis/peritoneal dialysis, chronic hemolysis,** paroxysmal nocturnal hemoglobinuria, hepatoma, **starvation,** infant diarrhea, homocystinuria, **hyperthyroidism,** hypothyroidism, diseases – (infant infectious d., **exfoliative skin d.,** myeloproliferative d.), liver disease connected with – (**alcoholism,** malabsorption sy), lactation, **leukemia, lymphoma, elder people, folate malabsorption, malnutrition, Crohn's disease, Whipple's disease, tumours, prematurity, insufficient folic acid intake, psoriasis, extensive intestinal resection,** scleroderma, **sprue,** febrile states, idiopathic steatorrhea, **pregnancy,** taeniasis, **excessive folate utilization by the body, protracted cardiac failure**

> **Interfering Factors:** infancy, medicaments – (acetylsalicylic acid, alcohol, aminopterin, aminosalicylic acid, ampicillin, antiepileptics, anticonvulsants, antimalarials, azulfadine, barbiturates, carbamazepine, chloramphenicol, cycloserine, erythromycin, estrogens, ethanol, isoniazid, metformin, methotrexate, nitrofurantoin, oral contraceptives, penicillin, pentamidine, phenobarbital, phenytoin, primidone, pyrimethamine, sulfasalazine, tetracyclines, triamterene, trimethoprim, valproic acid)

Analyte	Age/Gender	Reference Range	SI Units	Note
Folic Acid	Neonates	15.9–72.4	nmol/l	See ref.
	F + M	4.1–38	nmol/l	ranges note
		>4.3	nmol/l	

Galactokinase in RBC

Test Purpose. 1) to investigate increased levels of galactose, 2) to investigate a juvenile onset cataract.

Decreased Values
cataract, **galactosemia,** genetic galactokinase deficiency

Galactose-1-Phosphate in RBC

Test Purpose. 1) to investigate a neonate with suspected galactosuria, 2) to help in diagnosis of galactosemia in a baby with a positive neonatal screening test, 3) to help in diagnosis of classical galactosemia, 4) dietary monitoring of patients with galactosemia.

Increased Values
galactosemia

Glucose-6-Phosphate Dehydrogenase in RBC

(G6PD) G6PD is a red cell X-linked inheritance enzyme important to maintain reduced RBC proteins (reduced glutathione form, G-SH). Enzyme is involved in RBC saccharide NADPH metabolism production. In G6PD deficiency, NADPH is not produced, effecting protective glutathione function loss and hemolytic disorders.

Test Purpose. RBC metabolic disorders and hemolytic anemias differential diagnosis.

Increased Values
anemia – (megaloblastic a., pernicious a.), hyperthyroidism, myocardial infarction, hepatic coma, idiopathic thrombocytopenic purpura, chronic blood loss

Decreased Values
congenital nonspherocytic anemia, G6PD deficiency

Analyte	Age/Gender	Reference Range	SI Units	Note
Glucose-6-Phosphate Dehydrogenase in RBC		0.22–0.52	*	*mU/mol Hb
		0.10–0.23	**	**nU/10⁶ RBC

Glutathione in RBC

(syn: reduced glutathione in erythrocytes) RBC tripeptide is created from amino acid glycine, cystine and glutamic acid by enzyme glutathione synthase.
Function. Reduced RBC glutathione protects: a) enzyme and coenzyme – SH group against oxidation, b) membrane lipids against peroxidation, an enzyme involved in methemoglobin (Fe^{3+}) to hemoglobin (Fe^{2+}) reduction.
Test Purpose. RBC metabolism disorders and hemolytic anemias differential diagnosis.

Increased Values
pyrimidine-5'-nucleotidase deficiency, myelofibrosis

Decreased Values
strenuous exercise, deficiency of – (G6PD, gamma-glutamylsynthetase), diabetes mellitus, lead exposure

Glutathione Peroxidase in RBC

As a hexose-monophosphate shunt and glutathione cycle portion, enzyme is involved in RBC oxidative glycolysis (selenium-metalloenzyme which catalyzes hydrogen peroxide to water conversion).
Test Purpose. RBC metabolism disorders and hemolytic anemias differential diagnosis.

Increased Values
G6PD deficiency, acute lymphocytic leukemia, polyunsaturated fatty acids supplementation, alpha-thalassemia

Decreased Values
anemia – (sickle cell a., iron deficiency a.), selenium deficiency, lead exposure

Glutathione Reductase in RBC

(GR) Red cell enzyme. Its activity is chiefly a riboflavin nutrition state reflection.

Increased Values

strenuous exercise, G6PD deficiency, diabetes mellitus
   Interfering Factors: medicaments – (nicotinic acid)

Decreased Values

anemia – (congenital nonspherocytic hemolytic a., hypoplastic a., alpha-thalassemia a.)
Gaucher's disease, oligophrenia, pancytopenia, thrombocytopenia

---

Glycated Hemoglobin

(HbA_{1c}, HbAc, GHb, GHB, syn: glycohemoglobin, glycosylated hemoglobin, glycogenous hemoglobin, fast hemoglobin) Reaction product between glucose and N-terminal HbA valine. Glycohemoglobin is a minor hemoglobin (A_1 component). A_1 components (A_{1a}, A_{1b}, A_{1c}) which make up approximately 4–8% of the total hemoglobin are glycosylated. Blood glucose bound to hemoglobin is stored by the erythrocytes. Glycosylation is irreversible. GHb amount depends on the glucose amount available in the bloodstream over the RBC's 120-day life span. Because old RBCs are constantly being destroyed while new are being formed, GHb value determination reflects the average blood sugar level for the 100 to 120-day period before the test. With more glucose exposure there is greater GHb percentage. One important test advantage is that the sample can be drawn at any time, because it is not affected by short-term variations (food intake, exercise, stress, hypoglycemic agents, patient cooperation).
Test Purpose. 1) to assess diabetes mellitus control, 2) to check unstable IDDM and gestation DM therapies, 3) permanent hyperglycemia diagnosis.

Increased Values

alcohol, anemia – (sickle-cell a., thalassemia, **iron deficiency a.**), rheumatoid arthritis, iron deficiency, diabetes mellitus – (newly diagnosed d.m., **non-insulin dependent d.m., insulin dependent d. m.**, d. m. in pregnancy, poorly controlled diabetic patient), pheochromocytoma, cystic pancreatic fibrosis, fructosuria, galactosemia, **hemodialysis**, false elevated values – (when the RBC life span is lengthened – as in thalassemia), **chronic hyperglycemia,** intoxi-cation by – (lead, opiates), hyperlipoproteinemia, diseases – (d. with abnormal hemoglobin, d. with shortened survival erythrocyte rate), chronic renal insufficiency, diabetic neuropathy, tumours, **splenectomy, stress,** Cushing's syndrome, **chronic renal failure**
   Interfering Factors: TAG increase, medicaments – (hydrochlorothiazide, morphine, oral contraceptives, propranolol, salicylates)

Decreased Values

anemia – (**hemolytic a.,** congenital spherocytosis, **sickle cell a.**), shortened RBC life span (HbS, HbC, HbD presence), dialysis, phlebotomy, transfusion, acute caloric restriction, chronic blood loss, **pregnancy, chronic renal failure**
   Interfering Factors: medicaments – (galactose, salicylate, vitamin C, vitamin E)

Analyte	Age/Gender	Reference Range	SI Units	Note
Hemoglobin, Glycated (HbA_{1c})	Normal			See ref. ranges note
		0.036–0.058		
		0.042–0.063		
		0.050–0.080		
		0.050–0.080		
		0.033–0.056		

Analyte	Age/Gender	Reference Range	SI Units	Note
		0.044–0.057		
	Good compensation	0.06–0.07		
	Insufficient compensation	>0.08		

Haptoglobin

(Hp, HPT, syn: hemoglobin binding protein) Hemoglobin metabolism acute phase protein and antioxidative system portion, it is characterized with genetic polymorphism with three phenotypes (1-1, 2-1, 2-2). Phenotype 2-2 is an ischemic heart disease risk indicator. There are other haptoglobin subtypes used in forensic medicine.

Production. Transport glycoprotein (alpha-2-globulin) is synthesized in the liver.

Function. Protein carrier of released hemoglobin = irreversible free Hb binding mainly through the Hb and haptoglobin globin alpha-chain. Haptoglobin-hemoglobin complex is taken from circulation and catabolized by spleen and liver reticuloendothelial tissue phagocytic cells, thus ensuring iron and amino acid salvage. Haptoglobin concentration is inversely related to the hemolysis level. Hemoglobin-haptoglobin complexes preserve iron stores. Once the haptoglobin binding capacity has been exceeded, free Hb appears in the plasma. Since free Hb is a small molecule, it can be excreted in the urine. Hemoglobinemia and hemoglobinuria occur when the haptoglobin capacity for binding hemoglobin dimers is saturated.

Test Purpose. 1) to serve as an hemolysis index, 2) to distinguish between hemoglobin and myoglobin in plasma, as haptoglobin binds with free hemoglobin but does not bind with myoglobin, 3) to investigate hemolytic transfusion reactions, 4) to establish paternity proof, using genetic haptoglobin structure variations, 5) diagnosis of hemolytic anemia, 6) diagnosis of inflammatory disorders.

Increased Values – hyperhaptoglobinemia

amyloidosis, aplastic anemia, **rheumatoid arthritis**, dermatomyositis, **tissue destruction, diabetes mellitus, acute rheumatic fever**, diseases – (**arterial d.**, granulomatous d., **acute/chronic infectious d., acute/chronic inflammatory d.**), **cardiac infarction, collagenoses, colitis ulcerosa** (ulcerative colitis), **systemic lupus erythematosus,** Hodgkin's disease, lymphosarcoma, **tumours, nephritis,** nephrosis, **biliary ways obstruction, burns, pyelonephritis,** trauma, necrosis of tissue, scurvy, stress, pregnancy, **nephrotic sy, peptic ulcer**

> Interfering Factors: medicaments – (anabolic steroids, androgens, estrogens, fluoxymesterone, metandienone, methyltestosterone, nandrolone, oxymetholone)

Decreased Values – hypohaptoglobinemia

anemia – (**hemolytic a., autoimmune hemolytic a.,** sickle-cell a., **megaloblastic a., hereditary spherocytosis, thalassemia**), **liver cirrhosis**, G6PD deficiency, subacute bacterial endocarditis, **fetal erythroblastosis, hematoma,** paroxysmal nocturnal hemoglobinuria, intravascular hemolysis – (autoantibodies, immunohemolytic i. h. = cool autoantibodies + thermic autoantibodies, infectious i. h., medicamentous i. h., mechanical i. h.), chronic hepatitis, **hypertension, prosthetic heart valves,** liver diseases, **systemic lupus erythematosus,** chronic lymphadenosis, **malaria,** infectious mononucleosis, pancytopenia, **liver parenchyma disorders,** thrombotic thrombocytopenic purpura, **transfusion reactions,** malabsorption sy, **contact sports,** pregnancy, **uremia, congenital ahaptoglobinemia**

Interfering Factors: medicaments – (aminosalicylic acid, asparaginase, chlorpromazine, cisplatin, cortisone, dapsone, dextran, diphenhydramine, estrogens, furazolidine, indomethacin, isoniazid, methyldopa, nitrofurantoin, oral contraceptives, quinidine, streptomycin, sulfasalazine, tamoxifen, testosterone)

Analyte	Age/Gender	Reference Range	SI Units	Note
Haptoglobin	Adults	0.5–3.3	g/l	
	Hp 1–1	0.7–2.3	g/l	
	Hp 2–1	0.9–3.6	g/l	
	Hp 2–2	0.6–2.9	g/l	

Hematocrit

(Hct, HCT, Crit, PCV, syn: packed cell volume, packed red cell volume) Cellular blood constituent percentage in the total blood volume.

Test Purpose. 1) to aid in diagnosis of polycythemia, anemia or abnormal hydration conditions, 2) to aid in red cell indices calculation: mean corpuscular volume, mean corpuscular hemoglobin concentration, and mean corpuscular hemoglobin.

Increased Values
dehydration – (**hypotonic d., isotonic d.**), **eclampsia, erythrocytosis, hemoconcentration, diarrhea, congenital heart disease, surgery, polycythemia, polycythemia vera, polyglobulia, burns, shock, trauma, living in high altitudes,** profound diuresis
    Interfering Factors: medicaments – (androgens, nandrolone, oral contraceptives, spironolactone)

Decreased Values
anemia, rheumatoid arthritis, hepatic cirrhosis, idiopathic/infectious enterocolitis, hyperhydration – (hypertonic h., isotonic h.), **hyperthyroidism,** prosthetic heart valves, **hemorrhage** (recovery stage after acute h.), **leukemia,** malabsorption – (folic acid m., vitamin B_{12} m., iron m.), **malnutrition, Hodgkin's disease, plasmocytoma** (incl. multiple myeloma), burns, reaction to infectious/chemicals agents/medicaments, **hemolytic conditions, pregnancy,** incompatible blood transfusion, bone marrow failure due to – (radiation, toxins, fibrosis, tumor), transfusion reaction
    Interfering Factors: medicaments – (amphotericin B, azathioprine, cefalotin, chloramphenicol, chlorphenamine, hydralazine, ibuprofen, methyldopa, penicillin)

Analyte	Age/Gender	Reference Range	SI Units	Note
Hematocrit	Neonates	0.44–0.62		
	3 m–13 y	0.31–0.43		
	Adults M	0.42–0.52		
	Adults F	0.37–0.47		

Hemoglobin

(Hb, Hgb) Hb concentration is a measure of the total Hb peripheral blood amount. Red blood stain consists from hem (ferroprotoporphyrin complex) and globin (tetramer molecule composed from 4 globin chains). Hemoglobin proportion in adults: HbA (97% of total Hb, 2 alpha and 2 beta globin chains), HbA2 (2.5% of total Hb, 2 alpha and 2 delta globin chains), HbF (0.5%).

Production. Hemoglobin is produced by nucleated immature red blood cells.

Function. Main erythrocyte component, vehicle for O_2 and CO_2 transportation. Serves as one of primary extracellular fluid buffer substance, maintains acid-base balance by a process called chloride shift. The clinical test implications closely parallel those of the RBC count. Factors affecting hemoglobin oxygen affinity: 1) increased oxygen affinity: alkalosis (Bohr effect), ↓ RBC 2,3-DPG, ↓ temperature, carboxyhemoglobinemia, high-affinity hemoglobinopathies, 2) decreased oxygen affinity: acidosis (Bohr effect), ↑ RBC 2,3-DPG, ↑ temperature, hemoglobinopathies.

Test Purpose. 1) to measure anemia, polycythemia, blood loss severity and to monitor therapy response, 2) to obtain data for calculating mean corpuscular hemoglobin and mean corpuscular hemoglobin concentrations.

Increased Values

stroke, **dehydration**, encephalitis, **hemoconcentration**, diarrhea, **chronic obstructive pulmonary disease**, diseases – (**mitral valve d.**, **pulmonary d.**, **congenital heart d.**), tumours, **physical exertion**, intestinal obstruction, **polycythemia**, **polyglobulia**, burns, environment – (cold e., **high altitude e.**), loss of – (ions, body fluids), **symptomatic polyglobulia**, **congestive heart failure**, endocrine caused increase – (adrenaline, parathormone)

  Interfering Factors: medicaments – (adrenaline, gentamicin, glucocorticoids, hydralazine, oral contraceptives, methyldopa, pilocarpine)

Decreased Values

anemia – (**sickle cell a.**, thalassemia), rheumatoid arthritis, **hepatic cirrhosis**, deficiency of – (copper, iron), **glomerulonephritis**, hemoblastoses, **hemoglobinopathies**, paroxysmal nocturnal hemoglobinuria, **hyperhydration**, **hyperthyroidism**, adrenal hypofunction, artificial heart valves, diseases – (infectious d., acute renal d., chronic liver d., systemic d., acute inflammatory d.), **renal insufficiency**, chronic intoxication by – (benzene, copper, lead), carcinomatosis, leukemia, **systemic lupus erythematosus**, lymphoma, Crohn's disease, Hodgkin's disease, excess of – (ions, water), tumours, renal cortical necrosis, undernutrition, severe burns, X-rays therapy, reaction to chemicals/infectious agents/medicaments, **sarcoidosis**, splenectomy, splenomegaly, **hyper-IgM sy**, conditions – (**hemolytic c.**, **hemorrhagic c.**), **pregnancy**, incompatible blood transfusion, typhoid fever

  Interfering Factors: medicaments – (acetazolamide, acetylsalicylic acid, ACTH, aminosalicylic acid, amphetamine, amiodarone, amitriptyline, amphotericin B, ampicillin, antibiotics, antiepileptics, antineoplastic drugs, asparaginase, azapropazone, azathioprine, barbiturates, busulfan, captopril, carbimazole, cefalexin, cephalosporins, cefalotin, cefoxitin, cefuroxime, chlorambucil, chloramphenicol, chloroquine, chlorothiazide, chlorphenamine, chlorpromazine, chlorpropamide, chlortalidone, cholestyramine, cimetidine, cisplatin, clindamycin, cyclofenil, cyclophosphamide, cyclosporine, dactinomycin, dapsone, desipramine, diazepam, digitoxin, diclofenac, doxycycline, erythromycin, estrogens, ethanol, ethosuximide, fenoprofen, fluorouracil, gold salts, griseofulvin, hydralazine, ibuprofen, indomethacin, isoniazid, latamoxef, levodopa, mebendazole, mepacrine, mephenytoin, meprobamate, metamizole, metformin, methotrexate, meticillin, methyldopa, miconazole, nafcillin, naproxen, nomifensine, oral contraceptives, oxyphenbutazone, paracetamol, penicillamine, penicillin, phenacetin, phenazone, phenothiazines, phenylbutazone, phenytoin, probenecid, procainamide, procarbazine, propranolol, pyrazinamide, pyrimethamine, quinidine, rifampicin, streptomycin, sulfafurazole, sulfamethizole, sulfamethoxazole, sulfasalazine, sulfonylureas, sulindac, sulfonamides, tamoxifen, tetracyclines, thioridazine, thioguanine, tobramycin, tolazoline, tolbutamide, trimethadione, trimethoprim, valproic acid, vinblastine)

Analyte	Age/Gender	Reference Range	SI Units	Note
Hemoglobin	Neonates	145–225	g/l	
	2 m	90–140	g/l	
	6–18 y	115–155	g/l	
	Adults M	130–160	g/l	
	Adults F	120–160	g/l	
Hemoglobin, Free		0.01–0.05	g/l	

Hemoglobin A2

(HbA2) Hemoglobin A2 (2 alpha and 2 delta globin chains) is a minor normal adult blood component. HbA2 levels have special application to the diagnosis of beta-thalassemia trait, which may be present even though peripheral blood smear is normal.

Test Purpose. 1) to evaluate a HbA2 percentage from total Hb, 2) hemolytic anemias differential diagnosis, 3) to aid in the diagnosis of hemoglobinopathies and thalassemias.

Increased Values
megaloblastic anemia, beta-thalassemia, hyperthyroidism

Decreased Values
anemia – (sideroblastic a., alpha-thalassemia), **untreated iron deficiency, erythroleukemia, HbH disease**

Hemoglobin S

(HbS) Pathological Hb characterized with glutamic acid to valine change in the beta-globin chain 6th position. Hemoglobin S becomes more viscous, precipitating or bonding to cause sickle red cells. The abnormally shaped cells are unable to pass freely through the capillary system, this results in increased blood viscosity and sluggish circulation.

Test Purpose. 1) sickle cell anemia diagnosis, 2) hemolytic anemias differential diagnosis.

Increased Values – positive
sickle-cell anemia

Decreased Values
false negative values – (protein abnormalities, infants before 3 months, polycythemia)

Hemopexin

(Hx, Hpx) Hemopexin is a weak acute phase reactant. This polymorphic protein is synthesized by hepatocytes. Metheme is oxidized heme hemoglobin without globin and the hemopexin binds heme/metheme with high affinity after hemoglobin breakdown. The complex is cleared from the circulation by the liver, while the hemoglobin-haptoglobin complex is cleared by the reticuloendothelial system. Free carrier returns to the circulation and binds hematin from the methemalbumin complex. Hemopexin also binds other porphyrins. Once processed in the liver, the heme-hemopexin complex releases/returns hemopexin to the circulation; haptoglobin is destroyed once complexed with hemoglobin. Beta-migrating globulin hemopexin binds the heme released by hemoglobin degradation. By this means small iron atom porphyrin molecules are protected from urine excretion, thereby preserving body iron stores. Hemoglobin agents bonding to protein carriers protect body against renal impairment by excess Hb excretion.

Test Purpose. Hemolysis diagnosis.

Increased Values

diabetes mellitus, melanoma

Decreased Values

liver cirrhosis, malnutrition, intense hemolytic processes, nephrotic syndrome

Analyte	Age/Gender	Reference Range	SI Units	Note
Hemopexin	Total	0.50–3.3	g/l	
	fenotype 1–1	0.70–2.3	g/l	
	fenotype 2–1	0.90–3.6	g/l	
	fenotype 2–2	0.60–2.9	g/l	

Heparin Co-Factor II

(HC II) With dermatan sulphate plasmatic protein HC II inhibits thrombin selectively by creating a complex. Its activity is multiplied by heparin.

Test Purpose. 1) thrombotic conditions differential diagnosis, 2) inborn HC II defect identification.

Analyte	Age/Gender	Reference Range	SI Units	Note
Heparin Co-Factor II		90–105	mg/l	

Human Hematopoietic Growth Factors

- **SCF** (stem cell factor) – increases all hematopoietic cell type production, production of gonadal cells, mast cells, melanocytes.
  Production. Fibroblasts, hepatocytes, stromal cells, epithelial/endothelial cells.
- **IL-3** – increases neutrophil, monocyte, eosinophil, erythrocyte and basophil production.
  Production. T-lymphocytes.
- **IL-5** – increases eosinophil production.
  Production. T-lymphocytes
- **IL-11** – increases all hematopoietic progenitor and platelet production.
  Production. Stromal cells, fibroblasts.
- **GM-CSF** – increases neutrophil, dendritic cell, monocyte, eosinophil production.
  Production. T-lymphocytes, endothelial cells, fibroblasts, monocytes.
- **G-CSF** – increases neutrophil production.
  Production. Monocytes, fibroblasts.
- **M-CSF** – increases placental trophoblast cell and monocyte production.
  Production. Monocytes, fibroblasts, lymphocytes, epithelial/endothelial cells.
- **EPO** – increases erythrocyte production.
  Production. Kidney cells.
- **TPO** – increases platelet production.
  Production. Kidney, liver.

Left Side Shift

More neutrophilic sticks and metamyelocytes in peripheral blood smear (younger cells, juvenile neutrophils, immature neutrophil forms). Regenerative response indicator used in differential diagnosis of primary hemathological diseases and reactive blood stain changes.

Occurrence. Acidosis, actinomycosis, amebiasis, acute appendicitis, acute/chronic pelvic inflammatory disease, arthritis – (gonococcal a., suppurative a.), aspergillosis, balanitis, bartonellosis, blastomycosis, cellulitis, chronic pituitary adrenocortical insufficiency, dermatomyositis, diverticulitis, excessive hemolysis, thoracic empyema, chemotherapeutics, choledocholithiasis, cholera, diphtheria, diseases – (Chagas d., legionnaires' d., Lyme d.), disseminated intravascular coagulation, ulcerative colitis, echinococcosis, endometritis, epiglottitis, erysipelas, hantavirus infection, bacterial infections, acute hemorrhage, suppurative hidradenitis, chronic neutropenia in children, intoxications, leptospirosis, leukemia, listeriosis, lung anthrax, malaria, sepsis (toxemia), uremia, abscess – (brain a., breast a., kidney a., perinephric renal a., perianal a., gingival a., alveolar a., liver a., lung a., omentum a., pancreas a., parotid gland a., peritonsillar a., prostate a., scrotum a., spinal epidural a., spleen a., stomach a., subphrenic a., tonsil a., tubo-ovarian a.), acute myocarditis, bronchiectasis, diabetic ketoacidosis, acute/chronic sinusitis, acute/subacute bacterial endocarditis, purulent pericarditis, intestine perforation, acute fatty liver of pregnancy, puerperal infection, pyopneumothorax, pyoureter, cholangitis, cholecystitis, osteomyelitis, enterocolitis – (acute pseudomembranous e., necrotizing e.), acute epididymitis, peritonitis, pharyngitis, gonorrheal proctitis, pneumonia – (aspiration p., Hemophilus influenzae p., mycoplasmal p., acute interstitial p., tularemic p., Klebsiella p., staphylococcal p., streptococcal p., pneumococcal p.), polycythemia vera, acute prostatitis, oophoritis, acute pyelonephritis, toxoplasmosis, scarlet fever, herpes simplex infection in newborn, mesenteric venous thrombosis, meningitis – (bacterial m., meningococcal m., pneumococcal m.), shigellosis, rheumatic fever, septic shock

Leukocyte Antibodies

In recipient's blood, a positive result indicates presence of leukoagglutinins, identifying the transfusion reaction as a reaction to these antibodies. In donor's blood, a positive result indicates presence of leukoagglutinins.

Test Purpose. 1) to detect leukoagglutinins in blood recipeints who develop transfusion reactions, 2) to detect leukoagglutinins in blood donors after transfusion causes a reaction.

Increased Values
transfusion reactions
    Interfering Factors: i.v. contrast media, medicaments – (dextran)

Leukocytes

(WBC, syn: white blood cell count, WBC count, leukocyte count, total white count, white cell count, leucocytes) Leukocytes are colorless globe-shaped cells produced in bone marrow that always contain a nucleus. Peripheral blood smear (stained blood film, differential count, leucogram).

Function. To fight against infection, to defend the body against foreign organisms invasion by phagocytosis and transport/distribute antibodies in the immune response.

Production. Granulocytes, monocytes and lymphocytes are formed in the red bone marrow. Lymphocytes mature in the lymphatic tissue (spleen, thymus, tonsils).

Test Purpose. 1) to determine infection or inflammation, 2) to determine need for further tests, such as the WBC differential or bone marrow biopsy, 3) to monitor response to chemotherapy or radiation therapy.

- ■ **Leukocyte division**
  - ■ **basophils (basophilic segments):** blood dyscrasia, myeloproliferative diseases
  - ■ **eosinophils (eosinophilic segments):** parasitic diseases, allergic disorders
  - ■ **lymphocytes:** viral infections – (varicella, infectious mononucleosis, morbilli, rubella)
  - ■ **monocytes:** severe infections
  - ■ **neutrophils (neutrophilic sticks and neutrophilic segments):** diseases – (bacterial infectious d. , inflammatory d.), stress
  - ■ **agranulocytes – mononuclears (monocytes, lymphocytes)**
  - ■ **phagocytes** (microphages – granulocytes) + (macrophages – monocytes, histiocytes)
  - ■ **immunocytes** (lymphocytes – B-lymphocytes, T-lymphocytes, NK-cells) + (plasma cells)
- ■ **Leukocyte findings**
  - ■ **toxic granulation of neutrophils and metamyelocytes:** bacterial infections
  - ■ **atypical lymphocytes:** viral infections
  - ■ **giant cytoplasmic granules:** Chediak–Higashi sy
  - ■ **bilobed neutrophils:** Pelger–Huet anomaly
  - ■ **hypersegmented neutrophils:** pernicious anemia, folate deficiency, myeloproliferative diseases
  - ■ **myeloblasts, promyelocytes, myelocytes:** leukemia – (acute myeloblastic l., acute promyelocytic l., chronic myelocytic l.), myelofibrosis, polycythemia vera
  - ■ **large granular lymphocytes:** T-gamma proliferative disease (natural killer cells)
  - ■ **lymphoblasts:** leukemia – (acute lymphoblastic l., prolymphocytic l., chronic lymphocytic l.), malignant lymphoma, infectious mononucleosis
  - ■ **plasmablasts:** plasmocytoma (incl. multiple myeloma)

Increased Values – leukocytosis

abortion – (**spontaneous a., threatened a., septic a., missed a.**), **placental abruption, abscess, acidosis,** actinomycosis, allergy to – (mold, dust), dissecting aortic aneurysm, **amyloidosis, amebiasis,** anemia – (pernicious a., **sickle cells a., acute posthemorrhagic/posthemolytic a.**), anesthesia, **appendicitis, severe anoxia,** lung anthrax, arteritis – (**giant cell a., Takayasu's a.**), aspergillosis, pulmonary atelectasis, arthritis – (**rheumatoid a.**, gonococcal a., **suppurative a.**, psoriatic a., meningococcal a., syphilitic a., tuberculous a., viral a.), ascariasis, bronchial asthma, **balanitis,** bartonellosis, arachnid bite, neurogenic atonic bladder, **bronchitis,** berylliosis, **blastomycosis,** bronchiectasis, **bronchiolitis, subacromial bursitis, dehydratation,** cellulitis, **hepatic cirrhosis,** chronic bilateral obstructive uropathy, benign ovarian cyst, dermatitis herpetiformis, dermatomyositis, **acute gout,** diphtheria, **diverticulitis,** echinococcosis, **eclampsia,** embolism – (systemic arterial e., air e., cerebral e., **pulmonary e.**, coronary e., amniotic fluid e., fat e., paradoxical e., renal artery e.), acute disseminated encephalomyelitis, **endometritis,** enterocolitis – (**acute pseudomembranous e., necrotizing e., tuberculous e.**), tropical eosinophilia, **acute epididymitis, epiglottitis, erysipelas, erythema nodosum, HIV infection,** emotional disturbance, **thoracic empyema,** encephalitis – (St. Louis e., **herpes e.**, cytomegalovirus e.), **endocarditis, pharyngitis,** fasciitis – (**necrotizing f., eosinophilic f.**), fascioliasis, **Q fever, rheumatic fever,** smoking, cystic fibrosis, **gangrene,** viral gastroenteritis, granulomatosis – (lymphomatoid g., **Churg–Strauss g., Wegener's g.**), hepatitis – (**alcoholic h.**, chemical-induced h., viral h.), **febris rheumatica,** hidradenitis suppurativa, **malignant hyperthermia**, chloroma, **cholangitis, cholecystitis, choledocholithiasis, cholera, chorioamnionitis**, lymphocytic choriomeningitis, syphilitic chorioretinitis, immunodeficiency disorders, acute chorea, disease – (**legionnaire's d.**, cat-scratch d., Caroli's d., silo-filler d., Hodgkin's d., Wilson's d., **Still's d.**, Chagas d., **Lyme d.**, Crohn's d., **chronic granulomatous d.**, Brill-Zinsser d., Whipple's d., IgM heavy chain d.), diseases – (allergic d., endocrine d., **bacterial infectious d., chronic infectious d., parasitic i. d., fungal i. d.**, rickettsial i. d., **myeloproliferative d., inflammatory d.**), **cardiac infarction** (increase at 6–12 hrs, decrease at 3–7 d.), infarction – (**liver i., spleen i., omentum i., kidney i.**), insufficiency – (acute adrenocortical i., chronic pituitary adrenocortical i.), poisoning by – (chemicals, metals, medicaments, arsenic, benzene, beryllium, carbon monoxide, carbon tetrachloride, **ethylene glycol, venoms**, heavy metals, lead, mercury, nicotine, nickel, phosphorus, thallium, turpentine), **gonorrhea, diabetic ketoacidosis, pulmonary candidiasis**, disseminated intravascular coagulation, **coccidioidomycosis**, colitis – (**ulcerative c., granulomatous c.**), coma – (**diabetic c., uremic c.**, non-ketotic hyperosmolar c.), hereditary coproporphyria, cryptococcosis, **leptospirosis, listeriosis, acute/chronic leukemia, chronic lymphocytic leukemia, chronic myelocytic leukemia, progressive multifocal leukoencephalopathy, mesenteric lymphadenitis**, lupus erythematosus systemicus, **lymphangitis, lymphogranuloma venereum, lymphoma, Burkitt's lymphoma**, Waldenström's macroglobulinemia, **malaria, mastoiditis**, melioidosis, meningitis – (**pneumococcal m.**, aseptic m., **bacterial m., meningococcal m.**, Listeria m., Mollaret's m., tuberculous m.), **menstruation, tumor metastases, infectious mononucleosis, mumps, myelitis, acute myocarditis**, infectious myringitis, myelosclerosis, systemic mycosis, **myositis**, tumours of – (**bone, breast, colorectum**, esophagus, kidney, pancreas, liver, melanoma, gastrointestinal tract, lungs, stomach), **physical exertion**, nausea, necrosis – (**hepatic n., tissue n.**), lupus nephritis, **newborn, neonates with Down sy**, nocardiosis, response to – (**pain**, cold, **massage**, sunlight), **orchitis**, ornithosis, **osteomyelitis, pancreatitis**, paracoccidioidomycosis, paroxysmal nocturnal hemoglobinuria, **fatty liver, acute fatty liver of pregnancy, pelvic inflammatory disease**, bullous pemphigoid, **intestine perforation, pericarditis, periostosis, peritonitis**, pityriasis rosea, **pneumonia**, pneumomediastinum, **pertussis, plasmocytoma** (incl. multiple myeloma), **drug induced interstitial pneumonitis, polyarteritis nodosa**, polycythemia, **polycythemia vera, polymyositis, pre-eclampsia, premature labor, burns**, porphyria – (acute intermittent p., erythropoietic protoporphyria, erythropoietic p.), epidemic hemorrhagic fever, **prostatitis**, purpura – (**thrombocytopenic p.**, Henoch–Schoenlein p.), **pyelonephritis, pyoderma gangrenosum, pyometra, pyopneumothorax, pyoureter, rabies, radiotherapy**, reaction – (**leukemoid r., transfusion r.**), **leukemic reticuloendotheliosis, schistosomiasis**, silicotuberculosis, conditions – (allergic c., comatose c., **hemolytic c.**, febrile c., hypersensitivity c., **acute hemorrhagic c.**, convulsive c., **c. after surgery**, post splenectomy c. – early, **posthemorrhagic c., septic c., stress c., shock c.**), heat stroke, **electric shock, ectopic pregnancy, ruptured tubal pregnancy**, paroxysmal tachycardia, **pregnancy, miliary tuberculosis, uremia, vasculitis, acute/chronic sinusitis, toxic megacolon**, vomiting, ultraviolet irradiation, viral infectious diseases – (herpes zoster, poliomyelitis, **chicken pox**, measles, smallpox), **elderly people, otitis media**, ischemic damage to – (**extremities, abdominal viscera, heart**), pseudogout, **scarlet fever, shigellosis, syphilis, salpingitis, tonsillitis**, toxoplasmosis, **thrombangitis obliterans**, thrombocytemia – (**primary t.**, hemorrhagic t.), **thrombosis, thrombophlebitis, thyroiditis**, thyrotoxicosis, **trauma**, trichinosis, chronic morphine addiction, trypanosomiasis, **tularemia**, typhoid fever, typhus – (epidemic t., endemic t.), urticaria, **gonorrheal urethritis**, syndrome – (Waterhouse–Friederichsen sy, Sheehan's sy, Guillain–Barré sy, Mikulicz sy, hypereosinophilic sy, eosinophilia-myalgia sy, carcinoid sy, **Kawasaki sy, toxic shock sy, Cushing's sy**), occlusion of internal carotid artery, small intestine volvulus, **penetrating duodenal/gastric** ulcer, retinal artery occlusion, **puerperal infection**, ovary torsion, **acute**/chronic renal failure, acute liver failure, familial mediterranean fever

Interfering Factors: medicaments – (ACTH, adrenaline, aldesleukin, allopurinol, amphotericin B, ampicillin, atropine, azathioprine, carbamazepine, chlorambucil, chloroform, chloroquine, chlorpromazine, codeine, corticosteroids, dexmedetomidine, ethanol, ether, filgrastim, fluorouracil, fluphenazine, fosphenytoin, haloperidol, halothane, levodopa, lithium, mefloquine, melphalan, mycophenolate, naproxen, nitrofurantoin, norepinephrine, omeprazole, oral contraceptives, penicillamine, perphenazine, phenytoin, pilocarpine, piroxicam, prednisone, prochlorperazine, promethazine, quinidine, quinine, sargramostim, strychnine, sulfasalazine, sulfonamides, thioridazine, thiothixene, tretinoin, trifluoperazine, verteporfin)

Decreased Values – leukopenia

septic abortion, metabolic acidosis, **hereditary orotic aciduria**, **agranulocytosis**, **AIDS**, alcoholism, amebiasis, anaphylaxis, anemia – (aplastic a., megaloblastic a., pernicious a., hereditary spherocytosis, iron deficiency a., myelophthisic a., pyridoxine-responsive a.), **anorexia nervosa**, congenital red cell dysplasia, arthritis – (rheumatoid a., parvovirus a.), aspergillosis – (allergic pulmonary a., invasive a.), babesiosis, brucellosis, diabetes mellitus, diverticulitis, eclampsia, encephalitis – (herpes e., echo-encephalitis), epidemic myalgic encephalomyelitis, non-bacterial endocarditis, exanthema subitum, hemoglobinuria – (paroxysmal nocturnal h., paroxysmal h. following exercise), inhibited hemopoiesis, hepatitis – (infectious h., alcoholic h., acute h. type A, acute h. type B, chronic active h. B, acute h. type D, acute h. type E, autoimmune h.), herpes zoster, malignant histiocytosis, **histoplasmosis**, fever – (Dengue f., Colorado tick f., West Nile f., **yellow f.**, Rocky Mountain spotted f., epidemic hemorrhagic f., Q f., lassa f.), primary hyperparathyroidism, **hypersplenism**, hypopituitarism, disease – (legionnaires' d., Gaucher's d., Wilson's d., **Brill-Zinsser d.**, heavy chain d., light chain d., Letterer-Siwe d., graft-versus-host d.), diseases – (**autoimmune d.**, **liver d.**, spleen d.), infectious diseases – (protozoon i. d., **rickettsial i. d.**), viral infectious diseases – (**influenza**, varicella, measles, morbilli, parainfluenza, poliomyelitis, rubella), **immune mediated marrow suppression**, intoxication by – (acetaminophen, alcohol, **arsenic**, benzene, phenytoin, toluene), kala-azar, disseminated intravascular coagulopathy, **collagenoses**, leishmaniasis, leptospirosis, leukemia – (acute monocytic l., promyelocytic l., megakaryocytic l., acute lymphoblastic l., acute myeloblastic l., leukemic reticuloendotheliosis), **systemic lupus erythematosus**, angioimmunoblastic lymphadenopathy, intestinal lymphangiectasia, familial erythrophagocytic lymphohistiocytosis, **Waldenström's macroglobulinemia**, malaria, infantile malnutrition, systemic mastocytosis, **infectious mononucleosis**, mycosis fungoides, primary myelofibrosis, tumors – (small cell lung t., Hodgkin's d., neuroblastoma, rhabdomyosarcoma, thymoma), lupus nephritis, neutropenia – (**familial n.**, **idiopathic n.**, cyclic n.), ornithosis, panmyelopathy, paratyphus, parotitis, peritonitis, plasmocytoma (incl. multiple myeloma), pneumonia – (pneumococcal p., Klebsiella p., staphylococcal p., viral p.), bone marrow injuries – (**metastases**, **tumours**, **fibrosis**, **failure**), psittacosis, idiopathic thrombocytopenic purpura, **radiotherapy**, **sarcoidosis**, **septic conditions** (advanced), septic shock, neonatal sepsis, schistosomiasis, shigellosis, chronic congestive splenomegaly, hepatic steatosis, bone marrow suppression by – (heavy metals, medicaments), syndrome – (Felty's sy, **Chediak-Higashi sy**, myelodysplastic sy, preleukemic sy, Hand-Schueller-Christian sy, **Sjögren's sy**), toxoplasmosis, portal vein thrombosis, **miliary tuberculosis**, **tularemia**, **typhoid fever**, typhus – (endemic t., **epidemic t.**), radiation

Interfering Factors: prolonged rest, ageing, medicaments – (acetaminophen, acetazolamide, acetohexamide, acetylsalicylic acid, aciclovir, ajmaline, aldesleukin, allopurinol, amiloride, aminocaproic acid, aminoglutethimide, amlodipine, amoxapine, amoxicillin, amphotericin B, ampicillin, antazoline, antibiotics, antiepileptics, anticonvulsants, antihistamines, antimetabolites, antithymocyte globulin, arsenic, asparaginase, atenolol, azathioprine, barbiturates, benazepril, benzylpenicillin, bexarotene, bisoprolol, bumetanide, busulfan, candesartan, capecitabine, captopril, carbamazepine, carbidopa, carbimazole, carboplatin, carbutamide, carmustine, cefaclor, cefadroxil, cefalexin, cefalotin, cefamandole, cefazolin, cefdinir, cefixime, cefoperazone, cefotaxime, cefoxitin, cefprozil, cefradine, ceftazidime, ceftizoxime, ceftriaxone, cefuroxime, cephalosporins, chloral hydrate, chlorambucil, chloramphenicol, chlordiazepoxide, chloroquine, chlorothiazide, chlorphenamine, chlorpromazine, chlorpropamide, chlorprothixene, chlortetracycline, chlortalidone, cimetidine, cisplatin, cladribine, clofibrate, clomipramine, clozapine, cloxacillin, codeine, colchicine, corticosteroids, cyclophosphamide, cyclosporine, cysteamine, cytarabine, cytostatics, dacarbazine, dactinomycin, dapsone, daunorubicin, denileukin, desipramine, dexrazoxane, diazepam, diazoxide, dicloxacillin, didanosine, digitoxin, disopyramide, docetaxel, doxepin, doxorubicin, doxycycline, enalapril, epirubicin, erythromycin, estramustine, estrogens, ethanol, ethosuximide, ethotoin, etidronate, etoposide, felbamate, fenofibrate, flavoxate, floxuridine, flucytosine, fludarabine, fluorouracil, fluphenazine, flurbiprofen, fosinopril, fosphenytoin, furazolidine, furosemide, gabapentin, gatifloxacin, gemfibrozil, gemtuzumab, glipizide, glyburide, gold salts, grepafloxacin, haloperidol, heparin, hydralazine, hydrochlorothiazide, hydroxyurea, ibuprofen, idarubicin, ifosfamide, imipenem, imipramine, indomethacin, interferon alfa-2a, interferon alfa-2b, interferon alfa-n1, interferon alfa-n3, interferon alfacon-1, interferon beta-1b, irinotecan, isoniazid, lamotrigine, lansoprazole, leflunomide, leuprolide, levamisole, levetiracetam, levodopa, levofloxacin, levomepromazine, lomustine, loracarbef, mebendazole, mechlorethamine, meloxicam, melperone, melphalan, mepacrine, mephenytoin, meprobamate, mercaptopurine, meropenem, metamizole, metaxalone, methimazole, methocarbamol, methotrexate, meticillin, metolazone, metronidazole, mexiletine, mezlocillin, mitomycin, mitoxantrone, moxifloxacin, mycophenolate, nafcillin, nalidixic acid, naproxen, nitrofurantoin, nitrous oxide, nortriptyline, oral contraceptives, oxacillin, oxaprozin, oxyphenbutazone, paclitaxel, pamidronate, pantoprazole, paramethadione, penicillamine, penicillins, pentamidine, pentazocine, pentostatin, perindopril, perphenazine, phenazone, phenobarbital, phenothiazines, phenylbutazone, phenytoin, piperacillin, plicamycin, primaquine, primidone, probenecid, procainamide, procarbazine, prochlorperazine, promazine, promethazine, propylthiouracil, protriptyline, pyrimethamine, quinidine, rabeprazole, ranitidine, rifampicin, rifapentine, rituximab, samarium-153, silver sulfadiazine, sirolimus, sparfloxacin, streptomycin, streptozocin, strontium-89 chloride, sulfadiazine, sulfafurazole, sulfamethizole, sulfamethoxazole, sulfasalazine, sulfonamides, sulfones, sulfonylureas, sulindac, sultiame, tamoxifen, temozolomide, teniposide, thiazides, thioguanine, thioridazine, thiotepa, thiothixene, tobramycin, tocainide, tolazamide, tolazoline, tolbutamide, tolmetin, topiramate, topotecan, trastuzumab, trifluoperazine, trimethadione, trimethoprim, trovofloxacin, thyrostatics, valproic acid, valrubicin, vancomycin, verteporfin, vinblastine, vincristine, vinorelbine, warfarin, zalcitabine, zimeldine, zinc salts)

Analyte	Age/Gender	Reference Range	SI Units	Note
Leukocytes	Neonates	15–20*		*x 10^9/l
	Adults	4.1–10.9*		

Lipoxins

(LX) Eicosanoids formed from arachidonic acid (lipoxygenase interaction products). Lipoxin A4 (LXA4) effects: neutrophil chemotaxis, neutrophil chemokinesis, NK-cell activity inhibition, arteriolar dilatation, leukotriene antagonist, thromboxane 2 and PGI2 release, bronchial smooth muscle contraction, activates polymorphonuclears, stimulates prostaglandin (PG) formation. Lipoxin B4 (LXB4) effects: NK-cell activity inhibition, vasoconstriction, bronchial smooth muscle contraction.

Lymphocytes

(lym, T-lymphocytes + B-lymphocytes + non-T-, non-B-lymphocytes) Lymphocytes belong to a heterogenous leukocyte group created from mother stem cells in the bone marrow; they mature to progenitor lymphatic cells. Bone marrow and thymus are primary lymphatic tissues. B-/T-lymphocytes and NK-cells pass from bone marrow to blood circulation → lymphatic tissue and organs (secondary lymphatic tissues). Lymphocytes reproduce and are released into blood stream with proper stimulation (recirculation). Their primary function is to interact with antigens and mount an immune response. The latter may be: 1) antibody humoral production form, 2) cell mediated with lymphokines lymphocyte elaboration or 3) cytotoxic with cytotoxic killer lymphocyte production. T-lymphocytes (about 70% of lymphocytes) – migrate from bone marrow to the thymus → processed by the thymic epithelial cell hormone → transformed into immunocompetent cells: 1) T_H-helper lymphocytes 55% (enhance B-cells and macrophage activity, bearing the surface antigen CD4$^+$). T_H-1 subpopulation produces IL-2, TNF-beta, IFN-gamma, T_H-2 subpopulation produces IL-4, 5, 6, 10, 13; T_H-lymphocytes support antibody production (humoral, antibody immunity); 2) T_S – suppressor lymphocytes (carry CD8$^+$ surface antigen and inhibit other immune system cell activity); 3) T_C – cytotoxic lymphocytes (killers, carrying the CD8$^+$ surface antigen that are responsible for killing cells that express foreign antigens); 4) T_D - delayed hypersensitivity lymphocytes. T-cells distribution: a) CD4$^+$ (peripheral blood 35–60%, lymph nodes 35–60%, spleen 20–90%, thymus cortex 90%, thymus marrow 60–80%), b) CD8$^+$ (peripheral blood 20–30%, lymph nodes 20–40%, spleen 10–80%, thymus cortex 90%, thymus marrow 20–40%). B-lymphocytes (about 25%) – from the bone marrow-derived stem cell → transformed into plasma cells (plasmocytes). B-cells distribution: peripheral blood 15–30%, lymph nodes 70–95%, spleen 0–40%, thymus 0–10%.

Function of T-lymphocytes. Responsible for specific cell-mediated immunity, delayed hypersensitivity – cellular immune response, immunodefense against parasitic/intracellular microorganisms (acidfast bacteria, viral infections, fungal infections, protozoan infections), graft rejection reactions.

Function of B-lymphocytes. Responsible for humoral immunity and antibody production – serum immunoglobulins (specific antibody immunity) → protect against staphylococcus, streptococcus, hemophilus, pneumococcus reinfection. Neutralize viruses to prevent initial infection. Act as barriers along gastrointestinal and respiratory passages. Initiate microorganisms killing by macrophages and other cells bearing Fc receptors. Cause vasoactive amines secretion from mast cells and basophils. Active lyse autologous origin cells or engage in antigen-antibody complex diseases. Interfere with T-killer cell activity by directly/indirectly blocking the reaction. Immediate humoral immune response (primary immune response). Secondary (anamnestic, booster) immune response. Antibody synthesis is inhibited by T_S-cells. NK-cells (natural killer cells, 3–5 %) are responsible for nonspecific cell and antitumor immunity.

Serum lymphocyte suppression factors. a) proteins – albumin, immunoregulatory globulin, pregnancy associated globulins, alpha-1-acid glycoprotein, CRP, SAA, AFP, alpha globulins in inflammatory diseases, chronic infectious diseases, cancer, LDL-C, HLA antibodies, antigen-antibody complexes, T-cell antibodies, b) hormones – glucocorticoids, progesterone, estrogens, androgens, prostaglandins, c) drugs – ouabain, acetylsalicylic acid, chloroquine, d) others – interferon, cytokines, cyclic nucleotides.

Test Purpose. 1) to aid in primary and secondary immunodeficiency diseases diagnosis, 2) to distinguish benign from malignant lymphocytic proliferative diseases, 3) to monitor therapy response (antibiotics, chemotherapeutics), 4) to help in inflammatory disease diagnosis, mainly viral, 5) monitoring HIV infected pediatric/adult patients.

Increased Values – lymphocytosis, lymphocytic leukocytosis

anemia – (aplastic a., hereditary elliptocytosis, hereditary spherocytic hemolytic a., thalassemia major), angiostrongyliasis, syphilitic aortitis, arthritis – (rheumatoid a., syphilitic a., viral a.), **brucellosis**, dermatitis, dermatitis herpetiformis, dermatomyositis, encephalitis – (e. lethargica, herpes e.), enterocolitis – (tuberculous a.), viral exanthemas, heat exhaustion, mycoplasmal pharyngitis, acute hepatitis – (type A, type B, type D, type E), histoplasmosis, hyperthyroidism, **decreased adrenal function** (hypoadrenalism), **cytomegalovirus infection**, lymphocytic choriomeningitis, syphilitic chorioretinitis, disease – (**Addison's d., Hodgkin's d.**, heavy chain d., Graves' d., Chagas' d., Crohn's d.), diseases – (**autoimmune d.**, upper respiratory way d.), infectious diseases – (**acute/chronic i. d., chronic bacterial i. d.**), viral infectious diseases – (**parotitis, pertussis**, smallpox, **rubella**, varicella, **rubeola**), insufficiency – (chronic pituitary adrenocortical i., acute adrenocortical i.), intoxication by – (arsenicals, lead, tetrachlorethane), **ulcerative colitis**, progressive multifocal leukoencephalopathy, immunoblastic lymphadenopathy, infectious lymphocytosis – (**mycoplasmatic i. l., rickettsial i. l.**), leukemia – (**acute/chronic lymphatic l., chronic lymphocytic l.**, hairy cell l., monoblastic l., plasma cell l.), systemic lupus erythematosus, mesenteric lymphadenitis, lymphogranuloma venereum, **lymphosarcoma**, non-Hodgkin's lymphoma, malaria, meningitis – (aseptic m., tuberculous m.), **infectious mononucleosis**, mumps, tumors – (breast t., stomach t., uterine cervix t.), **neutropenia**, mumps orchitis, osteopetrosis, tuberculous pericarditis, graft rejection, **plasmocytoma** (incl. multiple myeloma), pneumonia – (**viral p.**, mycoplasmal p.), **polyarteritis nodosa, idiopathic thrombocytopenic purpura**, serum sickness, scleroderma, silicotuberculosis, stress, syndrome – (chronic fatigue sy, preleukemic sy, DiGeorge sy), **syphilis, toxoplasmosis**, trypanosomiasis, pituitary dwarfism, **tuberculosis**, typhoid fever, **thyrotoxicosis**, vasculitis, **Waldenström's macroglobulinemia**, acute liver failure

Interfering Factors: children (up to 5 years), high altitudes, medicaments – (p-aminosalicylic acid, chlorphenamine, dexamethasone, diphenylhydantoin, epinephrine, griseofulvin, interferon alfacon-1, isoprenaline, norepinephrine, oxacillin, phenothiazines, phenytoin, salbutamol, sulfonamides)

Increased Values of CD4+/CD8+ ratio

rheumatoid arthritis, primary biliary cirrhosis, atopic dermatitis, IDDM, systemic lupus erythematosus without kidney impairment, psoriasis

Decreased Values – lymphopenia, lymphocytopenia, lymphocytic leukopenia

AIDS (acquired immunodeficiency syndrome), antithymocyte antibodies, **aplastic anemia, bone marrow aplasia/suppression**, lymphocyte destruction by – (**antilymphocytic globulin, cytostatic chemotherapy, ionization**), thoracic duct drainage, hemodialysed patients, malignant histiocytosis, **hypogammaglobulinemia**, diseases – (**collagen vascular d., immunodeficiency d.**, cardiac d.), acute myocardial infarction, **renal insufficiency, severe cachexia**, cardiomyopathy, **leukemia, systemic lupus erythematosus**, intestinal lymphangiectasia, intestinal lymphangitis, irradiation therapy, lymphogranuloma, **Whipple's disease**, malignant histiocytosis, multiple sclerosis, **myasthenia gravis**, mycosis fungoides, tumors – (pituitary gland t., Burkitt's lymphoma, lymphomas, **Hodgkin's disease**, thymoma, constrictive pericarditis, burns, alkylating agents, radiotherapy, reticular dysgenesis associated with aleukocytosis, **sarcoidosis**, conditions – (**malabsorption c., septic c.**), **severe combined immunodeficiency disorders** (SCID), stress – (physical s., psychic s.), syndrome – (**ataxia–teleangi-**

ectasia sy, **Cushing's sy, DiGeorge sy,** Nezelof's sy, Guillain–Barré sy, lymphoproliferative sy linked to X-chromosome, **postradiation sy, Wiskott–Aldrich sy**), tuberculosis – (**miliary t.,** t. of lymphatic nodes – advanced), trauma, uremia, failure – (**renal f., congestive heart f.**), Waldenström's macroglobulinemia

    Interfering Factors: medicaments – (abacavir, ACTH, aldesleukin, alemtuzumab, antilymphocyte antibodies, capecitabine, chlorambucil, cladribine, corticosteroids, cyclosporine, denileukin, dexamethasone, gemtuzumab, hydrocortisone, immunosuppressives, irinotecan, kava kava, lithium, methotrexate, pamidronate, phenytoin, prednisone, rifapentine, steroids)

Decreased Values of CD4+/CD8+ ratio
systemic lupus erythematosus with kidney impairment, viral infectious diseases – (AIDS, cytomegalovirus v. i. d., herpetic v. i. d., measles), myelodysplastic diseases, infectious mononucleosis, burns, graft-versus-host reaction, vigorous exercise

Decreased Values of T-Lymphocytes CD3
bronchial asthma, cytostatics, eczema, irradiation disease, diseases – (atopic d., autoimmune d., chronic liver d., gastrointestinal tract d.), infectious diseases – (candidiasis, parasitic i. d., Pneumocystis carinii), viral infectious diseases – (herpetic v. i. d., influenza, morbilli, rubella), infectious mononucleosis, tumors, burns, postsurgery conditions

Analyte	Age/Gender	Reference Range	SI Units	Note
Lymphocytes	Neonates	<22	%	
	Infants	<60	%	
	Adults	12–40	%	
		0.12–0.40		
		1.2–3.1	x 10⁹/l	
Lymphocytic Surface Markers (T-cells)				
	CD3	0.84–3.06 *		*x 10⁹ cells/l
		0.57–0.85		
	CD4	0.49–1.74 *		
		0.30–0.61		
	CD8	0.18–1.17 *		
		0.12–0.42		
	CD4/CD8	0.86–5.00		

Mastocytes

(syn: mast cells) Mastocytes are lymphoreticular character cells with a small nucleus and dark-violet granules in cytoplasma which are water-soluble. Mastocyte granules are replete with substances (mediators, heparin and histamine mainly) that have the capacity to regulate microcirculation, leading to changes in vascular permeability. Their products influence cell traffic in/out of tissues, activate neural pathways and may severely constrict the airway smooth muscles. Thus massive mast cell and basophil products release mediate a violent hypersensitive immediate-type life-threatening reaction known as anaphylaxis. Mast cell mediators: a) preformed and eluted are histamine, eosinophil chemotactic factors, neutrophil chemotactic factors, superoxide, arylsulfatase A, elastase, hexosaminidase, glucosidase, galactosidase, kallikrein-like enzyme, interleukins 3, 4, 5, 6, 8, interferon gamma, and tumor necrosis factor alpha, b) preformed and granule associated are tryptase, carboxypeptidase, superoxide dismutase, catalase, arylsulfatase B, c) newly generated: leukotrienes LTC4, LTD4, LTE4, platelet-activating factor, and prostaglandins (PGD2).

Test Purpose. 1) to help in bone marrow suppression diagnosis, 2) to help in chronic inflammatory disorder diagnosis, 3) to confirm mastocytosis.

Increased Values – mastocytosis
macroglobulinemia, **mastocytosis**, bone marrow suppression

Mean Corpuscular Hemoglobin

(MCH) Auxiliary index obtained by multiplying blood hemoglobin concentration by ten and dividing by the red blood cell count (Hb:RBC) as an expression of the hemoglobin amount/ weight per single red blood cell.

Test Purpose. To aid in diagnosis and classification of anemias.

Increased Values (relatively)
macrocytic anemia, newborns, infants
    Interfering Factors: severe leukocytosis, cold agglutinins, in vivo hemolysis, monoclonal proteins, lipemia, medicaments – (ethanol)

Decreased Values
anemia – (**hypochromic a.**, **microcytic a.**, a. in infectious disease, sideroblastic a., sideropenic a., thalassemia)

Analyte	Age/Gender	Reference Range	SI Units	Note
Mean Corpuscular Hemoglobin	Neonates	0.48–0.57	fmol	
	<2m	0.40–0.53	fmol	
	2 m–2 y	0.35–0.48	fmol	
	2 y–6 y	0.37–0.47	fmol	
	6 y–12 y	0.39–0.51	fmol	
	12–18 y	0.39–0.54	fmol	
	Adults	0.40–0.53	fmol	
		27–34	pg	

Mean Corpuscular Hemoglobin Concentration

(MCHC) Auxiliary index obtained by dividing blood hemoglobin concentration by the hematocrit (Hb:HCT). The average hemoglobin concentration in single erythrocyte is conventionally expressed in percentage. When values are decreased, the cell has a hemoglobin deficiency and is said to be hypochromic; when values are normal, the anemia is said normochromic (normocytic), and when values are increased anemia is hyperchromic.

Test Purpose. To aid in anemias diagnosis and classification.

Increased Values (relatively)
anemia – (**hereditary spherocytosis**, pernicious a., **sickle cell anemia**), newborns, infants
    Interfering Factors: cold agglutinins, severe lipemia, medicaments – (heparin, oral contraceptives)

Decreased Values

anemia – (**hypochromic a.**, macrocytic a., a. in infectious diseases, pyridoxine-responsive a., sideroblastic a., **sideropenic a.**, **thalassemia**, chronic blood loss a., **iron deficiency a.**), hemoglobinopathies

   Interfering Factors: severe leukocytosis

Analyte	Age/Gender	Reference Range	SI Units	Note
Mean Corpuscular Hemoglobin Concentration	Neonates	4.65–5.58	*	*mmol Hb/l
	<2m	4.50–5.74	*	RBC
	2 m–2 y	4.65–5.58	*	
	2 y–18 y	4.81–5.74	*	
	Adults	4.84–5.74	*	
		30–35	g/dl	

Mean Corpuscular Volume

(MCV) Average single RBC volume is obtained by multiplying the HCT by 1 000 and dividing by the red cell count. When the MCV is increased, RBC is said to be abnormally large – macrocytic, when the MCV value is decreased RBC is said to be abnormally small – microcytic. RBC are normo-/micro-/macrocytic.

Test Purpose. To aid diagnosis and classification of anemias.

Increased Values

alcoholism, anemia – (**aplastic a.**, hemolytic a., macrocytic a. in hepatic diseases, megaloblastic a., **pernicious a.**, sideroblastic a., myelophthisic a.), deficiency – (**folate d., vitamin B$_{12}$ d.**), smoking, **hypothyroidism**, celiac disease, **liver diseases**, tumors – (stomach t.), **reticulocytosis**, sprue, myelofibrosis, conditions – (posthemorrhagic c., postsplenectomy c.), **myelodysplatic sy**, marrow suppression/aplasia, orotic aciduria, pregnancy, women after menopause, newborns, infants

   Interfering Factors: cold agglutinins, severe leukocytosis, hyperglycemia, medicaments – (aminosalicylic acid, anticonvulsants, azathioprine, carbamazepine, colchicine, cyclophosphamide, ethanol, ethotoin, hydroxyurea, isoniazid, metformin, methotrexate, neomycin, oral contraceptives, phenacetin, phenobarbital, phenytoin, primidone, pyrimethamine, sulfamethoxazole, sulfasalazine, triamterene, trimethoprim, zidovudine)

Decreased Values

anemia – (hypochromic a., microcytic a., **a. of chronic disease**, a. in infectious diseases, hereditary spherocytosis, **sideroblastic a.**, **sideropenic a.**, **thalassemia**, pyridoxine-responsive a., a. from chronic blood loss), **hemoglobinopathies**, hyperthyroidism, hemorrhage, tumors, posttraumatic splenectomy, blood transfusion, chronic renal failure, lead poisoning

   Interfering Factors: in vitro hemolysis

Analyte	Age/Gender	Reference Range	SI Units	Note
Mean Corpuscular Volume	1–3 d	95–121	fl	
	6 m–2 y	70–86	fl	
	6 y–12 y	77–95	fl	
	12 y–18 y	78–100	fl	
	Adults	80–94	fl	

Mean Platelet Volume

(MPV) Mean platelet volume means an average single PLT volume. With intense thrombopoietin stimulation, higher ploidy megakaryocytes proportion increases. These megakaryocytes produce larger PLT and thus elevate the PLT volume. MPV varies with total PLT production.

Test Purpose. Information about thrombocytopoiesis activity.

Increased Values
megaloblastic anemia, **May-Hegglin anomaly**, diabetes mellitus with retinopathy, hyperthyroidism, prosthetic heart valve, splenectomy, rheumatic heart disease, diseases – (**myeloproliferative d., valvular heart d.**), disseminated intravascular coagulation, acute/chronic myelogenic leukemia, systemic lupus erythematosus, idiopathic thrombocytopenic purpura in remission, **Bernard-Soulier sy**, vasculitis, massive hemorrhage

Decreased Values
anemia – (**aplastic a.**, megaloblastic a.), **hypersplenism, chemotherapy-induced myelosuppression, Wiskott-Aldrich sy**

Analyte	Age/Gender	Reference Range	SI Units	Note
Mean Platele Volume		7.8–11.0	fl	

Methemalbumin

(syn: Fairley's pigment, methem, hematin) Residual hematin overlaps transport protein hemopexin capacity, binds temporarily to albumin, and creates in large RBC breakdown. Methemalbumin (hematin bound to serum albumin) is formed in plasma during intravascular hemolysis when haptoglobin is depleted. Free metheme may be bound to other transport conservation proteins, hemopexin and transported to the liver for further catabolism. Oxidized heme is bound to hemopexin or to albumin (methemalbumin). Complex with albumin is retained in kidney until hemopexin from liver hematin releases. Methemalbumin remains stable in the plasma until more hemopexin is synthesized to activate transport molecules; hemopexin binds hematin from methemalbumin complex. Therefore, methemalbumin is more indicative of a chronic intravascular hemolysis.

Test Purpose. Sensitive chronic intravascular hemolysis indicator.

Increased Values – methemalbuminemia
hemoglobinuria – (paroxysmal cold h. – PCH, paroxysmal nocturnal h. – PNH), intravascular hemolysis, hemolytic newborn disease, falciparum malaria, acute hemorrhagic pancreatitis, hemolytic posttransfusion reaction

Methemoglobin

(MHb, MetHb, syn: hemiglobin) Blood stain in which the heme ferrous iron form has been ferric oxidized; it is incapable of combining with and transporting oxygen (oxygen and iron cannot combine). Reverse hemoglobin binding can be done via two reduction systems: NADH-methemoglobin reductase and NADPH-reduced glutathione. Methemoglobin causes oxyhemoglobin dissociation curve shift to the left. When high MetHb concentration is produced in the RBC, it reduces the RBC capacity to combine with oxygen → anoxia and cyanosis result.

Test Purpose. 1) acquired hemolytic anemia differential diagnosis, 2) to investigate unexplained central cyanosis, 3) to assess possible oxidant drug hemolysis.

Increased Values – methemoglobinemia
NADH-MetHb reductase deficiency, paroxysmal hemoglobinuria, **HbM hemoglobinopathy**, black water fever, clostridial infection, poisoning by – (aminoaromatic derivatives, aniline, dyes, nitrobenzene), hereditary methemoglobinemia, radiation

> **Interfering Factors:** increased water/food nitrates, smoking, ionizing radiation, medicaments – (acetaminophen, acetanilid, amyl nitrite, benzocaine, chlorates, chloroquine, dapsone, isoniazid, isosorbide dinitrate, isosorbide mononitrate, lidocaine, local anesthetics, metoclopramide, nitrates, nitric oxide, nitrites, nitrofurantoin, nitroglycerin, nitroprusside, phenacetin, phenazone, phenazopyridine, phenytoin, potassium chlorate, prilocaine, primaquine, sulfamethoxazole, sulfasalazine, sulfonamides, trimethoprim)

Analyte	Age/Gender	Reference Range	SI Units	Note
Methemoglobin		9.3–37.2	µmol/l	
	Infants	0.004–0.0115		
	Children	<0.02		
	Adults	<0.008		
	Smokers	<0.02		

Monocytes

(mono, syn: monomorphonuclear monocytes) Belong to heterogenous leukocyte group, created in the bone marrow from common monocyte and granulocyte stem cells (CFU-GM). Monocytes are washed to blood stream → enter into tissue → change to free/bound macrophages → become MPS portion (mononuclear phagocytic system) → differentiate to specific tissue macrophages.

Function. Immunodefense cells, macrophage system → enter the tissues to become the macrophages (e.g. histiocytes, liver Kuppfer's cells, spleen and lymph node sinusoidal macrophages, peritoneal macrophages, macrophages that line the pulmonary air spaces). They are particularly active and evident in subacute/chronic inflammations. Kill/phagocytize/remove injured/dead cells, microorganisms, insoluble particles, antigens. By phagocytosed material breakdown to antigen peptides → surface monocyte receptors bind antigen peptides to HLA system molecules and expose them to T-lymphocytes. Monocytes interact with antigen-antibody-complement complexes to promote phagocytosis. Antiviral agent production – interferon. They are responsible for antigen recognition and processing → presenting to responsive T- and B-lymphocytes → participate in immune reactions (T-lymphocytes proliferation induction) → initiate both cell-mediated and humoral immune responses. Monocytes have an antitumorous activity. Participate in hemopoiesis (growth factors production – extrarenal erythropoietin, inhibition factors production – prostaglandins). They secrete various soluble, biologically active substances: enzymes – (lysozyme, neutral proteases, plasminogen activator, collagenase, elastase, angiotensin convertase), acid hydrolases – (lipases, ribonucleases, glycosidases, phosphatases), vitamin D, arachidonic acid metabolites, complement components – (C1, 2, 3, 4, 5, properdin), binding proteins – (transferrin, transcobalamin II, fibronectin), monokines (e.g. interleukin 1, 6, 8, 10, 12), IFN-alpha, IFN-beta, GM-CSF, M-CSF, G-CSF, TNF-alpha, PDGF, PAF, TGF-beta, angiogenesis factors, factors B, D, I, H, coagulation factors (V, VII, IX, X, prothrombin, thromboplastin). Ligands bound by macrophage surface receptors: a) opsonins – complement components (C3, C4), immunoglobulins, carbohydrates and carbohydrate-binding proteins, b) chemotactic factors – oligopeptides, complement components (C5a), thrombin, fibrin, c) hormones and other mediators – insulin, histamine, epinephrine, calcitonin, parathyroid hormone, somatomedins, d) growth factors and cytokines – colony-stimulating factors (GM-CSF, M-CSF), interleukins (IL-1, 3, 6, 10), interferons (alpha, beta, gamma), tumor necrosis factors, transforming growth factor beta, e) miscellaneous – transferrin, lactoferrin, modified low-density lipoproteins, fibronectin. Tissue/other macrophages: 1) lung macrophages (alveolar) → phagocytose and retain dust particles, 2) liver macrophages (Kuppfer cells) → phagocytose iron excess and bile stains, 3) spleen macrophages → phagocytose disintegrated RBCs, 4) connective tissue macrophages (histiocytes), 5) bone marrow macrophages/precursors, 6) skin and tissue macrophages, 7) lymph node macrophages, 8) CNS macrophages (microglia), 9) blood – monocytes, 10) synovium – type A synovial cells, 11) bone – osteoclasts, 12) pleural cavity – pleural macrophages, 13) chronic inflammatory exudate – exudate macrophages, 14) peritoneal cavity – peritoneal macrophages.

Increased Values – monocytosis, monocytic leukocytosis
anemia, arteritis temporalis, **rheumatoid arthritis, brucellosis, bacterial endocarditis**, hepatitis, malignant histiocytosis, cytomegalovirus infection, diseases – (collagen vascular d., **acute/chronic infectious d., viral infectious d., myeloproliferative d.**), myocardial infarction in remission, protozoal and rickettsial diseases – (kala-azar, malaria, toxoplasmosis, trypanosomiasis, epidemic typhus, Rocky Mountain spotted fever), inflammatory bowel disease, chemical poisoning, collagenoses, **colitis ulcerosa**, leprosy, leukemia – (**monocytic l.**, myeloid l., acute/chronic myelomonocytic l.), radiation therapy, **systemic lupus erythematosus**, lymphogranuloma, **infectious mononucleosis**, tumours – (**Hodgkin's lymphoma**, non-Hodgkin's lymphoma, mammary gland t., ovarian t., stomach t.), disease – (**Crohn's d.**, Gaucher's d., Niemann–Pick d.), chronic idiopathic neutropenia, myeloid metaplasia, newborn, parotitis, plasmocytoma (incl. multiple myeloma), **polyarteritis nodosa**, polycythemia vera, thrombocytopenic purpura, **salmonellosis, sarcoidosis, postsplenectomy conditions**, sprue, **syphilis, myelodysplastic sy, tuberculosis**, bone marrow suppression
  Interfering Factors: medicaments – (griseofulvin, prednisone)

Decreased Values – monocytopenia, monocytic leukopenia
anemia – (aplastic a., lymphocytic a.), acute infectious diseases, leukemia – (acute myelogenous l., **hairy cell l.**), stress
  Interfering Factors: medicaments – (glucocorticoids, glucose, immunosuppressives, prednisone)

Analyte	Age/Gender	Reference Range	SI Units	Note
Monocytes	Neonates	<8	%	
	Infants	<10	%	
	Adults	2–11	%	
		0.02–0.11		
		0.15–0.58	x 10⁹/l	

Neutrophil Alkaline Phosphatase

(LAP, NAP, syn: leukocyte alkaline phosphatase, combined esterase) A constituent in mature granulocyte granules.

Test Purpose. 1) to examine the alkaline phosphatase in neutrophils, 2) differential diagnosis of myeloproliferative diseases (chronic myelocytic leukemia versus leukemoid reaction), 3) helpful parameter in acute leukemia and paroxysmal nocturnal hemoglobinuria diagnosis, 4) to aid in the evaluation of polycythemia vera, myelofibrosis with myeloid metaplasia.

Increased Values

agranulocytosis, **aplastic anemia**, **liver cirrhosis**, cardiac cirrhosis, hairy cell leukemia, myeloproliferative diseases, bacterial infectious diseases, thrombocytopenia infections, **obstructive jaundice**, reactive leukocytosis, neutrophilia, acute/chronic lymphoblastic leukemia, **Hodgkin's disease**, **myelofibrosis**, myeloid metaplasia, plasmocytoma (incl. multiple myeloma), **polycythemia vera**, **leukemoid reactions**, conditions – (**postoperative c.**, **stress c.**), syndrome – (Down sy, Klinefelter's sy), **pregnancy**, essential thrombocytemia
 Interfering Factors: medicaments – (corticosteroids, oral contraceptives)

Decreased Values

anemia – (aplastic a., pernicious a., sickle cell a., sideroblastic a.), hepatic cirrhosis, diabetes mellitus, progressive muscular dystrophy, gout, granulocytopenia, **paroxysmal nocturnal hemoglobinuria**, **hereditary hypophosphatasia**, diseases – (infectious d., collagen d.), leukemia – (**acute/chronic granulocytic l.**, **acute monocytic l.**, **acute myeloblastic l.**, **chronic myelogenous l.**), infectious mononucleosis, **idiopathic thrombocytopenic purpura**, sarcoidosis, syndrome – (nephrotic sy, nephrotic sy), congestive heart failure

Analyte	Age/Gender	Reference Range	SI Units	Note
Neutrophil Alkaline Phosphatase		<0.02		See ref.
		0.16–0.83		ranges note

Neutrophils

(neu, Pans, Segos, Ploys, syn: segmented neutrophils, polymorphonuclear neutrophils) Neutrophils are cells belonging to the leukocyte group created in bone marrow. Their mother cell is GFU-GM. Neutrophil sticks alive in blood stream only few hours before returning to tissues → disintegration.

Function. Responsible for primary non-specific defense (with NK-cells) against microbial invasion through phagocytosis. They are equipped with specific properties: a) WBC adhesion to endothelium, b) movement and chemotaxia, c) phagocytosis and degranulation, d) microorganism killing. Neutrophils are acute inflammation cells and bear surface receptors for IgA, IgG and complement components. Neutrophil antimicrobial systems: low pH, lysozyme, lactoferrin, defensin, cathepsin G, peroxide, superoxide radical, hydroxyl radical, singlet oxygen, myeloperoxidase, defensin.

Test Purpose. 1) to aid in inflammatory processes and intoxication diagnosis, 2) myeloproliferative diseases differential diagnosis, 3) to aid in myocardial infarction diagnosis, 4) leukopenia differential diagnosis.

Increased Values – neutrophilia, neutrocytosis, neutrophilic leukocytosis

acidosis, anemia – (pernicious a., **acute posthemorrhagic/posthemolytic a.**), anoxia, appendicitis, **rheumatoid arthritis**, hepatic cirrhosis, dermatitis, diphtheria, diverticulitis, **gout**, eclampsia, endocarditis, exposure to extreme heat/cold, gangrene, **rheumatic fever**, diseases – (**myeloproliferative d.**, **inflammatory d.**), infectious diseases – (**bacterial i. d.**, **parasitic i. d.**, **fungal i. d.**, rickettsial i. d.), viral infectious diseases – (herpes zoster, poliomyelitis, chicken pox, smallpox), **myocardial infarction**, intoxication by – (arsenic, benzene, carbon monoxide, ethylene glycol, venoms, heavy metals, lead, mercury, turpentine), disseminated intravascular coagulation, **diabetic/uremic coma**, gonorrhea, leukemia – (granulocytic l., chronic myelogenic l., **myelocytic l.**), **elderly people**, myelosclerosis, **myositis**, tumours – (bone marrow t., lymphoma, melanoma, liver t., gastrointestinal tract t.), **physical exertion** (physical exercise), **newborn, neonates with Down sy**, osteomyelitis, otitis media, **polycythemia vera**, **burns**, ischemic damage to – (extremities, abdominal viscera, heart), hemolytic transfusion reactions, salpingitis, septicemia, conditions – (allergic c., **hemolytic c.**, hemorrhagic c., **c. after surgery**, shock c.), **stress, Cushing's sy, electric shock**, pregnancy, **primary thrombocytemia, thrombosis, miliary tuberculosis, thyroiditis**, thyrotoxicosis, **trauma**, uremia, **vasculitis**, vomiting, chronic morphine addiction

   Interfering Factors: medicaments – (ACTH, adrenaline, chlorpropamide, corticoids, cortisone, dexamethasone, digitalis, erythromycin, glucocorticoids, heparin, histamine, hydrocortisone, lithium, norepinephrine, potassium chlorate, prednisone, procainamide, quinidine, sulfonamides, vaccines)

Decreased Values – neutropenia, neutrophilic leukopenia

agranulocytosis, acromegaly, **AIDS, aleukia**, alcoholism, anemia – (**aplastic a., megaloblastic a., myelophthisic a., pernicious a., iron deficiency a.**), anorexia nervosa, apergillosis, autoimmune neutropenia, autoimmune panleukopenia, bone radiation therapy, rheumatoid arthritis, **brucellosis**, hepatic cirrhosis, **congenital dysgranulopoietic neutropenia**, copper deficiency, cytomegalovirus infection, familiary neutropenia – (**benign f. n., severe f. n.**), severe folic acid or vitamin B_{12} deficiency, erythropoietin administration in children, renal dialysis, **paroxysmal nocturnal hemoglobinuria**, chronic active hepatitis, **infectious hepatitis**, hepatitis – (type B, type E), histoplasmosis, hypersensitivity, hypersplenism, portal hypertension, hyperthyroidism, hypopituitarism, hypothyroidism, diseases – (endocrine d., **severe infectious d.**, blood d., liver d., protozoal d., **acute viral infectious d.**), **influenza**, insufficiency – (chronic pituitary adrenocortical i., chronic primary adrenocortical i.), intravenous immunoglobulins injection in children, kala-azar, **varicella** (chickenpox), toxic agents, leukemia – (**acute lymphoblastic l., monocytic l.**), **systemic lupus erythematosus, lymphomas, Addison's disease**, m. haemolyticus neonatorum, malaria, malnutrition, **mucormycosis**, myelokathexia, myelofibrosis, myelophthisis, **infectious mononucleosis**, neuroblastoma, **tumors/metastases, idiopathic neutropenia**, extracorporeal circulation (heartlung machines), **measles, newborn alloimmune neutropenia**, neutropenia associated with agammaglobulinemia linked to X-chromosome, neutropenia associated with LGL-leukemia, newborn asphyxia, paratyphoid, **mumps** (parotitis), extracorporeal oxygenation, parvoviruses infection, **pneumonia, poliomyelitis**, polyarteritis nodosa, pre-leukemia, pulmonary microcirculation disorders, **radiotherapy**, rickettsial infections, **rubella**, scleroderma, septic conditions, neonatal sepsis, **splenomegaly**, drug-induced marrow suppression – (allopurinol, aminopyrine, antibiotics, oral antidiabetics, antineoplastic drugs, nonsteroid antirheumatics, azathioprine, cimetidine, phenothiazines, phenylbutazone, phenytoin, chloramphenicol, chlorothiazides, ibuprofen, isoniazid, carbamazepine, co-trimoxazol, propylthiouracil, sulfasalazine, sulfonamides, tolbutamide, gold), syndrome – (Blackfan-Diamond sy, Felty's sy, Chediak-Higashi sy, **hyper-IgM sy**, lazy leukocytes sy, Pearson's sy, Schwachmann's sy), **anaphylactoid shock**, trypanosomiasis, **tuberculosis, tularemia**, thyrotoxicosis, **typhoid fever**, inborn error of amino acid metabolism

   Interfering Factors: medicaments – (acetaminophen, acetazolamide, acetylsalicylic acid, ajmaline, alemtuzumab, allopurinol, alprenolol, altretamine, amiloride, aminoglutethimide, aminophenazone, aminosalicylic acid, amiodarone, amoxicillin, ampicillin, aprindine, asparaginase, auranofin, azathioprine, benzylpenicillin, busulfan, candesartan, capecitabine, captopril, carbamazepine, carbenicillin, carbimazole, carboplatin, carmustine, cefaclor, cefadroxil, cefalexin, cefalotin, cefamandole, cefazolin, cefoperazone, cefotamine, cefotaxime, cefotetan, cefoxitin, cefprozil, cefradine, ceftazidime, ceftizoxime, ceftriaxone, cefuroxime, cephalosporins, chlorambucil, chloramphenicol, chlordiazepoxide, chloroquine, chlorothiazide, chlorpromazine, chlorpropamide, chlortalidone, cidofovir, cimetidine, cisplatin, cladribine, clindamycin, clomipramine, cloxacillin, clozapine, cyclophosphamide, cytarabine, dacarbazine, dactinomycin, dapsone, daunorubicin, demeclocycline, desipramine, diazepam, diazoxide, dicloxacillin, didanosine, diltiazem, diphenylhydantoin, disopyramide, docetaxel, doxorubicin, doxycycline, enalapril, epirubicin, ethacrynic acid, ethosuximide, etoposide, fenoprofen, floxuridine, flucytosine, fludarabine, fluorouracil, fluphenazine, fomivirsen, foscarnet, fosphenytoin, furosemide, ganciclovir, gemcitabine, gemtuzumab, gentamicin, gold salts, griseofulvin, haloperidol, hydralazine, hydrochlorothiazide, hydroxychloroquine, hydroxyurea, ibuprofen, idarubicin, ifosfamide, imipenem, imipramine, indomethacin, interferon alfa-2a, interferon alfa-2b, interferon alfa-n1, interferon beta-1b, interferon gamma-1b, irinotecan, isoniazid, isotretinoin, itraconazole, lamivudine, lansoprazole, levamisole, levetiracetam, levodopa, lincomycin, lomustine, mebendazole, mechlorethamine, melphalan, meprobamate, mercaptopurine, metamizole, methazolamide, methimazole, methotrexate, methysergide, meticillin, metronidazole, methyldopa, methylthiouracil, mezlocillin, minocycline, mirtazapine, mitomycin, mitoxantrone, mycophenolate, nafcillin, naproxen, nevirapine, nitrofurantoin, novobiocin, olanzapine, omeprazole, oxacillin, oxyphenbutazone, paclitaxel, paracetamol, penicillamine, penicillins, pentazocine, pentazoline, pentostatin, perindopril, phenacemide, phenacetin, phenazone, phenothiazines, phenylbutazone, phenytoin, piperacillin, plicamycin, primidone, procainamide, procarbazine, prochlorperazine, promazine, propranolol, propylthiouracil, pyrimethamine, quinidine, quinine, ranitidine, retinol, rifabutin, rifampicin, rifapentine, rituximab, saquinavir, spironolactone, stavudine, streptomycin, streptozocin, strontium-89, sulfafurazole, sulfamethoxazole, sulfapyridine, sulfasalazine, sulfathiazole, sulfisoxazole, sulfonamides, sulindac, tamoxifen, temozolomide, teniposide, terbinafine, tetracyclines, thalidomide, thiamazole, thiamphenicol, thiazides, thiethylperazine, thioridazine, thiotepa, ticlopidine, tocainide, tolbutamide, topotecan, trandolapril, trimethadione, trimethoprim, trimetrexate, valrubicin, vancomycin, vinblastine, vinorelbine, zalcitabine, zidovudine, zinc salts, zomepirac)

Analyte	Age/Gender	Reference Range	SI Units	Note
Granulocytes				
neutrophilic sticks	Adults	3–5	%	
		0.03–0.05		
		0.6–1.2	x 10⁹/l	
neutrophilic g.	Neonates	<65	%	
	Infants	<25	%	
	Adults	47–79	%	
	Adults	0.47–0.79		
		2.5–5.6	x 10⁹/l	

Osmotic Resistance of Erythrocytes

(OF, syn: osmotic fragility, red cell fragility, erythrocyte fragility) The osmotic fragility test measures the susceptibility or RBC resistance to osmotic stress. By exposing erythrocytes to a hypotonic sodium chloride solution → the cell swells → erythrocytes rupture → hemolysis. Spherocytic RBCs, with a decreased surface-to-volume ratio, have a limited capacity to expand in hypotonic solutions, and thus lyse at a lesser osmotic stress level than do normal biconcave RBCs. Conversely, target cells, with a high surface to volume ratio, have an increased capacity to expand in hypotonic solutions, and have decreased susceptibility to osmotic lysis. Erythrocytes which burst in higher salt concentration have higher fragility; those that burst in lower salt concentration have decreased fragility. In healthy persons, unincubated blood RBC hemolysis begins at 0.45–0.50% sodium chloride and is complete by 0.35 % sodium chloride.

Test Purpose. 1) to aid in hereditary spherocytosis diagnosis, 2) to supplement stained cell examination to detect morphologic red cell abnormalities, 3) to evaluate hemolytic anemia and immune hemolytic conditions.

Increased osmotic resistance – decreased fragility, low fragility (<0.3% NaCl)
anemia – (**sickle-cell a., thalassemia, iron deficiency a.**, megaloblastic a.), **hemoglobinopathies, liver diseases, obstructive icterus**, leptocytosis associated with – (iron deficiency anemia, asplenia, liver diseases, reticulocytosis), early infancy, polycythemia vera, **splenectomy**

Decreased osmotic resistance – increased fragility, high fragility (>0.5% NaCl)
anemia – (**autoimmune hemolytic a.**, familial hemolytic a., **acquired hemolytic a., hereditary spherocytosis**), liver cirrhosis, infectious diseases – (malaria, syphilis, tuberculosis), severe pyruvate kinase deficiency, hereditary elliptocytosis, hemolytic newborn disease (erythroblastosis fetalis), hemolytic disease caused by Rh incompatibility, hemolytic icterus, **chemical/drug poisoning**, malignant lymphoma, leukemia, pregnancy, tumors, **burns**

Analyte	Age/Gender	Reference Range	SI Units	Note
Osmotic Resistance of Erythrocytes				
In 20 °C	Min	0.44–0.40		
	Max	0.32–0.30		
In 37 °C	Min	0.75–0.70		
	Max	0.40–0.30		

Pancytopenia

All blood cell counts decrease (red blood cells, white blood cells, platelets). Pancytopenia evaluation is used in bone marrow suppression differential diagnosis (aplastic anemia, myelodysplastic sy), pernicious anemia, osteomyelofibrosis and immunity disorders.

■ **Central causes:** anemia – (**aplastic a., megaloblastic a.**), vitamin B_{12}/folate deficiency, viral hepatitis, cytomegalovirus infection, infectious diseases, Epstein–Barr virus infection, primary bone marrow infiltration, medicaments – (chemotherapeutics, chloramphenicol, phenylbutazone), leukemia – (**acute l.**, hairy cell l.), lymphomas, Hodgkin's disease, **myelofibrosis** (myelosclerosis), tumours, **plasmocytoma** (incl. multiple myeloma), osteopetrosis, parvoviruses, irradiation, **myelodysplastic syndrome**, tuberculosis, bone marrow inhibition

■ **Peripheral causes:** AIDS, anorexia nervosa, rheumatoid arthritis, hepatic cirrhosis, hemodilution, **paroxysmal nocturnal hemoglobinuria**, hypersplenism, autoimmune diseases, kala-azar, chronic myelogenic leukemia, **systemic lupus erythematosus**, malaria, infectious mononucleosis, **Gaucher's disease**, Niemann–Pick disease, tumors, splenic/portal vein obstruction, Felty's sy, elevated right-sided heart pressure, tuberculosis

---

Partial Thromboplastin Time

(PTT, APTT, syn: activated partial thromboplastin time) APTT informs about intrinsic/common hemocoagulation activation pathway plasmatic factors initiated by negatively charged surface factor XII interaction. PTT evaluates factors I, II, V, VIII, IX, X, XI, XII, prekallikrein and high-molecular weight kininogen. Factor VII is not required for the PTT because it bypasses the extrinsic system. Sensitive screening test for internal (intrinsic) coagulation system and stage II clotting mechanism disorder detection. This test is performed on a citrated blood specimen. The PTT is more sensitive for detecting minor common pathway deficiencies than the prothrombin time.

Test Purpose. 1) to aid in preoperative screening of bleeding tendencies, 2) to screen for congenital/acquired coagulation deficiencies (clotting factors VIII, IX, X, XI, XII, prekallikrein and high molecular weight kininogen), 3) to monitor heparin therapy, 4) to screen for factor VIII, IX, XI inhibitors, 5) to determine lupus anticoagulant presence, 6) disseminated intravascular coagulation diagnosis, 7) differential diagnosis of thrombotic complications, 8) to detect classical hemophilia A, 9) to detect the presence of dysfibrinogenemia, liver failure, congenital hypofibrinogenemia.

Increased Values – prolonged PTT

amyloidosis, pyogenic liver abscess, **lupus anticoagulant, rheumatoid arthritis, liver cirrhosis**, primary/secondary biliary cirrhosis, chronic glomerulonephritis, **dysfibrinogenemia**, coagulant factors defects/deficiency – (prekallikrein, II, V, VIII, IX, X, XI, XII), **vitamin K deficiency**, glycogen storage disease – (type IV, VI), hemophilia – (**A, B**), hemochromatosis – (secondary h., idiopathic h.), **hyperfibrinolysis, hypofibrinogenemia, liver diseases**, hepatic coma, **disseminated intravascular coagulation**, leishmaniasis, **leukemia**, drug induced lupus erythematosus, systemic lupus erythematosus, malabsorption, malaria, disease – (**von Willebrand's d.**, Wilson's d.), fatty liver, drug reactions, hemorrhagic shock, syndrome – (Reye's sy, hepatorenal sy), massive blood transfusion, repeated plasma transfusions, tuberculosis, liver failure, congenital deficiency of Fitzgerald factor and high molecular weight kininogen, fibrin degradation products, typhoid fever, intoxication by – (**acetaminophen, coumarin, heparin**)

Interfering Factors: lipemia, positive rheumatoid factor, medicaments – (acetaminophen, antihistamines, anistreplase, argatroban, ascorbic acid, asparaginase, azlocillin, chlorpromazine, digitalis, heparin, oral anticoagulants, penicillin, phenothiazines, phenytoin, protamine, salicylates, tetracyclines, thrombolytics, valproic acid, warfarin)

Decreased Values – shortened PTT

early stage of disseminated intravascular coagulation, acute hemorrhage, polycythemia vera, **tumours**

Interfering Factors: medicaments – (oral contraceptives)

Analyte	Age/Gender	Reference Range	SI Units	Note
Partial Thromboplastin Time				
standard		60–85	s	
Activated Partial Thromboplastin Time (APTT)	Children	<90	s	
	Adults	25–35	s	

Phagocytes

Function. 1) chemotaxis, 2) phagocytosis – (direct, mediated by opsonines), 3) killing – (intracellular – non/dependent, extracellular – direct, mediated by antibody), 4) secretion – (monokines – IL-1, TNF-2).

Neutrophils, eosinophils, basophils, monocytes, tissue macrophages – (Kupffer's hepatic cells, alveolar macrophages, neuroglia).

Analyte	Age/Gender	Reference Range	SI Units	Note
Phagocytosis (NBT-test)	spontaneous ph.	0.60–0.80		
	stimulated ph.	0.80–1.00		

Phosphofructokinase in RBC

(PFK) Enzyme involved in RBC metabolism (anaerobic glycolysis) with fructose-6-phosphate to fructose-1,6-diphosphate change.

Test Purpose. RBC metabolic disorders and hemolytic anemias differential diagnosis.

Decreased Values
severe muscle dysfunction (type VII glycogen storage disease)

Plasmatic Coagulation Factors

Protein character factors involved in blood coagulation in the 2nd (plasmatic) coagulation phase, functioning as enzymes after activation.

■ Factor I
(syn: fibrinogen, F I). See fibrinogen.

■ Factor II
(F II, syn: prothrombin) Glycoprotein (alpha-1-globulin), vitamin K dependent, serine protease, when activated by catalytic prothrombin complex action (enzyme factor Xa, Va, Ca^{2+}, PF3, phospholipid tissue thromboplastin component) → thrombin (enzyme) production. Besides main substrate fibrinogen later thrombin activates factor V, VIII, XIII and platelets. Thrombin changes fibrinogen to fibrin. It adsorbs to $Al(OH)_3$, $BaSO_4$, $Ca_3(PO_4)_2$.

Production. Hepatocyte in liver reticuloendothelial system. Retains its potency in stored blood or plasma and remains in serum in trace amounts after plasma clotting.

Test Purpose. 1) differential diagnosis of thrombophilic conditions, 2) to aid in hepatic lesion stage assessment.

Increased Values – hyperprothrombinemia
hypercoagulation conditions
>**Interfering Factors:** medicaments – (estrogens, oral contraceptives)

Decreased Values – hypoprothrombinemia
vitamin K impaired absorption, anemia – (aplastic a., pernicious a.), lupus anticoagulant, **congenital deficiency of factor II, vitamin K deficiency,** gastrocolic fistula, gastroenteritis, **hereditary hypoprothrombinemia, liver diseases,** leucemia, newborns, biliary ducts obstruction, plasmocytoma, hepatic parenchyma injury, fat malabsorption, liver cirrhosis
>**Interfering Factors:** medicaments – (anabolic steroids, androgens, antibiotics, coumarin anticoagulants, heparin, latamoxef, paracetamol, salicylates, warfarin)

Analyte	Age/Gender	Reference Range	SI Units	Note
factor II		<100	mg/l	
		0.7–1.2		
		70–120	%	
		0.6–1.40	µmol/l	
		0.5–1.5	kU/l	
		60–150	AU	

- **Factor III**
  (F III, syn: tissue factor, thrombokinase, tissue thromboplastin) External coagulation way factor, injured tissue product (co-factor), with two components: a) lipoprotein component (tissue factor) for thrombin activation by F VII to VIIa activation, b) phospholipid component (tissue phospholipid), a prothrombinase complex component in the prothrombin to thrombin change. Clotting pathway: extrinsic system only.

Production. Thromboplastic activity in most tissues, especially active tissues are brain, lung and placenta.

- **Factor IV**
  (F IV, syn: calcium ions)

Function. Factor IX and X co-factor. Calcium ions are involved in hemostasis as a coagulation factor activation co-factor in all coagulation cascade stages except contact phase and fibrinogen to fibrin change. They are not in stabilized plasma, but are in serum. They are involved in the prothrombin to thrombin change. Anticoagulants (citrate, oxalate, ethylene diaminetetraacetic acid – EDTA) chelate calcium and anticoagulate blood, thus calcium is unable to participate in coagulation. See also blood calcium.

- **Factor V**
  (F V, syn: proaccelerin, platelet phospholipids and calcium ions, unstable factor, labile factor, Ac globulin, plasma accelerator globulin) Factor V is a glycoprotein.

Function. Activated proaccelerin form is a factor Xa co-factor, involved in the prothrombin to thrombin change. Platelet factor V is present in granules of platelets and is necessary to the binding of Xa to the platelet surface. Activated factor V–Va is a prothrombin converting complex component; proaccelerin is labile. It is involved in plasmin activation. The molecular characterization of Va, in particular identification of the structural determinants responsible for accelearation of prothrombin activation and those that bind to phospholipid surfaces have been described.

Production. Liver – hepatocytes, megakaryocytes, reticuloendothelial system histiocytes. F V is converted in the plasma from a single chain to a two chain molecule under the influence of thrombin activation. Activity is destroyed during coagulation process. F V is absent in serum.

Increased Values – hyperproaccelerinemia
    Interfering Factors: medicaments – (antiepileptics, estrogens, oral contraceptives)

Decreased Values – hypoproaccelerinemia
lupus anticoagulant, **congenital factor V deficiency, hereditary hypoproaccelerinemia, liver diseases, disseminated intravascular coagulation** (DIC), massive blood transfusion, liver cirrhosis, primary fibrinolysis
    Interfering Factors: medicaments – (anabolic steroids, androgens, antibiotics, asparaginase, dextran, heparin, methyltestosterone, salicylates)

Analyte	Age/Gender	Reference Range	SI Units	Note
factor V		<10	mg/l	
		0.7–1.2		
		70–120	%	
		0.6–1.40	μmol/l	
		0.5–2.0	kU/l	
		60–150	AU	

■ **Factor VII**
    (F VII, SPCA, syn: proconvertin, coenzyme, proconvertin stable factor, autoprothrombin I, serum prothrombin conversion accelerator) Vitamin K dependent glycoprotein, serine protease, external coagulation pathway factor, the only factor in factor X activation. Factor VII is directly activated by tissue thromboplastin lipoprotein component to VIIa. Active F VIIa form is a F X to F Xa change and F IX to F IXa catalyst. Clotting pathway: extrinsic system only.
    Production. Liver – hepatocytes. Retains its potency in stored stabilized blood or plasma and remains present in serum after plasma has clotted. It adsorbs to $Al(OH)_3$, $BaSO_4$, $Ca_3(PO_4)_2$. It is the first clotting factor decreasing after vitamin K antagonists administration, e.g. oral anticoagulants.
    Test Purpose. 1) differential diagnosis of inborn/acquired hypoproconvertinemia, 2) aids in liver dysfunction assessment and vitamin K deficiency.

Increased Values – hyperproconvertinemia
atherosclerosis
    Interfering Factors: medicaments – (estrogens, oral contraceptives)

Decreased Values – hypoproconvertinemia
lupus anticoagulant, deficiency – (**congenital factor VII d., vitamin K d.**), **hemorrhagic newborn disease, liver diseases, kwashiorkor,** fat malabsorption
    Interfering Factors: medicaments – (acetylsalicylic acid, anabolic steroids, androgens, antibiotics, coumarin anticoagulants, dextran, heparin, latamoxef, methyltestosterone, paracetamol, salicylates, tocopherol, warfarin)

Analyte	Age/Gender	Reference Range	SI Units	Note
factor VII		<0.5	mg/l	
		0.7–1.3		
		70–130	%	
		0.7–1.30	μmol/l	
		65–135	AU	

Factor VIII

(F VIII, AHG A, AHF A, syn: antihemophilic globulin A, antihemophilic factor A) Factor X and Xa activation co-factor by factor IXa. Clotting pathway: intrinsic system only. Factor VIII is an acute-phase reactant. Factor VIII deficiency is the most common hereditary bleeding disorder.

Production. Possibly liver – hepatocytes, possibly endothelial cells and megakaryocytes. Activity destroyed during coagulation process. Absent in serum; F VIII is labile, disappearing fairly rapidly from refrigerated plasma.

Test Purpose. Differential diagnosis of inborn/acquired hemorrhagic disorders.

Increased Values
atherosclerotic vascular disease, **congenital factor VIII deficiency, hyperthyroidism,** hypoglycemia, disease – (**coronary heart d., thromboembolic d.**), disseminated intravascular coagulation, diseases – (liver d., **acute inflammatory d.**), **macroglobulinemia, plasmocytoma** (incl. multiple myeloma), secondary fibrinolysis, **sudden coumarin therapy cessation, postoperative states,** Cushing's sy, **pregnancy** (3rd trimester), acute deep venous thrombosis

> Interfering Factors: medicaments – (epinephrine, oral contraceptives)

Decreased Values
lupus anticoagulant, **hemophilia A,** disseminated intravascular coagulation, **von Willebrand's disease, antibodies to factor VIII,** massive blood transfusion

> Interfering Factors: plasminogen activators, medicaments – (heparin, streptokinase)

Analyte	Age/Gender	Reference Range	SI Units	Note
factor VIII		<0.15	mg/l	
		0.6–1.5		
		60–150	%	
		0.5–2.0	μmol/l	
		60–145	AU	
factor VIII antigen		0.7–1.5		
		50–200	AU	

Factor IX

(F IX, syn: Christmas factor, antihemophilic globulin B – AHG B, antihemophilic factor B – AHF B, plasma thromboplastin component – PTC, autoprothrombin II, Christmas disease factor) Serine protease, vitamin K dependent single chain glycoprotein, a coagulation protein. It is about 18% carbohydrate, its complete amino acid sequence has been determined. Factor IX is activated to the F IXa by F XIa, tissue factor substance and calcium. Active F IXa form catalyzes F X to F Xa with F VIIIa as a co-factor. Clotting pathway: intrinsic system only.

Production. Liver – hepatocytes. Retains its potency in stored blood or plasma and remains in serum after the plasma has clotted; it is stable and adsorbable.

Test Purpose. 1) differential diagnosis of inborn/acquired hemorrhagic diseases, 2) liver dysfunction condition assessment.

Increased Values
> Interfering Factors: medicaments – (epinephrine, estrogens, oral contraceptives)

Decreased Values
congenital deficiency of factor IX, lupus anticoagulant, **decompensated hepatic cirrhosis, vitamin K deficiency, hemophilia B,** liver diseases, Gaucher's disease, **newborns, nephrotic sy,** fat malabsorption

> **Interfering Factors:** plasminogen activators, medicaments – (dextran, dicumarol, heparin, streptokinase, tocopherol, warfarin)

Analyte	Age/Gender	Reference Range	SI Units	Note
factor IX		<4	mg/l	
		0.6–1.5		
		60–150	%	
		0.6–1.40	μmol/l	
		60–140	AU	

■ **Factor X**
(F X, syn: Stuart–Prower factor, Stuart factor) Stable protease, vitamin K dependent glycoprotein. Its active form F Xa is directly involved in prothrombin (II) to thrombin (IIa) change with F Va, Ca^{2+} and PF 3 as co-factors. F X is involved in F VII to F VIIa change. Common coagulation pathway factor.
Production. Liver – hepatocytes. Retains potency in stabilized stored blood or plasma and remains in serum after plasma has clotted; it is adsorbable.
Test Purpose. 1) low-molecular weight heparin therapy monitoring, 2) differential diagnosis of hemorrhagic diathesis.

Increased Values
pregnancy

> **Interfering Factors:** medicaments – (antiepileptics, estrogens, oral contraceptives)

Decreased Values
lupus anticoagulant, **congenital factor X deficiency,** fat malabsorption, liver disease, vitamin K deficiency

> **Interfering Factors:** medicaments – (anabolic steroids, androgens, antibiotics, heparin, methyltestosterone, salicylates, tocopherol, warfarin)

Analyte	Age/Gender	Reference Range	SI Units	Note
factor X		<10	mg/l	
		0.7–1.3		
		70–130	%	
		0.7–1.30	μmol/l	
		60–130	AU	

■ **Factor XI**
(F XI, syn: Rosenthal's factor, plasma thromboplastin antecedent – PTA, antihemophilic factor C – AHF C) Plasmatic thromboplastin precursor, serine protease, a coagulation glycoprotein. Circulates in the plasma as a dimer, the two chains are held by disulfide bonds. Factor XI (to XIa) is activated by factor XIIa and the dimer is broken into two chains. Activation of F XI requires surfaces (usually phospholipid) and presence of prekallikrein and HMWK. Structural organization of the complete factor XI gene has been described. Activated form F XIa is involved with F VIIa in F IX to F IXa change. Clotting pathway: intrinsic system only.

Production. Liver – hepatocytes. Present in serum.
Test Purpose. 1) differential diagnosis of hemorhagic conditions, 2) F XI deficiency diagnosis.

Increased Values
Interfering Factors: medicaments – (epinephrine, oral contraceptives)

Decreased Values
lupus anticoagulant, **congenital factor XI deficiency**, **paroxysmal nocturnal hemoglobinuria**, diseases – (**liver d.**, **congenital heart d.**), **intestinal vitamin K malabsorption**, newborns
Interfering Factors: plasminogen activators, medicaments – (dextran, heparin, streptokinase)

Analyte	Age/Gender	Reference Range	SI Units	Note
factor XI		2–7	mg/l	
		0.6–1.4		
		60–140	%	
		0.6–1.40	µmol/l	
		65–135	AU	

■ **Factor XII**
(F XII, syn: Hageman's factor, factor of contact, contact factor) Plasmatic coagulation factor, serine protease which can be activated via active surfaces (in vivo: exposed subendothelium, activated platelet surface, some fatty acids, bacterial endotoxin, in vitro: a) glass, caolin, b) proteolytic activation – plasmin, kallikrein, trypsin). F XII to F XIIa activation starts F XI to F XIa change and gradual step-activation of other plasmatic factors; so-called intrinsic clotting pathway. Factor XII is the first protein adsorbed to negatively charged surfaces (collagen fibers, platelet membranes and other tissue surfaces) after endothelial damage. With XII to XIIa activation (by kallikrein), there is interaction with prekallikrein, HMWK and XIIa fragments in a complex circular reinforcement loop where activation also occurs in fibrinolytic system (plasminogen), complement system (C1), and vasoactive system (kinin pathway, HMWK to bradykinin activation). Clotting pathway: intrinsic system only.
Production. Liver – hepatocytes. Present in serum.
Test Purpose. 1) differential diagnosis of hemorrhagic diathesis and thrombotic conditions, 2) to identify F XII defect.

Increased Values
physical exercise
Interfering Factors: medicaments – (epinephrine, oral contraceptives)

Decreased Values
lupus anticoagulant, **congenital factor XII deficiency**, newborns, thrombophilic states, **nephrotic sy**, pregnancy
Interfering Factors: plasminogen activators, medicaments – (captopril, heparin, streptokinase)

Analyte	Age/Gender	Reference Range	SI Units	Note
factor XII		27–45	mg/l	
		0.6–1.4		
		60–140	%	

Analyte	Age/Gender	Reference Range	SI Units	Note
		0.6–1.40	µmol/l	
		65–150	AU	

■ **Factor XIII**

(F XIII, FSF, syn: fibrin stabilizing factor, fibrinoligase, Laki-Lorand factor) Transglutaminase. Activated factor XIII (by thrombin) stabilizes fibrin unstable monomer conversion to polymerized fibrin and a fibrin coagulum (in calcium presence, it causes covalent fibrin gamma-chain molecule cross-linkage → stable insoluble definite clot, making it resistant to the lytic action of plasmin). Factor XIII also promotes the cross-linking of alpha-2-antiplasmin to fibrin, increasing the resistance to fibrin degradation.

Production. Liver – hepatocyte, megakaryocytes or platelets. Activity destroyed during coagulation process. F XIII is stable in stabilized plasma; only a small rest remains in serum.

Test Purpose. 1) screening test for F XIII decreased values, 2) differential diagnosis of hemorrhagic diathesis, 3) to aid in keloid scar creation differentiation and wound healing disorders, 4) F XIII deficiency identification.

Decreased Values

agammaglobulinemia, anemia – (sickle cell a., pernicious a.), hyperfibrinogenemia, liver diseases, lead poisoning, plasmocytoma, Henoch-Schönlein purpura, postoperative states, pregnancy

Analyte	Age/Gender	Reference Range	SI Units	Note
factor XIII (fibrin stabilizing factor)		<10	mg/l	
		0.6–1.5		
		60–150	%	
		20–50	U/l	
		1–2	AU	

■ **Plasmatic Prekallikrein**

(syn: Fletcher's factor, prekallikrein assay) Serine protease that functions as factor XIIa co-factor in F XI to F XIa activation during the contact coagulation cascade phase. Prekallikrein is a coagulation protein involved in the bradykinin generation (vasoactive peptide) and one of the major factors required for contact activation (others are Hageman's factor and high-molecular weight kininogen). Clotting pathway: intrinsic system only. Fletcher's factor deficiency is associated with a clotting defect without bleeding. This factor is normally deficient in newborns.

Production. Liver.

Decreased Values

hereditary prekallikrein deficiency, severe liver diseases, nephrotic sy, uremia

Analyte	Age/Gender	Reference Range	SI Units	Note
prekallikrein		<50	mg/l	

■ **High-molecular Weight Kininogen**

(HMW-K, syn: Williams-Fitzgerald-Flaujeace factor) Plasmatic kininogen, contact factor, co-factor. It functions as factor XIIa co-factor in F XI to F XIa activation during the contact phase in coagulation cascade. HMWK is a protein required for bradykinin generation (a vasoactive peptide). Clotting pathway: intrinsic system only.

Production. Liver.

Decreased Values
hereditary HMW-K deficiency, acute myocardial infarction

Analyte	Age/Gender	Reference Range	SI Units	Note
High-Molecular Weight Kininogen		<60	mg/ml	

Plasmin

(syn: fibrinolysin) Plasmin is an effector fibrinolytic system enzyme; plasmin functions in fibrinolysis and fibrinogenolysis as well as in activated complement cascade. Plasmin inhibitors include: A2MG, alpha-2 plasmin inhibitor, AAT, antithrombin III.
Test Purpose. 1) plasmin deficiency identification, 2) fibrinolysis disorders differential diagnosis.

Increased Values
metastatic prostatic tumors, **intrauterine fetal death**
    Interfering Factors: medicaments – (oral contraceptives)

Plasminogen

(PMG, Pgn, syn: profibrinolysin) PMG is beta-2-globulin converted to plasmin by plasminogen activators (tPA, uPA).
Function. Plasminogen is inactive plasmin precursor having the ability to dissolve formed fibrin clots (fibrinolysis), fibrinogen, fibrin monomers, and factor II. It is useful parameter during streptokinase therapy; activates factor XII, factor VII, and induces platelet aggregation.
Test Purpose. 1) to assess fibrinolysis, 2) to detect congenital/acquired fibrinolytic disorders, 3) to monitor thrombolytic therapy, 4) to evaluate DIC.

Increased Values
exercise, **eclampsia**, inflammatory diseases, metastatic prostatic tumors, **intrauterine fetal death**, **pregnancy** (3rd trimester), arterial/venous clotting
    Interfering Factors: medicaments – (anabolic steroids, estrogens, ethanol, oral contraceptives)

Decreased Values
primary fibrinolysis, diabetic patients with thrombosis, Behcet's disease, liver cirrhosis, congenital deficiency of plasminogen, premature neonates, newborns, neonatal hyaline membrane disease, **liver diseases**, **disseminated intravascular coagulation** (DIC), pre/eclampsia, **hyperfibrinolytic states**
    Interfering Factors: medicaments – (streptokinase, urokinase)

Analyte	Age/Gender	Reference Range	SI Units	Note
Plasminogen		0.8–1.50		
		80–150	%	
		0.06–0.25	g/l	

Plasminogen Activator Inhibitor

(PAI, tPAi) Single chain plasma glycoprotein produced by different cells (endothelial cells, hepatocytes, fibroblasts), PAI-1 is stored in endothelial cells and platelet alpha-granules. It plays an important role in fibrinolysis regulation. It is a potent tissue-type (tPA) plasminogen activator inhibitor and urokinase/urokinase-type (uPA) plasminogen activator by stechiometric complex creation. PAI functions as a serine protease inhibitor and acute phase reactant. PAI-2 is synthesized by macrophages. Higher values are in the morning.

Test Purpose. 1) to evaluate deep vein thrombosis, myocardial infarction and postoperative thrombosis risk, 2) non-specific endothelial cell injury indicator.

Increased Values
atherosclerosis, diabetes mellitus, embolism, hyperlipoproteinemia, hypertriacylglycerolemia, disease – (**coronary artery d.**, hypertonic d.), infectious diseases, liver diseases, **myocardial infarction, tumors**, obesity, sepsis, **after surgery conditions**, preeclampsia, trauma, pregnancy (3rd trimester), **deep vein thrombosis**
   Interfering Factors: pregnancy

Decreased Values
inborn PAI-1 deficiency connected with bleeding conditions
   Interfering Factors: medicaments – (anabolic steroids)

Analyte	Age/Gender	Reference Range	SI Units	Note
Plasminogen Activator Inhibitor		<10	AU/ml	
		0.6–3.5	U/ml	

Plasmocytes

Plasmocytes are differentiated secretory lymphocytic B-stem cells which originate in lymphocyte with antigen contact.

Function. Antibody secretion in immune body response.

Test Purpose. 1) differential diagnosis of reactive plasmocytoses, 2) generalized plasmocytoma identification.

Increased Values – plasmocytosis
aplastic anemia, bone marrow aplasia, rheumatoid arthritis, liver cirrhosis, diseases – (acute/chronic infectious d., chronic renal d., liver d.), leukemia – (**plasma-cell l.**, chronic lymphytic l.), Hodgkin's disease, systemic lupus erythematosus, malaria, infectious mononucleosis, benign lymphocytic meningitis, rubella, measles, tumours – (liver t., kidney t., breast t., prostate t.), **plasmocytoma** (incl. multiple myeloma), rheumatism, syphilis, trichinosis, **tuberculosis**, varicella

Decreased Values – plasmocytopenia
inborn/acquired immunoglobulin decrease

Analyte	Age/Gender	Reference Range	SI Units	Note
Plasmocytes	Neonates	<0.25	%	
	Infants	<0.5	%	

Platelet-Activating Factor

(PAF) Allergic reaction mediator.

Production. Neutrophils, eosinophils, basophils, mast cells, monocytes, platelets, endothelial cells, renal medullary epithelial cells, glomerular mesangial cells.

Function. Platelet activation, amine secretion, neutrophil activation, enzyme release, prostaglandins and thromboxanes production by platelets. Increases vascular permeability and plasma extravasation. Mimics physiological and intravascular IgE-mediated human systemic anaphylaxis sequelae. Potent eosinophils/neutrophils chemotactic attraction/activation. Prolongs increase in bronchial hyperresponsiveness (bronchoconstriction). Hypotension, decreased cardiac output, vasoconstriction. Arachidonic acid release and eicosanoid production. Host cells and tissues damage.

Increased Values
atherosclerosis

Platelet Adhesion

(syn: platelet adhesiveness, platelet retention) Platelet are able to adhere to the damaged vessel surface, vascular wall collagen, through subendothelial structures (collagen is the most potent adhesion activator), physical factors (blood viscosity, platelet count, blood flow speed), plasmatic proteins (von Willebrand's factor is the most important) and platelet activation. Platelet adhesion is the first step of primary hemostatic plug production.

Test Purpose. 1) to evaluate platelet function, 2) to aid in von Willebrand's disease, Glanzmann's thrombasthenia, Bernard–Soulier syndrome diagnosis.

Increased Values
atherosclerosis, **diabetes mellitus**, homocystinuria, hyperfibrinogenemia, hyperlipidemia, ischemic heart disease, acute infections, increased factor VII levels, tumours, burns, sclerosis multiplex, after surgery, trauma

> **Interfering Factors:** elder people, diurnal variations, physical exertion, medicaments – (oral contraceptives)

Decreased Values
platelet defects, glycogenoses (glycogen storage disease), diseases – (myeloproliferative d., congenital heart d.), **von Willebrand's disease, Bernard-Soulier sy, Glanzmann's thrombasthenia**, uremia

> **Interfering Factors:** medicaments – (acetylsalicylic acid)

Analyte	Age/Gender	Reference Range	SI Units	Note
Platelet Adhesion		44.5–53.5		See ref.
		27.4–36.6		ranges note

Platelet Aggregation

Platelet aggregation and sticking is an important step in primary hemostatic plug production with acute blood vessel endothelium damage. Reciprocal platelet aggregation binding is mediated preferably by fibrinogen, which creates the linkage between neighbouring platelet membranes by receptor connection place created by specific membrane glycoproteins complex (GP IIb, GP IIIa). Many factors are involved in aggregation, e.g. thromboxane (TXA2), thrombin, epinephrine, platelet activating factor (PAF), collagen, arachidonic acid, ADP. Platelets have surface-binding sites for adenosine diphosphate (ADP), a natural biologically active platelet aggregating substance.

Test Purpose. 1) to assess platelet aggregation, 2) diagnosis/differential diagnosis of congenital/acquired platelet bleeding disorders, and other bleeding disorders (von Willebrand's disease, Glanzmann's disease, Bernard–Soulier sy, Raynaud's phenomenon), 3) to determine storage pool or platelet granule defects, 4) to determine an aspirin-like defect or defect of prostaglandin pathway.

Increased Values – shortened aggregation
diabetes mellitus, **smoking, hemolysis, familial hyperlipoproteinemia** (type II), thromboembolic disease, cardiovascular system diseases, von Willebrand's disease (type IIB), myocardial infarction, stress

> **Interfering Factors:** hyperbilirubinemia, hyperlipidemia, blood storage temperature, medicaments – (heparin, oral contraceptives)

Decreased Values – prolonged aggregation
afibrinogenemia, albinism, pernicious anemia, May–Hegglin anomaly, recent aortocoronary/dialysis bypass, liver cirrhosis, connective tissue defects, vitamin B_{12} deficiency, dysproteinemias, hypothyroidism, **von Willebrand's disease**, diseases – (**myeloproliferative d., liver d.**), **acute leukemia, systemic lupus erythematosus, infectious mononucleosis,** narcotics – (cocaine, marijuana), antiplatelet antibodies, polycythemia vera, idiopathic thrombocytopenic purpura, syndrome – (**Bernard–Soulier sy,** Chediak–Higashi sy, **Wiskott–Aldrich sy**), **Glanzmann's thrombasthenia,** thrombocytopenia, **uremia**

> **Interfering Factors:** medicaments – (acetylsalicylic acid, antibiotics, antihistamines, azlocillin, captopril, carbenicillin, chlordiazepoxide, chloroquine, chlorpromazine, clofibrate, corticosteroids, dextran, diazepam, diclofenac, dipyridamole, diuretics, furosemide, gentamicin, heparin, ibuprofen, indomethacin, ketoprofen, mezlocillin, nifedipine, nitrofurantoin, penicillin, phenothiazines, phentolamine, phenylbutazone, piperacillin, promethazine, propranolol, prostaglandin E1, pyridinol, pyrimidine, sulfinpyrazol, theophylline, tricyclic antidepressants, volatile general anesthetics, warfarin)

Analyte	Age/Gender	Reference Range	SI Units	Note
Platelet Aggregation		>0.60		

Platelet Antibodies

(PLA, syn: antiplatelet antibody, platelet-bound antibodies, platelet-specific antibodies, platelet-associated antibodies) Immune-mediated platelet destruction may be caused by autoantibodies directed against antigens located on the platelet membrane. To antibodies belong: a) autoantibodies, e.g. in infectious diseases, medicament influences, and lymphoproliferative diseases, b) allo-antibodies, e.g. in incompatible blood transfusion, and in bone marrow transplantation. Antibodies directed to platelets will cause early platelets destruction and subsequent thrombocytopenia.

Test Purpose. 1) to detect the antibodies that destroy platelets, 2) to diagnose and follow immune thrombocytopenia conditions, 3) to detect causes of clinical refractoriness to platelet transfusions.

Increased Values – positive
paroxysmal hemoglobinuria, diseases – (autoimmune d., lymphoproliferative d.), disseminated intravascular coagulation, systemic lupus erythematosus, Hodgkin's disease, purpura – (idiopathic thrombocytopenic p., posttransfusion p.), sepsis, neonatal thrombocytopenia, recovery from chemotherapy

Interfering Factors: medicaments – (acetaminophen, antabuse, cephalosporins, chlorothiazide, chlorpropamide, digoxin, heparin, oral hypoglycemic agents, penicillin, phenobarbital, quinidine, salicylates, gold salts, organic arsenicals)

Platelet-Associated Immunoglobulin G

Increased Values
immune-complex diseases, systemic lupus erythematosus, plasmocytoma (incl. multiple myeloma), acute/chronic immune thrombocytopenic purpura, septic thrombocytopenia

Platelet Factor 4

(PF 4, syn: endothelial cell growth inhibitor, heparin neutralizing protein) Specific thrombocytic protein composed of four identical subunits. It is synthesized in megakaryocytes and platelets. PF 4 is released from platelet alpha-granules after stimulation (platelet activation) in conjunction with proteoglycan. The synthesis of PF4 is enhanced by IL-1. It is stored in endothelial cells and not present in urine. PF4 is found also in mast cell granules and on the endothelium of human umbilical veins, but not arteries. It is chemotactic for inflammatory cells such as neutrophils and monocytes. It activates neutrophils and induces their degranulation. PF4 has a half-life in plasma less than 3 minutes, and its rapid clearance appears to be a function of binding to the vascular endothelium. Once bound to the endothelium, PF4 can be released by heparin in a time-dependent manner. It neutralizes the anticoagulatory activity of heparin sulfate in the extracellular matrix of endothelial cells. It inhibits local antithrombin III activity and thus promotes coagulation. It stimulates the activity of leukocyte elastase and inhibits collagenases. PF4 accelerates the generation of blood clots at the sites of injuries and initiates many cellular processes of wound healing. It may be useful in the treatment of tumors due to its marked anti-angiogenic activity. PF4 may be implicated in pathological and physiological processes of bone and has been found to inhibit the growth of human osteoblast-like osteosarcoma cells. Recombinant PF4 efficiently reverses heparin anticoagulation without adverse effects of heparin-protamine complexes and may be an appropriate substitute for protamine sulfate in patients undergoing cardiovascular surgery and other procedures that require heparin anticoagulation. It has been suggested that PF4 mRNA expression should be a marker of mature megakaryoblasts and that its expression in megakaryoblastic leukemia may indicate that a patient will have long survival and a good response to chemotherapy.

Test Purpose. Platelet activation indicator and an index of platelet aggregation and thromboembolic risk.

Increased Values
angina pectoris, diabetes mellitus, pulmonary embolism, diseases – (vascular d., infectious d., renal d., chronic cardiac d., thrombotic d., inflammatory d.), myocardial infarction, insufficiency – (pulmonary i., heart i.), tumors, extracorporal circulation, polycythemia vera, conditions – (c. after heart prostheses implantation, postsurgery c., shock c.)

Analyte	Age/Gender	Reference Range	SI Units	Note
Platelet Factor 4		<15	µg/l	

Platelet Serotonin

Test is used for carcinoid syndrome diagnostics.

Increased Values
oat cell carcinoma of lung, multiple endocrine neoplasia (types I and II), islet cell tumors of pancreas, medullary carcinoma of the thyroid, **carcinoid sy**

Platelet-Specific Alloantibodies

Increased Values – positive
purpura – (post-transfusion p., idiopathic thrombocytopenic p.), neonatal alloimmune thrombocytopenia

Platelets

(PLT, syn: thrombocytes, platelet count, thrombocyte estimation, thrombocyte count) Platelets are the smallest individual blood cells.
Function. Involved in primary hemostasis (blood coagulation/clotting), vascular integrity, vasoconstriction, adhesion and aggregation activity in primary platelet hemostatic plug formation that occludes small vessel breaks or obturates vessel by blood clot in pathological conditions (thrombogenesis) + stores/transports/releases vasoactive amines, platelet factor 3 and thromboxane A2. Platelets influence right endothelium cell function; they are involved in plasma coagulation factor activation and have phagocytic activity.
Production. In bone marrow by peripheral megakaryocyte cytoplasm cleavage during megakaryocytopoiesis and thrombocytopoiesis, 2/3 are in circulating blood, 1/3 in the spleen.
Production agonists. a) strong a.: thrombin, collagen, PGs, endoperoxides, TXA2, PAF, b) mild a.: ADP, epinephrine, vasopressin and serotonin.
Production antagonists. PGI2, PGD2, EDRF.
Platelet activating agents. a) indirect: collagen, b) direct: thrombin, epinephrine, ADP, TXA2.
Platelet inflammation mediators. Serotonin, ADP, ATP, histamine, fibrinogen, factor Va/VII, platelet factor 4, von Willebrand's factor, B-lysine, protease, cathepsin A, collagenase, elastase, PAF, TXA2, TGF-beta, galactosyl-transferase, P-selectin, PDGF, reactive oxygen products, glycoprotein Ib, thrombospondin.
Test Purpose. 1) to evaluate platelet production 2) to assess chemotherapy or radiation therapy platelet production effects, 3) to diagnose and monitor severe thrombocytosis or thrombocytopenia, 4) to confirm visual platelet number estimation and morphology from a stained blood film, 5) to evaluate, diagnose and/or follow up bleeding disorders, idiopathic thrombocytopenic purpura, disseminated intravascular coagulation, leukemia states, 6) to investigate purpura, petechiae, 7) to evaluate response to platelet transfusions, steroid or other therapy.

Platelet morphology. Megathrombocytes (platelet >2.5 μ): accelerated platelet production, compensation for increased platelet destruction, vitamin B$_{12}$ deficiency, myeloproliferative diseases, Bernard–Soulier syndrome

Increased Values – thrombocytosis, thrombocytemia

anemia – (hemolytic a., **posthemorrhagic a., sideropenic a.**), rheumatoid arthritis, asphyxia, celiac disease, **hepatic cirrhosis, strenuous exercise, iron deficiency,** acute rheumatic fever, hemophilia, diseases – (autoimmune d., **myeloproliferative d.,** rheumatic d., heart d., **inflammatory d.**), **acute/chronic infectious diseases,** colitis ulcerosa (ulcerative colitis), **acute hemorrhage,** collagenoses, leukemia – (chronic granulocytic l., megakaryocyte l., **chronic myelogenous l.**), treatment of – (folate deficiency, vitamin B$_{12}$ deficiency), lymphomas, Hodgkin's disease, Whipple's disease, **myelofibrosis with myeloid metaplasia, tumours, surgery, osteomyelitis, chronic pancreatitis, polycythemia, polycythemia vera, high altitudes,** conditions – (after surgery c., postpartum c., after blood loss c.), **splenectomy, stress,** pregnancy, **essential thrombocytemia, reactive thrombocytosis, tuberculosis, trauma,** recovery from – (bone marrow suppression, bleeding episode, thrombocytopenia), postpartum

    Interfering Factors: medicaments – (ceftazidime, ceftizoxime, ceftriaxone, cephalosporins, cytotoxic medicaments, enoxaparin, epinephrine, estrogens, glucocorticoids, isotretinoin, lithium, meropenem, methadone, metoprolol, miconazole, oral contraceptives, penicillamine, propranolol, rifampicin, ticlopidine, tocopherol, tolazamide)

Decreased Values – thrombocytopenia

AIDS, **alcoholism,** alloimmunization, **anaphylaxis,** anemia – (**aplastic a.,** dyserythropoietic a., autoimmune hemolytic a., **hemolytic a.,** microangiopathic hemolytic a., **megaloblastic a.,** pernicious a., iron deficiency a.), anesthesia, cold environment, **May–Hegglin anomaly, hepatic cirrhosis,** deficiency of – (folate, vitamin B$_{12}$, iron), eczematous dermatitis, eclampsia, **tumor emboli in microcirculation, erythroblastosis fetalis,** hyperbaric exposure, **hemangioma, paroxysmal nocturnal hemoglobinuria** (PNH), histoplasmosis, **hypersplenism,** hyperthyroidism, **chemotherapy, heart valve prostheses,** diseases – (hepatic d., cyanotic congenital heart d.), infectious diseases – (bacterial i. d., protozoan i. d., rickettsial i. d., **viral i. d.**), marrow infiltration (leukemia, lymphoma, fibrosis), intoxication by – (benzene, benzol, organic chemicals), isoimmunization, **disseminated intravascular coagulation,** collagenoses, post-delivery complications, leukemia – (acute/**chronic lymphocytic**/myeloid l., hairy cell l.), **lymphoma,** malaria, bone marrow metastases, microangiopathies, **Gaucher's disease, myelofibrosis** (myelosclerosis), myelophthisis, atrial myxoma, **tumors,** extracorporeal circulation, **pancytopenia in bone marrow failure, plasmocytoma** (incl. multiple myeloma), pneumonia, preeclampsia, purpura – (neonatal p., **posttransfusion p., idiopathic thrombocytopenic p., thrombotic thrombocytopenic p.**), **radiation, radiotherapy,** neonatal rubella, **sepsis,** spleen diseases – (congestive s. d., infectious s. d., tumorous s. d.), **splenomegaly, allergic conditions,** syndrome – (**aplastic sy,** Alport's sy, **Bernard-Soulier sy, adult respiratory distress sy** – ARDS, Ehlers-Danlos sy, Evans' sy, **Fanconi's sy,** Felty's sy, **hyper-IgM sy, hemolytic-uremic sy,** Hermansky-Pudlak sy, Chédiak-Higashi sy, **myelodysplastic sy, Wiskott-Aldrich sy,** thrombocytopenia – absent radius bones sy), toxoplasmosis, transfusion – (**massive blood t.,** exchange t.), grafts, Glanzmann's thrombasthenia, thrombocytopenia – (**idiopathic t., isoimmune neonatal t., secondary t., t. in HIV positivity**), drug induced thrombocytemia, immune thrombocytopenia – (lymphoproliferative i. t., **i. t. in systemic lupus erythematosus**), renal vein thrombosis, brain injury, **uremia,** vasculitis, heart bypass, failure – (renal f., congestive heart f.), fetal – maternal ABO incompatibility, bleeding conditions

Interfering Factors: medicaments – (abciximab, acetaminophen, acetazolamide, acetylsalicylic acid, aciclovir, ajmaline, aldesleukin, alemtuzumab, allopurinol, alprenolol, altretamine, aminophenazone, aminocaproic acid, aminosalicylic acid, amiodarone, amlodipine, amoxapine, amoxicillin, amphotericin B, ampicillin, amrinone, antazoline, antiepileptics, antihemophilic factor VIII, antihistamines, antirheumatics, antithymocyte globulin, apronal, ardeparin, asparaginase, atenolol, auranofin, aurothioglucose, azapropazone, azathioprine, barbiturates, benazepril, benoxaprofen, betamethasone, bisoprolol, H_2-blocking agents, bumetanide, busulfan, candesartan, capecitabine, captopril, carbamazepine, carbenicillin, carbidopa, carboplatin, carbutamide, carmustine, carvedilol, cefalexin, cefalotin, cefamandole, cefazolin, cefixime, cefoxitin, ceftizoxime, cephalosporins, chlorambucil, chloramphenicol, chloroquine, chlorothiazide, chlorphenamine, chlorpromazine, chlorpropamide, chlorprothixene, chlortalidone, cimetidine, cisplatin, cladribine, clindamycin, clometacin, clomipramine, clonazepam, clopamide, codeine, colchicine, cortisone, cotrimoxazole, cyclosporine, cyclophosphamide, cytarabine, cytostatics, dacarbazine, dactinomycin, dalteparin, danaparoid, daunorubicin, denileukin, desipramine, dexamethasone, dexrazoxane, diamorphine, diazepam, diazoxide, dicloxacillin, diflunisal, digitalis, digitoxin, digoxin, diltiazem, diphenylhydantoin, diuretics, enalapril, enoxaparin, epirubicin, erythromycin, estramustine, estrogens, ethacrynic acid, ethambutol, ethanol, ethosuximide, etoposide, felbamate, fenofibrate, fenoprofen, floxuridine, fluconazole, flucytosine, fludarabine, fluorouracil, fluphenazine, flurbiprofen, fomivirsen, fosphenytoin, furosemide, ganciclovir, gatifloxacin, glutethimide, gold salts, heparin, hydantoines, hydralazine, hydrochlorothiazide, hydroxyurea, ibuprofen, idarubicin, ifosfamide, imipenem, imipramine, inamrinone, indomethacin, interferon alfa-2a, interferon alfa-2b, interferon alfa-n1, interferon alfacon-1, irbesartan, irinotecan, isocarboxazid, isoniazid, isoprenaline, isotretinoin, kava kava, lamivudine, lamotrigine, lansoprazole, latamoxef, leflunomide, levamisole, levodopa, linezolid, lomustine, loracarbef, loxapine, measles/mumps/rubella vaccines, mebendazole, mechlorethamine, mefloquine, meloxicam, melphalan, meperidine, meprobamate, mercaptopurine, mercurial diuretics, meropenem, metamizole, methicillin, methimazole, methotrexate, methyldopa, methylprednisolone, mexiletine, miconazole, milrinone, minoxidil, mitomycin, mitoxantrone, moricizine, moxifloxacin, mycophenolate, myelosuppressives, nafcillin, nalidixic acid, nimodipine, nitrofurantoin, nitroglycerin, nortriptyline, omeprazole, oral contraceptives, oxacillin, oxaprozin, oxprenolol, oxyphenbutazone, paclitaxel, pantoprazole, paracetamol, penicillins, penicillamine, pentamidine, pentobarbital, pentosan, pentostatin, perphenazine, pethidine, phenacetin, phenazone, phenobarbital, phenothiazines, phenylbutazone, phenytoin, piroxicam, plicamycin, potassium iodide, prednisolone, prednisone, primidone, probucol, procainamide, procarbazine, propylthiouracil, pyrazinamide, pyrimethamine, quinidine, quinine, rabeprazole, ranitidine, reserpine, rifabutin, rifampicin, rituximab, salbutamol, salicylates, samarium-153, saquinavir, secobarbital, silver sulfadiazine, sirolimus, sparfloxacin, stavudine, stilbol, streptomycin, streptozocin, strontium-89 chloride, sulfadiazine, sulfamethizole, sulfamethoxazole, sulfasalazine, sulfizoxazole, sulfonamides, sulfonylureas, sulindac, tamoxifen, temozolomide, teniposide, terbinafine, tetracyclines, thiazide diuretics, thiethylperazine, thioguanine, thioridazine, thiotepa, thiothixene, ticarcillin, ticlopidine, tirofiban, tobramycin, tocainide, tolazamide, tolazoline, tolbutamide, topotecan, trandolapril, triamcinolone, triamterene, trifluoperazine, trimethadione, trimethoprim, trimetrexate, trovafloxacin, vancomycin, valproic acid, velacivlovir, verapamil, vinblastine, vincristine, vinorelbine, zidovudine, zimeldine)

Analyte	Age/Gender	Reference Range	SI Units	Note
Platelets	Neonates	290–350*		*x 10⁹/l
	Adults	130–370*		

Porphobilinogen Deaminase

(U-I-S, syn: uroporphyrinogen I synthase/cosynthetase, erythrocyte uroporphyrinogen I synthase, uroporphyrinogen decarboxylase) This enzyme converts porphobilinogen to uroporphyrinogen I; the enzyme is necessary for the RBC to produce heme which catalyzes 4 porphobilinogen molecules condensation → linear tetrapyrrole, hydroxymethylbilane creation. Enzyme is in RBC, fibroblasts, lymphocytes, liver cells and amniotic fluid cells.
Test Purpose. 1) acute intermittent porphyria carriers screening, 2) differential diagnosis of acute intermittent porphyria when compared to variegate porphyria.

Decreased Values
acute intermittent porphyria (AIP)

Porphobilinogen Synthase

(PBG-S, syn: DALA dehydratase)

Decreased Values
inborn PBG-S defect, plumboporphyria, **lead exposure**, **lead intoxication**

Potassium in RBC

Increased Values
congestive heart failure

Decreased Values
hyperaldosteronism, long-standing diuretic therapy

Prostacyclin

(6-keto-PG-F1a, PGI2) Prostacyclin is the main arachidonic acid product in vascular tissue (endothelial cells).
Function. Strong hypotensive agent in vascular beds vasodilation, including the pulmonary and cerebral circulation. Prostacyclin is the most potent endogenic platelet aggregation inhibitor; blocks fibrinogen ADP-induced bond to activated platelets; it is the most potent natural vascular wall antiaggregation principle.

Increased Values
dysmenorrhea, Graves' disease, tumors of – (prostate, breast), congestive heart failure

Decreased Values
atherosclerosis, diabetes mellitus, hypertension, conditions – (hypercoagulability c., thrombotic c.)

Protein C

(PC, syn: protein C antigen) Glycoprotein depending on vitamin K.

Production. By the liver.

Function. When activated, inhibits hemocoagulation. PC is a major key coagulation cascade co-factor, factors Va/VIIIa inhibitor in complex with protein S. Thrombomodulin is a protein C activation potentiator, an endothelial cell co-factor, and important to potentiate proteins C and S in thromboembolism prevention. It has both profibrinolytic and anticoagulant properties.

Test Purpose. 1) to investigate the otherwise unexplained thrombosis causes and to establish inheritance patterns, 2) to help the diagnostic evaluation for hypercoagulability.

Increased Values
nephrotic sy
> **Interfering Factors:** medicaments – (oral contraceptives, stanozolol)

Decreased Values
biliary obstruction, deficiency – (**inborn protein C d., vitamin K d.**), diseases – (autoimmune d., **severe liver d.**), **consumptional coagulopathy, liver parenchyma lesion,** malabsorption, tumors, **surgery,** gram-negative sepsis, **adult respiratory distress sy** (ARDS), nephrotic sy, **pregnancy, deep venous thrombosis**
> **Interfering Factors:** elder people, medicaments – (coumarin, L-asparaginase, oral contraceptives, warfarin)

Analyte	Age/Gender	Reference Range	SI Units	Note
Protein C		70–130	%	
		0.70–1.30		
		3–6	mg/l	

Protein S

A glycoprotein depending on vitamin K. A plasma factor essential for prevention of thrombosis, partly due to its activity as cofactor for the plasma anticoagulant protease-activated protein C.

Production. Synthesized by the liver.

Function. Coagulation inhibitor. Free protein S form as a protein C co-factor in stechiometric complex with activated protein C and inactivated F V leads to acceleration of F Va and F VIIIa inactivation. Protein S linked to C_{4b}-BP (C_{4b} binding protein) has no anticoagulation activity. The unbound fraction circulates in the plasma as the active form.

Decreased Values
biliary obstruction, deficiency – (congenital d. of protein S, **vitamin K d.**), diseases – (autoimmune d., **liver d.**), **disseminated intravascular coagulation,** malabsorption, surgery, diabetic nepropathy, acute-phase reaction, chronic renal failure, gram-negative sepsis, syndrome – (adult respiratory distress sy (ARDS), **nephrotic sy,** antiphospholipid sy), coumarin induced skin necrosis, **pregnancy, deep venous thrombosis**
> **Interfering Factors:** newborns, medicaments – (L-asparaginase, coumarin, oral contraceptives)

Analyte	Age/Gender	Reference Range	SI Units	Note
Protein S		70–140	%	
		0.70–1.40		
		418–600	mg/l	

Prothrombin Fragment 1+2

(F 1+2, syn: prothrombin fragment F1.2) Prothrombin fragment 1+2 is released by prothrombinase from prothrombin during thrombin formation, thus it is a prothrombin activation fragment.

Test Purpose. 1) to study hypercoagulable conditions, 2) to assess thrombotic risks, 3) to monitor anticoagulant therapy, 4) to assess patients with active and/or progressive thrombosis.

Increased Values
severe liver diseases, leukemia, postmyocardial infarction, **thrombosis**

Decreased Values
Interfering Factors: medicaments – (anticoagulants, antithrombin III)

Analyte	Age/Gender	Reference Range	SI Units	Note
Prothrombin Fragment 1+2		0.4–1.1	nmol/l	

Prothrombin Time

(PT, syn: Quick time, Quick test, Quick prothrombin time, thromboplastin time, pro time) PT measures the extrinsic coagulation cascade portion initiated by factor VII and tissue factor interaction. Stage II hemostasis evaluation (factors I, II, V, VII, IX, X). PT reagents are tissue thromboplastin and ionized calcium.

Test Purpose. 1) to provide overall extrinsic coagulation factors V, VII and X, prothrombin and fibrinogen evaluation, 2) to monitor oral anticoagulant therapy response, 3) screening test for vitamin K deficiency diagnosis, 4) disseminated intravascular coagulation diagnosis, 5) to diagnose factors II, V and X inhibitors, 6) to screen for hemostatic disorders involving fibrin formation, 7) to detect congenital deficiencies of factors II, V, VII, X.

Increased Values – >120% (1.2 INR), shortened PT
high fat diet, hypercoagulability, metastatic tumors, thrombophlebitis, **vitamin K supplementation**

Interfering Factors: medicaments – (anabolic steroids, antacids, antibiotics, barbiturates, chloral hydrate, cholestyramine, carbamazepine, clofibrate, diphenhydramine, digitalis, estrogens, glutethimide, griseofulvin, nafcillin, oral contraceptives – estrogen, rifampicin, salicylates – low dose, sulfonamides)

Decreased Values – <80% (0.8 INR), prolonged PT
afibrinogenemia, alcoholism, **impaired vitamin K intestinal absorption**, **liver cirrhosis**, **amyloidosis**, **vitamin K deficiency**, diverticulitis, hepatitis – (acute h. type A, **acute h. type B**, chronic active h. B, acute h. type E, cholestatic h., drug induced h., autoimmune h., acute

h. type D, **alcoholic h., chemical induced h.**), **hyperfibrinolysis, dysfibrinogenemia, hypervitaminosis** A, **hypofibrinogenemia**, idiopathic familial hypoprothrombinemia, **acute/chronic hepatic diseases**, renal insufficiency, intoxication by – (**salicylate, heparin, coumarin**), jaundice – (obstructive j., cholestatic j.), **disseminated intravascular coagulation** (DIC), ulcerative colitis, hepatic coma, passive congestion of liver, **systemic lupus erythematosus**, malnutrition, Crohn's disease, metastatic liver tumors, coagulant factors deficiency – (**I, II, V, VII, IX, X**), **biliary ducts obstruction, antibodies against coagulant factors**, scurvy, sprue, Reye's sy, premature infants, fistulas, steatorrhea, steatohepatitis, celiac disease, chronic diarrhea, acute liver failure, heat exhaustion

Interfering Factors: alcohol, diarrhea, vomiting, medicaments – (acetaminophen, acetylsalicylic acid – large doses, allopurinol, aminosalicylic acid, amiodarone, antacids, anabolic steroids, anistreplase, antibiotics, antihistamine, asparaginase, barbiturates, beta-lactam antibiotics, carbenicillin, cefalotin, cefoperazone, cefotetan, cefradine, ceftizoxime, ceftriaxone, cephalosporins, chloral hydrate, chloramphenicol, chlorpromazine, cholestyramine, cimetidine, clofibrate, colchicine, colestipol, coumarines, cyclophosphamide, diazoxide, diphenylhydantoin, disulfiram, erythromycin, estrogens, ethacrynic acid, ethylalcohol, fluconazole, glucagon, glutethimide, griseofulvin, halothane, heparin, heptabarbital, ibuprofen, indomethacin, interferon alpha-2b, ketoconazole, laxatives, loracarbef, MAO-inhibitors, mefenamic acid, meprobamate, mercaptopurine, methimazole, methotrexate, methyldopa, metronidazole, neomycin, niacin, nortriptyline, oral anticoagulants, oral contraceptives, phenylbutazone, phenytoin, plicamycin, propylthiouracil, pyrazinamide, quinidine, quinine, salicylates, sulfinpyrazone, sulfonamides, tamoxifen, theophylline, thiazides, ticarcillin, thyroid hormones, tolazamide, tolbutamide, tolmetin, vitamin E – large doses, warfarin)

Analyte	Age/Gender	Reference Range	SI Units	Note
Prothrombin Time		12–15	s	
		0.8–1.2	(INR)	
		80–120	%	

Pyrimidine-5'-Nucleotidase in RBC

(P-5'-NT, syn: pyrimidine-5'-nucleotide nucleotidase)

Decreased Values
anemia – (autosomal recessive hemolytic a., beta thalassemia), pyrimidine-5'-nucleotidase deficiency, occupational lead exposure, severe lead poisoning

Pyruvate Kinase

(PK, syn: pyruvate kinase assay) Red cell enzyme, takes part in the phosphoenolpyruvate to pyruvate anaerobic glucose metabolism.
Test Purpose. 1) to differentiate PK-deficient hemolytic anemia from other congenital hemolytic anemias or from acquired hemolytic anemia, 2) to detect PK deficiency in asymptomatic heterozygous inheritance.

Increased Values
Duchene's muscular dystrophy, muscular diseases, myocardial infarction, physical exercise

Decreased Values

congenital inherited nonspherocytic hemolytic anemia, anemias, aplasias, **pyruvate kinase deficiency**, metabolic liver diseases, leukemia, medicaments, myelodysplastic sy

---

Red Cell Distribution Width

(RDW) Main RBC population width in histogram by MCV. RDW measures size variability of RBC population.

Test Purpose. 1) information about the RBC anisocytosis stage, 2) to evaluate anemia, 3) to differentiate iron deficiency anemia from other microcytic anemias.

Increased Values

alcoholism, anemia – (megaloblastic a., immune hemolytic a., a. of chronic disease, myelo-dysplastic a., myelophthisic a., nutritional a., sickle cell a., sideroblastic a., sideropenic a., homozygous thalassemias), deficiency – (G6PD d., folate d., vitamin B_{12} d.), liver diseases, RBC fragmentation, HbH presence

    Interfering Factors: cold agglutinins, hyperglycemia, chronic lymphocytic leukemia, post red cell transfusion

Analyte	Age/Gender	Reference Range	SI Units	Note
Red Cell Distribution Width (index)		12.8–15.2		

Red Cell Mass Volume

(RCV) Total volume of body RBCs. At hematocrit values between 0.20 and 0.55, a linear relationship exists between HCT and RCV.

Test Purpose. 1) conditions with changed total blood volume without plasma to RBC ratio change (simple hypervolemia), 2) to evaluate untrue anemia in polyplasmia and spleno-megalia, 3) to evaluate polyglobulia as a dehydration result or hypervolemia „anemia", 4) to help in polycythemia vera diagnosis.

Increased Values

diseases – (pulmonary d., congenital cardiac d.), carboxyhemoglobinemia, methemoglobin-emia, newborn infants with HCT ↑ 0.55, tumors – (cerebellar hemangioma, hepatoma, uter-ine leiomyomas, kidney t.), polycythemia vera, right-left cardiac shunt, pregnancy, high altitude

Decreased Values

anemia, pheochromocytoma, starvation, chronic infectious diseases, acute/chronic hemor-rhage, obesity, bed rest, radiation, old age

---

Reptilase Time

Test giving information about qualitative/quantitative fibrinogen changes. Reptilase is a thrombin-like enzyme derived from Bothrops atrox venom that is not inhibited by heparin. It acts on fibrinogen to cleave fibrinopeptide A, leading to clottable fibrin monomer forma-tion.

Test Purpose. 1) differential diagnosis of hypo/dysfibrinogenemias, 2) fibrin polymerization disorders differential diagnosis, 3) to examine heparinized patient fibrinogen changes, 4) to investigate patients with prolonged thrombin time.

Increased Values – prolonged reptilase time
a/dys/hypofibrinogenemia, primary systemic amyloidosis, Waldenström's macroglobulinemia, plasmocytoma (incl. multiple myeloma)
   Interfering Factors: paraproteins, medicaments – (anistreplase)

Analyte	Age/Gender	Reference Range	SI Units	Note
Reptilase Time		15–22	s	

Reticulocyte Hemoglobin Content

Test Purpose. 1) to help in diagnosis of iron deficiency and iron-deficiency anemia, 2) to monitor the response to iron therapy in iron-deficiency anemia.

Decreased Values
anemia – (iron deficiency a., thalassemia), iron deficiency

Reticulocytes

(syn: reticulocyte count) Young, immature, erythrocyte non-nucleated cells series formed in the bone marrow, the last developmental erythropoiesis stage before the mature erythrocyte. Reticulocyte contains original structure remnants of some organels (ribosomes, endoplasmic reticulum) in cytoplasm after nucleus expelling; therefore, reticulocyte can still synthesize hemoglobin. The test is underutilized, especially when one considers it is at a pivotal decision making conjuncture. The reticulotyte production index will indicate whether one is working with a hyperproliferative or nonproliferative anemia, and thus what testing should be subsequently ordered.
Test Purpose. 1) to aid in distinguishing between hypoproliferative and hyperproliferative anemias, 2) to help assess blood loss, bone marrow response to anemia and anemia therapy response, 3) to evaluate erythropoietic activity.

Increased Values – reticulocytosis
abetalipoproteinemia, anemia – (**hemolytic a., sickle cell a.**, hereditary spherocytosis, thalassemia major, thalassemia minor, hereditary elliptocytosis, autoimmune hemolytic anemia, G6PD hemolytic a., pyruvate kinase deficiency hemolytic a., myelophthisic a., microangiopathic a.), babesiosis, bartonellosis, cirrhosis – (liver c., primary biliary c.), deficiency – (factor I, V, VII, VIII, IX, X, XI, vitamin E d.), **erythroblastosis fetalis, erythroleukemia**, hemoglobinopathy, hemoglobinuria – (paroxysmal nocturnal h., paroxysmal cold h., paroxysmal post-exercise h.), sickle cell crisis, acute hemolysis, hepatitis – (acute h. type A, acute h. type B, acute h. type D, acute h. type E), chronic hemorrhage, hypersplenism, **chronic hypoxemia**, disease – (hemoglobin C d., hemoglobin H d., Gaucher's d., von Willebrand's d., Hodgkin's d.), **acute hemorrhage** (3 to 4 days later), **leukemia**, lymphocytic lymphoma, malaria, specific anemia treatment – (**megaloblastic a., iron deficiency a.**), endocardial myxoma, nephropathy – (sickle cell n., chronic lead n.), metastatic tumors, post-anemia treatment – (folate supplementation, iron supplementation, vitamin B_{12} supplementation),

poisoning by – (arsenic, lead), **polycythemia vera**, thrombocytopenic thrombotic purpura, leukemoid reaction, scurvy, **splenectomy**, **hemolytic states**, syndrome – (hemolytic uremic sy, tropical splenomegaly sy), **pregnancy**

> Interfering Factors: medicaments – (ACTH, captopril, chlorphenamine, cisplatin, hydralazine, methyldopa, paracetamol, phenazone, quinidine, sulfasalazine)

Decreased Values – reticulocytopenia

alcoholism, anemia – (**aplastic a., megaloblastic a., a. of chronic disease, sideroblastic a., thalassemia**, macrocytic a., microcytic a., **folic acid deficiency a., iron deficiency a.**, vitamin B_{12} deficiency a.), **untreated pernicious anemia, hepatic cirrhosis**, hypofunction – (**anterior pituitary h., adrenocortical h.**), diseases – (endocrine d., liver d., **chronic infectious d.**, renal d.), **bone marrow infiltration**, bone marrow suppression – (sepsis, chemotherapy/radiotherapy), **aplastic crisis in hemolytic anemia**, polycythemia vera, blood transfusion, bone marrow replacement, **radiotherapy, myxedema**, myelodysplastic sy, **marrow failure**

> Interfering Factors: medicaments – (chloramphenicol, dactinomycin, methotrexate, vinblastine)

Analyte	Age/Gender	Reference Range	SI Units	Note
Reticulocytes	Neonates	0.02–0.06*		*x 10^{12}/l
		0.100–0.300		
	Adults	0.025–0.075*		
		0.005–0.015		

Right Side Shift

Hypersegmented, multilobulated neutrophils, polymorphonuclear cells, older cells in peripheral blood smear. Used in differential diagnosis of liver diseases, pernicious and megaloblastic anemias.

Occurrence. Anemia – (megaloblastic a., pernicious a.), gangrene, hemolysis, liver diseases, medicaments and chemicals – (ACTH, arsenic, benzene, digitalis, venoms, potassium chlorate, mercury, sulfonamides), myocardial infarction, tumours – (bone marrow t., liver t., gastrointestinal tract t.), burns, hemolytic transfusion reactions, after surgery conditions

Sulfhemoglobin

Sulfhemoglobin is a green monochrome formed through oxidative sulfation of 1 or 2 heme from 4 heme hemoglobin groups. It cannot be reduced to Hb (bond is irreversible) but it may be oxidized further and will contribute to Heinz bodies formation in some instances. Generally it is very stable in blood and is lost from the circulation only with erythrocytes breakdown. It is incapable of carrying oxygen and shifts the P50 to the right.

Test Purpose. To assess possible drugs exposure.

Increased Values – sulfhemoglobinemia
chronic constipation

> Interfering Factors: medicaments – (acetylsalicylic acid, nitrates, nitrites, phenacetin, sulfides, sulfonamides)

Analyte	Age/Gender	Reference Range	SI Units	Note
Sulfhemoglobin		negat.		

Terminal Deoxynucleotidyl Transferase

(TdT, syn: terminal transferase) Nuclear enzyme which is important in lymphocyte differentiaton with immature and less mature cellular forms.

Occurrence. Thymocytes, precursor cells of lymphocytes in bone marrow.

Test Purpose. 1) acute leukemia differential diagnosis, 2) acute lymphatic leukemia type determination.

Increased Values
active acute lymphoblastic leukemia, chronic myelogenous leukemia in blast crisis, **lymphomas**, neuroblastoma, idiopathic thrombocytopenic purpura

Thrombin Time

(TT, TCT, syn: thrombin clotting time, fibrin time, thrombin-fibrindex) The test is affected by the fibrinogen/plasmin concentrations and quality, FDP, and antithrombotic agents. Performed on citrated blood specimens; the test measures the time needed for plasma to clot (first fibrin fibre creation time) in the laboratory after calcium and thrombin are added – (fibrinogen → fibrin). TT is a test for the presence of sufficient amount of functional (clottable) fibrinogen. The test evaluates thrombin–fibrinogen interaction, bypassing the extrinsic and intrinsic pathways and assessing the terminal common pathway order (as a component of plasmatic coagulation).

Test Purpose. 1) to detect fibrinogen deficiency or defect, 2) to aid in disseminated intravascular coagulation and hepatic disease diagnosis and monitoring, 3) to monitor heparin, fibrinolytic or thrombolytic agent treatment effectiveness.

Increased Values – prolonged TT
afibrinogenemia, increased antithrombin activity, **dysfibrinogenemia**, hyperbilirubinemia, **hypofibrinogenemia**, diseases – (**liver d.**, inflammatory d.), **DIC**, systemic lupus erythematosus, paraproteinemia, plasmocytoma (incl. myeloma multiforme), polycythemia vera, pregnancy, systemic hyperfibrinolysis, **uremia**
   Interfering Factors: fibrin degradation products, fibrinogen, medicaments – (anistreplase, asparaginase, heparin, streptokinase, thrombolytics, urokinase)

Analyte	Age/Gender	Reference Range	SI Units	Note
Thrombin Time		18–22	s	

Beta-Thromboglobulin

(beta-TG) Beta-thromboglobulin is a specific platelet protein containing 4 identical subunits in PLT alpha-granules and released after stimulation (e.g. ADP, collagen, immune complexes, thrombin). It is synthesized in the cells as a biologically inactive precursor called platelet basic protein (PBP). Beta-TG is a platelet-specific protein released with PLT aggregation. It inhibits prostacyclin secretion (PGI2), a locally active anticoagulant modulating intravascular coagulation. Beta-TG is a strong chemoattractant for fibroblasts and is weakly chemotactic for neutrophils. It stimulates mitogenesis, extracellular matrix synthesis, glucose metabolism and plasminogen activator synthesis.

Test Purpose. 1) to evaluate prothrombotic conditions/hypercoagulability, 2) to aid in disseminated intravascular coagulation diagnosis, 3) to differentiate DIC from primary lysis, 4) to assess PLT hyperreactivity, 5) to evaluate the thrombolytic regimen effects (e.g. vascular occlusive disease, heart failure, coronary atherosclerosis).

Increased Values

atherosclerosis, diabetes mellitus, disseminated intravascular coagulation, acute myocardial infarction, systemic lupus erythematosus, tumors, vascular wall injury, preeclampsia, vulgar psoriasis, conditions – (c. after heart prostheses implantation, c. after surgery, thromboembolic c.), nephrotic sy, deep-vein thrombosis

Analyte	Age/Gender	Reference Range	SI Units	Note
Beta-Thrombo-Globulin		10–35	µg/l	

Thrombomodulin

(TM, syn: endothelial co-factor) Thrombomodulin is endothelial cell thrombin receptor. The thrombin-thrombomodulin complex activates protein C (anticoagulant influence). TM is an anticoagulant protein co-factor modulating thrombin specificity for receptor and activating the central enzyme protein C; involved in factor Va, VIIIa, and fibrinogen inactivation. Plasma thrombomodulin fragments reflect endothelial cell injury. TM activates platelets by thrombin and inhibits thrombin via antithrombin III.
Test Purpose. Endothelial cell damage assessment.

Increased Values

atherosclerosis, diabetes mellitus, diabetic microangiopathy, **endothelial injury**, ischemic heart disease, DIC, systemic lupus erythematosus, tumors, endothelial cell injury, thrombotic thrombocytopenic purpura, adult respiratory distress syndrome (ARDS), pulmonary thromboembolism, thrombosis, failure – (renal f., acute hepatic f.), **vasculitis**

Decreased Values

smoking, primary pulmonary hypertension

Thrombopoietin

(TPO, MGDF, c-mpl-ligand) TPO is highly glycated protein; the terminal portion is identical with erythropoietin.
Function. Main thrombopoiesis regulator involved in CD 34+ cell differentiation to megakaryocyte line; increases aggregation to many inductors: ADP, epinephrine, thrombin, and collagen; involved in platelet alpha-granule degradation with thrombin cooperation.
Production. Kidney, liver, spleen, and bone marrow.

Thromboxane A2

(TXA2) Belongs to the prostaglandins, synthesized from platelet arachidonic acid where its release has an opposite effect to prostacyclin. Allergic reactions mediator.

Function. Microvasculature constriction (arterial smooth muscle), bronchodilation. TXA2 stimulates platelet aggregation; it is the last prostaglandin metabolism stage in activated platelets; increases neutrophil adhesion. It has a very short half-life (about 30 s) and is rapidly converted to an inactive metabolite thromboxane B2.

Analyte	Age/Gender	Reference Range	SI Units	Note
Thromboxane B2		18–91	pg/ml	

Tissue Plasminogen Activator

(tPA) Plasma serine protease proteins stored in endothelial cells are released to blood circulation after stimulation. Initiates fibrinolytic process by plasminogen to plasmin transformation. Two tPA forms (tissue and vascular) are structurally identical but immunologically unlike uPA (urokinase) and scuPA precursor (single chain urokinase PA type).
Test Purpose. Endothelial cell injury marker.

Increased Values
atherosclerosis, inborn hyperfibrinolysis, diabetes mellitus, severe liver diseases, myocardial infarction, conditions – (septic c., shock c.)
> **Interfering Factors:** physical exertion, venous stasis, stress, elder age, medicaments – (antidiuretic hormone)

Decreased Values
fibrinolysis insufficiency

Total Blood Volume (TBV)

Sum of plasma volume plus red cell volume, small leukocyte and platelet volume.
Test Purpose. 1) information about blood volume condition changes, where the total blood volume changes without plasma to RBC ratio change (simple hypervolemia with normal hemogram), excessive plasma volume increase (polyplasmia with false anemia), RBC distribution change (false anemia in splenomegaly), in other conditions (e.g. dehydration polyglobulia, fluid retention „anemia", true polycythemia evidence), where direct total circulating RBC and plasma volume determination is needed, 2) to evaluate the blood volume change level.

Increased Values
acidosis, severe starvation, overhydration, diseases – (pulmonary d., congenital cardiac d.), renal insufficiency, recumbent posture, polycythemia vera, primary/secondary erythrocytosis, athletes, pregnancy, thyrotoxicosis, vasodilatation, cardiac failure

Decreased Values
severe anemias, chronic azotemia, physical exercise, salt deficiency, dehydration, diabetes mellitus, exposure to cold, pheochromocytoma, starvation, diarrhea, chronic infections, hemorrhage, recumbent posture, obesity, burns, prolonged bed rest, prolonged standing, old age, vomiting

Von Willebrand's Factor

(vWF) High-molecular plasma glycoprotein present physiologically in low concentrations. It is produced in endothelial cells and platelets, and stored in endothelial cells (Weibel–Paladie bodies), released after activation or endothelial cell damage.

Function. It is a coagulatory F VIII: C carrier circulating in blood as a complex, and playing an important role in primary hemostasis as platelet adhesion to endothelium mediator. Factor deficiency results in prolonged bleeding time.

Test Purpose. 1) hemorrhagic diatheses differential diagnosis, 2) von Willebrand's disease identification, 3) endothelial cell damage indicator.

Increased Values

rheumatoid arthritis, atherosclerosis, **diabetes mellitus**, smoking, hyperlipidemia, hypercholesterolemia, disease – (hypertonic d., **ischemic heart d.**), diseases – (renal d., **connective tissue d.**, liver d., **inflammatory d.**), **myocardial infarction**, **tumors**, vascular endothelium damage, arteriosclerosis obliterans, conditions – (febrile c., postsurgery c.), **vasculitides**

> **Interfering Factors:** blood group "O" carriers, stress, pregnancy, medicaments – (oral contraceptives)

Decreased Values

von Willebrand's disease

Analyte	Age/Gender	Reference Range	SI Units	Note
von Willebrand's Factor		<8	mg/l	
		0.6–1.5	IU/ml	

Pericardial Fluid

D. Mesko

Normal pericardial fluid is clear, pale yellow, and varies from 10 to 50 ml in volume. Most investigators agree that pericardial fluid is an ultrafiltrate of plasma, but it has been proposed by others that it is myocardial interstitial fluid overflow. Pericardial fluid is returned through lymphatic pathways to the venous circulation.

Test Purpose. To assist in identifying the cause of pericardial effusion and to help determine appropriate therapy.

Blood

Positive Values
dissecting aortic aneurysm, hemopericardium, diseases – (rheumatoid d., inflammatory d.), systemic lupus erythematosus, tumors, **metastatic tumors,** pericarditis – (bacterial p., **idiopathic hemorrhagic p.,** tuberculous p., **uremic p.**), **damage to blood vessels, myocardial rupture,** syndrome – (postmyocardial infarct sy, postpericardectomy sy), **trauma**

Exudate

rheumatoid diseases, acute myocardial infarction, systemic lupus erythematosus, tumors, pericarditis, tuberculosis

Glucose

Decreased Values
bacterial endocarditis, tumors, pericarditis – (bacterial p., malignant p., tuberculous p.)

Leukocytes

Increased Values
myocardial abscess, infective endocarditis, esophago-pericardial fistula, pericarditis – (bacterial p., mycobacterial p., parasitic p., p. after surgical procedures, malignant p., p. after penetrating trauma, protozoal p., rickettsial p., tuberculous p.), hepatic abscess rupture, septicemia, contiguous infection spread – (pneumonia)

Lymphocytes

Increased Values
pericarditis – (fungal p., tuberculous p.), tumors

Volume

Increased Values

myocardial abscess, infective endocarditis, rheumatoid diseases, myocardial infarct, antico-agulant therapy, systemic lupus erythematosus, lymphoma, metastatic tumors, myxedema, pericarditis – (bacterial p., mycoplasmal p., fungal p., p. after surgical procedures, malignant p., p. after penetrating trauma, tuberculous p., viral p.), leakage of aortic aneurysm, septi-cemia, tuberculosis, trauma, uremia

Peritoneal Fluid

D. Mesko

Peritoneal (ascitic) fluid is a plasma ultrafiltrate, formation depends on the balance between capillary hydrostatic pressure, capillary permeability, and lymphatic resorption. Transudates result from increased hydrostatic pressure or decreased plasma oncotic pressure; exudates are due to increased capillary permeability or decreased lymphatic resorption. Normal peritoneal fluid is clear, pale yellow, and scanty in amount (under 50 ml).

Ascites: fluid found within the peritoneal cavity. Development of ascites is secondary to renal sodium and water retention. The technique – paracentesis – is an invasive procedure entailing of needle insertion into the peritoneal cavity for ascitic fluid removal. Peritoneal fluid is usually evaluated for gross appearance, RBCs, WBCs, protein, glucose, amylase, ammonia, alkaline phosphatase, LD, cytology, bacteria, fungi, CEA and cytological examination.

Alkaline Phosphatase

Increased Values
infarcted intestines, perforation/strangulation of small intestine

Ammonia

Increased Values
perforated appendicitis, perforation of the viscera, small/large bowel strangulation, peptic ulcer

Amylase

Increased Values
pancreatic cyst/pseudocyst, biliary tract diseases, ovary tumors, metastatic tumors, **acute pancreatitis**, gastroduodenal perforation, peritonitis, ruptured ectopic pregnancy, **intestinal strangulation/necrosis/perforation/infarction**, acute mesenteric venous thrombosis, **pancreatic trauma**

Appearance

hemorrhagic: **tumors**, pancreatitis – (acute p., **hemorrhagic p.**), **ruptured ectopic pregnancy, tuberculosis, abdominal trauma**
milky (chylous, pseudochylous): hepatic cirrhosis, damage/blockage of the thoracic duct by – (adhesions, **lymphoma, tumors**, parasitic infestation, **tuberculosis**, trauma)

turbid (turbidity, cloudy): **appendicitis,** ascites, inflammatory diseases, tumors, **pancreatitis, primary bacterial peritonitis,** ruptured bowel following trauma, strangulated/infarcted intestine

Bacteria

Increased Values – positive
appendicitis, ovarian diseases, pancreatitis, primary peritonitis, ruptured intestine, tuberculosis

CA 125

Tumor marker.

Increased Values – positive
endometriosis, tumors of – (endometrium, ovary, fallopian tube)

Carcinoembryonic Antigen

Increased Values – positive
tumors of – (lung, breast, gastrointestinal tract, ovary)

Cholesterol

Decreased Values
organ congestion

Colour

- **chylous:** tumors, tuberculosis, nephrotic sy, diseases of pancreas
- **red: tumors,** pancreatitis – (acute p., **hemorrhagic p.**), **ruptured ectopic pregnancy, tuberculosis, abdominal trauma**
- **straw-coloured: liver cirrhosis,** hypoproteinemia, **tumors,** hepatic vein obstruction (Budd–Chiari sy), chronic pancreatitis, intraabdominal perforation, constrictive pericarditis, Meig's sy (ovarian tumour), tuberculosis
- **bile stained** (green): cholecystitis, **acute pancreatitis,** perforated – (**intestines,** duodenal ulcer, **gallbladder**)

Creatinine

Increased Values
extravasation of the urine into peritoneal cavity, rupture of the bladder

Cytological Picture

Positive
peritoneal carcinomatosis, tumors of – (colon, pancreas, ovary, stomach)

Eosinophils

Increased Values
chronic peritoneal dialysis, eosinophil enteritis, lymphoma, ruptured hydatid cyst, vasculitis, congestive heart failure

Erythrocytes (Blood)

Increased Values – positive
appendicitis, infectious/inflammatory diseases, cirrhosis of the liver, diseases – (liver d., pancreas d., kidney d., heart d.), endometriosis, **tumors, hemorrhagic pancreatitis, damage to blood vessels**, rupture/perforation – (**hepatic adenoma r., r. of aortic aneurysm**), mesenterial thrombosis, abdominal trauma – (**penetrating a. t., blunt a. t.**), **tuberculosis**

Exudate

appendicitis, infectious diseases, intestinal infarction, tumors – (hepatoma, lymphoma, metastatic t., mesothelioma), pancreatitis, peritonitis – (primary bacterial p., biliary p.), tuberculosis, trauma, myxedema, vasculitis

Fibronectin

Test Purpose. 1) metastases and peritoneal carcinomatosis diagnosis, 2) cardiac failure diagnosis, 3) pancreatic, peritoneal and reactive inflammatory diseases diagnosis, 4) liver cirrhosis diagnosis.

Decreased Values
diseases – (liver d., cardiac d.), organ congestion, tumor metastases, tumors, pancreatitis, peritonitis

Fungi

Positive
histoplasmosis, candidiasis, coccidioidomycosis

Glucose

Decreased Values
inflammatory diseases, peritoneal carcinomatosis, peritonitis – (**bacterial p., tuberculous p.**)
↑ serum to ascitic glucose: diseases – (infectious d., inflammatory d.), primary peritonitis
↓ serum to ascitic glucose: **peritoneal carcinomatosis, tumors, tuberculous peritonitis**

Hyaluronic Acid

Increased Values
mesothelioma

Lactate Dehydrogenase

A peritoneal fluid to serum LDH ratio of greater than 0.6 is typical of an exudate.

Increased Values
ascites – (**pancreatic a., tuberculous a.**), exudates, inflammatory diseases, **perforated viscus**, tumours, peritonitis – (**bacterial p.**, primary p.), **malignant effusion**

Lactic Acid

Increased Values
diseases – (**infectious d.**, inflammatory d.), tumors, **bacterial peritonitis**

Decreased Values
hepatic cirrhosis, tumors

Leucine Aminopeptidase

(LAP, syn: arylamidase, arylamidase naphthylamidase) Cellular peptidase used as a test of biliary excretory function.

Increased Values
malignant effusion

Leukocytes

Increased Values
abscess, **hepatic cirrhosis**, diseases – (**infectious d., inflammatory d.**), perforated viscus, peritonitis – (**bacterial p.**, primary p.), **tuberculosis**, tumors, **peritoneal carcinomatosis**

Lipase

Increased Values
pancreatitis

Lymphocytes

Increased Values
chylous ascites, tuberculous peritonitis

pH

Increased Values – alkaline pH
organ congestion

Decreased Values – acid pH
diseases – (infectious d., inflammatory d.), peritoneal tumor metastases, bacterial peritonitis

Polymorphonuclears

Increased Values
abscess, diseases – (infectious d., inflammatory d.), perforated viscus, primary peritonitis

Proteins

Levels greater than 30 g/l are characteristic of exudates, whereas transudates usually have a protein content of less than 30 g/l.

Increased Values – Exudates
abscess, cirrhosis of the liver, diseases – (gastrointestinal d., **infectious d.**, hepatic d., systemic d., pancreatic d.), pulmonary infarction, **collagenoses, lymphocytic lymphoma**, tumours – (**ovary adenocarcinoma**, ovary theca cell t., breast t.), **intestine obstruction**, perforated viscus, peritonitis – (**bacterial p., primary p.**, granulomatous p.), **pseudomyxoma peritonei**, syndrome – (Meigs' sy), trauma, tuberculosis, congestive heart failure

Decreased Values – Transudates
hepatic cirrhosis, **peritoneal dialysis, acute glomerulonephritis**, myxedema, **nephrotic sy, congestive heart failure**

Specific Gravity

Increased Values
tumors, tuberculosis, pyogenic peritonitis, congestive heart failure, diseases of pancreas

Transsudate

hepatic cirrhosis, hypoproteinemia, nephrotic sy, congestive heart failure, constrictive pericarditis, Budd–Chiari syndrome, inferior v. caval obstruction, nephrotic syndrome

Triacylglycerols

Increased Values
chronic chylous ascites, lymphoma

Urea

Increased Values
extravasation of the urine into peritoneal cavity, rupture of the bladder

Volume

Increased Values
hepatic cirrhosis, hepatoma, hypoproteinemia, lymphoma, mesothelioma, metastatic
tumors, pancreatitis, primary/secondary bacterial peritonitis, damage/obstruction to thoracic duct by – (parasitic infestation, tuberculosis, trauma), tuberculosis, trauma, congestive heart failure

Pleural Fluid

D. Mesko

Accumulation of fluid in the pleural space is called pleural effusion. Pleural fluid is removed for both diagnostic and therapeutic purposes. Thoracentesis (pleural puncture) is an invasive procedure that entails needle insertion into the pleural space for fluid removal. Pleural effusions result from hemostatic forces imbalance or disruption that control fluid movement across cell membranes. Pleural fluid is produced by the parietal pleura and absorbed by the visceral pleura (via capillaries and lymphatics) as a continuous process. Fluid is formed by plasma filtration through capillary endothelium, at a rate controlled by capillary pressure, plasma oncotic pressure and capillary permeability.

Transudate is fluid accumulation (ultrafiltrate of plasma) due to increased hydrostatic pressure in pleural capillaries, or decreased plasma oncotic pressure. Transudate ordinarily reflects changes in permeability of the filtering membranes.

Exudates are caused usually by increased capillary permeability or decreased lymphatic resorption, and result from infection or malignancy.

Pleural fluid is evaluated for gross appearance, cell counts, protein, lactic dehydrogenase, glucose, amylase, Gram's stain and bacteriological cultures, Mycobacterium tuberculosis, fungi, cytology and carcinoembryonic antigen levels.

Exudate	Transudate
increased protein concentration (>30 g/l)	proteins 2–6 g/l (<30 g/l)
pleural fluid/serum proteins >0.5	pleural fluid/serum proteins <0.5
positive fibrinogen	negative fibrinogen
positive coagulation	negative coagulation
decreased glucose concentration	glucose concentration as in blood
specific density (gravity) >1020 (1016)	specific density (gravity) <1012 (1016)
many cells	solitary cells
positive Rivalta's reaction	negative Rivalta's reaction
pleural fluid/serum LD >0.6	pleural fluid/serum LD <0.6
cholesterol concentration >1.55 mmol/l	cholesterol concentration <1.55 mmol/l
pleural fluid/serum cholesterol >0.32	pleural fluid/serum cholesterol <0.32
pH <7.30 (7.35–7.45)	pH >7.30 (7.40–7.50)
turbid/chylous appearance	clear/amber appearance

Acid Phosphatase

Increased Values
metastatic effusion from prostate cancer

Adenosine Deaminase

(ADA) Adenosine deaminase is an enzyme involved in purine catabolism, catalyzing adenosine to inosine conversion.

Increased Values
rheumatoid arthritis, empyema, lymphoproliferative diseases, lymphocytic pleuritis, sarcoidosis, tuberculosis

Albumin

Increased Values
transudate (in relation to globulins)

Alkaline Phosphatase

Increased Values
pulmonary infarction, malignant pleural effusion

Amylase

Increased Values
alcoholic hepatic cirrhosis, **pulmonary embolism, pulmonary infarction,** tumors – (**colon t.**, chronic lymphocytic leukemia, Hodgkin's disease, **pancreas t., prostate t., ovary t., stomach t.**), **amylase producing lung tumors, perforation of thoracic duct, induced pleuritis in acute pancreatitis** (P), **pancreatic pseudocyst** (P), **esophageal rupture into the pleural cavity** (S), tuberculosis, cardiac failure

Alpha-1-Antitrypsin

Increased Values
pulmonary embolism, exudates, inflammatory diseases, tumors

Decreased Values
liver cirrhosis, transudates, chronic cardiac failure

Appearance

- **thick puslike fluid** (purulent, presence of a foul odour): empyema, parapneumonic effusion
- **opaque**: empyema, chylothorax, damage/obstruction of the thoracic duct, pseudochylothorax, fatty degenerated malignant cells – (lymphoma)
- **admixtures**: cellular detritus – (exudate), erythrocytes – (pulmonary infarction, perforation of pulmonary and subphrenic abscess/cyst, pneumothorax, trauma, exudates in acute pancreatitis, exudates in uremia, malignant exudate, tuberculous exudates), fibrinous fibres – (exudate)

- **hyperviscous:** mesothelioma
- **turbid: empyema,** rheumatic fever, diseases – (**bacterial infectious d., rheumatoid d.,** autoimmune inflammatory d.), **tumors,** pancreatitis, tuberculosis

Bacteriological Picture

Non-specific and specific flora, anaerobic microorganisms and fungi.
- **Bacillus Koch** (Mycobacterium tuberculosis): pulmonary tuberculosis
- **non-specific flora:** bronchiectasis, acute/chronic bronchitis, bronchopneumonia, pulmonary empyema, lung tumors, pneumonia

Carcinoembryonic Antigen

Increased Values
empyema, **germ line tumors,** pancreatitis, **lung cancer, breast cancer, gastrointestinal tract tumors,** tuberculosis, parapneumonic effusion, pleural effusion secondary to tumors

Cellular Constituents

Increased Values
- **basophils:** leukemia
- **eosinophils:** allergic exogenous alveolitis (see also item eosinophils)
- **erythrocytes: pulmonary embolism,** asbestosis, empyema, exudate in – (**tumors,** acute pancreatitis, **tuberculosis,** uremia), diseases – (infectious d., rheumatoid d., inflammatory d.), **pulmonary infarction,** pancreatitis, perforation of – (lung/subphrenic abscess/cyst), pneumothorax, **damage to blood vessels, trauma,** pleural endometriosis, postcardiotomy sy, congestive heart failure
- **LE cells:** systemic lupus erythematosus
- **leukocytes: bacterial infectious diseases,** myocardial abscess, pneumonia, pulmonary infarction, pancreatitis, infective endocarditis, hepatic abscess rupture, tumors, postcardiotomy syndrome
- **lymphocytes:** exogenous allergic alveolitis, **rheumatoid arthritis, chylothorax,** systemic lupus erythematosus, **lymphomas, tumours,** rheumatoid pleuritis, **sarcoidosis, tuberculosis,** uremic effusion
- **malignant cells:** exudate of malignant etiology in – (lymphoma, lung t., breast t.)
- **mesothelial cells:** fluidothorax, inflammatory diseases, mesothelioma, tumors
- **neutrophils:** exogenous allergic alveolitis, **cryptogenic fibrosing alveolitis,** pulmonary embolism, **empyema,** pancreatic exudate, smokers, rheumatoid diseases, **pulmonary infarction,** systemic lupus erythematosus, **tumors, pancreatitis, pneumonia,** postmyocardial infarction sy, **tuberculosis,** parapneumonic effusion
- **mononuclear cells:** tumors, tuberculosis, rheumatoid diseases, transudates, lymphoma, uremia
- **polymorphonuclears:** pancreatitis, subphrenic abscess, pneumonia, pulmonary infarction

Decreased Values
alveolar macrophages: exogenous allergic alveolitis, cryptogenic fibrosing alveolitis, **sarcoidosis**

Cholesterol

Increased Values
exudate, chylous pleural fluid – (in malignant tumors, in trauma, congenital)

Circulating Immune Complexes

Increased Values
rheumatoid arthritis, collagen vascular diseases, systemic lupus erythematosus

Colour

- **white-yellow** (opaque): pus – (empyema), cholesterol effusion, chylothorax
- **red** (transparent): exudate in – (acute pancreatitis, uremia), pulmonary infarction, perforation of pulmonary/subphrenic abscess/cyst, pneumothorax, exudate in – (tumors, tuberculosis)
- **greenish**: biliopleural fistula
- **greenish-yellow**: rheumatoid effusion
- **red** (opaque): blood – (asbestosis, trauma, pleural endometriosis, pulmonary infarction, trauma, postcardiotomy sy, **tumor effusions**, uremia)
- **pale amber** (transparent): transudate/exudate of different etiology
- **white cream**: fatty degenerated malignant cells – (lymphoma), chylothorax, granulomatous diseases, trauma, pseudo-chylothorax, metastatic carcinoma
- **dark brown** (through black): older bleeding, hepatic amebiasis, aspergillosis

C 3, C4 Complement

Decreased Values
rheumatoid arthritis, systemic lupus erythematosus, tumors, bacterial pneumonia, tuberculosis

Complement CH50

Increased Values
congestive heart failure

Decreased Values
pleural effusion in systemic lupus erythematosus

Creatine Kinase

Increased Values
tumors

Eosinophils

Increased Values
allergic exogenous alveolitis, leaking aortic aneurysm, rheumatoid arthritis, asthma bronchiale, asbestosis, bronchitis, liver cirrhosis, allergic dermatitis, empyema, bacterial endocarditis, fever – (rheumatoid f., hay f.), chronic renal diseases, parasitic diseases – (amebiasis, ascariasis, filariasis, paragonimiasis), fungal diseases – (actinomycosis, histoplasmosis, coccidioidomycosis), pulmonary infarction, subhepatic infection, upper respiratory tract infection, systemic lupus erythematosus, tumors – (bronchogenic t., endothelioma, leukemia, Hodgkin's disease, pleural mesothelioma), ornithosis, pancreatitis, periarteritis nodosa, pneumonia, pneumothorax, polyarthritis, sarcoidosis, septicemia, syphilis, syndrome – (hypersensitivity sy, Löfler's sy), tuberculosis, thoracic trauma, uremia, effusion – (postoperative e., postpneumonic e.), congestive heart failure
Interfering Factors: medicaments – (bromocriptine, dantrolene, nitrofurantoin)

Erythrocytes (Blood)

Increased Values
asbestosis, diseases – (infectious d., inflammatory d.), **tumors**, **organ perforation**, tuberculosis, **trauma**, congestive heart failure, pleural endometriosis, **pulmonary infarction**, postcardiotomy sy, uremia

Exudate

abscess – (**lung a.**, **subphrenic a.**, liver a., spleen a.), rheumatoid arthritis, hepatic cirrhosis, **lung empyema**, hepatitis, diseases – (rheumatoid d., inflammatory d. of respiratory system, autoimmune inflammatory d.), familial recurrent polyserositis, infectious diseases – (fungal i. d., **respiratory system i. d.**), **pulmonary infarction**, subdiaphragmatic infections, **systemic lupus erythematosus**, tumors – (**pleural t., lung t.**, pleural endometriosis, mesothelioma, lymphoma, leukemia, gastrointestinal tract t.), **pancreatitis**, pseudocyst of pancreas, **asbestos pleurisy, pneumonia, parapneumonic processes, ruptured esophagus**, Wegener's granulomatosis, familial Mediterranean fever, sarcoidosis, syndrome – (Meig's sy, Churg–Strauss sy, Sjögren's sy), **tuberculosis, chest trauma**, rheumatoid pleurisy, collagen vascular diseases, **pulmonary embolism, hemothorax, chylothorax, postmyocardial infarction sy**, uremia, postradiation sy, **abdominal surgery**, hypothyroidism, urinothorax, chronic atelectasis, tumor metastases – (breast t., ovary t.), mixed connective tissue disease, vasculitis
Interfering Factors: medicaments – (methysergide, nitrofurantoin)

Fibrin Degradation Products

Increased Values
tumors

Decreased Values
congestive heart failure

Fibronectin

A glycoprotein found in body fluids, in free connective tissue matrix, and basement membranes. It is involved in cell aggregation, adhesiveness, locomotion and clearance by the reticuloendothelial system.

Increased Values
connective tissue diseases, rheumatoid pleurisy, tuberculosis

Gene Probes

DNA-DNA, DNA-RNA hybridization, amplification by speed polymerase chain reaction (PCR) – mainly to prove the tuberculosis mycobacteria evidence.

Positive
tuberculosis

Globulins

Increased Values
exudate (in relation to albumin)

Alpha Globulins

Decreased Values
tumors

Glucose

Decreased Values
rheumatoid arthritis, thoracic empyema, exudate of bacterial etiology, pleuritis – (lupus p., rheumatoid p.), esophageal rupture, tuberculosis, effusions – (parapneumonic e., in malignant tumors)

Beta-Glucuronidase

Increased Values
lung tumors

Glycosaminoglycans

(syn: mucopolysaccharides)

Increased Values
thoracic empyema, alveolar cell tumors, **mesothelioma**, tuberculosis

Haptoglobin

Increased Values
pulmonary embolism, exudates, inflammatory diseases, tumors

Decreased Values
liver cirrhosis, transudates, chronic cardiac failure

Hemopexin

Increased Values
pulmonary embolism, exudates, inflammatory diseases, tumors

Decreased Values
liver cirrhosis, transudates, chronic cardiac failure

Immunoglobulin A

Increased Values
inflammatory diseases, tumors, metastatic carcinoma effusions

Immunoglobulin G

Increased Values
inflammatory diseases, tumors, tuberculosis, metastatic carcinoma effusions

Lactate Dehydrogenase

Increased Values
thoracic empyema, bacterial exudate, **fibrosis**, hemothorax, diseases – (**collagen d., rheumatoid d.**, inflammatory d.), pulmonary infarction, **tumours**, massive necrosis of small bowels, pancreatitis, **paragonimiasis**, lupus pleuritis, **pancreatic pseudocyst, esophageal rupture**, tuberculosis, parapneumonic effusion

Lactic Acid

Increased Values
thoracic empyema, hepatic cirrhosis, rheumatoid diseases, nephrosis, trauma, effusion – (bacterial e., tuberculous e.), congestive heart failure

LE Cells

Increased Values
disseminated lupus erythematosus

Leukocytes

Increased Values
bacterial infectious diseases, myocardial abscess, **pneumonia,** pulmonary infarction, pancreatitis, **empyema,** infective endocarditis, **parapneumonic effusion,** hepatic abscess rupture, tumors, postcardiotomy syndrome

Lymphocytes

Increased Values
tuberculosis, exogenous allergic alveolitis, **rheumatoid arthritis, chylothorax,** systemic lupus erythematosus, **lymphomas, tumours,** rheumatoid pleuritis, **sarcoidosis,** uremic effusion

Lysozyme

Increased Values
acute myelocytic leukemia, tuberculosis

Alpha-2-Macroglobulin

Increased Values
pulmonary embolism, exudates, inflammatory diseases, tumors

Decreased Values
liver cirrhosis, transudates, chronic cardiac failure

Beta-2-Microglobulin

Increased Values
connective tissue disease, tumors – (lymphoma, plasmocytoma incl. multiple myeloma), tuberculosis, rheumatoid pleural effusion

Odour

- **ammonia:** urinothorax
- **putrid:** thoracic empyema

Orosomucoid

Increased Values
exudates, pulmonary embolism, inflammatory diseases, tumors – (lymphoma, pancreas t., lung t., breast t., ovary t.)

Decreased Values
liver cirrhosis, transudates, chronic cardiac failure

pH

Increased Values – basic, alkaline
liver cirrhosis, exudate of malignant etiology, transudates, congestive heart failure

Decreased Values – acid
fibrosing cryptogenic alveolitis, **rheumatoid arthritis**, echinococcosis, **empyema, exudates,** hemothorax, diseases – (**collagen d., rheumatoid d.**), **tumours**, massive necrosis of small bowels, **collagen vascular diseases**, pancreatitis, **systemic lupus erythematosus, pancreatic pseudocyst, esophageal rupture, tuberculosis**

Proteins

Increased Values ↑ 30 g/l – exudate
thoracic empyema, **drug hypersensitivity,** diseases – (gastrointestinal d., **infectious d.,** rheumatoid d., **connective tissue d.**), **pulmonary infarction,** systemic lupus erythematosus, **tumors, pancreatitis,** plasmocytoma (incl. multiple myeloma), **tuberculosis, trauma,** uremia

Decreased Values ↓ 30 g/l – transudate
liver cirrhosis, peritoneal dialysis, acute glomerulonephritis, myxedema, nephrotic sy, congestive heart failure

Rheumatoid Factor

Increased Values
rheumatoid diseases, bacterial pneumonia, effusion – (parapneumonic e., malignant e., tuberculous e.)

Transudate

cirrhosis – (**liver c.,** primary biliary c., cardiac c.), **hypoalbuminemia,** failure – (**congestive heart f.,** chronic renal f.), dengue, lymphocytic lymphoma, hypoalbuminemia, acute atelectasis, peritoneal dialysis, pericarditis – (constrictive p., acute p.), myxedema heart disease, obstruction of v. cava superior, pulmonary embolism, epidemic pleurodynia, urinothorax, misplaced subclavian catheter, myxedema, sarcoidosis, syndrome – (Meig's sy, nephrotic sy), early mediastinal malignancy, tumors – (lung t.)

Tumour Markers

Alpha-fetoprotein, beta-2-microglobulin, CA 19-9, CK-BB, ferritin, chorionic gonadotropin (hCG), carcinoembryonic antigen (CEA), CYFRA-21.

Positive
exudate of malignant etiology

Tumor Marker CA 125

Positive
exudate of malignant etiology, tumors – (ovarian t., breast t., lung t., gastrointestinal tract t.)

Volume

Increased Values
liver cirrhosis, tumors, tuberculosis, congestive heart failure

Saliva
D. Mesko

Saliva physiological contents: proteins, ammonia, IgA, IgG, IgM, glycoproteins, urea, uric acid, glucose, cholesterol, amylase, alkaline/acid phosphatase, lactate, AST, ALT, electrolytes, fatty acids, amino acids, lactoferrin, lysozyme, esterases, LD. About 90% of salivary secretion comes from the parotid and submandibular glands, 5% from the sublingual glands and up to 5% flows from the minor salivary glands (labial, lingual, buccal and palatal mucous glands).

Factors affecting salivary composition: diurnal variation, flow rate, age, sex, drugs, diet, duration and type of stimulus, hormones, salivary gland size. Functions of saliva: protective and antibacterial.

Indications for saliva examination: 1) therapeutic drug monitoring (e.g. dexamethasone, digoxin, lithium, phenobarbital, theophylline), 2) testing for abused drugs (e.g. amphetamines, barbiturates, benzodiazepines, cocaine, codeine, ethanol, heroin, marijuana).

Chloride

Increased Values
parotitis, Sjögren's sy

Immunoglobulin A

Increased Values
rheumatoid arthritis, infantile hypogammaglobulinemia, rheumatoid diseases, parotitis, Sjögren's sy

Immunoglobulin G

Increased Values
parotitis, Sjögren's sy

Lysozyme

Increased Values
Sjögren's sy

Beta-2-Microglobulin

Increased Values
Sjögren's sy

Natrium

Increased Values
rheumatoid arthritis, cystic fibrosis, parotitis, Sjögren's sy

Decreased Values
adrenal hyperfunction, congestive heart failure

Phosphorus

Decreased Values
parotitis, Sjögren's sy

Potassium

Increased Values
cystic fibrosis

Proteins

Increased Values
parotitis

Seminal Fluid

D. Mesko

Semen analysis is important in determining the spermatogenesis normalcy and the reproductive tract patency. Seminal fluid (seminal plasma) physiologically contents: proteins, albumin, alpha-1-glycoprotein, alpha-1-antitrypsin, ceruloplasmin, beta-1-globulin, transferrin, IgA, IgG, amino acids, sugars – (fructose, glucose, fucose, sorbitol, inositol, sialic acid, mannose, mannitol, galactose, ribose, glycerol), electrolytes – (sodium, potassium, calcium, magnesium, copper, zinc, iron, chloride, bicarbonate), acid phosphatase, pepsinogen, trypsin, lactate, neutral lipids, steroid hormones and prostaglandins. It is essential to analyze a fresh specimen (not more than one hour old) in order to obtain meaningful results for liquefaction and spermatozoa motility.

Normal findings in seminal fluid: white color, grayish, pale yellow, viscid consistency, coagulates promptly, liquefaction in 20–60 min, volume in 2–7 ml, spermatozoa motility >60% means good movement, present fructose, spermatozoa morphology of less than 30% is abnormal, pH 7.2–7.8.

Test Purpose. 1) to evaluate male fertility with infertile couples, 2) to substantiate the effectiveness of vasectomy, 3) to detect semen on the body/clothing in suspected rape or elsewhere at a crime scene, 4) to identify blood group substances when exonerating or incriminating a suspect, 5) to rule out paternity on grounds of sterility.

Sperm Analysis

(syn: semen analysis) Spermatogenesis, the germ cell to spermatozoa maturation, takes 72 days and requires intact hypothalamic-pituitary-testicular access. Luteinizing hormone causes synthesis of testosterone from the Leydig's cells, which diffuses to the tubular cells where it affects spermatogenesis directly/indirectly through Sertoli's cells function (as a matrix for the germ cells). Follicle-stimulating hormone also is required to produce spermatozoa and acts directly on the Sertoli's cells. Complete semen analysis consists of at least five determinants: volume, density/liquefaction, motility (quality, percent motile, total motile count), quantitative spermatozoa movement, and morphological characteristics. Other determinants are: pH, cytology, sperm concentration.

Antibodies Against Spermatozoa

(antisperm antibodies)
Test Purpose. To detect antibodies bound to heads of spermatozoa in semen in the investigation of infertility.

Increased Values – positive
male infertility, vasectomy, testicular trauma, viral orchitis, bacterial infectious diseases of genitourinary tract

Colour

- **red** (hemospermia): tumors of – (prostate, urethra, seminal vesicles), spermatocystitis, trauma
- **yellow-green** (pyospermia): purulent prostatitis, spermatocystitis, vesiculitis

Fructose

Decreased Values
congenital abnormalities in the male genital tract, patency disorders of ejaculatory ducts, absence/obstruction of vas deferens and seminal vesicles

Alpha-Glucosidase

Decreased Values
azoospermia, **male infertility**, varicocele, vasectomy

Odour

- **present**: absces of – (prostate, seminal vesicles), purulent inflammatory diseases
- **absent**: prostate atrophy

pH

Increased Values
acute inflammation of male adnexes

Decreased Values
contamination with urine, chronic male adnexes inflammation

Prostatic Acid Phosphatase

Increased Values
vaginal swabs from rape victims

Spermatozoa Count

- **azoospermia** (absence of spermatozoa): anabolic steroids abuse, germinal aplasia, testicular atrophy after mumps, ejaculation – (absent e., retrograde e.), obstruction of the ejaculatory system, orchitis, seminiferous tubule sclerosis, spermatozoa maturation arrest, primary testicular Leydig's cells failure

- **oligozoospermia** (lower spermatozoa count): testicular atrophy after mumps, hyperpyrexia, male hypogonadism, diseases – (genital infectious d., pituitary d., hypothalamic d., systemic d.), cryptorchism (cryptorchidism), medicaments – (anabolics, antineoplastics, azathioprine, chlorambucil, cimetidine, cyclophosphamide, estrogens, ketoconazole, methotrexate, methyltestosterone, nandrolone, nitrofurantoin, procarbazine, sulfasalazine, vincristine), obstruction of ejaculatory system, idiopathic oligospermia, orchitis, testicular radiation, damage to the germinal epithelium, postvasectomy conditions, varicocele, primary/secondary testicular failure
- **polyzoospermia** (increased spermatozoa count)
- **teratozoospermia** (less 60% of normally configurated spermatozoa)

Spermatozoa Motility

Decreased Values – asthenozoospermia
absence of the spermatozoal postacrosomal sheath, prolonged abstinence, myotonic dystrophia, male hypogonadism, cryptorchism, necrozoospermia (all spermatozoa avital), reduced fertility, spermatozoa – (acrosome-less s., macrocephalic s.), Kartagener's sy

Volume

- **aspermia** (absence of semen fluid): retrograde ejaculation, condition after retroperitoneal lymphadenectomy in testicular tumor, bilateral ductus deferens closure
- **hyperspermia** (increased volume of semen fluid): reduced fertility, acute prostatitis, medicaments – (finasteride, nandrolone)
- **hypospermia** (decreased volume of semen fluid): sexual abstinence (less 5 days), unilateral ductus deferens aplasia, myotonic dystrophia, smoking, hyperpyrexia, male hypogonadism, cryptorchidism, decreased levels of testosterone, chronic prostatitis, prostate tuberculosis, primary/secondary testicular failure

Sputum

D. Mesko

Mucus secretion is part of the normal broncho-pulmonary cleansing. Secretions form a layer about 5 μm thick, immediately overlaying the ciliated epithelium. By ciliary action this semisticky fluid mantle moves upward toward the oropharynx, carrying inhaled particles that have found their way down to the respiratory bronchioles. Besides mechanical cleansing, mucus attacks inhaled bacteria directly. The antibacterial effect of normal tracheo-bronchial mucus results largely from the antibody activity, although lysozymes and slightly acid pH conditions also help maintain sterility. The antibodies are predominantly IgA and enter the mucus by direct glandular secretion rather than by transudation from the plasma.

- Sampling techniques: fresh, early morning sputum after patient fasting – first sputum expectorated on arising, 1–2 hours sputum collection, 24 hours sputum collection. Major approaches for collection: spontaneous cough, induced cough, nasopharyngeal suctioning.
- Examinations: inspection, microscopical, bacteriological, cytological and culturing.
- Normally (physiological): the tracheo-bronchial tree produces 100 to 150 ml of mucus per day from goblet cells and mucous glands. Content: albumin, globulins, IgA, IgG, glykanes, glykoproteins, lactoferrin, kallikrein, lysozyme, carbohydrates, peptides, amino acids, minerals.

Sampling:
- collection of deep-cough sputum for 3 to 5 consecutive mornings
- transtracheal aspiration
- induced sputum (by inhalation of hypertonic NaCl)

Appearance

- **serous:** pulmonary edema
- **mucous:** acute/chronic bronchitis, acute tracheobronchitis (early), asthmatic attack
- **purulent:** pulmonary abscess, asthma bronchiale, bronchiectasis, purulent bronchitis, bronchopneumonia, find a vent of pulmonary empyema into a bronchus, pulmonary tuberculosis
- **putrid:** pulmonary abscess, bronchiectasis, anaerobic infection – (pulmonary gangrene, secondary in bronchogenic tumors)

Bacteriological Picture

Non-specific and specific flora, anaerobic microorganisms and fungi.
- **Bacillus Koch** (Mycobacterium tuberculosis): pulmonary tuberculosis
- **non-specific flora:** bronchiectasis, acute/chronic bronchitis, bronchopneumonia, pulmonary empyema, lung tumors, pneumonia

Blood

Hemoptysis means streaks/sanguineous admixture (bloody sputum, blood stained sputum). Hemoptoe means massive pulmonary bleeding (large hemorrhage).

Positive
- **general causes** (extrapulmonary origin): pernicious anemia, **hemorrhagic diathesis**, **hemophilia**, spurious hemoptysis – (bleeding of nose/nasopharynx), **coagulopathies**, leucemia, hemodynamics disorders – (mitral stenosis), thrombocytopathies, **thrombocytopenia**, **vasculopathies**, congestive heart failure
- **local causes** (pulmonary origin): **pulmonary abscess, bronchiectasis, acute/chronic/ venostatic bronchitis, pulmonary edema, pulmonary gangrene, pulmonary hemosiderosis, pulmonary infarction, pulmonary tumors, croupous pneumonia, pulmonary tuberculosis, trauma**
  Interfering Factors: acetylcysteine, alteplase, anistreplase, argatroban, bivalirudin, cilostazol, porfimer, rifapentine, streptokinase, tenecteplase, urokinase

Colour

- **white** (milky): asthma bronchiale, bronchitis, bronchioalveolar carcinoma
- **red** (blood): pulmonary abscess, vascular anomalies, bronchiectasis, acute/chronic/ venostatic bronchitis, pulmonary edema, pulmonary gangrene, pseudohemoptysis – (hematemesis, origin in ENT area, origin in stomatological area), pulmonary hemosiderosis, parasitic pulmonary diseases, pulmonary infarction, benign pulmonary tumours, pulmonary tumors, croupous pneumonia, complicated silicosis, pulmonary tuberculosis, trauma
- **red currant jelly:** Klebsiella pneumoniae
- **red** (other causes): dyes, rifampicin, Serratia marcescens
- **dark brown:** gangrene, amebic liver abscess rupture into bronchus
- **grey-black:** coal-miners, anthracosilicosis, Bacteroides melaninogenicus pneumonia
- **green:** bronchiectasis, acute/chronic bronchitis, pulmonary tumors, pneumonia, Pseudomonas infection
- **yellow:** bronchiectasis, bronchitis, bronchopneumonia, jaundice, pulmonary infectious diseases, eosinophilic pulmonary infiltrates, pneumonia

Cytological Picture

The looking for malignant cells on malignant lung tumours suspicion.
- **physiological:** alveolar macrophages, bronchial epithelial cells, lymphocytes, polymorphonuclear cells
- **tumorous cells:** bronchogenic tumors
- **altered polymorphonuclears:** pulmonary abscess, pulmonary diseases – (purulent p. d., inflammatory p. d.)

Macroscopically

colour, admixtures – (putrid, purulent, bloody, mucous, serous), amount, odour

Microscopical Picture

The looking for particulate matter. Fresh preparation, Gram's stain.

Cellular Constituents

- **alveolar epithelial cells and their fragments**: asthma bronchiale, acute infectious diseases
- **Bacillus Koch** (Mycobacterium tuberculosis): pulmonary tuberculosis
- **bronchial epithelial cells**: viral infections
- **eosinophils**: exogenous allergic alveolitis, asthma bronchiale, eosinophilic infiltrates
- **physiologically**: solitary – alveolar macrophages, bronchial epithelial cells, mononuclear cells, polymorphonuclear leucocytes
- **lymphocytes**: exogenous allergic alveolitis, sarcoidosis
- **macrophages**: alveolar proteinosis
- **neutrophils**: exogenous allergic alveolitis, cryptogenic fibrosing alveolitis, smokers
- **PMN leukocytes**: bronchiectasis, chronic bronchitis, inflammatory diseases, pneumonia

Decreased Values
alveolar macrophages: allergic exogenous alveolitis, cryptogenic fibrosing alveolitis, sarcoidosis

Non-Cellular Constituents

- **Charcot–Leyden crystals**: asthma bronchiale
- **Curschmann's spirals**: asthma bronchiale, obstruction of small bronchi
- **firm plugs**: bronchiolitis, fibrinous bronchitis, exacerbation of allergic bronchopulmonary aspergillosis
- **lipid droplets in macrophages**: pneumonia – (aspiration p., lipoid p.)
- **dense sputum, crystalline concretions**: broncholithiasis
- **asbestos particles**: asbestosis

Odour

- **putrid**: pulmonary abscess, bronchiectasis, putrid bronchitis, pulmonary gangrene
- **fishy**: paragonimiasis
- **sweet**: pulmonary gangrene

Volume

Increased Values
pulmonary abscess, bronchiectasis, bronchitis – (chronic b., purulent b.), bronchopneumonia, pulmonary empyema, cigarette smoking, pulmonary gangrene, pulmonary mycoses, acute tracheobronchitis

Stool

D. Mesko

Feces (stool) are composed of
- waste indigestible material residues such as food cellulose eaten over the previous 4 days
- bile (pigments and salts) – color is normally due to altered bile pigments by bacterial action
- intestinal secretions, including mucus
- leukocytes that migrate from the bloodstream
- shed epithelial cells
- bacteria make up at least one-third of total solids
- inorganic material (10–20 %) that is chiefly calcium and phosphates
- undigested/unabsorbed food

Stool examination:
size, shape, consistency, color, odor, presence/absence of blood, pH, mucus, pus, tissue fragments, food residues, bacteria/parasites, parasite fragments/eggs, biliary dyes, muscular fibres, starch, enzymes, proteins, carbohydrates, minerals

---

Alpha-1-Antitrypsin

Increased Values
exudative enteropathy

Bile

Normally the bile is never found in feces.

Increased Values – positive
diarrhea, severe liver diseases, hemolytic jaundice, complete biliary obstruction

---

Bile Pigments

Estimation of the total bile pigments excretion, breakdown products of hemoglobin. Bilirubin metabolism products → intestinal bacteria → urobilinogen, sterkobilinogen, urobilin, sterkobilin. Bilirubin in newborns → oxidizes to green biliverdin.

Decreased Values
block of bile flow into intestine

Blood

Upper gastrointestinal bleeding less than 50 ml is only registered biochemically (occult, hidden bleeding). Do not rely on digital rectal examination in hospital patients (high false positive rate). Avoid for three days prior testing: red meat, cantaloupe and other melon, broccoli, turnips, radishes, cauliflower, vitamin C, acetylsalicylic acid preparations, NSAIDs.

Test Purpose. 1) to detect gastrointestinal bleeding, 2) to aid early diagnosis of colorectal cancer, 3) to help in differential diagnosis of anemias, 4) suspicion of occult hemorrhage, 5) diagnosis of intestinal polypose and ulcerative colitis.

Positive, upper Gastrointestinal Tract Bleeding
duodenitis, esophagitis, gastritis – **(atrophic g., erosive g.),** hernia – (diaphragmatic h., hiatus h.), **gastric/duodenal ulcer disease,** tumors of – **(duodenum, esophagus, stomach),** bleeding from – **(pharynx),** varices of – **(esophagus, stomach), anastomotic ulcer**

Positive, lower Gastrointestinal Tract Bleeding
angiodysplasia, Meckel's diverticulum, **diverticulitis, diverticulosis, anal/anorectal fissure, colorectal hemangioma, hemorrhoids, inflammatory bowel diseases,** bacterial infections – (amebiasis, Campylobacter, Salmonella spp., Shigella spp.), colitis – **(ischemic c., radiation c., c. ulcerosa),** vascular malformations, **tumors of colorectum,** Crohn's disease, Rendu–Osler disease, polyarteritis nodosa, polyps of – **(colon, rectum),** proctitis, Henoch–Schönlein purpura, foreign body, mesenteric thrombosis, tuberculosis, typhoid fever, **gastrointestinal trauma, recent gastrointestinal surgery**

Positive – other causes
amyloidosis, aortic aneurysm, liver cirrhosis, hematobilia, nasal bleeding, pancreatic tumors, neurofibromatosis, pancreatitis, radiation, Kaposi's sarcoma, scurvy, Turner's sy, uremia

Positive – Interfering Factors
medicaments – (acetylsalicylic acid, antibiotics, bromides, ceftibuten, colchicine, corticosteroids, indomethacin, iodine, iron, meloxicam, methyldopa, NSAIDS, rauwolfia derivatives, rofecoxib, salicylates, steroids, vitamin C), peroxidases of bacterial origin, peroxidases of vegetable origin – (bananas, horse radish, lettuce), **high red meat/fish diet,** vigorous brushing of the teeth in increased hemorrhage of gums

Negative
false negative – (ascorbic acid, antacids)

Carbohydrates

Increased Values
diarrhea from disaccharidase deficiency

Chloride

Increased Values
idiopathic proctocolitis, ileostomy, cholera

Chymotrypsin

Decreased Values
pancreatic dysfunction, cystic fibrosis of the pancreas, pancreatic insufficiency, pancreatic duct obstruction, chronic pancreatitis

Analyte	Age/Gender	Reference Range	SI Units	Note
Chymotrypsin		>220	nkat/g	

Color

- **red:** surface blood – (anal abnormalities, hemorrhoids), lower GIT bleeding
- **black** (melena): bleeding of upper GIT, ferrous medicaments, bismuth intake, active charcoal
  Interfering Factors: red – (beet), black – (high meat diet, charcoal, cherries), light – (milky diet, low meat diet), green – (antibiotics, chlorophyll-rich green vegetables), yellow – (breast-fed infants, rhubarb, bowel sterilization by antibiotics)
- **medicaments:** whitish – (antacids, aluminium salts), red – (pyrvinium pamoate, phenolphthalein, tetracyclines, anticoagulants, salicylates), black – (iron drugs, bismuth salts, charcoal, phenbutazone, oxyphenbutazone), pink-red – (excessive dose of anticoagulants/salicylates), light – (barium), green – (indomethacin, mercurial salts), brown – (anthraquinones), green to blue – (diathiazine), orange-red – (phenazopyridine), yellow-brown – (senna)
- **grey** (gray, fatty): chocolate, cocoa, fat (steatorrhea)
- **grey-whitish** (acholic): high milk products diet, mechanic icterus (bile duct obstruction), barium ingestion
- **dark brown:** high meat diet, prolonged exposure to air
- **dark green:** hemolytic icterus
- **green:** diet high in spinach and other greens, severe diarrhea, antibiotic therapy
- **silver:** combination of jaundice and blood
- **yellow to yellow green:** diet high in spinach and other greens, severe diarrhea, vegetable laxatives, rapid transit time

Consistency

- **diarrhea mixed with erythrocytes:** amebiasis, cholera, large bowel tumors, typhoid fever
- **diarrhea with leukocytes:** regional enteritis, colitis ulcerosa, salmonellosis, shigellosis, intestinal tuberculosis
- **fatty – pasty** (grayish-white): celiac disease, cystic fibrosis, biliary duct obstruction, barium ingestion, sprue
- **thin** (diarrhea): decreased fluid absorption, amyloidosis, intestinal bypass, enzyme deficiency (lactase), high vegetable diet, diabetic enteropathy, bacterial enterotoxins – (Vibrio cholerae, E. coli, staphylotoxin), entero-enteric fistulas, watery diarrhea, hypokalemia, ischemic/inflammatory bowel diseases, diseases of pancreas – (insufficiency, tumors, inflammatory d.), lack of contact of intraluminal fluid with absorptive surface, calcitonin, carcinoid, ulcerative colitis, medicaments – (ampicillin, magnesium-containing antacids, cephalosporins, digitalis, glucagon, guanethidine, quinidine, potassium,

laxatives, lincomycin, mannitol, propranolol, secretin, sorbitol), lymphoma, Crohn's disease, Whipple's disease, malabsorption, maldigestion, medullary tumors of the thyroid, biliary obstruction, vasoactive intestinal polypeptide, motor disturbances, bowel resection, increased fluid secretion, sprue, syndrome – (irritable bowel sy, hypochlorhydria sy)

■ **dry**: high meat diet
■ **thick** (constipation): gastrointestinal tract abscesses, adhesions, dehydration, urinary bladder distension, diabetic enteropathy, intramural hematoma, hypothyroidism, psychiatric illnesses, prolonged bed immobility, decreased/altered gastrointestinal motility, opiates, spinal cord injury, Hirschsprung's disease, tumors of gastrointestinal tract, decreased bulk/intake of meals, extra/intraluminal obstruction, polyps, altered defecation reflex, scleroderma, secondary conditions to painful rectal/anal lesions, irritable bowel sy
■ **watery** (voluminous): disaccharidase deficiency, Escherichia coli, cholera, staphylococcal food poisoning, toxigenic

Elastase-1

(syn: pancreatic elastase)

Increased Values
chronic pancreatitis

Analyte	Age/Gender	Reference Range	SI Units	Note
Pancreatic Elastase-1		>200	*	*µg/g of stool

Fat

(syn: fecal fat, quantitative stool fat determination) Fat excretion by the stools is constant, not dependent on food intake. The source of stool fat is the intestinal mucosa cell residuum, which is a product of bacterial breakdown. To quantify fat excretion, there must be known dietary intake and timed stool collection. In feces, most lipids are present as fatty acids, both saturated and unsaturated, since neutral fats are hydrolyzed by lipases high in small intestine. Lipase deficiency, usually from pancreatic disease, usually increases neutral fat proportion. Normal lipid absorption requires bile from the gall bladder, enzymes from the pancreas and a normal intestines.

Test Purpose. 1) to confirm steatorrhea, 2) to help in the diagnosis of malabsorption sy, 3) to diagnose pancreatopathies, 4) to evaluate fat absorption as an indicator of liver, gall bladder, pancreas and intestinal functions.

Positive Values – steatorrhea
abetalipoproteinemia, pernicious anemia, **coeliac disease** (gluten-sensitive enteropathy), hepatic cirrhosis, deficiency – (pancreatic enzymes d., bile d.), cholelithiasis, diabetes mellitus, gastro-intestinal fistula, **cystic fibrosis**, viral hepatitis, **hepatopathy**, **diarrhea**, hyperlipoproteinemia, peptic ulcer disease, **diseases of pancreas**, malignant infiltration of the intestinal wall, carcinoid, malabsorption secondary to – (amyloidosis, **radiation enteritis**, **Crohn's disease**, **Whipple's disease**, scleroderma, **sprue**), maldigestion secondary to – (obstruction of the pancreatobiliary tree – **cancer**, **stricture**, gallstones), **malnutrition**, Addison's

disease, lymphatic passage obstruction, **pancreatic insufficiency,** pancreatic cancer, **pancreatitis,** accelerated passage of gastric contents, fat intake with saturated fatty acid prevailing, impaired fat resorption, resection of the intestine, sprue, multiple sclerosis, progressive systemic sclerosis, **idiopathic steatorrhea,** dumping sy, short-gut syndrome secondary to – (congenital anomaly, surgical bypass, **surgical resection), intestinal tuberculosis,** thyrotoxicosis

> Interfering Factors: mayonnaise, mineral oils, castor oil, suppositories, medicaments – (aminosalicylic acid, amphotericin B, azathioprine, cholestyramine, colchicine, colestipol, laxatives, kanamycin, methotrexate, neomycin, octreotide, orlistat, tetracyclines)

Hemoglobin

Increased Values – positive, upper Git Bleeding
duodenitis, esophagitis, gastritis – (**atrophic g., erosive g.**), hernia – (diaphragmatic h., hiatus h.), **gastric/duodenal ulcer disease, pharyngeal bleeding,** tumors – (**duodenum t., esophagus t., stomach t.**), varices of – (**esophagus, stomach**), **anastomotic ulcer**

Positive, lower Gastrointestinal Tract Bleeding
angiodysplasia, Meckel's diverticulum, **diverticulitis, diverticulosis, anal/anorectal fissure, colorectal hemangioma, hemorrhoids, inflammatory bowel diseases,** bacterial infections – (amebiasis, Campylobacter, Salmonella spp., Shigella spp.), colitis – (**ischemic c., radiation c., c. ulcerosa**), vascular malformations, **colorectum tumors,** Crohn's disease, Rendu–Osler disease, polyarteritis nodosa, polyps – (**colon p., rectum p.**), proctitis, Henoch–Schönlein purpura, foreign body, mesenteric thrombosis, tuberculosis, typhoid fever, **gastrointestinal trauma, recent gastrointestinal surgery**

> Interfering Factors: medicaments – (acetazolamide, amphetamine, amphotericin B, azapropazone, cefamandole, cyclophosphamide, diclofenac, ethanol, fenoprofen, phenylbutazone, griseofulvin, ibuprofen, indomethacin, ketoprofen, clindamycin, acetylsalicylic acid, aminosalicylic acid, lincomycin, methyldopa, naproxen, oxyphenbutazone, piroxicam, procarbazine, gold salts)

Hepatitis A Antigen

(HAAg)
Test Purpose. 1) Diagnosis of hepatitis A, 2) identification of infection before clinical symptoms (14 days) appear, 3) monitoring of patient infectiosity.

Leukocytes

Test Purpose. 1) To help in diagnosis of diarrheal diseases, 2) to detect conditions associated with marked fecal leukocytes, blood and mucus.

Increased Values
ulcerative colitis, salmonellosis, shigellosis, typhoid, infection caused by – (**Campylobacter jejuni, Escherichia coli infection** – enteroinvasive E. coli, enterohemorrhagic E. coli, **Yersinia enterocolitica,** Vibrio parahemolyticus, Clostridium difficile, Mycobacterium tuberculosis, rotaviruses), antibiotic associated colitis, amebiasis

Decreased Values

toxigenic bacteria – (Clostridium, Staphylococcus), diarrhea – (non-specific d., viral d., non-invasive E. coli d.), cholera, amebic colitis, parasites – (Entamoeba histolytica, Dientamoeba fragilis, Giardia lamblia)

Magnesium

Test Purpose. 1) To identify magnesium-containing laxatives as the cause of diarrhea, 2) to assess increased loss of magnesium from the gut as a cause of hypomagnesemia.

Increased Values

diarrhea due to magnesium-containing laxatives, magnesium loss from the gut

Microscopical Picture

- ■ **parasites and ova**
- ■ **starch granules:** starch intolerance, cystic pancreatofibrosis
- ■ **fatty drops**
- ■ **crystals:** calcium oxalate c., fatty acid c., triple phosphate c., hematoidin c. – (gastrointestinal tract hemorrhage), Charcot–Leyden c. – (parasitic infestation, amebiasis)
- ■ **epithelial cells:** gastrointestinal tract inflammation
- ■ **striated muscular fibres:** coeliac disease, pancreatic insufficiency, faster passage, disorder of gastrointestinal resorption
- ■ **inflammatory cells:** inflammatory bowel diseases, invasive bacterial infections – (amebiasis, Campylobacter, Salmonella spp., Shigella spp.)

Mucus

Mucus in stool appears in conditions of parasympathetic excitability.
- ■ **purulent-bloody m.:** acute diverticulitis, bacillary dysentery, colitis ulcerosa, colon tumors, intestinal tuberculosis
- ■ **copious m.:** villous adenoma of the colon
- ■ **bloody mucus on the stool surface:** amebae, rectum tumors, shigella, rectum inflammation
- ■ **gelatinous m. on the stool surface:** mucous colitis, excessive straining at stool, spastic constipation, irritable bowel sy, emotional influence

Natrium

Secretory diarrhea result in liquid feces with high sodium levels.
Test Purpose. To help in differentiation of secretory from non-secretory diarrhea.

Increased Values

diarrhea in – (pancreatic islet cell tumor, cathartics, enterotoxins, cholera), idiopathic proctocolitis, ileostomy

Non-Protein Nitrogen

Increased Values
gastrocolic fistula, severe diarrhea, pancreatic diseases, steatorrhea

Odour

Odour is caused by indole and skatole, formed by intestinal putrefaction and bacterial action fermentation.
- **putrid**: putrid dyspepsia
- **acid**: ferment dyspepsia, sweet food

Osmolality

Test is used to distinct osmotic from nonosmotic secretory diarrhea. A large deficit in the calculated osmolality from the measured stool osmolality indicates osmotic diarrhea.

Osmotic Gap

Increased Values
osmotic diarrhea

pH

Test detects carbohydrate and fat malabsorption and evaluates small intestinal disaccharidase deficienies. Stool pH is dependent in part on fermentation of sugars. Colonic fermentation of normal amounts of carbohydrate sugars and production of fatty acids accounts for the normally slightly acidic pH.
Test Purpose. To help in diagnosis of sugar intolerance.

Increased Values – alkaline pH
villous adenoma, coeliac disease, cystic fibrosis of pancreas, **increased protein breakdown**, secretory diarrhea, colitis, antibiotic usage

Decreased Values – acid pH
decreased absorption of – (carbohydrates, fat), intestinal lactase deficiency, fermenting dyspepsia, acute enteritis, **carbohydrate malabsorption**, sugar intolerance, high lactose intake

Physiological Finding

- **macroscopic**: color – (brown), consistency – (plastic), amount – (0–300 g/day), negative – (mucus, pus, blood, parasites), shape – (formed), odor (depends on pH of stool, bacterial fermentation)
- **microscopic**: negative – (yeasts, leukocytes, undigested food, meat fibers, starch, trypsin, eggs and segments of parasites), fat – (fatty acid crystals, neutral fat)

■ **chemical**: negative – (occult blood, bile), pH – (neutral, weakly alkaline), positive – (nitrogen, coproporphyrins, protoporphyrins, trypsin, uroporphyrins)

Porphyrins

(coproporphyrins + protoporphyrins)
Test Purpose. 1) differential diagnosis of variegate porphyria and hereditary coproporphyria from acute intermittent porphyria in acute stage, 2) to reveal latent forms of acute hepatic porphyrias, 3) to help in the diagnosis of erythropoietic porphyrias and protoporphyrias.

Increased Values
hemolytic anemia, **liver diseases, lead poisoning, hereditary coproporphyria**, porphyria – (**erythropoietic p.**, acute intermittent p.), **porphyria cutanea tarda, porphyria variegata** (variegate porphyria), **protoporphyria**

Analyte	Age/Gender	Reference Range	SI Units	Note
Coproporphyrins		600–1800	nmol/d	

Potassium

Test Purpose. To document fecal potassium loss as a cause of hypokalemia.

Increased Values
severe diarrhea, colon/rectum villous tumors

Decreased Values
ileostomy

Proteins

Increased Values
pancreatofibrosis

Pus

positive
localized abscesses, diverticulitis, chronic bacillary dysentery, fistulas – (anus f., sigmoid rectum f.), chronic ulcerative colitis, necrotic tumors, parasites

Reducing Sugars

(syn: reducing substances) Sugars should be rapidly absorbed in the upper small intestine. If not, they remain in the intestine causing osmotic diarrhea by the osmotic pressure of the unabsorbed intestinal sugar. The unabsorbed sugars are measured as reducing substances.

Test Purpose. 1) to detect deficiency of intestinal border enzymes, primarily sucrase and lactase (disaccharidases), 2) to help in diagnosis of sugar intolerance (lactose, sucrose, glucose/galactose).

Increased Values
disaccharidase deficiency, reduced digestion/absorption of sugars

Shape

- ■ **excessive hard**: increased absorption of fluid due to delayed transport
- ■ **ribbon-like**: decreased rectal elasticity, spastic bowel, rectal stricture
- ■ **scybala** (small, round, hard stools): constipation

Trypsin

Decreased Values
cystic fibrosis of pancreas, pancreatic insufficiency, obstruction of the pancreatic duct, loss of pancreatic exocrine function

Urobilinogen

Total bile pigments excretion as hemoglobin breakdown products are evaluated.
Test Purpose. 1) to aid in the diagnosis of hepatobiliary and hemolytic disorders, 2) to evaluate the function of liver and bile ducts.

Increased Values
anemia – (**hemolytic a.**, sickle cell a., pernicious a., thalassemia), **erythroblastosis fetalis**, hemolytic jaundice, pulmonary infarction, severe bruises

Decreased Values
aplastic anemia, primary biliary cirrhosis, **hepatic cirrhosis**, **depressed erythropoiesis**, hepatitis – (alcoholic h., toxic h., viral h.), **choledocholithiasis**, drug-induced cholestasis, **severe liver diseases**, **cachexia**, **antibiotic therapy**, Gilbert's disease, tumors of – (**pancreas head, Vater's papilla, bile duct**), hemolytic jaundice, thalassemia, complete biliary obstruction – (**calculi, tumors, scar tissue**), parenchymal hepatic injury, syndrome – (Crigler–Najjar sy, Dubin-Johnson sy, Rotor's sy)
    Interfering Factors: medicaments – (antibiotics)

Volume

Increased Values
laxative abuse, secretory diarrhea, malabsorption, increased carbohydrate intake, steatorrhea, vegetarian diet

Decreased Values
infectious diarrhea, inflammatory bowel diseases, increased intake of – (meat, proteins), syndrome – (irritable bowel sy, malabsorption sy)

Sweat

D. Mesko

Contains 0.5–1% soluble and inorganic materials (Na, Cl, Ca, Ni, Cu, Zn, Pb) and organic materials (urea, ammonia, amino acids, creatinine, protein, carbohydrates, steroids, glycoproteins).

Aluminium

Increased Values
cystic fibrosis

Chloride

Test Purpose. To detect cystic fibrosis. Indications to repeat the test for confirmation: positive test, suspected false negative test.

Increased Values
cystic fibrosis, **G6P-ase deficiency**, anorexia nervosa, nephrogenic diabetes insipidus, resistant diabetes mellitus, atopic dermatitis, **congenital ectodermal dysplasia**, fucosidosis, familial hypoparathyroidism, hypogammaglobulinemia, pseudohypoaldosteronism, congenital adrenal hyperplasia, **hypothyroidism**, familial cholestasis, **adrenal insufficiency**, **malnutrition**, **Addison's disease**, **mucopolysaccharidosis**, exercise, high temperature conditions, nephrotic sy, Klinefelter's syndrome, nephrosis, meconium ileus, renal failure, type I glycogen-storage disease

Decreased Values
false decreased values – (edema, hypoproteinemia, excessive sweating)

Color

- ■ **brown**: ochronosis
- ■ **red**: rifampin
- ■ **blue**: occupational exposure to copper
- ■ **blue-black**: idiopathic chromhidrosis

Natrium

Increased Values
cystic fibrosis, **G6P-ase deficiency**, anorexia nervosa, nephrogenic diabetes insipidus, resistant diabetes mellitus, atopic dermatitis, **congenital ectodermal dysplasia**, fucosidosis, familial hypoparathyroidism, hypogammaglobulinemia, pseudohypoaldosteronism, congenital adrenal hyperplasia, **hypothyroidism**, renal diseases, familial cholestasis, **adrenal insufficiency**, **malnutrition**, **Addison's disease**, **mucopolysaccharidosis**, alcoholic pancreatitis, exercise, high temperature conditions, nephrotic sy, Klinefelter's syndrome, nephrosis, meconium ileus, renal failure, type I glycogen-storage disease

Decreased Values
adrenocortical hyperfunction

Potassium

Increased Values
cystic fibrosis, hyperadrenalism, congestive heart failure

Synovial Fluid

D. Mesko

Synovial fluid (joint fluid, synovia) is a blood plasma dialysate with hyaluronic acid (0.2–0.5%), a mucopolysaccharide produced by synovial lining cells (B-type synoviocytes), which functions as a stable film of lubricant for joints. The high viscosity is due to the hyaluronan which polymerises to form large molecular weight complexes. Hyaluronan holds water and provides a liquid cushion for the cartilage, acts as a transport system for nutrients to the chondrocytes. Synovial fluid supplies nutrition to the synovial membrane. There are proteins within the synovial fluid, but the large molecular weight proteins are excluded from the synovial fluid. Synovial fluid is relatively acellular and has about 70% of monocytes and 30% lymphocytes. Synovia may be obtained readily from the larger joints by arthrocentesis. The normal knee joint contains only a few drops to a maximum of 4 ml of synovia. Normal/physiological findings: colorless/pale yellow, straw coloured, clear, highly viscous consistency, slightly alkaline liquid, does not clot, with electrolytes in amounts comparable to those found in blood, IgG, IgA, IgM, leucocytes, lymphocytes, monocytes, macrophages.

Test Purpose. 1) to aid differential diagnosis of arthritis, particularly septic or crystal-induced forms, 2) to identify the cause/nature of joint effusion, 3) to relieve the pain/distension resulting from accumulation of fluid within the joint, 4) to administer drugs locally.

Appearance

- ▪ **chylous** (fatty): rheumatoid arthritis, filariasis, subchondral fractures, hyperlipidemias, chronic infections, pancreatic disease-associated fat necrosis, systemic lupus erythematosus
- ▪ **milky** (pseudochylous): arthritis – (acute gouty a., chronic rheumatoid a., tuberculous a.), calcium hydroxyapatite arthropathy, systemic lupus erythematosus
- ▪ **turbid** (turbidity, cloudy): arthritis – (acute bacterial a., rheumatoid a., septic a., tuberculous a.), uratic arthritis, diseases – (bacterial infectious d., inflammatory d.), leukocytosis, systemic lupus erythematosus, osteoarthritis

Bacterial Antigens

Detection of bacterial antigens in synovial fluid is a potentially useful test in reactive arthritis, that occurs about 10 to 14 days following an enteric or genital infection (Salmonella, Shigella, Yersinia, Chlamydia).

Positive
reactive arthritis following enteric/genital infection

Ceruloplasmin

Increased Values
rheumatoid arthritis

Clot Formation

Normal synovial fluid does not clot because it lacks fibrinogen as well as prothrombin, factors V, VII, tissue thromboplastin and antithrombin.

Positive
arthritis – (**acute bacterial a.**, uratic a., **psoriatic a.**, **rheumatoid a.**, juvenile rheumatoid a., **septic a.**, **traumatic a.**, tuberculous a.), infectious arthritis – (mycobacterial i. a., **mycoplasmal i. a.**, fungal i. a., treponemal i. a.), reactive arthritis in – (subacute bacterial endocarditis, regional enteritis, Campylobacter/Yersinia infection, ulcerative colitis, postileal bypass, Reiter's sy, inflammatory bowel disease), viral arthritis in – (hepatitis, HIV, mumps, rubella), **febris rheumatica** (rheumatic fever), diseases – (**degenerative joint d.**, rheumatoid d., connective tissue d.), **systemic lupus erythematosus**, osteoarthritis, **osteochondritis dissecans**, trauma, crystal-induced synovitis – (hydroxyapatite s., corticosteroid injection, oxalosis, **villonodular s.**, pyrophosphate s.), vasculitis

Colour

Normal synovial fluid is colorless. It is likely that the diapedesis of RBCs and their subsequent breakdown release hemoglobin and through metabolization a bilirubin is produced, giving a yellow (xantochromic) colour to the fluid. The WBC render the fluid white, and the degree of whiteness is proportional to their concentration.

- ▪ **straw:** agammaglobulinemia, acromegaly, amyloidosis, sickle cell anemia, infectious arthritis – (bacterial i. a., mycobacterial i. a., mycoplasmal i. a., fungal i. a., viral i. a.), arthritis – (psoriatic a., juvenile rheumatoid a., traumatic a.), reactive arthritis – (postileal bypass r. a., regional enteritis, Campylobacter infection, ulcerative colitis, Reiter's sy, Yersinia), Charcot's arthropathy, erythema multiforme, hemochromatosis, febris rheumatica (rheumatic fever), hypersensitivity, serum sickness, diseases – (rheumatoid d., connective tissue d.), systemic lupus erythematosus, Gaucher's disease, Paget's disease, Whipple's disease, myxedema, avascular necrosis, ochronosis, osteoarthritis, osteochondritis dissecans, osteochondromatosis, polyarteritis, polychondritis, polymyalgia rheumatica, polymyositis, sarcoidosis, scleroderma, ankylosing spondylitis, crystal-induced synovitis – (gouty s., hydroxyapatite s., corticosteroid injection, villonodular s., pseudo-gouty s.), vasculitis
- ▪ **greenish:** arthritis – (chronic rheumatoid a., septic a.), acute synovitis due to gout/pseudogout
- ▪ **red, reddish:** trauma, neuroarthropathy, hemophilia, bleeding disorders, tumors, anticoagulants, chondrocalcinosis, thrombocytosis, sickle cell disease, joint prostheses
- ▪ **yellow:** amyloidosis, sickle-cell anemia, arthritis – (psoriatic a., rheumatoid a.), Lyme disease (borreliosis), joint inflammatory diseases, osteoarthritis, osteochondritis dissecans, osteochondromatosis, spondylitis ankylopoietica (ankylosing spondylosis), Reiter's sy, acute crystal synovitis, trauma

Complement

Increased Values
osteoarthritis

Decreased Values
rheumatoid arthritis, acute rheumatic fever, **systemic lupus erythematosus**

C3-Complement

Increased Values
rheumatoid arthritis, systemic lupus erythematosus, ankylosing spondylitis

C4-Complement

Increased Values
rheumatoid arthritis, systemic lupus erythematosus, ankylosing spondylitis

Copper

Increased Values
rheumatoid arthritis

Crystals

Five general types of endogenic crystals may precipitate in/around joints causing symptoms of clinical arthritis: monosodium urate, calcium pyrophosphate, apatite, lipids and calcium oxalate. To produce gout, the monosodium urate crystals must have been phagocytosed by neutrophils.

Increased – positive
- **hydroxyapatite**: hereditary arthritis, arthropathy – (**apatite a., destructive a.**), hereditary bursitis, calcific bursitis/tendinitis, dermatomyositis, long-term dialysis, hyperparathyroidism, hypervitaminosis D, hereditary tumoral calcinosis, systemic lupus erythematosus, **osteoarthritis**, sarcoidosis, systemic sclerosis, syndrome – (CREST sy, milk-alkali sy), hereditary tendinitis, chronic renal failure
- Charcot–Leyden: eosinophilic synovitis
- **calcium oxalate** (variable bipyramidal morphology, strongly positively birefringent): small bowel bypass, deficiency – (pyridoxine d., thiamine d.), **chronic dialysis**, diet rich in oxalate – (rhubarb), inflammatory bowel diseases, Aspergillus niger infections, ethylene glycol poisoning, ascorbic acid, primary oxalosis, small bowel resection, decreased renal excretion, **renal failure**
- **calcium phosphate** (basic, clumps, globules): calcific periarthritis

- **calcium pyrophosphate** (calcium pyrophosphate dihydrate crystals – CPPD, various shapes, usually rod/rhomboidal shape, weekly positive birefringent): pyrophosphate arthropathy, **hereditary disposition**, hemophilia, hemochromatosis, hyperparathyroidism, hypophosphatasia, hypomagnesemia, myxedematous hypothyroidism, meniscectomy, ochronosis, **osteoarthritis, pseudogout**, joint trauma
- **cryoprotein** (cryoglobulin, polygonal shaped, positively birefringent): peripheral erosive arthritis, cryoglobulinemia, plasmocytoma (incl. multiple myeloma), tendinitis, paraproteinemias
- **lipid**: acute arthritis
- **monosodium urate** (needle-shaped, frequently intracellular, strongly negatively birefringent, soluble in water): ethanol abuse, lactic acidosis, chronic hemolytic anemia, **uratic arthritis** (gouty arthritis), enzymatic defect of purine biosynthesis, starvation, **primary hyperuricemia**, diseases – (lymphoproliferative d., myeloproliferative d.), ketoacidosis, lead nephropathy, preeclampsia, increased production of uric acid, psoriasis, decreased renal excretion of uric acid – (cyclosporine, low-dose salicylates, diuretics, ethambutol, pyrazinamide), renal failure
- **miscellaneous crystals**: adenosine triphosphatase, allopurinol, alpha-1-antitrypsin, aluminium phosphate, amiodarone, amyloid, apatite, beclomethasone, bilirubin, biliverdin, cystine, guanine, calcium carbonate, hippuric acid, leucine, corticosteroids, contrast media, urea, myoglobin, porphyrin, leukemic proteins, bile salts, sulfonamides, triamterene, tyrosine

Cytophagocytic Mononuclear Cells

Large mononuclear cells which contain phagocytosed neutrophils. The neutrophils are apoptotic and there is a relationship between the number of cytophagocytic mononuclear cells and the number of apoptotic neutrophils.

Increased Values
arthritis – (rheumatoid a., **reactive a.**)

Eosinophils

Increased Values
allergy, angioedema, arthritis – (parasitic a., psoriatic a., reactive a. associated with Strongyloides infestation, **rheumatoid a.**, tuberculotic a.), **acute rheumatic fever, Lyme disease**, infectious/parasitic diseases, **intra-articular hemorrhage, irradiation therapy, metastatic tumors to synovium, post arthrography conditions**, syndrome – (atopic sy, **hypereosinophilic sy**), **urticaria**, contrast dye, idiopathic eosinophilic synovitis

Erythrocytes

Increased Values – positive (blood)
arthritis – (**hemophilic a.**, rheumatoid a., **septic a.**), arthropathy – (Charcot's a., neurogenic a.), arteriovenous fistulas, **hemangioma**, myeloproliferative disease with thrombocytosis, **anticoagulant therapy**, von Willebrand's disease, sickle cell disease, **tumours**, metastatic tumors, chondrocalcinosis, anticoagulants, osteoarthritis, ruptured aneurysm, **scurvy** (scorbutus), **villonodular synovitis, trauma of aspiration, thrombocytopenia**, thrombocytosis, **trauma, hemorrhagic effusion**

Glucose

Decreased Values
arthritis – (**rheumatoid a.**, septic a.), **crystal arthropathies, infectious/inflammatory joint diseases**

Lactic Acid

Increased Values
arthritis – (rheumatoid a., **septic a.**)

Lactate Dehydrogenase

Increased Values
gout, arthritis – (infectious a., rheumatoid a.)

Analyte	Age/Gender	Reference Range	SI Units	Note
Lactate Dehydrogenase		<5.3	µkat/l	

LE Cells

positive
rheumatic fever, systemic lupus erythematosus

Leukocytes

The total white cell count and differential is used to determine whether fluid is inflammatory or non-inflammatory. One of the problems with measuring WBC in synovial fluid is that its viscosity causes clumping of the cells producing a falsely low total white cell count.

Increased Values
agammaglobulinemia, acromegaly, amyloidosis, sickle cell disease, arthritis – (acute bacterial a., uratic a., **psoriatic a.**, **rheumatoid a.**, juvenile rheumatoid a., **septic a.**, **traumatic a.**, tuberculous a.), acute/chronic gout, infectious arthritis – (**bacterial i. a.**, mycobacterial i. a., **mycoplasmal i. a.**, **fungal i. a.**, treponemal i. a.), reactive arthritis in – (subacute bacterial endocarditis, regional enteritis, Campylobacter/Yersinia infection, ulcerative colitis, postileal bypass, Reiter's sy, inflammatory bowel disease), viral arthritis in – (hepatitis, HIV, mumps, rubella), Charcot's arthropathy, erythema – (e. multiforme, **e. nodosum**), Wegener's granulomatosis, hemochromatosis, **febris rheumatica** (rheumatic fever), hyperlipoproteinemia, hypersensitivity, serum sickness, diseases – (**degenerative joint d.**, rheumatoid d., connective tissue d.), carcinoid, **systemic lupus erythematosus**, Gaucher's disease, Paget's disease, Whipple's disease, myxedema, avascular necrosis, neuroarthropathy, ochronosis, osteoarthritis, **hypertrophic pulmonary osteoarthropathy**, **osteochondritis dissecans**, osteochondromatosis, polyarteritis, polychondritis, polymyalgia rheumatica, **polymyositis, pseudogout**, sarcoidosis, **scleroderma, ankylosing spondylitis**, syndrome – (Henoch-Schönlein sy, Sjögren's sy), trauma, crystal-induced synovitis – (hydroxyapatite s., corticosteroid injection, oxalosis, **villonodular s.**, pyrophosphate s.), vasculitis

Lymphocytes

Increased Values
arthritis – (**rheumatoid a.** – early stage, chronic lymphocytic a., **tuberculous a.** – early stage, **viral a.**), bacterial endocarditis, hemophilia, **systemic lupus erythematosus**, non-Hodgkin's lymphomas, poststreptococcal rheumatism, Sjögren's sy, eosinophilic fasciitis, pigmented villonodular synovitis

Macrophages

Increased Values – positive
rheumatoid arthritis, subchondral fractures, histiocytosis X, leprosy, lipidosis due to lysosomal storage defect – (Fabry's disease, Gaucher's disease, Niemann-Pick disease), systemic lupus erythematosus, osteoarthritis with subchondral bone cyst, pancreatitis associated with synovial fat necrosis, pigmented villonodular synovitis, tuberculosis, xanthochromatosis

Monocytes

Increased Values
sickle cell disease, **arboviruses**, arthritis – (juvenile rheumatoid a., viral a., varicella a.), chronic gout, **hepatitis**, **serum sickness**, **systemic lupus erythematosus**, Whipple's disease, osteoarthritis, **rubella**, scleroderma, connective tissue disease, systemic sclerosis, knee luxation

Mucin Clot

Test estimates the degree of polymerization of hyaluronic acid sufficiently to classify clots.

Firm
acromegaly, amyloidosis, sickle cell anemia, traumatic arthritis, Charcot's arthropathy, hemochromatosis, rheumatic fever, systemic lupus erythematosus, Gaucher's disease, Paget's disease, myxedema, avascular necrosis, ochronosis, osteoarthritis, osteochondritis dissecans, ostechondromatosis, scleroderma, villonodular synovitis, knee luxation

Friable
agammaglobulinemia, arthritis – (psoriatic a., juvenile rheumatoid a.), infectious arthritis – (bacterial i. a., mycobacterial i. a., mycoplasmal i. a., fungal i. a., viral i. a.), reactive arthritis in – (regional enteritis, Campylobacter/Yersinia infection, ulcerative colitis, post-ileal bypass, Reiter's sy), gout, erythema multiforme, febris rheumatica (rheumatic fever), hypersensitivity, serum sickness, diseases – (rheumatoid d., connective tissue d.), systemic lupus erythematosus, Whipple's disease, polyarteritis, polychondritis, polymyositis, polymyalgia rheumatica, pseudogout, sarcoidosis, scleroderma, ankylosing spondylitis, crystal-induced synovitis – (hydroxyapatite s., corticosteroid injection), vasculitis

5-Nucleotidase

(5-NT) A plasma membrane enzyme relevant to the biliary tract.

Increased Values
calcium pyrophosphate dehydrate deposition, metastatic neoplasia to the bone, osteoarthritis

Polymorphonuclears

Increased Values
agammaglobulinemia, arthritis – (Lyme a., psoriatic a., juvenile rheumatoid a.), acute bacterial arthritis – (a. pyogenic a., a. septic a., a. suppurative a.), infectious arthritis – (bacterial i. a., mycobacterial i. a., mycoplasmal i. a., fungal i. a., treponemal i. a.), reactive arthritis in – (subacute bacterial endocarditis, regional enteritis, Campylobacter/Yersinia infection, ulcerative colitis, postileal bypass, Reiter's sy), viral arthritis in – (hepatitis, HIV, mumps, rubella), gout, subacute bacterial endocarditis, erythema – (e. multiforme, e. nodosum), Wegener's granulomatosis, febris rheumatica, hyperlipoproteinemia, hypersensitivity, serum sickness, diseases – (rheumatoid d., connective tissue d.), carcinoid, leukemia, systemic lupus erythematosus, Whipple's disease, polyarteritis, polychondritis, polymyalgia rheumatica, polymyositis, pseudogout, sarcoidosis, scleroderma, ankylosing spondylitis, syndrome – (Henoch-Schönlein sy, Sjögren's sy), crystal-induced synovitis – (hydroxyapatite s., corticosteroid injection s., oxalosis), trauma, vasculitis

Proteins

Increased Values
arthritis – (gouty a., rheumatoid a., septic a.)

Analyte	Age/Gender	Reference Range	SI Units	Note
Proteins, Total		10–20	g/l	

Pus

positive
arthritis – (fungal a., psoriatic a., rheumatoid a., acute septic a., tuberculous a.), gout, Lyme disease, pseudogout, Reiter's sy

Ragocytes

Ragocytes are neutrophils or macrophages which contain distinctive granules. The granules are thought to consist of immune complexes and contain immunoglobulins, including antinuclear antibody, rheumatoid factor, DNA particles and fibrin.

Increased Values
arthritis – (gouty a., **rheumatoid a.**, **septic a.**), pseudogout

C-Reactive Protein

Increased Values
rheumatoid arthritis

Rheumatoid Factor

Increased Values
rheumatoid arthritis

Beta-Thromboglobulin

Platelet product.

Increased Values
rheumatoid arthritis

Viscosity

Viscosity is helpful in distinguishing between inflammatory and non-inflammatory synovial fluid. The low viscosity is due to reduced production of hyaluronan as well as a reduction in its polymerisation, with the resulting hyaluronan being of low molecular weight. The viscosity can be determined at the bedside. Normal synovial fluid has a positive "string test" where the fluid when dripped from the syringe forms a string of greater than 10–15 cm. Inflammatory synovial fluid drips like water, forming small drops.

Increased Values
acromegaly, **amyloidosis**, sickle-cell anemia, traumatic arthritis, Charcot's arthropathy, hemochromatosis, rheumatic fever, systemic lupus erythematosus, Gaucher's disease, Paget's disease, myxedema, avascular necrosis, ochronosis, **osteoarthritis**, **osteochondrosis dissecans**, **osteochondromatosis**, scleroderma, villonodular synovitis, knee derangement

Decreased Values
agammaglobulinemia, arthritis – (psoriatic a., **rheumatoid a.**, juvenile rheumatoid a., **septic a.**), infectious arthritis – (bacterial i. a., mycobacterial i. a., mycoplasmal i. a., fungal i. a., viral i. a.), pyrophosphate arthropathy, **Lyme borreliosis**, **uratic arthritis** (gouty arthritis), **enteritis regionalis**, erythema multiforme, febris rheumatica, serum sickness, diseases – (**joint inflammatory d.**, connective tissue d.), infections – (Campylobacter, Yersinia), corticosteroid injections, **colitis ulcerosa**, leukemia, **systemic lupus erythematosus**, Whipple's disease, polyarteritis, polychondritis, polymyalgia rheumatica, polymyositis, **pseudogout**, sarcoidosis, scleroderma, **spondylitis ankylopoietica**, postileal bypass conditions, **Reiter's sy**, synovitis – (hydroxyapatite s., acute crystal s.), vasculitis, rapid effusion following trauma

Analyte	Age/Gender	Reference Range	SI Units	Note
Viscosity		300	cP	

Volume

Increased Values

congestive heart failure, myxedema, anasarca, amyloidosis, osteoarthritis, arthritis – (acute bacterial a., uratic a., **psoriatic a.**, **rheumatoid a.**, juvenile rheumatoid a., **septic a.**, **traumatic a.**, tuberculous a.), hemophilia, fractures, **osteochondritis dissecans**, osteonecrosis, osteochondromatosis, crystal-induced synovitis – (hydroxyapatite s., corticosteroid injection, oxalosis, pyrophosphate s.), **systemic lupus erythematosus**, sickle cell disease, polyarteritis nodosa, fat droplet synovitis, acute/chronic gout, **pseudogout, scleroderma**, polymyalgia rheumatica, infectious arthritis – (**bacterial i. a.**, mycobacterial i. a., **mycoplasmal i. a., fungal i. a.**, treponemal i. a.), chondrocalcinosis, viral arthritis in – (hepatitis, HIV, mumps, rubella), **febris rheumatica** (rheumatic fever), disease – (Behcet's d.), reactive arthritis in – (subacute bacterial endocarditis, regional enteritis, Campylobacter/Yersinia infection, ulcerative colitis, postileal bypass, Reiter's sy, inflammatory bowel disease), **villonodular synovitis, trauma**, Charcot's arthropathy, tumors, diseases – (**degenerative joint d.**, rheumatoid d., connective tissue d.), joint prostheses, thrombocytosis, myeloproliferative diseases

Interfering Factors: medicaments – (anticoagulants, corticosteroids)

Tears

D. Mesko

Acid Beta-Galactosidase

Decreased Values
gangliosidosis GM1

Arylsulfatase A

Decreased Values
metachromatic leukodystrophy

Alpha-Fucosidase

Decreased Values
fucosidosis

Alpha-Galactosidase

Decreased Values
Fabry's disease

Alpha-1,4-Glucosidase

Decreased Values
glycogenosis (type II)

Hexosaminidase A

Decreased Values
disease – (**Sandhoff's d., Tay-Sachs d.**)

Alpha-Mannosidase

Decreased Values
mannosidosis

Volume

Decreased Values
decreased facial nerve function, dehydration, syndrome – (Horner's sy, Sjögren's sy)

Urine

D. Mesko, R. Pullmann

Freshly voided first morning specimens of urine are best, especially if it is infected, as composition changes occur when the urine is allowed to stand, basic sampling procedures should be followed.

The complete specimen should be well mixed, but not centrifuged or filtered before taking out a portion for testing. The specimen container should be absolutely clean, free from contaminants, nothing should be added to the specimen before analysis except when it is recommended, and it should be cooled if storage is needed.

If the examination is delayed, bacteria multiplication will result in pH alteration, cells may degenerate, and casts will often dissolve in alkaline urine.

Acetoacetic Acid

Increased Values
  Interfering Factors: medicaments – (acetylsalicylic acid, captopril, ethanol, ether, insulin, isoniazid, levodopa, metformin, methyldopa, nicotinic acid, phenytoin, rimiterol, salbutamol, valproic acid)

Acid Phosphatase

Increased Values
diseases – (kidney d., prostate d.)

Addison's Sediment

Quantitative evaluation of 3–24 hrs urine specimen.
- **increased leukocytes + erythrocytes + casts:** glomerulonephritis
- **increased leukocytes:** pyelonephritis

Alanine

Increased Values – hyperalaninuria
secondary lactic acidosis, rheumatoid arthritis, deficiency – (glycogen synthase d., pyruvate dehydrogenase d.), histidinemia, lead intoxication, increased level of pyruvic acid, Hartnup disease
  Interfering Factors: bacterial contamination

Beta-Alanine

Increased Values
hyperbetaalaninemia, rejection of kidney transplant

Alanine Aminopeptidase

Increased Values
immediately following renal transplant, glomerulonephritis, urinary tract diseases, acute/chronic pyelonephritis, tumors, proximal tubular injury
    Interfering Factors: medicaments – (cisplatin, gentamicin, mannitol, prednisolone)

Alanine Aminotransferase

Increased Values
hepatitis, hyperthyroidism, renal diseases, icterus

Aldosterone

Test Purpose. To aid in primary and secondary aldosteronism diagnosis.

Increased Values – hyperaldosteronuria
aldosterone-secreting adenoma of the adrenal cortex, aldosteronism – (**primary a., secondary a.**), adrenocortical hyperplasia, hypertension, edematous conditions
    Interfering Factors: medicaments – (ACTH, angiotensin, deoxycorticosterone, corticosterone, cortisone, ethacrynic acid, furosemide, hydrochlorothiazide, hydrocortisone, laxatives, lithium, oral contraceptives, progesterone, spironolactone, testosterone, thiazide diuretics, triamterene)

Decreased Values – hypoaldosteronuria
isolated aldosterone deficiency, diabetes mellitus, acute alcoholic intoxication, Addison's disease, syndrome – (sy of hypoaldosteronism due to renin deficiency, Turner's sy)
    Interfering Factors: medicaments – (clonidine, deoxycorticosterone, fludrocortisone, glucocorticoids, heparin, labetalol, metyrapone, propranolol, timolol)

Analyte	Age/Gender	Reference Range	SI Units	Note
Aldosterone				See ref.
free		130–810	pmol/d	ranges note
		70–450	ng/d	
		50–230	nmol/d	
		15–71	nmol/d	
		5–35	nmol/d	
aldosterone glucuronide		6.3–32	nmol/d	
tetrahydro-aldosterone		18–120	nmol/d	

Alkaline Phosphatase

Increased Values
hypoxia, renal diseases, kidney tumours, pregnancy
    Interfering Factors: medicaments – (acetylsalicylic acid, polymyxin B, streptomycin, sulfonamides)

Aluminium

Test Purpose. 1) intoxication diagnosis, 2) monitoring of aluminium exposed persons (industry, dialysis), 3) prolonged parenteral nutrition, 4) chronic renal insufficiency monitoring.

Increased Values
cystic fibrosis, aluminium intoxication, hemodialysis patients

Analyte	Age/Gender	Reference Range	SI Units	Note
Aluminium		0–1.2	µmol/d	

Amino Acids

(syn: total amino acids, amino acids screen, inborn errors of metabolism screen, metabolic screen for amino acids) Test commonly includes examination of: glycine, hydroxyproline, isoleucine, leucine, methionine, ornithine, phenylalanine, proline, tyrosine, valine.
Test Purpose. 1) to screen for renal aminoacidurias, 2) to confirm plasma test findings when tests results suggest overflow aminoacidurias, 3) prolonged parenteral nutrition monitoring.

Increased Values – aminoaciduria
acidemia – (**methylmalonic a., propionic a.**), **alkaptonuria**, aminoaciduria – (argininosuccinic a., dibasic a., dicarboxylic a., a. of normal newborn), argininemia, liver cirrhosis, citrullinuria, **cystathioninuria, cystinosis,** cystinuria, ornithine transcarbamylase deficiency, vitamin deficiency – (**B, C, D**), diabetes mellitus with ketosis, progressive muscular dystrophy, eclampsia, **phenylketonuria, galactosemia,** focal sclerosing glomerulonephritis, glycogenosis (type I), **viral hepatitis,** histidinemia, homocitrullinuria, **homocystinuria,** hyperammonemia, hyperphenylalaninemia, nonketotic hyperglycinemia, hyperornithinemia, **hyperparathyroidism,** hyperprolinemia, **hyperthyroidism,** hypophosphatasia, disease – (Canavan d., Hartnup d., **maple syrup urine disease, Wilson's d.**), connective tissue diseases, iminoglycinuria, intolerance – (**fructose i.,** lactose i.), intoxication by – (heavy metals, cadmium, lead), carnosinemia, malnutrition, liver necrosis, chronic lead nephropathy, **osteomalacia,** body irradiation, **plasmocytoma** (incl. multiple myeloma), burns, **congenital disorders of metabolism,** severe liver damage, prolinuria, **rickets,** renal transplant reaction, syndrome – (**Fanconi's sy,** Lowe's sy, nephrotic sy), shock, pregnancy, thalassaemia major, **tyrosinemia,** tyrosinosis, **acute/chronic renal failure**
    Interfering Factors: medicaments – (acetylsalicylic acid, ACTH, adrenaline, aminocaproic acid, amphetamine, ampicillin, bismuth salts, cephalexin, colistin, dopamine, ephedrine, gentamicin, glucocorticoids, hydrocortisone, insulin, kanamycin, levarterenol,

levodopa, metamphetamine, metanephrine, methyldopa, neomycin, normetanephrine, penicillamine, phenacetin, phenylephrine, polymyxin, salicylates, steroids, tetracyclines, triamcinolone)

Decreased Values
Interfering Factors: medicaments – (adrenaline, insulin)

Alpha-Aminoadipic Acid

Increased Values
aciduria – (alpha-aminoadipic a., alpha-ketoadipic a.), hyperlysinemia, Reye's sy, saccharopinuria

Beta-Aminoisobutyric Acid

Increased Values
beta-aminoisobutyric aciduria, hyperbetaalaninemia, lead poisoning, protein malnutrition, tumors, excessive tissue breakdown, Down sy

Delta-Aminolevulic Acid

(DALA, ALA, delta-ALA, syn: 5-aminolevulic acid, aminolevulinic acid) Porphyrin and heme biosynthesis metabolite (a heme synthesis intermediate) produced from succinyl-CoA and glycine. Porphobilinogen precursor in porphyrin metabolism. Two ALA molecules are condensed to form porphobilinogen.
Test Purpose. 1) to aid in the diagnosis of congenital or acquired porphyrias and certain hepatic disorders, such as hepatitis and hepatic tumors, 2) to screen for lead poisoning, lead exposure, 3) heavy metals poisoning screening.

Increased Values
alcohol abuse, **hepatitis**, diabetic ketoacidosis, **hereditary coproporphyria**, chemicals, poisoning by – (medicaments, **inorganic lead, iron**), **hepatic tumours**, **acute intermittent porphyria**, plumboporphyria, porphyria cutanea tarda, **porphyria variegata**, pregnancy, **hereditary tyrosinemia**
Interfering Factors: ammonia, medicaments – (barbiturates, griseofulvin, penicillin)

Decreased Values
alcohol liver diseases
Interfering Factors: medicaments – (cisplatin)

Analyte	Age/Gender	Reference Range	SI Units	Note
Delta-Aminolevulic Acid		<49	μmol/d	

Alpha-Aminonitrogen

(syn: amino acid nitrogen)

Test Purpose. 1) renal failure differential diagnosis, 2) nutrition monitoring in enteral/parenteral nutrition, 3) diet monitoring in patients with chronic renal insufficiency, 4) differential diagnosis of comatose conditions, 5) aminoaciduria diagnosis.

Increased Values
cirrhosis hepatis, renal diabetes, arthritis urica, acute hepatic dystrophy, eclampsia, hepatitis, PIH (pregnancy induced hypertension), cachexia, myeloid leukemia, energetic metabolism and nutrition monitoring, lung tumours, vitamin deficiency – (B_{12}, C), nephrosis, pneumonia, severe hepatic lesions, rachitis, pregnancy, typhoid fever

Analyte	Age/Gender	Reference Range	SI Units	Note
Alpha-Aminonitrogen		13.5–20.3	mmol/l	*mmol/creatinine
		0.98–1.5	*	**fraction
		0.03–0.04	**	excretion

Ammonia

Test Purpose. 1) pediatric and neonatal indications – encephalopathies, quality/quantity consciousness disorders, seizure conditions, 2) comatose conditions differential diagnosis, 3) tubular secretion evaluation mainly in unexplained loss of natrium and potassium iones.

Increased Values
acidosis, dyspepsia, exsicosis, physical exertion, febrile states
    Interfering Factors: medicaments – (glycine, methenamine)

Decreased Values
alkalosis, vegane diet, plant food
    Interfering Factors: medicaments – (acetazolamide)

Amylase

(syn: alpha-amylase total)

Test Purpose. 1) suspicion on macroamylasemia, 2) renal insufficiency diagnosis and monitoring, 3) to diagnose acute pancreatitis when serum amylase levels are normal or borderline, 4) to aid chronic pancreatitis and salivary gland disorders diagnosis, 5) suspect extra-pancreatic origin of increased amylase levels – cardiosurgery, anorexia, bulimia, alcoholism, lung diseases, ovarian cystadenocarcinoma.

Increased Values – hyperamylasuria
pancreatic abscess, **acute alcoholism**, aortic aneurysm with dissection, acute appendicitis, ascites, **pancreatic cyst/pseudocyst**, **perforated/necrotic/strangulated bowel**, ERCP, **postoperative hyperamylasemia**, **cholecystitis**, choledocholithiasis, diseases – (**biliary tract d.**, gall-

bladder d.), infarction – (mesenteric i., **pulmonary i.**), viral infections, renal insufficiency, **diabetic ketoacidosis, macroamylasemia,** tumors of – (**pancreas,** lung, ovary), **acute pancreatic necrosis** (early), obstruction – (salivary duct o., intestinal o., **pancreatic duct o.**), pancreatitis – (**acute p.,** chronic p.), **parotitis, peritonitis,** burns, **chronic pancreatitis relapse, ruptured ectopic pregnancy,** traumatic shock, **ectopic pregnancy,** trauma – (abdominal t., cerebral t., **pancreatic t.,** spleen t.), **penetrated/perforated peptic ulcer,** renal failure

Interfering Factors: medicaments – (captopril, glucagon, morphine, nitrofurantoin)

Decreased Values – hypoamylasuria
alcoholism, cachexia, diabetes mellitus, cystic fibrosis (mucoviscidosis), severe liver diseases, kidney disease, tumors – (pancreatic t., liver t.), toxemia of pregnancy, pancreatic insufficiency, total pancreatic necrosis, chronic pancreatitis, liver cirrhosis, hepatic abscess, hepatitis, pancreatectomy, chronic pancreatitis

Analyte	Age/Gender	Reference Range	SI Units	Note
Alpha-Amylase				See ref.
Total		<16.7	μkat/l	ranges note
		<15.0	μkat/d	
		<77	kU/mol *	*kU/mol creatinine
		<11.3	μkat/g *	*μkat/g creatinine
Pancreatic		<13.3	μkat/l	
		<53	kU/mol *	*kU/mol creatinine
		<7.8	μkat/g *	*μkat/g creatinine

Antibodies Against Legionella

Test detect antibodies to Legionella pneumophila and support the clinical diagnosis of legionnaires' disease.

Increased Values
legionnaires' disease

Antimony

Increased Values
industrial exposure – (lead i. e., paint i. e., glass i. e., weapons i. e.)

Arginine

Increased Values – hyperargininuria
dibasic aminoaciduria, cystinosis, cystinuria, infants, newborns

Arylsulfatase A

(ARSA) Arylsulfatase is a lysosomal enzyme found in every cell except the mature erythrocyte. Principally active in the liver, pancreas and kidneys, where exogenous substances are detoxified becoming ester sulfates.

Test Purpose. To aid in the diagnosis of bladder, colon or rectum cancer, of myeloid (granulocytic) leukemia, and of metachromatic leukodystrophy (an inherited lipid storage disease).

Increased Values
tumors – (t. of colorectum, leukemia, t. of bladder)

Decreased Values
metachromatic leukodystrophy

Asparagine

(Asn) Asparagine is the ammonia storage form in tissues.

Increased Values – hyperasparaginuria
cystinosis, Hartnup disease, burns

Aspartate Aminotransferase

Increased Values
infectious kidney diseases, toxic renal tubules lesions

Aspartic Acid

Increased Values
dicarboxylic aminoaciduria

Bacteria

Bacteria are common in urine specimens because of the abundant normal microbial flora of the vagina or external urethral meatus and because of their ability to rapidly multiply in urine standing at room temperature. Therefore, microbial organisms found in all collected urines should be interpreted in view of clinical symptoms. Diagnosis of bacteriuria in a case of suspected urinary tract infection requires culture. A colony count may also be done to see if significant numbers of bacteria are present. Multiple organisms reflect contamination. However, the presence of any organism in catheterized or suprapubic tap specimens should be considered significant.

Positive – bacteriuria

urinary tract anomalies, cystitis – (acute c., chronic interstitial c.), fungi, urinary tract infections, parasites, urinary tract tuberculosis, renal perinephric abscess, acute/chronic prostatitis, pyelonephritis – (acute p., chronic p.), ureteral calculus, chronic urethritis, subacute bacterial endocarditis, Crohn's disease, benign prostate hypertrophy, pelvis abscess, typhoid fever, urethra tumors

Analyte	?	Age/Gender	Reference Range	SI Units	Note
Bacteria		Children	$<10^9$	l	
		Adults	$<10^{11}$	l	

Bacterial Antigens

The value of urinary antigen tests is limited.
Tests are available for: Haemophilus influenzae type b, Neisseria meningitidis, Streptococcus pneumoniae, Group B streptococcus, Legionella pneumophila.

Bilirubin

Tests for bilirubin should be made on fresh urine. Different strip colors may indicate that other bile pigments are present in the sample. Bilirubin is formed in the spleen reticuloendothelial cells and in bone marrow from hemoglobin breakdown; then is transported to the liver. Bilirubin is excreted in the urine, if there is conjugated bilirubin (direct bilirubin) in the blood stream. Normally, small amounts of urobilinogen, not bilirubin, are found in the urine.
Test Purpose. To help identify jaundice causes.

Increased Values – positive, conjugated bilirubinuria
hepatic cirrhosis, false positive values – (chlorpromazine, acetylsalicylic acid metabolites, urobilin, urobilinogen), hepatitis – (alcoholic h., **drug induced h.**, **toxic h.**, **viral h.**), **transient familial hyperbilirubinemia in infants**, hypothyroidism, **cholangitis**, **cholelithiasis**, **extra/ intrahepatic cholestasis**, diseases – (**liver d.**, **inflammatory d. of biliary ducts**), icterus – (hemolytic i., hepatocellular i., neonatal physiological i., **obstructive i.**), fructose intolerance, **gallstones**, **Gilbert's disease**, tumors of – (**liver**, pancreas, **biliary ways**), **efferent biliary ways obstruction**, **surgical biliary ways trauma**, **acute/chronic hepatic parenchymatous lesion**, **biliary ways stricture**, syndrome – (Crigler-Najjar sy, **Dubin-Johnson sy**, breast-milk jaundice sy, **Rotor's sy**)

> **Interfering Factors:** medicaments – (acetophenazine, allopurinol, antibiotics, barbiturates, chlorpromazine, diuretics, ethoxazene, nitrate, oral contraceptives, phenazopyridine, phenothiazines, pyridium, steroids, sulfonamides, vitamin C)

Negative Bilirubin
false negative values – (indomethacin, high nitrite levels, ascorbic acid, bilirubin oxidation in delayed examination)

Bladder Tumor Antigen

(BTA) Test detects basement membrane proteins.

Increased Values – positive
nephritis, nephrolithiasis, gastrointestinal tract injury, prostate biopsy/resection, renal/bladder calculi, sexually transmitted diseases, tumors of – (**kidney, bladder**, penis, ovary, endometrium, cervix)

Blood

Hematuria – blood in the urine, (erythrocyturia + hemoglobinuria), (macro + microhematuria), (gross hematuria + microscopic hematuria). Chemical testing for blood in the urine is based on peroxidase hemoglobin activity, myoglobin and some degradation products. Chemicals will react to free hemoglobin and reagent lysed RBCs used in the test. An alternative test is microscopy, which counts the erythrocytes in a set volume, where sediment has been concentrated by centrifugation. This test does not detect free hemoglobin, whether excreted as such or lysed from excreted erythrocytes in standing urine. Thus, free hemoglobin in the absence of intact urine erythrocytes causes positive results in chemical testing and negative results in microscopy. Urine for blood testing should be stirred immediately before the testing and microscopy should be utilized with fresh urine. In microscopic hematuria, number of RBCs is not related to the significance of the causative lesion. Presence of blood clots virtually rules out glomerular origin of blood. Large thick clots suggest bladder origin, small stringy clots suggest upper tract. RBC casts or Hb casts indicates blood is of glomerular origin, but their absence does not rule out glomerular disease.

Test Purpose. 1) to aid in urinary tract bleeding diagnosis, 2) to aid in hemolytic anemias diagnosis, infection or severe intravascular hemolysis from a transfusion reaction.

Positive – prerenal hematuria (erythrocyturia + hemoglobinuria)
sickle cell anemia, arteriosclerosis, primary amyloidosis, abdominal aortic aneurysm, hypersensitivity angiitis, deficiency of factor – (VII, X, XI), babesiosis, strenuous exercise, subacute bacterial endocarditis, **hemorrhagic diathesis**, hypertensive encephalopathy, endometriosis, idiopathic retroperitoneal fibrosis, Wegener's granulomatosis, **hemophilia, nocturnal hemoglobinuria**, hemoglobin S-related diseases, true hermaphroditism, malignant hypertension, hyperparathyroidism, disease – (legionnaire's d., mixed connective tissue d., von Willebrand's d., Whipple's d.), renal infarction in endocarditis, **transfusion incompatibility**, intoxication by – (arsenic, phenol, snake venom, carbon disulfide, carbon tetrachloride, glycol, heavy metals, methanol, copper, naphthalene, phosphorus, trichloroethylene, turpentine), disseminated intravascular coagulation, **coagulopathy**, collagenoses, leishmaniasis, leptospirosis, leukemia, lymphocytic lymphoma, systemic lupus erythematosus, malaria, myiasis, plasmocytoma (incl. multiple myeloma), Pneumocystis carinii pneumonia, abortion – (incomplete a., septic a.), polycythemia, erythropoietic porphyria, rhabdomyosarcoma, scleroderma, scurvy, fever – (scarlet f., familial Mediterranean f., epidemic hemorrhagic f.), schistosomiasis, serum sickness, sepsis, **hemolytic conditons**, venomous snake bite, arachnid bite, syndrome – (hemangioma-thrombocytopenia sy, Goodpasture's sy, Kawasaki's sy, hyperviscosity sy, hemolytic-uremic sy, toxic shock sy, Reiter's sy), syphilis, hereditary hemorrhagic teleangiectasia, transfusion, hemorrhagic thrombocytemia, **thrombocytopenia**, thrombosis – (systemic arterial t., renal vein t.), **vasculitis**, inborn error of amino acid metabolism

Interfering Factors: medicaments – (abciximab, acetylsalicylic acid, aldesleukin, allopurinol, alteplase, amphotericin B, anagrelide, analgesics, anistreplase, anticoagulants, ardeparin, argatroban, ascorbic acid, Bacillus Calmette–Guerin vaccine, bacitracin, bivalirudin, bromfenac, bromides, busulfan, cephalosporins, colchicine, cyclophosphamide, dalfopristin, danaparoid, denileukin, diclofenac, diflunisal, enoxaparin, eptifibatide, erythromycin, etodolac, fenoprofen, flurbiprofen, gatifloxacin, gemcitabine, gemtuzumab, gold salts, heparin, hydrocodone, ibuprofen, ifosfamide, indinavir, indomethacin, iodides, isotretinoin, kava kava, ketoprofen, ketorolac, lepirudin, levodopa, mebendazole, meclofenamate, methenamine, methocarbamol, methotrexate, mitomycin, mycophenolate, nabumetone, naproxen, nitrates, oxaprozin, penicillamine, penicillin, phenylbutazone, piroxicam, polymyxin B, potassium chloride, primaquine, probenecid, reteplase, rifampin, rifapentine, samarium, somatropin, streptokinase, sulfamethoxazole, sulfizoxazole, sulfonamides, sulindac, tenecteplase, tirofiban, tolcapone, tolmetin, topiramate, urokinase, valrubicin, warfarin)

Positive – renal hematuria (erythrocyturia + hemoglobinuria)

abscess – (kidney a., perinephric a.), renal tubular acidosis, **renal cystic degeneration**, **renal embolism**, **glomerulonephritis**, renal hemangioma, hematuria – (benign familial h., essential h.), nocturnal paroxysmal hemoglobinuria, **hydronephrosis**, renovascular hypertension, **inflammatory diseases**, **renal infarction**, **renal infections**, acute/chronic renal insufficiency, systemic lupus erythematosus, **vascular malformations**, tumours of kidney – (nephroblastoma – Wilms' tumor, papilloma, squamous cell t.), nephrocalcinosis, nephropathy – (IgG-IgA n., hypercalcemic n., analgesic n., obstructive n.), nephritis – (acute n., chronic n., lupus n., radiation n., **interstitial n.**), lipoid nephrosis, **nephrolithiasis**, malignant nephrosclerosis, **nephrotoxins**, necrosis – (cortical adrenal n., **acute tubular n.**), ectopic kidney, medullary sponge kidney, perinephritis, **polycystic kidney**, renal artery occlusion, oxaluria, necrotizing papillitis, polyarteritis nodosa, purpura – (**Henoch–Schönlein p., renal p.**, idiopathic thrombocytopenic p., thrombotic thrombocytopenic p., secondary thrombocytopenic p.), **pyelonephritis**, **physical stress**, renal transplant rejection, syndrome – (Alport's sy, nephrotic sy), **renal tuberculosis**, tubulopathies, **trauma**, acute renal failure, xanthinuria

Positive – postrenal hematuria (erythrocyturia + hemoglobinuria)

abscess – (pelvic a., periurethral a., retroperitoneal a.), acute appendicitis, **cystitis**, cystocele, congenital urinary tract defects, diverticula of – (colon, ureter), **bladder fistula, prostate diseases** – (abscess, hyperplasia, hypertrophy, calculus, **tumours, prostatitis**), **inflammatory diseases**, urinary tract infections, **catheterization**, vascular malformations, **urogenital tract tumours, urinary tract obstruction**, polyp of ureter/urethra, **purpura**, uterus rupture in pregnancy, acute salpingitis, urethra/ureter stricture, **foreign bodies, tuberculosis**, intestine ulceration – (dysentery, tuberculosis), tuberculosis of genito-urinary system, ureterocele, foreign body in bladder, **urethritis**, urethrorrhagia, **urolithiasis, trauma**

False positive hematuria

menstruation, bladder catheterization trauma, bacteriuria, beets, blackberries, rhubarb

False negative hematuria

formalin urine preservation, ascorbic acid (vitamin C)

Macroscopic hematuria

concrements, urinary tract tumors, cystic kidney, urogenital tuberculosis, trauma

Microscopic Hematuria

strenuous exercise, glomerulonephritis, infectious diseases, collagenoses, interstitial nephritis, pyelonephritis, uretherolithiasis

Cadmium

(Cd) Cadmium accumulates in tissue, concentrating primarily in the kidneys and liver. More than 95% of blood Cd is in the erythrocytes.

Test Purpose. 1) Cd toxicity proof in industry exposure (vapours), 2) Cd toxicity proof in non-industry exposure (e.g. food and low pH fluids storage in metal can).

Increased Values

exposure – (inhalation in industrial settings, orally), smokers
    Interfering Factors: medicaments – (EDTA)

Decreased Values (relatively)

    Interfering Factors: medicaments – (antacids, antibiotics, antituberculotics)

Analyte	Age/Gender	Reference Range	SI Units	Note
Cadmium	non-smokers	<9	µmol/l	
	intoxication	88–180	µmol/l	

Calcium

(syn: urine calcium, quantitative calcium)

Test Purpose. 1) to evaluate calcium and phosphate metabolism and excretion, 2) to monitor calcium or phosphate deficiency treatment, 3) differential diagnosis of metabolic osteopathies and osteoporosis, 4) urolithiasis metaphylaxia, 5) Ca metabolism assessment, if serum Ca is increased/decreased/normal, but these clinical syndromes are present: bone pain, renal insufficiency, chronic diarrhea and steatorrhea, prolonged corticoid therapy, conditions after arteficially provoked menopause.

Increased Values – hypercalciuria

acidosis, **renal tubular acidosis**, **acromegaly**, bone atrophy, **diabetes mellitus**, starvation, **idiopathic hypercalcemia/hypercalciuria**, **hyperparathyroidism**, **hyperthyroidism**, adrenal hypofunction, hypervitaminosis D, diseases – (**osteolytic bone d.**, renal d.), **immobilization**, **vitamin A, D intoxication**, ulcerative colitis, leukemia, lymphoma, disease – (Crohn's d., **Paget's d.**, Wilson's d.), **malignant tumours metastases**, **glucocorticoids excess**, tumours of – (lung, breast), osteomalacia, **osteoporosis**, **plasmocytoma** (incl. multiple myeloma), **sarcoidosis**, syndrome – (**Cushing's sy**, **Fanconi's sy**, milk/alkali sy), tuberculosis, fractures, **increased calcium intake**, excess milk intake, medullary sponge kidney
    Interfering Factors: adult people, high milk intake, high calcium/sodium/magnesium intake, medicaments – (acetazolamide, amiloride, ammonium chloride, anabolic steroids, androgens, antacids, anticonvulsants, ascorbic acid, caffeine, calcipotriene, calcitriol, carbonic anhydrase inhibitors, cholestyramine, corticosteroids, dihydrotachysterol, diuretics, dopamine, doxercalciferol, etidronate, furosemide, glucocorticoids, phosphates, sodium phytate, steroids, thiazides, viomycin, vitamin D)

Decreased Values – hypocalciuria

alkalosis, **vitamin D deficiency, familial hypocalciuric hypercalcemia, hypoparathyroidism,** hypothyroidism, renal diseases, insufficiency – (kidney i., parathyroid gland i., thyroid gland i.), malabsorption, **acute/chronic nephritis, acute/chronic nephrosis, renal osteodystrophy, osteomalacia,** low calcium diet, preeclampsia, **pseudohypoparathyroidism, rhachitis** (vitamin D resistant rickets), **steatorrhea, malabsorption sy,** renal failure, metastatic carcinoma of prostate

> **Interfering Factors:** alkaline urine, increased phosphate intake, medicaments – (corticosteroids, etidronate, indapamide, lithium, oral contraceptives, phenytoin, sodium phytate, thiazide diuretics)

Analyte	Age/Gender	Reference Range	SI Units	Note
Calcium	M	<7.5	mmol/d	
average diet intake	F	<6.2	mmol/d	
non-calcium diet		0.13–1.0	mmol/d	See ref. ranges note
lower calcium diet *		1.25–3.8	mmol/d	

Calculi

(kidney stones, renal stones). A typical urinary calculus is composed of crystalline substances precipitated in the body.
Components: ammonium acid urate, calcium bilirubinate, calcium carbonate, calcium hydrogen phosphate, calcium oxalate dihydrate, calcium oxalate monohydrate, calcium phosphate, carbonate apatite, cellular material, cholesterol, core composition, cystine, dried blood, hydroxyapatite, magnesium ammonium phosphate, magnesium hydrogen phosphate, sodium uric acid, sodium acid urate monohydrate, triamterene, uric acid, uric acid dihydrate, xanthine

Cannabinoids

(syn: Cannabis, Marijuana) A positive test for cannabinoids indicates the presence of cannabinoid metabolites, 11-nor-9-carboxy-delta-9-THC is the major one (carboxy THC) in urine, but is not related to source, time of exposure, amount or impairment. Urine may contain carboxy THC for a week or 10 days after light or moderate use and as long as a month to 7 weeks after heavy use. Rapid storage of THC tetrahydrocannabinol metabolites in body fat occurs after use. These substances are then released from storage sites slowly over time. Test evaluates drug abuse and assesses toxicity.

Increased Values
marijuana abuse

Carnitine

(syn: L-carnitine, total carnitine)

Decreased Values
severe renal diseases

Carnosine

(Car) Carnosine is present in the skeletal muscles.

Increased Values
high-meat diet, carnosinemia

Casts

(syn: cylinders) Casts are clumps of material or cells formed in the renal collecting duct (distal nephron) and in the distal convoluted tubule, which have the tubule shape, thus the term cast. The proximal convoluted tubule and loop of Henle are not locations for cast formation. When cellular casts remain in the nephron for some time before they are flushed into the bladder urine, the cells may degenerate to become a coarsely granular cast, later a finely granular cast and ultimately, a waxy cast. In end-stage kidney disease of any cause, the urinary sediment often becomes very scant because few remaining nephrons produce dilute urine.

- **mucoprotein matrix:** hyaline casts (mucoprotein matrix – Tamm–Horsfall protein – secreted by the tubules precipitates and gels)
- **protein matrix:** granular casts (tubular protein in hyaline cast, cellular material disintegration – red and white blood cells), hemoproteinic c., waxy c. (final granular casts step when urine flow is reduced and renal failure progresses, waxy casts may be cellular and hyaline formed in distal nephron). The factors which favor protein cast formation are low flow rate, high salt concentration, low pH, all of which favor protein denaturation and precipitation.
- **protein matrix + cells:** epithelial (tubular cells), erythrocytic c., leucocytic c.
- **other:** pseudocasts (composed of clumped urates, leukocytes, bacteria, artifacts), lipidic c. = fatty c. (free fat droplets in protein matrix), mixed c. (hyaline cast with various cells), miscellaneous c. – (crystals or bacteria)

Positive – cylindruria
- **epithelial casts: amyloidosis, eclampsia, glomerulonephritis**, viral diseases, **cytomegalovirus infection**, poisoning by – (nephrotoxic drugs, **ethylene glycol, heavy metals, salicylate**), **nephrosis, tubular necrosis, acute tubular injury, renal allograft rejection**, nephrotic syndrome
- **erythrocytic casts** (red blood cell casts, RBC casts, Erc casts, sticked RBC's): amyloidosis, **sickle cell anemia, strenuous physical exercise, glomerulonephritis, malignant hypertension, renal infarction**, collagenoses, **systemic lupus erythematosus, acute interstitial nephritis**, IgA nephropathy, lupus nephritis, cystic kidney, polyarteritis nodosa, **acute tubular injury, acute pyelonephritis, kidney impairment in subacute bacterial endocarditis**, scurvy (scorbutus), **Goodpasture's sy, renal vein thrombosis, vasculitis**
- **granular + hyaline casts:** amyloidosis, dehydration, pure carbohydrate diets, **glomerulonephritis**, malignant hypertension, infectious diseases – (**urinary tract d., viral d.**), **renal diseases, chronic lead poisoning**, medicaments – (amphotericin, calcitonin, cephaloridine, diuretics, indomethacin, kanamycin), acid urine, exertion, nephritis, **diabetic nephropathy**, proteinuria, **pyelonephritis, renal transplant rejection**, conditions – (febrile c., **c. after exercise**), **stress, nephrotic sy**, failure – (chronic renal f., congestive heart f.), tubular interstitial disease

- **hemoglobin and myoglobin casts**: hemoglobinuria, crush sy
- **hyaline casts**: **glomerulonephritis**, hypertension, concentrated urine – (physiologically in healthy people), kidney palpation, low urine flow, **proteinuria, pyelonephritis**, postural reaction, **febrile states, stress, psychic/strenuous exercise**, failure – (**chronic renal f., congestive heart f.**)
- **leucocytic casts** (WBC, Lkc casts, white cell casts): **glomerulonephritis**, tubular diseases – (**interstitial nephritis**), renal parenchymal infection, **lupus nephritis, pyelonephritis**, nephrotic sy
- **lipidic (fatty) casts**: tubular degeneration, chronic glomerulonephritis, glomerulosclerosis, diseases – (**chronic renal d.**, tubular inflammatory d.), nephritis, nephrosis, shock kidney, proteinuria, **nephrotic sy**, severe muscular trauma
- **waxy casts**: amyloidosis, **tubular degeneration, glomerulonephritis, malignant hypertension, renal tubular inflammatory diseases, acute/chronic renal insufficiency, diabetic nephropathy**, nephrosclerosis, nephrosis, **renal allograft rejection, nephrotic sy, acute/chronic renal failure**
- **mixed casts**: proliferative glomerulonephritis, tubulointerstitial diseases
- **miscellaneous casts** (crystals, bacteria): bacterial pyelonephritis
  Interfering Factors: medicaments – (amikacin, gentamicin, neomycin, streptomycin, tobramycin)

Catalase

Increased Values
pernicious anemia, hematuria, proteinuria, pyuria

Catecholamines

Hormones and substances of adrenal medulla excreted by urine: adrenaline, noradrenaline, vanilmandelic acid, metanephrine, normetanephrine.
Test Purpose. 1) to aid in pheochromocytoma diagnosis in unexplained hypertension, 2) to aid diagnosis of neuroblastoma and ganglioneuroma, 3) to help to confirm disorders of the autonomic nervous system.

Increased Values
adrenal medullary hyperplasia, **diabetic ketoacidosis**, progressive muscular dystrophy, encephalopathy, **pheochromocytoma, ganglioblastoma, ganglioneuroma**, ganglioneuroblastoma, hypoglycemia, **hypothyroidism**, renal diseases, **myocardial infarction**, CNS infarction, CNS hemorrhage, **myasthenia gravis, neuroblastoma, malignant hypertension**, CNS tumors, paragangliomas, acute psychosis, polytrauma, acute intermittent porphyria, syndrome – (Guillain–Barré sy, carcinoid sy), manic depressive disorders, **after surgery conditions, severe stress**, thyrotoxicosis
  Interfering Factors: tea, formaldehyde, nicotine, **vigorous physical exercise**, medicaments – (acetylsalicylic acid, adrenaline, alcohol, alpha-1-blockers, aminophylline, amphetamine, ampicillin, ascorbic acid, beta-blockers, caffeine, calcium channel blockers, chloral hydrate, chlorpromazine, clonidine, contrast media, diazoxide, disulfiram, ephedrine, erythromycin, hydralazine, imipramine, insulin, isoproterenol, labetalol, levodopa, MAO inhibitors, methenamine, methyldopa, minoxidil, niacin, nicotinic acid, nitroglycerin, nitroprusside, phenacetin, phenothiazines, quinidine, quinine, reserpine, riboflavin, theophylline, tetracyclines, tricyclic antidepressants, vitamin B-complex)

Decreased Values

diabetes mellitus (autonomic neuropathy), parkinsonism

Interfering Factors: radiographic dyes, medicaments – (acetylsalicylic acid, alpha-2-agonists, anileridine, bretylium, bromocriptine, calcium channel blockers, chlorpromazine, cimetidine, clofibrate, clonidine, disulfiram, guanethidine, imipramine, isoproterenol, levodopa, MAO inhibitors, mephenesin, methocarbamol, methyldopa, metyrosine, nalidixic acid, ouabain, penicillins, phenazopyridine, prazosin, propranolol, reserpine, salicylates, thyroxine)

Analyte	Age/Gender	Reference Range	SI Units	Note
Catecholamines total,				
free	0–1 y	10–15	µg/d	
	1–5 y	15–40	µg/d	
	6–15 y	20–80	µg/d	
	Others	30–100	µg/d	
Catecholamines				
Norepinephrine	0–1 y	0–59	nmol/d	
	1–2 y	0–100	nmol/d	
	2–4 y	24–171	nmol/d	
	4–7 y	47–266	nmol/d	
	7–10 y	77–384	nmol/d	
	Others	87–473	nmol/d	
Epinephrine	0–1 y	0–13.6	nmol/d	
	1–2 y	0–19.1	nmol/d	
	2–4 y	0–32.7	nmol/d	
	4–7 y	1.1–55	nmol/d	
	7–10 y	2.7–76	nmol/d	
	Others	2.7–109	nmol/d	
Dopamine	0–1 y	0–555	nmol/d	
	1–2 y	65–914	nmol/d	
	2–4 y	261–1697	nmol/d	
	Others	424–2611	nmol/d	

Chloride

Indicator of electrolyte balance in connection with sodium and fluid changes (rising and falling in tandem). Urine electrolyte values must be interpreted together with their serum concentrations, acid-base balance status, urine pH and ammonia excretion in indicated cases. Urine ammonia gap determination is used in differential diagnosis of hyperchloremic metabolic acidosis.

Test Purpose. 1) to help evaluate fluid and electrolyte imbalance, 2) to monitor the low-salt diet effects, 3) to help evaluate renal and adrenal disorders, 4) water-salt and acid-base balance disorders (abnormal water and NaCl balance diagnosis in hyponatremia, differential diagnosis of extra/renal causes in hypo/hyperkalemia, differential diagnosis of extra/renal hyperchloremic metabolic acidosis causes).

$AGu\ (mmol/l) = Na^+ + K^+ - Cl^-$	if urine pH is about 5–5.5
$AGu\ (mmol/l = Na^+ + K^+ - Cl^- - HCO_3^-$	if urine pH is about 6.5

AGu – anion gap

negative AGu	ammonia excretion more than 80 µmol/l
positive AGu	ammonia excretion less than 30 µmol/l

If in the case of hyperchloremic metabolic acidosis a negative AGu value is present, then a renal cause can be excluded; it is necessary to find extrarenal causes (e.g. loss of HCO_3^-).

Increased Values

diabetic acidosis, **dehydration**, vegane diet, **starvation, adrenal hypofunction, salicylate intoxication,** Addison's disease, **salt-losing nephritis**, rachitis, convalescence, Bartter's syndrome, exudate resorption, **adrenal failure**

  Interfering Factors: increased salt intake, medicaments – (bromides, corticosteroids, diuretics – chlorothiazides, mercurial d., salicylates, steroids)

Decreased Values

colonic villous adenoma, **primary aldosteronism,** hypochloremic metabolic alkalosis, **emphysema,** starvation, **diarrhea,** acute exudative diseases, cachexia, **Addison's disease,** nephritis, **pyloric obstruction, prolonged gastric suction,** pneumonia, **excessive diaphoresis,** febrile states, **malabsorption sy,** scarlatina (scarlet fever), typhoid fever, **prolonged vomiting,** failure – **(acute renal f., congestive heart f.)**

  Interfering Factors: decreased salt intake, medicaments – (diuretics)

Analyte	Age/Gender	Reference Range	SI Units	Note
Chloride		85–170	mmol/d	
		46–168	mmol/l	

Chromium

It is necessary to test a possible increased Cr food intake (multivitamins + trace elements) or to exclude latent diabetes mellitus firstly, if the urine Cr values are 2–3 times higher. **Test Purpose.** 1) to evaluate industrial exposure, suspected toxicity, 2) in conjunction with serum levels, to attempt suspect chromium deficiency detection, especially in recent glucose intolerance onset.

Increased Values

heavy exercise, diabetes mellitus (IDDM), **professional** (occupational) **exposure,** increased sugar intake, Turner's sy, physical trauma

Analyte	Age/Gender	Reference Range	SI Units	Note
Chromium		<1	µg/d	

Chylus

Test Purpose. To help in diagnosis of injury/obstruction of lymphochylous system.

Increased Values – chyluria

trauma to chest/abdomen, **obstruction of the lymphochylous system, filariasis,** abdominal tumors, lymph node enlargement, pyelonephritis

Citric Acid

(syn: citrate, citrate excretion) Citrate in urine inhibits crystal formation. Replacement drug therapy with potassium citrate is useful in delaying and preventing further stone formation.

Decreased Values – hypocitraturia
idiopathic calcium urolithiasis, enteric hyperoxaluria, high sodium intake, nephrolithiasis

Analyte	Age/Gender	Reference Range	SI Units	Note
Citrates		2–4	mmol/dU	

Citrulline

Increased Values – hypercitrullinuria
citrullinemia, Hartnup disease

Cobalt

Increased Values
professional (occupational) exposure

Colour

- **whitish opalescent** (turbidity): bacteria, phosphates, pus, chyles, leukocytes, urates, lipuria, polymorphonuclears, primary hyperoxaluria
- **red**: aniline dyes, bromsulphophthalein, beets, blackberries, food dyes, hemoglobin, blood, medicaments – (amidopyrine, ampicillin, chlorzoxazone, dantrone, deferoxamine, ethoxazene, ibuprofen, mannose, oxamniquine, phenacetin, phenothiazines, phenytoin, pyridium, quinine, rifampicin), myoglobin, porphobilinogen, porphyrins, tomatoes, rhubarb, senna, toxins – (aniline, naphthalene, lead, mercury), uroporphyrin, water-melon
- **physiologically**: amber, can vary from pale straw (dilute urine) to brown (concentrated urine) – pigments urochrome (yellow), urorosein – uroerythrin (red)
- **brown through black**: alkaptonuria, bilirubin, glomerulonephritis, indicans, homogentisic acid, medicaments – (chloroquinone, dantrone, furazolidine, hydroquinone, iron compounds, levodopa, methocarbamol, methyldopa, metronidazole, nitrofurantoin, primaquine, phenacetin, phenazopyridine, phenothiazines, phenytoin, quinine, sulfonamides), melanin, melanoma, methemoglobin, myoglobin, porphyrins, rhubarb, toxins – (aloe, benzene, phenols, cresols, naphthalene, naphthol, nitrobenzene, lead, mercury), tyrosinosis, urobilin, bile pigments
- **blue**: medicaments – (amitriptyline, boric acid, methocarbamol, nitrofurantoin), tryptophan metabolism disorders
- **orange (bilirubin, urobilin)**: excessive sweating, fever, concentrated urine, medicaments – (butazopyridine, chlorzoxazone, dantrolene, ethoxazene, mannose, methyldopa, oxamniquine, phenazopyridine, phenothiazines, phensuximide, phenytoin, pyridium, riboflavin, rifampicin, senna, sulfasalazine, triamterene, warfarin), myoglobinuria, food – (beets, blackberries, food coloring dyes, carrots, paprika, rhubarb), porphyrins, restricted fluid intake, toxins – (heavy metals, naphthalene, lead, mercury)
- **various shades**: drugs
- **pink (to red)**: beets, blackberries, RBC, hemoglobin, food coloring dyes, medicaments – (amidopyrine, ampicillin, antipyrine, deferoxamine, diphenylhydantoin, doxorubicin, ibuprofen, methyldopa, phenacetin, phenazopyridine, phenolphthalein, phenothiazines,

phensuximide, phenytoin, pyridium, quinine, rifampicin), myoglobin, porphobilin, porphyrins, tomatoes, rhubarb, toxins – (aniline, naphthalene, lead, mercury), urates, watermelon, bile presence

- **dark brown:** alkaptonuria, bilirubin, hematin, Addison's disease, melanin, methemoglobin, medicaments – (chloroquine, deferoxamine, ethoxazene, ibuprofen, levodopa, methyldopa, metronidazole, pamaquine, phenacetin, phenazopyridine, phenothiazines, phensuximide, phenytoin, quinine), myoglobin, porphyrin, rhubarb, resorcin, tanine, urological tea
- **dark yellow** (through brown): bilirubin, carrots, blood, medicaments – (anthraquinone laxatives, nitrofurantoin, pamaquine, primaquine, phenacetin, sulfamethoxazole), multivitamins, insufficient fluid intake, riboflavin, urobilin, highly concentrated urine, rhubarb
- **very pale amber:** alcohol, diabetes insipidus, diabetes mellitus, diuretics, chronic interstitial nephritis, polyuria, excessive water intake, stress, hypercalcemia
- **smoky or pale reddish:** blood
- **yellow-orange:** medicaments – (aminopyrine, anisindione, phenazopyridine, sulfasalazine, warfarin), urobilin, bilirubin, carrots, vitamin K, dehydration
- **darkening on standing, alkalinization, oxygenation:** melanogen, hemoglobin, indican, porphyrins, salicylate metabolites, metronidazole, tyrosinosis, sickle cell crisis, urobilinogen, phenols, homogentisic acid
- **greenish-blue** (blue-green): bacteria, biliverdin, pseudomonas infection, medicaments – (amitriptyline, boric acid, chlorophyll, guaiacol, indomethacin, magnesium salicylate, triamterene, thymol, vitamin B-complex), methylene blue, poisoning by – (phenols, indigo blue, crezol, methocarbamol, methylene blue), pyuria, thymol
- **greenish-orange:** bilirubin, cresol, phenol, methocarbamol, resorcinol, biliverdin

Concentration Test

14–36 hrs without fluids → urine collection → specific gravity >1028 (855–1335 osmol/kg according to age).

Copper

Test Purpose. 1) to help detect Wilson's disease, Menkes' sy, 2) to screen infants with a family history of Wilson's disease, 3) to help detect acute or chronic copper toxicity.

Increased Values
rheumatoid arthritis, biliary cirrhosis, chronic active hepatitis, acute/chronic copper intoxication, Wilson's disease, proteinuria, syndrome – (**Menkes' sy, nephrotic sy**)
    Interfering Factors: medicaments – (captopril, D-penicillamine)

Decreased Values
nutritional deficiency, hypothyroidism, Addison's disease, protein malnutrition

Analyte	Age/Gender	Reference Range	SI Units	Note
Copper		0.16–0.94	µmol/dU	

Coproporphyrins

Test Purpose. To aid in congenital or acquired porphyrias diagnosis.

Increased Values – coproporphyrin I
congenital erythropoietic porphyria

Increased Values – coproporphyrin III
exposure – (arsenic e., chronic ethanol e., mercury e.), liver diseases, **lead poisoning, heredi-tary coproporphyria**, dietary brewers yeast, tumors, **porphyria cutanea tarda**, **porphyria variegata** (variegate porphyria), chronic renal failure
   Interfering Factors: medicaments – (barbiturates, oral contraceptives)

Analyte	Age/Gender	Reference Range	SI Units	Note
Coproporphyrins		51–351	nmol/d	

Cortisol

(UFC, syn: urinary-free cortisol, urinary free corticoids, hydrocortisone, urine cortisol)
Test Purpose. To aid in Cushing's sy diagnosis.

Increased Values
adrenal hyperplasia, tumors of – (**pituitary, adrenals**), **stress**, syndrome – (**ectopic ACTH sy, Cushing's sy**), **pregnancy** (3rd trimester)
   Interfering Factors: medicaments – (amphetamines, carbamazepine, estrogens, oral contraceptives, spironolactone, tricyclic antidepressants, vasopressin)

Decreased Values
congenital adrenal hyperplasia, hypopituitarism, Addison's disease, adrenogenital syn-drome
   Interfering Factors: medicaments – (danazol, ephedrine, glucocorticoids, hydrochloro-thiazide, ketoconazole, levodopa, lithium, oxazepam)

Analyte	Age/Gender	Reference Range	SI Units	Note
Cortisol, Free	1–14 y	<74	nmol/d	
	Puberty	<138	nmol/d	
	Adults	27–276	nmol/d	

Cotinine

The test may remain positive for some days after the last cigarette. Passive smoking does not give rise to high levels.
Test Purpose. Detection of nicotine intake, usually in patients on a non-smoking program.

Increased Values
smokers

Creatine

Increased Values – hypercreatinuria
muscular atrophy/dystrophy, acute paroxysmal myoglobinuria, acromegaly, diabetes mellitus, muscular tissue destruction, diet without carbohydrates, **starvation**, healing fractures, eunuchoidism, diseases – (endocrine d., infectious d.), **hyperthyroidism, myopathies,** Addison's disease, burns, leukemia, conditions – (severe febrile c., c. after pregnancy), children growth, raw meat diet, systemic lupus erythematosus, myasthenia gravis, crush injury, excessive water depletion, tetanus, pregnancy, Cushing's syndrome, congenital amyotonia, poliomyelitis
> **Interfering Factors:** medicaments – (ACTH, cortisone)

Decreased Values – hypocreatinuria
congenital amyotonia, **hypothyroidism**, renal diseases

Creatinine

Creatinine is by-product of muscular energetic metabolism, it is a breakdown product of creatine. By far the most important source of energy inside cells are the high-energy phosphate bonds of the ATP molecule. When one of these bonds is broken, energy is released and ATP becomes ADP. Creatine phosphate represents a backup energy source for ATP, because it can quickly re-convert ADP back to ATP. The creatinine is a waste product, that cannot be used by cells for any constructive purpose. Creatinine is excreted from the body entirely by the kidneys.

Test Purpose. 1) to help assess glomerular filtration, 2) to check the accuracy of 24-hour urine collection, based on a relatively constant creatinine excretion levels, 3) to evaluate kidney function, 4) with plasma creatinine, to estimate plasma creatinine clearance, 5) with another urine analyte, to calculate the analyte/creatinine ratio, 6) with plasma creatinine and another analyte present in both plasma and serum, to calculate a fractional excretion rate of that analyte.

Increased Values – hypercreatininuria
acromegaly, acute tubular necrosis, muscular tissue destruction, dehydration, **diabetes mellitus,** diabetic nephropathy, gigantism, glomerulonephritis, muscular dystrophy, starvation, hypothyroidism, hepatic insufficiency, myasthenia gravis, pneumonia, **increased protein ingestion** (meat meals), pyelonephritis, febrile conditions, tetanus, typhoid fever, serious physical exertion/exercise, failure – (congestive heart f., renal f.), rhabdomyolysis, urinary tract obstruction, Cushing's sy, reduced renal blood flow, shock conditions
> **Interfering Factors:** hyperglycemia, ketoacidosis, large musculature, medicaments – (aminoglycosides, cephalosporins, cephalotin, cefamandole, cefazolin, cefoxitin, captopril, cimetidine, cisplatin, corticosteroids, gentamicin, ascorbic acid, fructose, levodopa, methyldopa, nitrofurans, probenecid, trimethoprim)

Decreased Values – hypocreatininuria
amyloid, anemia, muscular atrophy, vegetarian diet, muscular dystrophy, **impaired kidney function, acute/chronic glomerulonephritis, starvation,** hyperthyroidism, diseases – (advanced renal d., inflammatory d. of muscles), **leukemia, polycystic kidney, urinary tract obstruction, paralysis,** polymyositis, **pyelonephritis**

Interfering Factors: hyperbilirubinemia, small musculature, medicaments – (anabolic steroids, androgens, phenacetin, thiazides)

Analyte	Age/Gender	Reference Range	SI Units	Note
Creatinine	M	5–18	mmol/d	
	F	8–27	mmol/d	
	M 20–29 y	190–230	µmol/kg/d	
	70–79 y	100–152	µmol/kg/d	
	F 20–29 y	140–207	µmol/kg/d	
	70–79 y	81–123	µmol/kg/d	

Crystals

Positive – crystaluria

■ **alkaline urine:** amorphous phosphates, magnesium-ammonium phosphate, calcium phosphates, cholesterol, triple phosphates, calcium carbonate, ammonium urate

■ **phosphates (calcium-phosphate):** renal tubular acidosis, primary hypercalciuria, hyperparathyroidism, intoxication, alkali ingestion

■ **other:** cystine – (congenital cystinuria, cystinosis, cystine storage disease, severe liver disease), cholesterol, leucine – (severe liver disease, Fanconi's sy, maple syrup urine disease), leucine/tyrosine – (acute yellow atrophy, terminal cirrhosis, maple syrup urine disease, severe liver diseases), tyrosine – (congenital tyrosinosis, tyrosinemia, severe liver impairment), xanthine – (xanthinuria), orotic acid – (orotic aciduria)

■ **calcium oxalate:** idiopathic hypercalciuria, primary hyperoxaluria, primary hyperparathyroidism, severe chronic renal diseases, vitamin D intoxication, concentrated urine, osteoporosis, increased intake of fruits and vegetables – (garlic, tea, cabbage, oranges, tomatoes, rhubarb, spinach), sarcoidosis, milk–alkali sy, oxalosis

■ **acid urine:** bilirubin, cysteine, calcium oxalate, uric acid, urates

■ **urates/uric acid:** antituberculotics – (pyrazinamide), atherosclerosis generalisata, gout (uratic arthritis, gouty arthritis), **hyperuricemia**, cardiac infarction, **renal insufficiency**, leukemia, cytostatic therapy, tumours, **increased purine intake**, febrile diseases, Lesch–Nyhan sy

Interfering Factors: medicaments – (acetazolamide, aciclovir, erythromycin, methenamine, methotrexate, metyrosine, sulfadiazine, sulfamethoxazole, sulfizoxazole, sulfonamides, thiabendazole, xanthines)

Cyclic Adenosine Monophosphate

cAMP urine levels are determined by glomerular filtration rate and by direct production in kidney. cAMP amount depends on tubules number and PTH concentration. PTH stimulates an adenylate cyclase activity in renal cortex.

Test Purpose. 1) to aid in the diagnosis and differential diagnosis of pseudohypoparathyroidism, 2) to determine pseudohypoparathyroidism type (I or II), 3) suspect primary hyperparathyroidism, 4) hypercalcemia differential diagnosis in tumors, if there is suspect paraneoplastic PTH secretion.

Increased Values

vitamin D deficiency, familial Mediterranean fever, **hypercalcemia of malignancy**, **hyperparathyroidism**, calcium malabsorption, osteomalacia, pseudohypoparathyroidism (type II), manic states, calcium urolithiasis

Decreased Values

depression, hypoparathyroidism, pseudohypoparathyroidism

Analyte	Age/Gender	Reference Range	SI Units	Note
Cyclic Adenosine Monophosphate		<1000	nmol/d	*nmol/ mmol
		330–660	*	creatinine

Cyclic Guanosine Monophosphate

(cGMP) cGMP is present in urine as a result of blood filtrate and a direct renal secretion of cGMP. There is no direct correlation between blood and urine cGMP.

Analyte	Age/Gender	Reference Range	SI Units	Note
Cyclic Guanosine Monophosphate		30–200	*	*nmol/ mmol creatinine

Cystathione

Increased Values – hypercystathioninuria

methylmalonic aciduria, cystathioninuria, hepatoblastoma, homocystinuria, neuroblastoma, premature infants, secondary to pyridoxine deficiency

Cystatine C

It is a low molecular weight protein, its stable level of production is used in GFR measurement and is a better indicator of GFR than creatinine.

Increased Values – hypercystatinemia

acromegaly, **acute tubular necrosis**, muscular tissue destruction, dehydration, **diabetes mellitus**, **diabetic nephropathy**, diseases – (autoimmune systemic d., **renal d.**), diseases connected with a very high bilirubin levels, gigantism, **glomerulonephritis**, muscular dystrophy, starvation, hypothyroidism, hepatic insufficiency, myasthenia gravis, pneumonia, **increased protein ingestion** (meat meals), **pyelonephritis**, febrile conditions, tetanus, typhoid fever, serious physical exertion/exercise, failure – (congestive heart f., **renal f.**), rhabdomyolysis, urinary tract obstruction, Cushing's sy, reduced renal blood flow, shock conditions

Analyte	Age/Gender	Reference Range	SI Units	Note
Cystatine C		<0.01	mg/l	

Cysteine

Increased Values – hypercysteinuria

cystinosis, cystinuria – (increased arginine, cystine, lysine, ornithine excretion), pregnancy (1st trimester)

Interfering Factors: medicaments – (cycloleucine, histidine, progesterone)

severe burns

Interfering Factors: medicaments – (ascorbic acid, penicillamine)

Analyte	Age/Gender	Reference Range	SI Units	Note
Cysteine		<317	µmol/d	

Deoxypyridinoline

(DPD) About 90% of organic bone matrix is composed of collagen I. This collagen is inter-linked with specific molecules which are responsible for bone toughness and strength. Molecules in matured collagen I are of three types: pyridine, pyridinoline (PID) and deoxy-pyridinoline (DPD). DPD is produced by enzyme lysine catalysis with lysyl oxidase, released into blood stream during bone resorption, excreted by urine in original form without food influence. In bone there is a permanent metabolic process called remodelation composed from degradation, bone resorption mediated by osteoclast action and osteolysis, and formation process mediated by osteoblasts. There is resorption formation balance in physiological conditions. In pathological conditions these contrary processes are divided; resorption and bone tissue loss prevail. Specific bone matrix degradation products determination gives analytic data about bone metabolism level. DPD urine excretion results are counted to creatinine values.

Test Purpose. 1) to assess bone remodelation, 2) to assess metabolic osteoporosis activity.

Increased Values

false increased values – (adrenal diseases, thyroid diseases, immobilization, hyperparathyroidism, malabsorption, kidney transplantation, tumors with metastases, tumor associated hypercalcemia, rheumatic diseases, nanismus, hyperthyroidism, lactation, body growth period, pregnancy), osteoporosis, Paget's disease, osteomalacia medicaments – false increased values – (gonadotropin-releasing hormone analogues, anticonvulsants, heparin, thyroid hormones, corticosteroids)

Decreased Values

Interfering Factors: medicaments – (biphosphonates, calcitonin, estrogens substitution in postmenopause)

Analyte	Age/Gender	Reference Range	SI Units	Note
Deoxypyridinoline	M	2.3–5.4	*	*
	F	3.0–7.4	*	nmol DPD/ mmol creatinine

Dilution Test

Drink 20 ml of fluid/kg of body weight → within 3 hrs 50% of volume drunk should be excreted → then urine specific gravity <1003.

Eosinophils

Test Purpose. To help to distinguish acute interstitial nephritis from acute tubular necrosis.

Increased Values – eosinophiluria
chronic pyelonephritis, acute glomerulonephritis, IgA nephropathy, Henoch-Schönlein purpura, cholesterol embolization to kidney, renal atheroemboli, Schistosoma hematobium infestation, bladder cancer, acute rejection of renal allograft, obstructive uropathy, prostatitis, **eosinophilic cystitis, interstitial nephritis**

Estrogens

Total estrogens, estradiol + estriol. Estradiol is the most active endogenic estrogen, significantly increasing in 3rd trimester of pregnancy. Serial urine and blood estriol excretion studies provide objective means of assessing placental function and fetal well-being. Placenta synthesizes estrogens from precursors (mainly 16-alpha-OH DHEAS) which are created in fetal adrenals. Placental estriol is excreted in mother urine by complex mechanism. Continuous monitoring from 28th pregnancy week is of clinical importance. Basal level is best evaluated from three sampling days. Urine estriol levels about 40 µmol/dU during four weeks can be assessed as alarming. There is a very high fetal death risk with values less 20 µmol/l. Rising values indicate an adequately functioning fetoplacental unit.

Test Purpose. 1) to evaluate ovarian activity and help determine causes of amenorrhea and female hyperestrogenism, 2) to aid in the diagnosis of ovarian, adrenocortical or testicular origin tumors, 3) to assess fetoplacental status, especially in high-risk pregnancy (such as maternal hypertension, diabetes mellitus, preeclampsia, PIH – pregnancy induced hypertension, or stillbirth history), this is the main test purpose; serum and urine estrogens examinations are equivalent in this indication.

Increased Values – estrogens
cirrhosis hepatis, corpus luteum cyst, **adrenal cortex hyperplasia,** liver diseases, tumours – **(t. of adrenal cortex, testicular t., ovarian t. producing estrogens),** precocious puberty, Stein–Leventhal sy, pregnancy
> **Interfering Factors:** medicaments – (acetazolamide, ACTH, chlorpromazine, clomiphene, cortisone, gonadotropin, hydrochlorothiazide, levodopa, meprobamate, methenamine, testosterone)

Increased Values – estriol
glycosuria, congenital adrenal hyperplasia, **urinary tract infections,** tumors of – **(adrenals, testes, ovary), multiple pregnancy**
> **Interfering Factors:** medicaments – (ACTH, ampicillin, barbiturates, corticosteroids, estrogen-containing drugs, oxytocin, phenothiazines, tetracyclines)

Decreased Values – estrogens
ovarian agenesis, inadequate luteal phase, pituitary/adrenal glands hypofunction/dysfunction, anovulatory bleeding, **primary/secondary ovarian malfunction/insufficiency, menopause,** congenital anomalies, failing pregnancy, fetal death, fetal distress, placental insufficiency, preeclampsia/eclampsia, syndrome – (adrenogenital sy, Stein-Leventhal sy, Turner's sy)

Interfering Factors: medicaments – (acetazolamide, ACTH, ampicillin, cyclophospha-mide, dexamethasone, fructose, galactose, glucose, hydrochlorothiazide, insulin, neomy-cin, oral contraceptives, penicillin, phenothiazines)

Decreased Values – estriol
anemia, **anencephaly, congenital anomalies, anorexia nervosa**, fetal adrenal aplasia/hypo-plasia, **complicated diabetes mellitus**, sulfatase deficiency, **fetal distress** (fetoplacental de-terioration), **dysmaturity, hemoglobinopathy**, hydatidiform mole, **hypopituitarism**, diseases – (intestinal d., renal d., severe liver d.), **placental insufficiency**, Rh isoimmunization, mal-nutrition, **menopause, fetal death, pre/eclampsia**, placental infarction, placental dysfunc-tion, pyelonephritis, syndrome – (**adrenogenital sy**, Stein–Leventhal sy, **Turner's sy**), failing pregnancy, high-altitudes

Interfering Factors: medicaments – (ampicillin, clomiphene, corticosteroids, dexam-ethasone, diuretics, erythromycin, estrogens, glutethimide, meprobamate, neomycin, oral contraceptives, penicillin, phenazopyridine, phenolphthalein, probenecid, senna)

Analyte	Age/Gender	Reference Range	SI Units	Note
Estrogens, Total	Children	<10	µg/d	
	M	5–25	µg/d	
	F Follicular phase	5–25	µg/d	
	Ovulatory phase	28–100	µg/d	
	Luteal phase	22–80	µg/d	
	Pregnancy	<45000	µg/d	
	30 w	17.4–55.5	µmol/d	
	35 w	34.7–97.1	µmol/d	
	40 w	52–140	µmol/d	
	Menopause	<10	µg/d	
Estriol, Total	Pregnancy 30 w	21–62	µmol/d	
	35 w	31–97	µmol/d	
	40 w	45–146	µmol/d	

Ethanolamine

(EA) Relatively high concentrations are found in the brain, lungs and liver.

Increased Values
ethanolaminosis, primary hepatoma, hyperlysinemia

Fibrin Degradation Products

Decreased Values
kidney diseases, **bladder tumors**, renal transplant rejection

Fluorides

Increased Values
occupational exposure, intoxication

Follicle-Stimulating Hormone + Luteinizing Hormone

Function. In women FSH promotes maturation of the ovarian follicle → the maturing follicles produce estrogen → as estrogen levels rise LH is produced. FSH and LH induce ovulation. In men FSH promotes spermatogenesis, LH stimulates androgens secretion and increased testosterone synthesis. LH in women acts on the interstitial cells → synthesis of androgens, estrogens and progesterone.

Test Purpose. 1) cycle disorders diagnosis, 2) sterility diagnosis.

Increased Values FSH
ovarian/testicular agenesis, **alcoholism**, climacterium praecox, gonadal dysgenesis, peripheral hypogonadism, primary ovarian insufficiency, **castration**, **menopause**, **orchitis**, precocious puberty – (idiopathic p. p., secondary p. p.), states after cytostatic therapy, syndrome – (**Klinefelter's sy**, complete testicular feminization sy, Turner's sy), **gonadal failure**
   Interfering Factors: medicaments – (clomiphene)

Increased Values FSH + LH
primary gonadal insufficiency, precocious puberty, complete testicular feminization sy

Decreased Values FSH
acromegalia, sickle-cell anemia, **anorexia mentalis** (nervosa), **hemochromatosis**, **anterior pituitary hypofunction**, central hypogonadism, selective hypopituitarism, **several illnesses**, secondary ovarian insufficiency, ovarian tumours – (feminizing o. t., masculinizing o. t.), androgens/estrogens producing tumours – (adrenal glands t., testes t.), **polycystic kidney**, panhypopituitarism, pituitary/hypothalamic lesions caused by – (**tumours**, **trauma**), **pregnancy**
   Interfering Factors: medicaments – (digitalis, estrogens, oral contraceptives)

Decreased Values FSH + LH
hypopituitarism, panhypopituitarism, failure of pituitary/hypothalamus

Fructose

Increased Values – fructosuria
hepatic cirrhosis, **essential fructosuria**, hepatitis, severe infectious diseases, fructose intolerance, mercury intoxication, Wilson's disease, food, **hepatic failure**
   Interfering Factors: ingestion of honey, fruits, sucrose, syrups

Galactose

Increased Values – galactosuria
newborn biliary atresia, children – (premature ch., ch. with high milk consumption), **galactokinase-deficient galactosemia**, **hepatitis**, severe infectious diseases, newborn icterus, monosaccharide intolerance, **neonates up to 6 days**, severe hepatic lesion, pregnancy (3rd trimester)
   Interfering Factors: lactose

Analyte	Age/Gender	Reference Range	SI Units	Note
Galactose	Neonates	<3.33	mmol/l	
	Children	<0.08	mmol/dU	

Globulins

Increased Values
multiple myeloma, macroglobulinemia, primary amyloidosis, Fanconi's syndrome (adults)

Glucose

Increased urine glucose levels appear with increased blood glucose. Glucose is filtered into primary urine by glomerules from plasma → resorption in proximal tubules. Less than 0.1% of glucose normally filtered by the glomerulus appears in urine. Dipsticks employing the glucose oxidase reaction for screening are specific for glucose but can miss other reducing sugars (galactose, fructose).

Test Purpose. 1) glucose tolerance disorders screening, 2) diabetes mellitus therapy control, 3) glycosuria in pregnancy and renal function disorders.

Increased Values – positive, glycosuria, glucosuria
abscess of pancreas, acidosis, incomplete abortion, **acromegaly**, adenoma of – (**pituitary**, adrenal cortex, **pancreas**), anoxia, apoplexia, asphyxia, hepatic cirrhosis (advanced), cystinosis, **diabetes mellitus, renal diabetes, renal tubular dysfunction**, acute hepatic dystrophy, emotions, encephalitis, false positive results – (phenazopyridine, ascorbic acid, levodopa, nalidixic acid, cephalosporins, probenecid), **pheochromocytoma**, diabetic gangrene, **gigantism**, glucagonoma, acute glomerulonephritis, cystic fibrosis of pancreas, **alimentary glycosuria**, hemochromatosis, hyperaldosteronism, infectious hepatitis, false positive results – (heavy meal, lactation, x-ray contrast media, increased carbohydrate intake, stress, excitement), adrenal hyperfunction, **hyperthyroidism**, hypokalemia, diseases – (renal tubular d., chronic liver d.), **acute/chronic infectious diseases, myocardial infarction**, intoxication – (lead i., cadmium i., mercury i., carbon monoxide i.), diabetic ketoacidosis, non-ketotic hyperosmolar coma, **diabetic coma**, subarachnoid hemorrhage, Basedow's disease, tumors of – (adrenal cortex t., central nervous system, pancreas), **chronic interstitial nephritis**, nephrosis, nephropathy – (toxic n.), diabetic neuropathy, obesity, potassium deficiency, shock kidney, **pancreatitis**, pancreatectomy, severe burns, brain injury/hemorrhage, hepatic toxic lesions, **low renal threshold, pyelonephritis**, rabies, sepsis, conditions – (painful c., **hyperglycemic c.**), syndrome – (**Cushing's sy, Fanconi's sy**, Mauriac sy), shock, **pregnancy**, uremia

> **Interfering Factors:** medicaments – (acetazolamide, ACTH, adrenaline, aminosalicylic acid, ammonium chloride, ascorbic acid, asparaginase, cephalosporins, cephalotin, chloral hydrate, chloramphenicol, chlorothiazide, chlorpromazine, chlortalidone, cidofovir, cimetidine, clobetasol, corticosteroids, desonide, dexamethasone, dextrothyroxine, diazoxide, diuretics, edetate calcium disodium, ephedrine, estrogens, ethacrynic acid, ether, flurandrenolide, furosemide, glucagon, glucocorticoids, glucose infusion, homogentisic acid, hydrochlorothiazide, indapamide, isoniazid, lactose, levodopa, lithium, metolazone, nafcillin, nalidixic acid, nicotinic acid, nitrofurantoin, oral contraceptives, phenothiazines, polythiazide, salicylates, somatropin, streptomycin, sulfonamides, thiazides, triamcinolone, triamterene)

Analyte	Age/Gender	Reference Range	SI Units	Note
Glucose		0.3–1.1	mmol/l	

Glucuronic Acid

Increased Values
    Interfering Factors: medicaments – (acetylsalicylic acid, chloral hydrate, sulfonamides)

Gamma-Glutamyltransferase

Decreased Values
chronic nephritis

Glutamine

Increased Values
generalized aminoaciduria, rheumatoid arthritis, **Hartnup disease**

Glycine

Increased Values – hyperglycinuria
acidemia – (methylmalonic a., propionic a.), **generalized aminoaciduria**, rheumatoid arthritis, cystinuria, **glycinuria**, non-ketotic hyperglycinemia, hyperprolinemia, hypoglycemia, **Hartnup disease**, burns, vitamin D resistant rickets, pregnancy
    Interfering Factors: medicaments – (niacinamide)

Decreased Values – hypoglycinuria
    Interfering Factors: medicaments – (ascorbic acid – large doses, niacin)

Beta-2-Glycoprotein I

Increased Values
renal tubular diseases, breast tumors

Glycosaminoglycans

(syn: GAG, mucopolysaccharides) Glycosaminoglycans are any of several high molecular weight linear heteropolysaccharides having disaccharide repeating units containing an N-acetylhexosamine and a hexose or hexuronic acid. Glycosaminoglycans are freely dispersed within many tissues and body fluids. Glycosaminoglycans which accumulate in disorders and produce positive screening urine reactions are dermatan sulfate, heparan sulfate, keratan sulfate, chondroitin sulfate and hyaluronic acid.
Test Purpose. To diagnose mucopolysaccharidoses in infants with family disease history.

Increased Values
syndromes – (Hurler's sy, Hunter's sy, Sanfilippo's sy A, B)

Analyte	Age/Gender	Reference Range	SI Units	Note
Glycosamino-Glycans	0–1 y	10.0–27.2	*	*mg/mmol
	1–2 y	7.8–13.4	*	creatinine
	2–4 y	7.6–12.0	*	
	4–6 y	6.5–8.3	*	
	6–10 y	4.9–7.7	*	
	10–15 y	3.4–5.6	*	
	15–20 y	1.9–3.9	*	
	20–50 y	0–1.6	*	

Hallucinogens

Test Purpose. To detect presence of hallucinogens, such as LSD, marijuana, mescaline and other drugs in the body.

Increased Values
hallucinogens

Hemoglobin

Hemoglobinuria can be a hemolysis result, if the serum haptoglobin capacity (1–2 g/l) and renal tubular resorption threshold (0.9–1.4 g/l) are exceeded. Hemoglobin is catabolized in renal tubular cells and iron is stored as hemosiderin.
Test Purpose. 1) proteinuria differential diagnosis (prerenal proteinuria marker), 2) to help confirm diagnosis of hemolytic anemia or severe RBC destruction from a transfusion reaction or other causes.

Positive values – hemoglobinuria
anthrax, anemia – (**acquired hemolytic a.**, sickle-cell a., hereditary spherocytosis, thalassemia), **necrotizing arteriolitis**, fava bean sensitivity, **cystitis**, deficiency – (G6PD d., pyruvate kinase d.), gas gangrene, **acute**/chronic **glomerulonephritis**, hemoglobinuria – (**paroxysmal cold h.**, march h., **paroxysmal nocturnal h.**), **hematuria**, hemochromatosis, **hemolysis**, hemodialysis, malignant hypertension, **cardiac valve prostheses**, **infectious diseases**, **kidney infarction**, infusions, **transfusion incompatibility**, poisoning by – (arsenic, snake venom, copper, naphthalene), **renal calculi**, **disseminated intravascular coagulation**, menstrual blood, **malaria**, myoglobinuria, **tumors**, lupus nephritis, poisonous snake/spider bites, polyarteritis, **burns**, **transurethral prostatectomy**, **pyelonephritis**, puerperium, purpura – (**Henoch–Schönlein p.**, thrombotic thrombocytopenic p.), **hemolytic transfusion reaction**, severe aortic regurgitation, salmonellosis, syndrome – (Goodpasture's sy, **hemolytic-uremic sy**), scarlatina, **urethritis**, pregnancy, **hemolyzed blood transfusion**, **typhoid fever**, **urinary tract trauma**, tuberculosis, **physical exercise**
> **Interfering Factors:** medicaments – (acetaminophen, acetylsalicylic acid, aciclovir, aminoglycosides, aminosalicylic acid, amoxicillin, amphotericin B, anticoagulants, bacitracin, capreomycin, captopril, carmustine, cephalosporins, ciprofloxacin, cisplatin, cyclophosphamide, cyclosporine, erythromycin, fenoprofen, gold salts, hydralazine, levodopa, lithium, mebendazole, methotrexate, methoxyflurane, meticillin, neomycin, oxacillin, penicillamine, penicillin, pentamidine, phenacetin, phenazone, plicamycin, polymyxin B, primaquin, probenecid, quinine, rifampin, salicylates, streptozocin, sulfonamides, suprofen, tetracyclines, thiazides, vancomycin, viomycin, vitamin C)

False positive hemoglobinuria
oxidizing agents, peroxide

False negative hemoglobinuria
formaldehyde, ascorbic acid

Hemosiderin

Hemosiderin in the urine indicates a recent or chronic free hemoglobin release into the circulating plasma and hemopexin or haptoglobin depletion. Hemosiderin is usually attributable to intravascular hemolysis. Hemoglobin in glomerular filtrate is reabsorbed by renal tubular cells and broken down to hemosiderin. Hemosiderin stained urine sediment is a screening test for increased iron excretion.
Test Purpose. 1) to aid in hemochromatosis, hemolytic anemia and nephrotic syndrome diagnosis, 2) to help in diagnosis of possible chronic intravascular hemolysis.

Increased Values – hemosiderinuria
anemia – (**hemolytic a.**, chronic hemolytic a., sickle-cell a., severe megaloblastic a., **microangiopathic hemolytic a.**, pernicious a., thalassemia major), Clostridial exotoxemia, hemoglobinuria – (paroxysmal cold h., **paroxysmal nocturnal h.**), **hemochromatosis**, hemolysis – (due to body burns, heart valve h.), cold hemagglutinin disease, excessive intake of iron – (**dietary, injections**), hemolytic transfusion reactions, multiple blood transfusions

Hexosaminidase

Increased Values
stroke, rheumatoid arthritis, aortocoronary bypass, diabetes mellitus, active phase of acute tubular necrosis, acute glomerulonephritis, glomerulopathies, hypertension, diseases – (degenerative joint d., chronic liver d., urinary tract infectious d.), myocardial infarction, heavy metal poisoning, analgesic nephropathy, plasmocytoma (incl. multiple myeloma), burns, renal injury due to hypotension/anoxia, chronic pyelonephritis, acute renal transplant rejection, after surgery conditions, renal artery stenosis in hypertensives, syndrome – (Goodpasture's sy, nephrotic sy), thrombosis of donor renal artery/vein as a result of ischemia/nephrotoxicity, carotid thrombosis
    Interfering Factors: medicaments – (amphotericin, aminoglycosides, cisplatin, immunosuppressives)

Histamine

Test is used to measure histamine that was released in vivo prior to collection of the specimen and to evaluate possible systemic mastocytosis.

Increased Values
systemic mastocytosis

Histidine

Increased Values – histidinuria
generalized aminoaciduria, histidinemia, Hartnup disease, pregnancy

Homocysteine

Increased Values – homocysteinuria
generalized aminoaciduria, homocystinuria

Homogentisic Acid

Test Purpose. Test is used for diagnosis of alkaptonuria.

Increased Values
alkaptonuria
   Interfering Factors: medicaments – (aminosalicylic acid, levodopa, phenothiazines, salicylates)

Homovanilic Acid

(HVA, syn: homovanilate) Homovanilic acid is a major terminal metabolite of the dopamine pathway; dopamine is a precursor to epinephrine and norepinephrine. Synthesized primarily in the brain, the liver breaks down most dopamine to HVA for excretion.
Test Purpose. 1) to aid in neuroblastoma and ganglioneuroma diagnosis, 2) to help to rule out pheochromocytoma.

Increased Values
pheochromocytoma, **ganglioblastoma**, ganglioneuroblastoma, **neuroblastoma**, excessive physical exercise, emotional stress
   Interfering Factors: medicaments – (acetylsalicylic acid, disulfiram, levodopa, MAO inhibitors, methocarbamol, pyridoxine, reserpine)

Analyte	Age/Gender	Reference Range	SI Units	Note
Homovanilic Acid	0–1 y	<20	*	*mmol/mol
	2–4 y	<14	*	creatinine
	5–19 y	<8	*	
	Adults	<8	*	
		<45	µmol/d	

Human Chorionic Gonadotropin

(hCG, syn: beta-hCG, beta-human chorionic gonadotropin, human choriongonadotropin) Placental trophoblast hormone. The test becomes positive 6–10 days following ovulation, if pregnancy occurs. The normal doubling time for the hormone in early pregnancy is 36 hours. Low levels for gestational age and/or a low rate of increase may indicate threatened abortion or ectopic pregnancy.

Test Purpose. 1) to detect and confirm pregnancy, including ectopic, 2) to aid in diagnosis and treatment monitoring of hydatidiform mole or trophoblast tumor diagnosis, 3) to help in diagnosis of threatened abortion, or ectopic pregnancy.

Increased Values

erythroblastosis fetalis, tumors – (colon t., embryonic t., **melanoma, pancreas t., liver t., plasmocytoma** – incl. multiple myeloma, **lung t., mammary gland t., seminoma, teratoma, teratoid testes t., ovary t., teratoid ovary t., stomach t.**), placental tumours – (**mola hydatidosa, choriocarcinoma, chorioepithelioma**), **pregnancy, multiple pregnancy**
> Interfering Factors: hematuria, proteinuria, bacteriuria, medicaments – (anticonvulsants, antiparkinsons, chlorpromazine, chlorprothixene, fluphenazine, hypnotics, methadone, phenothiazines, promethazine, tranquillisers)

Decreased Values – false negative

abortus imminens (threatened abortion), fetal death, **graviditas extrauterina** (ectopic pregnancy)
> Interfering Factors: medicaments – (carbamazepine, promethazine)

5-Hydroxyindoleacetic Acid

(5-HIAA, syn: indoleacetic acid) A denatured serotonin product (metabolite) vasoconstricting hormone produced by the gastrointestinal tract argentaffin cells. Regulates smooth muscle contraction and peristalsis. Highest values are in winter and 50% lower are in summer.

Test Purpose. To aid in carcinoid tumors diagnosis.

Increased Values

severe pain – (sciatica, spasms of smooth/skeletal muscle), cystic fibrosis, smoking, hemorrhage, malabsorption, **Whipple's disease**, tumours – (**oat cell t. of bronchus, carcinoid**, t. of larynx, t. of thyroid, t. of gastrointestinal tract), sprue – (**non-tropical s., tropical s.**), pregnancy, thrombosis
> Interfering Factors: pineapple, avocado, bananas, mushrooms, kiwi, coffee, tomatoes, plums, walnuts – they contain serotonin, medicaments – (acetamide, acetanilid, atenolol, fluorouracil, guaiphenesin, melphalan, methocarbamol, pindolol, phenacetin, phenothiazines, reserpine)

Decreased Values

depressive illnesses, phenylketonuria, Hartnup disease, malabsorption, mastocytosis, small intestine resection, Down sy
> Interfering Factors: medicaments – (ACTH, chlorpromazine, ethylalcohol, heparin, imipramine, isoniazid, levodopa, MAO inhibitors, methenamine, methyldopa, promethazine, ranitidine, salicylates, tricyclic antidepressants)

Analyte	Age/Gender	Reference Range	SI Units	Note
5-Hydroxyindole-acetic Acid		3–47	µmol/d	

4-Hydroxy-3-Methoxymandelic Acid

(HMMA, syn: 4-hydroxy-3-methoxymandelate)
Test Purpose. 1) to investigate hypertension, particularly paroxysmal hypertension and hypertension in young adults, 2) investigation of suspected neuroblastoma or related tumors.

Increased Values
pheochromocytoma, neuroblastoma, severe stress conditions, heart failure

Hydroxyproline

(total hydroxyproline) Amino acid. Hydroxyproline constitutes about 10–13% of the collagen molecule; more than 50% of collagen is in bones. Urinary hydroxyproline excretion is a useful measure of total collagen turnover. There is diurnal hydroxyproline excretion rhythm with greater excretion overnight. Hydroxyproline excretion reflects bone resorption. If the urine sampling is correct, the hydroxyproline determination has a higher sensitivity than in serum determination.
Test Purpose. 1) diagnosis and evaluation of primary hyperparathyroidism, 2) evaluation of bone metabolism in osteoporosis, 3) evaluation of bone metabolism in dialyzed patients, 4) evaluation of clinical bone metastases course, 5) evaluation of clinical acromegalia course and therapy control.

Increased Values
growth spurt, **acromegaly, hereditary hydroxyprolinemia, hyperparathyroidism**, hyperthyroidism, **Paget's disease**, myeloma, **bone tumours**, metastatic bone tumors, orchiectomy, bone diseases, osteomalacia, acute osteomyelitis, osteoporosis, psoriasis, severe burns, rickets, sarcoidosis, syndrome – (Klinefelter's sy, Marfan's sy), pregnancy (3rd trimester), extensive fractures
    Interfering Factors: high protein diet, bed rest, postpartum, medicaments – (glucocorticoids, growth hormone, parathyroid hormone, phenobarbital, sulfonylurea, thyroxine, vitamin D)

Decreased Values
muscular dystrophy, hypoparathyroidism, hypopituitarism, hypothyroidism, malnutrition
    Interfering Factors: medicaments – (acetylsalicylic acid, antineoplastics, ascorbic acid, estradiol, estriol, calcitonin, calcium gluconate, corticosteroids, glucocorticoids, mithramycin, propranolol, salicylates)

Analyte	Age/Gender	Reference Range	SI Units	Note
Hydroxyproline				
total		362–458	µmol/d	
free		36–190	*	*µmol/d x BSA

Hydroxyproline, free

Amino acid. Hydroxyproline urinary excretion reflects bone resorption and collagen metabolism. Collagen has a very high hydroxyproline content.

Test Purpose. 1) to monitor treatment for disorders characterized by bone resorption, including Paget's disease, metastatic bone tumors and certain endocrine disorders, 2) to aid in bone resorption disorders diagnosis.

Increased Values
growth spurt in childhood, acromegaly, **hereditary hydroxyprolinemia**, hyperparathyroidism – (primary h., secondary h.), malignant tumors metastases into bone, **Paget's disease**, bone tumours, osteomalacia, **osteoporosis**, plasmocytoma, prolonged bed-rest, rickets, syndrome – (Klinefelter's sy, Marfan's sy), **pregnancy**

Immunoglobulin A

Increased Values
IgA nephropathy, severe nephrotic sy

Interleukin 6

Increased Values
graft-versus-host disease

Iron

Test Purpose. To assess response to iron chelation therapy.

Increased Values
iron overload

Analyte	Age/Gender	Reference Range	SI Units	Note
Iron		<1.8	µmol/d	

Isoleucine

Increased Values
generalized aminoaciduria, maple syrup urine disease, Hartnup disease, hepatic failure

17-Ketogenic Steroids

(17-KGS) 17-KGS are composed of four groups of compounds: group 1 includes cortisol and cortisone, group 2 includes cortisols and cortolones, 3 includes pregnanetriol and derivatives and group 4 includes 17-OH progesterone and 17-OH pregnenolone.

Test Purpose. 1) to evaluate adrenocortical function, 2) to aid in Cushing's syndrome and Addison's disease diagnosis.

Increased Values
smoking, **hyperadrenalism**, infections, **adrenal tumors**, obesity, surgery, burns, **severe stress**, syndrome – (**adrenogenital sy, adrenocortical sy, Cushing's sy**), pregnancy
   Interfering Factors: medicaments – (ampicillin, cephalotin, digitoxin, glucocorticoids, meprobamate, penicillin, phenothiazines, spironolactone)

Decreased Values
hypopituitarism, **cretinism, Addison's disease**, malnutrition, **panhypopituitarism**
   Interfering Factors: medicaments – (ACTH, ampicillin, dexamethasone, estrogens, glucose, hydrocortisone, oral contraceptives, phenytoin, prednisone, prednisolone)

Analyte	Age/Gender	Reference Range	SI Units	Note
17-Ketogenic Steroids	F <55 y	10–52	µmol/d	
	M <60 y	17–80	µmol/d	

Alpha-Ketoglutaric Acid

Increased Values
renal diseases, exertion – (physical e., psychic e.)

Ketones

(syn: ketones, ketone bodies, ketobodies, ketone body) Catabolic products. The purpose of catabolism is to provide an energy source when glucose cannot be transferred to cells because of insulin insufficiency. Abnormal metabolites (end-product of fatty-acid breakdown in liver) found in urine as a result of ketoacidosis are beta-hydroxybutyric acid, acetoacetic acid and acetone. Urine ketones are unstable – chilling the specimen is best if there must be a delay before ketone testing. Positive results may be interpreted as small, moderate or large ketonuria.

Test Purpose. 1) to screen and evaluate ketonuria, 2) to detect ketoacidosis, to identify diabetes mellitus that is out of control, 3) to identify carbohydrate deprivation, 4) to monitor diabetes mellitus, low-carbohydrate diets and treatment of uncontrolled diabetes mellitus.

Positive Values – ketonuria
diabetic ketoacidosis, primary lactic acidosis, acromegaly, **alcoholism**, anemia (severe), **anesthesia, anorexia, dehydration, uncontrolled diabetes mellitus**, diet – (carbohydrate free d., **weight reduction d.**), hypoglycemic encephalopathy, **glycogenoses**, renal glycosuria, **starvation, diarrhea**, hyperinsulinism, PIH (pregnancy induced hypertension), **hyperthermia, hyperthyroidism**, intoxication by – (acetone, ethanol, methanol), **ketoacidosis**, lactation, **diabetic coma, increased lipid metabolization**, catecholamine excess, **fasting**, decreased carbohydrate intake, inborn error of amino acid metabolism, increased intake of – (proteins, **fat**), **febrile states**, Mauriac syndrome, typhoid fever, pregnancy, trauma, **acetonemic vomiting**

Interfering Factors: medicaments – (acetylcholine, acetylcysteine, acetylsalicylic acid, ACTH, bromsulfophthalein, captopril, cysteine, dimercaprol, ether, glucocorticoids, growth hormone, inositol, insulin, isoniazid, isopropanol, levodopa, metformin, methionine, nicotinic acid, paraldehyde, penicillamine, phenazopyridine, phenformin, phenolsulfophthalein, pyridium, salicylates, valproic acid)

Analyte	Age/Gender	Reference Range	SI Units	Note
Ketobodies (as OH-butyrate)		<50	mg/l	

17-Ketosteroids + 17-Hydroxycorticosteroids

(17-KS, 17-OHCS, syn: 17-hydroxysteroids) 17-KS – adrenal medulla hormones and testicular androgens precursors and metabolites (dehydroepiandrosterone, DHEAS, androsterone, androstenedione, etiocholanolone). In men, approximately 1/3 of hormone metabolites come from the testes and 2/3 from the adrenal cortex; in women and children all the excreted hormones (androgens) are derived from the adrenal cortex. 17-OHCS are adrenal steroids metabolites (cortisol, 11-deoxycortisol). 17-KS levels are highest in AM and lowest at night.

Test Purpose. 1) to assess adrenocortical function, 2) to aid in adrenal and gonadal dysfunction diagnosis, 3) to aid in adrenogenital sy diagnosis, 4) to monitor cortisol therapy in adrenogenital sy treatment.

Increased Values 17-KS

adrenal adenoma, premature infants, diabetes mellitus, **hyperpituitarism, congenital adrenal hyperplasia** (virilizing forms), diseases – (chronic d., **severe infectious d.**), Cushing's disease, non-malignant virilizing adrenal tumours, tumours – (**androgenic arrhenoblastoma, t. of adrenals, t. from testicular interstitial cells, t. from ovarian luteal cells**), **obesity,** ectopic ACTH-producing tumors, **female pseudohermaphroditism,** syndrome – (**adrenogenital sy, Cushing's sy, Stein–Leventhal sy**), **pregnancy**

> **Interfering Factors:** exercise, stress, medicaments – (ACTH, ampicillin, androgens, antibiotics, cephalotin, chloramphenicol, chlorpromazine, danazol, dexamethasone, erythromycin, gonadotropins, meprobamate, penicillin, phenothiazines, quinidine, secobarbital, spironolactone, testosterone)

Decreased Values 17-KS

rheumatoid arthritis, liver cirrhosis, **gout,** eunuchoidism, smoking, infectious hepatitis (early), adrenal hypofunction, gonadal hypofunction, secondary female hypogonadism (pituitary), **hypopituitarism, hypothyroidism,** chronic diseases, cachexia, **men castration,** cretinism, **Addison's disease, myxedema, nephrosis, ovarectomy, panhypopituitarism,** Klinefelter's sy, **thyrotoxicosis,** women after menopause

> **Interfering Factors:** medicaments – (ACTH, anabolic steroids, androgens, carbamazepine, corticosteroids, dexamethasone, estrogens, morphine, opiates, oral contraceptives, phenothiazines, phenytoin, probenecid, promazine, propoxyphene, pyrazinamide, reserpine, salicylates, thiazide diuretics, tiaprofenic acid)

Increased Values 17-OHCS

acromegaly, eclampsia, **severe hypertension,** hyperthyroidism, acute diseases, **Cushing's disease, tumours,** obesity, acute pancreatitis, syndrome – (**ectopic ACTH sy,** Cushing's sy), pregnancy, **thyrotoxicosis,** virilism

Interfering Factors: physical stress, medicaments – (acetazolamide, cephalotin, cefoxitin, chloral hydrate, chlordiazepoxide, chlorpromazine, colchicine, diethylstilbestrol, digitalis, erythromycin, estrogens, fructose, glucocorticoids, glutethimide, hydrocortisone, iodides, meprobamate, methenamine, methicillin, oleandomycin, paraldehyde, phenothiazines, quinidine, quinine, reserpine, spironolactone)

Decreased Values 17-OHCS
surgical adrenal removal without appropriate steroid replacement, hypopituitarism, hypothyroidism, adrenal infarction, Addison's disease, myxedema, adrenal suppression after prolonged exogenic steroid ingestion, adrenogenital sy

Interfering Factors: medicaments – (barbiturates, dexamethasone, estrogens, chlorpromazine, carbamazepine, corticosteroids, meperidine, morphine, narcotic analgesics, oral contraceptives, pentazocine, phenothiazines, phenytoin, prednisone, promethazine, propoxyphene, reserpine)

Analyte	Age/Gender	Reference Range	SI Units	Note
17-Hydroxycorti-costeroids		0.9–2.5	*	*mmol/mol creatinine
	F	9.5–28	µmol/d	
	M	12–35	µmol/d	
17-Ketosteroids	F <55 y	21–44	µmol/d	
	M <60 y	28–55	µmol/d	

Lactate Dehydrogenase

Increased Values
diseases – (renal d., inflammatory d.), acute glomerulonephritis, **systemic lupus erythematosus, urogenital tract tumours,** nephritis, nephrosclerosis – (**diabetic n.,** malignant n.), renal infarction, nephrotic syndrome, acute myocardial infarction, acute tubular necrosis, acute pyelonephritis, cystitis

Interfering Factors: retrograde pyelography, medicaments – (acetylsalicylic acid, cephalosporins, cytostatics, gentamicin, neomycin, phenylbutazone)

Lactose

Increased Values
hiatal hernia, diarrhea, lactation, **congenital lactosuria, high milk intake,** neonatal sepsis, steatorrhea, pregnancy

Lead

Urinary lead excretion indicates excessive lead exposure, regardless of clinical presentation. Urine lead determination is valuable in determining the efficacy of chelation therapy. Urine lead levels are not recommended for monitoring exposure as, at these low concentrations, results are highly variable even when corrected for creatinine concentration.

Increased Values
lead intoxication/exposure

Analyte	Age/Gender	Reference Range	SI Units	Note
Lead		<0.39	μmol/d	

Leucine

Increased Values
generalized aminoaciduria, maple syrup urine disease, Hartnup disease, severe burns, pregnancy (1st trimester)

Leucine Aminopeptidase

Increased Values
chronic alcohol abuse, disordered glomerular filtration, renal hypoxia, acute inflammatory renal diseases, tumour lysis, urogenital tract tumours, toxic renal lesions, **hepatic cirrhosis**, hepatitis – (**acute h.**, **chronic active h.**), gallstones, **cholestasis**, **obstructive hepatobiliary diseases**, acute alcohol intoxication, hepatic ischemia, tumors of – (**pancreas**, **liver**), pancreatitis, severe preeclampsia
   Interfering Factors: medicaments – (kanamycin, streptomycin, sulfonamides)

Leukocyte Esterase

(syn: WBC esterase) Screening test used to detect leukocytes (whole cells or as lysed cells) in the urine. A negative leukocyte esterase test means that an infection is unlikely and that, without additional evidence of urinary tract infection, microscopic exam and/or urine culture need to be done to rule out significant bacteriuria.

Increased Values – positive
urinary tract infectious diseases, false positive results– (specimens contamined with vaginal secretions)

Leukocytes

Pyuria refers to the presence of abnormal numbers of WBC's in urine. Usually, the WBC's are granulocytes. White cells from the vagina or the external urethral meatus in men and women may contaminate the urine.

Increased Values – positive, leukocyturia
cystitis, glomerulonephritis, **infectious diseases of urinary tract**, **collagenoses**, tumors – (**bladder t.**, **kidney t.**, **prostate t.**, leukemia), nephritis – (**interstitial n.**, **lupus n.**), analgetic nephropathy, burns, **pyelonephritis**, **vesicoureteral reflux**, **lues**, renal tuberculosis, urethral trauma caused by – (cystoscopy, catheterization, intercourse), urolithiasis
   Interfering Factors: medicaments – (acetylsalicylic acid, allopurinol, ampicillin, capreomycin, heroin, isotretinoin, kanamycin, levodopa, methicillin, phenazone)

Light Chains

Increased Values
increased immunoglobulin catabolism, nephrotoxic agents, systemic lupus erythematosus, renal tubular disorders

Analyte	Age/Gender	Reference Range	SI Units	Note
Light Chains kappa and lambda		<10	mg/l	

Lipids

Increased Values – positive (lipiduria)
fat embolism, polycystic kidney disease, severe diabetes mellitus, severe eclampsia, intoxication by – (ethylene glycol, mercury, phosphorus, carbon monoxide), extensive trauma with bone fractures, acute/chronic interstitial nephritis, renal tubular necrosis, **nephrotic sy**

Lysine

Increased Values – lysinuria
dibasic aminoaciduria, cystinurias, hyperlysinemia, burns, pregnancy (1st trimester)

Lysozyme

Granulocytes and monocytes degradation product.
Test Purpose. 1) to aid in diagnosis of acute monocytic or granulocytic leukemia and to monitor the disease progression, 2) to evaluate proximal tubular function and diagnose renal impairment, 3) to detect rejection or infarction in kidney transplantation.

Increased Values
regional enteritis, diseases – (**chronic infectious d.**, renal d.), infarction of kidney, leukemia – (**monocytic l.**, **chronic myeloid l.**, **acute myelomonocytic l.**), nephrosis, **polycythemia vera**, burns, renal tubules lesions, acute pyelonephritis, **renal homograft rejection**, sarcoidosis, nephrotic sy, **kidney tuberculosis**

Decreased Values
bone marrow hypoplasia, lymphocytic leukemia

Analyte	Age/Gender	Reference Range	SI Units	Note
Lysozyme		<0.3	mg/l	

Magnesium

Test Purpose. 1) to rule out magnesium deficiency when there are central nervous system irritation symptoms, 2) to detect excessive urinary magnesium excretion, 3) to help evaluate renal disease glomerular function.

aldosterone, chronic alcoholism, chronic renal diseases, Addison's disease, **Bartter's sy**
   Interfering Factors: medicaments – (aldosterone, ammonium chloride, amphotericin B, caffeine, cisplatin, corticosteroids, cyclosporine, dextrose, diuretics, ethacrynic acid, ethanol, furosemide, gentamicin, lithium, magnesium antacids, mannitol, platinum, thiazides, urea)

Decreased Values – hypomagnesiuria
diabetic acidosis, primary aldosteronism, **magnesium deficiency**, dehydration, **acute/chronic diarrhea**, renal diseases, malabsorption, pancreatitis, **decreased magnesium intake, advanced renal failure**
   Interfering Factors: medicaments – (clopamide, nifedipine, oral contraceptives)

Analyte	Age/Gender	Reference Range	SI Units	Note
Magnesium		2.5–8.5	mmol/d	
		0.70–1.05	mmol/l	
		0.93–0.98	*	*tubular resorption
		0.02–0.07	**	**fraction excretion

Manganese

Test Purpose. 1) to confirm manganese exposure/toxicity/poisoning by documenting excess urine excretion, 2) to individualize manganese dosage in long-term parenteral nutrition.

Increased Values
chronic manganese poisoning (professional, occupational – industrial exposure), mineral supplements

Melanogens

Melanogens (colorless) are oxidized to melanin if the urine is exposed to air for several hours. Urine becomes brown through black.

Increased Values – melanogenuria
malignant melanoma, Addison's disease, hemochromatosis

Mercury

Increased Values
industrial exposure, mercury poisoning, excessive therapeutic intake

Metanephrines

Epinephrine and norepinephrine immediate metabolites.

pheochromocytoma, malignant tumors metastases, **neuroblastoma**, sepsis, **severe stress**, shock

Interfering Factors: medicaments – (amphetamines, antihypertensive drugs, caffeine, chlorpromazine, dopamine, hydrazines, levodopa, MAO inhibitors, phenothiazines, prochlorperazine)

Decreased Values
Interfering Factors: medicaments – (levodopa)

Methionine

Increased Values – hypermethioninuria
cystinuria, methionine adenosyltransferase deficiency, homocystinuria, methionine malabsorption sy, tyrosinosis

Decreased Values – hypomethioninuria

severe burns

3-Methylhistidine

Increased Values
multiple trauma, severe burns

Decreased Values

malnutrition

Methylmalonic Acid

Increased Values
congenital methylmalonic aciduria, pernicious anemia, vitamin B_{12} deficiency

Analyte	Age/Gender	Reference Range	SI Units	Note
Methylmalonic Acid	6–12 w	0–55	*	*mmol/mol creatinine

Alpha-1-Microglobulin

Test Purpose. To aid in the diagnosis of renal tubular damage.

Increased Values
diabetic nephropathy, heavy metal exposure, renal tubular damage, nephritis, nephrotoxic medications, urinary tract infectious diseases

Analyte	Age/Gender	Reference Range	SI Units	Note
Alpha-1-Microglobulin		<12	mg/l	
		<20	mg/d	
	<40 y	<20	*	*g/mol creatinine
	>40 y	<2.2	*	

Beta-2-Microglobulin

Test Purpose. The investigation of renal tubulointerstitial disorders and degree of tubular dysfunction.

Increased Values

tubulointerstitial disorders, pyelonephritis, poisoning by – (mercury, cadmium), hepatitis, sarcoidosis, Fanconi's syndrome, tumors, Wilson's disease, renal allograft rejection, nephrocalcinosis, cystinosis, Crohn's disease, vasculitis
> **Interfering Factors:** medicaments – (aminoglycosides, cefalotin, cisplatin, gentamicin, lithium, nifedipine, tobramycin)

Analyte	Age/Gender	Reference Range	SI Units	Note
Beta-2-Microglobulin		<0.30	mg/l	
		0.5–2.0	µl/s*	*clearance

Myoglobin

Oxygen-binding protein of the striated muscle. Indicates recent necrosis of skeletal or cardiac muscle. In acute myocardial infarction myoglobin occur within 1-2 hours, test has 100% sensitivity, but is less specific than CK-MB elevation.
Test Purpose. 1) to aid in muscular disease diagnosis, 2) to detect extensive muscle tissue infarction, 3) to assess muscular damage extent from crushing trauma, 4) to aid in suspected rhabdomyolysis diagnosis, 5) to differentiate myoglobinuria from hemoglobinuria in patients with coloured urine.

Increased Values – myoglobinuria

phosphorylase deficiency (McArdle's disease), alcoholism, **dermatomyositis, march hemoglobinuria with myoglobinuria**, malignant hypertension, **hyperthermia**, hypophosphatemia, hypokalemia, hypomagnesemia, diseases – (acute/chronic muscular d., **progressive muscular d.**), infectious diseases – (coxsackie, Epstein-Barr virus, herpes simplex, influenza A), **myocardial infarction**, intoxication by – (benzene, **CO**, ethanol, hexachloride, **snake venom**, copper, nicotine, opiates, strychnine, toluene, zinc), **diabetic ketoacidosis**, systemic lupus erythematosus, **hereditary paroxysmal myoglobinuria, arterial occlusion**, decreased muscle oxygenation, **alcoholic polymyopathy, polymyositis, burns**, injuries – (**crush i., muscle i.**), conditions – (septic c., convulsive c., seizure c.), decreased/**increased** muscle energy consumption, **status epilepticus, febrile conditions, electrical shock**, toxins, trichinosis, thromboembolism, heat stroke, **strenuous/prolonged exercise**
> **Interfering Factors:** alcoholism, methadone, heroin, cocaine, medicaments – (aminocaproic acid, amphetamines, amphotericin B, barbiturates, diazepam, ethanol, halothane, hypnotics, isopropanol, opiates, phencyclidine, sedatives, strychnine, succinylcholine, tricyclic antidepressants)

Analyte	Age/Gender	Reference Range	SI Units	Note
Myoglobin		<0.3	mg/l	

Natrium

Natrium is a primary regulator of water excretion and acid-base balance maintenance – in combination with chloride and bicarbonate. Natrium helps maintain electrolyte balance in intra/extracellular fluids in combination with potassium. Important in nerve conduction and irritability of muscles, nerves and the heart.

Test Purpose. 1) to help evaluate fluid/electrolyte balance, 2) to monitor the effects of a low-salt diet, 3) to help evaluate renal and adrenal disorders, 4) to work up volume depletion.

Increased Values – hypernatriuria
alkalosis, **dehydration, diabetes mellitus**, glycosuria, **starvation**, PIH, **hypoaldosteronism, hypothyroidism, adrenal cortex insufficiency, salicylate intoxication, ketoacidosis**, salt losing nephritis, syndrome – (**SIADH**, Schwartz–Bartter sy), failure – (**adrenal cortex f., chronic renal f.**)

> **Interfering Factors:** increased salt intake, medicaments – (antibiotics, antitussives, caffeine, calcium gluconate, captopril, chlorothiazide diuretics, cisplatin, cyclophosphamide, diltiazem, dopamine, ethacrynic acid, furosemide, laxatives, lithium, nifedipine, steroids, thiazides, triamterene)

Decreased Values – hyponatriuria
aldosteronism, hypochloremic metabolic alkalosis, hepatic cirrhosis, **pulmonary emphysema, diarrhea**, diseases of liver, nephritis, pyloric obstruction, pancreatitis, **diaphoresis**, after surgery conditions, prolonged gastric suctioning, stress, syndrome – (**Cushing's sy, malabsorption sy, nephrotic sy**), **vomiting**, failure – (**acute renal f., congestive heart f.**)

> **Interfering Factors:** decreased salt intake, medicaments – (clopamide, diuretics, naproxen, ramipril, steroids)

Analyte	Age/Gender	Reference Range	SI Units	Note
Natrium		30–300	mmol/dU	

Neopterin

Neopterin is a pteridine derivative, a pyrazinopyrinidine compound. It is produced by macrophages after induction by interferon gamma and serves as a marker of cellular immune system activation.

Test Purpose. To assess prognosis of HIV infection.

Increased Values – positive
HIV infection, rheumatoid arthritis, systemic lupus erythematosus, viral infectious diseases, **tumors**, tetrahydrobiopterin biosynthesis disorders, graft rejection, viral infection in transplant patients, conditions with impaired – (cellular immunity, renal function), autoimmune diseases

Analyte	Age/Gender	Reference Range	SI Units	Note
Neopterin	<25 y F	<208	nmol/l	
	<25 y M	<195	nmol/l	

Analyte	Age/Gender	Reference Range	SI Units	Note
	26–35 y F	<240	nmol/l	
	26–35 y M	<182	nmol/l	
	36–55 y F	<229	nmol/l	
	36–55 y M	<197	nmol/l	
	55–65 y F	<250	nmol/l	
	55–65 y M	<218	nmol/l	
	>65 y F	<250	nmol/l	
	>65 y M	<230	nmol/l	

Nickel

(Ni) Serum and urine levels are useful indices of chronic environmental exposure and industrial exposure.

Increased Values
industrial exposure

Nicotinic Acid

Decreased Values
alcoholism, hepatic cirrhosis, dietary deficiency, diarrhea, **Hartnup disease**, **pellagra**, excessive dietary leucine intake, carcinoid sy
  Interfering Factors: medicaments – (glibenclamide, isoniazid, valproic acid)

Analyte	Age/Gender	Reference Range	SI Units	Note
Nicotinic Acid		2.43–12.17	μmol/d	

Nitrites

Nitrite production from nitrate ions in urine results from the activity of many common bacteria species. Nitrite production depends also on the amount of nitrate available in the urine and bacteria working time since the bladder was last emptied. Thus, while nitrite in a urine specimen implies bacterial infection, it does not indicate the degree of infection; conversely absence of nitrite does not imply absence of bacterial infection.
Test Purpose. 1) to detect potentially significant bacteriuria, 2) to aid in the cystitis diagnosis, pyelonephritis, and urinary tract infection.

Increased Values – positive
cystitis, **urinary system infection**, gross hematuria, pyelonephritis

False Positive Values
bacterial metabolism (if delayed examination), red urine from any cause, dye metabolites

False Negative Values
vegetarian diet, medicaments – (antibiotics, ascorbic acid – high doses)

Nuclear Matrix Protein 22

(NMP 22) Test measures nuclear mitotic apparatus protein in urine, a component of the nuclear matrix. Test is used to aid in the management of patients with transitional cell carcinoma of the urinary tract. Factors, that may affect assay results include use of the wrong stabilizer or unstabilized urine, recent invasive procedures, presence of some benign urinary tract conditions and administration of systemic chemotherapy to patients with malignancy.

Increased Values – positive
transitional cell carcinoma of the urinary tract

Odour

- ■ **acetonic:** diabetes mellitus, starvation, diabetic ketoacidosis, ketonuria
- ■ **ammoniacal:** urinary tract infectious diseases
- ■ **garlic:** food, poisoning by – (arsenic, phosphorus, selenium, toluene) fresh urine in
- ■ **aromatic:** fresh urine in healthy persons
- ■ **brewery, oasthouse:** oasthouse disease, methionine malabsorption
- ■ **flavin:** multivitamins, vitamin B_{12}
- ■ **foetor hepaticus:** hepatic coma
- ■ **putrid:** putrid bacteria
- ■ **maple syrup, burned sugar:** maple syrup urine disease
- ■ **cabbage:** methionine malabsorption, tyrosinemia
- ■ **cat like urine:** carboxylase multideficiency
- ■ **maggi:** isoleucine, leucine, valine, methylmalonic acid
- ■ **almond:** cyanide poisoning
- ■ **sweaty feet:** methylmalonic, propionic, isovaleric, butyric/hexanoic acidemia
- ■ **sulfurous:** cystinuria, homocytinuria
- ■ **unpleasant:** cystitis
- ■ **musty, mousy:** phenylketonuria
- ■ **sweet:** ketosis
- ■ **rotting fish:** trimethylaminuria
- ■ **fishy:** tyrosinemia

Opacity

- ■ **whitish:** alkaline materials – (phosphates), bacteria, emulgated fat, pus, yeast, leucocytes
- ■ **physiologically:** clear or slightly hazy
- ■ **pinkish curdy deposit:** acid materials – (uric acid, oxalates, urates)

Ornithine

Increased Values – ornithinuria
dibasic aminoaciduria, cystinurias

Osmolality

(syn: urine osmolality) Osmolality is the measurement of dissolved particles. Depends on the number of particles in volume solute unit. 12 hrs fluid restriction → osmolality 850 osmol/kg. Osmolality is a better measurement than specific gravity. Osmolality is a measure of renal tubular concentration, depending on the state of hydration. Simultaneous determination of urine and serum osmolalities facilitates interpretation of results. The urine osmolar gap is described as the sum of urinary concentrations of sodium, potassium, bicarbonate, chloride, glucose and urea compared to measured urine osmolality. Determination of the urine osmolal gap is used to characterize metabolic acidosis.

Test Purpose. 1) osmolality is used in precise kidney concentrating ability evaluation, 2) to monitor electrolyte, water balance, and dehydration, 3) to help in diagnosis of renal disease, syndrome of inappropriate ADH secretion, diabetes mellitus, 4) to evaluate glycosuria and proteinuria.

Increased Values – hyperosmolality
acidosis, hepatic cirrhosis, dehydration, glycosuria, **high protein diet, hypernatremia, Addison's disease, postsurgery conditions**, SIADH (syndrome of inappropriate ADH secretion), **shock, congestive heart failure**
   Interfering Factors: medicaments – (anesthetics, carbamazepine, chlorpropamide, cyclophosphamide, metolazone, sodium i.v., vincristine)

Decreased Values – hyposmolality
aldosteronism, acute renal insufficiency, glomerulonephritis, **diabetes insipidus, hypercalcemia, hypokalemia, renal tubular necrosis, primary polydipsia, excessive water drinking, severe pyelonephritis**
   Interfering Factors: muscular exercise, starvation, medicaments – (glucose, lithium, methoxyflurane, tolazamide, urea)

Analyte	Age/Gender	Reference Range	SI Units	Note
Osmolality		>850	*	*mOsm/kg H$_2$O

Oxalates

Oxalates are an oxalic acid salts and end-products of metabolism excreted almost exclusively in the urine.

Test Purpose. 1) to detect primary hyperoxaluria in infants, 2) to rule out renal insufficiency hyperoxaluria.

Increased Values – hyperoxaluria
methoxyflurane anesthesia, **celiac disease, hepatic cirrhosis, vitamin B$_6$ deficiency, diabetes mellitus, primary hyperoxaluria**, diseases – (small bowel d., pancreatic d., **biliary tract d.**), pancreatic insufficiency, **ethylene glycol poisoning, Crohn's disease**, malabsorption, calcium-oxalate nephrolithiasis, excessive intake of vitamin C, **ileal resection, sarcoidosis, jejunoileal shunt** (jejunoileal bypass for morbid obesity), **steatorrhea due to pancreatic insufficiency**, vegetarianism
   Interfering Factors: animal proteins, beets, tea, chocolate, beans, strawberries, cocoa, pepper, tomatoes, rhubarb, spinach, gelatin, medicaments – (ascorbic acid – large doses, calcium, vitamin C)

Decreased Values – hypooxaluria
renal failure
  Interfering Factors: medicaments – (nifedipine, pyridoxine)

Analyte	Age/Gender	Reference Range	SI Units	Note
Oxalates		<4.4	μmol/d	

Para-Aminobenzoic Acid

Increased Values
  Interfering Factors: medicaments – (acetaminophen, benzocaine, furosemide, chloramphenicol, lidocaine, multivitamins, pancreatic enzymes, phenacetin, procaine, procainamide, sulfonamides, thiazide diuretics)

Decreased Values
severe hepatic dysfunction, impaired renal function, malabsorption

Pentoses

Reducing sugars.

Increased Values – pentosuria
allergy, liver cirrhosis, pentosuria – (alimentary p., essential p.), febrile conditions
  Interfering Factors: cherries, grapes, plums, medicaments – (antipyretics, cortisone, morphine, thyroid hormones)

pH

pH expresses exact urine strength as a dilute acid or base solution and measures the urine free hydrogen ion concentration. The glomerular filtrate of blood plasma is usually acidified by renal tubules and collecting ducts from a pH of 7.4 to about 6 in the final urine. The change to the acid side of 7.4 is accomplished in the distal convoluted tubule and the collecting duct. pH indicates renal tubules ability to maintain normal hydrogen ion concentrations in the plasma and extracellular fluid. Kidneys maintain normal acid-base balance primarily through the sodium reabsorption and tubular hydrogen secretion and ammonia in exchange. It should be read immediately after dipping the strip. Estimate alkaline, neutral and acid pH. Mixed food pH is 5–6.5, vegetarian food has a pH >7.0. Uric acid, cystine, and calcium oxalate stones precipitate in acid urine.

Increased Values – basic, alkaline pH
renal tubular acidosis, alkalosis – (**metabolic a., respiratory a.**), **vegetarian diet, respiratory diseases with hyperventilation and respiratory alkalosis, urinary tract infections,** salicylate intoxication, pyloric obstruction, **gastric suction,** postprandial (shortly after meals), excessive alkali ingestion, plant food, Fanconi's sy, **vomiting, chronic renal failure**
  Interfering Factors: citrus fruits, **standing urine with urea-splitting bacteria action, producing ammonia,** medicaments – (acetazolamide, adrenaline, aldosterone, amiloride, amphotericin B, antibiotics, diuretics, kanamycin, neomycin, niacinamide, phenacetin, potassium citrate, sodium bicarbonate, streptomycin)

Decreased Values – acid pH

acidosis – (**diabetic a.**, **metabolic a.**), metabolic alkalosis, alkaptonuria, ascites, dehydration, diabetes mellitus, **pulmonary emphysema**, phenylketonuria, **starvation, diarrhea**, hydrothorax, renal bacterial infectious diseases, **respiratory diseases with CO_2 retention and respiratory acidosis**, renal tubular insufficiency, cachexia, **nephritis**, digestion disorders, **sleep, febrile states**, food intake of – (protein, **meat**), **renal tuberculosis**, vomiting, chronic renal failure, septic conditions

> **Interfering Factors:** medicaments – (ACTH, ammonium chloride, ascorbic acid, diazoxide, methionine, thiazide diuretics)

Phenylalanine

Test Purpose. 1) to help in hyperalaninemia detection, including phenylhydroxylase and tetrahydrobiopterin co-factor deficiency, 2) tyrosyluria as a result of transient tyrosinemia in premature newborns with immature hepatic metabolism, 3) primary test purpose is nutrition adherence monitoring in known cases.

Increased Values – phenylalaninuria

cystinosis, hepatolenticular degeneration, **phenylketonuria**, hyperphenylalaninemia, **Hartnup disease**, pregnancy (1st trimester)

Phosphoethanolamine

(PEA) Highest levels are at night and lowest are in AM.

Increased Values

high-protein diet, **hypertension**, hypophosphatasia, bone disorders

> **Interfering Factors:** medicaments – (ascorbic acid)

Phosphorus

(syn: phosphates) Isolated determination of urine phosphates excretion is insufficient for phosphorus metabolism assessment. Clearance methods are used: a) phosphate clearance (Cp), b) tubular reabsorption percentage (TRP%), c) tubular maximum of phosphate reabsorption (TmP/GFR) or phosphate threshold indicates maximum phosphate concentration in glomerular filtrate; below this concentration all filtrated phosphate is reabsorbed in tubules.

Test Purpose. Phosphate clearance and tubular reabsorption percentage: 1) diagnosis of tubular syndromes with phosphates loss, 2) primary and secondary parathyroid glands disorders. Tubular maximum of phosphate reabsorption is used in tubular reabsorption disorders diagnosis, 3) to evaluate calcium/phosphorus balance.

Increased Values – hyperphosphaturia

acidosis, amyloidosis, cystinosis, **phosphate diabetes, hyperparathyroidism, hyperthyroidism, plasmocytoma** (incl. multiple myeloma), intoxication by – (cadmium, lead), conditions after – (acute tubular necrosis, transplantation), severe hepatic impairment, **glucose intake, rachitis, febrile states**, syndrome – (**Fanconi's sy**, nephrotic sy), Wilson's disease, vitamin D deficiency, renal tubular acidosis, thalassemia, pregnancy

Interfering Factors: medicaments – (acetazolamide, acetylsalicylic acid, alanine, androgens, asparaginase, bicarbonate, calcitonin, cidofovir, corticosteroids, diuretics, estrogens, hydrochlorothiazide, metolazone, phosphates, PTH, tryptophan, valine, vitamin D)

Phosphate Clearance – Increased Values
renal tubular acidosis, phosphate diabetes, primary hyperparathyroidism, secondary hyperparathyroidism in – (vitamin D deficiency, malabsorption)
    Interfering Factors: increased phosphate and NaCl food intake

Decreased Values – hypophosphaturia
alkalosis, narcosis, acute liver dystrophy, **hypoparathyroidism,** hypothyroidism, acute infectious diseases, **renal insufficiency,** diarrhea, vitamin D intoxication, **nephritis, acute/chronic nephrosis, osteomalacia,** rachitis, sarcoidosis, glucose administration, febrile states, **steatorrhea,** milk–alkali sy, pregnancy, vomiting, pseudohypoparathyroidism
    Interfering Factors: medicaments – (alanine, aluminium-containing antacids, mannitol)

Phosphate Clearance – Decreased Values
acromegaly, hypoparathyroidism, renal insufficiency – (acute r. i., chronic r. i.)
    Interfering Factors: lactation, body growth, pregnancy

Tubular Reabsorption Percentage – Decreased Values
renal tubular acidosis, phosphate diabetes, primary hyperparathyroidism

Tubular Maximum of Phosphate Reabsorption – Decreased Values
hyperparathyroidism – (primary h., secondary h.), tubular syndromes

Analyte	Age/Gender	Reference Range	SI Units	Note
Inorganic Phosphorus		11–32	mmol/d	
		0.11–0.45	ml/s *	*clearance
		0.07–0.20	**	**fraction excretion

Porphobilinogen

(syn: PBG) Porphobilinogen production from DALA is realized in all body cells that are able to synthesize a heme. By means of TS-porphobilinogen deaminase → uroporphyrinogen I is produced, and TL-uroporphyrinogen III-cosynthase → uroporphyrinogen III. Porphyrinogens are produced in liver, bone marrow, and kidney cell cytosol.
Test Purpose. 1) to help in diagnosis of acute intermittent porphyria, variegate porphyria, lead poisoning, chronic hepatic porphyria, hereditary coproporphyria, 2) to help in chronic hepatic injury differential diagnosis (alcohol, medicaments, toxins).

Increased Values – hyperporphobilinogenuria
lead and heavy metals poisoning, **hereditary coproporphyria,** tumors, **acute intermittent porphyria, variegate porphyria,** halogenated solvents poisoning
    Interfering Factors: urobilinogen, medicaments – (aminophenazone, barbiturates, carbamazepine, chlorpropamide, danazol, dapsone, diphenylhydantoin, diclofenac, glutethimide, griseofulvin, hydantoins, mephenytoin, meprobamate, methyldopa, oral contraceptives, pentazocine, phenothiazines, phenylbutazone, primidone, pyrazinamide, pyrazolone, sulfonamides, sulfonylureas, tolazamide, tolbutamide, trimethadione, valproic acid)

Interfering Factors: medicaments – (cisplatin, methyldopa)

Analyte	Age/Gender	Reference Range	SI Units	Note
Porphobilinogen		0–8.8	μmol/d	quantitatively
		negat		qualitatively

Porphyrins

Test includes uroporphyrins, coproporphyrins and porpholbilinogens measurement. Porphyrins are cyclic compounds formed from delta-aminolevulinic acid. Proteins used in the hemoglobin heme synthesis. Normally, insignificant amounts are excreted in the urine.
Test Purpose. 1) to aid in congenital or acquired porphyrias diagnosis, 2) acute and chronic lead poisoning, 3) toxic porphyria, porphyrinuria, 4) chronic liver injury with toxins, 5) blood diseases, 6) iron metabolism disorders, 7) tumor diagnosis.

Increased Values – porphyrinuria
anemia, vitamin deficiency, **hepatic cirrhosis**, hemochromatosis, **infectious hepatitis, liver diseases, obstructive icterus,** pancreatic insufficiency, intoxication by – (barbiturates, ethanol, petrol, **heavy metals, acute/chronic lead,** tetrachlormethane), **hereditary coproporphyria,** leukemia, **Hodgkin's disease,** tumours, **pellagra,** porphyria – (**congenital erythropoietic p., p. cutanea tarda, p. variegata, acute intermittent p.**), **central nervous system disorders,** patients on dialysis, pregnancy
Interfering Factors: menstruation, medicaments – (acriflavine, aminophenazone, aminosalicylic acid, barbiturates, carbamazepine, chloral hydrate, chlorpropamide, dapsone, estrogens, ethoxazene, ethylalcohol, glutethimide, griseofulvin, meprobamate, methyldopa, morphine, oral contraceptives, pentazocine, phenazopyridine, phenylbutazone, procaine, pyrazinamide, rifampin, sulfamethoxazole, sulfonamides, sulfonylurea, tetracycline)

Analyte	Age/Gender	Reference Range	SI Units	Note
Porphyrins				
total		<120	nmol/dU	
uroporphyrin		4–29	nmol/dU	
coproporphyrin		20–120	nmol/dU	
carboxyporphyrin				
(penta-, hexa-, hepta-)		<12	nmol/dU	
porphyrin				
(dicarboxy-, tricarboxy-)		<3	nmol/dU	

Potassium

Potassium acts as a part of the body's buffer system and of electrolyte balance maintenance.
Test Purpose. Differential diagnosis of hyper/hypokalemia caused by renal/extrarenal disorders. See also urine chloride.

Increased Values – hyperkaluria

acidosis – (**diabetic a.**, metabolic a., **renal tubular a.**), **primary/secondary aldosteronism, alkalosis, dehydration, diabetes mellitus,** vegane diet, **starvation** (early), diarrhea, adrenal hyperfunction, **renal ischemia,** diabetic coma, **Cushing's disease,** physical exertion, **interstitial nephritis, renal disorders, pyelonephritis,** febrile states, syndrome – (**Bartter's sy,** Cushing's sy, Fanconi's sy, hypercalcemic sy), salicylate intoxication, vomiting, **chronic renal failure**

> **Interfering Factors:** medicaments – (acetazolamide, ACTH, aldosterone, amphotericin B, benzylpenicillin, calcitonin, carbenicillin, carbenoxolone, corticosteroids, deoxycorticosterone, diuretics, dopamine, ethacrynic acid, gentamicin, glucocorticoids, levodopa, nafcillin, penicillin, salicylates, saluretics, streptozocin, sulfanilamide, thiazides, ticarcillin)

Decreased Values – hypokaluria

ascites, dehydration, dialysis, **gastrointestinal drainage, gastrointestinal fistula, glomerulonephritis,** starvation, **diarrhea,** hypokalemia, adrenal cortex insufficiency, **Addison's disease,** oliguric nephropathies, **nephrosclerosis, pyelonephritis, malabsorption sy,** decreased intake of kalium, vomiting, **acute renal failure**

> **Interfering Factors:** medicaments – (alanine, amiloride, anesthetics, clopamide, dextrose, diazoxide, epinephrine, growth hormone, indomethacin, laxatives, levarterenol, potassium sparing diuretics, ramipril)

Analyte	Age/Gender	Reference Range	SI Units	Note
Potassium		35–80	mmol/l	

Pregnanediol

Principal progesterone metabolite, influencing ovarian and placental function. Normally, urine pregnanediol levels reflect variations in progesterone secretion during the menstrual cycle and during pregnancy. In women, increases markedly after ovulation and peaking in midluteal phase. 50% day-to-day levels variation.

Test Purpose. 1) to evaluate placental function in pregnant females, 2) to evaluate ovarian function in nonpregnant females.

Increased Values

ovary arrhenoblastoma, luteal ovary cyst, **hyperadrenocorticism, adrenocortical hyperplasia,** congenital adrenal hyperplasia due to 17-alpha hydroxylase and 11-beta-hydroxylase deficiency, **chorioepithelioma, metastatic ovarian cancer,** diffuse thecal luteinization, luteinized granulosa, theca-cell tumors, biliary tract obstruction, **ovulation,** precocious puberty in girls, **pregnancy**

> **Interfering Factors:** medicaments – (ACTH, ampicillin, gonadotropins)

Decreased Values

menstrual abnormalities, **amenorrhea, anovulation,** essential hypertension in pregnancy, **ovarian hypofunction,** liver diseases, fetal distress, hydatidiform mole, tumors of – (**breast, ovary**), chronic nephritis in pregnancy, **fetal death, threatened abortion, preeclampsia,** failure – (**placental f., ovarian f.**)

> **Interfering Factors:** medicaments – (ampicillin, estrogens, oral contraceptives, phenothiazines, progesterone)

Pregnanetriol

Pregnanetriol is a compound substance reflecting one adrenocortical activity segment. A precursor in adrenal corticoid synthesis, arising from 17-OH progesterone, pregnanetriol is not a ketosteroid, but a ketogenic steroid.

Test Purpose. 1) to aid in adrenogenital sy diagnosis, 2) to monitor cortisol replacement.

Increased Values
physical exercise, 21-hydroxylase deficiency, congenital adrenal enzymopathies, **congenital adrenocortical hyperplasia**, tumors of – (adrenals, ovary), syndrome – (**adrenogenital sy**, Stein–Leventhal sy)

  Interfering Factors: medicaments – (gonadotropin)

Decreased Values
17-alpha-hydroxylase deficiency sy, ovarian failure

Analyte	Age/Gender	Reference Range	SI Units	Note
Pregnanetriol	Children			
	2 w–2 y	0.06–0.6	μmol/d	
	5 y	<1.5	μmol/d	
	15 y	<4.5	μmol/d	
	Adults	<5.9	μmol/d	

Proline

Increased Values – prolinuria
hepatolenticular degeneration, **hyperprolinemia**, iminoglycinurias, **severe prolinuria**, carcinoid sy

Proteins

Proteins in urine – proteinuria (persistent, transient, intermittent). Quantitative analysis – physiological protein urine excretion is <0.3 g a day. Normally, only small plasma proteins filtered at the glomerulus are reabsorbed by the renal tubule. However, a small amount of filtered plasma proteins and protein secreted by the nephron (Tamm–Horsfall protein) can be found in normal urine. Proteinuria (>0.3 g/24 hr.) means protein in urine, which are mainly albumin, but globulins also may be present. Proteinuria >3.5 g/24 hr is severe. Dipstick screening for protein is done on whole urine, but semi-quantitative tests for urine protein should be performed on the supernatant of centrifuged urine since the cells suspended in normal urine can produce a falsely high estimation of protein. Precipitation by heat is a better semi-quantitative method, but overall, it is not a highly sensitive test. The sulfo-salicylic acid test is a more sensitive precipitation test. It can detect albumin, globulins and Bence–Jones protein (immunoglobulin light chains) at low concentrations. Electrophoretic glomerular proteinuria 1) selective: primarily albumin and transferrin (diabetes mellitus, immune complex disease, minimal change disease), 2) nonselective: pattern resembles serum (diabetes mellitus, primary/secondary glomerulonephritis, amyloidosis, collagen diseases). Tubular proteinuria: principally alpha-1, alpha-2, beta and gamma globulins (chronic pyelonephritis, interstitial tubular nephritis, congenital tubular nephropathies, polycystic kidneys, acute tubular necrosis due to ischemia, hypercalcuria). Mixed glomerular-tubular proteinuria: (chronic renal failure, chronic pyelonephritis).

Test Purpose. 1) to aid in pathological conditions diagnosis characterized by proteinuria, mainly in renal disease, 2) Bence Jones protein – to confirm plasmocytoma presence (incl. multiple myeloma) in patients with characteristic clinical signs.

Qualitative analysis

■ **Strip test (dipstick)** – estimate colour blocks – (negative, trace, 1, 2, 3 crosses). Clinical judgement must determine "trace" results significance, particularly in high specific gravity urine. The test area may most closely match "trace" despite only physiological protein concentrations. False positive results are obtained from alkaline and/or highly buffered urine.

■ **Salicylsulfonic acid test** – if the urine is cloudy, filter some for this test. Shake the tube with urine and acid, then look for urine cloudiness which indicates protein.

■ **Protein loss selectivity** – (electrophoresis, immunodiffusion, immunoelectrophoresis) to characterize the immunoglobulins.

Quantitative analysis

■ <2 g/day: renal polycystic degeneration, chronic pyelonephritis
■ >2 g/day: glomerular diseases
■ >5 g/day: nephrotic syndrome

Increased Values – positive proteinuria, extrarenal causes

anemia, primary aldosteronism, hypersensitivity angiitis, rheumatoid arthritis, ascites, babesiosis, cystinosis, acute cystitis, LCAT deficiency, dermatomyositis, diabetes mellitus, hypertensive encephalopathy, fever – (epidemic hemorrhagic f., rheumatic f., typhoid f., yellow f., familial Mediterranean f., Lassa f.), gout, **subacute bacterial endocarditis, galactosemia**, idiopathic monoclonal gammopathy, pulmonary gangrene, Wegener's granulomatosis, hepatitis – (h. type B, peliosis h., chemical induced h.), infantile idiopathic hypercalcemia, hyperlordosis, **benign/malignant hypertension**, benign prostate hypertrophy, hyperthyroidism, disease – (Fabry's d., Gaucher's d., light chain d., heavy chain d., Wilson's d., Whipple's d., legionnaire's d.), diseases – (acute infectious d., **convulsive d.**, bladder d., ureter d., liver d., prostate d., urethra d., heart d.), hereditary fructose intolerance, **cardiac insufficiency**, diabetic ketoacidosis, poisoning by – (phosphorus, arsenic, glycol, carbon disulfide, carbon tetrachloride, heavy metals, sulfosalicylic acid, lead, opiates, mercury, cadmium, trichloroethylene, turpentine), colitis – (ulcerative c., granulomatous c.), leishmaniasis, leptospirosis, **leukemia**, insulin lipodystrophy, systemic lupus erythematosus, lymphoma, Waldenström's macroglobulinemia, **malaria**, hydatidiform mole, infectious mononucleosis, **tumors**, intestinal obstruction, ornithosis, **orthostatic proteinuria** (positive in upright patient – extreme renal vasoconstriction, negative in supine or recumbent patient – clearing with recumbency), oxalosis, acute fatty liver of pregnancy, plasmocytoma (incl. multiple myeloma), constrictive pericarditis, polyarteritis nodosa, **preeclampsia**, pneumonia, purpura – (Henoch–Schönlein p., thrombotic thrombocytopenic p.), rabies, rhabdomyolysis, sarcoidosis, scleroderma, venomous snake bite, scorpion sting, syndrome – (**Goodpasture's sy**, Kimmelstiel–Wilson sy, Kawasaki's sy, Fanconi's sy, hemolytic–uremic sy, sweet's sy, oculo-cerebral-renal sy, HELLP sy, Alport's sy, hypereosinophilic sy), **shock conditions**, heat stroke, syphilis, **toxemia**, tuberculosis, tularemia, trauma, pheochromocytoma, common cold, **cold baths**, extreme cold weather, **febrile states**, psychic conditions – (emotional stress), **pregnancy, strenuous exercise, congestive heart failure**, urethritis, thrombosis of – (inferior vena cava, renal vein)

Interfering Factors: radiographic contrast media, medicaments – (acetaminophen, acetazolamide, acetylsalicylic acid, aldesleukin, amikacin, aminoglycosides, aminosalicylic acid, amphotericin B, ampicillin, antimony compounds, arsenicals, auranofin, aurothioglucose, bacitracin, benzylpenicillin, bismuth salts, bromfenac, capreomycin, captopril, carbutamide, cefaloridine, cephaloridine, cephalosporins, cephalotin, chloral hydrate, chlorpromazine, chlorpropamide, chlortalidone, cidofovir, clofibrate, colchicine, colistin, corticosteroids, cotrimoxazole, cyclosporine, diclofenac, diflunisal, dithiazine, EDTA, enalapril, ethambutol, etodolac, fenoprofen, gemcitabine, gentamicin, gold salts, griseofulvin, hydralazine, hydrocodone, ibuprofen, indomethacin, interferon alfa-2a, interferon alfa-2b, interferon alfa-n1, interferon beta-1b, iodine compounds, isoniazid, isotretinoin, ketoprofen, ketorolac, lithium, meclofenamide, mercurial compounds, methicillin, mitomycin, modafinil, nabumetone, nafcillin, naproxen, neomycin, nephrotoxic medicaments, netilmicin, non-steroidal anti-inflammatory drugs, oxacillin, paracetamol, paromomycin, penicillamine, penicillins, phenacetin, phenazopyridine, phenylbutazone, phenytoin, piroxicam, plicamycin, polymyxin B, prednisone, promazine, rifampicin, rifapentine, salicylates, sodium bicarbonate, streptomycin, streptozocin, sulfamethoxazole, sulfisoxazole, sulfonamides, sulfones, sulindac, sulphizoxazol, suprofen, tetracyclines, tobramycin, tolbutamide, tolmetin sodium, viomycin)

Increased Values – positive proteinuria, renoparenchymatous causes

amyloidosis, acute/chronic glomerulonephritis, glomerulosclerosis – (diabetic g., hypertonic g.), essential hematuria, kidney contusion, kidney infarction, **PIH, tumors of urinary tract,** nephritis – **(interstitial n.,** lupus n., radiation n.), nephropathy – **(diabetic n.,** Balkan n., phenacetin-induced n., hypokalemic n., chronic lead n., IgA n.), **nephrosclerosis, lipoid nephrosis, polycystic kidney, pyelonephritis, renal transplant rejection, nephrotic sy, tubulopathy,** acute tubular necrosis, renal tubular acidosis, medullary cystic disease

Positive Proteinuria – renovascular causes

polyarteritis nodosa, **thrombosis v. renalis,** vasculitis – (allergic v., renal v.), renal artery stenosis

Positive Proteinuria in systemic diseases

amyloidosis, benign monoclonal gammopathy, **collagenosis, systemic lupus erythematosus,** Waldenström's disease, paraproteinemia, **plasmocytoma** (incl. multiple myeloma), sarcoidosis

Bence Jones Protein – paraproteinuria

amyloidosis, rheumatoid arthritis, Wegener's granulomatosis, cold agglutinins disease, liver diseases, **lymphoproliferative disorders, Waldenström's macroglobulinemia, tumour metastases to the bone, plasmocytoma** (incl. multiple myeloma), **plasma cell leukemia, light chain myeloma,** polymyositis, sarcoma, monoclonal gammopathies, connective-tissue disease, renal insufficiency, tumors, cryoglobulinemia, lymphocytic lymphoma, syndrome – (Fanconi's sy, Schnitzler's sy), chronic renal failure, hyperparathyroidism, **IgM heavy chain disease**

Bence Jones Protein – false paraproteinuria

rheumatoid arthritis, systemic lupus erythematosus, scleroderma, polymyositis, chronic renal insufficiency, **lymphomas, chronic lymphocytic leucemia,** metastatic carcinoma of – (lung, gastrointestinal tract, genitourinary tract), medicaments – (aminosalicylic acid, penicillin), radiographic contrast media

Interfering Factors: specimen contamination with – (menstrual blood, prostatic secretions, semen)

False Positive Proteinuria

contamination of the urine – (bacteria, blood, quaternary ammonia compounds), radiocontrast agents, medicaments – (cephalosporins, penicillin, sulfonamide derivatives, tolbutamide), highly alkaline urine, highly concentrated urine

False Negative Proteinuria

very high salt concentration, highly buffered alkaline urine, highly diluted urine

Decreased Values

Interfering Factors: highly alkaline urine, medicaments – (indomethacin, sulindac)

Protein markers use in diagnosis

- ■ **albumin:** mid-molecular substances marker, semiquantitative evidence from 150 mg/l sensitivity. Isolated albumin increase testifies for selective glomerular filtration. It is a typical finding in diabetic and hypertensive nephropathies.

- ■ **albumin + globulin:** markers of mid/high-molecular substances, indicators of nonselective glomerular proteinuria mainly in glomerulonephritides, pre/eclampsia, systemic connective tissue diseases, nephrotic sy.

- ■ **beta-2-microglobulin** (alpha-1-microglobulin resp.): marker of low-molecular substances, it testifies tubulopathies. Total proteinuria less 1.5 g/d. Typical finding mainly in medicament damage (analgesics, antibiotics, cytostatics, tuberculostatics), toxic damage (Pb, Cd), interstitial nephritides, pyelonephritides, acute renal failure, posttransplantation conditions, hypokalemic nephropathies, congenital tubulopathies.

- ■ **albumin + IgG + beta-2-microglobulin:** markers of low/mid/high-molecular substances, it testifies a mixed glomerular-tubular proteinuria. Total proteinuria less 3.5 g/d. Typical finding mainly in advanced glomerulonephritis with renal insufficiency, advanced nephrosclerosis in diabetes mellitus and hypertension, toxic nephrosclerosis and pyelonephritis.

- ■ **alpha-2-macroglobulin + IgG + albumin:** standard set in differential diagnosis of renal/postrenal microhematuria in connection with RBC dysmorphism determination.

Analyte	Age/Gender	Reference Range	SI Units	Note
Proteins		<70	mg/l	
		<80	mg/d	
Albumin (MAU)		<20	mg/l	
		<30	mg/d	*See ref. ranges note
		<2.26	g/mol*	

Pterins

Test Purpose. To help in diagnosis of malignant hyperphenylalaninemia, a rare variant of phenylketonuria. Classical phenylketonuria shows predominance of tetrahydrobiopterin.

Increased Values

malignant hyperphenylalaninemia

PUS

(positive urine pus) Indicates leukocytes in the urine.

Positive Values – pyuria
abscess – (**appendicular a., colon diverticulum a., bladder a., renal a., pelvic a., periappendical a., prostate a., psoas a.**), **balanitis with fimosis, cystitis,** bladder diverticula, glomerulonephritis, collagenoses, leucorrhea, megaureter, tumors of – (**caecum, colon, rectum, uterus**), interstitial nephritis, renal papillary necrosis, **acute/chronic prostatitis, pyelitis, pyelonephritis, pyonephrosis, pyosalpinx,** urinary tract stricture, **foreign body in urinary tract,** trichomoniasis, renal tuberculosis, small intestine ulceration – (dysentery, tuberculosis), urethritis, **urolithiasis, seminal vesiculitis**
> **Interfering Factors:** medicaments – (amikacin, denileukin, gentamicin, neomycin, rifapentine, ropinirole, streptomycin, tobramycin)

Reducing Substances

Normally neither glucose nor galactose are found in the urine. Although glucose is the most common reducing sugar found in urine, sometimes galactose, lactose, fructose, pentose and maltose may be found. If the urine gives a positive reducing sugars result, but a negative glucose result, further investigation may be needed to find the non-glucose reducing substance.
Test Purpose. To help in detection of non-glucose reducing substances that are not detected by specific tests for glucose.
Arabinose, cysteine, formaldehyde, fructose, galactose, isoniazid, ketone bodies, creatinine, ascorbic acid, glucuronic acid, hippuric acid, homogentisic acid, uric acid, oxalic acid, lactose, maltose, ribose, salicylates, sulfanilamide, xylose.

Increased Values
alkaptonuria, cirrhosis hepatis, infants on artificial diets, lactase deficiency, diabetes mellitus, muscular dystrophy, fructosemia, **essential fructosuria, galactosemia,** galactosuria, glomerulonephritis, **glycosuria,** hepatitis, hiatal hernia, hyperglycemia, diarrhea, diseases – (severe infectious d., pituitary d., adrenal d., thyroid d., liver d., CNS d.), hereditary fructose intolerance, lactose intolerance, neonatal icterus, monosaccharide intolerance, intoxication by – (mercury, lead), **lactation,** neonatal sepsis, neonatal gastroenteritis, neonatal hepatitis, phenylketonuria, congenital lactosuria, Wilson's disease, nephrosis, pentosuria, severe hepatic lesions, food, neonatal sepsis, steatorrhea, pregnancy (3rd trimester), Fanconi's syndrome, tyrosinosis
> **Interfering Factors:** rhubarb, medicaments – (ACTH, aminosalicylic acid, anesthetics, ascorbic acid, cephalosporins, chloral hydrate, corticosteroids, EDTA, epinephrine, fructose, galactose, glucuronic acid, homogentisic acid, isoniazid, lactose, lithium, morphine, nicotinic acid, oxalates, phenothiazines – long term, salicylates, streptomycin, thiazides, thyroxine, tranquilizers)

Retinol Binding Protein

Test Purpose. To detect various renal disorders.

chronic renal diseases, proximal tubular dysfunction

Analyte	Age/Gender	Reference Range	SI Units	Note
Retinol Binding Protein		<0.5	mg/l	

Sarcosine

(Sar) An amino acid occurring as an intermediate in kidney and liver choline metabolism.

Increased Values – sarcosinuria
severe folate deficiency, sarcosinemia

Sediment

(syn: urine sediment) Urinary sediment exam: casts, cells, bacteria, ova, parasites, yeast, tumor cells, crystals, fat.

Analyte	Age/Gender	Reference Range	SI Units	Note
Urine Sediment				
Erythrocytes		0–1	per field	
Leukocytes		1–4	per field	
Squamous epithelial cells		5–15	per field	
Renal epithelial cells		0		
Casts				
hyaline		occas.		
epithelial		0		
erythrocyte		0		
granular		0		
leukocyte		0		
Bacteria		0		
Yeast		0		
Trichomonads		0		
Salts		0		

Selenium

Urinary selenium content varies markedly in normals and is subject to feeding and clearance effects that confound its use in either exposure or deficiency.

Increased Values
industrial intoxication – (electro-industry, glass-industry), renal failure

Decreased Values
smoking, hemodialysis, cardiomyopathies, catabolism, **decreased selenium dietary intake, stress conditions, pregnancy, long-term parenteral nutrition**, renal failure

Serine

Increased Values
burns, poultry ingestion

Silver

(Ag, syn: argentum)
Test Purpose. To monitor an exposure to silver through dermal contact and inhalation.

Increased Values
silver exposure

Specific Gravity

Specific gravity – which is roughly proportional to urine osmolality which measures solute concentration – measures urine density, or the ability of the kidney to concentrate or dilute the urine over that of plasma. Specific gravity is a measure of urine particle concentration (including wastes and electrolytes). As a general rule, greater urine volume passage lowers specific gravity (dilute urine), and in diminished urine volume, as in febrile states, concentration will be higher (concentrated urine). The specific gravity is used to evaluate concentrating and excretory kidney functioning. Dipsticks are available that also measure specific gravity in approximations. Occasionally, as in diabetes mellitus, there is increased urine volume with high specific gravity. If specific gravity is not >1022 after a 12 hour period without food or water, renal concentrating ability is impaired and the patient either has generalized renal impairment, or nephrogenic diabetes insipidus. In the finalstage renal disease, specific gravity tends to become 1007–1010.

eusthenuria	1020–1040
hypersthenuria	↑ 1040
hyposthenuria	↓ 1020
isosthenuria	= 1010
physiologically	1015–1025

Increased Values – increased specific gravity – hypersthenuria
dehydration, diabetes mellitus, glomerulonephritis, glycosuria, diarrhea, PIH, hypotension, pituitary tumors, nephrosis, adrenal insufficiency, **excessive sweating, proteinuria, water restriction, febrile states, renal artery stenosis, excessive water loss,** syndrome – (nephrotic sy, **sy of inappropriate antidiuretic hormone secretion**), shock, **pituitary trauma, vomiting,** failure – (liver f., **heart f.**), **renal blood flow decrease**
  Interfering Factors: radiographic contrast media (x-ray contrast dye, radioopaque contrast media), normal morning specimen, medicaments – (antibiotics, dextran, diuretics, isotretinoin, mannitol)

Decreased Values – decreased specific gravity – hyposthenuria
kalium deficiency, diabetes insipidus – (**idiopathic d. i., nephrogenic d. i., psychogenic d. i.**), **glomerulonephritis, hyperhydration,** malignant hypertension, **hypothermia,** chronic renal insufficiency, **acute tubular necrosis, severe renal damage, pyelonephritis, renal failure,**

acute renal diseases, hypercalcemia due to sarcoidosis, hyperparathyroidism, diseases – (bone d., renal d.), intoxication by – (lithium – chronic, vitamin D), sickle-cell nephropathy, plasmocytoma (incl. multiple myeloma), excessive fluid intake

Interfering Factors: medicaments – (amikacin, aminoglycosides, amphotericin B, carbenoxolone, colistin, cyclosporine, gentamicin, lithium, methoxyflurane, neomycin, streptomycin, tobramycin)

Analyte	Age/Gender	Reference Range	SI Units	Note
Specific Gravity	Neonates	1012		
	First few days	1002–1006		
	Adults	1002–1030		
		>1025		See ref.
		1015–1025		ranges note

Styrene Metabolite Profile

Test includes measurement of creatinine, mandelic acid, mandelic acid/creatinine ratio. Test is used to monitor exposure to styrene. Mandelic acid in urine represents approximately 85% of the styrene dose. Urine mandelic acid levels indicate the extent of chronic ethyl benzene and styrene exposures, which are typically associated with industry.

Sucrose

(syn: saccharose) Non-reducing sugar.

Increased Values
congenital lactose intolerance, increased sucrose intake

Taurine

Increased Values
pernicious anemia, folic acid deficiency, hyperbetaalaninemia, severe burns, pregnancy (1st trimester)
Interfering Factors: medicaments – (progesterone)

Decreased Values
Interfering Factors: medicaments – (acetylsalicylic acid, phenylbutazone)

Telopeptides

This proces leads to Ca, P, enzyme and matrix degradation products washout, which have variable bone specificity and are used to bone resorption determination. Telopeptides belong to collagen matrix degradation products (hydroxyproline, hydroxylysine glycosides, pyridine derivatives and so-called cross-link type I C-terminal telopeptides (ICTP, or CTx) and type I N-terminal telopeptides (INTP, or NTx). a) CTx – is used mainly in urine determination (so-called cross-labs). Antibodies (cross-labs ELISA) are directed against beta isomers. b) INTP – is used in urine determination. Its specificity is increasing, because do not react peptides, which have collagen II origin (rheumatoid arthritis, osteoarthritis, Paget's disease), collagen III (synovia) and II (cartilage).

Analyte	Age/Gender	Reference Range	SI Units	Note
N-Terminal Telo-peptide Fragment Type I (NTx)	M 20–79 y	<79	*	*nmol/ mmol crea-tinine
	F 21–55 y	<79	*	
	49–79 y	<140	*	

Tetrahydrodeoxycortisol

(THS, syn: tetrahydro-11-deoxycortisol, tetrahydro-compound S)

Increased Values
eclampsia, congenital adrenal hyperplasia due to 11-beta-hydroxylase deficiency, pancreatitis, severe stress

Decreased Values
hypopituitarism, Addison's disease

Thallium

(Th) Test is used to monitor exposure to thallium. Thallium exposure is associated with industrial inhalation and/or dermal absorption of metallic thallium or thallium salts. Thallium compounds are employed in semiconductor research, optical systems and photoelectric cells. Thallium salts are used as insecticides and rodenticides. Poisoning from occupational exposure to thallium can occur in the manufacture of optical instruments, rodenticides, dyes and certain alloys. Environmental exposure may follow emissions from smelters, cement plants and coal-fired plants.

Increased Values
exposure to thallium

Threonine

Increased Values – hyperthreoninuria
hepatolenticular degeneration, Hartnup disease, severe burns, pregnancy
Interfering Factors: medicaments – (ascorbic acid – large doses, tetracyclines)

Decreased Values – hypothreoninuria
rheumatoid arthritis

Transferrin

Test Purpose. 1) to aid in the differential diagnosis of malnutrition, acute inflammatory diseases and infectious diseases, 2) to assess renal function, 3) to evaluate the RBC disorders, 4) to monitor the therapy.

Increased Values – hypertransferrinemia
anemia – (**aplastic a., posthemorrhagic a., sideropenic a.**), hepatitis – (**acute h., viral h.**), polycythemia, **inadequate iron intake**
   Interfering Factors: pregnancy (3rd trimester), medicaments – (estrogens, ethanol, oral contraceptives)

Decreased Values – hypotransferrinemia
anemia – (sickle-cell a., pernicious a., **thalassemia**), rheumatoid arthritis, **congenital atransferrinemia**, hepatic cirrhosis, diabetes mellitus, **hemochromatosis**, chronic hepatitis, hypertension, diseases – (**acute/chronic infectious d., renal d., liver d., inflammatory d.**), **iron poisoning, kwashiorkor, malnutrition, tumors, nephrosis**, plasmocytoma (incl. multiple myeloma), septic conditions, **protein loss, nephrotic sy**, uremia, **systemic lupus erythematosus**

Analyte	Age/Gender	Reference Range	SI Units	Note
Transferrin		<1.2	mg/l	

Trichloroacetic Acid

(TCA) Test is used to monitor exposure to perchloroethylene, trichloroethane and trichloroethylene. Urine trichloroacetic acid accounts for 32% of absorbed trichloroethylene.

Increased Values
perchloroethylene, trichloroethane, trichloroethylene

Tryptophan

Increased Values – tryptophanuria
Hartnup disease

Tubulo-Epithelial Cells

Increased Values – positive
inflammatory urinary tract diseases – (pyelonephritis), poisoning by – (ethylene glycol, heavy metals), malignant nephrosclerosis, **acute tubular necrosis**, necrotizing papillitis, tubular injuries, renal transplant rejection
   Interfering Factors: medicaments – (salicylates)

Tyrosine

Increased Values – tyrosinuria
galactosemia, hyperthyroidism, hypertyrosinemia, Hartnup disease, severe burns, pregnancy (1st trimester), hepatic failure

Urea

(syn: urea nitrogen)
Test Purpose. To assess total renal function.

Increased Values
proteins destruction, pheochromocytoma, hyperthyroidism, phosphorus poisoning, tumours, **increased protein intake,** conditions – (febrile c., postoperative c.)
  Interfering Factors: medicaments – (quinine, salicylates)

Decreased Values
acidosis, advanced hepatic cirrhosis, dehydration, low protein diet, acute hepatic dystrophy, **acute/chronic glomerulonephritis,** diseases – (renal d., severe hepatic d.), parenchymatous icterus, renal insufficiency, malnutrition, **tumors,** nephritis, **nephrosclerosis, acute tubular necrosis, polycystic kidney, renal artery obstruction,** pyelonephritis, **shock,** pregnancy, toxemia, renal tuberculosis, uremia, **congestive heart failure**
  Interfering Factors: medicaments – (growth hormone, insulin, testosterone)

Analyte	Age/Gender	Reference Range	SI Units	Note
Urea		170–580	mmol/dU	

Uric Acid

(syn: urate) A nucleic acid metabolite, uric acid concentration is a de novo synthesis and dietary sources product. 75% of urate is eliminated through the kidney and 25% through the intestine. Renal urate excretion involves reabsorption by the proximal tubules, secretion by the proximal tubules distal part and further reabsorption by the distal tubules.
Test Purpose. 1) to detect enzyme deficiencies and metabolic disturbances that affect uric acid production (e.g. stones, gout), 2) to help measure renal clearance efficiency, 3) to measure body's production and excretion of uric acid.

Increased Values – uricosuria, hyperuricosuria, hyperuricaciduria
anemia – (sickle-cell a., **pernicious a.**), **hepatic cirrhosis, high purine diet, gout,** glycogenoses, starvation, PIH, diseases – (infectious d., **liver d.**), lead poisoning, cachexia, **ulcerative colitis, lymphatic leukemia during radiotherapy, chronic myeloid leukemia, lymphosarcoma,** Wilson's disease, **plasmocytoma** (incl. multiple myeloma), severe pneumonia, **polycythemia vera, tubular resorption defects, febrile states,** oxidative stress, syndrome – (**Fanconi's sy, Lesch–Nyhan sy**), renal calculi, **nephrolithiasis,** Crohn's disease, jejunoileal bypass
  Interfering Factors: chronic alcoholism, **radiographic contrast media,** medicaments – (alcohol, cytostatics, thiazide diuretics, antiinflammatory preparations, salicylates, vitamin C, warfarin)

Decreased Values – hypouricosuria
chronic alcoholism, anemia, **uratic arthritis**, folic acid deficiency, diabetes mellitus, **eclampsia**, chronic glomerulonephritis, **diabetic glomerulosclerosis**, **renal insufficiency**, **lead poisoning**, collagenoses, **nephritis**, urinary obstruction, xanthinuria, renal failure, hypertension

Analyte	Age/Gender	Reference Range	SI Units	Note
Uric Acid		1.2–6.0	mmol/d	See ref.
		<3.6	mmol/d	ranges note
		<1.78	mmol/l	
		0.07–0.72	ml/s*	*clearance
		0.044–0.122	**	**fraction excretion

Urinary Gonadotropin Peptide

Urinary gonadotropin peptide (glycoprotein) is the core beta-hCG fragment.

Increased Values – positive
tumors of – (cervix, endometrium, ovary)

Urobilinogen

Formed from hemoglobin metabolism → liver → bile → intestine → transformation through bacterial action into urobilinogen; part is excreted with the feces, another portion is absorbed into the portal blood-stream → liver → metabolization → excretion in the bile. Bilirubin is changed into urobilinogen in the duodenum by intestinal bacteria. Urobilinogen traces that escape removal from the blood by the liver are carried by the blood to the kidneys and excreted in the urine. Urobilinogen is even less stable than urine bilirubin which has been left to stand; it oxidizes to urobilin, which does not react in some urobilinogen tests.
Test Purpose. 1) to aid in extrahepatic obstruction diagnosis such as common bile duct blockage, 2) to aid in hepatic and hematologic disorders differential diagnosis.

Increased Values – positive – urobilinogenuria
anemia – (**hemolytic a.**, pernicious a.), bananas, **primary biliary cirrhosis, hepatic cirrhosis**, erythroblastosis fetalis, hepatitis – (alcoholic h., infectious h., toxic h., **viral h.**), false positive values – (5-hydroxyindoleacetic acid, porphobilinogen), **cholangitis**, diseases – (**severe infectious d., liver d.**), **hemolytic icterus, pulmonary infarction**, heart insufficiency, liver infarction, liver metastases, intoxication by – (acetone, formaldehyde, chloroform), tumors of pancreas, malaria, Gilbert's disease, infectious mononucleosis, constipation, **biliary efferent ducts obstruction with infection**, parenchymal hepatic injury, hemolytic conditions, severe bruises, febrile states, syndrome – (Dubin-Johnson sy, Rotor's sy), **congestive heart failure**
    Interfering Factors: medicaments – (adrenaline, aminosalicylic acid, chlorpromazine, methyldopa, phenothiazines, procaine, sulfonamides, tetracyclines)

Decreased Values

primary biliary cirrhosis, hepatic cirrhosis, hepatitis – (alcoholic h., toxic h., viral h.), **severe diarrhea**, cholelithiasis, drug-induced cholestasis, **severe inflammatory diseases, renal insufficiency**, Gilbert's disease, acid urine, pancreas head tumors, nitrites, biliary efferent ducts obstruction without infection caused by – (**calculi, tumors, scar tissue**), parenchymal hepatic injury, syndrome – (Crigler-Najjar sy, Dubin-Johnson sy, Rotor's sy)

Interfering Factors: medicaments – (antibiotics)

Uropepsin

Increased Values
ulcus bulbi duodeni

Decreased Values
pernicious anemia

Uroporphyrin

Test Purpose. To aid in congenital or acquired porphyrias diagnosis.

Increased Values – uroporphyrin I
congenital erythropoietic porphyria

Increased Values – uroporphyrin III
tumors, **acute intermittent porphyria**, **porphyria cutanea tarda**, **variegate porphyria**, chronic renal failure

Valine

Increased Values
generalized aminoaciduria, maple syrup urine disease, Hartnup disease, severe burns, pregnancy (1st trimester)

Interfering Factors: medicaments – (ascorbic acid – large doses)

Vanilmandelic Acid

(VMA) Major catecholamine metabolite, the result of both carboxy-o-methyl transferase and monoamine oxidase action. VMA levels reflect endogenous epinephrine and norepinephrine production.

Test Purpose. 1) to help detect pheochromocytoma, neuroblastoma, ganglioneuroblastoma and ganglioneuroma, 2) to evaluate adrenal medulla function, 3) to evaluate hypertension.

Increased Values
nicotine abuse, **acute anxiety**, asthma bronchiale, **pheochromocytoma**, ganglioblastoma, **ganglioneuroblastoma, ganglioneuroma**, hypertension, **hyperthyroidism**, myocardial infarction, heart insufficiency, **carcinoid**, meningitis, **tumors, neuroblastoma**, polyneuritis, porphyria, **sepsis, shock conditions, stress, sympatoblastoma**, uremia, **vigorous exercise**

Interfering Factors: bananas, candy, tea, chocolate, dressing, jam, fruit juice, starvation, gelatin foods, cocoa, coffee, carbonated drinks, cheese, vanilla, chewing gum, medicaments – (acetylsalicylic acid, adrenaline, ajmaline, aminosalicylic acid, caffeine, dopamine, glucagon, guanethidine, histamine, insulin, labetalol, levodopa, lithium, methenamine, methyldopa, nitroglycerin, oxytetracycline, phenothiazines, reserpine)

Decreased Values
severe shock conditions

Interfering Factors: radiographic iodine contrast agents, alkaline urine, uremia, medicaments – (acetylsalicylic acid, chlorpromazine, clofibrate, clonidine, disulfiram, guanethidine, imipramine, MAO inhibitors, methyldopa, morphine, phenothiazines, reserpine)

Analyte	Age/Gender	Reference Range	SI Units	Note
Vanilmandelic Acid		18–33	μmol/d	

Vitamin B₁

Test Purpose. 1) to help confirm vitamin B_1 deficiency, 2) to help distinguish vitamin B_1 deficiency from other causes of polyneuritis.

Decreased Values
beriberi, poor diet, hyperthyroidism, alcoholism, severe liver diseases, chronic diarrhea, prolonged diuretic therapy

Analyte	Age/Gender	Reference Range	SI Units	Note
Thiamine	Children 1–3 y	75–85	*	*μmol/mol creatinine
	Adults	28–55	*	

Vitamin C

Test Purpose. To aid in the diagnosis of scurvy, scurvy-like conditions, and metabolic disorders such as malnutrition interferring with oxidative processes.

Decreased Values
infectious diseases, prolonged i.v. therapy, **malabsorption**, **malnutrition**, **tumors**, **burns**, **scurvy**, **stress conditions**, renal diseases, vitamin C deficiency

Volume

(syn: urine volume, diuresis) Urine output (void) in normal adults averages between 1200–1500 ml (500–2000 ml) over 24 hours – 4/5 of volume in day, 1/5 at night, depending on fluid intake and fluid lost by routes other than the kidneys such as perspiration or sweating. The volume excreted can also vary in anxiety/stress/hysterical conditions, in various diseases, through climatic conditions and after drug ingestion.

Changes in Micturition

- **anuria (<100 ml/day, <5 ml/h):** amyloidosis, urinary ways blockage by uric acid crystals, intravascular hemolysis, polycystic kidney disease, acute renal diseases, acute/chronic renal insufficiency, poisoning by – (arsenic, bismuth, bromates, CO, DDT, dinitrophenols, ethylene glycol, formaldehyde, phosphorus, mushrooms, copper, methanol, naphthalene, lead, mercury, oxalates, paraquat, organic solvents, thallium, turpentine, trinitrotoluene, gold, iron), calculus in kidney or ureter, severe collapse with low blood pressure, both ureters ligature, systemic lupus erythematosus, tumors – (infiltrating uterine t., t. of bladder), acute/chronic nephritis, acute tubular necrosis, efferent urinary ways obstruction, pyelonephritis, conditions – (febrile c., c. after septic abortion, c. after blood transfusion), crush sy, both kidneys tuberculosis, acute/chronic renal failure

  Interfering Factors: medicaments – (acetaminophen, acetylsalicylic acid, acyclovir, aldesleukin, allopurinol, aminocaproic acid, aminoglycosides, amphotericin B, ascorbic acid, bacitracin, benazepril, boric acid, captopril, carbamazepine, cefalosporins, celecoxib, cephalotin, clomiphene, clotrimazol, colchicine, colistin, cyclosporine, deferoxamine, dexmedetomidine, dextran, dicloxacillin, diltiazem, diphenhydramine, disopyramide, enalapril, enflurane, erythromycin, fenoprofen, follitropin, fosinopril, furosemide, gold salts, halothane, hydralazine, hydrochlorothiazide, ibuprofen, indapamide, indomethacin, interleukin 2, iodine preparations, isoniazid, mannitol, menotropins, methotrexate, metrizimide, mitomycin, moexipril, nifedipine, nonsteroidal anti-inflammatory drugs, opioids, paraldehyde, penicillamine, penicillins, pentamidine, perindopril, phenacetin, phencyclidine, phenylbutazone, polymyxins, retinol – high doses, rifampicin, ropivacaine, streptokinase, sulfamethizol, sulfonamides, theophylline – high doses, thiazides, thiopental, tolmetin, torsemide, triamterene, warfarin, zomepirac)

- **nycturia** (nocturia, frequent nocturnal urination): sickle cell anemia, **liver cirrhosis,** diabetes insipidus – (pituitary d. i., nephrogenic d. i.), diabetes mellitus (uncontrolled), postobstructive diuresis, interfering factors – (advanced age), recovery phase of acute tubular necrosis, hypercalcemia, prostate hyperplasia, hypokalemia, diseases – (infectious d. of urinary tract, chronic renal d.), insufficiency – (renal i., hepatic i., cardiac i.), bladder calculi, medicaments – (amphotericin B, beta-blockers, diuretics, glucose infusion, lithium, mannitol, methoxyflurane), malnutrition, radiocontrast media, prostate tumors, nephropathy – (obstructive n., analgesic n.), psychogenic water drinking, pyelonephritis, conditions – (edematous c., hypercatabolic c., polyuric c., c. after renal transplantation), urethral stricture, urinary tract infection, **nephrotic sy, congestive heart failure**

- **oliguria (<300 ml/day, <13 ml/h** – decreased urine volume): acidosis, alcohol, ascites, dehydration, dermatomyositis, dysentery, massive edema, eclampsia, acute glomerulonephritis, Wegener's granulomatosis, hemolysis, malignant hypertension, hypokalemia, hyponatremia, hypotension, cholera, diseases – (bladder d., acute renal d., prostate d.), **myocardial infarction, acute/chronic renal insufficiency,** intoxication by – (bismuth, bromates, CO, DDT, dinitrophenols, ethylene glycol, formaldehyde, inorganic phosphorus, mushrooms, heavy metals, copper, methanol, naphthalene, lead, mercury, oxalates, paraquat, organic solvents, thallium, turpentine, trinitrotoluene, iron), ischemia, disseminated intravascular coagulation, coma, sickle cell crisis, hemorrhage, systemic lupus erythematosus, protein malnutrition, myositis, tumours, interstitial nephritis caused by – (infections, heavy metals), nephrolithiasis, analgesic nephropathy, **acute tubular necrosis, obstruction of efferent urinary ways,** periarteritis nodosa (polyarteritis nodosa), crush injuries, septic abortion, pyelonephritis, rhabdomyolysis, post-transfusion reaction, sarcoidosis, sepsis, scleroderma, after surgery conditions, **shock,** pregnancy, typhus, **heat stroke,** trauma

Interfering Factors: medicaments – (ACE inhibitors, acetaminophen, acetylsalicylic acid, ACTH, acyclovir, aldesleukin, allopurinol, aminocaproic acid, aminoglycosides, amphotericin B, antibiotics, ascorbic acid, bacitracin, benazepril, boric acid, captopril, carbamazepine, cefalosporins, cephalotin, celecoxib, cidofovir, clomiphene, clotrimazol, colchicine, colistin, cyclosporine, deferoxamine, dexmedetomidine, dextran, diphenhydramine, dicloxacillin, diltiazem, disopyramide, enalapril, enflurane, erythromycin, etidronate, fenoprofen, follitropin, fosinopril, furosemide, gold salts, halothane, hydralazine, hydrochlorothiazide, ibuprofen, indapamide, indomethacin, interleukin 2, iodine preparations, isoniazid, kanamycin, lisinopril, mannitol, menotropins, methotrexate, metrizimide, mitomycin, moexipril, morphine, neomycin, nifedipine, nonsteroidal antiinflammatory drugs, opioids, paraldehyde, penicillamine, penicillins, pentamidine, perindopril, phenacetin, phencyclidine, phenylbutazone, polymyxins, retinol – high doses, rifampicin, ropivacaine, somatostatin, streptokinase, streptozocin, sulfamethizol, sulfonamides, sulfonylurea, theophylline – high doses, thiazides, thiopental, tolmetin, torsemide, triamterene, vasopressin, warfarin, zomepirac)

■ **polacisuria** (frequent urination with small amount of urine expelled): diabetes insipidus, diabetes mellitus, prostate hyperplasia, urinary tract infections – (cystitis, prostatitis, urethritis), tumors

■ **polyuria (>2 500 ml/day** – increased urine volume): **alcohol, amyloidosis**, sickle-cell anemia, **diabetes insipidus, diabetes mellitus,** osmotic diuresis caused by – (glucose, mannitol, urea), postobstructive diuresis, encephalitis, **renal glycosuria, hyperhydration, hypercalcemia,** hyperparathyroidism, hyperthyroidism, **hypokalemia,** histiocytosis X, diseases – (endocrinous d., hypothalamic d.), **chronic renal insufficiency,** Cushing's disease, protein malnutrition, meningitis, edema mobilization – (renal e. m., hepatic e. m., cardiac e. m.), tumors – (craniopharyngioma, lymphoma, t. of breast), interstitial nephritis, nephropathy – (analgesic n., salt-losing n.), **polyuric phase of acute tubular necrosis,** plasmocytoma (incl. multiple myeloma), psychogenic polydipsia, cerebrovascular accident, excessive water intake, chronic pyelonephritis, sarcoidosis, postmenstruation conditions, renal artery stenosis, syndrome – (adrenogenital sy, Bartter's sy, Conn's sy, Sjögren's sy), end-stage renal diseases, **pregnancy** (3rd trimester), renal transplantation, tuberculosis, high altitude, **polyuric phase of acute renal failure**

Interfering Factors: medicaments – (acetylsalicylic acid, alosetron, amiloride, amphotericin B, bicarbonate, bumetanide, caffeine, carbidopa, carbinoxamine, chlorpromazine, chlorthalidone, cidofovir, cisplatin, citalopram, clotrimazol, clozapine, demeclocycline, dexfenfluramine, digitalis, diltiazem, diuretics, dopamine, ethacrynic acid, ethanol, furosemide, glucocorticoids, halothane, hydrochlorothiazide, indapamide, levodopa, lithium, mannitol, methoxyflurane, metolazone, nifedipine, oral hypoglycemic agents, phenytoin, pramipexole, probenecid, propoxyphene, saluretics, spironolactone, thiazides, torsemide, triamterene, vincristine, xanthines)

Analyte	Age/Gender	Reference Range	SI Units	Note
Urine Volume	1–2 d	0.03–0.06	l/d	
	3–10 d	0.10–0.30	l/d	
	11 d–2 m	0.25–0.45	l/d	
	3 m–1 y	0.40–0.50	l/d	
	2–3 y	0.50–0.60	l/d	
	4–5 y	0.60–0.70	l/d	
	6–8 y	0.65–1.00	l/d	
	9–14 y	0.80–1.40	l/d	
	Adults	1.00–1.60	l/d	

Xylose

(syn: xylose absorption test) About 55–60% of an oral xylose intake is passively absorbed in the proximal small intestine. The accuracy of the measurement depends on the absorption rate and the excretion rate of xylose by the kidneys. To avoid misinterpretations as a result of renal retention, a blood determination of xylose should be assayed with a concurrent urine. In patient with renal insufficiency, rely on the serum test only.

Test Purpose. To evaluate mucosal absorption efficiency.

Decreased Values – decreased xylose absorption

ascariasis, ascites, blind loops syndrome, dehydration, disease – (celiac d., Crohn's d., renal d., thyroid d.), immunoglobulin deficiency, intestinal malabsorption, pellagra, postsurgery conditions, pregnancy, radiation enteritis, stomach emptying disorders, tropical sprue, tumors, vomiting

> **Interfering Factors:** medicaments – (acetylsalicylic acid, atropine, colchicine, digitalis, indomethacin, MAO inhibitors, nalidixic acid, neomycin, opium alkaloids, phenelzine)

Analyte	Age/Gender	Reference Range	SI Units	Note
Xylose		0.16–0.33	abs.	

Zinc

Zinc is utilized as an alloying agent in brass and other metals, as well as in metal plating. Zinc chloride is often produced in the chemical smoke generators that are employed in industry. Zinc chloride is also used in soldering fluxes and wood preservatives. Zinc excretion gives an indication of the loosely bound or exchangeable zinc in the body but does not necessarily reflect body stores.

Test Purpose. 1) to evaluate zinc exposure, 2) to evaluate low serum zinc levels, 3) to evaluate compliance in oral zinc therapy of Wilson's disease.

Increased Values

alcoholism, arthritis, **hepatic cirrhosis**, **viral hepatitis**, hyperparathyroidism, **inflammatory diseases**, systemic lupus erythematosus, **tumors**, post surgery conditions, hemolytic anemia, sickle cell disease, diabetes mellitus, chronic renal diseases, zinc poisoning, acute phase response, catabolism

> **Interfering Factors:** medicaments – (ethacrynic acid, furosemide, isotonic sodium chloride, thiazide diuretics)

Decreased Values

hypogonadal dwarfism, zinc deficiency

Analyte	Age/Gender	Reference Range	SI Units	Note
Zinc		0.77–23	μmol/l	
		0.15–1.47	*	*mmol/mol creatinine

II

Biochemical/Laboratory Findings in Clinical Units and Conditions

Biochemical/Laboratory Findings in Clinical Units and Conditions

D. Mesko, R. Pullmann

Abetaglobulinemia
    ↓ ✶ beta globulins, proteins

Abetalipoproteinemia
    ↑ ✶ acanthocytes
    ↓ Apo A-I, ✶**Apo B**, ✶**beta-LPs**, Bil, **ESR**, Hb, HCT, **HDL-C**, **cholesterol**, **chylomicrons**, LDL-C, LPs, PL, **TAG**, ✶ vitamin – (A, E), **VLDL-C**
    ■ *Stool* ↑ ✶ fat

Ablatio of Placenta
    ↓ RBC, **fibrinogen**, Hb, HCT

Abortion
  incomplete abortion
    ↑ ALT, WBC
  missed abortion
    ↑ **WBC**
    ↓ **hCG**
  septic abortion
    ↑ CRP, bacteria (culture), elastase (PMN), **ESR**, PCT, PT, **WBC**
    ↓ WBC
    ■ *Urine* ↓ volume
  spontaneous abortion
    ↑ AFP, APLA, **WBC**
    ↓ fibrinogen, hCG
  threatened abortion (imminens)
    ↑ AFP, ALP, anti-HCV, euglobulin lysis time, ✶ **ESR**, ✶ **hCG**, hPL, **WBC**, progesterone
    ↓ AAP, fibrinogen, estriol, hCG, **hPL**, **progesterone**
    ■ *Urine* ↓ estriol, hCG, **pregnanediol**
    ■ *Amniotic Fluid* ↑ AFP

Abruptio of Placenta
    ↑ **ESR, WBC**
    ↓ RBC, **fibrinogen**, Hb, HCT

Abscess
    ↑ ALT, Bil, Bil conjugated, Bil unconjugated, **CRP, ESR, WBC**, ✶ **neopterin**, neu, ✶ **PCT**, ✶ **PMN-elastase**, SAA
    ↓ albumin, **RBC, Hb**, HCT, PLT
  appendix abscess
    ↑ **ESR, WBC**
    ↓ albumin
  Brodie's abscess
    ↑ **ESR, WBC**

cerebral abscess

↑ ALT, **ESR, WBC**

- *Cerebrospinal Fluid* ↑ **bacteria** (+ culture), **proteins, RBC,** G, cholesterol, CHS, LA, LD, **WBC, lym,** macrophages, **neu, pleocytosis, PMN, pressure**
  ↓ G, **chloride**

– cerebral epidural abscess

- *Cerebrospinal Fluid* ↑ bacteria (+ culture), **proteins,** WBC, lym, neu, pressure

Douglas' space abscess

↑ **ESR, WBC**

intraperitoneal abscess

↑ **ESR, WBC**

- *Peritoneal Fluid* ↑ bacteria (+ culture), proteins, WBC

kidney abscess

↑ **ESR, WBC**
↓ WBC

- *Urine* ↑ **albumin,** * **bacteria** (+ culture), **proteins, RBC,** Hb, **pus**
  ↓ volume

liver abscess

↑ AFP, * **ALP,** ALP (WBC), **ALT,** AMS, APTT, **AST,** * **Bil, conjugated Bil,** unconjugated Bil, CEA, ceruloplasmin, **ESR,** * **globulins,** GMT, granulocytes, Hb (free), **ICD,** LD, **LAP, WBC, neu,** 5-nucleotidase, **OCT,** PT

↓ * **albumin,** AMS, **RBC,** G, **Hb, HCT,** CHS, **PLT**

- *Urine* ↓ sulfate
- *Pleural Fluid* ↓ WBC

– amebic liver abscess

↑ **ALP, ALT, AST, Bil, ESR, GMT, LAP, 5-NT, WBC**
↓ **albumin,** Hb, HCT, microcytes

lung abscess

↑ **ADH,** bacteria (early) (culture), **ESR,** uric acid, **WBC,** neopterin (TB, HIV), **neu**
↓ albumin, RBC, Hb, HCT

- *Sputum* ↑ * **bacteria** (+ culture), * **pus,** blood, * **volume, viscosity**
- *Urine* ↑ **albumin,** proteins
- *Pleural Fluid* ↑ adenosine deaminase, proteins, eos, **RBC,** LA, LD, WBC, mucopolysaccharides, **neu,** TM – (CEA), **PMN**
  ↓ G, **pH**
- *Bronchoalveolar Lavage Fluid* ↑ bacteria (+ culture), PMN

myocardial abscess

↑ **CRP, ESR, WBC**

- *Pericardial Fluid* ↑ WBC
- *Pleural Fluid* ↑ WBC

omentum abscess

↑ **ESR, WBC**
↓ albumin

pancreatic abscess

↑ ALP, ALT, AMS, **ESR, WBC**
↓ albumin

- **Urine** ↑ AMS
- **Peritoneal Fluid** ↑ proteins, WBC

pelvic abscess
↑ ESR, WBC
↓ albumin

periappendical abscess
↑ ESR, WBC
↓ albumin
- **Urine** ↑ pus
- **Peritoneal Fluid** ↑ bacteria (+ culture), proteins, WBC

perinephric abscess
↑ bacteria (culture), ESR, PMN, WBC

peritonsillar abscess
↑ ESR, WBC

prostatic abscess
↑ ESR, WBC
- **Urine** ↑ bacteria (+ culture), RBC, pus, WBC

spinal epidural abscess
- **Cerebrospinal Fluid** ↑ proteins, WBC, lym, pressure
↓ pressure

tubo-ovarian abscess
↑ ESR, WBC
↓ albumin

Abuse, Androgen
↑ LDL-C, PLT aggregation, PLT, RBC
↓ FSH, HDL-C, LH, testosterone
- **Urine** ↑ **androgens**

Achlorhydria
↑ gastrin
↓ Fe, pepsinogen, secretin, vitamin – (B_{12})
- **Gastric Fluid** ↓ pepsin

Acidosis
↑ AB, **acetoacetate**, **acetone**, epinephrine, ALT, ammonia, AMS (S), AST, **BHBA**, proteins, CK, ESR, G, glucagone, Hb, HTC, **K**, catecholamines, **ketones**, creatinine, uric acid, lactate, LD, WBC, MAC, Mg, neu, norepinephrine, plasma volume, osmolality, pyruvate, FFA, urea
↓ AB, AST, BE, 2,3-DPG, GPD (RBC), HCO_3^-, chloride, K, lym, Mg, Na, pCO_2, pH, TBG
- **Urine** ↑ acetone, ammonia, AMS, Ca, DALA, G, chloride, K, catecholamines, ketones, creatinine, Na, volume, **osmolality**, P
  ↓ Mg, pH, urea

diabetic ketoacidosis
↑ * acetoacetate, * acetone, * anion gap, epinephrine, ALT, ammonia, AMS, AST, BHBA, proteins, CK, CK-MB, ESR, * G, **glucagon**, GD, **Hb**, HCT, **chloride**, ICD, K, **catecholamines**, * **ketones**, cortisol, * **creatinine**, uric acid, * **LA**, **LD**, lipids, WBC, * **MAC**, MD, **Mg**, Na, **neu**, norepinephrine, * **osmolality**, * **P**, PRL, **pyruvate**, GH, SD, **TAG**, tri-iodothyronine resin uptake, **FFA**, **urea**
↓ albumin, **AST**, BE, Ca^{2+}, CO_2, **eos**, G6PD (RBC), HCO_3^-, CHS, **chloride**, K, creatine (false), **lym**, **Mg**, Na, P, * pCO_2, * pH, T3

- *Urine* ↑ acetone, ammonia, **AMS**, proteins, DALA, **G**, chloride, **K**, catecholamines, ∗ **ketones**, creatinine, Mb, **Na**, **volume**, specific gravity
  - ↓ Mg, **pH**
- *Synovial Fluid* ↑ crystals – (urate)
- *Saliva* ↑ GMT

hyperkalemic metabolic acidosis
↑ BHBA, chloride, **K**, LA
↓ AB, BE, HCO_3^-, chloride, pCO_2, pH

lactic acidosis
↑ **acetone**, ALT, AMS, anion gap, **AST**, BHBA, G, **K**, **ketobodies**, ∗ **LA**, **uric acid**, **LD**, **WBC**, ∗ **MAC**, P, pyruvate
↓ BE, G, ∗ HCO_3^-, chloride, ∗ **pH**, pO_2, urea
- *Urine* ↑ alanine, G, ketones
- *Synovial Fluid* ↑ crystals – (urate)

metabolic acidosis
↑ anion gap, AST, BHBA, Ca, CO_2, chloride, cholesterol, K, ketobodies, LA, LD, P, **uric acid**, WBC
↓ AB, ∗ **BE**, 2,3-DPG (RBC), ∗ **HCO_3^-**, chloride, WBC, Mg, **pCO_2**, ∗ **pH**
- *Urine* ↑ Ca, K
  - ↓ AB, BE, **pH**

– compensated metabolic acidosis
↑ BHBA, chloride, K, LA
↓ HCO_3^-, chloride, **pCO_2**

renal tubular acidosis
– distal renal tubular acidosis (type 1)
↑ ALP, ∗ **chloride**, ∗ **MAC**, PTH
↓ albumin, ∗ **HCO_3^-**, ∗ **K**, carbonic anhydrase, P, pH, vitamin D_3
- *Urine* ↑ proteins, **Ca**, G, HCO_3^-, **K**, crystals – (∗ **Ca-phosphate**), uric acid, WBC, **Na**, volume, ∗ **P**, ∗ **pH**
  - ↓ citrate, pH

– proximal renal tubular acidosis (type 2)
↑ aldosterone, anion gap, ∗ **chloride**, K, ∗ **MAC**
↓ albumin, aldosterone, Ca, ∗ **HCO_3^-**, ∗ **K**, carbonic anhydrase, uric acid, Mg, **Na**, osmolality, P, ∗ **pH**
- *Urine* ↑ **amino acids**, ammonia, Ca, ∗ **G**, ∗ **HCO_3^-**, K, crystals – (Ca-phosphate), uric acid, lysozyme, **Na**, **volume**, ∗ **P**, ∗ **pH**
  - ↓ specific gravity, pH

– renal tubular acidosis (type 4)
↑ ALP, **chloride**, K, MAC
- *Urine* ↑ **Na**
  - ↓ ammonium, pH

respiratory acidosis
– acute respiratory acidosis
↑ Ca, HCO_3^-, K, P, **pCO_2**
↓ AB, BE, chloride, O_2, **pH**

– chronic respiratory acidosis
↑ Ca, **HCO_3^-**, K, **pCO_2**
↓ chloride, pH

– compensated respiratory acidosis
↑ AB, BE, Ca, **HCO_3^-**, K, **pCO_2**

Aciduria

    L-glyceric aciduria

        ■ *Urine* ↑ * L-glyceric acid, oxalic acid

    hereditary orotic aciduria

        ↑ **aldolase, anisocytes,** basophilic stippling, Bil, **unconjugated Bil, homo-**
               cysteine, RBC Howell-Jolly bodies, **macrocytes, megalocytes**

        ↓ Hb, HCT, RTC, WBC

        ■ *Urine* ↑ * orotic acid

Acrodermatitis Enteropatica

        ↑ Ni

        ↓ Zn

Acromegaly

        ↑ ALP, Ca, CK, CK-MB, FSH, * G, * GH-RH, glucagon, cholesterol,
             * ILGF-I, IGFBP-3, * insulin, IRI, K, ketobodies, creatine, **creatinine,**
             acetoacetic acid, uric acid, LH (early), Na, osteocalcin, P, PRL, * GH,
             somatomedin C, T3, T4, triiodothyronine resin uptake, **urea,** FFA,
             VLDL-C

        ↓ * estradiol, * FSH, IGFBP-1, cortisol, LD, neu, * SHBG, T4, TBG, TSH,
             * testosterone, uric acid, Zn

        ■ *Urine* ↑ Ca, G, GFR, hydroxyproline – (**total, free**), ketones, 17-KGS,
             17-ketosteroids, 17-OHCS, creatine, creatinine

          ↓ 17-KS, FSH, specific gravity

        ■ *Cerebrospinal Fluid* ↑ proteins

        ■ *Synovial Fluid* ↑ WBC, pyrophosphate, viscosity

Adnexitis

        ↑ ESR, WBC, neu

Afibrinogenemia

        ↑ **PLT aggregation, APTT, BT,** clotting time, **PT, TT**

        ↓ * **fibrinogen,** ESR

Agammaglobulinemia (linked to X-chromosome)

        ↑ T-lym

        ↓ **proteins,** * **B-lym,** factor XIII, * **gamma globulins,** * **IgA,** IgE, * **IgG,**
          * **IgM,** lym

        ■ *Synovial Fluid* ↑ WBC, PMN

          ↓ viscosity

Agenesis

    ovarian agenesis

        ↑ FSH

        ■ *Urine* ↑ FSH

          ↓ estrogens

    renal agenesis

          ↓ volume

    testicular agenesis

        ↑ FSH

        ■ *Urine* ↑ FSH

Agranulocytosis

        ↑ ESR, lym (relat), **mono** (relat)

        ↓ * **granulocytes,** * WBC, neu

Alcoholism

        ↑ acetone, AFP, ALP, ALT, AMS, anion gap, Apo – (A-I, A-II, B), APTT,
          * **AST, mAST,** Bil, BHBA, Ca, **carbohydrate-deficient transferrin,** Cd,
          CEA, **CK,** CK-MB, Cu, estradiol, estrogens, ferritin, PL, **FSH,** * GMT,

HDL-C, haptoglobin, HbA$_{1c}$, hexosaminidase B, * **cholesterol**, **chy-lomicrons, IgA, ketones**, * **uric acid**, **cortisol**, **LA**, LAP, **LD**, **LH**, lipase, MAC, * **macrocytes**, * **MCV**, Ni, **OCT**, osmolality, **P**, Pb, PT, PTH, PL, sideroblasts, spherocytes, GH, * **TAG**, tropomyosin, 5-OH tryptophan, VDRL (false), **VLDL-C, FFA**, Zn

↓ albumin, aldosterone, ALT, AMS, AST (later), delta-aminolevulinic de-hydratase, **Ca**, CK, Cr, **G, G tolerance**, HDL-C, **K**, WBC, lipoprotein lipase, **Mg**, Mn, Na, P, pCO$_2$, pH, porphyrins, PRL, PT, T4, testoster-one, **PLT**, urea, vitamin – (**A, B$_6$, B$_{12}$, C, folate, niacin, riboflavin, thia-mine**), **Zn**

- *Urine* ↑ **AMS, FSH, ketones**, coproporphyrin III, creatine, lipids, DALA, uric acid, **Mb**, Mg, Zn
  ↓ **Ca**, * **uric acid, niacin**
- *Cerebrospinal Fluid* ↑ lym, mono, pressure
- *Amniotic Fluid* ↑ FSH
- *Synovial Fluid* ↑ crystals – (urate)

Alkalosis

↑ AB, BE, HCO$_3^-$, Na, pCO$_2$, pH, urea
↓ AB, BE, Ca, ESR, HCO$_3^-$, chloride, K, Na, P, pCO$_2$, PTH
- *Urine* ↑ **K, Na**, pH
  ↓ ammonia, Ca, chloride, pH

metabolic alkalosis

↑ AB, BE, CO$_2$, **HCO$_3^-$**, Na, **pCO$_2$, pH**, urea
↓ Ca, Ca$_{2+}$, **chloride**, K, Na, P, PTH
- *Urine* ↑ AB, **K**, **pH**
  ↓ ammonia, BE, Ca, chloride, pH

– **chronic metabolic alkalosis**

↑ **HCO$_3^-$, pCO$_2$, pH**

respiratory alkalosis

↑ **chloride**, K, P, **pH**
↓ Ca, HCO$_3^-$ (chronic stage), K, **pCO$_2$** (acute stage)
- *Urine* ↑ pH
- *Cerebrospinal Fluid* ↑ LA

– **compensated respiratory alkalosis**

↓ AB, BE, Ca, **HCO$_3^-$, pCO$_2$**

Alkaptonuria

↑ * **homogentisic acid**, uric acid
- *Urine* ↑ * **homogentisic acid**
  ↓ pH

Allergy

↑ ASLO, bas, * **C3 complement**, CIC, * **eos**, eosinophil cationic protein, fibrinogen, fibronectin, ESR, haptoglobin, IgA, * **IgE**, * **IgE specific Ab**, IgG, alpha-1 proteinase inhibitor, cryoglobulins, WBC, neu, pCO$_2$, PMN, RAC, RAL, RF, T-lym
↓ albumin, bas, RBC, HCT, IgA, complement – (C2, C3, C4), WBC, neu, pO$_2$, **PLT**, transferrin
- *Urine* ↑ proteins, RBC, Hb, pentoses, casts – (RBC)
- *Bronchoalveolar Lavage Fluid* ↑ eos, IgG, IgM, lym, neu, T-lym
- *Pleural Fluid* ↑ eos, lym, neu
  ↓ alveolar macrophages
- *Sputum* ↑ eos, lym, neu, PMN, viscosity
  ↓ alveolar macrophages

■ *Synovial Fluid* ↑ eos, WBC, PMN

Alopecia Areata

■ *Gastric Fluid* ↑ pH
↓ HCl

Alveolitis

allergic exogenous alveolitis

↑ * **Ab against Thermoactinomyces candidus, * Ab against Thermo-monospora viridis,** ANA, anti-DNA, aspergillus precipitins, **CIC,** Eo, ESR, IgA, IgE specific, IgG, WBC, pCO_2, PMN, RF, T-lym (CD8)

↓ ACE, **pO_2, PLT**

■ *Bronchoalveolar Lavage Fluid* ↑ eos, IgG, IgM, lym, mastocytes, neu, **PMN, T-lym** (CD4, CD8)

↓ macrophages

■ *Pleural Fluid* ↑ eos, lym, neu
↓ alveolar macrophages

■ *Sputum* ↑ eos, lym, neu
↓ alveolar macrophages

fibrosing cryptogenic alveolitis

↑ ACE, **ANA, * CIC,** EPO, RBC, **ESR, * gamma globulins, * IgA, * IgG** (IgG1, IgG3), IgM, *** cryoglobulins,** WBC, pCO_2, **RF,** T-lym

↓ proteins, lipase, macrophages, pO_2, FFA

■ *Bronchoalveolar Lavage Fluid* ↑ alveolar macrophages, D-dimers, eos, histamine, IgG (IgG1, IgG3), IL-8, IGF, collagenase, LTB4, lym, **neu,** PDGF-B, PMN, TNF-alpha, transforming growth factor beta, free oxygen radicals, mucin-like high-molecular glycoprotein

↓ macrophages, FFA

■ *Pleural Fluid* ↑ LD, **neu**
↓ alveolar macrophages, **pH**

■ *Sputum* ↑ blood, neu
↓ alveolar macrophages

Amenorrhea

primary amenorrhea

↑ beta-carotene, DHEAS, estradiol, *** FSH,** LH, PRL

↓ **estradiol,** progesterone

■ *Urine* ↓ pregnanediol

secondary amenorrhea

↑ PRL, DHEAS

↓ FSH, T3, T4, TSH

Aminoacidemia

isovaleric aminoacidemia

↑ ammonia, glycine, MAC

↓ G

■ *Urine* ↑ ketones

methylmalonic aminoacidemia

↑ ammonia, **glycine,** isoleucine, MAC, *** methylmalonic acid**

↓ G

■ *Urine* ↑ **glycine,** ketones, *** methylmalonic acid**

■ *Cerebrospinal Fluid* ↑ methylmalonic acid

propionic aminoacidemia

↑ **ammonia, glycine, MAC,** ketones, isoleucine

↓ biotin, G, gamma globulins, neu, PLT

■ *Urine* ↑ **glycine**, ketones, methylcitrate, propionate

Aminoaciduria

beta-aminoisobutyric acid aminoaciduria
■ *Urine* ↑ ✱ **beta-aminoisobutyric acid**

argininosuccinic acid aminoaciduria
↑ ALP, ALT, **ammonia**, AST, citrulline, ✱ **argininosuccinic acid**
↓ arginine
■ *Urine* ↑ ✱ **argininosuccinic acid**, orotic acid
■ *Cerebrospinal Fluid* ↑ citrulline, **argininosuccinic acid**

dibasic aminoaciduria
■ *Urine* ↑ arginine, lysine, ornithine

dicarboxylic aminoaciduria
■ *Urine* ↑ aspartic acid, glutamic acid

generalized aminoaciduria
■ *Urine* ↑ arginine, **glutamine**, **glycine**, histidine, homocystine, isoleucine, leucine, valine

glutamic acid aminoaciduria
↑ Bil, ✱ **glutamic acid**
↓ RBC, Hb, HCT
■ *Urine* ↑ **glutamic acid**

glutaric acid aminoaciduria
↑ glutaric acid, MAC
■ *Urine* ↑ glutaric acid

isovaleric aminoaciduria
↑ ammonia, glycine, **isovalerylglycine**, **isovaleric acid**, MAC
↓ gamma globulins, K, neu, PLT
■ *Urine* ↑ isovalerylglycine, isovaleric acid

methylmalonic aminoaciduria
↑ **ammonia**, **glycine**, isoleucine, **ketones**, **acetoacetic acid**, **methylmalonic acid**, MAC
↓ RBC, G, gamma globulins, Hb, HCT, **neu**, PLT
■ *Urine* ↑ cystathionine, **glycine**, **ketones**, **methylmalonic acid**
■ *Amniotic Fluid* ↑ **methylcitric acid**, **methylmalonic acid**

propionic aminoaciduria
↑ ammonia, **glycine**
↓ biotin, gamma globulins, neu, PLT
■ *Urine* ↑ **glycine**, methylcitrate, propionate

Amyloidosis, Primary
↑ ACE, **ALP**, AST, **beta globulins**, ✱ **Bence Jones protein** (lambda light chains, kappa light chains), **proteins**, Bil, conjugated Bil, **B2M**, BT, **ESR**, gamma globulins, haptoglobin, K, complement – (C3), creatinine, uric acid, **WBC**, lipids, **paraproteins**, PT, PLT, ✱ **SAA**, urea, viscosity
↓ **albumin**, proteins, RBC, factor X, fibrinogen, ✱ **gamma globulins**, Hb, HCT, IgG, IgM, **folate**, PT
■ *Urine* ↑ ✱ **Bence Jones protein** (lambda light chains), ✱ **proteins**, RBC, volume, casts – (**epithelial**, RBC, granular, hyaline, waxy)
↓ creatinine, specific gravity, volume
■ *Stool* ↑ blood, fat
■ *Synovial Fluid* ↑ volume, WBC, **viscosity**

Analbuminemia

↑ alpha-2-globulins, beta globulins, CCK-PZ, gamma globulins

↓ * **albumin, proteins**

Anastomosis, Portocaval

↑ ammonia, Fe

Anemia

↑ ACP, aldolase, anisocytes, anulocytes, AST, bas, RBC stippling, Bil, conjugated Bil, unconjugated Bil, ceruloplasmin, **Cu**, BT, delta Bil, clotting time (Lee–White), 2,3-DPG, echinocytes, elliptocytes, **EPO**, Fe, ferritin, **ESR** (severe), gastrin, glutathione peroxidase, haptoglobin, HbA$_{1c}$, HbA2, HbF, HbS, Heinz bodies (RBC), RBC Howell–Jolly bodies, cold agglutinins, **chloride**, cholesterol, ICD, IgA, IgG, calcitonin, catalase, sickle cells, cryoglobulins, uric acid, LA, LD, WBC, lipids, MAC, macrocytes, MCHC, MCV, MD, megalocytes, microcytes, mono, plasma volume, RBC osmotic fragility, RBC osmotic resistance, ovalocytes, plasmocytes, poikilocytes, porphyrins, **clot retraction**, RTC, transferrin satur., spherocytes, schistocytes, siderocytes, somatostatin, target cells, TIBC, PLT, transferrin, urea, Zn

↓ albumin, **ALP**, proteins, Bil, ceruloplasmin, Co, Cu, eos, EPO, **RBC**, estriol, factor – (II, V, VII, IX, XI, XIII), Fe, ferritin, ESR, glutathione peroxidase, haptoglobin, **Hb**, HbA2, HbA$_{1c}$, HbF, HDL-C, hemopexin, **HCT**, cholesterol, **CHS**, catalase, complement – (C3, C4), creatinine, uric acid, LA, LCAT, LDL-C, WBC, lipids, lym, MCH, MCHC, MCV, mono, MPV, Neu, NBB, RBC osmotic fragility, RBC osmotic resistance, pO$_2$, PRA, pyruvate kinase, RTC, transferrin satur., secretin, TAG, TIBC, T-lym, PLT, transferrin, vitamin – (B$_1$, B$_6$, B$_{12}$, **C**, folic acid), Zn

- *Urine* ↑ proteins, RBC, haptoglobin, Hb, hemosiderin, catalase, ketones, coproporphyrin I, blood, methylmalonic acid, uric acid, volume, porphyrins, UBG, urobilin, uropepsin, casts – (RBC)

  ↓ estriol, FSH, creatinine, uric acid, volume
- *Stool* ↑ porphyrins, SBG, UBG
- *Gastric Fluid* ↑ pH

  ↓ HCl, intrinsic factor, MAO, volume, pepsin, pH

anemia in chronic diseases

↑ AAT, anisocytes, ceruloplasmin, CRP, * **ferritin**, fibrinogen, **ESR**, gamma globulins, haptoglobin, HbF, IL-1, C3-complement, WBC, macrocytes, **microcytes**, orosomucoid, poikilocytes, RDW, TNF, **free RBC protoporphyrin**, zinc protoporphyrin

↓ **EPO, RBC**, * **Fe**, * **Hb**, HDL-C, HCT, LDL-C, MCH, MCHC, MCV, **RTC**, **transferrin satur.**, * **TIBC, transferrin**

- *Urine* ↑ RBC, Hb

– anemia in chronic liver diseases

↑ * **macrocytes, MCV, RTC**, target cells, stomatocytes, WBC

↓ **Hb, HCT**, MCHC

– anemia in chronic renal diseases

↑ MAC, P, 2,3-DPG (RBC)

↓ EPO, Fe, folic acid, **Hb, HCT**

aplastic anemia (hypoproliferative)

↑ ALP, Bil, CCK-PZ, ceruloplasmin, **Cu**, **BT**, 2,3-DPG (RBC), **EPO**, Fe, ∗ **ferritin**, haptoglobin, **HbF**, HLA – (DPw3), capillary fragility, LAP (WBC), LD, lym, **macrocytes**, MCV (RBC), plasmocytes, protoporphyrin (RBC), sTfR, **transferrin satur.**, TIBC, **transferrin**

↓ eos, Bil, **RBC**, factor II, **Hb**, **HCT**, **WBC**, **lym**, **mono**, **MPV**, ∗ **neu**, ∗ **RTC**, **TIBC**, ∗ **PLT**, T-lym, transferrin receptor, vitamin – (B$_{12}$)

■ *Urine* ↑ EPO
■ *Stool* ↓ UBG

autoimmune anemia

↑ **ADA**, cold agglutinins, cryoglobulins

↓ RBC, **Hb**, **HCT**, complement – (C1, CH50), RBC osmotic resistance

– autoimmune hemolytic anemia

↑ ACP, **ADA**, adenylate kinase (RBC), aldolase, ALT, **anti-RBC**, **antimicrosomal Ab**, antithyroglobulin Ab, **antithyroidal Ab**, **AST**, baso, Bil, ∗ **unconjugated Bil**, conjugated Bil, delta Bil, Ca, 2,3-DPG (RBC), ferritin, **ESR**, haptoglobin, Hb (free), ∗ **cold agglutinins**, complement – (C$_3$, C$_4$), creatinine, ∗ **cryoglobulins**, IgG, uric acid, **LD**, LD – (1, 2), **WBC**, **MCV**, MD, methemalbumin, microspherocytes, mono, neu, osmotic fragility (RBC), P, RDW, **spherocytes**, RTC, PLT, **urea**

↓ RBC, ∗ **haptoglobin**, **Hb**, HbA$_{1c}$, GHb, **HCT**, **folate**, complement – (C1, C1r, C1s, C2, **C3**, C4, CH50), WBC, neu, ∗ **RBC osmotic resistance**, RTC, PLT

■ *Urine* ↑ coproporphyrin, iron, **Hb**, **UBG**
  ↓ volume
■ *Stool* ↑ porphyrins, SBG, **UBG**

dyserythropoietic anemia

↓ Hb, HCT, PLT

fetal anemia

■ *Amniotic Fluid* ↑ volume, rT3

hemolytic anemia

– acute hemolytic anemia

↑ ACP, ACHE (RBC), ADA, aldolase, AST, **Bil**, conjugated Bil, **unconjugated Bil**, delta Bil, ∗ **ferritin**, cryoglobulins, uric acid, **LD**, LD – (1, 2), MCV, MD, PLT, ∗ **sTfR**, urea

↓ HCT

■ *Urine* ↑ haptoglobin, Hb, **hemosiderin**, UBG
■ *Stool* ↑ porphyrins, UBG

– chronic hemolytic anemia

↑ aldolase, ANA, ALT, AST, bas, RBC stippling, **Bil**, ∗ **unconjugated Bil**, delta Bil, elliptocytes, ∗ **Fe**, ∗ **ferritin**, HbF, RBC Heinz bodies, RBC Howell–Jolly bodies, cold agglutinins, IgA, IgG, ∗ **nucleated RBC**, sickle cells, cryoglobulins, uric acid, lipids, **LD**, LD – (1, 2), **WBC**, macrocytes, MCV, MD, porphyrins, protoporphyrin, pyknocytes, **RTC**, transferrin satur., ∗ **transferrin receptor**, schistocytes, siderocytes, stomacytes, ∗ **TIBC**, PLT, urea

↓ Apo B, **RBC**, Fe, **haptoglobin**, **Hb**, GHb, hemopexin, HDL-C, **HCT**, **cholesterol**, LCAT, LDL-C, **PLT**, RTC, transferrin satur., **TIBC**, PLT, vitamin – (E, **folate**), transferrin

■ *Urine* ↑ **hemosiderin**, Hb, **UBG**
■ *Stool* ↑ porphyrins, SBG, UBG
■ *Synovial Fluid* ↑ crystals – (urate)

- familial nonspherocytic hemolytic anemia

⟶ ↑ ACP, ANA, **RBC basophilic stippling, Bil,** unconjugated Bil, ellipto-cytes, **RBC Heinz bodies, RBC Howell–Jolly bodies, LD,** MCV, MD, RBC osmotic fragility, porphyrins, pyknocytes, **RTC,** stomacytes, urea

⟶ ↓ RBC, G6PD (RBC), **Hb, HCT,** RBC osmotic resistance, **pyruvate kinase, PLT**

■ *Urine* ↑ UBG

- microangiopathic hemolytic anemia

⟶ ↑ ALT, ANA, Hb, ✳ **helmet cells,** LD, ✳ **microspherocytes,** poikilocytes, pyknocytes, ✳ **schistocytes,** stomacytes

⟶ ↓ RBC, Fe, **haptoglobin, Hb, HCT,** PLT

■ *Urine* ↑ Fe, Hb, **hemosiderin**

hereditary anemia

- hereditary elliptocytic anemia

⟶ ↑ Bil, unconjugated Bil, ✳ **elliptocytes,** HbF, lym, **RBC osmotic fragility,** RTC

⟶ ↓ **Hb, HCT,** RBC osmotic resistance

- hereditary spherocytic anemia

⟶ ↑ aldolase, **ALT,** ACHE (RBC), **AST, anisocytes,** baso, **Bil, unconjugated Bil,** Ca (RBC), **Fe,** HbF, Heinz bodies, uric acid, **LD, WBC, lym,** MCH, **MCHC,** MCV, microcytes, ✳ **microspherocytes,** P, plasmocytes, **poikilocytes, RBC Howell–Jolly bodies,** ✳ **RBC osmotic fragility, RTC, spherocytes,** siderocytes, **PLT,** TIBC, viscosity

⟶ ↓ CK, **RBC,** folic acid, **haptoglobin, Hb, HCT,** cholesterol, **WBC,** lipids, LPs, **MCV, RBC osmotic resistance, PL,** PLT, **TAG**

■ *Urine* ↑ **Hb,** coproporphyrin, N-formiminoglutamic acid, **UBG**

■ *Stool* ↑ **UBG**

hypochromic anemia (maturation disorders)

⟶ ↑ anulocytes, HbA2, target cells, **TIBC**

⟶ ↓ **Bil, RBC, Fe, Hb,** HbA2, **HCT, MCHC, MCH, MCV, transferrin satur.**

macrocytic anemia

⟶ ↑ unconjugated Bil, gastrin, LD, ✳ **macrocytes, MCH,** ✳ **MCV**

⟶ ↓ RBC, **Hb, HCT,** WBC, MCHC, PLT, vitamin – (B_{12}, folate)

megaloblastic anemia

⟶ ↑ ACP, **aldolase, anisocytes,** APA, RBC basophilic stippling, Bil, **unconjugated Bil,** elliptocytes, eos, **Fe,** ✳ **ferritin,** gastrin, G6PD (RBC), HbA2, HbF, ✳ **homocysteine,** RBC Howell–Jolly bodies, ICD, LA, **LD,** LD – (1, 2), **macrocytes,** ✳ **MCH,** ✳ **MCV,** MD, **megalocytes,** ✳ **methyl-malonic acid,** MPV, ovalocytes, PMN, poikilocytes, schistocytes, ✳ **RDW,** transferrin receptor, ✳ **sTfR**

⟶ ↓ Fe, RBC, haptoglobin, **Hb, HCT,** cholesterol, WBC, MPV, **neu,** RTC, **PLT,** vitamin – (B_1, ✳ B_{12}, folate)

■ *Urine* ↑ hemosiderin, methylmalonic acid

■ *Gastric Fluid* ↓ HCl, intrinsic factor, pepsin

myelophthisic anemia

⟶ ↑ nucleated RBC, RBC basophilic stippling, RTC

⟶ ↓ RBC, Hb, HCT, WBC, PLT

normochromic anemia

⟶ ↑ creatinine

⟶ ↓ **HCT,** Fe, TIBC

pernicious anemia

↑ **AMA**, ANA, **anisocytes**, **APA**, antimicrosomal Ab, **antithyroglobulin Ab**, **antithyroidal Ab**, **Bil**, **unconjugated Bil**, stippled RBC, eos, **Fe**, **ferritin**, **gastrin**, G6PD (RBC), **HbF**, HLA – (DR2, DR5), **homocysteine**, RBC Howell–Jolly bodies, nucleated RBC, **calcitonin**, **methylmalonic acid**, LD, LD – (1,2), WBC, macrocytes, **MCH**, MCHC, **MCV**, megaloblasts, **neu**, **poikilocytes**, * **anti-intrinsic factor Ab**, transferrin satur. (untreated), schistocytes, siderocytes, **TIBC**, transcobalamin II, transketolase, UBBC, * **antiparietal cell Ab**

↓ Al, **ALP**, **Bil**, **RBC**, factor – (II, XIII), **Hb**, **HCT**, cholesterol, CHS, lipids, uric acid, WBC, **neu**, pepsinogen, PL, PRA, RTC, transferrin satur. (early treatment), secretin, **TIBC**, transferrin, **PLT**, vitamin – (B_{12}, folate), Zn

■ *Urine* ↑ hemosiderin, catalase, **coproporphyrin I**, **methylmalonic acid**, uric acid, taurine, **UBG**, uropepsin

■ *Stool* ↑ fat, **UBG**

■ *Gastric Fluid* ↑ pH

↓ * **HCl**, intrinsic factor, **MAO**, volume, pepsin

■ *Sputum* ↑ blood

posthemorrhagic anemia

↑ **WBC** (2–5 hrs after), **neu**, * **RTC** (1–2 days after, peak 4–7 day), **PLT** (2–6 hrs after), * **transferrin**, * **sTfR**, * **transferrin satur.**

↓ albumin, proteins, * **ferritin**, clotting time, **RBC** (later), **Hb** (3–72 hrs after), **HCT** (3–72 hrs after), transferrin satur.

sickle-cell anemia

↑ ACHE (RBC), **ALP** (crisis), ALT, **Bil**, unconjugated Bil, **drepanocytes**, elliptocytes, **ESR**, **Fe**, glycated Hb, HbA2, **HbF**, * **HbS**, RBC Howell–Jolly bodies, hPL, CHS, nucleated RBC, * **sickle cells**, uric acid, LD, LD – (1, 2), **WBC**, MCV, MD, **neu**, **RBC osmotic resistance**, osmolality, P, **poikilocytes**, **RTC**, **siderocytes**, * **target cells**, **PLT**, urea, viscosity

↓ albumin, **ALP** (WBC), RBC, factor B, factor XIII, FSH, **ESR**, glutathione peroxidase (RBC), haptoglobin, **Hb**, **GHb**, **HCT**, MCV, **RBC osmotic fragility**, PL, TIBC, transferrin, Zn

■ *Urine* ↑ **proteins**, RBC, Hb, **hemosiderin**, **blood**, uric acid, volume, casts – (RBC)

↓ FSH

■ *Stool* ↑ UBG

■ *Synovial Fluid* ↑ WBC, **mono**, RBC, viscosity, volume

sideroblastic anemia

↑ **anisocytes**, elliptocytes, **Fe**, **ferritin**, **HbF**, hemosiderin, macrocytes, MCH, **MCV**, microcytes, **mono**, poikilocytes, **RDW**, RTC, **transferrin satur.**, **sideroblasts**, **siderocytes**, stippled RBC, target cells, PLT, free protoporphyrin (RBC), zinc protoporphyrin

↓ ALP (WBC), **RBC**, Fe, **Hb**, HbA2, HCT, **folate**, WBC, MCH, MCHC, MCV, neu, osmotic fragility (RBC), **RTC**, TIBC, **PLT**, **free protoporphyrin** (RBC), transferrin, vitamin – (B_6), volume (RBC)

sideropenic anemia

↑ * **anisocytes**, **anulocytes**, APA, * **elliptocytes**, EPO, **GHb**, * **microcytes**, RBC osmotic resistance, PMN, poikilocytes, porphyrins, * **RDW**, **target cells**, * **TIBC**, PLT, * **transferrin**, **transferrin receptor**, **free protoporphyrin** (RBC), zinc protoporphyrin

↓ * RBC, * Fe, * ferritin, glutathione peroxidase (RBC), * Hb, HbA2, HCT, catalase (RBC), WBC, * MCHC, * MCH, * MCV, neu, RBC osmotic fragility, RTC, * transferrin satur., TIBC, * PLT

thalassemia
– alpha thalassemia

↑ anisocytes, Fe, ferritin, glutathione peroxidase (RBC), HbF, microcytes, RBC, siderocytes, target cells

↓ RBC, haptoglobin, Hb, HbA2, HbF, HbH, HCT, MCH, MCHC, MCV, RTC, TIBC, transferrin, vitamin – (folic acid, B_{12})

– beta thalassemia major

↑ ADA, ACHE (RBC), ALT, * anisocytes, AST, RBC basophilic stippling, Bil, unconjugated Bil, Cu, elliptocytes, Fe, ferritin, GHb, * HbA2, *HbF, Hb (free), RBC Heinz bodies, nucleated RBC, sickle cells, uric acid, LD, WBC, pre-beta-LP, lym, microcytes, mono, RBC osmotic resistance, * poikilocytes, protoporphyrin (RBC), RBC, RTC, transferrin satur., transferrin receptor, transferrin satur., schistocytes, spherocytes, siderocytes, PLT, target cells, TAG, TIBC

↓ RBC, factors – (V, VII, IX, XI), G tolerance, haptoglobin, â Hb, HbA, HbA$_{1c}$, HbF, hemopexin, * HCT, cholesterol, folate, WBC, lipids (+RBC), MCH, MCHC, MCV, microcytes, P, RBC osmotic fragility, pyrimidine-5 nucleotidase (RBC), RTC, TIBC, transferrin, PLT, Zn

- ■ *Urine* ↑ amino acids, proteins, hemosiderin, UBG, urobilin
- ■ *Stool* ↑ UBG
  - ↓ UBG

– beta thalassemia minor

↑ ALT, anisocytes, RBC basophilic stippling, Bil, unconjugated Bil, Cu, Fe, ferritin, * HbA2, HbF, RBC Heinz bodies, catalase (RBC), sickle cells, microcytes, osmotic resistance (RBC), poikilocytes, RBC, RDW, RTC, transferrin receptor, transferrin satur., schistocytes, siderocytes, target cells

↓ RBC, folic acid, haptoglobin, Hb, HbA, HbA2, HCT, free protoporphyrin (RBC), cholesterol, MCH, MCHC, MCV, transferrin

- ■ *Urine* ↑ UBG
- ■ *Stool* ↑ UBG

– beta thalassemia trait

↑ anisocytes, Fe, HbA2, microcytes, ovalocytes, poikilocytes, RBC, RBC basophilic stippling, RTC, target cells, transferrin satur.

↓ Hb, MCV, RBC osmotic fragility

vitamin B$_{12}$/folate deficiency anemia

↑ aldolase, anisocytes, anti-intrinsic factor Ab, Bil, Bil unconjugated, BT, Cu, elliptocytes, eos, Fe, * ferritin, G6PD (+RBC), HbF, * homocysteine, RBC Howell–Jolly bodies, ICD (+RBC), LD, LD5, lysozyme, macrocytes, * MCH, * MCV, MD (+RBC), megalocytes, * methylmalonic acid, poikilocytes, RDW, * sTfR, UBBC

↓ ACHE, ALP, * Fe, * RBC, * Hb, HCT, cholesterol, CHS, complement – (C3), K, uric acid, WBC, neu, osmotic fragility (RBC), RTC, PLT, TIBC, vitamin – (B$_6$, * B$_{12}$, * folate)

- ■ *Urine* ↑ amino acids, N-forminio-glutamic acid, methylmalonic acid, taurine
  - ↓ uric acid

Anencephaly

↑ **AFP**

↓ estriol

- *Urine* ↓ **estriol**
- *Amniotic Fluid* ↑ acetylcholinesterase, * **AFP**, **volume**
  ↓ DHEAS, estriol, cortisol, GH

Anesthesia

spinal anesthesia

- *Cerebrospinal Fluid* ↑ WBC

total anesthesia

↑ G, HCO_3^-, cholesterol, acetoacetic acid, **ketobodies**, WBC, lipids, pCO_2

↓ chloride, pO_2, PLT, testosterone

- *Urine* ↑ **ketones**
  ↓ P

Aneurysm, Dissecting Aortic

↑ AMS, * **AST**, * **CK**, CRP, LD, cTnI, Mb, * **WBC**

↓ RBC, Hb, HCT

- *Urine* ↑ AMS
- *Pericardial Fluid* ↑ RBC, volume

Angina, Pectoral

↑ ALT, Apo B-100, AST, factor IV, G, GMT, **cholesterol**, creatinine, LDL-C, WBC, uric acid, Mb, cTnI

↓ ESR

unstable pectoral angina

↑ ALT, * **AST**, CRP, GP-BB, LD, * **WBC**, cTnI, cTnT

Angiocardiography

↑ **AST**, CK, CK-MB

Angioedema

acquired angioedema

↓ C1-esterase inhibitor, complement – (C1q)

hereditary angioedema

↑ AAT

↓ * **C1-esterase inhibitor**, complement – (C2, C3, **C4**)

- *Synovial Fluid* ↑ eos

Angioplasty, Percutaneous Transluminal Coronary

↑ AST, CK, CRP, CK-MB, fibrinogen, GP-BB, H-FABP, cTnT, cTnI

Angiitis, Hypersensitivity

↑ eos

↓ albumin

Anovulation

↑ **PRL**

↓ estradiol

- *Urine* ↓ estrogens, pregnanediol

Anorexia Nervosa

↑ aldosterone, AMS, Apo B, * **beta-carotene**, BT, **cholesterol**, K, ILGF-I, * **cortisol**, **creatinine**, * **ketobodies**, acetoacetic acid, **LDL-C**, **MAC**, **osmolality**, **PRL**, SHBG, **GH**, rT3, TAG, **urea**, vitamin – (D)

↓ ACE, **albumin**, AMS, **proteins**, Ca, RBC, **estradiol**, estrone, estrogens, FSH, ESR, **G**, Hb, HCT, chloride, **cholesterol**, IgG, IgM, IGF-I, **K**, creatinine, uric acid, **WBC**, LH, **Mg**, **Na**, norepinephrine, osteocalcin, P, pH, * **T3**, **T4**, testosterone, TIBC, **PLT**, urea, vitamin – (B_2, **folate**)

- *Urine* ↑ ketones, cortisol
  - ↓ estriol, FSH, 17-KS, 17-KGS
- *Sweat* ↑ chloride, Na

Anoxia

↑ G, catecholamines, * LA, LD, WBC, **neu**, pCO_2, troponin I
↓ eos, * pH, * pO_2

Aplasia

congenital pure RBC aplasia

↑ **adenosine deaminase** (RBC), **EPO**, PLT, **purine nucleoside phosphorylase** (RBC), transferrin satur.
↓ **Hb, HCT, RTC,** WBC

germinal aplasia

- *Urine* ↑ gonadotropin
  - ↓ 17-KS
- *Seminal Fluid* ↓ spermatozoa

lymphoid aplasia

↓ **IgA,** IgG, IgM

Apoplexy, Cerebral (stroke)

↑ Ab against beta-2 GP I, ACLA, ALT Apo E-IV, BT, **fibrinogen,** ESR, **G, Hb, uric acid, LD,** Lp(a), Na, **Ni, TAG**
↓ cholesterol
- *Urine* ↑ G, volume
- *Cerebrospinal Fluid* ↑ AST, albumin CFS/serum, * **proteins,** * **RBC,** * **G,** Hb, ICAM CSF/serum, IDH, * **blood,** * **LA,** LD, WBC, MBP, PG
  - ↓ G

Appendicitis, Acute

↑ AMS, * **CRP,** ESR, HCT, * **WBC,** neu, * **elastase** (PMN), PCT, SAA, urea
- *Urine* ↑ AMS, RBC, Hb, WBC
- *Peritoneal Fluid* ↑ RBC

Argininemia

↑ ammonia (after meals), * **arginine**
- *Urine* ↑ arginine, cystine, ornithine

Arrest, Cardiopulmonary

↑ AST, CK, K, * **LA,** MAC, MAL, * **mAST,** * pCO_2, * **pH,** pyruvate, RAC, RAL, troponin – (I, T)
↓ * **pH,** * pO_2, * O_2 satur.

Arteriosclerosis

↑ PLT adhesiveness, Apo – (B, C-III), Apo E (2/2, 4/4 phenotypes), antibody against Chlamydia pneumoniae, Cd, **ceruloplasmin,** CO_2, CRP, **Cu,** RBC, factor – (VII, VIII), **fibrinogen,** G, glycoprotein IIIa (PLA1/2), HCO_3^-, **homocysteine, cholesterol,** uric acid, **creatinine, LDL-C, lipids,** Lp(a), A2MG, MDA, P, pCO_2, PAI-1, PDGF, **TAG, urea,** volume (RBC), Zn
↓ Apo – (AI, AII), **HDL-C,** cholesterol, Leiden's factor, LCAT (early), lipase, Mg, paraoxonase, prostacyclin, Se, volume (RBC)
Note: gene polymorphism – (ACE D/D, angiotensinogen, Apo B XbaI, CBS, factor Leiden, MTHFR)
- *Urine* ↑ RBC, Hb, crystals – (urate)
- *Cerebrospinal Fluid* ↑ proteins, LA

Arteritis

cranial arteritis

↑ * ESR

Takayasu's arteritis

↑ **alpha-2-globulins**, CIC, fibrinogen, **ESR**, **gamma globulins**, HLA – (**Bw2**, **Bw52**, **DQ**, **DR4**), IgA, IgG, **IgM**, **WBC**, **LE cells**, lym, **neu**

↓ albumin, **Hb**, **HCT**

■ *Urine* ↑ **estrogens** (females)

temporal arteritis (giant cell a.)

↑ AAT, ACLA, alpha-1-globulins, **alpha-2-globulins**, **ALP**, **ALT**, ANA, ANCA, p-ANCA, **AST**, CIC, **CRP**, **ESR**, haptoglobin, **HLA** – (**B8**, **DR4**), IgG, IgM, IL-6, **WBC**, mono, PLT

↓ albumin, B-lym, RBC, **Hb**, **HCT**, complement – (C3), T-lym (CD8+)

Arthritis

arthritis associated with hemochromatosis

↑ ADA, **AFP**, **ALT**, **AST**, **Ca**, Cu, D-dimers, * **Fe**, * **ferritin**, G, HLA – (**A3**, **B7**, **B14**), CHS, WBC, PTH, * **transferrin satur.**, siderocytes, GH, TIBC

↓ ACTH, Cu, **FSH**, LH, P, PTH, GH, testosterone, * **TIBC**, **transferrin**, TSH

■ *Urine* ↑ **Fe**, G, Hb, **hemosiderin**, porphyrins

■ *Synovial Fluid* ↑ crystals – (calcium pyrophosphate), WBC, viscosity, volume

chronic arthritis

↑ ceruloplasmin, Cu, D-dimers, uric acid, mucoproteins

↓ cholesterol

■ *Urine* ↑ 17-KS

■ *Synovial Fluid* ↑ ALP

↓ aldolase, arylsulfatase, LD, N-acetylglucosaminidase, pH

fungal arthritis

■ *Synovial Fluid* ↑ **clot formation**, WBC, **volume**

gonorrheal arthritis

↑ **WBC**

■ *Synovial Fluid* ↑ * **bacteria** (+ culture), **WBC**, **neu**, volume

↓ **G**

hemophilic arthritis

■ *Synovial Fluid* ↑ volume, **RBC**, **volume**

infectious arthritis

↑ alpha-1-globulins, alpha-2-globulins, * **A2MG**, **bacteria** (culture), conjugated Bil, D-dimers, **ESR**, uric acid, **WBC**, urea

↓ complement – (CH50), transferrin satur.

■ *Synovial Fluid* ↑ * **bacteria** (+ culture), A2MG, proteins, alpha-2-globulins, clot formation, gamma globulins, LA, LD, **WBC**, **PMN**, **volume**

↓ albumin, G, viscosity

Lyme arthritis

↑ ALP, ALT, * **Ab against B. burgdorferi**, **AST**, **treponemal antibodies** (false), CIC, CK-MB, D-dimers, **ESR**, GMT, **HLA** – (**DR2**, **DR4**), IgG, **IgM**, **cryoglobulins**, LAP, LD, 5-NT, **WBC**

↓ RBC, ESR, Hb, HCT, WBC

■ *Synovial Fluid* ↑ C3, C4, CIC, eos, pus, WBC, PMN

↓ viscosity

psoriatic arthritis

↑ alpha-2-globulins, ceruloplasmin, **CRP, ESR,** RF, **HLA** – (**A2, B7, B13, B16, B27, BW17, Bw38, Bw39, CW6, DR4, DR7**), complement – (**C3, C4**), **WBC,** uric acid

↓ RBC, Hb

■ *Synovial Fluid* ↑ ✱ **ALP, C3,** ✱ **WBC, clot formation, volume,** PMN
  ↓ G, viscosity

pyogenic arthritis

↑ **bacteria** (culture), **CRP, ESR, mucoproteins,** RF, **WBC**

↓ G

■ *Synovial Fluid* ↑ ✱ **bacteria** (+ culture), **clot formation,** proteins, volume, WBC

rheumatoid arthritis

↑ **AAT,** Ab against salivary duct, **ACA, ACE, AGP, alpha-1-globulins, alpha-2-globulins, ALP,** ALT, **A2MG, AMA, ANA,** ANCA, **p-ANCA, anti-ss-DNA, anti-ds-DNA,** antiendothelial Ab, anti-HSP 65, alpha-1-anti-chymotrypsin, **antikeratine Ab, antimicrosomal Ab,** anti-p 56, anti-poly (ADP-ribose), anti-RA33, **anti-RNP,** anti-Scl-70, anti-Ro/SSA, anti-La, Ha/SSB, antithyroglobulin Ab, **antithyroidal Ab, APF, ASLO,** ASMA, **betaglobulins,** B2M, **proteins,** Ca, CEA, **ceruloplasmin, CIC, CRP, Cu,** D-dimers, **elastase, eos, ESR,** ferritin, **fibrinogen,** phospholipase A2, **gamma globulins, gastrin,** glycated Hb, **GMT, haptoglobin,** hexosaminidase, HLA – (B27, DPw4, DQ7, DQw7, DR1, DR4, DR6, Dw4, Dw10, Dw13, Dw14, Dw15), h-sICAM-1, h-sVCAM-1, **IgA,** IgD, IgE, **IgG, IgM,** IFN-gamma, IL – (1, 6, 8), complement – (Ba, Bb, C1q, C2, C3, C4, C4d, C9), **creatine, uric acid, cryoglobulins, glutamic acid,** bile acids, **WBC, LD, LE cells,** lupus inhibitor, lym, **Mn, mono, mucoproteins,** 5-NT, neopterin, **neu,** osteocalcin, PT, **anti-DNA-histone complex Ab,** RANA, RF – (✱ **IgA,** ✱ **IgM**), N-telopeptides, TNF-alpha, transferrin, **PLT,** urea, VDRL (false), **viscosity**

↓ **albumin,** ALP, A2MG, **amino acids, arginine,** AT III, beta-galactosidase, beta-2-glycoprotein I, **CK,** proteins, EPO, **RBC, Fe,** glutamine, glycoproteins, G tolerance, **Hb, HCT,** HDL-C, histidine, **cholesterol,** complement – (**C1r,** C1s, C2, **C3, C4, CH50**), LDL-C, lipids, **WBC,** Mb, MCV, neu, osteocalcin, pCO_2, **transferrin satur., TIBC,** transferrin, vitamin – (C, D), Zn

■ *Urine* ↑ **alanine,** albumin, **Cu, glutamine, glycine, hexosaminidase,** hydroxyproline
  ↓ catecholamines, cysteine, glutamic acid, pyridoxine, threonine, tyrosine

■ *Synovial Fluid* ↑ ✱ **aldolase,** AAT, **ACP,** ANA, ✱ **ALP,** alpha-1-antichymotrypsin, B2M, ✱ **N-acetyl-beta-D-glucosaminidase, proteins, ceruloplasmin, clot formation,** Cu, eos, RBC, pus, IFN-gamma, IgM, IL – (1, 2, **6,** 8), trypsin inhibitor, complement – (**C3**), LA, ✱ **LD, WBC, lym,** lymphokines, macrophages, **neu,** 5-NT, PG, PMN, **ragocytes, RF,** TNF-alpha, beta-thromboglobulin, volume

↓ complement – (C3, C4), **G,** factor B, chylomicrons, pH, **viscosity,** ✱ **mucin clotting**

■ *Pericardial Fluid* ↑ proteins, cholesterol, gamma globulin, LD
  ↓ complement – (C4), G

- **Pleural Fluid** ↑ adenosine deaminase, **proteins**, CIC, CSF – (GM, M), eos, epithelial cells, RBC, crystals – (cholesterol), LD, WBC, **lym**, mono, mononuclear cells, neu, PMN, **RF**
  ↓ **C3, C4, G, pH**, viscosity
- **Bronchoalveolar Lavage Fluid** ↑ lym
- **Gastric Fluid** ↑ pH
  ↓ HCl
- **Saliva** ↑ IgA, Na

juvenile rheumatoid arthritis (Still's disease)

↑ alpha globulins, **ALT, ANA, anti-ds-DNA, anti-ss-DNA, anti-RNP, ASLO, AST**, complement – (**C3, C4**), CIC, **CRP, ESR, gamma globulins, ferritin**, GMT, **haptoglobin**, HLA – (**B27**, Dpw2, DR1, DR4, DR5, DR8, DRw6, DRw8, Dw4, Dw14, Dw5, Dw52), immunoglobulins, **WBC**, LE cells, **neu, RF, PLT**

↓ **albumin**, A2MG, **RBC**, ESR, **Fe, Hb, HCT**, IgG, WBC, PLT, TIBC, vitamin – (C)

- **Synovial Fluid** ↑ **WBC**, C3, clot formation, lym, mono, plasmocytes, volume, PMN
  ↓ complement – (**C3, C4**), **G**, viscosity

septic arthritis

↑ **ESR, WBC, PMN**

- **Synovial Fluid** ↑ proteins, **clot formation**, RBC, **pus**, LA, LD, WBC, **neu, PMN, ragocytes, volume**
  ↓ **G**, pH, WBC, **viscosity**

syphilitic arthritis

↑ WBC, lym

- **Synovial Fluid** ↑ clot formation, WBC, PMN

traumatic arthritis

↑ WBC

- **Synovial Fluid** ↑ **clot formation, volume**

tuberculous arthritis

↑ WBC

- **Synovial Fluid** ↑ eos, clot formation, pus, **WBC, lym**, macrophages, **neu**, PMN, volume
  ↓ **G**, viscosity

uratic arthritis (gouty a.)

↑ **ADA, alanine**, Apo E, **AST**, ✶ **CRP**, ✶ **ESR** (attack), RF, **cholesterol**, IDL-C, IgG, complement (total), **glutamic acid** (+RBC), ✶ **uric acid**, creatinine, WBC (attack), **neu**, ✶ **TAG, urea**

↓ alpha-1-globulins, alpha-2-globulins, **glycine**, complement (total), P, serine

- **Urine** ↑ alpha-aminonitrogen, albumin, **proteins**, ✶ **urate crystals**, ✶ **uric acid**
  ↓ GFR, **17-KS**, 17-OHCS, 17-KGS, pH, uric acid
- **Synovial Fluid** ↑ aldolase, **proteins**, complement – (**C3**, total c.), clot formation, phagocytes, pus, ragocytes, crystals – (✶ **monosodium urate**), uric acid, LD, ✶ **WBC**, mono, **neu**, PMN, volume
  ↓ **G**, viscosity

viral arthritis

↑ neopterin, WBC, lym, RF

- ■ *Synovial Fluid* ↑ clot formation, WBC, **lym**, mono
  ↓ viscosity

Arthropathy

Charcot's arthropathy

- ■ *Synovial Fluid* ↑ RBC, WBC, viscosity, crystals – (hydroxyapatite), volume

crystal arthropathy

- ■ *Synovial Fluid* ↑ cholesterol, crystals – (hydroxyapatite, cholesterol, drugs, uric acid), volume, WBC, PMN
  ↓ **G, viscosity**

destructive arthropathy

- ■ *Synovial Fluid* ↑ crystals – (hydroxyapatite)

Asbestosis

↑ ACA, ACE, RF, ANA, ESR, gamma globulins
↓ pO_2

- ■ *Pleural Fluid* ↑ eos, RBC, WBC, lym, CD4/CD8, B-lym, LTB4
- ■ *Sputum* ↑ ✻ asbestos particles
- ■ *Bronchoalveolar Lavage Fluid* ↑ ✻ asbestos particles

Ascites

↑ AMS, AMS (P), conjugated Bil, **TAG** (chylous)
↓ **albumin, proteins**

- ■ *Urine* ↑ **AMS**, proteins
  ↓ K, pH
- ■ *Peritoneal Fluid* ↑ ALP, AMS, bacteria (+ culture), **proteins**, GMT, HCO_3^-, RBC, blood, K, LD, WBC, metHb, neu, P, PMN, **volume, TAG**, turbidity, color changes
  ↓ cholesterol, HCO_3^-, pH

Asphyxia

↑ catecholamines, PLT

- ■ *Urine* ↑ G

Asplenia

↑ acanthocytes

Assault, Sexual (rape)

- ■ *Vaginal Fluid* ↑ ✻ ACP, ✻ spermatozoa, ✻ spermatozoa motility

Asthma, Bronchial

↑ AAT, **ADH, ASMA**, AST, CIC, CK, Cu, 2,3-DPG, **eos, eosinophil cationic protein**, G, h-sICAM-1, Hb, HCT, HCO_3^-, uric acid, LA, LD, LD5, WBC, neu, ✻ pCO_2, ✻ **pH** (early stage of attack), pyruvate, MAC (later), RF, ✻ **RAC, RAL** (early)
↓ K, HCO_3^-, cortisol, complement – (C4), Na, pCO_2 (early stage of attack), pH, pO_2, pH, vitamin – (B_6)

- ■ *Urine* ↑ VMA
- ■ *Pleural Fluid* ↑ eos
- ■ *Sputum* ↑ **Curschmann's spirals, eos, Charcot–Leyden crystals**
- ■ *Bronchoalveolar Lavage Fluid* ↑ IL-2
- ■ *Sweat* ↑ chloride

allergic bronchial asthma

↑ ADH, CIC, **eos**, ✻ **eosinophil cationic protein**, IgE, IgE specific Ab, WBC, pCO_2, **pH** (early stage of attack), MAC (later), **RAC, RAL**
↓ Na, pCO_2 (early stage of attack), pO_2, PLT, vitamin – (B_6)

- ■ *Sputum* ↑ bacteria (+ culture), **Curshmann's spirals**, **eos**, **histiocytes**, mucus, **Charcot–Leyden crystals**, **PMN**, **viscosity**, color changes
- ■ *Urine* ↑ VMA
- ■ *Pleural Fluid* ↑ eos

Ataxia Teleangiectasia

- ↑ **∗ AFP**, ALT, ALP anti-EBV Ab, **B-lym**, **∗ CEA**, beta-LP, FSH, G, **IgM**, LH, **phytanic acid**, T-lym (CD8), vitamin – (E)
- ↓ IgA, IgE, IgG, beta-LP, 17-KS, **lym**, **T-lym (CD4)**, vitamin – (E)

Note: mitochondrial DNA (molecular genetic analysis), decreased cellular imunity

Atelectasis, Pulmonary

- ↑ WBC
- ↓ pO$_2$

Atherosclerosis

- ↑ Apo A, Apo – (B, C-III), Apo E (2/2, 4/4 phenotypes), antibody against Chlamydia pneumoniae, PLT adhesiveness, ceruloplasmin, CRP, Cu, factor – (VII, VIII), **fibrinogen**, G, glycoprotein IIIa (PLA1/2), HCO$_3^-$, **homocysteine**, **cholesterol**, **uric acid**, **creatinine**, **LDL-C**, **lipids**, Lp(a), MDA, P, PF4, PAI-1, PDGF, **TAG**, beta-thromboglobulin, **urea**, Zn
- ↓ HDL-C, LCAT (early), Leiden's factor, lipase, Mg, paraoxonase, prosta-cyclin, vitamin – (B$_{12}$, folate)
- ■ *Urine* ↑ RBC, Hb, crystals – (urate)
- ■ *Cerebrospinal Fluid* ↑ proteins, LA

Note: gene polymorphism – (ACE D/D, angiotensinogen, Apo B XbaI, CBS, factor Leiden, MTHFR)

Atopy

- ↑ eos, **IgE**
- ■ *Sweat* ↑ chloride, Na

Atransferrinemia

acquired atransferrinemia

- ↑ transferrin satur., **sTfR**
- ↓ **Fe**, **TIBC**, **∗ transferrin**

congenital atransferrinemia

- ↑ Fe, transferrin satur., **sTfR**
- ↓ **∗ beta globulins**, RBC, Fe, Hb, HCT, TIBC, **∗ transferrin**

Atresia

biliary atresia

- ↑ alpha-1-globulins, **ALP**, **ALT**, **AST**, **Bil**, **conjugated Bil**, unconjugated Bil, **CK-BB**, clotting time, CRP, elastase, fibrinogen, GMD, **GMT**, **hapto-globin**, ICD, bile acids, **PT**, LP-X
- ↓ factor II, vitamin – (**E**, B$_2$)
- ■ *Urine* ↑ galactose, **conjugated Bil**, pH, pregnanediol, **UBG** (infection)
- ■ *Stool* ↓ **Bil**, UBG

duodenal atresia

- ↑ **AFP**
- ■ *Amniotic Fluid* ↑ AFP, volume

esophageal atresia

- ↑ **AFP**
- ■ *Amniotic Fluid* ↑ AFP, volume

urethral atresia

- ■ *Amniotic Fluid* ↓ volume

Atrophy, Muscular

      ↑ CK, CK-mass, Mb, **＊ myokinase, ＊ mitochondrial DNA**
- *Urine* ↑ **creatine**
      ↓ creatine, creatinine

Azoospermia

- *Seminal Fluid* ↓ ACP, citrate, alpha-glucosidase, Mg, fructose, Zn

Bacteremia

      ↑ **ESR, IL-6, WBC**

Balanitis

      ↑ **CRP, ESR, WBC**
- *Urine* ↑ **pus**

Berylliosis

      ↑ **ACE**, Ca, **RBC, gamma globulins**, Hb, WBC, uric acid
- *Urine* ↑ **＊ beryllium**, Ca

Biopsy of Prostate

      ↑ PAP, PSA

Bladder Catheterisation

      ↑ PSA
- *Urine* ↑ RBC, Hb, WBC

Blockage, Subarachnoid Spinal

- *Cerebrospinal Fluid* ↓ **pressure**

Bronchiectasis

      ↑ proteins, WBC
      ↓ **＊ AAT, ＊ alpha-1-globulins**, proteins, RBC, Hb, HCT, **＊ immunoglobu-lins**, pO_2
- *Sputum* ↑ bacteria (+ culture), **pus, blood, volume**, PMN, viscosity, color changes

Bronchiolitis

      ↑ RAC, **WBC**

Bronchitis

   acute bronchitis

      ↑ AAT, ammonia, **＊ CRP**, eos, **＊ fibrinogen, ＊ ESR**, LA, **＊ WBC, ＊ muco-proteins**, Na
      ↓ AMS
- *Sputum* ↑ **＊ bacteria** (+ culture), pus, **blood**, volume, **viscosity**
- *Pleural Fluid* ↑ eos
- *Bronchoalveolar Lavage Fluid* ↑ bacteria (+ culture)

   chronic bronchitis

      ↑ **＊ ACE, ＊ CEA, ＊ eos**, RBC, ESR, Hb, HCT, LA, **＊ WBC, ＊ pCO_2**, RAC
      ↓ **＊ AAT**, AMS, Hb, HCT, pO_2
- *Sputum* ↑ **＊ bacteria** (+ culture), eos, blood, volume, **Charcot–Leyden crystals**, PMN
- *Bronchoalveolar Lavage Fluid* ↑ bacteria (+ culture)

Bronchopneumonia

      ↑ AAT, ANA, **＊ CRP**, eos, **＊ fibrinogen, ＊ ESR**, LA, LD, **＊ WBC**, mucopro-teins, **neu**, NSE, orosomucoid, **＊ pCO_2, RAL**
      ↓ **albumin**, proteins, **＊ chloride**, IgA, WBC, Na, neu, P, **pO_2**
- *Pleural Fluid* ↑ eos, WBC, neu
- *Sputum* ↑ bacteria (+ culture), pus, blood, WBC, volume, PMN, vis-cosity

- *Urine* ↑ alpha-aminonitrogen, **proteins**, ketones, creatinine, uric acid, WBC, casts – (granular, hyaline)
  ↓ chloride

Bulimia

↑ AMS, HCO_3^- (vomiting), ketobodies, **cortisol**, **MAC** (laxatives), **MAL** (vomiting), P, pH (vomiting)

↓ FSH, HCO_3^- (laxatives), **chloride**, **K**, LH, **Na**, pH (laxatives), PRL, progesterone, serotonin, T3

- *Urine* ↑ pH

Burns

↑ **PLT adhesion**, AGP, albumin (early stage), **aldolase**, aldosterone, **alpha-1-globulins**, **alpha-2-globulins**, ALT, amino acids, AMS, **AST**, proteins (early), CK, CRP, RBC, factor – (V, VIII), **FDP**, phenylalanine, ferritin, fibrinogen (later), **ESR**, glucagon, glycine, **haptoglobin**, **Hb**, **HCT**, chloride, IgE, K, carboxy-Hb (inhalation), complement – (C3a, C5a), **creatinine**, LD 5, WBC, Na, **neu**, Ni, norepinephrine, ornithine, osmolality, RBC osmotic fragility, P, pCO_2, pemphigus Ab, PLT, proline (2nd day), schistocytes, spherocytes, **urea**, **viscosity**, VLDL-C

↓ **albumin** (later stage), **AMS**, Apo B, AT III, **proteins** (later), **Ca**, Ca^{2+}, Cr, Cu, **eos**, **FDP**, fibrinogen (acute), G, Hb, HCT, **chloride**, cholesterol, CHS, **IgA**, **IgG**, **IgM**, isoleucine, K, complement – (C1r, C1s, C2, C3, C4, C5, C6, C7, C8, C9, CH50), LDL-C, leucine, lym, **Mg**, Mn, Na, osmolality, plasma volume, **RBC osmotic resistance**, pH, **pO_2**, proline (4th day), TAG, valine (4th day), **Zn**

- *Urine* ↑ amino acids, AMS, asparagine, cystathionine, RBC, G, glycine, **Hb**, hemosiderin, hexosaminidase, total hydroxyproline, 17-KGS, leucine, WBC, lysozyme, **Mb**, 3-methylhistidine, serine, taurine, threonine, tyrosine, valine
  ↓ methionine, vitamin C
- *Sputum* ↑ casts – (mucin + fibrin + WBC + cell debris during inhalation burns)
- *Cerebrospinal Fluid* ↑ leucine

Bursitis

- *Synovial Fluid* ↑ crystals – (hydroxyapatite)

Bypass

aortocoronary bypass

↑ cTnT, cTnI, APTT, CK-MB (mass)

↓ uric acid

- *Urine* ↑ hexosaminidase

Cachexia

↑ acetone, alpha-1-globulins, amino acids, AMS, beta globulins, BHBA, Bil, unconjugated Bil, Ca, gamma globulins, **ESR** (advanced), glucagon, K, creatinine, uric acid, MAC, Na, urea

↓ albumin, ALP, AMS, **proteins**, Ca, C-peptide, EPO, Fe, ESR, **fibrinogen**, G, HCO_3^-, **cholesterol**, CHS, **insulin**, K, LDL-C, lipase, **lym**, Mg, osmolality, P, **T3**, **TAG**, TBG, TIBC, urea

- *Urine* ↑ acetone, alpha-aminonitrogen, Ca, chloride, creatine, creatinine, uric acid, Na, volume, VMA
  ↓ chloride, creatinine, uric acid, 17-KS, osmolality, pH
- *Stool* ↓ UBG

Cardiomyopathy

↑ ALT, AST, **antimyocardial Ab**, BSP retention, **CK**, CK-MB, Co, creatinine, eos, ESR, RBC, LA, LD, **NT-pro-ANP**

↓ Ca, carnitine, Fe, Hb, HCT, lym, P, **Se**

■ *Urine* ↓ Se

■ *Pericardial Fluid* ↑ RBC, WBC

■ *Ascitic Fluid* ↑ RBC, WBC

Carnosinemia

↑ * carnosine

■ *Urine* ↓ * homocarnosine, * carnosine

■ *Cerebrospinal Fluid* ↑ homocarnosine, carnosine

Castration

female castration

↑ FSH

■ *Urine* ↑ FSH

male castration

↓ ACP

■ *Urine* ↓ 17-KS

Catabolism

↑ ALA, BHBA, Glu, K, **ketones**, creatinine, Mg, osmolality (acute), **urea**, FFA

↓ G, lipids, osmolality (chronic), TAG

■ *Urine* ↓ Se

Cellulitis

↑ D-dimers, WBC

Chloridorrhea, Congenital

↑ * MAC

↓ * chloride, * K

■ *Stool* ↑ * volume, * chloride
    ↓ pH

Cholangiopancreatography, Endoscopic, Retrograde (ERCP)

↑ * AMS, * lipase, trypsin

Cholangitis

↑ **ALP**, ALP (isoenzymes), * **ALT**, **AST**, AMS, **Bil**, conjugated Bil, Bil unconjugated, eos, **ESR**, chenodeoxycholic acid, cholic acid, cholesterol, **GMT**, granulocytes, IgG, **LAP**, LD, lipase, lipids, neu, 5-NT, **TAG**, **bile acids**, **WBC**

↓ G, PLT

■ *Urine* ↑ **AMS, conjugated Bil**, UBG

■ *Stool* ↓ UBG

primary sclerosing cholangitis

↑ **ALP**, **ALT**, **ANA**, * **ANCA**, ASMA, **AST**, **Bil** (later), conjugated Bil, **ceruloplasmin**, **gamma globulins**, **GMT**, HLA – (DR52), * **IgG**, IgM, **antineutrophil nuclear Ab**

↓ albumin

Cholecystitis

↑ alpha-1-globulins, alpha-2-globulins, **ALP**, ALP (isoenzymes), **ALT**, **AMS**, **AST**, **Bil**, BSP retention, **CA 19-9**, **CEA**, **ESR**, gamma globulins, **GMT**, cholesterol, LAP, **lipase**, neu, 5-NT, OCT, **WBC**

↓ **albumin**, AMS, **proteins**

■ *Urine* ↑ **AMS**, conjugated Bil, **UBG**

■ *Saliva* ↑ GMT

acute cholecystitis

↑ alpha-1-globulins, alpha-2-globulins, **ALP, ALT, AMS, AST, Bil, conjugated Bil**, unconjugated Bil, CK-MB, CRP, clotting time, elastase, fibrinogen, **ESR**, gamma globulins, GMD, **GMT, haptoglobin**, hexosaminidase, **cholesterol**, IgA, LAP, 5-nucleotidase, **lipase, PT**, TAG, **WBC**

↓ factor II, vitamin – (B_2)

■ *Urine* ↑ **AMS, conjugated Bil, pH, UBG**

■ *Stool* ↓ **Bil, UBG**

chronic cholecystitis

↑ alpha-1-globulins, alpha-2-globulins, **ALP, ALT, AMS, AST, Bil**, conjugated Bil, unconjugated Bil, **CA 19-9, CEA**, CRP, clotting time, elastase, fibrinogen, **ESR**, gamma globulins, **GMT**, cholesterol, **lipase**, WBC

↓ **albumin, proteins**

Cholecystopathy

↑ AMS, cholesterol, lipase

Choledocholithiasis

↑ * **ALP**, ALP (WBC), **ALT**, * **AMS, Bil**, * **Bil conjugated**, Bil unconjugated, ceruloplasmin, * **GMT**, cholesterol, chenodeoxycholic acid, cholic acid, * **LAP**, * **WBC**, lipase, lipids, * **LP-X, TAG, bile acids**

■ *Urine* ↑ **AMS, Bil, conjugated Bil**, UBG

■ *Stool* ↓ UBG

Cholelithiasis

↑ * **ALP, ALT**, AMS, AST, **Bil**, * **Bil conjugated**, CA 19-9, * **GMT**, chenodeoxycholic acid, cholic acid, cholesterol, immunoreactive trypsin, **LAP, WBC**, LD, * **lipase**, * **5-nucleotidase**, somatostatin, **TAG, bile acids, trypsin**

■ *Urine* ↑ conjugated Bil
   ↓ UBG

■ *Stool* ↑ fat

■ *Cerebrospinal Fluid* ↑ AMS

Cholestasis

↑ * **ALP**, ALP (isoenzyme, WBC), * **ALT, AMA**, * **AMS**, Apo E, AST, **beta globulins** (later), **Bil**, * **Bil conjugated, Bil unconjugated**, ceruloplasmin, **Cu**, delta Bil, Fe, ESR, * **GMT**, HDL-C, **cholesterol, IgM**, * **chenodeoxycholic acid, cholic acid**, * **LAP**, LDL-C, lipase, lipids, * **LP-X**, * **5-nucleotidase**, PT, PL, * **TAG**, * **bile acids**

↓ albumin (later), Apo A-I, AT III, RBC, Fe, Hb, HDL-C, HCT, prothrombin, vitamin – (B_{12}, E)

■ *Urine* ↑ **conjugated Bil**, UBG

■ *Sweat* ↑ chloride

familial intrahepatic cholestasis

↑ conjugated Bil

Chondrocalcinosis

↑ PTH

■ *Synovial Fluid* ↑ complement – (**C3**), pus, crystals – (* **calcium pyrophosphate**), WBC, PMN, RBC, volume

   ↓ **viscosity**

Chorea Huntington's

↑ FFA

↓ alanine, amino acids, isoleucine, leucine, proline, tyrosine, valine

---

Chorioamnionitis

↑ **CRP**, elastase, **WBC**

Choriomeningitis, Lymphocytic

↑ ✱ **antibodies against arenavirus** (IgG, IgM), lym, **WBC**

↓ WBC (early), PLT

■ *Cerebrospinal Fluid* ↑ ✱ **antibodies against arenavirus** (IgG, IgM), proteins, **lym**

Chorioretinitis

↑ **anti-toxocara Ab**, lym, **WBC**

Chylothorax

↓ **lym**

■ *Pleural Fluid* ↑ cholesterol, blood, lipids, **lym**, TAG

Circulation, Extracorporeal

↑ euglobulin lysis time, complement – (C3a, C5a), LA

↓ A2MG, neu, PLT

Cirrhosis

alcoholic cirrhosis

↑ **AAT, ACE**, ACP, ACP (prostatic), **AFP, acanthocytes**, albumin, aldolase, ✱ **aldosterone**, ✱ **ALP**, ALP (isoenzymes), alpha-2-globulins, ✱ **ALT**, AMA, A2MG, amino acids, ✱ **ammonia, AMS**, ANA, ✱ **anti-HCV Ab**, anti-HBc, Apo – (A-I, A-II, B), **ASMA**, ✱ **AST**, ✱ **Bil**, conjugated Bil, unconjugated Bil, BSP retention, CA 19-9, **carbohydrate-deficient transferrin**, CEA, ✱ **ceruloplasmin**, CK, CK-MB, estrogens, factor – (VIII), **FDP, Fe, ESR**, G, **gamma globulins** (later), **globulins**, glucagon, **GMT**, HBsAg, HBcAg, HBV-DNA, HCV-RNA, cold agglutinins, **cholesterol**, ✱ **IgA**, ✱ **IgG**, IgM, IL-6, insulin, **calcitonin**, creatinine, LA, uric acid, **LD**, LD5, lecithin (RBC), lipase, **WBC**, LPs, beta-LPs, MAC+RAL, MCV, NT-pro-ANP, **5-NT, OCT**, orosomucoid, osmolality, Pb, **PT, PL**, RAL, RF, rT3, RTC, SHBG, somatostatin, T4, ✱ **TAG**, transferrin saturation, triiodothyronine resin uptake, tropomyosin, TSH, urea, bile acids

↓ **albumin** (later), ALT, AST, C3, **Ca**, CHS, carbohydrate-deficient transferrin (false), CK, Cr, **RBC**, Fe, **G**, G tolerance, haptoglobin, **Hb, HCT**, cholesterol, C1-INH, **K**, complement – (C3, C4), uric acid, WBC, **Mg** (+RBC), Mn, **Na**, osteocalcin, P, porphyrins, prealbumin, RBP, RTC, T3, PLT, TIBC, transferrin, urea, vitamin – (B₁, B₆, folate)

■ *Urine* ↑ **aldosterone**, amino acids, AMS, K, Mg, P, bile acids

↓ volume

■ *Pleural Fluid* ↑ AMS

■ *Peritoneal Fluid* ↑ WBC

↓ proteins, specific gravity

■ *Cerebrospinal Fluid* ↑ amino acids

cardiac cirrhosis

↑ ACP, **AST**, Bil, conjugated Bil, unconjugated Bil

hepatic cirrhosis

↑ **AAT, ACE**, ACP, ACP (prostatic), **ADA, ADH, AFP, acanthocytes, aldolase**, ✱ **aldosterone**, ✱ **ALP**, ✱ **ALT**, AMA, A2MG, aminotripeptidase, ✱ **ammonia**, AMS, ANA, ✱ **anti-HCV Ab**, anti-HBc, Apo – (A-I, A-II, B), anti-thyroglobulin, arginase, APTL, **ASAL, ASMA**, ✱ **AST**, ATPase, bas, **beta-glucuronidase, proteins** (early, compensated), ✱ **Bil, conjugated Bil, unconjugated Bil**, B2M, BSP retention, BT, CA 19-9, CA

125, CEA, **carbohydrate-deficient transferrin**, ✱ **ceruloplasmin**, CHE, CK, CK-MB, C-peptide, **Cu**, euglobulin lysis time, **estradiol**, **estrogens**, factor – (VIII), **FDP**, Fe, phosphohexoisomerase, **FSH**, fumarase, **ESR**, FTI, G, ✱ **gamma globulins**, **gastrin**, G-6-PD, **glucagon**, glutathione reductase, glycerol, GMD, **GMT**, guanase, hCG, Hb (free), HBsAg, HBcAg, HBV-DNA, HCV-RNA, **hexosaminidase**, hydroxyproline, **cold agglutinins**, chloride, cholesterol, **ICD, IgA**, ✱ **IgG**, IgM, IL-6, **calcitonin**, immunoreactive proinsulin, insulin, chenodeoxycholic acid, cholic acid, **uric acid**, creatinine, **cryoglobulins**, LA, **LAP**, **LD, LD5**, LE cells, **LH, WBC**, lipase, **lipids**, lipoprotein lipase, lym, MAL (later), MCV, MD, Mn, Na, neu, NT-pro-ANP, **5-nucleotidase**, orosomucoid, osmolality, plasma volume, **OCT, PT, PRA, PRL, RF, RTC**, SD, **SHBG**, somatostatin, GH, T3, rT3, **T4**, ✱ **TAG**, TBG, transferrin satur., triiodothyronine resin uptake, tropomyosin, trypsin, PLT, TSH, tyrosine, **urea, VIP**, viscosity, vitamin – (B$_{12}$), vitamin B$_{12}$ binding capacity, **bile acids**

↓ **AAT**, ✱ **albumin**, alpha-2-antiplasmin, A2MG, AMS, Apo AI, AT III, **proteins, Ca**, ceruloplasmin, Cu, **RBC**, factor – (V, IX), Fe, **fibrinogen, G**, G tolerance, haptoglobin, **Hb, HDL-C, HCT**, chloride, **cholesterol**, cholesterol esterase, **CHS**, IgG, **ILGF-I**, IGFBP-3, **C1-INH**, K, complement – (C3, C4), uric acid, **LDL-C, WBC, Mg** (+RBC), **mucoproteins, Na** (later), neu, Ni, orosomucoid, osmolality, **oxalate**, P, pentoses, plasmocytes, **prealbumin**, RBP, **RTC**, transferrin satur., Se, somatomedin C, T3, T4, **TBG, testosterone**, TIBC, transferrin, **PLT**, UBBC, **urea**, vitamin – (A, D, E, folate, niacin), volume (RBC), **Zn**

■ *Urine* ↑ alpha-aminonitrogen, aldosterone, amino acids, AMS, **Bil, conjugated Bil**, RBC, estrogens, fructose, **G**, K, coproporphyrin, crystals – (leucine, tyrosine), **uric acid**, bile acids, WBC, **osmolality**, PBG, **porphyrins**, reducing sugars, **UBG**, urobilin, casts – (granular, hyaline), **Zn**

　↓ 17-KS, Na, niacin, volume, pH, sulfate, UBG, urea

■ *Cerebrospinal Fluid* ↑ amino acids, proteins, **glutamine, tryptophan**
　↓ Zn

■ *Stool* ↑ blood, **fat**
　↓ UBG

■ *Pleural Fluid* ↑ AMS, eos, LA, mononuclear cells, pH, volume, WBC
　↓ A2MG, **proteins**, haptoglobin, hemopexin, LD, orosomucoid, specific gravity, WBC

■ *Peritoneal Fluid* ↑ **proteins**, chylomicrons, **RBC, WBC**
　↓ ✱ **proteins**, cholesterol, specific gravity, LA

■ *Saliva* ↑ GMT

posthepatitic cirrhosis
　　　↑ ALP, ALT, **IgG**, IgM

primary biliary cirrhosis
　　　↑ AAT, **ACE**, ACP (prostatic), alpha globulins, ✱ **ALP**, ✱ **ALT**, ✱ **AMA**, ✱ **ANA**, ✱ **ANCA**, anti-ds-DNA, **anti-ss-DNA**, antimitochondrial Ab, anti-Scl-70, anti-Ro/SSA, anti-La/SSB, antithyroidal Ab, **ASGP-R**, ✱ **ASMA**, AST, **beta globulins**, ✱ **Bil**, ✱ **conjugated Bil**, C3, ceruloplasmin, ✱ **CIC**, Cu, ESR, gamma globulins (later), ✱ **GMT**, HLA – (DRB8), HDL-C (early), ✱ **cholesterol**, IgA, IgG,

* **IgM**, **cryoglobulins**, chenodeoxycholic acid, cholic acid, LDL-C, WBC, **lipids**, **LP-X**, MAC, MAC+RAL, **5-nucleotidase**, PT, * **PL**, T4, **TAG** (later), **TBG**, transferrin satur., VLDL-C (early), **bile acids**

↓ **albumin** (later), Apo – (AI, AII, E), fibrinogen, **G**, complement – (**C3**, **C4**), **HDL-C** (later), **IGFBP-3**, C1-INH, **uric acid**, **lym**, **Na**, osteocalcin, PL, * **prothrombin**, RBP, TAG, **testosterone**, TIBC, **transferrin**, tri-iodothyronine resin uptake, PLT, vitamin – (A, D, E, K)

■ *Urine* ↑ amino acids, **Bil**, **conjugated Bil**, **Cu**, **UBG**
  ↓ UBG
■ *Stool* ↑ **fat**
  ↓ UBG

Citrullinemia

↑ **alanine**, **ammonia**, * **citrulline**, aspartic acid, glutamine
↓ arginine
■ *Urine* ↑ * **citrulline**, **glutamine**, orotic acid
■ *Cerebrospinal Fluid* ↑ * **citrulline**

Citrullinuria

↑ citrulline, glutamine, glycine, homocitrulline, hydroxyproline, aspartic acid, methionine, serine, valine
■ *Urine* ↑ alanine, arginine, * **citrulline**, cystathionine, cysteine, cystine, ethanolamine, glutamine, glycine, histidine, homocitrulline, hydroxylysine, hydroxyproline, aspartic acid, glutamic acid, lysine, ornithine, serine, threonine

Climacterium, Precoccious

↑ FSH, LH
■ *Urine* ↑ FSH

Coagulation, Disseminated Intravascular

acute disseminated i. coagulation

↑ **ACP**, **PLT Ab**, **APTT**, **beta-thromboglobulin**, unconjugated Bil, **BT**, * **D-dimers**, **platelet factor 4**, tissue factor, * **FDP**, fibrinogen, fibrinolytic activity, * **fibrinopeptide A**, cryofibrinogen, prothrombin factor 1+2, LD, WBC, MPV, neu, **PT** (acute form), RTC, **schistocytes**, thrombomodulin, **TT**, urea, vWF

↓ A2MG, alpha-2-antiplasmin, **AT III**, RBC, euglobulin fibrinolysis, factor B, factors – (II, V, VII, **VIII**, X, XIII), * **fibrinogen**, **fibrinopeptide A**, fibronectin, ESR, haptoglobin, Hb, HCT, complement – (**C3**, **CH50**), WBC, **PT** (subacute form), **plasminogen**, proaccelerin, protein C, protein S, * **PLT**

■ *Urine* ↑ RBC, FDP, Hb

chronic disseminated i. coagulation

↑ D-dimers, FDP, fibrinogen, fibrinolytic activity, PT, TT
↓ APTT, fibrinogen, plasminogen, PLT

Colitis

↑ Hb, HCT, G, chloride, Na, neu, pH
↓ albumin, proteins, chloride, lym, Mg, Na, pH, pCO$_2$
■ *Urine* ↓ specific gravity

collagenous colitis

↑ eos, ESR

pseudomembranous colitis

↑ **WBC**
↓ albumin
■ *Stool* ↑ **blood**, * **cytotoxins**, **Hb**, pH, **RBC**, **WBC**

ulcerative colitis

↑ AAT, Ab against Saccharomyces cerevisiae, alpha-1-globulins, alpha-2-globulins, alpha-1-antichymotrypsin, **ALP**, ALP (WBC), **ALT**, ANA, **ANCA, c-ANCA, p-ANCA**, atypical-ANCA, anti-La/SSB, **AST, bas**, CCK-PZ, eos, phospholipase A2, **ESR**, GM-CSF, **GMT, haptoglobin**, hCG, HLA – (B5, B8, DR2), IL – (1, 6, 8, 10), **C1-INH**, catecholamines, complement – (**C3**, C4), cryoglobulins, uric acid, LD, **WBC**, lupus inhibitor, lym, lysozyme, **mono**, motilin, neu, pH, **PT**, serotonin, somatostatin, TBG, TIBC, TM – (CA 19-9, **CEA**, M2-PK), TNF-alpha, **PLT**

↓ **albumin, proteins,** beta globulins, Ca, **RBC, Fe, Hb, HCT,** chloride, **cholesterol, K,** carotene, **WBC,** MCH, MCHC, MCV, **Mg, Na,** prealbumin, PT, PL, **PLT,** T3, transferrin satur., vitamin – (B$_6$, B$_{12}$), volume (plasma), Zn

- *Urine* ↑ Ca, catecholamines, **uric acid**
- *Stool* ↑ RBC, **frequency, Hb,** cholesterol, **mucus, pus, blood,** pH, **WBC, volume, fat**
- *Synovial Fluid* ↑ WBC, clot formation, PMN, volume
  ↓ viscosity

Collagenosis

↑ AAT, alpha-1-globulins, alpha-2-globulins, **AMA, ANA,** ANCA, p-ANCA, anti-ss-DNA, anti-ds-DNA, ASLO, proteins, CEA, CK-MB, Cu, fibrinogen, **ESR,** gamma globulins, **haptoglobin,** IgM, cryoglobulins, **LD,** LD- (2, 3, 4), mono, OCT, PLT

↓ **albumin,** proteins, WBC, **lym, PLT**

- *Urine* ↑ **proteins,** RBC, Hb, pus, **WBC,** casts – (RBC)
  ↓ uric acid
- *Cerebrospinal Fluid* ↑ proteins, pressure
- *Peritoneal Fluid* ↑ protein
- *Pleural Fluid* ↑ CIC, **LD**
  ↓ pH

Colonoscopy

↑ ACP

Coma

coma in acute insufficiency of adrenal cortex

↑ Ca^{2+}, HCT, K, MAC
↓ G, chloride, MCV, Na

diabetic coma

– hypoglycemic diabetic coma

↑ ACTH, epinephrine, RBC, glucagon, K, creatinine, WBC, Na, neu
↓ G

- *Cerebrospinal Fluid* ↓ G

– hyperglycemic ketoacidotic diabetic coma

↑ **acetone,** ammonia, AMS, **BHBA,** RBC, glucagon, **G,** HCT, chloride, K, catecholamines, **creatinine,** acetoacetic acid, **uric acid, WBC, MAC,** Mg, Na, **neu, osmolality,** P, urea, FFA

↓ Ca^{2+}, HCO$_3^-$, K, **Na,** P, pCO$_2$, pH

- *Urine* ↑ **acetone,** protein, **G,** K, **ketones,** creatinine, **volume**
- *Cerebrospinal Fluid* ↑ CK, G
  ↓ pressure

– hyperosmolar non-ketoacidotic diabetic coma

   ↑ ALT, ✳ **G**, K, WBC, **Na**, ✳ **osmolality**, **urea**

   ↓ HCO_3^-, K, Na

   ■ *Urine* ↑ acetone, **G**, K

hepatic coma

– endogenous hepatic coma

   ↑ **ALT**, ammonia, anion gap, APTT, **AST**, Bil, unconjugated Bil, **gamma globulins**, **glutamine**, **GMT**, creatinine, **LA**, **MAC**, PT

   ↓ albumin, cholesterol, PT

   ■ *Cerebrospinal Fluid* ↑ **glutamine**

– exogenous hepatic coma

   ↑ **ALT**, ✳ **ammonia**, APTT, anion gap, **AST**, Bil, **glutamine**, GMT, G6PD (RBC), creatinine, LA, WBC, MAL, Na, **PT**, vitamin – (B_{12})

   ↓ albumin, cholesterol, PT

   ■ *Cerebrospinal Fluid* ↑ **glutamine**

myxedematous coma

   ↑ ALT, epinephrine, cholesterol, ✳ **CK**, CK-MB, **CK-MM**, catecholamines, creatine, **creatinine**, ESR, ✳ **cholesterol**, ✳ **IDL-C**, **LD**, ✳ **LDL-C**, **uric acid**, WBC, pCO_2, RAC, TAG, ✳ **TBG**, TSH, urea

   ↓ ALP, G, RBC, Fe, ✳ **FT4**, FT4 index, Hb, HCT, HDL-C, chloride, K, **Na**, neu, osmolality, pO_2, SHBG, GH, T3, ✳ **T4**, **triiodothyronine resin uptake**, TSH

pituitary coma

   ↓ G, cortisol, MAC, Na, pCO_2, GH, T4, TSH

uremic coma

   ↑ Al, alpha-aminonitrogen, ✳ **ALP**, **AMS**, **ammonia**, ✳ **B2M**, **BT**, Ca, **Ca$_{2+}$**, CK, CK-MB, CK-BB, G, **glucagon**, ✳ **chloride**, **cholesterol**, insulin, ✳ **K**, **calcitonin**, catecholamines, cortisol, ✳ **creatinine**, ✳ **uric acid**, LA, LD, WBC, **MAC**, **Mg**, **Na**, neu, plasma volume, **osmolality**, P, PT, **PRA**, **PRL**, ✳ **PTH**, pyruvate, **GH**, **TAG**, thrombomodulin, **trypsin**, cTnT, TT, PLT, ✳ **urea**

   ↓ ✳ **albumin**, AST, **proteins**, Ca, ✳ **Ca^{2+}**, **RBC**, factors - (II, VII, IX, X, XIII), ✳ **Fe**, G, **haptoglobin**, Hb, HCT, HDL-C, HCO_3^-, cholesterol, K, cortisol, glutamic acid, WBC, lym, **Na**, **pH**, PRA, **T3**, T4, TAG, **testosterone**, **PLT**, Zn

   ■ *Urine* ↑ ✳ **proteins**, ✳ **RBC**, G, **pus**, **K**, ✳ **blood**, WBC, **Na**, casts – (cellular, granular, hyaline, **waxy**), **VMA**

   ↓ ✳ **specific gravity**, Mg, ✳ **volume**, oxalate, pH, Se urea, VMA

Complex, AIDS Dementia

   ↑ urea

   ■ *Cerebrospinal Fluid* ↑ B2M, proteins, IgG, p24 antigen, neopterin, WBC

   ↓ G

Conditions

convulsive conditions (seizure)

   ↑ ALT, anion gap, ✳ **AST**, ✳ **CK**, CK-BB, ✳ **WBC**, pCO_2, PRL

   ↓ eos, Mn

   ■ *Urine* ↑ protein

   ■ *Cerebrospinal Fluid* ↑ bas, **LA**

febrile conditions

   ↑ ACP, ✳ **CRP**, G, creatinine, **acetoacetic acid**, ✳ **ESR**, ✳ **uric acid**, ketobodies, ✳ **WBC**, Na, osmolality, pCO_2, PCT, RAL, ✳ **urea**

          ↓ albumin, beta-carotene, G, K, pCO_2, proteins, vitamin – (A, B, folic
          acid), Zn
     ■ *Urine* ↑ ammonia, ＊ **proteins**, ＊ **cAMP**, ＊ **K**, **ketones**, creatine, creati-
          nine, crystals – (＊ **urate**), **uric acid**, ＊ **specific gravity**, ＊ **P**, pentoses,
          ＊ **UBG**, urea, casts – (＊ **granular**, ＊ **hyaline**)
          ↓ ＊ **chloride**, **volume**, **pH**
     ■ *Seminal Fluid* ↓ volume, spermatozoa count
     ■ *Gastric Fluid* ↓ pH

hemolytic conditions

          ↑ ACP, ACHE (RBC), **ADA**, adenylate kinase (RBC), aldolase, ALP, ALT,
          ammonia, **anti-RBC**, **antimicrosomal Ab**, antithyroglobulin Ab, **an-
          tithyroid Ab**, AST, basophilic stippling (RBC), bas, **Bil**, Bil delta,
          unconjugated Bil, CK, elliptocytes, Fe, ferritin, **ESR**, gamma globu-
          lins, GMT, haptoglobin, HbF, Heinz bodies (RBC), Howell–Jolly
          bodies (RBC), **cold agglutinins**, IgA, IgG, K, calcitonin, **cryoglobu-
          lins**, uric acid, **LD**, LD – (1, 2), **WBC**, lipids, macrocytes, **MCV**, MD,
          methemalbumin, Mg, **neu**, NSE, RBC osmotic fragility, porphyrins,
          protoporphyrin, RTC, transferrin satur., **spherocytes**, **RTC**, schisto-
          cytes, TIBC, PLT, urea
          ↓ Apo B, ceruloplasmin, Cu, RBC, Fe, G, G6PD (RBC), **haptoglobin**, **Hb**,
          HbA_{1c}, HDL-C, hemopexin, **HCT**, cholesterol, complement – (C1, C1r,
          C1s, C2, **C3**, C4, CH50), LCAT, LDL-C, WBC, **RBC osmotic resistance**,
          pyruvate kinase, RTC, transferrin satur., TIBC, PLT, vitamin – (E, K,
          folic acid)
     ■ *Urine* ↑ ALT, conjugated Bil, RBC, Hb, hCG, hemosiderin, UBG
          ↓ volume
     ■ *Stool* ↑ porphyrins, SBG, UBG
     ■ *Amniotic Fluid* ↑ anti-Rh factor, Bil, RBC, hCG, placental lactogen
          ↓ estriol

hemorrhagic conditions

          ↑ aldosterone, ALT, BT, catecholamines, MAC, neu, PRA, TIBC
          ↓ albumin, bas, proteins, Fe, Hb, HCT, chloride, cortisol, Na, PT, vitamin
          – (K)

hypercoagulable conditions

          ↑ APTT, **anti-phospholipid Ab**, ＊ **PLT aggregation**, ＊ **beta-thrombo-
          globulin**, factor Leiden, ＊ **fibrinogen**, fibrinopeptide A
          ↓ APTT, ＊ **AT III**, fibrinogen, plasminogen, protein – (C, S), TT

hypoxic conditions

– acute hypoxic conditions

          ↑ **ALT**, K, ＊ **LA**, ＊ **MAC**, RAC
          ↓ pH, ＊ pO_2

– chronic hypoxic conditions

          ↑ ＊ **AST**, 2,3-DPG, ＊ **EPO**, RBC, FDP, Hb, K, ＊ **LA**, ＊ **LD**, ＊ **MAC**, pCO_2, RAC
          ↓ BE, ＊ **pH**, ＊ pO_2

immunodeficient conditions

          ↑ ASLO, bas, ＊ **B-lym**, ＊ **C3 complement**, ＊ **CIC**, eos, fibrinogen, fibro-
          nectin, ESR, haptoglobin, ＊ **IgA**, ＊ **IgE**, ＊ **IgE specific Ab**, IgG, ＊ **al-
          pha-1-proteinase inhibitor**, cryoglobulins, WBC, neu, pCO_2, PMN,
          RAC, RAL, RF, T-lym
          ↓ albumin, anti-EBV VCA IgG (false), bas, B-lym, **RBC**, **Hb**, **HCT**, **IgA**, IgD,
          IgG, **IgM**, complement – (C1q, C2, C3, C4), WBC, **lym**, **neu**, pO_2, **PLT**,
          T-lym, transferrin

- ■ *Urine* ↑ proteins, RBC, Hb, pentoses, casts – (RBC)
- ■ *Bronchoalveolar Lavage Fluid* ↑ eos, IgG, IgM, lym, neu, T-lym
- ■ *Pleural Fluid* ↑ eos, lym, neu
  - ↓ alveolar macrophages
- ■ *Sputum* ↑ eos, lym, neu, PMN, viscosity
  - ↓ alveolar macrophages
- ■ *Synovial Fluid* ↑ eos, WBC, PMN

painful conditions
- ↑ * **G**, * **WBC**
- ↓ Na, osmolality
- ■ *Urine* ↑ G, 5-HIAA

postartrography conditions
- ■ *Synovial Fluid* ↑ **eos**

postlabor conditions
- ↑ beta-endorphins, WBC, PLT
- ↓ PLT
- ■ *Urine* ↑ creatine

post-myocardial infarction conditions
- ↑ AAT, AGP, alpha-1-globulins, alpha-2-globulins, ALT, antimyocardial Ab, AST, CK, CRP, fibrinogen, ESR, HBD, catecholamines, uric acid, LD, LD – (1, 2), WBC, L-myosin, prothrombin fragment 1.2, troponin I, tro-ponin T
- ■ *Pleural Fluid* ↑ neu

postsurgery conditions
- ↑ * **AAT**, **ADH**, PLT adhesion, * **epinephrine**, * **aldosterone**, alpha-1-globulins, ALP (WBC), ALT, unconjugated Bil, * **CEA**, CK-MM, * **CRP**, euglobulin lysis time (after 48 hrs), elastase, **factor VIII**, FDP, * **fibrinogen**, * **ESR**, plasminogen activator inhibitor, * **K**, catecholamines, cortisol, LA, **WBC**, mucoproteins, * **neu**, norepinephrine, PCT, PRL, taurine, TPA, PLT, urea
- ↓ albumin, arginine, **proteins**, Ca^{2+}, **Cr**, euglobulin lysis time (first 48 hrs), factor XIII, G, cholesterol, **CHS**, Mn, Na, ornithine, osmolality, proline, PTH, vitamin C (WBC), Zn
- ■ *Urine* ↑ **AMS**, hexosaminidase, catecholamines, osmolality, urea, Zn
  - ↓ Na

posttransfusion conditions
- ↑ antiplatelet Ab, **Bil**, neu
- ↓ **haptoglobin**, Hb, HCT, methemalbumin, PLT
- ■ *Urine* ↑ Hb, casts – (Hb)

prelabor hemorrhagic conditions
- ↑ BT, euglobulin lysis time

psychic conditions

– acute psychosis
- ↑ ADH, aldolase, **CK**, FT4, cortisol, T3, T4, TSH

– anxious psychic conditions
- ↑ epinephrine, CHS, FDP, norepinephrine, * **serotonin**, * **FFA**
- ↓ oxytocin, pCO_2
- ■ *Urine* ↑ **PABA**, VMA

– depressive psychic conditions
- ↓ norepinephrine, serotonin, taurine
- ■ *Urine* ↑ catecholamines

    ↓ cAMP, 5-HIAA
- ■ *Cerebrospinal Fluid* ↑ CRH
– manic psychic conditions
    ↑ * norepinephrine
    ↓ 5-OH-tryptamine (serotonin)
    ■ *Urine* ↑ * cAMP

septic conditions

↑ epinephrine, alanine, alpha-1-globulins, **ALP**, ALP (WBC), **ALT**, ASLO, AST, anti-PLT, **beta globulins**, proteins, Bil, conjugated Bil, CK, **CRP**, Cu, **cystine**, D-dimers, elastase, **FDP**, phenylalanine, **fibrinogen**, phospholipase A2, **ESR**, **G**, **globulins**, glucagon, **glycine**, IFN-gamma, **IgA**, IgD, IgG, IgM, IL – (1-beta, 6), insulin, plasminogen activator inhibitor, **catecholamines**, ketobodies, complement – (C3a, C4a, C5a), **creatinine**, **uric acid**, **LA**, lactoferrin, **LD**, **WBC**, lym, **MAC**, **methionine**, **mono**, **neu**, NSE, 5-NT, osmolality, PAF, **PCT**, PGE2, pH, phenylalanine, PMN, PT, **RAL**, **TAG**, taurine, TT, tryptophan, tyrosine, **urea**

↓ alanine, **albumin**, aldosterone, A2MG, Apo – (AI, B), **arginine**, AT III, Ca, Ca^{2+}, CBG, RBC, factor – (II, XII), **Fe**, **fibrinogen**, G, G tolerance, **gamma globulins**, G6PD (RBC), **Hb**, **HCT**, HCO_3^-, **cholesterol**, **CHS**, IgA, IgG, IgM, complement – (**C3**, C4, total), **WBC** (advanced), lipids, **lym**, Mg, neu, **P**, pCO_2, pO_2, protein C, protein S, **PLT**, RTC, TBG, TIBC, Zn

■ *Urine* ↑ proteins, RBC, **G**, Hb, 17-KGS, 17-OHCS, catecholamines, Mb, metanephrines, casts (RBC), **VMA**
    ↓ volume, osmolality
■ *Cerebrospinal Fluid* ↑ proteins, glutamine
■ *Synovial Fluid* ↑ proteins, RBC, pus, LA, WBC, neu, PMN
    ↓ G, viscosity

Constipation

↑ Ca, sulfhemoglobin
■ *Urine* ↑ UBG

Contusion, Myocardial

↑ * CK-MB, * troponin I

Cor Pulmonale

↑ ALT, ammonia, **BNP**, eos, **RBC**, ESR, Hb, HCT, LA, WBC, **pCO_2**, RAC
↓ albumin, pO_2, satur. O_2

Cretinism

↑ cholesterol, **TSH**
↓ ALP, **FT4**, iodine, T4
■ *Urine* ↓ 17-KGS, 17-KS

Crisis, Acute Adrenocortical

↑ cortisol, eos, **K**, lym
↓ G, cortisol, **Na**

Cryofibrinogenemia

↑ AAT, A2M, fibrinogen, haptoglobin

Cryoglobulinemia

↑ ANA, **CIC**, IgG, * IgM, * **cryoglobulins**, paraproteins, RF, **urea**, * viscosity
↓ albumin, IgM, complement – (C1, C1q, C1r, C2, **C3**, **C4**, CH50)
■ *Urine* ↑ **proteins**, RBC, Hb

	↓ **volume**
	■ *Synovial Fluid* ↑ crystals – (cryoglobulin)
Cryptorchism	
	↑ FSH
	↓ testosterone
	■ *Seminal Fluid* ↓ volume, spermatozoa count
Cycle, Anovulatory	
	↑ **PRL**
	↓ estradiol
	■ *Urine* ↓ pregnanediol
Cyst	

Cyst

ovarian cyst

↑ AMS, CA 27-29, CA 125, hCG, WBC, progesterone, testosterone
■ *Urine* ↓ FSH

pancreatic cyst

↑ AMS, AMS (P), elastase, **lipase**
↓ elastase
■ *Urine* ↑ AMS
■ *Peritoneal Fluid* ↑ AMS

renal cyst

↑ AFP, **RBC**, Na
■ *Urine* ↑ **proteins, RBC, Hb**

Cystathioninuria

↑ * **cystathionine**
↓ RBC, Hb, PLT
■ *Urine* ↑ cystathionine
■ *Cerebrospinal Fluid* ↑ cystathionine

Cystinosis

↑ ALP, chloride, * **cystine**, ESR, K, creatinine, MAC, P, urea
↓ **Ca, CO₂, Hb, HCT**, K, **uric acid**, P, pCO₂, pH, **PLT**
■ *Urine* ↑ alanine, albumin, **amino acids**, ammonia, arginine, asparaginase, cystathionine, * **cystine**, phenylalanine, RBC, **G**, globulins,
glycine, histidine, hydroxyproline, isoleucine, K, glutamic acid, uric
acid, leucine, lysine, methionine, ornithine, proline, **proteins**, pyruvate, **volume, P**, pH, serine, threonine, tryptophan, tyrosine, valine,
casts – (granular c.)
↓ GFR
■ *Stool* ↑ P

Cystinuria

■ *Urine* ↑ * **arginine**, Ca, cystathionine, cysteine, * **cystine, cystine
crystals**, glycine, histidine, hydroxylysine, * **lysine**, methionine,
* **ornithine**
↓ pH

Cystitis

↑ alpha-1-globulins, gamma globulins, **WBC, neu**
■ *Urine* ↑ **bacteria** (+ culture), eos, **RBC**, Hb, **pus, WBC**, nitrites
↓ volume

Cystoscopy

↑ PSA, chromogranin A

Death, Fetal

↑ FDP, euglobulin lysis time, plasmin, **plasminogen**
↓ CBG, progesterone

■ *Urine* ↓ estriol, pregnanediol
■ *Amniotic Fluid* ↑ AFP

Defect
   neural tube defect
        ■ *Amniotic Fluid* ↑ AFP
   tubular renal defect
        ↑ K, **creatinine, MAC, urea**
        ↓ uric acid
        ■ *Urine* ↑ amino acids, proteins, G, **uric acid**, Na, P
          ↓ GFR, osmolality, pH

Defibrillation
        ↑ AST, **CK**, CK-MB

Deficiency
   adenine phosphoribosyltransferase deficiency
        ■ *Urine* ↑ adenine, 8-hydroxyadenine, 2,8-dihydroxyadenine
   adenosine deaminase deficiency
        ■ *Urine* ↑ adenosine, deoxyadenosine
   alpha-1-antitrypsin deficiency
        ↑ A2MG, ALT, AST, conjugated Bil, GMT
        ↓ * **AAT, alpha-1-globulins**, complement – (C4)
   L-carnitine deficiency
        ↑ ammonia, uric acid
        ↓ G, * **L-carnitine**
        ■ *Urine* ↑ Mb
   cholesterol desmolase deficiency
        ↑ K, PRA
        ↓ * **aldosterone**, * **androgens**, * **cortisol**, DHEA, 17-OH progesterone, **Na**,
          * **testosterone**
        ■ *Urine* ↓ * **aldosterone**, 17-KS, * **17-OHCS**, pregnanetriol
   coagulation factor II deficiency
        ↑ APTT, BT, coagulation time, **PT**
        ↓ * **factor II**, vitamin – (K)
        Note: molecular genetics
   coagulation factor V deficiency
        ↑ **APTT**, coagulation time, **PT**
        ↓ * **factor V**
        Note: molecular genetics (Leiden's factor)
   coagulation factor VII deficiency
        ↑ coagulation time, **PT**
        ↓ * **factor VII**
   coagulation factor X deficiency
        ↑ APTT, coagulation time, **PT**, TGT
        ↓ * **factor X**
   coagulation factor XI deficiency
        ↑ **APTT**, BT, coagulation time, **PT**, TGT
        ↓ * **factor XI**
   coagulation factor XII deficiency
        ↑ APTT, **coagulation time**, PT, TGT
        ↓ * **factor XII**
   cobalamin deficiency causing neuropsychiatric disorders
        ↑ * **homocysteine**, * **methylmalonic acid**

copper deficiency

    ↑ cholesterol, uric acid

    ↓ * **ceruloplasmin**, * **Cu**, RBC, Hb, HCT, WBC, neu

17-OH dehydrogenase deficiency

    ↑ androstenedione

    ↓ testosterone

18-OH dehydrogenase deficiency

    ↑ **17-OHCS, PRA**

    ↓ **aldosterone**

    ■ *Urine* ↑ **17-OHCS**

disaccharidase deficiency

    ↑ **LA**

    ↓ **lym, pH**

2,3-DPG deficiency

    ↑ **RBC**

    ↓ * **2,3-DPG**

C1-esterase inhibitor deficiency

    ↓ * **C1-INH**, complement – (C2, C4, CH100)

folate deficiency

    ↑ aldolase, anisocytes, **Bil**, Bil unconjugated, BT, Cu, **Fe**, G6PD (+RBC), HbF, homocysteine, ICD (+RBC), **LD, LD5**, lysozyme, macrocytes, **MCH**, **MCV**, MD, ovalocytes, RBC Howell–Jolly bodies, **UBBC**

    ↓ ACHE (RBC), **ALP, RBC, Hb, HCT**, * **Fe**, **cholesterol**, CHS, complement – (C3), **K**, **WBC**, **neu**, osmotic fragility (RBC), **RTC**, **PLT**, TIBC, **uric acid**, vitamin – (B$_{12}$, * **folate**)

    ■ *Urine* ↑ amino acids, N-forminio-glutamic acid, taurine

       ↓ **uric acid**

fructose-1,6-diphosphatase deficiency

    ↑ uric acid, lipids

    ↓ **F-1,6DP**, G

    ■ *Urine* ↑ **ketones**

deficiency of glucose-6-phosphate dehydrogenase in RBC

    ↑ unconjugated Bil, glutathione peroxidase (RBC), glutathione reductase (RBC), **Heinz bodies** (RBC), nucleated RBC, **uric acid**, **lipids**, WBC, poikilocytes, RTC, spherocytes

    ↓ G, * **G6PD** (RBC), glutathione (RBC), haptoglobin, **Hb**, **HCT**, WBC

    ■ *Urine* ↑ **ketones**

    ■ *Sweat* ↑ chloride

glucuronyl transferase deficiency

    ↑ unconjugated Bil

glycogen-synthase deficiency

    ↓ G

    ■ *Urine* ↑ alanine

growth hormone deficiency

    ↓ ACTH, ALP, G, * **GH**, P, * **PRL**, TSH

hexokinase deficiency (RBC)

    ↑ unconjugated Bil

21-hydroxylase deficiency

    ↑ ACTH, * **androgens**, * **androstenedione**, * **DHEA**, K, MAC, * **17-OH progesterone**, * **pregnanetriol**, PRA, * **progesterone**, * **testosterone**

    ↓ * **aldosterone**, cortisol, corticosterone, Na, 11-deoxycorticosterone

- ■ *Urine* ↑ aldosterone, androsterone, DHEA, DHEAS, ✳ **17-KS**, 17-OHCS, ✳ **pregnanetriol**, free cortisol, Na, chloride
  - ↓ aldosterone, 17-OHCS

17-alpha-hydroxylase deficiency
- ↑ ACTH, ✳ **11-deoxycorticosterone**, ✳ **18-OH corticosterone**, Na, progesterone
- ↓ ✳ **aldosterone**, deoxycortisol, DHEA, HCT, ✳ **17-OH progesterone**, K, cortisol, ✳ **PRA**, ✳ **testosterone**
- ■ *Urine* ↓ aldosterone, ✳ **17-KS**, ✳ **17-OHCS**, pregnanetriol

11-beta-hydroxylase deficiency
- ↑ ACTH, androgens, **androstenedione**, ✳ **11-deoxycorticosterone**, ✳ **11-deoxycortisol**, DHEA, cortisol, ✳ **17-OH progesterone**, **testosterone**
- ↓ **aldosterone**, HCT, K, **cortisol**, corticosterone, PRA
- ■ *Urine* ↑ androsterone, DHEA, DHEAS, 17-KS, 17-OHCS, pregnanetriol, **tetrahydro-deoxycorticosterone**, **tetrahydro-deoxycortisol**, free cortisol
  - ↓ aldosterone

3-beta-hydroxysteroid dehydrogenase deficiency
- ↑ **DHEA**, DHEAS, 17-OH progesterone, **17-OH pregnenolone**, ✳ **pregnenolone**, PRA, testosterone
- ↓ ✳ **aldosterone**, ✳ **androstenedione**, ✳ **cortisol**
- ■ *Urine* ↑ **17-KS**
  - ↓ aldosterone, **17-OHCS**, pregnanetriol

17-beta-hydroxysteroid dehydrogenase deficiency
- ↑ **pregnanetriol**, **17-OH progesterone**
- ■ *Urine* ↑ **17-KS**, **pregnanetriol**

IgA deficiency
- ↑ **anti-IgA Ab**, HLA – (DR3), IgG, IgD, IgE, IgM
- ↓ ✳ **IgA**

iodine deficiency
- ↑ TSH
- ↓ ✳ **iodine**, **T4**
- ■ *Urine* ↓ iodine

lactase deficiency
- ↓ **lactase**
- ■ *Urine* ↑ **lactose**

lecithin-cholesterol acyltransferase deficiency
- ↑ **cholesterol**, target cells, **TAG**
- ↓ Apo A-I, Hb, HCT, HDL-C, ✳ **LCAT**, PL, RBC
- ■ *Urine* ↑ proteins

lipoprotein lipase deficiency
- ↑ chylomicrons, **TAG**
- ↓ ✳ **LP lipase**

ornithine carbamoyltransferase deficiency
- ↑ ammonia, orotic acid
- ↓ citrulline
- ■ *Urine* ↑ orotic acid

phosphorylase deficiency
- ↓ G
- ■ *Urine* ↑ **ketones**, Mb

potassium deficiency

    ↑ G

    ↓ proteins, chloride, **K**

    ■ *Urine* ↓ specific gravity

purine-nucleoside phosphorylase deficiency

    ↓ uric acid

    ■ *Urine* ↑ inosine, deoxyinosine, guanosine, deoxyguanosine, uric acid

pyruvate kinase deficiency in RBC

    ↑ acanthocytes, 2,3-DPG, unconjugated Bil, echinocytes, Fe, **macrocytes**, RBC osmotic fragility, poikilocytes, **RTC**

    ↓ Hb, HCT, RBC osmotic resistance, * **pyruvate kinase** (RBC)

thyroxine-binding globulin deficiency

    ↓ T3, T4, * **TBG**

xanthine oxidase deficiency

    ↑ **hypoxanthine, xanthine**

    ↓ * **uric acid**

    ■ *Urine* ↑ **hypoxanthine, xanthine**

    ↓ uric acid

Dehydratation

    ↑ ADH, **albumin**, * **proteins**, Ca, * **RBC**, * **Hb**, * **HCT**, **chloride**, K, creatinine, uric acid, Mg, * **Na**, * **osmolality**, P, urea, WBC

    ↓ ESR, **HCO₃⁻**, Na, plasma volume, osmolality

    ■ *Urine* ↑ chloride, creatinine clearance, **K**, * **specific gravity**, * Na, casts – (granular, hyaline)

    ↓ K, Mg, **volume, pH**, urea

    ■ *Cerebrospinal Fluid* ↑ proteins, **ketones**

    ↓ pressure

hypertonic dehydratation

    ↑ **proteins, G, Hb, Na, osmolality, urea, MAC**

    ↓ **Ca**

    ■ *Urine* ↑ **specific gravity**

hypotonic dehydratation

    ↑ **proteins, RBC, Hb, HCT**, chloride, **MAC, urea**

    ↓ HCO₃⁻, **Na**, chloride, **osmolality**

    ■ *Urine* ↑ chloride, K, ketones, **specific gravity, Na**, pH, casts – (granular, hyaline)

    ↓ K, urea

isotonic dehydratation

    ↑ **proteins, RBC, Hb, HCT**, MAC, **urea**

    ↓ HCO₃⁻

    ■ *Urine* ↑ chloride, K, ketones, **specific gravity**, casts – (granular, hyaline)

    ↓ K, urea

Delirium Tremens

    ↑ **aldolase**, ALT, **CK**, catecholamines, **LD**

    ↓ K, vitamin – (B₁, folic acid, B₁₂)

Dementia

dialysis dementia

    ↑ **Al**, ALP, urea

    ■ *Cerebrospinal Fluid* ↑ WBC

senile dementia

    ↑ urea

$\downarrow$ vitamin – (B_{12})
■ *Cerebrospinal Fluid* $\uparrow$ WBC

Demyelination

$\uparrow$ E selectin
■ *Cerebrospinal Fluid* $\uparrow$ CK, enolase

Dermatitis

$\uparrow$ antiendomysial Ab, antireticulin Ab, CIC, eos, HLA – (B8, DQw2, DR3, Dw3, Dw5), IgE, WBC, lym, neu
$\downarrow$ albumin, proteins, Fe, CHS, vitamin – (B_2, B_{12}, folic acid)

allergic dermatitis (contact d., photoallergic d.)

$\uparrow$ CIC, **IgE**, lym

exfoliative dermatitis

$\uparrow$ eos, lym, B2M
$\downarrow$ * **albumin**, proteins, * **Fe**, folic acid, CHS

herpes dermatitis

$\uparrow$ **antiendomysial Ab**, antireticulin Ab, **eos**, HLA – (B8, DQw2, DR3, Dw3, Dw5), WBC, lym
$\downarrow$ albumin, **folate**

seborrheic dermatitis

$\downarrow$ Se, Zn, vitamin – (**B_2**, B_{12})

Dermatomyositis

$\uparrow$ ACA, ACE, **aldolase**, alpha-2-globulins, **ALT, ANA**, anti-ds-DNA, anti-aminoacyl-tRNA synthetase Ab – (anti-EJ, anti-OJ, anti-PL-7, anti-PL-12), **anti-histidyl-tRNA synthetase Ab**, * **anti-Jo-1**, anti-Jo-2, anti-cardiolipin Ab, anti-Ku Ab, **anti-Mi-2 Ab**, anti-RNP, **anti-Scl 70**, anti-SRP, **anti-Ro/SSA, anti-La,Ha/SSB**, * **antisynthetase Ab**, ASMA, **AST, CK**, CK-MB, **CK-MM**, Cu, **eos, ESR**, globulins, **haptoglobin**, HLA – (DR5, DR7, DRw52, DRw53), IgD, **LD, LD5**, LE cells, lym, **WBC, Mb**, MD, **non-histone ANA**, PM-1 antigen, **RF**, thymic antinuclear Ab, Ab against coxsackie
$\downarrow$ albumin, RBC, **Hb, HCT, CHS**, complement – (C2, C3, C4), plasmocytes
■ *Urine* $\uparrow$ **creatine, Mb**
■ *Synovial Fluid* $\uparrow$ crystals – (hydroxyapatite)

Dermatosis

$\downarrow$ vitamin – (B_2, B_{12})

Diabetes Insipidus

central diabetes insipidus

$\uparrow$ albumin, proteins, **chloride, uric acid, Na, osmolality**
$\downarrow$ * **ADH**
■ *Urine* $\uparrow$ **volume**
$\downarrow$ * **specific gravity**, * **osmolality**

nephrogenic diabetes insipidus

$\uparrow$ **ADH**, albumin, chloride, uric acid, **Na, osmolality**
$\downarrow$ ADH
■ *Urine* $\uparrow$ ADH, alpha-aminonitrogen, **G, volume**
$\downarrow$ * **specific gravity**, * **osmolality**
■ *Sweat* $\uparrow$ chloride, Na

psychogenic diabetes insipidus

■ *Urine* $\uparrow$ **volume**
$\downarrow$ **specific gravity**

Diabetes Mellitus

↑ AAT, **ACE**, acetone, **ACP**, PLT adhesion, alpha-aminonitrogen, PLT aggregation, albumin, aldolase, aldosterone, **alpha-2-antiplasmin, alpha-2-globulins, ALP**, ALT, **A2MG, amino acids, AMS**, amylin, ANA, Apo B, ASAL, **AST**, AT III, bas, **beta-carotene, beta globulins, beta-glucuronidase**, proteins, Ca, CK, 2,3-DPG (RBC), ESR, factor – (VIII), FDP, fibrinogen, **glucagon**, ✱ **G**, GIP, glutathione reductase (RBC), glycerol, ✱ **glycated Hb (HbA$_{1c}$)**, glycated protein, **GMT**, haptoglobin, hemopexin, **hexosaminidase**, hexosaminidase A, **cholesterol, chylomicrons**, CHS, IDL-C, IgG, IGFBP-1, inositol, insulin, **K**, ketobodies, complement – (C3), **uric acid**, creatine, cryofibrinogen, **creatinine, LA**, LD, **LDL-C**, lipase, **lipids**, beta-LP, MAC, **Mg**, MPV, O$_2$ satur., **osmolality**, P, PG, **PL**, PP, proinsulin **anti-beta cells Ab, pyruvate**, secretin, selectin – (E, P), **GH, TAG, PLT**, TPA, throm-bomodulin, **urea**, vitamin – (A, B$_{12}$), **VLDL-C, FFA**, vWf

↓ ACE, **PLT adhesion**, Al, alanine, **albumin, aldosterone**, alpha-2-globulins, AMS, amylin, AST, AT III, **proteins**, Ca, CO$_2$, C-peptide, euglobulin lysis time, estriol, G tolerance, glutathione (RBC), glycine, **HDL-C, chloride**, ILGF-I, IGFBP-1, immunoreactive trypsin, **insulin**, K, carnitine, catecholamines, uric acid, LH, lipase, lipoprotein lipase, lym, **Mg, Na**, norepinephrine, **plasma volume**, P, pCO$_2$, pH, **PRA**, prealbumin, prostacyclin, T3, transketolase, **trypsin**, vitamin – (B$_1$, B$_6$, folate), Zn

■ *Urine* ↑ **acetone**, aldosterone, **amino acids**, ammonia, **AMS**, **proteins**, Ca, Cr, ✱ **G**, 2,3-DPG, FDP, hexosaminidase, chloride, **K, ketones**, 17-ketosteroids, creatine, creatinine, lipids, lysozyme, **specific gravity**, Mb, Mg, **Na**, volume, **oxalate**, pH, casts – (granular c.)

↓ aldosterone, AMS, **estriol**, 17-OHCS, 17-KGS, **catecholamines**, uric acid, pH

■ *Cerebrospinal Fluid* ↑ **G**, proteins
↓ AMS

■ *Amniotic Fluid* ↑ **creatinine, volume**, rT3

■ *Sweat* ↑ chloride, Na

■ *Stool* ↑ **fat**

■ *Hair* ↑ Mn
↓ Cr, Zn

insulin-dependent diabetes mellitus (IDDM, type I)

↑ ANA, ✱ **G**, ✱ **IAA, HLA** – (Bw15, B8, **DQw8, DR2, DR3, DR4**), antityrosine-phosphatase Ab – (IA-2A, IA-2-beta-A), IgA, IGFBP-1, ✱ **anti-GAD Ab**, antiintrinsic factor Ab, ✱ **HbA$_{1c}$**, ✱ **ICA**, E selectin

↓ **C-peptide, insulin, IRI**, vitamin – (D)

Note: MODY (maturity onset diabetes of the young)

non-insulin-dependent diabetes mellitus (NIDDM, type II)

↑ amylin, C-peptide, ✱ **HbA$_{1c}$, IRI**, proinsulin
↓ C-peptide, **Cr**, IGFBP-1, insulin

Diabetes, Phosphate

↑ **ALP**, Ca, cAMP, osteocalcin, **PTH**, vitamin D
↓ **Ca**, Ca^{2+}, osteocalcin, P, vitamin – (D)

■ *Urine* ↑ **amino acids**, Ca, cAMP, G, hydroxyproline – (total, free), **P**
↓ Ca, Ca^{2+}, hydroxyproline, P

Dialysis

↑ **B2M**, Ca, Cu, ferritin, **cholesterol**, K, **creatinine**, **Mg**, Na, Ni, E selectin, TAG, TPA, urea

↓ Ca, ferritin, GHb, K, Mg, Mn, Na, neu, P, Se, vitamin – (B$_6$, folate)

■ *Urine* ↓ K

hemodialysis

↑ PLT adhesion, PLT aggregation, ALP, ALP (intestinal isoenzyme), Apo B-100, AT III, ∗ **B2M**, ∗ **Ca**, cTnT, cTnI, RBC, ferritin, **GHb**, cholesterol, IDL-C, **K**, complement – (C3a, C5a), **creatinine**, LDL-C, **Mg**, **Na**, selectin – (E, P), TAG, PLT, thrombomodulin, VCAM-1, VLDL-C, vWF

↓ ∗ **albumin**, ALT, alpha-2-antiplasmin, Apo A-I, AST, AT III, proteins, Ca^{2+}, BT, EDRF, endothelin 1, eos, Fe, ∗ **ferritin**, FT4, **HDL-C**, **K**, lym, Mg, Mn, **Na**, PGI2, plasminogen, protein – (C, S), Se, vitamin – (B$_6$, B$_{12}$, C, ∗ **folate**)

■ *Urine* ↑ Al

↓ K, Se

■ *Synovial Fluid* ↑ crystals – (hydroxyapatite, calcium oxalate)

peritoneal dialysis

↑ G, Mg

↓ albumin, **folate**

■ *Peritoneal Fluid* ↑ eos

↓ protein

■ *Pleural Fluid* ↓ **protein**

■ *Synovial Fluid* ↑ crystals – (hydroxyapatite, calcium oxalate)

Diarrhea

↑ albumin, ALP, **proteins** (early), Ca, RBC, **Hb**, **HCT**, chloride, K, **creatinine**, WBC, MAC, motilin, **Na**, osmolality, PT, **urea**

↓ albumin, proteins (later), Ca, CO$_2$, Cu, RBC, Fe, G, Hb, HCO$_3^-$, **chloride**, **K**, Mg, **Na**, **plasma volume**, osmolality, P, **pCO$_2$**, **pH**, vitamin – (B$_1$, B$_2$, K, folate, niacin)

■ *Urine* ↑ ammonia, K, ketones, lactose, LD, specific gravity, reducing sugars

↓ **chloride**, **K**, Mg, **Na**, niacin, **volume**, **pH**, **UBG**

■ *Stool* ↑ Bil, **mucus**, **pus**, chloride, **blood**, Mg, Na, pH, **WBC**, **volume**, **muscle fibres**, **fat**, **water**

↓ pH

acute diarrhea

↑ HCT, chloride, MAC, Na, proteins, creatinine, osmolality, WBC

↓ HCO$_3^-$, chloride, **K**, **pH**

■ *Urine* ↑ UBG

■ *Stool* ↑ **mucus**, **pus**, **blood**, **WBC**, **volume**, **muscle fibres**, **fat**, **water**

↓ pH

chronic diarrhea

↑ albumin, ALP, Ca, RBC, Hb, HCT, chloride, K, creatinine, WBC, motilin, Na, osmolality, PT, urea

↓ albumin, proteins (later), Ca, Cu, RBC, Fe, G, Hb, HCO$_3^-$, chloride, K, Mg, Na, plasma volume, P, pH, vitamin – (B$_1$, B$_2$, K, folate, niacin)

■ *Urine* ↑ K, ketones, lactose, LD, specific gravity, reducing sugars

↓ chloride, K, Mg, Na, niacin, volume, pH, UBG

- **Stool** ↑ mucus, pus, blood, WBC, volume, muscle fibres, fat, water
  - ↓ pH

diarrhea due to laxative abuse

↑ **chloride, MAC**

↓ K, HCO$_3^-$

- **Urine** ↓ K
- **Stool** ↑ K

osmotic diarrhea

- **Stool** ↑ osmotic gap

Diet

high purine diet

- **Urine** ↑ uric acid

non-carbohydrate diet

↓ porphyrins

- **Urine** ↑ ketones, creatine

pure carbohydrate diet

↑ TAG

↓ Apo A-I

- **Urine** ↑ casts – (granular, hyaline)

vegane diet

↑ Bil, folate, PTH, SOD, GP

↓ Ca, Ca^{2+}, Cu, G, Hb, cholesterol, uric acid, LDL-C, lipids, Mg, PL, Se, TAG, urea, vitamin – (B$_{12}$), VLDL-C

- **Urine** ↑ chloride, K, oxalate, pH
  - ↓ ammonia, creatinine
- **Stool** ↑ volume

weight reduction diet

↑ Apo A-I, HDL-C, **acetone, acetoacetic acid**, aldosterone, **amino acids**, BHBA, Bil, unconjugated Bil, Ca, gamma globulins, GIP, **glucagon**, **ketobodies, uric acid, MAC, fatty acids**, Na, rT3, secretin, **GH, urea**, FFA

↓ ACTH, aldosterone, **ACE, albumin**, ALP, AMS, **proteins**, estradiol (F), Ca, C-peptide, EPO, **Fe, folate**, G, **Hb**, HDL-C, HCT, **HCO$_3^-$**, cholesterol, **ILGF-I, insulin, K** (later), LDL-C, LH, **lipids, Mg**, osmolality, P, **pH, T3**, TAG, TIBC, **urea**, LA, vitamin B$_{12}$

- **Urine** ↑ **acetone**, Ca, **chloride, K, ketones**, creatine, creatinine, uric acid, Mg, **Na**, volume, **VMA**
  - ↓ chloride, K, **creatinine, uric acid**, osmolality, **pH**

Disease

Alzheimer's disease

↑ alpha-1-antichymotrypsin, Apo – (E-IV - later)

↓ beta-amyloid precursor protein

- **Urine** ↑ blood, proteins, pus, casts – (RBC)
- **Cerebrospinal Fluid** ↑ glial fibrillary acidic protein, pyruvic acid, taurine
  - ↓ ADH, somatostatin

Note: molecular biology – presenilin-1, presenilin-2 polymorphsim

Behcet's disease

- **Cerebrospinal Fluid** ↑ proteins, WBC

Berger's disease

↑ IgA

- *Urine* ↑ **blood**, proteins, **RBC**

Bornholm disease
- ↑ trypsin

celiac disease
- ↑ * **ALP, ANCA,** * **antiendomysial Ab,** * **antigliadin Ab,** antireticulin Ab, anti-tissue transglutaminase autoantibodies, CEA, G tolerance, GIP, HLA – (B5, **B8,** DQ2, **DR3,** DR7), **CHS, IgA,** uric acid, LD, MCV, mono, **PT,** PTH, serotonin, **PLT,** TIBC
- ↓ * **albumin,** ALP, **beta-carotene, proteins,** Ca, Ca^{2+}, **ceruloplasmin,** CO_2, Cu, * **RBC,** * **Fe,** ferritin, * **Hb, HCT,** chloride, CHE, **cholesterol,** IgG, * **IgM,** K, complement – (* **C3,** * **C4),** uric acid, LD, WBC, **lipids,** lym, MCH, MCHC, MCV, **Mg,** Na, P, pCO_2, PT, * **prothrombin, secretin–cholecystokinin,** STH, T3, T4, TBG, transferrin satur., urea, uric acid, vitamin – (A, B_2, B_6, B_{12}, **D,** E, K, * **folic acid),** Zn
- *Urine* ↑ **5-HIAA, oxalate,** P
  - ↓ 17-OHCS, 17-KS
- *Stool* ↑ Ca, * **fat,** HCO_3^-, volume, pH
  - ↓ pH
- *Hair* ↓ Zn

chronic granulomatous disease
- ↑ antithyroglobulin Ab, AST, **ESR, gamma globulins, WBC**
- ↓ Hb, HCT

chronic obstructive pulmonary disease
- ↑ aldosterone, BNP, CK-MB (exac.), **eos,** EPO, RBC, **Hb,** HCO_3^-, K, WBC, MAC+RAC, MAL+RAC, pCO_2, AAT, Apo B, Hb, HCT, chloride, **cholesterol,** LDL-C, pH, pO_2, TAG

cold agglutinin disease
- ↑ * **cold antibodies,** * **MCH,** * **MCV,** spherocytes
- ↓ **Hb, HCT**
- *Urine* ↑ Bence Jones protein, hemosiderin

coronary artery disease
- ↑ Apo B, CK, **factor VIII, fibrinogen,** homocysteine, **cholesterol, plasminogen activator inhibitor, LDL-C, TAG,** Zn
- ↓ Apo A-I, **HDL-C,** vitamin – (B_{12}, folate)

Crohn's disease (regional enteritis)
- ↑ **Ab against Saccharomyces cerevisiae,** AGP, **ALP,** ALP (WBC), alpha-1-glycoprotein, alpha-1-antichymotrypsin, ALT, ANA, ANCA, p-ANCA, atypical-ANCA, anti-reticulin Ab, **B2M, CEA, CRP, ESR, gamma globulins,** globulins, GM-CSF, haptoglobin, hCG, HLA-B27, IFN-gamma, **IgA,** IL – (1, 2, 6, 8), uric acid, **LD, WBC,** lym, lysozyme, **MAC, mono,** motilin, mucoproteins, Na, **neu,** PT, T3, TBG, TIBC, TNF-alpha, **PLT**
- ↓ ACE, **albumin,** beta-carotene, **proteins, RBC,** Fe, globulins, **Hb, HCT,** K, MCH, MCHC, MCV, **Mg, Na,** pH, prealbumin, PT, transferrin satur., **tryptophan,** vitamin – (B_2, B_{12}, **folate),** Zn, bile acids
- *Urine* ↑ **Ca,** lysozyme, uric acid, **oxalate**
- *Stool* ↑ blood, WBC, **fat**
- *Synovial Fluid* ↑ clot formation, WBC, PMN, volume
  - ↓ **viscosity**

Cushing's disease
- ↑ ACTH, alanine, **DHEA,** DHEAS, **G,** calcitonin, cortisol, MAL, PRL, tri-iodothyronine resin uptake

↓ albumin, ALP, aldosterone, CK, **K**
- *Urine* ↑ K, **17-OHCS**, 17-KS, volume

duodenal ulcer disease

↑ ACE, ALP, **alpha-1-globulins, alpha-2-globulins**, AMS, **Ca, CEA**, CO$_2$, ESR, **gastrin**, haptoglobin, hCG, IgA-specific Ab, IgG-specific Ab, immunoreactive trypsin, cryofibrinogen, **WBC, lipase**, norepinephrine, **pepsinogen**, pH, PP, secretin, somatostatin, TIBC, trypsin, **urea**

↓ albumin, A2MG, **Fe, proteins**, G, G tolerance, Hb, HCT, chloride, K, MCH, MCHC, MCV, Na, transferrin satur., vitamin C (WBC)

- *Urine* ↑ uropepsin
- *Gastric Fluid* ↑ **BAO, basal secretion, HCl, blood**, LD, lysolecithin, **MAO, volume, PAO**, pH
  ↓ **pH**
- *Peritoneal Fluid* ↑ ammonia, AMS
- *Stool* ↑ **blood**, fat

Fabry's disease

↓ alpha-galactosidase (+ WBC)
- *Urine* ↓ alpha-galactosidase
- *Tears* ↓ alpha-galactosidase

Gamstorp's disease

↑ ✳ K (attack)

Gaucher's disease

↑ ACE, ✳ **ACP**, ALP, ALT, anisocytes, **AST**, conjugated Bil, **nucleated RBC**, beta-glucuronidase, beta-glucosidase (+RBC), **GMT**, lym, lysozyme, uric acid, **LD, mono**, 5-NT, PAP, poikilocytes, RTC, vitamin B$_{12}$ binding protein, VLDL-C

↓ albumin, ✳ **beta-glucosidase** (WBC), **RBC, factor IX**, Fe, **glucocerebrosidase, Hb, HCT**, cholesterol, **WBC**, O$_2$ satur., pO$_2$, PLT

- *Cerebrospinal Fluid* ↑ AST
- *Synovial Fluid* ↑ WBC, macrophages, viscosity

Gilbert's disease

↑ **Bil**, ✳ **Bil unconjugated**, delta Bil, GMT, **CHS**
↓ UDPGT
- *Urine* ↑ conjugated Bil, UBG
  ↓ UBG
- *Stool* ↓ UBG

graft-versus-host disease, acute

↑ ✳ **ALP**, ✳ **AST**, ALT, **B2M**, ✳ **Bil**, IL – (2, 6), 5-nucleotidase, TNF-alpha
↓ WBC, lym, PLT
- *Stool* ↑ **blood**

graft-versus-host disease, chronic

↑ ✳ **ALP**, ALT, **B2M**, ✳ **Bil**, IL – (2, 6), 5-nucleotidase, TNF-alpha
↓ **B lym**, catalase, WBC, lym, ✳ **PLT**

Graves' disease

↑ ACE, ALP, ALT, ANA, **antimicrosomal Ab**, antithyroglobulin Ab, antithyroid Ab, antithyroid peroxidase Ab, **thyroxine autoantibodies**, AST, Ca, Ca^{2+}, ferritin, ✳ **FT4, FTI, G**, HLA – (**B8**, B27, **DR3**, Dw3), IgG, IgM, **creatine, LATS**, lym, P, prostacyclin, **anti-TSH receptor Ab**, ✳ **T3**, ✳ **T4, thyroglobulin**

↓ albumin, **cholesterol, Hb**, lipids, **PTH, TIBC**, ✳ **TSH**, vitamin – (**D3**)

- *Urine* ↑ Ca, creatine, **G**

■ *Stool* ↑ Ca

Hartnup disease

↓ **amino acids**, niacin, tryptophan

■ *Urine* ↑ **alanine**, arginine, asparagine, citrulline, cystathionine, cysteine, cystine, ethanolamine, **phenylalanine, glutamine, glycine, histidine,** homocitrulline, hydroxylysine, hydroxyproline, **isoleucine,** aspartic acid, **leucine,** lysine, methionine, ornithine, proline, serine, **threonine, tryptamine,** tryptophan, **tyrosine, valine**

↓ 5-HIAA, **niacin**

■ *Cerebrospinal Fluid* ↑ leucine

hemoglobin C disease

↑ Bil, ∗ **HbC,** HbF, RTC, target cells

↓ Hb, HCT, osmotic fragility

hemoglobin D disease

↑ ∗ **HbD,** spherocytes, target cells

↓ Hb, HCT

hemoglobin E disease

↑ ∗ **HbE, RBC, microcytes**

↓ Hb, HCT, **MCV**

Hurler's disease

■ *Urine* ↑ **dermatan sulfate, heparan sulfate**

immune-complex disease

↓ complement – (C1r, C1s, C2, **C3, C4,** C5, C6, C7, C8, C9, CH50)

inflammatory bowel disease

↑ TM – (CA 19-9, CA 125, M2-PK), p-ANCA

↓ albumin

■ *Synovial Fluid* ↑ clot formation, WBC, volume

ischemic cerebral disease

↑ A2MG, antiphospholipid Ab, AST, CK, Cu

■ *Cerebrospinal Fluid* ↑ **CK,** Cu, G, GMT, **LA,** LD, WBC, MBP

↓ Mg, pH

ischemic heart disease

↑ PLT adhesion, AST, CEA, CK, CK-MB, fibrinogen, **homocysteine, cholesterol,** uric acid, **LDL-C,** Lp(a), mAST, P-selectin, **TAG,** thrombomodulin, troponin I, troponin T, vWf

↓ Cu, **HDL-C,** IDL-C, vitamin – (B$_{12}$, folate), Zn

Jacobs-Creutzfeld disease

■ *Cerebrospinal Fluid* ↑ **enolase**

Note: molecular biology – PRNP gene polymorphism. CSF – 14-3-3 BP (p 130/131)

Krabbe's disease

↓ ∗ **beta-glucosidase** (+ WBC)

■ *Cerebrospinal Fluid* ↑ albumin, alpha-globulin

↓ beta-globulin, gamma-globulin

Leterer-Siwe disease

↑ ALT

↓ WBC

maple syrup urine disease

↑ **alloisoleucine** (attack), isoleucine, uric acid, **leucine** (attack), **MAC,** Mn, valine

↓ G
- *Urine* ↑ **amino acids**, citrulline, glutamine, glycine, hydroxyproline, ✳ **isoleucine**, crystals – (leucine, tyrosine), ✳ **leucine**, WBC, methionine, proline, serine, ✳ **valine**, branched-chain keto acids
- *Cerebrospinal Fluid* ↑ leucine

Ménétrier's disease
↓ albumin
- *Gastric Fluid* ↑ pH
  ↓ HCl

mixed connective tissue disease (MCTD)
↑ aldolase, **ANA**, ANCA, **anti-ds-DNA**, **anti-ss-DNA**, anti-RA33, **anti-RNA Ab**, ✳ **antinucleolar-RNP Ab**, anti-Ro/SSA, anti-Scl-70 Ab, ASMA, CIC, **CK**, **ESR**, **gamma globulins**, HLA – (DR2, DR4), complement – (C3, C4), **LE cells**, **RF**, VDRL (false)
↓ CK, **RBC**, **Hb**, complement – (C3, C4), **WBC**, **PLT**
- *Urine* ↑ proteins, RBC, blood, casts
- *Synovial Fluid* ↑ mono, WBC, RBC, PMN, volume
  ↓ viscosity

neonatal hemorrhagic disease
↑ BT, **coagulation time**, **PTT**, **PT**
↓ anisocytes, RBC, Fe, Hb, HCT, poikilocytes

Niemann-Pick disease
↑ ACE, ACP, aldolase, **ALP**, **ALT**, anisocytes, **AST**, elliptocytes, **nucleated RBC**, WBC, lipids, mono, PAP, poikilocytes, vitamin B_{12} binding protein, VLDL-C
↓ beta-glucosidase, **RBC**, **Hb**, **HCT**, cholesterol, **WBC**, ✳ **sphingomyelinase** (WBC), **PLT**
- *Cerebrospinal Fluid* ↑ **aldolase**, AST
- *Urine* ↓ ✳ **sphingomyelinase**
- *Synovial Fluid* ↑ macrophages

oasthouse urine disease
↑ phenylalanine, tyrosine, methionine, valine, leucine, isoleucine
- *Urine* ↑ phenylalanine, tyrosine, methionine, valine, leucine, isoleucine

Paget's disease
↑ **ACP**, ACP (prostatic), ✳ **ALP**, **Ca**, Ca^{2+}, calcitonin, **osteocalcin**, P, PICP, N-telopeptides
↓ Mg, osteocalcin
- *Urine* ↑ **Ca**, Ca^{2+}, hydroxyproline – (**total, free**), P, **pyridinoline**
- *Synovial Fluid* ↑ WBC, viscosity

Parkinson's disease
↓ dopamine, serotonin
- *Urine* ↓ **dopamine**, catecholamines

pelvic inflammatory disease
↑ CRP, mucoproteins, **ESR**, **WBC**
↓ albumin

polycystic kidney disease
↑ AFP, **EPO**, **RBC**, **HCT**, factor D, HLA – (B5), **creatinine**, **uric acid**, WBC, **urea**
↓ amino acids, RBC, HCT, IGFBP-1, osmolality, tyrosine
- *Urine* ↑ albumin, **proteins**, **RBC**, **Hb**, **pus**, **blood**, WBC, **volume**, fat, casts – (RBC)

    ↓ creatinine, specific gravity, volume, **urea**

Raynaud's disease
    ↑ **ANA**, anti-histidyl-tRNA synthetase Ab

Refsum's disease
    ↑ **phytanic acid, phytanate, pipecolic acid, FA** (very long chain)
    ↓ cholesterol
    ■ *Cerebrospinal Fluid* ↑ **proteins**

Rendu-Osler disease
    ↓ RBC, Hb, HCT
    ■ *Stool* ↑ blood

Rh-null disease
    ↑ HbF, osmotic fragility, stomatocytes
    ↓ **Hb, HCT**

serum disease (serum sickness)
    ↑ CIC, eos, ESR, WBC, lym, plasmocytes
    ↓ complement – (C3, C4), **WBC**
    ■ *Urine* ↑ proteins, blood
    ■ *Synovial Fluid* ↑ WBC, mono, PMN
      ↓ viscosity

silo-filler disease
    ↑ ASLO, bas, C3 complement, CIC, **eos**, fibrinogen, ESR, haptoglobin, IgA,
      IgE, IgE specific Ab, WBC
    ↓ complement – (C2, C3, C4), WBC, T-lym

stomach ulcer disease
    ↑ ACE, **alpha-1-globulins, alpha-2-globulins**, ALP, **AMS, APA, Ca**, CCK-
      PZ, **CEA**, CO_2, echinocytes, ESR, **gastrin**, haptoglobin, hCG, IgA-spe-
      cific Ab, IgG-specific Ab, immunoreactive trypsin, cryofibrinogen,
      lipase, WBC, MAL, norepinephrine, pepsinogen, pH, TIBC, trypsin,
      urea
    ↓ Al, **albumin**, A2MG, bas, **proteins, Fe**, G, G tolerance, Hb, HCT, chloride,
      K, MCH, MCHC, MCV, Na, vitamin C (WBC)
    ■ *Urine* ↑ AMS
    ■ *Gastric Fluid* ↑ **HCl, blood**, LD, lysolecithin, pH
      ↓ basal secretion, HCl, pH
    ■ *Peritoneal Fluid* ↑ AMS, proteins
    ■ *Stool* ↑ **blood**, fat

Tangier disease
    ↑ RTC, TAG
    ↓ alpha-1-globulins, Apo – (A-I, A-II, C-I, C-II, C-III), **HDL-C, cholesterol,**
      LDL-C, PL, pre-betalipoproteins, PLT

Weber-Christian disease
    ↑ ANA, IgA, IgG, IgM

Whipple's disease
    ↑ ALT, **ESR**, WBC, MAC
    ↓ **albumin, proteins, RBC, gamma globulins, Hb**, HCT, **cholesterol**, folate,
      lym
    ■ *Urine* ↑ 5-HIAA
    ■ *Stool* ↑ **fat**
    ■ *Synovial Fluid* ↑ WBC, mono, PMN
      ↓ viscosity

von Willebrand's disease

↑ APTT, BT, PT

↓ PLT, **PLT adhesion, PLT aggregation, factor VIII, clot retraction, ✳ von Willebrand's factor**

■ *Synovial Fluid* ↑ RBC

Wilson's disease

↑ **ALP, ALT, AST, Bil,** BSP retention, Ca^{2+}, Cu, ESR, G, **gamma globulins,** GMT, Hb (free), chloride, IgG, IgM, creatinine, LAP, LD, 5-NT, PT, pyruvate, urea

↓ **alpha-1-globulins, albumin, ALP, proteins,** Bil, unconjugated Bil, Ca, ✳ **ceruloplasmin, ✳ Cu,** RBC, G, G tolerance, haptoglobin, **Hb, HCT,** cholesterol, IgA, **IgG,** K, creatinine, **uric acid,** WBC, P, PTH, **PLT,** urea

■ *Urine* ↑ alpha-aminonitrogen, alanine, **amino acids,** proteins, **Ca, Cu,** RBC, phenylalanine, phosphates, fructose, **G,** 5-HIAA, homocysteine, isoleucine, **uric acid,** P, pH, proline, reducing sugars, threonine, tryptophan, tyrosine, valine

↓ creatinine clearance, GFR, specific gravity

■ *Cerebrospinal Fluid* ↑ Cu

■ *Synovial Fluid* ↑ pyrophosphate

Wolman's disease

↓ Hb, HCT

Diseases

allergic diseases

↑ ASLO, bas, C3 complement, CIC, **eos,** fibrinogen, fibronectin, ESR, **haptoglobin,** IgA, **IgE, IgE specific Ab,** IgG, alpha-1 proteinase inhibitor, cryoglobulins, WBC, neu, pCO_2, PMN, RAC, RAL, RF, T-lym

↓ albumin, bas, RBC, HCT, IgA, complement – (C2, C3, C4), WBC, neu, pO_2, T-lym, **PLT,** transferrin

■ *Urine* ↑ proteins, RBC, Hb, pentoses, casts – (RBC)

■ *Bronchoalveolar Lavage Fluid* ↑ eos, IgG, IgM, lym, neu, T-lym

■ *Pleural Fluid* ↑ eos, lym, neu

↓ alveolar macrophages

■ *Sputum* ↑ eos, lym, neu, PMN, viscosity

↓ alveolar macrophages

■ *Synovial Fluid* ↑ eos, WBC, PMN

arterial diseases

↑ AAT, ACLA, alpha-1-globulins, **alpha-2-globulins, ALP, ALT,** ANA, ANCA, **AST, CIC, CRP,** fibrinogen, **ESR, gamma globulins, haptoglobin,** cholesterol, **HLA** – (**B8, Bw2, Bw52, DQ, DR4**), IgA, IgG, **IgM,** IL-6, **WBC, LE cells,** lym, **neu**

↓ B-lym, RBC, **Hb, HCT**

■ *Urine* ↑ **estrogens** (females)

autoimmune diseases

↑ ACTH, **ADA,** AMA, **ANA,** anti-ds-DNA (double stranded) Ab, anti-Sm Ab, **PLT Ab,** antithyroglobulin Ab, unconjugated Bil, B2M, soluble CD4, phospholipase A2, h-sICAM-1, IgG, IgM, IL-6, sIL-2R, complement – (C4a), **cryoglobulins,** lupus inhibitor, **lym,** neopterin, orosomucoid, PLT

↓ ACTH, **albumin,** ceruloplasmin, IgG, factor – (VIII), IgG, complement – (C1, C1q, C1r, C1s, C2, C3, CH50), cortisol, lipids, protein C, protein S, **PTH**

biliary tract diseases

↑ AFP, Al, alpha-1-globulins, alpha-2-globulins, ALP, ALT, AMA, AMS, AST, beta globulins, Bil, Bil conjugated, Bil unconjugated, B2M, CA 15-3, CA 19-9, CA 50, CA 125, CEA, ceruloplasmin, **Cu**, delta Bil, Fe, ferritin, ESR, gamma globulins, GMD, GMT, HDL-C, cholesterol, chymotrypsin, IgM, chenodeoxycholic acid, cholic acid, LAP, LDL-C, WBC, lipase, lipids, MCA, Mn, 5-nucleotidase, PT, PL, TAG, trypsin, bile acids

↓ albumin, Apo A-I, AT III, beta-carotene, proteins, RBC, Fe, Hb, HDL-C, HCT, prothrombin, vitamin – (B_{12}, E)

- *Urine* ↑ AMS, Bil, Bil conjugated, oxalate, UBG
- *Peritoneal Fluid* ↑ AMS, protein
- *Stool* ↓ UBG

bone diseases

↑ ACP, aldolase, ALP, Ca, Ca^{2+}, cAMP, deoxypyridinoline, fibrinogen, ESR, hyaluronate, hydroxyproline, calcitonin, keratan sulfate, mucoproteins, Ne, TM – (ACP), 5-nucleotidase, osteocalcin, P, PTH, pyridinolone, Tr

↓ Ca, fluoride, cholesterol, osteocalcin, P, vitamin – (D)

- *Urine* ↑ amino acids, Ca, deoxypyridinoline, phosphoethanolamine, glycosaminoglycans, hydroxyproline, P
  ↓ Ca, hydroxyproline, specific gravity, P
- *Synovial Fluid* ↑ RBC, complement – (C3), crystals – (hydroxyapatite, calcium pyrophosphate), WBC, viscosity

cardiac diseases

↑ AAT, Ab against beta-2 GP I, ACLA, ACP, epinephrine, AGP, **aldolase, alpha-1-globulins, alpha-2-globulins**, alpha-HBD, ALP, **ALT, antimyocardial Ab**, Apo – ((a), B-100), **ALT, ANA**, antienterovirus Ab, **antiviral Ab, ASLO, AST**, beta-glucuronidase, Bil, **BNP, cGMP, CK, ✱ CK-MB, CK-MM, CRP**, Cu, **elastase**, enolase, **FDP, fibrinogen**, phosphohexoisomerase, phospholipase A2, fructose-1,6-diphosphate aldolase, **ESR, fibrinogen, G**, glutathione reductase, **glycogen phosphorylase BB**, GMT, **G6PD** (RBC), **haptoglobin, HBD**, hexosaminidase, HMWK, HCT, cholesterol, IgA, IgG, IgM, **plasminogen activator inhibitor**, catecholamines, complement – (C3), creatinine, uric acid, **LA, LD, LD1**, LD2, LD1:LD2, **LP(a)**, LDL-C, lym, **WBC, mAST, MD, Mn**, mono (remission), **mucoproteins, myoglobin**, L-myosin, **neu**, Ni, norepinephrine, OCT, PL, PMN, pyruvate kinase, ribonuclease, serotonin, **TAG, tropomyosin, ✱ troponin I, ✱ troponin T**, TSH, **urea**, VLDL-C, FFA

↓ albumin, bas, eos, Fe, HDL-C, **CHS**, K, LDL-C, lym, Na, orosomucoid, pH, **pO₂**, prealbumin, **transferrin satur.**, **T3**, vitamin – (B_6), Zn

- *Urine* ↑ **G**, hexosaminidase, catecholamines, crystals – (urate), **Mb**, VMA
- *Cerebrospinal Fluid* ↑ G
- *Pericardial Fluid* ↑ volume

central nervous system diseases
– infectious c. n. s. diseases

↑ ADH, alpha-2-globulins, CK, CRP, fibrinogen

- *Cerebrospinal Fluid* ↑ gamma globulins (chronic stage), IgG (chronic stage)

– inflammatory c. n. s. diseases

↑ alpha-1-globulins, alpha-2-globulins, AMS, CK

- *Cerebrospinal Fluid* ↑ A2MG, bas, CRP, IgG, acid proteinases, plasmocytes

– parasitic c. n. s. diseases

- *Cerebrospinal Fluid* ↑ bas, eos, **lym**, mono, plasmocytes

congenital heart diseases

↑ RBC, **FDP**, Hb, **HCT**, nucleated RBC, PLT

↓ PLT adhesion, albumin, estriol, **factor XI**, G, pO$_2$, free estriol

– cyanotic c. h. diseases

↑ RBC, LA

↓ PLT

connective tissue diseases

↑ ACE, **AMA**, anti-ds-DNA, anti-ss-DNA, ASLO, CK-MB, cryoglobulins, Cu, eos, **IgD**, anti-RNP Ab, LE cells, OCT

↓ albumin, CK

- *Cerebrospinal Fluid* ↑ IgG
- *Pleural Fluid* ↑ B2M, CIC, **proteins**, fibronectin

  ↓ pH
- *Synovial Fluid* ↑ WBC, clot formation, mono, PMN, volume

  ↓ viscosity

immunologically mediated diseases

↑ anti-GBMAb, anti-TBMAb, eos, HLA – (Bw35, B12, DR2, Dr4), IgA

- *Urine* ↑ **proteins**, **epithelial cells**, RBC, blood, WBC, casts – (**cellular**)

inflammatory diseases

– acute inflammatory diseases

↑ **AAT, AD, AGP, A2MG, alpha-1-antichymotrypsin,** alpha-2-antiplasmin, **alpha-1-globulins, alpha-2-globulins,** amyloid A, Apo E, AT III, **proteins, B2M,** CA 19-9, CA 50, CEA, **ceruloplasmin, CRP, Cu,** D-dimers, **elastase,** factor I, factor H, **factor VIII, ferritin, fibrinogen,** phospholipase A2, **ESR,** G, gamma globulins, **haptoglobin,** hemopexin, heme oxygenase, h-sVCAM-1, IgA, IgG, IL-6, C1-esterase inhibitor, kininogenase, complement – (C2, C3, C4, C5, C9, CH50), cryofibrinogen, WBC, Lp(a), **mucoproteins, neu, orosomucoid,** plasminogen, lipopolysaccharide binding protein, RF, serotonin, superoxide dismutase, TT, TPA, **PLT,** von Willebrand's factor, zinc protoporphyrin

↓ **albumin,** proteins, CBG, Fe, fibrinogen, Hb, cholesterol, IgA, IgG, interalpha-trypsin inhibitor, complement – (C3), prealbumin, **TIBC,** transferrin, transferrin sat., Zn

- *Urine* ↑ RBC, Hb, **Zn**

  ↓ UBG
- *Cerebrospinal Fluid* ↑ plasmocytes
- *Pericardial Fluid* ↑ RBC
- *Peritoneal Fluid* ↑ proteins, RBC, IgA, IgG, LA, LD, WBC

  ↓ G, pH
- *Pleural Fluid* ↑ AAT, A2MG, RBC, haptoglobin, hemopexin, LD, orosomucoid
- *Sputum* ↑ PMN

– chronic inflammatory diseases

↑ **AAT, AD,** AGP, **alpha-1-globulins, alpha-2-globulins,** amyloid A, anti-La/SSB, bas, proteins, **B2M,** C3, CA 19-9, CA 50, CBG, CEA, **ceruloplasmin, CRP, Cu,** D-dimers, **elastase, ferritin, fibrinogen, ESR,** gamma globulins, haptoglobin, IgA, **IgG**, mucoproteins, **neu**, **oroso-mucoid**, plasminogen, serotonin, TT, TIBC, TPA, **PLT**, zinc protopor-phyrin

↓ **albumin**, **RBC**, **Fe**, Hb, inter-alpha-trypsin inhibitor, complement – (C₃), prealbumin, **TIBC**, **transferrin**, transferrin sat., vitamin – (B₆, C), Zn

- ■ *Urine* ↑ RBC, Hb, **Zn**
  ↓ UBG
- ■ *Peritoneal Fluid* ↑ RBC, LA, WBC
  ↓ G, pH

gastrointestinal tract inflammatory diseases

↑ AAT, AFP, AGP, **alpha-1-globulins**, alpha-2-globulins, A2MG, ANCA, B2M, CEA, **CRP**, Cu, elastase, fibrinogen, phospholipase A2, ESR, gamma globulins, **haptoglobin**, hCG, HLA – (B27), IgA, IgG, **keto-bodies**, complement – (CH50), WBC, MAC, mono, motilin, muco-proteins, Na, OCT, alpha-1-acid glycoprotein, PT, serotonin, TPA, **PLT**

↓ albumin, beta-carotene, proteins, RBC, Fe, gamma globulins, Hb, HCT, CHS, IgA, IgG, IgM, K, lym, Mg, Na, pH, TBG, TIBC, transferrin, tryp-tophan, urea, vitamin – (B₂, **B₁₂**, **folate**, K), Zn

- ■ *Urine* ↑ Ca, lysozyme, oxalate
  ↓ estriol
- ■ *Peritoneal Fluid* ↑ proteins, WBC, volume
  ↓ pH
- ■ *Stool* ↑ AAT, albumin, mucus, blood, fat
- ■ *Synovial Fluid* ↑ crystals – (calcium oxalate)
  ↓ viscosity

intestine diseases

↑ AAT, AFP, alpha-1-globulins, alpha-2-globulins, ALP, A2MG, ammonia, AMS, CEA, CK, Cu, elastase, Eo, gamma globulins, gastrin, haptoglo-bin, IgA, IgG, complement – (CH50), **ketobodies**, LD, WBC, MAC, MAL, serotonin, TPA, Tr, urea

↓ albumin, ALP, A2MG, Ca, ceruloplasmin, Cu, factor II, Fe, G, GIP, Hb, HDL-C, chloride, cholesterol, CHS, IgA, K, LDL-C, Mg, Na, PT, TAG, TBG, TIBC, transferrin, urea, vitamin – (A, B₂, B₆, B₁₂, beta-carotene, C, D, E, K, folic acid), Zn

- ■ *Urine* ↑ oxalate
  ↓ estriol, K
- ■ *Stool* ↑ pus, blood, volume, fat
- ■ *Peritoneal Fluid* ↑ AMS, proteins, WBC, volume
  ↓ pH

joint diseases

↑ AAT, ACE, ADA, alanine, alpha-1-globulins, alpha-2-globulins, ALP, A2MG, ASLO, AST, proteins, beta globulins, Bil conjugated, cerulo-plasmin, CIC, CRP, Cu, elastase, eos, ferritin, fibrinogen, ESR, gam-ma globulins, GMT, haptoglobin, HLA, cholesterol, IDL-C, IFN-gamma, IgA, IgG, IgM, IL – (1, 6), complement – (Ba, Bb, C3, C4, C9), creatinine, creatine, glutamic acid, uric acid, cryoglobulins, WBC, LE cells, lupus inhibitor, lym, mono, mucoproteins, neu, orosomucoid, osteocalcin, RF, TAG, TNF-alpha, PLT, transferrin, urea, viscosity

↓ albumin, alpha globulins, ALP, A2MG, proteins, RBC, Fe, glutamine, Hb, HCT, cholesterol, complement – (C1r, C1s, C2, C3, C4, CH50), LDL-C, WBC, Mb, neu, osteocalcin, TIBC, transferrin, vitamin – (C, D), Zn

- **Urine** ↑ alanine, proteins, Cu, glutamine, glycine, hexosaminidase, hydroxyproline, crystals – (urate), uric acid
  - ↓ 17-KS, uric acid
- **Synovial Fluid** ↑ proteins, ceruloplasmin, clot formation, Cu, eos, RBC, pus, IFN-gamma, IL – (1, 2, 6, 8), complement – (C3), crystals – (urate), LA, LD, WBC, lym, lymphokines, macrophages, mono, neu, PMN, TNF-alpha, **volume**
  - ↓ C3 complement, RBC, G, crystals – (hydroxyapatite, calcium pyrophosphate), WBC, mono, neu, viscosity
- **Pleural Fluid** ↑ adenosine deaminase, proteins, eos, crystals – (cholesterol), LD, WBC, lym, PMN, RF
  - ↓ G, complement – (C3, C4), viscosity

– degenerative diseases of joints
  - ↑ complement – (C9)
  - **Urine** ↑ hexosaminidase
  - **Synovial Fluid** ↑ WBC

liver diseases

↑ AAT, ACE, **ACP**, ADA, **ADH**, acanthocytes, **aldolase, aldosterone**, alpha globulins, **ALP, ALT**, AMA, **A2MG**, aminotripeptidase, ammonia, **AMS, ANA**, APTT, arginase, **ASAL**, ASMA, **AST**, ATPase, bas, beta globulins, **beta-glucuronidase, proteins** (early, compensated), **Bil, Bil conjugated, Bil unconjugated**, B2M, BNP, ceruloplasmin, C-peptide, **Cu**, euglobulin lysis time, enolase, **estradiol**, estrogens, FDP, Fe, ferritin, fibrinogen, phosphoglucomutase, phosphohexoisomerase, fructose-1,6-diphosphate aldolase, **FSH**, fumarase, **ESR**, G, **gamma globulins**, gastrin, **glucagon**, glutathione reductase, glycerol, GMD, **GMT**, guanase, HBD, hCG, HDL-C, hexosaminidase, hydroxyproline, **cold agglutinins**, chloride, cholesterol, ICD, **IgA, IgG**, IgM, immunoreactive proinsulin, complement – (C2, C3, C4), **ketobodies, uric acid**, creatinine, **cryoglobulins**, LA, **LAP**, LD, LD5, LDL-C, LE cells, **LH**, lipase, lipids, lipoprotein lipase, lym, macrocytes, MAL (later), mAST, MD, microcytes, Mn, mono, Na, TM – (**AFP**, CA 15-3, CA 19-9, CA 27-29, CA 50, CA 125, CA 549, **CEA**, MCA, SCCA), neu, NT-pro-ANP, **5-nucleotidase**, plasma volume, **OCT**, orosomucoid, **PT, PL, PRA**, PRL, proconvertin, prothrombin, pyruvate kinase, RBP, RDW, **RF**, RTC, SD, serotonin, **SHBG**, somatostatin, GH, T3, T4, **TAG**, TBG, TIBC, TPA, PLT, transferrin, transketolase, TSH, TT, urea, **VIP**, viscosity, vitamin – (B$_{12}$), **bile acids**

↓ AAT, **albumin**, alpha-1-globulins, alpha-2-globulins, A2MG, AMS, Apo – (B-48, B-100), AST, **AT III**, beta globulins, **proteins**, C3, Ca, ceruloplasmin, Cu, **RBC**, factor IX, **fibrinogen**, G, granulocytes, haptoglobin, **Hb**, HDL-C, hemopexin, **HCT**, chloride, **cholesterol**, cholesterol esterase, **CHS**, IgG, IgM, **ILGF-I, K**, acid uric, **WBC**, Mg, mucoproteins, **Na** (later), neu, orosomucoid, osmolality, **oxalate**, P, pentoses, PICP, porphyrins, **prealbumin**, pseudocholinesterase, RBP, **RTC**, transferrin satur., Se, T3, T4, **TBG, testosterone**, TIBC, transferrin, **PLT**, UBBC, **urea**, vitamin – (D, E, folate, niacin), **Zn**

- **Urine** ↑ alpha-aminonitrogen, ALT, amino acids, **conjugated Bil**, RBC, estrogens, fructose, **G**, K, crystals – (leucine, tyrosine), DALA, fructose, G, galactose, **uric acid**, WBC, **osmolality, porphyrins**, reducing sugars, transferrin satur., T3, transferrin, **UBG**, urobilin, casts – (epithelial, granular, hyaline), **Zn**

      ↓ 17-KS, Na, niacin, volume, pH, UBG, urea
- ■ *Stool* ↑ blood, fat
    ↓ UBG
- ■ *Cerebrospinal Fluid* ↑ proteins, glutamine, lym, tryptophan
- ■ *Pleural Fluid* ↑ AMS, eos, LA, volume
    ↓ A2MG, **proteins**, haptoglobin, hemopexin, orosomucoid
- ■ *Peritoneal Fluid* ↑ proteins, RBC, **WBC**
    ↓ proteins, LA

– acute liver diseases

    ↑ ACP, Al, aldolase, ALP, ALT, **AMS**, AST, beta globulins, BHBA, proteins, B2M, ceruloplasmin, citrulline, FDP, **ferritin**, glycerol, GMD, GMT, chymotrypsin, **IgD**, IgE, immunoreactive trypsin, IRI, **LA**, LD, LD5, LDL-C, **mAST**, MD, Mn, OCT, **PT**, PRA, PTH, RF

    ↓ **alpha-2-antiplasmin**, AMS, factor II, **fibrinogen**, G, gc-globulin, haptoglobin, cortisol, uric acid, LCAT, **WBC**, neu, RBP, PLT

- ■ *Urine* ↑ proteins, conjugated Bil, estrogens, **uric acid**, porphyrins, UBG
    ↓ AMS, estriol, pregnanediol, urea
- ■ *Peritoneal Fluid* ↑ RBC

– chronic liver diseases

    ↑ **AAP**, AAT, acanthocytes, **ACE**, ACP, AFP, Al, aldolase, ALP, **AMS**, ANA, Apo B, beta globulins, BHBA, B2M, BNP, Ca, CA 15-3, CA 19-9, CA 50, CA 125, CA 549, CEA, ceruloplasmin, citrulline, estradiol, **FDP**, **ferritin**, **ESR**, G, **gamma globulins**, glycerol, GMD, GMT, hPL (F), chymotrypsin, IgA, **IgD**, IgE, IgG, IgM, immunoreactive trypsin, IRI, **LA**, LD, LD5, **LDL-C**, LH, MAC, macrocytes, MCA, **MCV**, methionine, Mn, 5-nucleotidase, NT-pro-ANP, OCT, **RBC osmotic resistance**, **PT**, PRA, PRL, prothrombin fragment 1.2, PTH, RF, rT3, SHBG, **GH**, target cells, TAG, TBG, **TT**, trypsin, VIP, vitamin – (B$_{12}$)

    ↓ AAT, **alpha-2-antiplasmin**, alpha-1-globulins, AMS, AT III, **beta globulins**, beta-carotene, **proteins**, Ca, CBG, euglobulin lysis time, factors – (II, V, VII, IX, X, XI, XII, XIII), Fe, **fibrinogen**, **haptoglobin**, G, Hb, **HDL-C**, **CHS**, ILGF-I, complement – (C4, C5, C6, C7, C8, C9, CH50), **cortisol**, uric acid, LCAT, **WBC**, neu, Ni, **RBC osmotic fragility**, osteocalcin, **plasminogen**, prekallikrein, **protein C**, **protein S**, pyruvate kinase, RBP, **T4**, **TBG**, testosterone, TIBC, **transferrin**, PLT, vitamin – (A, B$_1$, B$_2$, B$_{12}$, **D**, K, **folate**), Zn

- ■ *Urine* ↑ proteins, Bence Jones protein, conjugated Bil, estrogens, G, hexosaminidase, coproporphyrin III, crystals – (leucine, tyrosine), **uric acid**, porphyrins, UBG
    ↓ estriol, pregnanediol, urea
- ■ *Peritoneal Fluid* ↑ protein
- ■ *Stool* ↓ UBG

lymphoproliferative diseases

    ↑ cold agglutinins, paraproteins, uric acid, UBBC, viscosity
    ↓ IgM, C1-esterase inhibitor, lym
- ■ *Pleural Fluid* ↑ adenosine deaminase
- ■ *Synovial Fluid* ↑ crystals – (urate)

muscular inflammatory diseases

    ↑ ACA, AHBD, aldolase, **alpha-1-globulins**, alpha-2-globulins, ALP, ALT, ANA, anti-ds-DNA, anti-histidyl-tRNA synthetase Ab, anti-Ku, anti-Mi-2, anti-RNP, anti-Scl 70, anti-Sm, anti-SRP, anti-Ro/SSA, anti-

La,Ha/SSB, antisynthetase Ab, ASMA, AST, beta globulins, ceruloplasmin, CK, CK-MB, CK-MM, Cu, elastase, enolase, eos, ESR, HLA – (B8, DR3, DR5, DR7, DRw6, DRw52, DRw53), gamma globulins, IL-2, LD, LD5, WBC, LE cells, **Mb**, MD, mono, mucoproteins, neu, antithyroid Ab, pCO_2, pyruvate kinase, RF, T-lym, PLT

↓ RBC, gamma globulins, Hb, HCT, CHS, complement – (C2, C3, C4)

- *Urine* ↑ creatine, Mb
  ↓ creatinine
- *Synovial Fluid* ↑ crystals – (hydroxyapatite), WBC, PMN
  ↓ viscosity

myeloproliferative diseases

↑ ACP, **PLT aggregation**, ALP (WBC), **bas**, **eos**, HbF, **uric acid**, LD, **WBC**, macrocytes, megalocytes, **mono**, **MPV**, **neu**, transcobalamin II, **PLT**, UBBC, urea, vitamin – (B_{12})

↓ PTL adhesion, HDL-C, folate, LDL-C

- *Synovial Fluid* ↑ RBC, crystals – (urate), volume

pancreatic diseases

↑ **AAP**, ACA, ADH, aldolase, ALP, **AMS**, AST, beta-glucuronidase, Bil, Bil conjugated, Ca, Ca^{2+}, CCK-PZ, CEA, CRP, euglobulin lysis time, elastase, endorphins, enkephalins, Fe, ferritin, fibrinogen, ESR, G, glucagon, glucocorticoids, **GMT**, Hb, HCT, cholesterol, chymotrypsin, ILGF-II, immunoreactive trypsin, calcitonin, catecholamines, creatinine, glutamic acid, LAP, LD, LDL-C, lipase, WBC, lipids, MAC, MAL, methemalbumin, TM – (CA 15-3, CA 19-9, CA 125), pancreatic ribonuclease, PP, PTH, somatostatin, GH, GH-RH, TAG, thrombomodulin, trypsin, trypsinogen, urea, VLDL-C

↓ albumin, alpha-2-globulins, A2MG, AMS, proteins, Ca, Ca^{2+}, RBC, Fe, fibrinogen, glucagon, Hb, HCT, chloride, immunoreactive trypsin, insulin, K, complement – (C3), lipase, lipoprotein lipase, Mg, Na, P, pH, pO_2, trypsin, vitamin – (A, B_{12}, D, E, K)

- *Urine* ↑ AMS, G, 17-OHCS
  ↓ Mg, volume
- *Peritoneal Fluid* ↑ * **AMS**, proteins, RBC, lipase, methemalbumin, specific gravity
  ↓ pH
- *Pleural Fluid* ↑ AMS, proteins, RBC, LD, WBC, lipase, neu, orosomucoid
- *Stool* ↑ volume, fat

peripheral vessels diseases

↑ cold agglutinins, P-selectin

pleural diseases

↑ AAT, alpha-1-globulins, alpha-2-globulins, ceruloplasmin, **CRP**, fibrinogen, **ESR**, gamma globulins, **WBC**, lym, mucoproteins, **neu**

↓ proteins

- *Bronchoalveolar Lavage Fluid* ↑ globulins, IL, tumor-necrosis factor alpha, free oxygen radicals
- *Pleural Fluid* ↑ AAT, adenosine deaminase, albumin, A2MG, AMS, ANA, anti-DNA, bacteria (culture), beta-glucuronidase, B2M, proteins, CK, eos, RBC, FDP, fibronectin, haptoglobin, Hb, hemopexin,

cholesterol, IgA, IgG, creatinine, blood, LA, LD, WBC, LE cells, lipase, lym, lysozyme, specific gravity, mucopolysaccharides, neu, volume, orosomucoid, pH, PMN, RF, TAG

↓ alpha globulins, proteins, G, cholesterol, complement – (C3, C4, CH50), LD, WBC, lipids, lym, pH

■ *Sputum* ↑ volume, PMN

prostate diseases

↑ ACP, AMS, CK, ESR, G, creatinine, WBC, Na, TM – (CA 549, PSA), PAP, plasmin, plasminogen, PRL, urea

↓ RBC, Hb, HCT

■ *Urine* ↑ ACP, bacteria (+ culture), proteins, RBC, Hb, pus, blood, WBC

↓ pH

psychiatric diseases

↑ ADH, aldolase, **CK**, FT4, HLA – (A28), index FT4, cortisol, norepinephrine, serotonin, T3, **T4**, TSH

↓ epinephrine, CHS, norepinephrine, oxytocin, pCO_2, serotonin, taurine, FFA

■ *Urine* ↑ cAMP, catecholamines, **PABA**, VMA

↓ cAMP, 5-HIAA

■ *Cerebrospinal Fluid* ↑ CRH

pulmonary diseases

↑ **AAT**, ACE, ACTH, ADH, albumin, aldolase, **alpha-1-globulins**, alpha-2-globulins, ALP, AMS, ANA, anti-DNA, ASAL, **ASLO**, AST, bacteria (culture), proteins, Bil, Ca, ceruloplasmin, **CIC**, CK, CK-BB, CK-MB, CK-MM, CRH, **CRP**, Cu, euglobulin lysis time, elastase, **eos**, RBC, FDP, ferritin, **fibrinogen**, **ESR**, G, gamma globulins, gastrin, glucagon, GMT, haptoglobin, **Hb**, hPL, cold agglutinins, IgA, IgE, IgE specific antibodies, IgG, complement – (C3), uric acid, LA, lactoferrin, LD, LD3, **WBC**, lipase, lym, **MAC**, macrocytes, mono, **mucoproteins**, **neu**, NSE, TM – (AFP, aldolase, CA 15-3, CA 19-9, CA 50, CA 72-4, CA 549, CEA, CYFRA 21-1, DU-PAN-2, hCG, hPL, sialic acid, NSE, orosomucoid, oxytocin, PRL, PSA, PTH, ribonuclease, SCCA, sialyltransferase, TPA, VIP), pCO_2, PT, gastrin releasing peptide, pH, **RAC**, **RAL**, RF, somatostatin, GH, GH-RH, T-lym, PLT

↓ AAT, ACE, ADH, AMS, albumin, alpha-aminonitrogen, Apo B, proteins, RBC, fibrinogen, Hb, HCT, chloride, cholesterol, IgA, cortisol, complement – (C3, C4), LDL-C, WBC, Na, P, pCO_2, **pO_2**, prealbumin, T3, T4, PLT, transferrin, Zn

■ *Bronchoalveolar Lavage Fluid* ↑ alveolar macrophages, proteins, eos, RBC, globulins, IL, lipids, lym, mastocytes, mesothelial cells, neu, PMN, T-lym, TNF-alpha, free oxygen radicals

■ *Pleural Fluid* ↑ AAT, adenosine deaminase, albumin, A2MG, AMS, ANA, anti-DNA, bacteria (culture), beta-glucuronidase, B2M, proteins, CK, eos, RBC, FDP, fibronectin, haptoglobin, Hb, hemopexin, cholesterol, IgA, IgG, creatinine, blood, LA, LD, WBC, LE cells, lipase, lym, lysozyme, specific gravity, mucopolysaccharides, neu, volume, orosomucoid, pH, PMN, RF, TAG

↓ alpha globulins, proteins, G, cholesterol, complement – (C3, C4, CH50), LD, WBC, lipids, lym, pH

- **Sputum** ↑ asbestos particles, bacteria (+ culture), Curschmann's spirals, eos, histiocytes, mucus, pus, Charcot–Leyden crystals, blood, WBC, lym, macrophages, neu, volume, PMN, viscosity
  ↓ alveolar macrophages
- **Urine** ↑ albumin, alpha-aminonitrogen, AMS, proteins, Ca, hCG, ketones, creatinine, uric acid, WBC, UBG, casts – (granular, hyaline)
- **Peritoneal Fluid** ↑ RBC, TM – (CEA)

inflammatory pulmonary diseases

↑ AAT, **alpha-1-globulins**, alpha-2-globulins, CA 15-3, CA 19-9, CEA, ceruloplasmin, **CRP**, Cu, elastase, ferritin, **ESR**, G, gamma globulins, GMT, haptoglobin, **Hb**, IgG, **WBC**, mucoproteins, **neu**, NSE, orosomucoid, TPA, PLT

↓ AAT, proteins, IgA, complement – (C3), prealbumin, transferrin

- **Bronchoalveolar Lavage Fluid** ↑ globulins, IL, tumor-necrosis factor alpha, free oxygen radicals
- **Pleural Fluid** ↑ AAT, A2MG, haptoglobin, hemopexin, WBC, neu, volume, orosomucoid
- **Sputum** ↑ PMN

renal diseases

↑ AAT, ACP, ACTH, epinephrine, Al, aldosterone, alpha-aminonitrogen, ALP, ALT, **A2MG**, **ammonia**, AMS, amylin, ANF, Apo B, AST, beta-endorphins, beta globulins, BHBA, B2M, BNP, proteins, Ca, Ca^{2+}, CA 27-29, CEA, ceruloplasmin, **CIC**, CK, CK-MB, CK-MM, C-peptide, CRP, **Cu**, CYFRA 21-1, cystine, BT, enkephalins, eos, estriol, factor D, RBC, FDP, Fe, ferritin, fibrinogen, fructosamine, **ESR**, G, gamma globulins, gastrin, GIP, glucagon, glycerol, glycine, glycated albumin, glycated Hb, GMT, haptoglobin, histamine, HCO$_3^-$, chloride, cholesterol, CHS, chymotrypsin, IDL-C, ILGF-I, immunoreactive proinsulin, immunoreactive trypsin, insulin, K, calcitonin, carnitine, catecholamines, complement – (C3, C4), cortisol, creatine, **creatinine**, **uric acid**, **cryoglobulins**, LA, LD, LD1, LD2, LDL-C, WBC, LH, lipase, lipids, LPs, lysozyme, MAC, MAL, Mb, Mg, Na, neu, neurotensin, Ni, norepinephrine, NT-pro-ANP, plasma volume, osmolality, osteocalcin, P, PT, porphyrins, PP, PRA, PRL, PSA, PTH, **RF**, RTC, SCCA, Se, secretin, somatostatin, GH, TAG, thrombomodulin, trypsin, trypsinogen, TSH, urea, vitamin – (A, B$_{12}$, D, E)

↓ AAT, **albumin**, aldosterone, alpha-2-globulins, alpha-aminonitrogen, ALT, amino acids, Apo A-I, AST, AT III, beta globulins, proteins, Ca, Ca^{2+}, CBG, ceruloplasmin, Cu, EPO, RBC, estrogens, Fe, fibrinogen, FT3, FT4, G, **globulins**, HBA$_{1c}$, Hb, HDL-C, HCT, HCO$_3^-$, chloride, ILGF-I, K, carbonic anhydrase, complement – (C1r, C1s, C2, C3, C4), cortisol, glutamic acid, LCAT, WBC, lipoprotein lipase, lym, Mg, Na, Ni, volume, ornithine, osmolality, P, pH, PRA, progesterone, RTC, Se, serotonin, T3, T4, TBG, testosterone, TIBG, PLT, **transferrin**, tyrosine, vitamin – (B$_1$, B$_6$, B$_{12}$, D, folate), Zn

- **Urine** ↑ AAP, ACP, albumin, alpha-aminonitrogen, ALP, ALT, ammonia, AMS, bacteria (+ culture), beta-2-glycoprotein I, proteins, Ca, Ca^{2+}, cAMP, cystine, eos, RBC, G, Hb, hexosaminidase, pus, HCO$_3^-$, hydroxyproline, K, blood, crystals – (Ca-phosphate, Ca-oxalate, urate, waxy), alpha-ketoglutaric acid, uric acid, LD, WBC, lysozyme, Mb, specific gravity, Na, volume, osmolality, oxalates, P, pH, lipids, uroporphyrin, casts – (epithelial, RBC, **granular**, **hyaline**, WBC, Mb, lipid, waxy)

↓ Ca, FDP, chloride, K, carnitine, 17-KS, uric acid, specific gravity, Mg, Na, volume, osmolality, oxalates, P, pH, UBG, urea

- *Peritoneal Fluid* ↑ RBC
- *Sweat* ↑ Na

– acute renal diseases

↑ epinephrine, alpha-1-globulins, alpha-2-globulins, A2MG, ASLO, Ca, CIC, **CRP**, elastase, eos, **ESR**, gamma globulins, GMT, haptoglobin, chloride, cholesterol, IgA, IgE, IgG, IgM, K, creatinine, uric acid, cryoglobulins, LA, LD, LD5, WBC, lipase, lysozyme, MAC, Na, neu, orosomucoid, osmolality, P, urea

↓ albumin, RBC, estriol, Hb, HCT, HCO$_3^-$, chloride, K, complement – (C1q, C3, C4, C6, CH50), Mg, Na, pCO$_2$, PT, pH, PLT

- *Urine* ↑ AAP, amino acids, bacteria (+ culture), proteins, Ca, eos, RBC, G, Hb, hexosaminidase, pus, HCO$_3^-$, K, blood, WBC, lysozyme, specific gravity, nitrates, volume, pH, PO$_4^-$, tubular cells, casts – (epithelial, RBC, granular, hyaline, WBC, lipid, mixed)

↓ Ca, estriol, chloride, K, creatinine, specific gravity, volume, osmolality, P, urea

– chronic renal diseases

↑ epinephrine, albumin, alpha-1-globulins, alpha-2-globulins, A2MG, BNP, CIC, CRP, CYFRA 21-1, elastase, FDP, ferritin, **ESR**, G, gamma globulins, GMT, haptoglobin, HbF, chloride, cholesterol, IgA, IgE, IgG, IgM, K, **creatinine**, **uric acid**, LA, LD, lipase, lipids, lysozyme, MAC, MAL, Mg, Na, norepinephrine, orosomucoid, osmolality, P, PT, plasmocytes, **PTH**, **RBP**, urea, vitamin – (A, beta-carotene)

↓ alanine, albumin, proteins, **Ca**, **Ca^{2+}**, EPO, RBC, estriol, Fe, Hb, HCT, CHS, K, complement – (C1r, C1s, C2, C3, C4, CH50), WBC, Mg, Na, Ni, pH, RTC, **transferrin**, vitamin – (A)

- *Urine* ↑ AAP, amino acids, bacteria (+ culture), proteins, Ca, eos, RBC, G, Hb, hexosaminidase, pus, K, creatinine, blood, crystals – (Ca-oxalate), WBC, lipids, nitrates, volume, retinol binding protein, fat, casts – (epithelial, RBC, granular, hyaline, WBC, lipid, waxy, mixed)

↓ Ca, estriol, GMT, chloride, K, creatinine, uric acid, specific gravity, volume, P, urea

– infectious renal diseases

↑ AAT, alpha-aminonitrogen, alpha-1-globulins, alpha-2-globulins, A2MG, ASLO, proteins, CIC, **CRP**, elastase, Fe, **ESR**, G, gamma globulins, haptoglobin, chloride, cholesterol, IgA, IgG, IgM, K, creatine, creatinine, uric acid, cryoglobulins, LA, LD, LD5, **WBC**, lipids, lysozyme, MAC, mucoproteins, Na, orosomucoid, osmolality, P, urea

↓ albumin, proteins, estriol, HCO$_3^-$, chloride, K, complement – (C1r, C1s, C2, C3, C4, C6, CH50), LD, Na, osmolality, PT, pH, PLT, urea, vitamin – (A)

- *Urine* ↑ AAP, AST, bacteria (+ culture), proteins, estriol, **RBC**, **G**, **Hb**, hexosaminidase, pus, K, blood, LAP, LD, **WBC**, lysozyme, specific gravity, nitrates, pH, casts – (epithelial, RBC, granular, hyaline, WBC)

↓ Ca, estriol, chloride, K, creatinine, uric acid, specific gravity, Na, volume, osmolality, P, pH, urea

rheumatic diseases

↑ **AAT**, ACA, ACE, AGP, alpha-1-antichymotrypsin, alpha-1-globulins (acute period), alpha-2-globulins (acute period), ALP, A2MG, AMA, **ANA**, ANCA, anti-ds-DNA, anti-ss-DNA, anti-endothelial Ab, anti-HSP 65, antikeratin Ab, antimicrosomal Ab, antimyocardial Ab, anti-RNP, anti-Scl-70, anti-Ro/SSA, anti-La,Ha/SSB, APF, **ASLO**, ASMA, proteins, beta globulins, ceruloplasmin, CIC, CRP, Cu, elastase, eos, ESR, ferritin, fibrinogen, gamma globulins (chronic stage), gastrin, glycated Hb, GMT, **haptoglobin**, HLA – (B27, DPw4, DQ7, DQw7, DR1, DR4, DR6, Dw4, Dw10, Dw13, Dw14, Dw15), IgA, IgE, IgG, IgM, IFN-gamma, IL – (1, 6), complement – (Ba, Bb, C3, C4, C4d, C9), creatine, uric acid, cryoglobulins, glutamic acid, LE cells, **WBC** (acute stage), lupus inhibitor, lym, Mn, mono, mucoproteins, neu, osteocalcin, PT, anti-DNA-histone complex Ab, antithyroglobulin Ab, antithyroid Ab, RANA, RF – (IgA, IgM), TNF-alpha, PLT, transferrin, viscosity

↓ albumin, ALP, A2MG, amino acids, arginine, beta-2-glycoprotein I, proteins, **RBC**, Fe, glutamine, Hb, HCT, cholesterol, complement – (C1r, C1s, C2, C3, C4, CH50), WBC, Mb, neu, osteocalcin, transferrin satur., TIBC, PLT, transferrin, vitamin – (C, D), Zn

- *Urine* ↑ alanine, Cu, glutamine, glycine, hexosaminidase, hydroxyproline
  ↓ threonine
- *Pericardial Fluid* ↑ RBC, volume
- *Pleural Fluid* ↑ adenosine deaminase, B2M, proteins, CSF – (GM, M), eos, RBC, crystals – (cholesterol), LA, **LD**, WBC, lym, neu, PMN, **RF**
  ↓ C3, C4, G, pH, viscosity
- *Bronchoalveolar Lavage Fluid* ↑ lym
- *Synovial Fluid* ↑ ceruloplasmin, Cu, eos, RBC, pus, IFN-gamma, IL – (1, 2, 6, 8), LA, LD, WBC, lym, lymphokines, macrophages, mono, neu, PMN, TNF-alpha, volume
  ↓ C3, G, viscosity
- *Saliva* ↑ IgA, Na

skin diseases

↑ antiendomysial Ab, antireticulin Ab, CIC, eos, HLA – (B8, DQw2, DR3, Dw3, Dw5), IgE, IgG, WBC, lym, neu, RF

↓ Al, albumin, proteins, Fe, CHS, vitamin – (B$_2$, B$_{12}$, folic acid)

spleen diseases

↓ WBC, PLT

thyroid gland diseases

↑ AAT, ADH, epinephrine, ALP, AMA, ANA, antiadrenal Ab, anti-ds-DNA, antimicrosomal Ab, antithyroglobulin Ab, **antithyroid Ab**, antithyroxine Ab, **APA**, bas, beta-carotene, proteins, Ca, cAMP, ceruloplasmin, CK, Cu, DPD, endorphins, enkephalins, FT3, FT4, ESR, G, histaminase, HLA – (Bw35, B37, DR5), cholesterol, CHS, IgA, IgM, iodine, calcitonin, catecholamines, complement – (C3), acetoacetate acid, uric acid, LATS, LD, WBC, lym, macrocytes, neu, TM – (**ACTH**, AFP, **beta-lipotropin**, CA 50, CEA, hCG, NSE, TPA), norepinephrine, plasma volume, P, PP, antibodies against thyroid peroxidase, anti-TSH receptors Ab, PTH, SHBG, somatostatin, substance P, **T3**, **T4**, TAG, **TSH**, **thyroglobulin**, VIP

↓ albumin, ALP, AMS, Ca, Ca^{2+}, RBC, Hb, HCT, cholesterol, IgA, iodine, K, complement – (C3), WBC, neu, pepsinogen, PRL, T3, T4, TBG, TSH, vitamin – (D3)

- **Urine** ↑ cAMP, 5-HIAA, 17-OHCS
  ↓ Ca, cAMP, 17-OHCS, 17-KS, P
- **Stool** ↑ fat
- **Cerebrospinal Fluid** ↑ proteins

urinary tract diseases

↑ alpha-1-globulins, alpha-2-globulins, AMS, CRP, **ESR**, gamma globulins, **WBC**, neu

↓ albumin

- **Urine** ↑ acetone, alanine, albumin, ammonia, AMS, bacteria (+ culture), **proteins**, Ca, DALA, Eo, **RBC**, estriol, G, **Hb**, hexosaminidase, **pus**, HCO_3^-, chloride, K, catecholamines, ketones, creatinine, crystals – (Ca-phosphate), uric acid, **WBC**, leukocyte esterase, Mb, Na, nitrites, **volume**, osmolality, P, pH, casts – (**granular, hyaline**)
  ↓ estriol, hCG, Mg, volume, pH, pregnanediol, urea

– infectious urinary tract diseases

↑ alpha-1-globulins, alpha-2-globulins, CRP, ferritin, **ESR**, **WBC**, neu

- **Urine** ↑ bacteria (+ culture), **proteins**, RBC, G, Hb, **WBC**, **volume**, casts – (**granular, hyaline**)

Diseases, Infectious

actinomycosis (Actinomyces israelii)

↑ ESR, WBC, IgA, **IgG, IgM**

↓ albumin, Hb, HCT

- **Sputum** ↑ * **bacilli** (+ culture)
- **Pleural Fluid** ↑ * **bacilli** (+ culture)

acute infectious diseases

↑ AAT, AD, PLT adhesion, **AGP**, ALP, ALT, AMS, alpha-aminonitrogen, **alpha-1-antichymotrypsin**, alpha-1-globulins, **alpha-2-globulins**, **ASLO**, AST, BHBA, conjugated Bil, **B2M**, B-lym, **ceruloplasmin, CIC, CRP, Cu**, D-dimers, **elastase**, eos, **FDP**, ferritin, **fibrinogen, ESR**, gamma globulins, IFN-gamma, **glucagon, haptoglobin**, IgA, IgE specific antibodies, IgG, **IgM**, IL – (2, 4, 6), K, complement – (C3, C4), cortisol, creatinine, cryoglobulins, uric acid, LA, LD, **WBC, lym**, lysozyme, MAC, **mono, mucoproteins, neu**, orosomucoid, RF, TNF, **PLT**, tropomyosin, trypsin, urea, viscosity

↓ ACE, albumin, proteins, carbohydrate-deficient transferrin (false), ceruloplasmin, Cu, eos, **Fe**, RBC, fibronectin, **G6PD** (RBC), Hb, HDL-C, HCT, chloride, cholesterol, **CHS**, complement – (C1r, C1s, C3, CH50), lym, neu, pH, pO_2, **transferrin satur.**, PLT, transferrin, vitamin – (A, C), Zn

- **Urine** ↑ bacteria (+ culture), proteins, Ca, RBC, fructose, **G**, galactose, Hb, hemosiderin, pus, ketobody, 17-KGS, **17-KS**, uric acid, WBC, lysozyme, Mb, volume, reducing sugars, **UBG**, casts – (granular, hyaline, WBC)
  ↓ P
- **Cerebrospinal Fluid** ↑ proteins, **IgG**, LA, WBC, lym, MBP, PMN, pressure
  ↓ G

- *Sputum* ↑ eos, mucus, Charcot–Leyden crystals, blood
- Peritoneal Fluid ↑ LA, RBC, **WBC**
  ↓ **pH**
- *Pleural Fluid* ↑ AMS, B2M, proteins, RBC, fibronectin, IgG, LD, lym, lysozyme, mucopolysaccharides, neu, volume
- *Stool* ↑ proteins, heme, mucus, pus, blood
- *Synovial Fluid* ↑ CIC, eos, pus, complement – (C3, C4), crystals – (calcium oxalate), WBC, macrophages, PMN
  ↓ viscosity

AIDS (HIV positivity)

↑ **ACE**, ALP, **ALT**, ANA, ANCA, c-ANCA, atypical-ANCA, anti-CMV Ab, anti-EBV Ab, anti-RBC, **p24 antigen, anticardiolipin Ab, ✶ anti-HIV Ab** (IgG), antilymphocyte Ab, anti-PLT Ab, APA, ASMA, **AST, B2M,** B-lym, soluble CD4, CD8-lym (suppressant), ceruloplasmin, **CIC, CRP, elastase, ESR,** ferritin, **gamma globulins**, G, GM-CSF, GMT, ✶ **HIV antigen,** ✶ **HIV-1 RNA,** ✶ **HIV** (culture), ✶ **HIV DNA** (PCR), HBcAg, h-sICAM-1, **IgA, IgD,** IgE, IgG, **IgM, IFN-alpha** (acid labile), IFN-gamma, cortisol, IL – (2, 4, 6), sIL-2R, sIL-6R, IL2 receptors, LD, **WBC, lysozyme, neopterin,** antibrain Ab, RF, **T4,** TAG, alpha-1-thymosin, TNF-alpha, PLT, VDRL (false)

↓ aldosterone, albumin, anti-EBV-VCA (false), **CD4-lym (helper),** EPO, **RBC,** G, **Hb, HDL-C, HCT,** cholesterol, **IgD,** IgG, IL-2, complement – (C1r, **C3**), cortisol, **WBC, lym,** Na, neu, protein S, Se, serotonin, T-lym (T4, CD4+), T4/T8 ratio, **PLT,** vitamin B$_{12}$

- *Urine* ↑ proteins, **anti-HIV Ab**
- *Cerebrospinal Fluid* ↑ ✶ **anti-HIV, proteins,** B2M, WBC, MBP
- *Synovial Fluid* ↑ clot formation, WBC, PMN, volume

amebiasis (Entamoeba histolytica)

↑ ALP, **ALT, ✶ antibodies against E. histolytica** (IgG, IgM), **AST,** Bil, eos, **ESR, GMT, LAP,** LD, neu, **5-NT, WBC**

↓ albumin, CHS, **Hb, HCT,** WBC, microcytes

- *Cerebrospinal Fluid* ↑ **proteins, RBC,** lym, **WBC, PMN, pressure**
  ↓ G
- *Pleural Fluid* ↑ proteins, specific gravity
  ↓ pH
- *Stool* ↑ proteins, ✶ **entamoebal antigen,** heme, **mucus,** Charcot–Leyden crystals, **blood, ✶ protozoans,** WBC

anthrax (Bacillus anthracis)

↑ ✶ **bacilli,** ESR, WBC, PMN

- *Urine* ↑ Hb
- *Cerebrospinal Fluid* ↑ **bacilli, proteins,** RBC, PMN
  ↓ G
- *Peritoneal Fluid* ↑ bacilli
- *Pleural Fluid* ↑ bacilli
- *Stool* ↑ bacilli

ascariasis (Ascaris lumbricoides)

↑ eos, WBC, IgE

- *Stool* ↑ ✶ **parasite ova**

aspergillosis (Aspergillus fumigatus + species)

↑ ADH, ALT, **∗ antibodies against aspergillus** (IgG, IgM), **∗ aspergillus antigen, eos, IgE, IgE specific Ab**, WBC, urea

↓ albumin, HCO_3^-, WBC, pH, **pO_2**, pCO_2

■ *Sputum* ↑ **Curshmann's spirals, ∗ fungi, eos, mucus,** Charcot–Leyden crystals, mycelia, casts, **color changes**

■ *Bronchoalveolar Lavage Fluid* ↑ macrophages

■ *Synovial Fluid* ↑ crystals – (calcium oxalate)

babesiosis (Babesia microti)

↑ ALT, AST, **∗ protozoans** (+ RBC), **∗ babesia antigen, ∗ babesia DNA** (PCR), Bil, GMT, LD

↓ **RBC, Hb, HCT**, WBC, **PLT**

■ *Urine* ↑ Hb

bacterial infectious diseases

↑ unconjugated Bil, CK-MB, CRP, elastase, **ESR**, complement – (C3), **WBC,** neu, PCT, tropomyosin

↓ albumin, complement – (C1r, C1s, C4, C5, C6, C7, C8, C9, CH50), C1-INH

■ *Pleural Fluid* ↑ **WBC**

■ *Bronchoalveolar Lavage Fluid* ↑ neu

– acute bacterial infectious diseases

↑ AAT, ADA, ADH, aldolase, alpha-1-antichymotrypsin, alpha-1-globu-lins, A2MG, ANA, antimyocardial Ab, Apo E, **ASLO**, AT III, beta globulins, unconjugated Bil, proteins, Ca, ceruloplasmin, CIC, **CRP, elastase,** eos, RBC, **fibrinogen, ESR,** G, gamma globulins, haptoglo-bin, Hb, cold agglutinins, IgA, IgG, kininogenase, complement – (C2, C3, C4, C5, C9), uric acid, LA, lactoferrin, **WBC,** lipase, lym, lysozyme, MAC, mono, mucoproteins, neu, orosomucoid, pCO_2, PT, plasmino-gen, plasmocytes, RF, febrile agglutinins, tropomyosin, urea, VDRL (false)

↓ ACE, albumin, proteins, RBC, G, Hb, HCT, cholesterol, IgM, comple-ment – (C1r, C1s, C5, C6, C7, C8, C9, CH50), cortisol, pH, PLT

■ *Urine* ↑ proteins, Ca, RBC, Hb

■ *Sputum* ↑ bacteria (+ culture), RBC, blood

■ *Pleural Fluid* ↑ ADA, B2M, proteins, RBC, fibronectin, IgG, LD, lym, lysozyme, mucopolysaccharides, neu, **WBC,** volume

■ *Stool* ↑ mucus, blood, WBC

– chronic bacterial infectious diseases

↑ ASLO, CIC, CRP, ESR, complement – (C3, C4), WBC, **lym,** RF, urea

↓ complement – (C1r, C1s, C5, C6, C7, C8, C9, CH50)

balantidiasis (Balantidium coli)

■ *Stool* ↑ **∗ protozoans**

bartonellosis (Bartonella quintana)

↑ **∗ bacilli, ∗ antibodies against Bartonella quintana** (IgG), nucleated RBC, WBC

cat scratch disease (Bartonella henselae)

↑ **∗ bacilli** (PCR), **∗ antibodies against Bartonella henselae** (IgG, IgM), eos, **ESR,** WBC

■ *Cerebrospinal Fluid* ↑ **∗ bacilli** (PCR)

bejel (T. pallidum, subspecies endemicum)

↑ syphilis Ab (false), **treponemal antibodies** (false), VDRL

blastomycosis (Blastomyces dermatitidis, Paracoccidioides brasiliensis)
    ↑ ALP, ✻ **antibodies against B. dermatitidis**, ESR, WBC
    ↓ albumin, Hb, HCT
    ■ *Sputum* ↑ ✻ **fungi** (+ culture)
borreliosis, Lyme (Borrelia burgdorferi)
    ↑ ALP, ALT, ✻ **Ab against B. burgdorferi**, AST, treponemal antibodies
      (false), CIC, CK-MB, **ESR**, GMT, **HLA – (DR2, DR4)**, HCT, IgG, IgM,
      cryoglobulins, LAP, LD, 5-NT, **WBC**
    ↓ RBC, ESR, Hb, HCT, WBC
    ■ *Synovial Fluid* ↑ C3, C4, CIC, eos, pus, WBC, PMN
      ↓ viscosity
    ■ *Cerebrospinal Fluid* ↑ ✻ antibody against B. burgdorferi, proteins, IgG,
      lym, PMN, pressure, **WBC**
      ↓ G
brucellosis (Brucella melitensis, B. suis, B. abortus)
    ↑ ✻ **Ab against brucella**, ALP, **ALT**, **AST**, ESR, IgG, IgM, LAP, WBC, **lym**,
      mono, febrile agglutinins, 5-NT, RF, syphilis Ab (false), VDRL (false)
    ↓ albumin, RBC, ESR, Hb, HCT, **WBC**, neu
    ■ *Cerebrospinal Fluid* ↑ proteins, lym
      ↓ G, chloride
campylobacteriosis (Campylobacter jejuni + species)
    ↑ ✻ **bacteria** (culture)
    ■ *Stool* ↑ ✻ **bacteria** (culture)
    ■ *Synovial Fluid* ↑ clot formation, volume
candidiasis (moniliasis) (Candida albicans)
    ↑ ✻ **antibodies against C. albicans**, ✻ **fungi** (culture), Ca, IgE, **WBC**
    ↓ complement – (C3), WBC
    ■ *Nails* ↑ ✻ **fungi** (culture)
cholera (Vibrio comma)
    ↑ ✻ **antitoxin Ab**, ASLO, **proteins**, **RBC**, Hb, **HCT**, chloride, **creatinine**, uric
      acid, LA, **WBC**, **MAC**, **Na**, neu, P, specific gravity, **urea**, ✻ **vibriocidal**
      Ab, viscosity
    ↓ HCO_3^-, chloride, K, Na, pH
    ■ *Urine* ↓ volume
    ■ *Stool* ↑ HCO_3^-, chloride, Na
chronic infectious diseases
    ↑ **AD**, **AGP**, alpha-1-globulins, ALP, ALT, AMS, **ASLO**, AST, BHBA, conju-
      gated Bil, **ceruloplasmin**, **CIC**, **CRP**, **Cu**, D-dimers, **elastase**, eos, FDP,
      ESR, ferritin, **fibrinogen**, **gamma globulins**, **glucagon**, **haptoglobin**, IgA,
      IgD, **IgG**, **K**, complement – (C3, C4), cortisol, uric acid, LA, LD, **WBC**,
      lym, lysozyme, **mono**, **mucoproteins**, **neu**, TBG, TPA, **PLT**, tropo-
      myosin, urea
    ↓ albumin, proteins, Cu, eos, RBC, **Fe**, galactose, **G6PD** (RBC), Hb, HCT,
      HDL-C, cholesterol, **CHS**, complement – (C3, C4, C5, C6, C7, C8, C9,
      CH50), LDL-C, WBC, lym, neu, plasma volume, RTC, **transferrin**
      satur., PLT, TIBC, **transferrin**, vitamin – (A, B_{12}, C)
    ■ *Urine* ↑ bacteria (+ culture), proteins, G, Hb, hemosiderin, 17-KGS,
      17-KS, WBC, lysozyme, volume, reducing sugars, casts – (granular,
      hyaline, WBC)
clonorchiasis (Clonorchis sinensis)
    ■ *Stool* ↑ ✻ parasite ova, ✻ Clonorchis sinensis antigen

- *Duodenal Content* ↑ ✳ parasite ova

clostridial infectious diseases (Clostridium perfringens)
- ↑ **Bil,** CK-MB, **WBC,** creatinine, spherocytes, osmotic fragility (RBC), MHb
- ↓ **Hb, HCT, PLT**
- *Urine* ↑ **proteins, Hb,** hemosiderin, **casts**
  - ↓ volume
- *Stool* ↑ WBC

coccidioidomycosis (Coccidioides immitis)
- ↑ ✳ **Ab against Coccidioides immitis** (IgG, IgM), ✳ **fungi** (culture), ACE, Ca, **eos,** ESR, IgE, **WBC**
- ↓ ACE, albumin, G
- *Sputum* ↑ ✳ **fungi** (+ culture)
- *Bronchoalveolar Lavage Fluid* ↑ ✳ **fungi** (+ culture)
- *Cerebrospinal Fluid* ↑ **proteins,** ✳ **Ab against Coccidioides immitis** (IgG, IgM), ✳ **fungi** (culture), eos, WBC, **pressure**
  - ↓ G
- *Stool* ↑ ✳ **fungi** (culture)
- *Urine* ↑ ✳ **fungi** (culture)

coccidiosis (Isospora hominis, I. belli, Cryptosporidium parvum)
- *Stool* ↑ ✳ **protozoan oocysts**

cryptococcosis (Cryptococcus neoformans)
- ↑ ALT, ✳ **cryptococcal antigen,** ✳ **fungi** (culture), ✳ **antibodies against C. neoformans** (IgG, IgM), WBC
- *Cerebrospinal Fluid* ↑ **proteins,** ✳ **fungi** (culture), ✳ **cryptococcal antigen,** ✳ **antibodies against C. neoformans** (IgG, IgM), **WBC, lym, pressure**
  - ↓ G
- *Sputum* ↑ ✳ **fungi** (culture)
- *Urine* ↑ ✳ **fungi** (culture)
- *Stool* ↑ ✳ **fungi** (culture)

cryptosporidiosis (Cryptosporidium)
- ↑ ✳ **cryptosporidial antigen**
- *Stool* ↑ ✳ **protozoans**

cysticercosis (Cysticercus cellulosae, larva of Taenia solium)
- ↑ CK-MB, proteins, mono
- ↓ G
- *Cerebrospinal Fluid* ↑ proteins, WBC, pressure
  - ↓ G

dengue (flaviviruses)
- ↑ ✳ **antibodies against flavivirus** (IgM), ✳ **flavivirus DNA** (PCR)
- ↓ WBC, PLT

diphtheria (Corynebacterium diphtheriae)
- ↑ globulins, **neu, toxoid antibodies, WBC, urea**
- ↓ **G, Hb, HCT,** WBC
- *Urine* ↑ **albumin,** blood, **casts**
- *Cerebrospinal Fluid* ↑ **proteins,** mono

disease, legionnaires' (Legionella pneumophila)
- ↑ ALP, ALT, AST, ✳ **antibodies against Legionella** (IgG, IgM), ✳ **bacilli** (culture), **Bil,** ESR, LD, **WBC,** ✳ **PCR** (Legionella), **PMN**
- ↓ albumin, WBC, **Na, P,** pCO_2, pO_2

- *Urine* ↑ * bacillus Ag, * PCR (Legionella), **proteins**, RBC, blood
- *Sputum* ↑ * bacilli (culture), PMN, **positive DNA probe**
- *Bronchoalveolar Lavage Fluid* ↑ **positive DNA probe**, * PCR (Legionella)
- *Pleural Fluid* ↑ * bacilli (culture), **bacillus Ag, positive DNA probe**

dysentery, bacillary (Shigella species)

↑ chloride, ↑ RBC, Hb, K, **WBC**, MAC, neu, Na, urea

↓ chloride, **proteins**, G, **Hb, HCT**, K, WBC, **Na**, pCO_2, pH, PLT

- *Stool* ↑ * bacteria (culture), **RBC, mucus, blood**, WBC, **pus**

ehrlichiosis (rickettsial-like coccobacillus)

↑ * **Ehrlichia DNA** (PCR), ALT,AST, * **antibodies against Ehrlichia** (IgG, IgM)

↓ Hb, HCT, WBC, PLT

- *Cerebrospinal Fluid* ↑ * **Ehrlichia DNA** (PCR), proteins, lym

erysipelas (Str. pyogenes)

↑ ESR, WBC

erythema infectiosum (fifth disease) (Parvovirus B19)

↑ * **antibodies against parvovirus B19** (IgG, IgM), eos

exanthema subitum (human herpesvirus 6)

↑ * **HHV-6**, * **early viral antigen**, * **antibodies against HHV-6**, * **HHV-6 DNA** (PCR), WBC (early), lym

↓ WBC (later)

fascioliasis (Fasciola hepatica)

↑ **ALT, AST**, eos, * **antibodies against F. hepatica** (IgG, IgM), IgE, WBC

- *Stool* ↑ * **parasite ova**, * **F. hepatica antigen**
- *Duodenal Content* ↑ * **parasite ova**

fever, Colorado tick (reoviridae)

↑ * **antibodies against orbivirus** (IgG, IgM), * **orbivirus antigen** (RBC)

↓ WBC, PMN

fever, hemorrhagic

↑ APTT, * **antibodies against hantavirus** (IgG, IgM), Hb, HCT, **LD**, WBC, Na, PT, WBC, urea

↓ **albumin**, proteins (total), WBC, **PLT**

- *Urine* ↑ **proteins**
  ↓ volume

Hantavirus pulmonary syndrome

↑ * **antibodies against hantavirus** (IgG, IgM), Hb, HCT

↓ PLT

fever, paratyphoid (Salmonella paratyphi A or B)

↑ * **bacteria** (culture), lym, WBC

↓ eos, Hb, HCT, WBC, neu

fever, Rocky Mountain, spotted (Rickettsia rickettsii)

↑ ALT, * **Ab against R. rickettsii** (IgG, IgM), **AST**, * **R. rickettsii DNA** (PCR), CK-MB, WBC, **mono**, urea

↓ **albumin**, proteins, Ca, factor – (II, V, XII), fibrinogen, Hb, HCT, **WBC**, Na, neu, PLT

- *Urine* ↑ **casts**
  ↓ volume
- *Cerebrospinal Fluid* ↑ * **Ab against R. rickettsii** (IgG, IgM)

fever, typhoid (Salmonella typhi)

    ↑ **ADA**, Ag H, Ag O, **ALP**, ALP isoenzymes, ALT, **AST**, ✻ **bacteria** (culture), ✻ **anti-typhoid Ab**, Bil, **CK**, **Cu**, ESR, globulins, IgA, complement – (C3), **LD**, **WBC** (early), **lym**, MD, T4

    ↓ **eos**, ESR, Fe, **Hb**, HCT, **WBC**, **neu**, T3, TBG, Zn

    ■ *Urine* ↑ albumin, alpha-aminonitrogen, ✻ **bacteria** (culture), **proteins**, **Hb**, ketones, creatinine

       ↓ chloride, volume

    ■ *Stool* ↑ blood, ✻ **bacteria** (culture)

fever, yellow (flaviviruses)

    ↑ ALT, ✻ **anti-arbovirus Ab**, Bil

    ↓ G, **WBC**, **lym**, neu

    ■ *Urine* ↑ proteins

       ↓ **volume**

    ■ *Stool* ↑ blood

filariasis (Wuchereria bancrofti, Brugia malayi)

    ↑ ✻ **Ab against filaria**, ✻ **filaria antigen**, ✻ **parasite**, ALT, **eos**, **IgE**, RF

    ■ *Urine* ↑ chylus, ✻ **filaria antigen**

    ■ *Cerebrospinal Fluid* ↑ ✻ **parasite** (non-lymphatic filariasis)

    ■ *Peritoneal Fluid* ↑ **proteins**, TAG

fungal infectious disease

    ↑ ACE, Ca, CK-MB, IgA, **IgM**, **WBC**, neu, PCT

    ↓ RBC

    ■ *Synovial Fluid* ↑ clot formation, volume

giardiasis (Giardia lamblia)

    ↑ **antibodies against G. lamblia** (IgG, IgM)

    ■ *Stool* ↑ ✻ **protozoans**, ✻ **Giardia antigen**

gonorrhea (Neisseria gonorrhoeae)

    ↑ WBC, neu

    ■ *Urine* ↑ ✻ **bacteria** (+ culture), ✻ **gonococcal antigen**

    ■ *Stool* ↑ ✻ **bacteria** (+ culture)

herpes simplex (Herpes simplex virus)

    ↑ ✻ **anti-Herpes simplex virus 1,2 Ab** (IgG, IgM), ✻ **HSV DNA** (PCR)

    ■ *Cerebrospinal Fluid* ↑ proteins, **WBC**, **lym**

herpes zoster (Herpes zoster virus)

    ↑ ✻ **antibodies against Herpes zoster virus**, ALP, ALT, AST, B2M, creatinine, LD, **WBC**, mono, neu, PRL, urea

    ↓ albumin, **Hb**, HCT, WBC

    ■ *Cerebrospinal Fluid* ↑ **proteins**, 5-HIAA, HVA, **WBC**, **lym**, mono, pleocytosis, pressure

    ■ *Urine* ↑ Mb

histoplasmosis (Histoplasma capsulatum)

    ↑ ALT, ✻ **Ab against H. capsulatum** (IgG, IgM), ✻ **fungi** (+ culture), ✻ **histoplasma antigen**, ACE, Ca, lym, WBC

    ↓ RBC, Fe, **Hb**, HCT, **WBC**, neu, PLT

    ■ *Sputum* ↑ ✻ **histoplasma antigen**, ✻ **fungi** (+ culture)

    ■ *Urine* ↑ ✻ **histoplasma antigen**

    ■ *Cerebrospinal Fluid* ↑ ✻ **histoplasma antigen**

    ■ *Bronchoalveolar Lavage Fluid* ↑ ✻ **histoplasma antigen**

hookworm disease (Necator americanus, Ancylostoma duodenale)

↑ anisocytes, bas, **eos**, cholesterol, IgE, IgM, **WBC**, poikilocytes, TIBC

↓ **albumin, proteins, Fe, RBC, Hb, HCT,** iron, MCH (RBC), MCHC (RBC), MCV (RBC), **microcytes,** transferrin satur.

■ *Urine* ↑ proteins

■ *Stool* ↑ ✴ **parasite ova, blood**

i. d. caused by adenoviruses

↑ ✴ **antibodies against adenoviruses,** ESR

↓ WBC

i. d. caused by cestodes

↑ eos, IgE

↓ folic acid

i. d. caused by chlamydia

↑ ✴ **bacteria** (culture), ✴ **antibodies against chlamydia** (IgG, IgM), ✴ **chlamydia antigen,** VDRL (false)

i. d. caused by coxsackie

↑ ✴ **Ab against coxsackie,** trypsin

■ *Urine* ↑ Mb

■ *Cerebrospinal Fluid* ↑ proteins, lym, PMN

i. d. caused by cytomegalovirus

↑ ✴ **anti-CMV Ab** (IgG, IgM), ✴ **CMV DNA** (PCR), ✴ **CMV antigen,** ALP, ALT, ANA, anti-EBV-VCA IgG (false), AST, Bil, **CRP,** h-sVCAM-1, ✴ **cytomegalovirus** (PCR, WBC), cold agglutinins, IgE, **IgG,** IgM, complement – (C3), **cryoglobulins, lym,** mono, RF

↓ albumin, Hb, HCT, complement – (C4), neu, PLT

■ *Urine* ↑ ✴ **CMV antigen,** ✴ **cytomegalovirus** (culture), ✴ **CMV DNA** (PCR), casts – (epithelial)

■ *Stool* ↑ ✴ **CMV antigen**

■ *Amniotic Fluid* ↑ ✴ **cytomegalovirus** (culture)

■ *Bronchoalveolar Lavage Fluid* ↑ ✴ **anti-CMV Ab** (IgG, IgM), ✴ **CMV antigen**

■ *Cerebrospinal Fluid* ↑ proteins, ✴ **CMV DNA** (PCR), ✴ **anti-CMV Ab** (IgG, IgM), **pp65 antigen** (WBC)

i. d. caused by Haemophilus influenzae

↑ ✴ **bacteria** (culture), WBC, PMN

■ *Urine* ↑ ✴ **bacterial capsular Ag** (type B)

■ *Cerebrospinal Fluid* ↑ ✴ **bacterial capsular Ag** (type B)

i. d. caused by Helicobacter pylori

↑ ✴ **antibodies against H. pylori** (IgG)

■ *Stool* ↑ ✴ **H. pylori antigen**

■ *Urine* ↑ antibodies against H. pylori (IgG)

■ *Saliva* ↑ antibodies against H. pylori (IgG), PCR

■ *Gastric Fluid* ↑ PCR

i. d. caused by Neisseria

↓ complement – (C5, C6, C7, C8)

i. d. caused by Parainfluenza virus

↑ ✴ **Ab against Parainfluenza virus**

↓ WBC

i. d. caused by parvoviruses

↑ ✴ **Ab against Parvovirus B19**

↓ neu

i. d. caused by Pneumocystis carinii
> ↑ **✶ P. carinii DNA** (PCR), **antibodies against P. carinii** (IgG, IgM), LD, pCO$_2$
> ↓ Hb, HCT, lym, pO$_2$
> ■ *Bronchoalveolar Lavage Fluid* ↑ **✶ fungi**
> ■ *Sputum* ↑ **✶ fungi**

i. d. caused by Pseudomonas aeruginosa
> ↑ **✶ bacteria** (culture), ESR, WBC, pCO$_2$
> ↓ WBC, pO$_2$

i. d. caused by respiratory syncytial virus
> ↑ **✶ Ab against respiratory syncytial virus** (IgG, IgM), **✶ respiratory syncytial virus antigen**, ESR, WBC

i. d. caused by Yersinia pestis
> ↑ ALT, AST, **✶ bacteria** (+ culture), **✶ antibodies against Yersinia pestis**, FDP, **WBC**, PT, **PMN**
> ■ *Sputum* ↑ **✶ bacteria**
> ■ *Cerebrospinal Fluid* ↑ proteins, PMN
>   ↓ G
> ■ *Synovial Fluid* ↑ clot formation, volume

i. d. caused by Yersinia enterocolitica
> ↑ **✶ antibodies against Yersinia enterocolitica**
> ■ *Stool* ↑ RBC, blood, WBC, **✶ bacteria** (culture)

influenza
> ↑ **✶ Ab against Influenza virus** (IgG, IgM), **B2M**, CRP, **cold agglutinins**, WBC, **lym**, RF
> ↓ **WBC**, lym, pCO$_2$, **neu**
> ■ *Urine* ↑ Mb

intra-amniotic i. d.
> ↑ **CRP, IL-6, WBC, PMN**
> ■ *Amniotic Fluid* ↑ **✶ bacteria** (culture), **WBC**, acid – (acetic, propionic, butyric, succinic)
>   ↓ **✶ G**

leishmaniasis (kala-azar) (Leishmania donovani)
> ↑ **✶ protozoans** (+ culture), **gamma globulins**, ESR, complement – (C1q), **IgG**, cryoglobulins, mono
> ↓ albumin, RBC, Hb, HCT, WBC, neu, PLT
> ■ *Urine* ↑ **proteins, blood**

leprosy (Mycobacterium leprae)
> ↑ ACE, ANA, Ca, CIC, CRP, **ESR**, fibrinogen, **globulins**, histamine, IgA, IgE, IgG, **IgM**, complement – (C3, total), **cryoglobulins**, LE cells, **WBC**, mono, plasmocytes, **RF**, T$_H$-**lym**, syphilis Ab (false), VDRL (false)
> ↓ albumin, alpha-1-globulins, **Ca**, FDP, RBC, T-lym, **cholesterol**, **Hb**, **HCT**, Mg
> ■ *Synovial Fluid* ↑ macrophages

leptospirosis (Leptospira icterohaemorrhagiae, L. canicola, L. pomona)
> ↑ ALP, ALT, AST, **✶ antibodies against leptospira** (IgG, IgM), **✶ bacteria** (culture), Bil, **CK**, ESR, IgM, IL – (6, 8), **✶ leptospira DNA** (PCR), **WBC, neu**, TNF, **urea**, VDRL (false)
> ↓ ESR, Hb, HCT, WBC, pCO$_2$, PLT
> ■ *Urine* ↑ proteins, **✶ bacteria** (culture), RBC, **WBC, casts**
>   ↓ volume

- *Cerebrospinal Fluid* ↑ proteins, **∗ bacteria** (culture), WBC, **lym**, mono, PMN, pressure

listeriosis (Listeria monocytogenes)
↑ **∗ bacteria** (+ culture), **ESR**, **WBC**
- *Cerebrospinal Fluid* ↑ **proteins**, **∗ bacteria** (+ culture), **WBC**, **PMN**

Lymphogranuloma venereum (Chlamydia trachomatis)
↑ **∗ antibodies against Chlamydia trachomatis** (L1, L2, L3), **ESR**, VDRL (false), lym (relat), mono (relat), **WBC**
↓ Hb, HCT

malaria (Plasmodium vivax, P. malariae, P. falciparum, P. ovale)
↑ ALT, ALP, AST, **∗ antibodies against Plasmodium** (IgG, IgM), Bil, conjugated Bil, **unconjugated Bil**, **CRP**, **ESR**, **DNA probe** (P. falciparum), gamma globulins, GMT, **cold agglutinins**, **IgM**, creatinine, **LA**, **WBC**, lym, methemalbumin, **mono**, **∗ parasite**, **∗ plasmodium DNA** (PCR), **PT**, **RF**, urea, syphilis Ab (false), VDRL (false), **viscosity**
↓ albumin, AT III, Ca, RBC, **fibrinogen**, G, granulocytes, **haptoglobin**, **Hb**, HCT, HCO$_3^-$, complement − (**C3, C4**), **WBC**, Na, neu, P, **pH**, **PLT**
- *Urine* ↑ **proteins**, RBC, **Hb**, **WBC**, UBG
  ↓ volume
- *Cerebrospinal Fluid* ↑ proteins, LA, WBC, lym, pressure
  ↓ G

measles (rubeola) (paramyxoviruses)
↑ **∗ Ab against rubeola virus** (IgG, IgM), B2M, cold agglutinins, ESR, WBC, lym
↓ complement − (C3), WBC (later), **lym, neu**, PLT (early)
- *Sputum* ↑ giant cells
- *Urine* ↑ rubeola antigen (sediment cells)
- *Cerebrospinal Fluid* ↑ **proteins**, WBC, lym, mono, pressure

mononucleosis, infectious (Epstein-Barr virus)
↑ ACP (WBC), ADA, **aldolase, ALP, ∗ ALT**, AMA, aminotripeptidase, AMS, **ANA, anti-ss-DNA, ∗ anti-EBV Ab, ASMA, AST, Bil**, B2M, BSP retention, CRP, **EBNA Ab** (IgG, IgM), **early antigen anti-D Ab, early antigen anti-R Ab**, eos, phosphohexoisomerase, fructose-1,6-diphosphate aldolase, globulins, **GMT**, guanase, Hb, HCT, HBD, **cold agglutinins, ICD, IgA, IgE, IgG, IgG-VCA, IgM-VCA, IgM, uric acid, cryoglobulins, LAP, LD**, LD − (2, 3, 4, 5), **WBC** (later), **∗ lym, mono, neu**, plasmocytes, **RF**, syphilis Ab (false), VDRL (false)
↓ PLT aggregation, albumin, eos, RBC, **ESR**, haptoglobin, **Hb, HCT**, cholesterol, CHS, WBC (early), **neu, PLT**
- *Urine* ↑ albumin, RBC, coproporphyrin, Mb, **UBG**

mucormycosis (Zygomycetes species)
↑ antibodies against Zygomycetes species (IgG, IgM)
- *Cerebrospinal Fluid* ↑ **∗ fungi** (culture)

mycoplasmosis (Mycoplasma pneumoniae)
↑ **∗ Ab against Mycoplasma pneumoniae** (IgG, IgM), **∗ bacteria** (+ culture), CRP, **ESR**, WBC, **cold agglutinins, lym**, VDRL (false), **∗ mycoplasma antigen**
- *Synovial Fluid* ↑ **clot formation, volume**

mycosis fungoides
↑ ALT
↓ lym, WBC

nocardiosis (Nocardia asteroides)

↑ * **antibodies against N. asteroides** (mycobacteriaceae), WBC
- *Sputum* ↑ * **fungi** (culture)
- *Bronchoalveolar Lavage Fluid* ↑ * **fungi** (culture)

opisthorchiasis (Opisthorchis felineus)

↑ * **antibodies against O. felineus** (IgE, IgG), * **opisthorchis antigen**
- *Stool* ↑ * **parasite ova**
- *Duodenal Content* ↑ * **parasite ova**

paragonimiasis (Paragonimus westermani)

↑ * **antibodies against P. westermani**, * **paragonimus antigen**, eos
- *Stool* ↑ * **parasite ova**, blood
- *Sputum* ↑ * **parasite ova**, blood

parasitic infectious diseases

↑ AFP, aldolase, ALP, ALT, AST, proteins, CIC, **eos**, cold agglutinins, IFN-gamma, **IgE**, IgG, IgM, IL-2, LD, **WBC**, mono, neu, PCT, poikilocytes, RF

↓ albumin, proteins, RBC, Fe, Hb, HCT, CHS, complement – (C3), WBC, vitamin – (B$_{12}$, folate), PLT, Zn
- *Urine* ↑ proteins, RBC, Hb, blood
- *Cerebrospinal Fluid* ↑ bas, eos
- *Synovial Fluid* ↑ eos
- *Stool* ↑ proteins, blood, WBC

– acute parasitic infectious diseases

↑ eos, IgG, neu

↓ Zn

parotitis, epidemic (mumps) (paramyxoviruses)

↑ AMS, * **antibodies against mumps virus** (IgG, IgM), B2M, cold agglutinins, ESR, **lipase**, WBC, **lym**, mono, trypsin

↓ **WBC, neu**
- *Urine* ↑ AMS, G, blood, * **mumps virus antigen**
- *Cerebrospinal Fluid* ↑ proteins, * **antibodies against mumps virus** (IgG, IgM), G, IgG, IgM, oligoclonal immunoglobulins, WBC, **lym**, mono, PMN, pressure
  - ↓ G
- *Synovial Fluid* ↑ WBC, clot formation, PMN, volume

pertussis (Bordetella pertussis)

↑ * **Ab against B. pertussis** (IgG, IgM), * **bordetella antigen**, WBC, **lym**
- *Sputum* ↑ * **bacteria** (+ culture)

pinta

↑ syphilis Ab (false), **treponemal antibodies** (false), VDRL

poliomyelitis, acute anterior (poliovirus)

↑ ALT, * **anti-poliovirus Ab**, AST, B2M, creatine, LA, WBC, mucoproteins, neu, pCO$_2$, PMN (early)

↓ chloride, WBC, mono (later), **neu** (later), pO$_2$
- *Cerebrospinal Fluid* ↑ AST, proteins, G, LD, LD2, LD3, **WBC, lym**, mono, PMN, **pressure**
  - ↓ vitamin C
- *Stool* ↑ * **poliovirus** (culture)

protozoan infectious diseases

↑ unconjugated Bil

↓ WBC, PLT

pseudomalleus (Burkholderia pseudomallei)
>↑ * Ab against Burkholderia pseudomallei

psittacosis (Chlamydia psittaci) (+ornithosis)
>↑ ALT, * antibodies against Chlamydia psittaci (IgG, IgM), ESR, cold ag-
>glutinins, VDRL (false), WBC
>↓ WBC (early)
>- *Urine* ↑ albumin, proteins
>- *Cerebrospinal Fluid* ↑ WBC
>- *Sputum* ↑ * bacteria (culture)
>- *Pleural Fluid* ↑ * bacteria (culture)

Q-fever (Coxiella burnetii)
>↑ ALT, * antibodies against C. burnetii (IgG, IgM), WBC
>↓ WBC

rabies (hydrophobia) (rhabdoviruses)
>↑ * Ab against Rabies virus, WBC, mono, PMN
>- *Urine* ↑ albumin, proteins, G, ketone bodies, casts – (hyaline)
>- *Cerebrospinal Fluid* ↑ proteins, * Ab against Rabies virus, * Rabies
>virus RNA (PCR), lym, WBC, PMN
>- *Saliva* ↑ * Rabies virus RNA (PCR), * Rabies virus (culture)

rickettsiosis
>↑ * Ab against Rickettsia species (IgG, IgM), ESR, lym, mono, neu, febrile
>agglutinins, WBC (later), urea, VDRL (false)
>↓ albumin, proteins, WBC (early), Hb, HCT, Na, neu, PLT
>- *Urine* ↑ albumin, Hb, blood, casts – (granular)
>- *Cerebrospinal Fluid* ↑ eos, WBC

rubella (German measles) (Rubella virus)
>↑ * Ab against rubella virus (IgG, IgM), unconjugated Bil, B2M, IgM,
>WBC (acute stage), lym, plasmocytes
>↓ WBC (later), neu, PLT
>- *Amniotic Fluid* ↑ * rubella virus
>- *Synovial Fluid* ↑ WBC, clot formation, mono, PMN, volume

salmonellosis
>↑ mono, febrile agglutinins
>- *Urine* ↑ Hb
>- *Stool* ↑ blood, WBC

scabies (Sarcoptes scabei)
>↑ eos

scarlatina (scarlet fever) (Streptococci A)
>↑ * ASLO, * bacteria (+ culture), CRP, eos, ESR, cold agglutinins, WBC,
>VDRL (false)
>- *Urine* ↑ proteins, albumin, RBC, Hb, casts
>↓ chloride

schistosomiasis (Schistosoma species)
>↑ * Ab against Schistosoma species, AFP, ALP, ALT, eos, CIC, CK-MB,
>ESR, IgE, IgG, IgM, WBC, RF
>↓ WBC
>- *Urine* ↑ proteins, * parasite ova (chronic), RBC, Hb, blood
>- *Sputum* ↑ * parasite ova
>- *Stool* ↑ * parasite ova (chronic)

sporotrichosis (Sporothrix schenckii)
>↑ * antibodies against Sporothrix schenckii (IgG, IgM)

- ■ *Cerebrospinal Fluid* ↑ ✳ antibodies against Sporothrix schenckii (IgG, IgM)

streptococcal infectious diseases
- ↑ antimyocardial Ab, ✳ **ASLO**, ✳ **bacteria** (+ culture), **CRP**, eos, **ESR**, **WBC**
- ■ *Urine* ↑ **albumin**, **RBC**, **Hb**, **casts**

strongyloidiasis (Strongyloides stercoralis)
- ↑ ✳ **antibodies against S. stercoralis**, **eos**, **WBC**
- ■ *Stool* ↑ ✳ **larvae**
- ■ *Sputum* ↑ ✳ **larvae**
- ■ *Duodenal Content* ↑ ✳ **larvae**

syphilis (Treponema pallidum)
- ↑ ALP, AMA, unconjugated Bil, ESR, **cold agglutinins**, cryoglobulins, **WBC**, **lym**, **mono**, **RF**, ✳ **syphilis Ab**, ✳ **treponemal antibodies**, ✳ **VDRL**
- ↓ LH
- ■ *Urine* ↑ **proteins**, **WBC**
- ■ *Cerebrospinal Fluid* ↑ proteins, lym, WBC, pressure, ✳ **treponemal DNA** (PCR), ✳ **VDRL**
  - ↓ G
- ■ *Synovial Fluid* ↑ volume

– neurosyphilis
- ↑ globulins, cold agglutinins, cryoglobulins, RF, ✳ **syphilis antibodies**, **VDRL**
- ↓ ADH
- ■ *Cerebrospinal Fluid* ↑ **proteins**, **G**, gamma globulins, IgG, WBC, **lym**, MBP, mono, RBC, **pressure**, VDRL
  - ↓ G

tapeworm infestation
– tapeworm infestation caused by Diphyllobothrium latum
- ■ *Stool* ↑ ✳ **parasite ova**

– tapeworm infestation caused by Echinococcus granulosus (echinococcosis)
- ↑ ALT, **eos**, IgE, ✳ **antibodies against echinococcus**, WBC
- ↓ albumin
- ■ *Pleural Fluid* ↓ pH

– tapeworm infestation caused by Hymenolepis nana
- ↑ **eos**, **WBC**
- ↓ Hb, HCT, macrocytes
- ■ *Stool* ↑ ✳ **parasite ova**

– tapeworm infestation caused by Taenia saginata
- ↑ eos
- ■ *Stool* ↑ ✳ **parasite ova**

– tapeworm infestation caused by Taenia solium
- ↑ eos, ✳ **antibodies against taenia**, ESR
- ■ *Cerebrospinal Fluid* ↑ eos, ✳ **antibodies against taenia**, proteins
  - ↓ G
- ■ *Stool* ↑ ✳ **parasite ova**

tetanus (Clostridium tetani)
- ↑ aldolase, ALT, ✳ **anti-tetanus toxin Ab**, AST, CK, ESR, catecholamines, **WBC**, **neu**, pH, pCO_2
- ↓ CO_2, CHS, **lym**, pCO_2, pH
- ■ *Urine* ↑ albumin, catecholamines, creatine, creatinine, WBC
- ■ *Cerebrospinal Fluid* ↑ pressure

toxocariasis (visceral larva migrans) (Toxocara caninum, T. cati)

↑ * anti-toxocara Ab, eos, gamma globulins, IgE, WBC

toxoplasmosis (Toxoplasma gondii)

↑ ALT, * **anti-toxoplasma Ab** (IgA, IgG, IgM), AST, unconjugated Bil, CK-MB, eos, ESR, **gamma globulins**, GMT, IgM, LD, **lym**, MAC, mono, * **toxoplasma antigen**, WBC

↓ **Hb**, HCT, PLT, WBC

■ *Cerebrospinal Fluid* ↑ proteins, * **toxoplasma antigen**, * **anti-toxoplasma Ab** (IgG, IgM), eos, * **protozoans**, WBC, mono, * **toxoplasma DNA** (PCR), **pressure**

■ *Urine* ↑ * **toxoplasma antigen**

■ *Amniotic Fluid* ↑ * **toxoplasma DNA** (PCR)

trachoma (Chlamydia trachomatis)

↑ * **antibodies against Chlamydia trachomatis** (A, B, C) (IgG, IgM), * **chlamydia antigen**

trichinosis (Trichinella spiralis)

↑ **aldolase**, alpha-2-globulins, ALT, * **anti-trichinella Ab**, * **trichinella antigen**, AST, CK, CK-MB, **eos**, ESR, **gamma globulins**, IgE, IgM, **LD**, **WBC, neu**

↓ albumin, **proteins**, ESR, **Hb**, HCT, CHS

■ *Urine* ↑ **albumin**, creatine, Mb, casts – (hyaline c., granular c.)

■ *Cerebrospinal Fluid* ↑ proteins, * **anti-trichinella Ab**, eos, lym, WBC

trichomoniasis (Trichomonas vaginalis)

■ *Urine* ↑ pus

trichostrongylosis (Trichostrongylus spp.)

↑ eos, WBC

■ *Stool* ↑ * **parasite ova**

trichuriasis (Trichuris trichiura)

↑ eos, WBC

↓ Hb, HCT, microcytes

■ *Stool* ↑ * **parasite ova**

trypanosomiasis (Trypanosoma rhodesiense, T. gambiense)

↑ ALT, AST, * **antibodies against Trypanosoma**, cold agglutinins, ESR, gamma globulins, GMT, **IgM**, WBC, lym, **mono**, * **protozoans**, RF, VDRL (false)

↓ Hb, HCT, complement – (C3), neu

■ *Cerebrospinal Fluid* ↑ proteins, * **protozoans**, IgM, WBC, **lym**, plasma cells

– Chagas' disease (T. cruzi)

↑ * **protozoans**, * **antibodies against Trypanosoma** (IgG), * **DNA probe** (Trypanosoma), lym, WBC

■ *Cerebrospinal Fluid* ↑ * **protozoans**

tuberculosis (Mycobacterium tuberculosis)

↑ ADA, ADH, aldolase, alpha-1-globulins, **ALP, ALT**, ANA, * **mycobacterial antigen**, * **anti-mycobacteria Ab**, ASLO, AST, Bil, beta globulins, proteins, **Ca, CRP**, Cu, * **mycobacterial DNA** (PCR), eos, **fibrinogen, ESR**, gamma globulins, **GMT, IgA, IgG**, uric acid, LA, LAP, LD, **WBC**, lipase (early), lipids, lym, **lysozyme**, MAC+RAL, microcytes, **mono**, mucoproteins, **neu**, 5-NT, **pCO₂**, PT, plasmocytes, PRL, **RF**, E selectin, **PLT**, VDRL (false), vitamin – (D3)

↓ ACE, **albumin**, **proteins**, **RBC**, Hb, HCT, cholesterol, IgM, **cortisol**, WBC, LH, **Na**, PLT, T-lym, vitamin – (A)

- **Urine** ↑ arylsulfatase, proteins, **＊ bacteria** (+ culture), Ca, blood, pus
- **Sputum** ↑ blood, **＊ bacteria** (+ culture)
- **Pleural Fluid** ↑ adenosine deaminase, AMS, **＊ bacteria** (+ culture), B2M, **proteins**, **RBC**, fibronectin, IgG, LD, **lym**, lysozyme, mucopolysaccharides, **neu**, TM – (CEA), volume
  - ↓ C3, C4, G, **pH**
- **Bronchoalveolar Lavage Fluid** ↑ RBC, **＊ bacteria** (+ culture)
- **Cerebrospinal Fluid** ↑ **proteins**, **＊ bacteria** (+ culture), eos, LA, **WBC**, **lym**, lysozyme, macrophages, **mono**, P, plasmocytes, RBC, pressure
  - ↓ G, chloride
- **Gastric Fluid** ↑ **＊** bacteria **(+ culture)**
- **Peritoneal Fluid** ↑ proteins, **RBC**, lym, WBC, mono, specific gravity
  - ↓ G
- **Synovial Fluid** ↑ clot formation
- **Pericardial Fluid** ↑ cholesterol

– **adrenal tuberculosis**
  - ↑ ACTH
  - ↓ cortisol

– **CNS tuberculosis**
  - **Cerebrospinal Fluid** ↑ **proteins**, WBC, lym, PMN, pressure
    - ↓ G

– **lung tuberculosis**
  - ↑ **ACE**, **ADH**, **ALP**, AMS, ANA, ASLO, **AST**, **bas**, proteins, Ca, CEA, CO$_2$, **CRP**, Cu (+RBC), eos, **fibrinogen**, **ESR**, gamma globulins, globulins, **IgA**, **IgG**, **uric acid**, **WBC**, **lym**, lysozyme, MAC+RAL, microcytes, **mono**, mucoproteins, **neu**, pCO$_2$, PT, **RF**, **PLT**, vitamin – (D3)
  - ↓ ACE, ADH, AMS, **albumin**, **proteins**, RBC, Hb, HCT, **cholesterol**, IgM, cortisol, **Na**, neu, O$_2$ satur., T-lym, **Zn**
  - **Urine** ↑ arylsulfatase, proteins, Ca
  - **Sputum** ↑ blood, **mycobacteria**
  - **Pleural Fluid** ↑ adenosine deaminase, **AMS**, B2M, **proteins**, CEA, **RBC**, fibronectin, cholesterol, IgG, **LD**, WBC, **lym**, lysozyme, mono, mononuclear cells, mucopolysaccharides, **neu**, pH, specific gravity, TM – (CEA), volume
    - ↓ C3, C4, **G**, lym, pH
  - **Bronchoalveolar Lavage Fluid** ↑ RBC
  - **Peritoneal Fluid** ↑ proteins, lym, mono
    - ↓ G

– **miliary tuberculosis**
  - ↑ ALT, ESR, **nucleated RBC**, **neu**, syphilis Ab (false)
  - ↓ WBC, **lym**, vitamin – (A)

– **prostate tuberculosis**
  - ↑ ESR
  - ↓ RBC, Hb, HCT
  - **Urine** ↑ pus
    - ↓ pH

– **renal tuberculosis**
  - **Urine** ↑ albumin, proteins, Ca, **RBC**, pus, blood, WBC, **lysozyme**, volume
    - ↓ pH, urea

tularemia (Francisella tularensis)

  ↑ * Ab against Fr. Tularensis (IgG, IgM), ALT, **AST**, eos, **ESR**, **WBC**, febrile
      agglutinins

  ↓ WBC, neu

typhus, epidemic (exanthematous t., Brill-Zinsser d.) (Rickettsia prowazekii)

  ↑ ALT, * antibodies against R. prowazekii (IgG, IgM), Bil, ESR, GMT, WBC,
      mono, PT, VDRL (false), **urea**

  ↓ albumin, proteins, **eos**, RBC, **fibrinogen**, **Hb**, **HCT**, chloride, **WBC**, Na,
      neu, PLT

  ■ *Urine* ↓ volume

varicella (chickenpox) (Varicella-zoster virus)

  ↑ B2M, * antibodies against Varicella-zoster virus (IgG, IgM), CRP, **WBC**,
      lym, neu

  ↓ WBC, **neu**

  ■ *Cerebrospinal Fluid* ↑ * antibodies against varicella-zoster virus

variola vera (smallpox) (orthopoxviruses)

  ↑ bas, B2M, * antibodies against orthopoxvirus, WBC, lym, neu

  ↓ WBC, PLT

viral infectious diseases

  ↑ ASMA, **B2M**, unconjugated Bil, BT, **CRP**, **elastase**, h-sICAM-1, **cold
      agglutinins**, LD – (2, 3, 4), lupus inhibitor, **lym**, **mono**, RF, thymidine
      kinase, tropomyosin, trypsin

  ↓ ADH, albumin, RBC, complement – (C1r, C1s), **PLT**

  ■ *Urine* ↑ AMS, casts – (epithelial)

– acute viral infectious diseases

  ↑ Ab against Influenza virus, ASMA, **B2M**, **CRP**, **elastase**, **cold agglutinins**, RF, thymidine kinase, tropomyosin, trypsin

  ↓ albumin, complement – (C1r, C1s), lupus inhibitor, neu

yaws (Treponema pertenue)

  ↑ Ab against B. burgdorferi, syphilis Ab (false), **treponemal antibodies**
      (false), VDRL

Diuresis

  – forced diuresis

  ↑ aldosterone, MAL, Na, pH, PRA,

  ↓ Ca, K, Mg

  – osmotic diuresis

  ↑ Na

  ↓ K, Na, osmolality

  ■ *Urine* ↑ volume

Diverticulitis

  ↑ CEA, CRP, elastase (PMN), **ESR**, **WBC**, neu

  ↓ RBC, **Fe**, Hb, HCT, WBC

  ■ *Urine* ↑ RBC, Hb

  ■ *Stool* ↑ mucus, pus, Hb, **blood**

Drainage, Ileostomic

  ↑ MAC

  ↓ K, pH, HCO$_3^-$

  ■ *Urine* ↓ K

Drowning, Near

freshwater drowning

  ↑ **Hb**, **K**, **MAC**, urea

                    ↓ **chloride** (severe), Hb, HCT, RBC, **Na** (severe), **pO₂, pH**
              ■ *Urine* ↑ proteins, Hb
                    ↓ volume
  seawater drowning
                    ↑ **chloride, MAC, Na**
                    ↓ K, Hb, HCT, **pO₂, pH, plasma volume**
Dysautonomia, Familial
              ■ *Urine* ↑ HVA
                    ↓ VMA
Dysfibrinogenemia
                    ↑ **APTT, PT, TT**
                    ↓ **fibrinogen**
Dysgammaglobulinemia
                    ↑ Apo B, IgA, IgG, IgM, LDL-C
                    ↓ **IgM**
Dysgenesis, Reticular, With Aleukocytosis
                    ↓ lym, **WBC**
Dysmenorrhea
                    ↑ FSH, LH, PRL, prostacyclin
                    ↓ estradiol, FSH, progesterone
              ■ *Urine* ↓ pregnanediol
Dysproteinemia
                    ↑ BT, IgG, lupus inhibitor, **TAG**, PLT, viscosity, VLDL-C
                    ↓ alpha-1-globulins, alpha-2-globulins, beta globulins, Cu
Dysrrhythmia
                    ↑ ALT, CK, LA, FFA
                    ↓ Hb, HCT, K, Mg, **pO₂**
Dystrophy
  acute hepatic dystrophy
                    ↑ **ALP, ALT**, aminonitrogen, **ammonia, AST, Bil**, GMD, GMT, vitamin B₁₂
                    ↓ **fibrinogen, CHS, cholesterol**, LD, **urea**
              ■ *Urine* ↑ alpha-aminonitrogen, **Bil**, G, leucine, tyrosine
                    ↓ P, urea
  muscular dystrophy
                    ↑ aldolase, **ALT, AST, CK, CK-MB, creatinine**, LD, pyruvic acid
              ■ *Urine* ↑ cystine
  – Duchenne's muscular dystrophy
                    ↑ **aldolase, AST, CK, CK-MB**, GMT, **LD, Mb**
                    ↓ IgG, testosterone
              ■ *Urine* ↑ **creatine**
                    ↓ creatinine
  – progressive muscular dystrophy
                    ↑ **aldolase, ALT, AST, CK, CK-MB**, phosphohexoisomerase, fructose-1,6-
                         diphosphate aldolase, GMT, IRI, creatine, **creatinine, LD**, LD5, **Mb**,
                         norepinephrine, pyruvate kinase, urea
                    ↓ CHS, IgG, creatinine, testosterone
              ■ *Urine* ↑ alpha-aminonitrogen, amino acids, catecholamines, **creatine,
                         creatinine**, cystine, Mb, reducing sugars
                    ↓ hydroxyproline, 17-ketosteroids, creatine, creatinine
  – progressive muscular dystrophy (limb-girdle)
                    ↑ aldolase, AST, **CK, LD**

　　　　　　　　　　　　■ *Urine* ↑ creatine
　　　　　　　　　　　　　　↓ creatinine
　　myotonic dystrophy
　　　　　　　　　　　　↑ aldolase, ALT, AST, **CK**, CK-MB
　　　　　　　　　　　　■ *Urine* ↑ creatine
　　　　　　　　　　　　　　↓ 17-ketosteroids

Ecchymoses

　　　　　　　　　　　　↑ BT, unconjugated Bil

Eclampsia

　　　　　　　　　　　　↑ aldosterone, alpha-aminonitrogen, alpha-1-globulins, alpha-2-globu-
　　　　　　　　　　　　　lins, ADH, **ALP**, **amino acids**, **AST**, proteins, **Bil**, fibrinogen, **G**, hCG,
　　　　　　　　　　　　　HCT, **chloride**, creatinine, **uric acid**, LA, beta-LP, **WBC**, Mg, neu, P, PAI-I,
　　　　　　　　　　　　　PAPP-A, **plasminogen**, PRA, PT, viscosity
　　　　　　　　　　　　↓ **albumin**, AMS, CO_2, estrogens, **fibrinogen**, G tolerance, globulins, GFR,
　　　　　　　　　　　　　chloride, immunoglobulins, LD, WBC, Mg, Na, pCO_2, plasma vol-
　　　　　　　　　　　　　ume, plasminogen, **PLT**, PRA, progesterone, **urea**
　　　　　　　　　　　　■ *Urine* ↑ alpha-aminonitrogen, albumin, amino acids, proteins, hCG,
　　　　　　　　　　　　　17-OHCS, 17-KGS, catecholamines, lipids, tetrahydrodeoxycortisol,
　　　　　　　　　　　　　casts – (**epithelial c.**)
　　　　　　　　　　　　　↓ proteins, **estriol, uric acid**, Na, pregnanediol
　　　　　　　　　　　　■ *Cerebrospinal Fluid* ↑ proteins, RBC
　　　　　　　　　　　　　↓ Mg

Eczema

　　　　　　　　　　　　↑ eos, eosinophil cationic protein, IgE, IgE (specific)
　　　　　　　　　　　　↓ proteins

Edema

　　cardiac edema
　　　　　　　　　　　　↑ **aldosterone**, ANP, BNP, PRA
　　　　　　　　　　　　↓ albumin, chloride
　　cerebral edema
　　　　　　　　　　　　■ *Cerebrospinal Fluid* ↑ LA, **pressure**
　　hepatic edema
　　　　　　　　　　　　↑ aldosterone, PRA
　　　　　　　　　　　　↓ albumin, chloride, K (RBC)
　　pulmonary edema
　　　　　　　　　　　　↑ **CK**, MAC, MAC+RAC, MAC+RAL, pCO_2
　　　　　　　　　　　　↓ chloride, pO_2
　　　　　　　　　　　　■ *Sputum* ↑ **blood**
　　　　　　　　　　　　■ *Pleural Fluid* ↑ IL-8
　　renal edema
　　　　　　　　　　　　↑ **aldosterone**, PRA

Effusion

　　　　　　　　　　　　↑ ALT, AST
　　　　　　　　　　　　↓ albumin
　　　　　　　　　　　　■ *Peritoneal Fluid* ↑ LAP, LD, volume
　　　　　　　　　　　　■ *Pleural Fluid* ↑ ACP, albumin, A2MG, ALP, proteins, B2M, **blood**, CEA,
　　　　　　　　　　　　　CK, eos, FDP, haptoglobin, hemopexin, RBC, IgA, IgG, LA, LD, lym,
　　　　　　　　　　　　　WBC, volume, mononuclear cells, mucopolysaccharides, neu, PMN,
　　　　　　　　　　　　　RF
　　　　　　　　　　　　　↓ alpha globulins, AAT, A2MG, C3, C4, G, haptoglobin, hemopexin,
　　　　　　　　　　　　　orosomucoid, pH

bacterial edema

- *Pleural Fluid* ↑ eos, proteins, LA, LD, lym, **WBC,** neu, PMN, RBC, RF, volume
- ↓ C_3, C_4, G, pH

malignant edema

- *Peritoneal Fluid* ↑ AMS, bacteria (culture), blood, ∗ **cholesterol, ∗ CEA, ∗ fibronectin,** LA, LAP, LD, lym, neu, proteins, pus, RBC, ∗ WBC, PMN, volume, TM – (CEA)
- ↓ G, pH
- *Pleural Fluid* ↑ ACP, albumin, A2MG, AMS, beta-glucuronidase, **blood, proteins,** eos, RBC, FDP, IgA, IgG, LA, LD, lym, WBC, mononuclear cells, mucopolysaccharides, TM – **(CEA, CA-125),** orosomucoid, volume, RF
- ↓ alpha globulins, C_3, C_4, G, **pH**

pericardial edema

- *Peritoneal Fluid* ↑ bacteria (+ culture), RBC, WBC, volume
- ↓ G

peritoneal edema

- *Peritoneal Fluid* ↑ AMS, bacteria (+ culture), blood, LA, LD, lym, methemalbumin, neu, proteins, pus, RBC, ∗ WBC, PMN, volume, TM – (CEA)
- ↓ **G, pH**

pleural edema

↑ ALT

↓ Na

- *Pleural Fluid* ↑ ACP, adenosine deaminase, AMS, ANA, bacteria (+ culture), albumin, ALP, A2MG, **blood, proteins,** B2M, CEA, eos, RBC, FDP, G, IgA, IgG, LA, LD, LE cells, **WBC,** creatinine, **lipids,** lym, volume, mononuclear cells, mucopolysaccharides, neu, pH, PMN, specific gravity, RF
- ↓ alpha globulins, AAT, A2MG, C_3, C_4, G, haptoglobin, hemopexin, cholesterol, WBC, orosomucoid, pH

rheumatoid edema

- *Pleural Fluid* ↑ adenosine deaminase, **proteins,** CSF – (GM, M), eos, epithelial cells, crystals – (cholesterol), **LD,** WBC, **lym,** mononuclear cells, PMN, **RF**
- ↓ C_3, C_4, **G, pH,** viscosity

traumatic edema (blunt)

- *Peritoneal Fluid* ↑ ∗ AMS, ∗ RBC, ∗ WBC
- ↓ RBC

traumatic edema (penetrating)

- *Peritoneal Fluid* ↑ ALP, AMS, bacteria (+ culture), ∗ **RBC,** ∗ **WBC**

tuberculous edema

- *Pleural Fluid* ↑ adenosine deaminase, AMS, ∗ **bacteria** (+ culture), B2M, **proteins, RBC,** fibronectin, IgG, LA, LD, **lym,** lysozyme, mucopolysaccharides, **neu,** RF, TM – (CEA), volume
- ↓ C_3, C_4, G, **pH**
- *Peritoneal Fluid* ↑ bacteria (+ culture), proteins, RBC, fibronectin, neu, volume

Electroacupuncture

- *Cerebrospinal Fluid* ↑ enkephalins

Electromyography

↑ CK, CK-mass, CK-MM, Mb

Embolism

↑ ACE, ACP, ACP (prostatic), ALP, ALT, AST, Bil, CK, CRP, D-dimers, elastase, **factor VIII, FDP**, fibrinopeptide A, ESR, cold agglutinins, LA, LD, LD – (1, 2, 3, 4), **WBC**, lipase, pH, RAL, TAG, thrombomodulin, FFA
↓ AGP, AT III, Ca, factor – (II), fibrinogen, Hb, CHS, pCO_2, **pO_2, sat. O_2**, PLT
- *Urine* ↑ ALP, RBC, Hb, blood, LD, Mb, fat
- *Cerebrospinal Fluid* ↑ proteins, RBC, blood, WBC, PMN
- *Pleural Fluid* ↑ AAT, A2MG, **AMS, RBC**, haptoglobin, hemopexin, neu, orosomucoid
- *Sputum* ↑ fat
- *Bronchoalveolar Lavage Fluid* ↑ fat

air embolism

↑ RAC, WBC

amniotic fluid embolism

↑ euglobulin lysis time, WBC
↓ fibrinogen

cerebral embolism

↑ WBC
- *Cerebrospinal Fluid* ↑ **proteins**, CK, RBC, blood, lym, WBC, PMN, **pressure**

fat embolism

↑ **lipase, TAG**, WBC, **FFA**
↓ **Ca**, Hb, pCO_2, pO_2, **PLT**
- *Urine* ↑ **fat**
- *Sputum* ↑ fat
- *Bronchoalveolar Lavage Fluid* ↑ fat

mesenteric artery embolism

↑ ACP, **ALP**, ALP (isoenzymes), ALT, **AMS, AST, CK**, HCT, **LA, LD**, lipase, **WBC, MAC, P**, PT, **urea**
↓ **albumin**, pH, proteins, cholesterol
- *Urine* ↑ AMS
- *Peritoneal Fluid* ↑ AMS
- *Stool* ↑ fat

paradoxical embolism

↑ AST, WBC

pulmonary embolism

↑ **ACE**, ACP, ALP, ALT, AST, Bil, unconjugated Bil, CK, **CRP, ✱ D-dimers, elastase, FDP**, fibrinopeptide A, **ESR**, GMT, cold agglutinins, **LA, LD**, LD – (1, **2**, 3, 4), **WBC**, pH, RAL
↓ AGP, fibrinogen, CHS, pCO_2, **pO_2, sat. O_2**, PLT
- *Pleural Fluid* ↑ AAT, A2MG, **AMS**, blood, **RBC**, haptoglobin, Hb, hemopexin, mononuclear cells, neu, orosomucoid, PMN, WBC

renal artery embolism

↑ **ALP, AST, LD**, WBC
- *Urine* ↑ **ALP, RBC, Hb, blood**, LD

Emphysema, Pulmonary

↑ AAT, ADH, **A2MG, ammonia**, CEA, EPO, **RBC, Hb, HCO_3^-**, HCT, plasma volume, **pCO_2**, RAC
↓ **AAT, alpha-1-globulins, chloride**, pH, pO_2, sat. O_2
- *Urine* ↓ chloride, Na, pH

Empyema, Pleural

- *Pleural Fluid* ↑ adenosine deaminase, proteins, eos, **RBC**, **ESR**, LA, LD, **WBC**, mucopolysaccharides, **neu**, TM – (CEA), **PMN**
  ↓ **G, pH**
- *Sputum* ↑ volume

subdural empyema

↑ **WBC**

- *Cerebrospinal Fluid* ↑ **proteins, WBC, PMN**, pressure

Encephalitis

↑ ADH, anti-arbovirus Ab, anti-enterovirus Ab, anti-Hu Ab, **CK, ESR**, G, Hb, **WBC**, Na

↓ WBC

- *Urine* ↑ volume
- *Cerebrospinal Fluid* ↑ proteins, **G**, chloride, LD, WBC, lym, MBP, mono, Na, PMN, pressure
  ↓ G, chloride, WBC, vitamin C

acute hemorrhagic encephalitis

- *Cerebrospinal Fluid* ↑ proteins, WBC, PMN, pressure

aseptic encephalitis

- *Cerebrospinal Fluid* ↑ **lym, mono**

bacterial encephalitis

- *Cerebrospinal Fluid* ↓ G

cytomegalovirus encephalitis

↑ WBC
↓ albumin

encephalitis lethargica

↑ ALT, lym

herpetic encephalitis

↑ lym
↓ WBC

Japanese B encephalitis

↑ ALT, anti-arbovirus Ab, AST

- *Cerebrospinal Fluid* ↑ MBP, proteins, WBC

postinfectious encephalitis

- *Cerebrospinal Fluid* ↑ WBC

postvaccinal encephalitis

- *Cerebrospinal Fluid* ↑ WBC

St. Louis encephalitis

↑ ALT, ✳ anti-St. Louis encephalitis virus Ab (IgM, IgG), lym, WBC
↓ WBC

- *Cerebrospinal Fluid* ↑ proteins, ✳ **anti-St. Louis encephalitis virus Ab** (IgM, IgG), WBC

viral encephalitis

- *Cerebrospinal Fluid* ↑ proteins, **lym**, MBP, **mono**, Na, plasmocytes, pressure

Encephalocele

↑ **AFP**

- *Amniotic Fluid* ↑ AFP, ACHE

Encephalomyelitis

acute disseminated encephalomyelitis

↑ ALT

- *Cerebrospinal Fluid* ↑ lym, proteins

acute viral encephalomyelitis
- *Cerebrospinal Fluid* ↑ **proteins** (later), WBC, PMN (early), **lym** (later)

amebic encephalomyelitis
- *Cerebrospinal Fluid* ↑ **proteins**, RBC, lym, **WBC, PMN, pressure**

epidemic myalgic encephalomyelitis
↑ ALT
↓ WBC

Encephalopathy

arsenical encephalopathy
- *Cerebrospinal Fluid* ↑ pressure, lym

drug encephalopathy
↑ AMS, AST, ALT, CK, eos, HBsAg, LD, lym, Mb, T$_4$
↓ c-AMP, cholesterol, O$_2$ satur., pO$_2$, testosterone
- *Urine* ↑ Mb
- *Cerebrospinal Fluid* ↑ **lym**, mono

hepatic encephalopathy
↑ **amino acids, ammonia**, Bil, phenylalanine, MAL, Na, pH, **RAL**, tryptophan, **FFA**
↓ albumin, isoleucine, K, leucine, Na, valine
- *Cerebrospinal Fluid* ↑ **glutamine**, WBC, tryptophan

hypertensive encephalopathy
- *Cerebrospinal Fluid* ↑ **proteins, pressure**

lead encephalopathy
- *Cerebrospinal Fluid* ↑ proteins, WBC, lym, **pressure**

septic encephalopathy
- *Cerebrospinal Fluid* ↑ glutamine

Wernicke's encephalopathy
↑ ALT, G, **pyruvic acid**
↓ **transketolase**

Endocarditis

bacterial endocarditis
↑ alpha-1-globulins, ALT, ANA, ANCA, c-ANCA, atypical-ANCA, antimyocardial Ab, ASLO, AST, **bacteria** (culture), ✳ **CIC**, ✳ **CRP**, ✳ **ESR**, **fibrinogen, gamma globulins**, globulins, IgG, IgM, ✳ **creatinine, cryoglobulins**, ✳ **teichoic acid antibodies** (Sta. aureus endocarditis), LA, **WBC**, macrophages, **mono**, ✳ **mucoproteins, neopterin, neu**, ✳ **PCT**, pH, RF, SAA, **urea**, VDRL (false)
↓ albumin, AMS, **RBC, factor B, Fe**, haptoglobin, **Hb, HCT**, cholesterol, IgA, complement – **(C3, C4), WBC**, pCO$_2$, **PLT**
- *Urine* ↑ **albumin, proteins, RBC, Hb, blood**, casts – (RBC c.)
- *Cerebrospinal Fluid* ↑ **proteins, WBC**, lym, PMN, pressure
- *Pericardial Fluid* ↑ bacteria (culture), WBC, volume
  ↓ G
- *Pleural Fluid* ↑ eos, WBC
- *Synovial Fluid* ↑ WBC, clot formation, lym, PMN, volume

Löffler's parietal fibroplastic endocarditis
↑ **eos, WBC**

rheumatic endocarditis
↑ alpha-1-globulins, **ASLO**, AST, CIC, **CRP, ESR**, gamma globulins, haptoglobin, complement – (C3), LE cells, **WBC**, mucoproteins, **neu, RF**, PLT

     ↓ albumin

     ■ *Urine* ↑ **proteins, RBC**

subacute endocarditis

     ↑ alpha-1-globulins, antimyocardial Ab, gamma globulins, cryoglobulins, LA, **WBC, RF**

     ↓ **RBC,** factor B, haptoglobin, complement – (C3)

     ■ *Urine* ↑ proteins, RBC, blood

     ■ *Cerebrospinal Fluid* ↑ proteins, pressure

     ■ *Synovial Fluid* ↑ WBC, PMN, volume

Endometriosis

     ↑ hCG, TM – (CA 15-3, CA 27-29, CA 125)

     ■ *Pleural Fluid* ↑ RBC

Enteritis

     ↑ ALP, MAC, OCT

     ↓ pH, vitamin – (B_2, beta-carotene)

     ■ *Stool* ↓ pH

Enterocolitis

idiopathic enteritis

     ↑ **WBC**

     ↓ beta-carotene, HCT

infectious enteritis

     ↑ beta-carotene, CRP, **WBC, urea**

     ↓ **albumin**, HCT

     ■ *Stool* ↑ mucus, blood, pH

necrotizing enteritis in infancy

     ↑ WBC, MAC

     ↓ Hb, HCT, Na, neu

     ■ *Stool* ↑ mucus, Hb, pH, **blood**

     ■ *Urine* ↓ volume

tuberculous enteritis

     ↑ **WBC**

     ↓ albumin

Enteropathy

necrotic enteropathy

     ↑ conjugated Bil, unconjugated Bil, PT

     ↓ Hb, Na

protein-losing enteropathy

     ↑ A2MG, **alpha-1-globulins, alpha-2-globulins,** beta-carotene, **eos, fibrinogen**

     ↓ AAT, **albumin,** beta-carotene, **proteins, Ca,** CBG, RBC, factor B, **gamma globulins, globulins,** Hb, **HCT,** CHS, **IgA, IgG, IgM,** K, complement – (C2), lym, TAG, T4, **TBG,** vitamin – (E)

     ■ *Stool* ↑ AAT, albumin, **fat**

Eosinophilia, Tropical

     ↑ **eos,** WBC

Epididymitis

     ↑ CRP, **ESR, WBC**

     ■ *Urine* ↑ **WBC, pus**

Epiglottitis (Croup)

     ↑ ESR, neu, **WBC**

Epilepsy
↑ anion gap, K, LA, MAC, urea
↓ Mg, Mn
- *Cerebrospinal Fluid* ↑ proteins, CK

Error, Inborn, of Amino Acid Metabolism
↑ ALT, anion gap, AST, G, MAC
↓ neu
- *Urine* ↑ RBC, Hb, ketones

Erythema
erythema multiforme
↑ eos
- *Synovial Fluid* ↑ WBC, PMN
↓ viscosity

erythema nodosum
↑ anti-Mycoplasma pneumoniae Ab, **WBC**, IgE
- *Synovial Fluid* ↑ WBC, PMN

Erythroblastosis, Fetal
↑ aldolase, **ammonia**, anisocytes, **Bil**, ∗ **unconjugated Bil**, BT, Hb, **nucleated RBC**, **MCV**, **MCH**, macrocytes, **WBC**, methemalbumin, **neu**, **RTC**, osmotic fragility, **spherocytes**
↓ fibrinogen, **G**, **haptoglobin**, Hb, **HbF**, **HCT**, **RBC**, RBC osmotic resistance, proconvertin, RTC, **PLT**, vitamin – (K)
- *Amniotic Fluid* ↑ anti-Rh factor, **Bil**, **RBC** (nucleated), hCG, placental lactogen
- *Amniotic Fluid* ↑ estriol
- *Urine* ↑ hCG, **UBG**
- *Stool* ↑ **UBG**

Erythrocytosis, Familial
↑ unconjugated Bil, ∗ **RBC**, **HCT**, **EPO**
↓ 2,3-DPG

Eunuchoidism
↑ PRL, SHBG
↓ androstenedione, EPO, **estradiol**, estrogens, **FSH**, ∗ **GRH**, **LH**, **progesterone**, ∗ **testosterone**, free testosterone, **Zn**
- *Urine* ↓ FSH, **17-KS**

Exanthema, Viral
↑ B2M, lym

Exudate
↓ albumin
- *Bronchoalveolar Lavage Fluid* ↑ proteins
- *Pericardial Fluid* ↑ AAT, A2MG, proteins, cholesterol
- *Peritoneal Fluid* ↑ proteins, fibrinogen, cholesterol, LD, specific gravity
↓ *G, LD*
- *Pleural Fluid* ↑ AAT, A2MG, proteins, RBC, fibrinogen, globulins, haptoglobin, hemopexin, cholesterol, specific gravity, orosomucoid, TM – (CA-125)
↓ G, LD, **pH**

Factors, Interfering – Age
adolescents
↑ **ACE**, estrone, ILGF-I, osteocalcin

children

↓ Fe, T4

↑ ALP, cAMP, 5-nucleotidase, P, PSA, SHBG, TIBC, transferrin, vitamin – (D2)

↓ AGP, Fe, fructosamine, complement – (C1q, C4), **ILGF-I**, urea, vitamin – (B₁₂)

■ *Urine* ↑ arginine

elder people

↑ PLT adhesion, **ALP**, ANA, antithyroglobulin Ab, APA, ASMA, **Cu**, euglobulin lysis time, **ferritin, fibrinogen**, gastrin, **glucose, cholesterol, IgM, creatinine**, cryoglobulins, **uric acid, WBC**, macrocytes, Na, **neu, norepinephrine**, 5-nucleotidase, osteocalcin, PP, **PTH**, RF, **TAG, urea**, vitamin – (D2, D3), VDRL (false)

↓ **albumin**, aldosterone, **Ca**, Cr, **DHEA, Fe, ILGF-I**, creatinine, LD, plasma volume, **P, Se, T3, testosterone**, vitamin – (**B₁**, B₆, B₁₂, **C, D**, E, **folate**), **Zn**

healthy adult people

↑ AAT, ANA, antithyroid Ab, anti-myelin Ab, antireticulin Ab, ASMA, delta Bil, lupus inhibitor

■ *Urine* ↑ Ca

■ *Gastric Fluid* ↑ HCl

newborns

↑ ACE, ACTH, angiotensin I, angiotensin II, beta-endorphins, unconjugated Bil, DHEA, Hg, calcitonin, **WBC**, macrocytes, mono, neu, PRL, pyknocytes, schistocytes, siderocytes, **GH, T4**, TBG

↓ ceruloplasmin, Cu, euglobulin lysis time, factor – (II, **IX**, XI, XII), Mg, T3, vitamin – (K)

■ *Urine* ↑ arginine, **galactose** (till 6th day)

■ *Cerebrospinal Fluid* ↑ glutamine

postmenopause female

↑ albumin, ALP, ALT, AST, G, gonadotropins, cholesterol, uric acid, Na, osteocalcin, P, PL

↓ euglobulin lysis time, SHBG

■ *Urine* ↓ estrogens, gonadotropins, 17-KS

smaller of twins

↓ G

Factors, Interfering – Body Posture

supine body posture

↑ ANF, plasma volume

↓ aldosterone, PSA (prolonged)

upright body posture

↑ aldosterone, angiotensin I, II, catecholamines, **PRA**

↓ plasma volume

Factors, Interfering – Diurnal Variations

↑ PLT adhesion, osteocalcin, PRA

↓ osteocalcin

early morning

↑ Ca, Ca²⁺, DHEA, DHEAS, DOC, Fe, histamine, ILGF-I, K, cortisol, uric acid, MSH, osteocalcin, PRA, 17-OH progesterone, PTH, testosterone, vitamin C, Zn

↓ ACP, Apo A, Cu, enkephalins, progesterone, GH, TIBC

evening

↑ ACP, Apo A, Ca, Cu, enkephalins, estradiol, creatinine, PTH, SHBG, TIBC

↓ androstenedione, beta-endorphins, DHEA, DHEAS, DOC, Fe, histamine, uric acid, LH, MSH, PRA, 17-OH progesterone, transferrin satur., TSH, Zn

morning

↑ androstenedione, beta-endorphins, cAMP, DHEAS, DOC, enkephalins, gastrin, insulin, K, cortisol, PRA, TSH

sleep

↑ angiotensin I, creatinine, LH, osteocalcin, PRL, progesterone, GH, TSH

↓ cAMP, estradiol, Fe, gastrin, ILGF-I, cortisol, SHBG

Factors, Interfering – Environment

cold environment

↑ epinephrine, G, Hb, catecholamines, WBC, neu, GH

↓ eos, PLT

■ *Urine* ↑ protein

heat environment

↑ ALT, AST, CK-MM, G, Hb, HCT, Na, neu, GH, LD, lym, WBC

↓ Na

■ *Urine* ↑ proteins, Mb

■ *Sweat* ↑ chloride, Na

high altitude environment

↑ **RBC**, EPO, FT3, **Hb, HCT**, K, **pCO$_2$**, PRL, RAL, T3, transferrin receptor, **PLT**

↓ aldosterone, estriol, LH, **pO$_2$**

■ *Urine* ↑ HCO$_3^-$, volume
   ↓ estriol

■ *Cerebrospinal Fluid* ↑ pressure

Factors, Interfering – Exertion

active athletes (predominantly aerobic activities)

↑ ACTH, ADH, PLT adhesion, **epinephrine**, A2MG, cAMP, androstenedione, Apo A-I, AST, **CK**, COHb, euglobulin lysis time, **beta-endorphins**, enkephalins, EPO, FDP, Hb, **HDL-C**, IgA, IGF-I, IGF-II, K, catecholamines, cortisol, acetoacetic acid, ketobodies, **LA**, LD, WBC, MAC, Mb, MSH, neu, NT-pro-ANP, blood volume, osteocalcin, plasminogen, PRL, pyruvate kinase, secretin, testosterone, TIBC, VIP, FFA, Zn

↓ Apo B-100, estradiol (F), G, HbA$_{1c}$, IgA, **insulin**, calcitonin, progesterone, PTH, SHBG, vitamin – (B$_1$)

■ *Urine* ↑ creatinine, casts – (RBC, granular, hyaline), VMA
   ↓ *osmolality*

■ *Sweat* ↑ chloride, Na

physical exertion generally

↑ ACTH, ADH, PLT adhesion, **epinephrine**, A2MG, ammonia, androstenedione, Apo A-I, AST, **beta-endorphins**, cAMP, **CK**, COHb, euglobulin lysis time, enkephalins, EPO, Hb, IgA, ILGF-I, ILGF-II, K, catecholamines, cortisol, **ketobodies**, acetoacetic acid, **LA**, LD, WBC, MAC, melatonin, myoglobin, neu, NT-pro-ANP, osteocalcin, plasminogen, PRL, pyruvate kinase, secretin, testosterone, TIBC, VIP, FFA, Zn

↓ Apo B-100, estradiol (F), G, **insulin**, calcitonin, progesterone, PTH, SHBG

- *Urine* ↑ ammonia, proteins, **Hb**, K, catecholamines, creatinine, alpha-ketoglutaric acid, casts – (RBC, granular, hyaline), VMA
- *Sweat* ↑ chloride

prolonged physical exertion

↑ ACTH, A2MG, Apo A-I, AST, beta-endorphins, cAMP, **CK**, DHEA, enkephalins, EPO, RBC, FDP, glucagon, Hb, HDL-C, HCT, ILGF-II, calcitonin, catecholamines, **ketobodies**, acetoacetic acid, **LA**, LD, LD – (4, 5), myoglobin, neu, osteocalcin, secretin, **GH**, VIP

↓ estradiol (F), G, IgA, IgG, Na, progesterone, PTH, SHBG, testosterone, vitamin – (B$_1$)

- *Urine* ↑ pregnanetriol
- *Sweat* ↑ chloride

strenuous exertion

↑ ACTH, **aldolase**, **epinephrine**, A2MG, Apo A-I, **AST**, **beta-endorphins**, **unconjugated Bil**, cAMP, ceruloplasmin, **CK**, **CK-MB**, COHb, enkephalins, factor XII, **FDP**, glucagon, glutathione reductase (RBC), Hb, IgA, catecholamines, **ketobodies**, acetoacetic acid, **uric acid**, **LA**, **LD**, LD – (4, 5), WBC, **Mb**, **MD**, melatonin, neu, norepinephrine, osteocalcin, plasminogen, pO$_2$, pyruvate kinase, secretin, testosterone, PLT, VIP

↓ Cu, estradiol (F), **G**, glutathione (RBC), haptoglobin, Hb, IgA, IgG, **insulin**, LH, **P**, progesterone, PTH, SHBG, T4, vitamin B$_1$

- *Urine* ↑ ammonia, proteins, Cr, **Hb**, K, **catecholamines**, creatinine, blood, alpha-ketoglutaric acid, **Mb**, pregnanetriol, casts – (**RBC**, **granular**, **hyaline**), VMA
  ↓ osmolality
- *Sweat* ↑ chloride

fasting

↑ beta-endorphins, ferritin, glucagon, **ketobodies**, **acetoacetic acid** (later), SHBG, GH, uric acid

↓ ILGF-I, insulin, melatonin, PRL, T3

- *Urine* ↑ ketones

hyperventilation

↑ euglobulin lysis time, pH

Factors, Interfering – Nutrition (increased intake of)

animal lipids (fats)

↑ Apo B, **ketobodies**, **acetoacetic acid**, LDL-C, **TAG**, urea

↓ PT

- *Urine* ↑ ketones

avocado

- *Urine* ↑ 5-HIAA

banana

↑ serotonin

- *Urine* ↑ 5-HIAA, UBG, VMA
- *Stool* ↑ blood

beans

- *Urine* ↑ oxalate

beets

- ■ *Urine* ↑ oxalate

cabbage

- ■ *Urine* ↑ crystals – (**Ca-oxalate**)

caffeine

- ↑ beta-endorphins

calcium

- ↑ Ca

carbohydrates

- ↑ **TAG**
- ↓ Apo A-I, HDL-C, LD
- ■ *Urine* ↑ **G**, P
- ■ *Stool* ↑ volume

cheese

- ■ *Urine* ↑ VMA

cherries

- ■ *Urine* ↑ pentoses

chewing gum

- ■ *Urine* ↑ VMA

chloride

- ↑ chloride

chocolate

- ■ *Urine* ↑ oxalate, VMA

cholesterol

- ↑ Apo B, **cholesterol, LDL-C**

cocoa

- ■ *Urine* ↑ **oxalate, VMA**

coffee

- ↓ uric acid
- ■ *Urine* ↑ 5-**HIAA, VMA**

dressings

- ■ *Urine* ↑ VMA

fatty acids

– polyunsaturated fatty acids

- ↑ HDL-C
- ↓ LDL-C, TAG

– polysaturated fatty acids

- ↑ LDL-C, urea
- ↓ HDL-C

fibres

- ↑ TAG
- ↓ HDL-C, cholesterol, LDL cholesterol, TAG

garlic

- ↓ fibrinogen, cholesterol, TAG
- ■ *Urine* ↑ crystals – (Ca-oxalate)

gelatin

- ■ *Urine* ↑ oxalate, VMA

glucose

- ■ *Urine* ↑ Cr, P
- ■ *Stool* ↑ volume

grapes

- ■ *Urine* ↑ pentoses

horse radish

  ■ *Stool* ↑ blood

kalium

  ↑ aldosterone, K

kiwi

  ■ *Urine* ↑ 5-HIAA

legumes

  ↑ uric acid

lettuce

  ■ *Stool* ↑ blood

leucine

  ■ *Urine* ↓ niacin

meal (postprandial)

  ↑ ALT, Apo A-IV, AST, G, K, uric acid, P, proinsulin, PTH, secretin, soma-
    tostatin, trypsin, FFA
  ↓ progesterone

meat

  ↑ carnosine, **creatinine**, uric acid
  ■ *Urine* ↓ pH
  ■ *Stool* ↑ volume

milk

  ↓ PTH
  ■ *Urine* ↑ Ca, **lactose**

– milk in children

  ↓ **Fe**
  ■ *Urine* ↑ galactose, LD

mushrooms

  ■ *Urine* ↑ 5-HIAA

nuts

  ↑ serotonin
  ■ *Urine* ↑ 5-HIAA

oil

– fish oil

  ↑ Apo A-I, Apo B, BT, G, HbA$_{1c}$, HDL-C, cholesterol, plasminogen activa-
    tor inhibitor, LDL cholesterol
  ↓ Apo B, PLT aggregation, fibrinogen, HDL-C, cholesterol, insulin, LDL
    cholesterol, Lp(a), norepinephrine, renin, GH, TAG, PLT, VLDL-C

– olive oil

  ↓ LDL cholesterol, TAG, VLDL-C

– soya oil

  ↓ HDL-C, cholesterol, LDL cholesterol

– sunflower oil

  ↓ Apo A-I, Apo B, HDL-C, cholesterol

orange

  ■ *Urine* ↑ crystals – (Ca-oxalate)

pepper

  ■ *Urine* ↑ oxalate

pineapple

  ↑ serotonin
  ■ *Urine* ↑ 5-HIAA

plums

  ■ *Urine* ↑ 5-HIAA, pentoses

proteins

↑ ammonia, cAMP, uric acid, **GH, urea**
↓ ALP, uric acid, PTH
- *Urine* ↑ phosphoethanolamine, **ketones, creatinine**, osmolality, oxalate, urea
- *Stool* ↓ volume

rhubarb

- *Urine* ↑ crystals – (Ca-oxalate), oxalate, reducing sugars
- *Synovial Fluid* ↑ crystals – (calcium oxalate)

salt

↓ PRA

spinach

- *Urine* ↑ crystals – (Ca-oxalate), oxalate

tea

↓ uric acid, vitamin – (B_1)
- *Urine* ↑ crystals – (Ca-oxalate), oxalate, VMA

tomatoes

↑ serotonin
- *Urine* ↑ crystals – (Ca-oxalate), 5-HIAA, oxalate

water

↓ albumin, osmolality
- *Urine* ↑ volume

yeast

↑ uric acid

Factors, Interfering – Nutrition (insufficient intake of)

calcium

↓ **Ca, Ca^{2+}**

cholesterol

↓ Apo B

chromium

↓ **Cr**

iron

↑ anisocytes, carbohydrate-deficient transferrin, GHb, microcytes, porphyrins, **TIBC, PLT**, zinc protoporphyrin
↓ albumin, **Fe, ferritin, Hb**, WBC, RTC, transferrin satur., PLT, **transferrin**, vitamin – (B_{12})
- *Urine* ↑ **hemosiderin**

magnesium

↑ ALP, Ca^{2+}, K

phosphorus

↑ Ca, **P**

proteins

↓ **ferritin, LD**, urea
- *Urine* ↓ urea

salt

↑ PRA

selenium

↑ AST, macrocytes, CK
↓ glutathione peroxidase (RBC)

total parenteral nutrition

    ↑ Al, ALP, ALT, AST, ammonia, Bil, conjugated Bil, Ca, Ca²⁺, eos, G, gluta-
       mine, GMT, HCT, chloride, cholesterol, K, creatine, LA, LD, MAC, Na,
       osmolality, pCO_2, TAG, urea

    ↓ Apo A-IV, biotin, Ca, Ca²⁺, **ceruloplasmin, Cr,** Cu, FA, folate, G, HCT,
       HCO_3^-, chloride, cholesterol, K, uric acid, LD, **Mg,** Na, osmolality, P,
       prealbumin, **Se,** urea, transthyretin, Zn

    ■ *Urine* ↑ Hb

vitamin A

    ↓ RBC, Hb, cholesterol, **carotene, retinol**

vitamin B₁

    ↑ **pyruvic acid**
    ↓ AST, RBC, Hb, HCT, ✳ **thiamine, RBC transketolase**
    ■ *Urine* ↓ **thiamine**
    ■ *Synovial Fluid* ↑ crystals – (calcium oxalate)

vitamin B₂

    ↓ RBC, glutathione (RBC), Hb, HCT, ✳ **riboflavin**
    ■ *Gastric Fluid* ↑ pH

vitamin B₆

    ↑ anisocytes, **Fe,** Hb, mono, poikilocytes, RBC basophilic stippling, RTC,
       PLT, protoporphyrin (RBC), **transferrin satur.**

    ↓ ALP (WBC), **ALT, AST,** RBC, folate, haptoglobin, HCT, CHS (RBC), WBC,
       MCH, MCHC, MCV, neu, RBC osmotic fragility, ✳ **pyridoxine,** PLT,
       RTC, TIBC

    ■ *Urine* ↑ cystathionine, cystine, homocystine, oxalate
      ↓ ✳ pyridoxic acid
    ■ *Synovial Fluid* ↑ crystals – (calcium oxalate)

vitamin B₁₂

    ↑ anisocytes, **Bil, Fe, gastrin,** HbA2, **HbF,** RBC Howell–Jolly bodies,
       ✳ **homocysteine,** LD, **macrocytes,** megaloblasts, ✳ **methylmalonic
       acid**

    ↓ ALP, **neu,** PLT, vitamin B₁₂
    ■ *Urine* ↑ alpha-aminonitrogen, methylmalonic acid

vitamin C

    ↑ haptoglobin, MCV, RTC
    ↓ albumin, **ALP, Fe,** fibrinogen, **folate,** Hb, HCT, ✳ **ascorbic acid,** MCH,
       MCHC, TIBC

    ■ *Urine* ↑ blood, RBC, alpha-aminonitrogen
      ↓ ascorbic acid
    ■ *Stool* ↑ blood

vitamin D

    ↑ **ALP, PTH,** vitamin – (D2, **D3)**
    ↓ ALP, **Ca,** Ca²⁺, **citrate,** ✳ **1,25-(OH)₂D3,** P
    ■ *Urine* ↑ cAMP, hydroxyproline, P
      ↓ **Ca,** Ca²⁺

vitamin E

    ↑ **CK, RTC, PLT**
    ↓ RBC, **haptoglobin, HCT,** ✳ **tocopherol**

vitamin K

    ↑ APTT, BT, **coagulation time,** PT
    ↓ factor – (VII, **IX,** X), proconvertin, **protein C, protein S,** prothrombin

water
- ↑ **chloride**, osmolality

zinc
- ↓ ALP, RBP, vitamin – (A), **Zn**
- ■ *Urine* ↑ **Zn**
  - ↓ Zn
- ■ *Hair* ↓ **Zn**

Factors, Interfering – Psychic Conditions

– emotions
- ↑ Apo B, epinephrine, beta-endorphins, G, cortisol, WBC, VLDL-C

– fear
- ↑ epinephrine

radiation therapy
- ↑ CEA, MHb, mono, neu, **uric acid**
- ↓ bas, gamma globulins, Hb, HCT, IgE, lym, **neu**, **RTC**, **PLT**, vitamin – (B$_{12}$), **WBC**
- ■ *Synovial Fluid* ↑ eos

radiographic contrast media
- ↑ AMS, unconjugated Bil, eos, histamine, catecholamines, creatinine, T4, TSH, urea
- ↓ albumin, GFR, uric acid, T3, PLT
- ■ *Urine* ↑ proteins, G, 17-KGS, crystals, **uric acid**, specific gravity
  - ↓ catecholamines, VMA
- ■ *Cerebrospinal Fluid* ↑ proteins, eos, WBC, macrophages, pressure
- ■ *Synovial Fluid* ↑ eos

Factors, Interfering – Variations, Seasonal

spring
- ↑ AST, cAMP, hydroxyproline, TAG
- ↓ ALT, beta-carotene, G, T3, T4, urea

summer
- ↑ Ca, creatinine, uric acid, LD, LH, P, PTH, vitamin C
- ↓ albumin, ALT, FT4, cholesterol, Mg, T3, T4, TSH, urea

autumn (fall)
- ↑ albumin, beta-carotene, Ca, G, hydroxyproline, urea
- ↓ AST, TAG

winter
- ↑ ALT, FT4, cholesterol, Mg, T3, T4, TAG, TSH
- ↓ Ca, cAMP, hydroxyproline, creatinine, uric acid, LD, LH, P, PTH, vitamin – (C, D3)

Failure

adrenal failure
- ↑ * **ACTH**, Ca, K, PRL
- ↓ androstenedione, HCO$_3^-$, * **chloride**, * **cortisol**, * **Na**
- ■ *Urine* ↑ Na, pH
  - ↓ K, 17-OHCS, volume, * **free cortisol**
- ■ *Saliva* ↓ cortisol

bone marrow failure
- ↓ RBC, **HCT**, **WBC**, **RTC**

gonadal failure (female)
- ↑ * **FSH**, **LH**, PRL, SHBG
- ↓ androstenedione, **dihydrotestosterone**, EPO, * **estradiol**, estrogens, FSH, LH, progesterone, * **testosterone**, free testosterone, Zn

- *Urine* ↑ ✳ FSH, ✳ LH
  - ↓ estradiol, estrogens, FSH, 17-KS, pregnanediol, pregnanetriol

gonadal failure (male)
- ↑ **anti-testicular Ab**
- ↓ LH, **testosterone**
- *Urine* ↑ 17-KS
- *Seminal Fluid* ↓ volume, spermatozoa count

heart failure
- ↑ ACA, **ADA**, ADH, **aldosterone**, alpha-aminonitrogen, **ALP**, ALP (isoenzymes), ✳ **ALT**, amino acids, ammonia, ✳ **ANF**, ASAL, **AST**, Bil, ✳ **conjugated Bil**, BNP, ✳ **unconjugated Bil**, BSP retention, CK, Cu, D-dimers, **RBC**, phosphohexoisomerase, fructose-1,6-diphosphate aldolase, ESR, FSH, **G**, gamma globulins, **cGMP, GMT, Hb**, HBD, HCO_3^-, CHS, ICD, **K**, K (RBC), **creatinine, uric acid, LA, LAP, ✳ LD**, LD – (2,3,4, ✳ 5), LH, ✳ **mAST**, MAL, MCV, MD, Mg, Na, norepinephrine, **NT-pro-ANP, plasma volume**, OCT, PT, pCO_2, **pH**, ✳ **PRA**, prostacyclin, pyruvate, ribonuclease, **urea**, vitamin – (B_{12})
- ↓ ADH, **albumin**, AMS, **proteins**, CO_2, eos, ESR, **fibrinogen**, G, **HCT, chloride, cholesterol**, cholinesterase, K, **lym, ✳ Mg, Na**, osmolality, **pH**, pCO_2, pO_2, O_2 satur., plasmocytes, PLT, testosterone, vitamin – (B_1, folate)
- *Urine* ↑ **albumin, Bil, proteins, RBC, WBC, specific gravity, osmolality, UBG**, casts – (RBC, **granular, hyaline**, WBC)
  - ↓ **chloride**, GFR, LD, **Na**, specific gravity, **volume**
- *Cerebrospinal Fluid* ↑ **pressure**
- *Sputum* ↑ blood
- *Pleural Fluid* ↑ **AMS**, eos, complement – (CH50), LA, LD, lym, mono, mononuclear cells, pH, **RBC**, volume
  - ↓ AAT, A2MG, proteins, haptoglobin, hemopexin, WBC, orosomucoid, pH
- *Peritoneal Fluid* ↑ proteins, RBC, G, WBC, specific gravity
  - ↓ **albumin**, proteins, **eos**
- *Seminal Fluid* ↓ **volume**
- *Sweat* ↑ K
- *Saliva* ↑ K, Na
  - ↓ chloride, Na
- *Synovial Fluid* ↑ volume

Note: hCG test, GnRH, karyotype, molecular biology (Y-chromosome long arm deletion)

– fetal heart failure
- *Amniotic Fluid* ↑ volume

liver failure
- ↑ **alpha-aminonitrogen**, AFP, ALP, ✳ **ALT**, ✳ **ammonia**, APTT, ✳ **AST**, ✳ **Bil**, ✳ **BT**, BNP, BSP retention, CO_2, D-dimers, ✳ **FDP**, globulins, glucagon, **GMT**, HDL-C, **creatinine**, LD, **WBC**, lym, **MAC**, MAL, pCO_2, ✳ **PT**, RAL, thrombomodulin, **TT**, **urea**
- ↓ ✳ **albumin**, ALT (later), AST (later), AT III, **beta-glucuronidase, proteins, euglobulin lysis time**, RBC, factor – (**II, ✳ V, VII, IX, X**), ✳ **fibrinogen, G**, G tolerance, haptoglobin, CHS, **cholesterol, HDL-C, LDL-C**, G, Hb, HCT, ILGF-I, complement – (C3), K (early), Mg, **Na**, Ni, P, pCO_2, pH, somatomedin C, T4, TBG, **PLT, urea**, vitamin – (A)
- *Urine* ↑ amino acids, **fructose**, RBC, hydroxyproline, hippuric acid, leucine, WBC, Na, specific gravity, ✳ **tyrosine**, casts – (hyaline)
  - ↓ GFR, Na

- **■** *Peritoneal Fluid* ↑ ALP, AMS, bacteria (culture), **proteins**, GMT, HCO$_3^-$, RBC, blood, K, LD, WBC, metHb, neu, P, PMN, **volume**, TAG, turbidity, color changes
  ↓ cholesterol, HCO$_3^-$, pH
- **■** *Cerebrospinal Fluid* ↑ leucine

lung failure

↑ AB, aldosterone, ammonia, BE, Ca, eos, EPO, RBC, ESR, Hb, HCT, HCO$_3^-$, K, LA, WBC, MAC, ✳ **pCO$_2$** ✳ **RAC**

↓ AAT, AB, ACE, **BE**, Hb, HCT, HCO$_3^-$, chloride, K, pH, ✳ **pO$_2$**, ✳ **satur. O$_2$**, PLT

– acute lung failure

↑ LA, WBC, ✳ **pCO$_2$**, ✳ **PCT**, RAC

↓ **Hb, HCT**, K, **WBC**, pH, pO$_2$

ovary failure

↑ anti-ovarian Ab, FSH, LH

↓ androstenedione, estradiol, **estrogens**, FSH, LH, progesterone

■ *Urine* ↑ FSH

↓ **estrogens**, FSH, gonadotropins, pregnanediol

pituitary failure

↑ eos, K, WBC

↓ **aldosterone**, estradiol, ✳ **FSH**, Hb, HCT, cortisol, ✳ **LH**, Na, ✳ **PRA**, ✳ **GH, T$_4$**

placental failure

↑ Hb, HCT, IgA, IgM, viscosity

↓ ALP, estriol, hPL, IgG, pregnancy-associated plasma protein – (A, B), pregnancy specific beta-1-glycoprotein

■ *Urine* ↓ **estriol**, pregnanediol

■ *Amniotic Fluid* ↑ AFP, creatinine, uric acid, PL, urea

↓ LAP

renal failure

– acute renal failure

↑ ACP, AGBMA, Al, ALP, AMS, ✳ **ANA**, ✳ **ANCA**, anti-Sm Ab, ANF, Apo B, ASLO, AST, beta-endorphins, BHBA, ✳ **B2M**, BNP, proteins, Ca, CIC, **CK**, CK-MM, **C-peptide**, ✳ **cystatine C, BT**, D-dimers, enkephalins, eos, factor D, fructosamine, G, GIP, glucagon, glycated albumin, cGMP, HCO$_3^-$, IDL-C, IGFBP-3, **chloride, chymotrypsin**, insulin, ✳ **K**, ✳ **uric acid**, creatine, ✳ **creatinine**, cryoglobulins, LA, LD, LDL-C, LH, lipase, **WBC, MAC**, MAL, Mb, **Mg**, Na (recovery phase), neurotensin, NT-pro-ANP, plasma volume, osmolality, **P**, PT, PRL, PSA, PTH, RF, thrombomodulin, **trypsin**, trypsinogen, ✳ **urea**

↓ ALT, **proteins**, ✳ **Ca** (early), ✳ **Ca^{2+}**, calcitriol, folic acid, PLT aggregation, PLT adhesiveness, ✳ **EPO, RBC**, G, **Hb** (later), HCT (later), HCO$_3^-$, chloride, K (diuretic phase), complement – (✳ **C3**, C4), cortisol, lipoprotein lipase, **lym**, Mg, **Na**, volume, osmolality, P (recovery phase), **pH**, Se, serotonin, T4, **PLT**

■ *Urine* ↑ ✳ **AMS, proteins**, eos, **RBC**, pus, K (diuretic phase), **WBC**, creatinine, creatinine urine/serum, blood, specific gravity, ✳ **Na** (early), ✳ **volume** (polyuric phase), ✳ **osmolality, tubular cells**, casts – (**RBC, granular**, hyaline, WBC, myoglobin, **tubular cells, waxy**)

↓ chloride, **K**, creatinine, specific gravity, Mg, **Na**, ✳ **volume** (early), osmolality, oxalate

■ *Sweat* ↑ chloride, Na
– **chronic renal failure**

↑ ACE, ACP (+RBC), ACTH, epinephrine, ✳ Al, aldosterone, ✳ **alpha-aminonitrogen,** ✳ **ALP,** alpha-1-globulins, alpha-2-globulins, **ALT,** amino acids, ammonia, **AMS,** ANA, ANF, anion gap, Apo B, beta-endorphins, BHBA, ✳ **B2M,** BNP, Ca, ✳ **Ca$_{2+}$** (stage dependent), cAMP, CA 19-9, **CEA, CK,** CK-MB, Co, **C-peptide,** BT, ✳ **cystatine C, cystine,** D-dimers, 2,3-DPG (RBC), EPO, estriol, factor VIII, FDP, Fe, fibrinogen, fluoride, fructosamine, **ESR, G, gastrin,** GIP, **glucagon, glycerol,** glycine, glycated albumin, GHb, cGMP, G6Pase, HbF, Hb (free), histamine, **HCO$_3^-$,** homocysteine, ✳ **chloride, cholesterol, chymotrypsin,** ILGF-I, IGFBP-3, immunoreactive proinsulin, immunoreactive trypsin, **insulin,** ✳ **K, K** (RBC), **calcitonin, catecholamines,** ketobodies, cortisol, **creatine,** ✳ **creatinine, uric acid,** LA, **LD,** ✳ **LDL-C,** LH, lipids, pre-beta-LPs, beta-LPs, **LPs, WBC, MAC,** MCV, melatonin, **Mg** (+RBC), **Na** (+RBC), **neu,** neurotensin, Ni, norepinephrine, NT-pro-ANP, plasma volume, ✳ **osteocalcin,** P, PT, **PP, PRA, PRL,** protoporphyrin (RBC), ✳ **PTH,** RTC, schistocytes, Se, secretin, somatostatin, sulfate, **GH,** ✳ **TAG,** cTnT, thrombomodulin, PLT, **trypsin,** TSH, ✳ **urea,** vitamin – (A, B$_{12}$, D, E), **VLDL-C,** vWF

↓ PLT adhesion, PLT aggregation, alanine, ✳ **albumin,** aldosterone, ALT, ammonia, Apo A-I, **arginine, proteins,** B2M, Ca, ✳ **Ca^{2+}** (stage dependent), Cd, CO$_2$, **RBC,** ✳ **EPO,** estrogens, factor – (II, V, **VII,** IX, X, XIII), ✳ **Fe,** FT3, FT4, G, **Hb, GHb,** HDL-C, **HCT,** HCO$_3^-$, **chloride,** ILGF-I, **K,** complement – (C3, C4), cortisol, **glutamic acid,** LCAT, WBC, lipoprotein lipase, **lym,** Mg, MCHC, MCV, **Na** (+RBC), ornithine, pCO$_2$, **pH,** plasma volume, plasmocytes, **PRA,** progesterone, RTC, Se, serotonin, **T3, T4, testosterone, PLT,** transferrin, transferrin receptor, threonine, **tyrosine,** vitamin – (B$_1$, B$_6$, **D$_3$,** folate), FFA, Zn

■ *Urine* ↑ ACP, alanine, albumin, aldosterone, ALP, amino acids, **AMS,** ✳ **proteins,** B2M, ✳ **RBC, G, pus,** hexosaminidase, insulin, **K,** coproporphyrin III, ✳ **blood,** uric acid, LD, **WBC,** lysozyme, mono, **Na, volume** (early), **pH,** Se, GH, uroporphyrin, casts – (**cellular, granular,** hyaline, **waxy**)

↓ ammonia, Ca, GFR, ✳ **specific gravity,** 17-OHCS, 17-KGS, Mg, Na, osmolality, ✳ **volume** (later), oxalate, pH, Se

■ *Cerebrospinal Fluid* ↑ proteins, creatine, WBC
■ *Pleural Fluid* ↑ pH
    ↓ LD, specific gravity
■ *Gastric Fluid* ↑ pH
    ↓ HCl
■ *Saliva* ↑ urea
■ *Seminal Fluid* ↓ spermatozoa count
■ *Synovial Fluid* ↑ crystals – (hydroxyapatite, urate)
■ *Sweat* ↑ chloride, Mg, Na, phosphate
■ *Stool* ↑ K

Fasciitis
eosinophilic fasciitis
↑ **eos, WBC**
necrotizing fasciitis
↑ ESR, **WBC**

Feeding, Breast
> ↓ Cr, Mn

Feminization
  adrenal feminization
> ■ *Urine* ↑ ✳ estrogens, 17-KS

  feminization in children
> ↑ estradiol

  testicular feminization
> ↑ estradiol, LH, **testosterone**

Fever
  familial Mediterranean fever
> ↑ **eos** (attack), **ESR** (attack), **fibrinogen, alpha-2-globulins, glycoprotein, WBC**
> ↓ Hb, HCT
> ■ *Urine* ↑ cAMP

  rheumatic fever
> ↑ ADA, alpha-1-globulins, alpha-2-globulins, ALT, ANA, ✳ antideoxy-ribonuclease B, anti-DNAase, ✳ **antihyaluronidase, antimyocardial Ab**, antistreptokinase, ✳ **ASLO, AST, proteins, CIC**, cold agglutinins, ✳ **CRP**, Cu, **elastase, fibrinogen**, ✳ **ESR, gamma globulins**, globulins, **haptoglobin, IgA, IgG**, immunoglobulins, complement – (C3, total), cryofibrinogen, **sialic acid, LD**, LE cells, ✳ **WBC**, MPV, **mucoproteins, neu**, plasma volume, PLT, ✳ **troponin** – (I, T)
> ↓ **albumin**, RBC, Hb, HCT, complement – (C3, CH50, total)
> ■ *Urine* ↑ **albumin**, epinephrine, **proteins, RBC**, homocystine, catechol-amines, coproporphyrin, **WBC**, norepinephrine, casts
>   ↓ G
> ■ *Synovial Fluid* ↑ **eos**, clot formation, LE cells, **WBC, neu**, PMN, viscos-ity, **volume**
>   ↓ complement – (C3, total), **viscosity**
> ■ *Pleural Fluid* ↑ eos

Fibrinolysis, Primary
> ↑ **APTT, D-dimers, FDP, PT**, schistocytes
> ↓ A2MG, euglobulin lysis time, **fibrinogen**, coagulation factor – (V, VIII), **plasminogen**

Fibrosis
  cystic pancreatic fibrosis
> ↑ Al, ALP, ALT, **alpha-1-antichymotrypsin**, atypical-ANCA, conjugated Bil, CA 19-9, elastase, G, gamma globulins, GMT, **glucagon**, GHb, chymotrypsin, **IgA**, IgE, **IgG**, IgM, IL-8, immunoreactive trypsin, WBC, MAC, **MAL**, pCO_2, serotonin, **trypsin**, bile acids
> ↓ **albumin**, AMS, beta-carotene, **proteins**, Cu, RBC, Hb, HCT, chloride, cholesterol, CHS, **K**, lipase, lipids, pO_2, prealbumin, prothrombin, **RBP**, vitamin – (A, B_{12}, **D, E, K**)
> ■ *Urine* ↑ Al, G, 5-HIAA
>   ↓ AMS
> ■ *Amniotic Fluid* ↑ ALP
>   ↓ alpha-glucosidase
> ■ *Sweat* ↑ ✳ **chloride**, K, ✳ **Na**
> ■ *Saliva* ↑ AMS, proteins, K, Na
> ■ *Bronchoalveolar Lavage Fluid* ↑ **neu, PMN**

- **Seminal Fluid** ↓ spermatozoa
- **Stool** ↑ albumin, protein, pH, **fat**
  ↓ **chymotrypsin, trypsin**
- **Gastric Fluid** ↓ pepsin

pulmonary cystic fibrosis

↑ ACE, ALT, **alpha-1-globulins, alpha-2-globulins,** atypical-ANCA, EPO, **gamma globulins, IgA, IgG,** IgM, IL-8, WBC, MAL, pCO$_2$

↓ **albumin,** beta-carotene, essential fatty acid, cholesterol, K, carotenoids, pO$_2$, vitamin – (A, E)

- **Urine** ↑ G
- **Gastric Fluid** ↑ **viscosity**
  ↓ **enzyme activity, HCO$_3^-$**
- **Sweat** ↑ Al, **chloride,** K, **Na**
- **Bronchoalveolar Lavage Fluid** ↑ neu, PMN
- **Stool** ↑ **fat**

retroperitoneal fibrosis

↑ **ESR,** eos, gamma globulins, **WBC**

↓ proteins, **Hb, HCT**

Fissure, Anal

- **Stool** ↑ **blood**

Fistula

arterio-venous fistula

↓ plasma volume
- **Synovial Fluid** ↑ RBC

esophago-pericardial fistula

- **Pericardial Fluid** ↑ WBC

gastric-duodenal fistula

↑ ALP, CEA, HCT, pH, WBC

↓ proteins, chloride, CO$_2$, Hb, HCT, K, Na, pH, pCO$_2$,

- **Stool** ↑ **fat**

intestinal fistula

↑ chloride, MAC, osmolality

↓ albumin, chloride, **K, Mg,** Na

- **Urine** ↓ K
- **Stool** ↑ pus, fat

lymphatic fistula

↓ albumin

pancreatic fistula

↑ MAC

- **Urine** ↓ K

Fluorosis

↑ fluoride, PTH

Fractures, Healing

↑ **ALP,** beta globulins, **LD,** lipids, osteocalcin, P

↓ P

- **Urine** ↑ Ca, hydroxyproline, creatine, **creatinine, lipids**

Fructosuria

↑ **fructose,** GHb

- **Urine** ↑ **fructose,** reducing sugars

Galactorrhea

↑ PRL

↓ estradiol, FSH, LH

Galactosemia

↑ **ALT, AST**, Bil, conjugated Bil, unconjugated Bil, phenylalanine, ∗ **galactose, galactose-1-phosphate** (RBC), GHb, inositol

↓ albumin, G, ∗ **GPUT** (RBC), galactokinase (RBC), **uric acid**

■ *Urine* ↑ **albumin, amino acids, proteins**, ∗ **galactose**, galactose-1-phosphate, **reducing sugars**, tyrosine

Gammopathy

monoclonal gammopathy

– benign monoclonal gammopathy

↑ alpha-2-globulins, ANCA, c-ANCA, gamma globulins, cholesterol, **LDL-C, paraproteins** (IgA, IgD, IgE, IgG, IgM), **monoclonal M-chain, L-chain kappa/lambda Ig**, prealbumin, viscosity

↓ IgG, IgM

■ *Urine* ↑ **proteins**, monoclonal light chain kappa/lambda Ig, Bence Jones protein

– malignant monoclonal gammopathy

↑ alpha-1-globulins, alpha-2-globulins, ANCA, c-ANCA, beta globulins, **proteins, ESR, gamma globulins**, HbF, cholesterol, chylomicrons, IDL-C, **creatinine, LDL-C, paraproteins**, prealbumin, VLDL-C

↓ **albumin, Hb**, IgM

■ *Urine* ↑ Bence Jones protein, proteins

–– heavy-chain disease

↑ eos, ESR, prealbumin, **uric acid**, lym, **plasmocytes, urea**

↓ albumin, Ca, RBC, gamma globulins, globulins, Hb, HCT, IgA, IgG, IgM, PLT, **WBC**

■ *Urine* ↑ **proteins**, Bence Jones protein

■ *Stool* ↑ K, **fat**

––– heavy-chain alpha disease

↑ **monoclonal heavy chain alpha Ig**, lym

■ *Urine* ↑ Bence Jones protein

––– heavy-chain gamma disease

↑ eos, ESR, **lym** (relative), **monoclonal heavy chain gamma Ig, plasmocytes**, prealbumin, **urea, uric acid**

↓ albumin, Ca, RBC, ∗ **gamma globulins**, globulins, Hb, HCT, IgA, IgG, IgM, WBC, PLT

■ *Urine* ↑ proteins, Bence Jones protein

■ *Stool* ↑ K, **fat**

––– heavy-chain Mu disease

↑ lym, **monoclonal heavy chain Mu Ig, monoclonal light chain kappa/ lambda Ig**

■ *Urine* ↑ Bence Jones protein, monoclonal light chain kappa/lambda Ig

–– plasmocytoma (incl. multiple myeloma)

↑ ACE, ACP, ACTH, albumin, alpha-1-globulins, ALP, ALP (WBC), A2MG, AMS, AST, Bence Jones protein, beta globulins, beta-lipotropin, **proteins, Ca**, BT, endorphins, enkephalins, eos, **factor VIII, ferritin, fibrinogen, ESR**, nucleated RBC, **gamma globulins**, globulins, HbF, **hexosaminidase, cold agglutinins, chloride**, cholesterol, chylomicrons, IDL-C, **IgA, IgD, IgE, IgG**, IgM, IL-6, sIL-6R, nucleated RBC, **uric acid, creatinine**, cryofibrinogen, **cryoglobulins**, LD, beta-LP, lupus inhibitor, **lym**, **WBC**, lysozyme, **macrocytes**, MCV, Mg, Mo, mono, TM – (**B2M**, **ferritin**, **fibronectin**), plasma volume, **osteocalcin**, P, ✳ **paraproteins**, **monoclonal M-chain**, **L-chain kappa/lambda Ig**, plasma volume, **plasmocytes**, prealbumin, pyroglobulins, RF, N-telo-peptides, T_S-lym (CD8), TT, UBBC, **urea**, VDRL (false), **viscosity**, **VLDL-C**

↓ ACE, **albumin**, alpha-1-globulins, alpha-2-globulins, **A2MG**, Apo B, EPO, **RBC**, factor – (II, XIII), gamma globulins, globulins, **Hb**, **HCT**, cholesterol, IgA, IgG, IgM, complement – (C3), **K**, **uric acid**, LDL-C, WBC, **Mg**, **Na**, **neu**, P, pO_2, T_H-lym (CD4), transferrin, vitamin – (B_{12}), **PLT**

- *Urine* ↑ albumin, **amino acids**, ✳**Bence Jones protein**, **proteins**, Ca, G, **globulins**, hexosaminidase, hydroxyproline – (total, free), K, crys-tals – (uric acid), **monoclonal light chain kappa/lambda Ig**, uric acid, TM – (hCG, hydroxyproline), volume, **P**, casts
  ↓ GFR, osmolality, specific gravity, volume
- *Cerebrospinal Fluid* ↑ albumin, **proteins**, globulins, IgG
- *Pleural Fluid* ↑ B2M, **proteins**
- *Synovial Fluid* ↑ crystals – (cryoglobulin)

--- IgA plasmocytoma (light-chain disease)

↑ Bence Jones protein, IgA, monoclonal heavy chain alpha Ig, monoclo-nal light chain kappa/lambda Ig, viscosity

↓ IgA, IgG, IgM, WBC

- *Urine* ↑ ✳ Bence Jones protein

--- IgD plasmocytoma (light-chain disease)

↑ IgD, monoclonal heavy chain delta Ig, monoclonal light chain lambda Ig

↓ WBC

- *Urine* ↑ ✳ Bence Jones protein

--- IgG plasmocytoma (light-chain disease)

↑ IgG, monoclonal heavy chain gamma Ig, monoclonal light chain kap-pa/lambda Ig, viscosity

↓ IgA, IgM, WBC

- *Urine* ↑ ✳ Bence Jones protein

--- solitary plasocytoma

↑ monoclonal light chain kappa Ig, paraproteins

- *Urine* ↑ Bence Jones protein
- *Cerebrospinal Fluid* ↑ albumin, IgG, proteins

-- Waldenstrom's macroglobulinemia

↑ ACP (WBC), **ANA**, alpha-1-globulins, beta globulins, ✳ **proteins**, B2M, BT, **eos**, factor VIII, ESR, **gamma globulins**, **cold agglutinins**, choles-terol, **chylomicrons**, IDL-C, IgG, ✳ **IgM**, cryofibrinogen, **cryoglobu-lins**, uric acid, WBC, **lym**, **macroglobulins**, mastocytes, **mono**, plas-ma volume, **paraproteins**, **monoclonal Mu-chain**, **L-chain kappa/lambda Ig**, PT, plasmocytes, prealbumin, RF, TT, urea, **viscosity**, **VLDL-C**

↓ **albumin**, **RBC**, ESR, factor – (II, V, VII, X), fibrinogen, **Hb**, **HCT**, IgA, IgG, IgM, complement – (total), **WBC**, lym, **neu**, **clot retraction**, PLT

- *Urine* ↑ ✳ Bence Jones protein, **monoclonal light chain kappa/lamb-da Ig**, proteins

polyclonal gammopathy

↑ alpha-1-globulins, alpha-2-globulins, gamma globulins, LDL-C, WBC, paraproteins, prealbumin

- *Urine* ↑ protein

Gangliopathy

↑ anti-Hu Ab

Gangliosidosis GM1 (Landing's disease)

↓ ✳ acid beta-galactosidase (WBC)

Gangliosidosis GM2

Sandoff's disease

↓ ✳ **hexosaminidase A** (+ WBC), ✳ **hexosaminidase B** (+ WBC)

- *Urine* ↓ ✳ hexosaminidase A, ✳ hexosaminidase B
- *Tears* ↓ ✳ hexosaminidase A, ✳ hexosaminidase B

Tay-Sachs disease

↑ AST, hexosaminidase B, **LD**

↓ ✳ **hexosaminidase A** (+ WBC), fructose 1-phosphate aldolase

- *Urine* ↓ ✳ hexosaminidase A
- *Cerebrospinal Fluid* ↑ AST
- *Tears* ↓ ✳ hexosaminidase A

Gangrene

↑ **aldolase, ALP, ALT, AST, CK**, CO_2, CRP, **ESR**, cryoglobulins, **LD, pCO_2,** pH, **WBC, neu**

↓ Hb, HCT, **chloride, Na,** pO_2, pCO_2

- *Urine* ↑ proteins

diabetic gangrene

↑ ALP, ALT, AST, G

- *Urine* ↑ G

gaseous gangrene

↑ WBC

- *Urine* ↑ Hb

muscular gangrene

↑ ALT, AST, ESR, neu, WBC

penis gangrene

↑ ALT, WBC

pulmonary gangrene

↑ **ESR, WBC, neu**

↓ Hb, HCT

- *Urine* ↑ protein
- *Sputum* ↑ **blood**, volume

Gastrectomy

↑ AMS, ASAL, CCK-PZ, TIBC (subtotal)

↓ Ca, Cr, Fe, G, Mn, transferrin satur., vitamin – (B_{12}, D, folate), Zn

Gastritis

↑ APA, **AST, eos, gastrin**, neu, **WBC**, TIBC, Ab against H. pylori

↓ **albumin**, proteins, CEA, RBC, Fe, **Hb, HCT**, MCH, MCHC, pepsinogen, transferrin satur., vitamin – (B_{12})

- *Urine* ↓ uropepsinogen
- *Gastric Fluid* ↑ HCl, mucus, **blood**, pH

  ↓ HCl, intrinsic factor, MAO, pepsin, **pH**
- *Stool* ↑ proteins, Hb, **blood**

atrophic gastritis

↑ **APA**
↓ **Fe, pepsinogen**
- *Gastric Fluid* ↑ pH
  ↓ intrinsic factor
- *Stool* ↑ blood

– chronic atrophic gastritis

↑ antiintrinsic factor Ab, **APA**, CEA, **gastrin**
↓ RBC, Fe, gastrin, Hb, HCT, pepsinogen, vitamin – (B$_{12}$)
- *Gastric Fluid* ↓ hydrochloric acid, MAO

Gastroenteritis

↑ eos, G, **Hb**, **HCT**, chloride, WBC, **MAL** (during vomiting), **MAC** (during diarrhea), Na, **neu**, pH
↓ **albumin**, A2MG, proteins, beta-carotene, CO$_2$, factor II, G, **chloride** (during vomiting), **K**, lym, Mg, Na, pCO$_2$
- *Urine* ↑ specific gravity
- *Cerebrospinal Fluid* ↓ G

eosinophilic gastroenteritis

↑ eos, WBC, **MAL** (during vomiting), **MAC** (during diarrhea)
↓ albumin, A2MG, beta-carotene, factor II, chloride (during vomiting), **K**, Na

Gastroenteropathy, Allergic

↑ CIC, eos, IgE
↓ albumin, RBC, HCT, PLT
- *Stool* ↑ Charcot–Leyden crystals, blood

Gastropathy, Hypertrophic Hypersecretory

- *Gastric Fluid* ↑ HCl
  ↓ pH

Gigantism

↑ ALP, Ca, Ca^{2+}, **G**, GH-RH, ✱ **IGF-I**, insulin, **creatinine**, P, **PRL**, ✱ **GH**, urea
↓ neu, SHBG
- *Urine* ↑ Ca, hydroxyproline, creatinine

Glomerulonephritis

cute glomerulonephritis (streptococcal)

↑ alpha-2-globulins, A2MG, amino acids, ✱ **AGBMA**, ANA, ✱ **ANCA**, ✱ p-ANCA, c-ANCA, **anti-DNAase B**, antihyaluronidase, anti-MPO, anti-streptokinase, ✱ **ASLO**, beta globulins, Ca, ✱ **CIC**, C-3 nephritic factor, CRP, ✱ **FDP**, ✱ **fibrinogen**, ✱ **ESR**, gamma globulins, HLA – (DR2), chloride, cholesterol, **IgA**, ✱ **IgG**, ✱ **IgM**, IL-6, ✱ **creatinine**, uric acid, ✱ **cryoglobulins**, LD, WBC, lipids, MAC+RAL, orosomucoid, P, plasmin, PMN, RF, schistocytes, **urea**
↓ **albumin, proteins**, factor B, RBC, **Hb**, HCT, **C1-INH**, complement – (✱ **C1q**, ✱ **C1r**, ✱ **C2**, ✱ **C3**, ✱ **C4**, ✱ **CH50**), creatinine clearance, Mg, PLT
- *Urine* ↑ AAP, ✱ **proteins**, RBC (dysmorphous), FDP, Hb, hexosaminidase, pus, blood, WBC, ✱ **specific gravity**, casts – (**epithelial**, ✱ **RBC**, ✱ **granular**, ✱ **hyaline**, WBC, lipid, mixed)
  ↓ aldosterone, GFR, K, creatinine, uric acid, **volume**, osmolality, **urea**

– membranoproliferative glomerulonephritis

↑ ✱ C-3 nephritic factor
↓ factor B, complement – (✱ **C3**, ✱ **CH50**)

- postinfectious glomerulonephritis (non-streptococcal)
  - ↑ **alpha-2-globulins, anti-DNAase B,** anti-diphosphopyridine nucleotidase, antinicotinamide adenine dinucleotidase, * **antihyaluronidase Ab, antikidney Ab, antistreptokinase Ab,** * **ASLO,** beta globulins, CIC, C-3 nephritic factor, CRP, factor – (VIII), **FDP,** fibrinogen, **ESR,** gamma globulins, cholesterol, **IgG,** creatinine, **cryoglobulins, WBC,** plasmin, **PMN, RF, urea**
  - ↓ albumin, **RBC,** factor B, **Hb, HCT,** complement – (**C3,** CH50), **PLT**
  - ▪ *Urine* ↑ aldosterone, **proteins, RBC,** FDP, **Hb, blood, WBC, specific gravity,** casts – (epithelial, **RBC,** granular, **WBC,** fatty)
    - ↓ aldosterone, **GFR,** Na, **volume,** urea
- rapidly progressive glomerulonephritis
  - ↑ **ESR, creatinine, urea**
  - ▪ *Urine* ↑ **proteins, Hb, blood, RBC, WBC,** casts – (hyaline, granular, RBC, WBC)
    - ↓ **volume**

chronic glomerulonephritis
  - ↑ albumin, A2MG, c-ANCA, **alpha-2-globulins,** * **CIC,** * **FDP, ESR,** * **cholesterol,** * **IgA,** * **IgG,** * **IgM, creatinine,** uric acid, LD, lipids, MAC, orosomucoid, P, **PT, urea**
  - ↓ albumin, **proteins,** RBC, **Hb, HCT,** * complement – (**C3, C4, CH50**)
  - ▪ *Urine* ↑ AAP, **amino acids,** * **proteins** (+ non-selective), * **RBC** (dysmorphous), G, Hb, pus, **blood, volume,** * casts – (**epithelial, RBC, granular, hyaline, lipid, waxy, mixed**)
    - ↓ K, creatinine, **uric acid, volume,** urea

subacute glomerulonephritis
  - ↑ A2MG, **anti-DNAase B,** * **AGBMA,** antihyaluronidase, antistreptokinase, **ASLO, Ca,** CIC, factor VIII, **ESR, chloride,** cholesterol, **IgA,** IgG, IgM, **creatinine,** urid acid, **cryoglobulins,** LD, orosomucoid, P, **urea**
  - ↓ **albumin,** complement – (**C1q, C3, C4, CH50**)
  - ▪ *Urine* ↑ AAP, **proteins, RBC, Hb,** hexosaminidase, pus, **blood, WBC,** tubular cells, specific gravity, casts – (**epithelial, RBC, granular, hyaline, WBC,** lipid, **mixed**)
    - ↓ creatinine, **volume, osmolality,** urea
  - ▪ *Peritoneal Fluid* ↓ protein
  - ▪ *Pleural Fluid* ↓ protein

Glomerulosclerosis, Diabetic
  - ↑ **cholesterol**
  - ↓ **albumin**
  - ▪ *Urine* ↑ **proteins,** microalbumin, oligopeptides, casts – (lipid)

Glycogenosis
  - ↑ **acetoacetic acid, ketobodies, uric acid,** LA, LDL-C, **MAC, TAG, VLDL-C**
  - ↓ PLT adhesion, **G, WBC**
  - ▪ *Urine* ↑ **ketones,** uric acid

type I (von Gierke's disease)
  - ↑ ALT, AST, **cholesterol,** chylomicrons, GMT, **ketones,** acetoacetic acid, **uric acid,** LA, LDL-C, lipids, **MAC,** PL, pyruvate, **TAG, VLDL-C, FFA**
  - ↓ ALP, RBC, **G, G6Pase,** Hb, HCT, LP lipase, **P,** pH, PLT
  - ▪ *Urine* ↑ **acetone,** amino acids, **G, ketones, proteins,** P
  - ▪ *Sweat* ↑ chloride, Na

type II (Pompe's disease)

    ↑ **cholesterol**, chylomicrons, acetoacetic acid, **ketobodies, uric acid, LA**, LDL-C, pyruvate, **TAG**, VLDL-C, FFA

    ↓ G, G6Pase, ∗ **alpha-1,4-glucosidase**, Hb, HCT, LP lipase, P

    ■ *Urine* ↑ acetone, amino acids, G

    ■ *Sweat* ↑ chloride, Na

    ■ *Amniotic Fluid* ↑ CK

       ↓ ∗ **alpha-1,4-glucosidase**

    ■ *Tears* ↓ ∗ **alpha-1,4-glucosidase**

type III (Forbes' disease, Cori's disease)

    ↑ ALT (children), AST (children), cholesterol, CK, ketobodies, uric acid, TAG

    ↓ G

    ■ *Urine* ↑ **acetone**

type IV (Andersen's disease)

    ↑ AST, Bil, globulins, ketobodies, WBC

    ↓ Hb, HCT, cholesterol

type V (McArdle's disease)

    ↑ aldolase, **CK**, K, LA, LD, LDL-C, myoglobin

    ↓ albumin, ∗ **phosphorylase** (WBC)

    ■ *Urine* ↑ **Mb**

type VI (Hers' disease)

    ↑ ALT, cholesterol, ketones, uric acid, TAG

    ↓ G, ∗ **phosphorylase** (WBC)

type VII (Lewis-Thompson disease)

    ↑ aldolase, CK, K, LA, LD, LDL-C

    ↓ G, ∗ **phosphofructokinase** (RBC)

    ■ *Urine* ↑ **Mb**

type VIII (Tar-rui disease)

    ↓ G

    ■ *Urine* ↑ epinephrine, norepinephrine

Glycosuria

    ↓ P

    ■ *Urine* ↑ estriol, specific gravity, volume, Na, **reducing sugars**

Goiter

    ↑ ∗ **antimicrosomal Ab**, ∗ **antithyroglobulin Ab, AGBMA**, antithyroid Ab, thyroxine autoantibodies, **FT4**, iodine, ∗ **TSH**, thyroglobulin

    ↓ iodine

adenomatous goiter

    ↑ **antimicrosomal Ab**, antithyroidal Ab

nodular goiter

    ↑ **antimicrosomal Ab**, antithyroglobulin Ab, **antithyroidal Ab**, thyroxine autoantibodies, T3, T4

Granulomatosis, Wegener's

    ↑ ANCA, ∗ **c-ANCA**, ∗ **p-ANCA**, antiendothelial Ab, antithyroglobulin Ab, ALT, AST, ∗ **CIC, CRP, eos, ESR**, gamma globulins, **IgA, IgG**, complement – (C3, C4), **creatinine**, cryoglobulins, HLA – (DR2, DR4, DRw7), **WBC**, MAC+RAL, **RF**, PLT, **urea**

    ↓ albumin, ∗ **RBC, Hb**, HCT, complement – (∗ **C3**), WBC, **PLT**

- *Urine* ↑ **proteins, RBC, Hb, blood,** casts – (**RBC**, granular, WBC)
- *Cerebrospinal Fluid* ↑ ANCA
- *Synovial Fluid* ↑ WBC, PMN

Growth

physiological body growth
↑ ACP, Ca, ILGF-I
↓ Zn

physiological bone growth
↑ ACP, ALP

Gynecomasty
↑ estradiol, PRL

Hematoma
↑ AAT, ALT, unconjugated Bil
↓ **haptoglobin**

subdural hematoma
- *Cerebrospinal Fluid* ↑ proteins, RBC, blood, pressure

Hemochromatosis
↑ ADA, **AFP, ALT, AST,** Ca, Cu, ✱ **Fe,** ✱ **ferritin,** G, HLA – (**A3, B7, B14**), CHS, PTH, ✱ **transferrin satur.,** siderocytes, GH, TIBC
↓ albumin, ACTH, Cu, **FSH,** LH, P, PTH, GH, testosterone, ✱ **TIBC,** **transferrin,** uric acid, TSH
- *Urine* ↑ ✱ **Fe,** G, Hb, ✱ **hemosiderin,** ✱ **porphyrins**
  ↓ FSH
- *Sputum* ↑ blood
- *Synovial Fluid* ↑ crystals – (calcium pyrophosphate), WBC, viscosity

neonatal hemochromatosis
↑ acanthocytes, **AFP, Bil**
↓ **albumin,** ALT, AST, **G,** Hb, HCT, PLT

primary idiopathic hemochromatosis
↑ **ALT,** AST, Bil, **Fe,** ferritin, **gamma globulins,** HLA – (A3, B7, B14), **PT,** transferrin satur.
↓ albumin, WBC, **TIBC,** PLT
- *Urine* ↑ protein

Hemoconcentration
↑ **albumin,** beta-carotene, **proteins,** Ca, **Hb, HCT,** oxytocin
↓ ESR

Hemodilution
↑ ESR

Hemoglobin F, Hereditary Persistence
↑ ✱ **HbF**
↓ **MCV, MCHC**

Hemoglobinopathy
↑ microcytes, unconjugated Bil, RBC Heinz bodies, uric acid, **RBC osmotic resistance,** sickle cells, target cells
↓ **RBC,** estriol, **Hb,** MCV, osmotic fragility
- *Urine* ↓ estriol

Hemoglobinuria

march hemoglobinuria
- *Urine* ↑ Hb, Mb

paroxysmal cold hemoglobinuria

↑ * **anisocytes**, Bil, * **cold autohemolysin**, cold agglutinins, LD, MCV, methemalbumin, MHb, nucleated RBC, * **poikilocytes**, * **sphero-cytes**

↓ RBC, Hb, HCT

■ *Urine* ↑ * **Hb, hemosiderin**, casts – (Hb, Mb)

paroxysmal nocturnal hemoglobinuria

↑ **PLT Ab, AST, Bil**, unconjugated **Bil, Hb**, Hb (free), HbF, complement – (C3), **LD**, WBC, macrocytes, **methemalbumin**, MCV, **MHb**, osmotic fragility, **RTC**

↓ ACHE (RBC), ALP (WBC), RBC, factor B, **factor XI, Fe, haptoglobin, Hb, HCT, CHS**, folate, complement – (C3), **WBC**, MCV, **neu**, pancyto-penia, pH, schistocytes, **PLT**

■ *Urine* ↑ albumin, **Fe**, RBC, **Hb, hemosiderin, UBG**, casts – (**Hb**, Mb)

■ *Stool* ↑ UBG

Hemolysis

acute hemolysis

↑ **ACP, AST**, Bil, unconjugated Bil, **K**, uric acid, **LD**, lipoprotein lipase, WBC, MD, Mg, NSE, RTC, urea, zinc protoporphyrin

↓ alpha-2-globulins, RBC, haptoglobin, Hb, HCT, hemopexin, vitamin – (E)

■ *Urine* ↑ Hb, hemosiderin

infectious hemolysis

↑ ACP, AST, Bil, unconjugated Bil, **CRP, K**, uric acid, **LD**, WBC, MD, Mg, ornithine, P, urea

↓ RBC, haptoglobin, transferrin satur.

■ *Urine* ↑ Hb

intravascular hemolysis

↑ AAT, ACP, **PLT aggregation**, AST, **Bil**, unconjugated Bil, COHb, delta Bil, nucleated RBC, Hb, **K**, uric acid, **LD**, lipoprotein lipase, **macrocytes**, MD, methemalbumin, ornithine, * **RTC**, urea

↓ alpha-2-globulins, **RBC**, * **haptoglobin**, * **Hb**, HCT, hemopexin

■ *Urine* ↑ **Bil, Hb, hemosiderin**, methemalbumin, UBG

↓ volume

■ *Stool* ↑ UBG

mechanic hemolysis

↑ cTnI, cTnT, ornithine, urea

↓ ACP, alpha-2-globulins, Bil, unconjugated Bil, * **proteins**, * **ferritin**, haptoglobin, Hb, uric acid, **LD**

medicamentous hemolysis

↑ ornithine, urea

↓ ACP, alpha-2-globulins, Bil, unconjugated Bil, haptoglobin, Hb, uric acid, **LD**

Hemoperfusion

↓ Ca, G, WBC

Hemophilia

hemophilia A

↑ anti-La/SSB, * **APTT**, AST, **BT**, * **clotting time** (Lee White), HBsAg, * **PT**, TGT

↓ **✱ factor VIII**, cholesterol, Hb, HCT
- *Urine* ↑ RBC, Hb, cystine
- *Gastric Fluid* ↑ blood
- *Sputum* ↑ blood
- *Synovial Fluid* ↑ crystals – (calcium pyrophosphate), lym, volume

hemophilia B
↑ anti-La/SSB, ✱ **APTT**, AST, **BT**, **clotting time** (Lee White), **PT**, TGT
↓ **✱ factor IX**, cholesterol
- *Urine* ↑ RBC, Hb, cystine
- *Gastric Fluid* ↑ blood
- *Sputum* ↑ blood
- *Synovial Fluid* ↑ crystals – (calcium pyrophosphate), lym, volume

hemophilia C
↑ coagulation time, **PT**, TGT
↓ **✱ factor XI**

Hemorrhage
↑ ADH, **aldosterone**, ALT, ammonia, AST, BT, CK, EPO, fibrinogen, ESR, glutamine, K, LA, **WBC**, neu, **PRA**, RTC, TIBC, PLT, transferrin, urea
↓ **albumin**, **proteins**, **RBC**, Fe, ferritin, G6PD, Hb, **HCT**, chloride, **catecholamines**, **cortisol**, MCV, Na, plasma volume, porphyrins, PT, transferrin satur.
- *Urine* ↑ G, 5-HIAA, cholesterol
- *Cerebrospinal Fluid* ↑ adenylate kinase, proteins, CK, eos, RBC, IgG, blood, LA, LD, WBC, Ly, pressure
  ↓ G, pH
- *Stool* ↑ blood

acute hemorrhage
↑ **RTC** (3-4 days later), transferrin, **PLT**
↓ **Fe**, **ferritin** (2 weeks later), plasma volume, PT, transferrin satur.

anovulatory hemorrhage
- *Urine* ↓ estrogens

cerebral hemorrhage
↑ AST, BT, **ESR**, glutamine, **WBC**
- *Urine* ↑ G, cholesterol
- *Cerebrospinal Fluid* ↑ **proteins**, CK, eos, RBC, IgG, blood, LA, lym, WBC, **pressure**

chronic hemorrhage
↑ TIBC, transferrin
↓ **Fe**, ferritin, G6PD (RBC), HCT, transferrin satur.

esophageal varices hemorrhage
↑ ammonia, **urea**
↓ proteins, HCT
- *Stool* ↑ blood

gastrointestinal tract hemorrhage
↑ ammonia, gastrin, **urea**
↓ proteins, HCT, Na
- *Stool* ↑ blood

intraamniotic hemorrhage
- *Amniotic Fluid* ↑ blood

intracranial hemorrhage
↑ AST

- **Cerebrospinal Fluid** ↑ RBC, IgG, **blood**, LA, LD, WBC, **macrophages**, pressure
  - ↓ cAMP

neonatal hemorrhage
– internal neonatal hemorrhage
  - ↑ unconjugated Bil
  - ↓ Hb, HCT
– twin-to-twin neonatal hemorrhage (recipient twin shows)
  - ↑ * unconjugated Bil, * Hb, * HCT
– twin-to-twin neonatal hemorrhage (donor twin shows)
  - ↑ nucleated RBC, RTC
  - ↓ * Hb, HCT

subarachnoid hemorrhage
  - ↑ ADH, CK
  - **Cerebrospinal Fluid** ↑ adenylate kinase, **proteins**, CK, CRP, eos, cholesterol, **blood, LA**, LD, **RBC, WBC**, lym, **pressure**
    - ↓ **G**, pH

subdural hemorrhage
  - **Cerebrospinal Fluid** ↑ blood, lym, pressure

Hemorrhoids
  - ↓ RBC, **Fe**, Hb, HCT
  - **Stool** ↑ **blood**

Hemothorax
  - ↑ pCO_2
  - ↓ Hb, pH, pO_2
  - **Pleural Fluid** ↑ blood, LD, RBC
    - ↓ pH

Hepatitis
acute hepatitis
  - ↑ AAT, ACP, ADA, AFP, **aldolase**, alpha globulins, **ALP**, ALP (hepatic isoenzyme), **ALT**, ammonia, AMS, anti-DNA, ASMA, **AST**, beta globulins, **B2M, Bil, conjugated Bil**, unconjugated Bil, C3, **CEA, ceruloplasmin**, enolase, **Fe**, ferritin, fibrinogen, **ESR**, gamma globulins, **GD, GMT**, IgA, **IgG, IgM**, uric acid, **LAP, LD**, LD5, LE cells, lipids, **lym**, macrocytes, **Mn**, mono, 5-nucleotidase, orosomucoid, **PT**, PRA, RBP, serotonin, SHBG, T4, TBG, **TIBC**, TPA, **transferrin**, PLT, vitamin – (B_{12}), bile acids
  - ↓ AAT, **albumin**, AMS, Apo A-IV, G, Hb, HCT, **HDL-C**, hemopexin, cholesterol, **CHS, IgM, C1-INH**, prealbumin, Se, triiodothyronine resin uptake, urea
  - **Urine** ↑ alpha-aminonitrogen, ALT, **conjugated Bil**, DALA, fructose, G, **galactose**, reducing sugars, UBG, urobilin, casts – (epithelial, granular)

– acute fulminant hepatitis with hepatic failure
  - ↑ ACP, AFP, **aldolase, ALP, ALT, ammonia**, anti-HBc Ab, anti-HBc IgM, ASMA, **AST, Bil, conjugated Bil, unconjugated Bil**, B2M, CEA, **Fe, ESR**, gamma globulins, **GMT, HBsAg**, HBcAg, **HBeAg**, ICD, IgA, IgG, IgM, **LAP**, LD, WBC, **mAST, PT**, PL, serotonin, T3, T4, TBG, **TIBC**, transferrin
  - ↓ **albumin**, alpha-1-globulins, alpha-2-globulins, AST (later), beta globulins, **proteins**, RBC, **G**, Hb, HCT, **cholesterol, CHS**, WBC, neu, PL, T3, transferrin, PLT

- ■ *Urine* ↑ amino acids, **Bil**, UBG
  - ↓ UBG
- ■ *Stool* ↑ fat
  - ↓ UBG
- ■ *Cerebrospinal Fluid* ↑ proteins, lym
- – acute hepatitis A
  - ↑ * **anti-HAV-IgM**, * **anti-HAV-IgG**, * **anti-HAV**, * **HAV-RNA**
  - ↓ WBC
- – acute hepatitis B (high infectivity)
  - ↑ **anti-HBc-IgM, anti-HBc**, * **HBeAg**, * **HBsAg**, * **HBV-DNA**
  - ↓ WBC
- – acute hepatitis B (late, low infectivity)
  - ↑ **anti-HBc, anti-HBc-IgG, anti-HBe, HBeAg, HBsAg**
- – acute hepatitis B (serologic gap)
  - ↑ **anti-HBc, anti-HBc-IgM**
- – acute hepatitis B (convalescence)
  - ↑ **anti-HBe, anti-HBc, anti-HBc**, * **anti-HBs -IgM**
- – acute hepatitis B (recovery)
  - ↑ * **anti-HBe, anti-HBc**, * **anti-HBs, anti-HBc-IgG**
- – acute hepatitis C
  - ↑ * **anti-HCV**
- – acute hepatitis D
  - ↑ * **anti-HDV-IgM, anti-HDV**, * **HDAg**
  - ↓ WBC
- – acute hepatitis E
  - ↑ * **anti-HEV**
  - ↓ WBC
- – acute viral hepatitis (hepatitis A, B, C, D, E)
  - ↑ AAP, AAT, **ACP, ADA, AFP, aldolase, ALP**, ALP (WBC), alpha-1-glycoprotein, alpha-2-globulins, * **ALT**, AMA, AMS, ANA, anti-DNA, **anti-HAV, anti-HAV-IgG, anti-HAV-IgM, anti-HBc, anti-HBe, anti-HBs, anti-HBc-IgG, anti-HBc-IgM, anti-HBe, anti-HBsAg, anti-HBs-IgG, anti-HBV, anti-HCV, anti-HDV, anti-HEV, ASAL, ASMA, AST, beta globulins, beta-glucuronidase, B2M, Bil, conjugated Bil, un-conjugated Bil**, BSP retention, **CEA, ceruloplasmin**, CRP, Cu, **Fe**, phenylalanine, folate, **ESR, gamma globulins**, GMD, **GMT**, guanine deaminase, **HAV-RNA, HBsAg, HBcAg, HBeAg, HBV-RNA, HCV-RNA, HDAg, HDV-RNA, HEV-RNA**, hexosaminidase, chenodeoxycholic acid, cold agglutinins, cholic acid, **ICD**, IgA, IgG, IgM, **isoleucine**, complement – (C3), cryoglobulins, **uric acid, LAP, LD**, LD5, LDL-C, lecithin (RBC), leucine, WBC, **lym**, MD, Mn, **mono**, neu, **5-nucleotidase, OCT**, phenylalanine, **PT, PL**, PRA, **RF**, RTC, serotonin, T3, **T4, TAG**, TBG, **TIBC, transferrin**, thymidine kinase, tyrosine, valine, **VLDL-C, bile acids**
  - ↓ **albumin, alpha-1-globulins, alpha-2-globulins**, beta globulins, beta-carotene, **proteins**, RBC, **G**, G tolerance, glycoproteins, Hb, HCT, **cholesterol, CHS**, complement – (C3), LD (isoenzymes), lipase, **WBC**, lym, Mg, mono, mucoproteins, **neu**, Ni, pCO$_2$, PL, plasmocytes, PLT, prealbumin, RBP, Se, T3, transferrin, vitamin – (A), Zn
  - ■ *Urine* ↑ **albumin**, alpha-aminonitrogen, ALT, **amino acids**, proteins, **conjugated Bil**, DALA, fructose, G, **galactose**, coproporphyrin, blood, **porphyrins, UBG**, urobilin, casts – (epithelial, **granular**), **Zn**

    ↓ 17-KS, specific gravity, UBG
- ■ *Stool* ↑ **fat**
  ↓ **Bil,** UBG
- ■ *Cerebrospinal Fluid* ↑ proteins, lym
- ■ *Synovial Fluid* ↑ clot formation, WBC, PMN, volume

alcoholic hepatitis

    ↑ ACP, **AFP, ALP,** ALP (hepatic isoenzyme), **ALT,** ammonia (later), ANA, Apo – (A-I, A-II, B), **AST, Bil, conjugated Bil, unconjugated Bil,** B2M, **carbohydrate-deficient transferrin,** ceruloplasmin, CK-MB, ferritin, gamma globulins, **GMT,** Hb, **cholesterol, IgA,** IL-8, **WBC,** MAL, mAST, MCH, **MCV,** Ni, 5-nucleotidase, OCT, osmolality, Pb, pH, **PT,** PRA, serotonin, T4, **bile acids**

    ↓ **albumin,** ALT, AST (later), proteins, Ca, CK, Cr, **RBC,** Fe, **Hb, HCT, CHS,** K, LD (later), WBC, Mg, Mn, Na, osteocalcin, pH, **PLT,** porphyrins, urea, vitamin – (B$_2$, B$_{12}$, folate)

- ■ *Urine* ↑ ALT, conjugated Bil, DALA, fructose, **galactose,** K, UBG
  ↓ UBG
- ■ *Stool* ↓ UBG

autoimmune chronic active hepatitis

    ↑ * **ALP,** * **ALT,** ANA, * **anti-LKM-1, anti-soluble liver Ag** (anti-SLA), anti-actin Ab, antimicrosomal Ab, antimitochondrial Ab, antithyroidal Ab, * **ASMA,** * **AST,** Bil, CIC, * **gamma globulins,** globulins, HLA – (A1, B1, B8, DRw3, DRw4, DW3), **IgG,** complement – (C2, C4), PT, liver specific sialoglycoprotein receptor Ab, RF

    ↓ albumin, C3 complement, WBC

chronic hepatitis
– chronic active hepatitis B (progressive)

    ↑ **AAT,** ACP, **AFP, ALP,** ALT, A2MG, AMA, ANA, anti-ds-DNA, **anti-ss-DNA, anti-HBc, anti-HBe,** antimicrosomal Ab, anti-Salmonella Ab, **ASMA, AST, Bil, conjugated Bil, unconjugated Bil,** B2M, **BSP retention,** CA 15-3, CBG, **CEA, ceruloplasmin,** FDP, **gamma globulins,** glycoproteins, GMD, **GMT,** * **HBeAg,** * **HBsAg,** * **HBV-DNA,** HDL-C, HLA – (B8, DR3), **cholesterol, CHS, IgA, IgG, IgM,** cortisol, cryoglobulins, chenodeoxycholic acid, cholic acid, **LAP, LE cells,** Mn, **PT,** plasmocytes, anti-DNA-histone complex Ab, antihepatocyte membrane Ab, PRA, **RF,** SHBG, **T3,** T4, TBG, TIBC, TSH, viscosity, **VLDL-C, bile acids,** FFA

    ↓ **albumin,** Apo AI, AT III, ceruloplasmin, **G,** haptoglobin, **Hb, HCT,** HDL-C, **cholesterol, CHS,** IGFBP-3, IgM, complement – (C3, total), **WBC,** T-lym, Mg (+RBC), neu, pCO$_2$, RBP, PLT, Se, FFA. Zn

- ■ *Urine* ↑ Bil, Cu, **UBG**

– chronic hepatitis B (high infectivity)

    ↑ ALT, **anti-HBc-IgG,** * **anti-HBc,** AST, Bil, * **HBeAg,** * **HBsAg,** * **HBV-DNA,** PT

    ↓ albumin

– chronic hepatitis B (late, low infectivity)

    ↑ **anti-HBc-IgG,** anti-HBc, anti-HBe, HBeAg, * **HBsAg**

– chronic hepatitis B (chronic persistent)

    ↑ ACE, ACP, ADA, **AFP, aldolase,** alpha-aminonitrogen, A2MG, **ALP, ALT,** AMA, aminotripeptidase, **ANA,** anti-LKM-1, **anti-HBe, anti-HBc, APTT,** arginase, ASMA, **AST,** ATPase, beta-glucuronidase, **Bil,** B2M, CA 15-3, CEA, ceruloplasmin, enolase, FDP, Fe, **ferritin,** phosphoglu-

comutase, phosphohexoisomerase, fructose-1,6-di-phosphate aldolase, fumarase, gamma globulins, glutathione reductase, GMD, **GMT**,
guanase, HBD, **HBeAg**, ✳ **HBsAg**, HDL-C, cholesterol, **ICD**, IgA, **IgG**,
IgM, cortisol, LAP, LD, LD5, LDL-C, LE cells, lipoprotein lipase, lym,
MD, mono, 5-nucleotidase, OCT, **PT**, PRA, pyruvate kinase, RF, serotonin, SHBG, T4, TIBC, TPA, transferrin, transketolase, vitamin –
(B$_{12}$), bile acids

↓ **albumin**, AT III, beta globulins, C3, ceruloplasmin, Cu, fibrinogen, granulocytes, **haptoglobin**, HDL-C, hemopexin, **CHS**, IgM, Mg, **prealbumin**, pseudocholinesterase, Se, transferrin, PLT, urea

■ *Urine* ↑ alpha-aminonitrogen, ALT, Bil, DALA, fructose, G, galactose,
UBG

– chronic hepatitis C

↑ ALT, ✳ **anti-HCV, anti-LKM-1**, AST, Bil, HCV RNA, PT

– chronic hepatitis D

↑ ALT, anti-HBc-IgG, anti-HBc-IgM, ✳ **anti-HDV**, anti-LKM-3, AST,
HBsAg, **HDAg, HDV-RNA**

hepatitis B (HBV)

↑ ACE, ACP, ADA, **AFP, aldolase, ALP**, ✳ **ALT**, alpha-aminotripeptidase,
aminonitrogen, A2MG, **AMA, ANA**, anti-ds-DNA, **anti-ss-DNA**, anti-
LKM-1, **anti-HBc, anti-HBe**, antimicrosomal Ab, anti-Salmonella Ab,
APTT, arginase, **ASMA**, AST, **Bil**, B2M, beta-glucuronidase, CBG,
CEA, ceruloplasmin, enolase, FDP, Fe, **ferritin**, phosphoglucomutase, phosphohexoisomerase, fructose-1,6-diphosphate aldolase, fumarase, **gamma globulins**, GMD, **GMT**, HBD, ✳ **HBeAg**, ✳ **HBsAg**,
✳ **HBV-DNA**, HDL-C, HLA – (**B8**, DR3), **cholesterol, CHS, ICD**, IgA,
IgG, IgM, cortisol, cryoglobulins, **LAP**, LD, LD5, LDL-C, LE cells, lipoprotein lipase, lym, **MD**, mono, 5-nucleotidase, OCT, **PT**, anti-DNA-
histone complex Ab, antihepatocyte membrane Ab, PRA, pyruvate
kinase, **RF**, serotonin, SHBG, **T3**, T4, TBG, TIBC, TPA, transferrin,
transketolase, TSH, viscosity, bile acids

↓ **albumin**, AT III, beta globulins, C3, ceruloplasmin, Cu, fibrinogen, granulocytes, **haptoglobin**, HDL-C, hemopexin, **CHS**, IGFBP-3, IgM,
complement – (**C3**), Mg, neu, **prealbumin**, pseudocholinesterase,
RBP, Se, transferrin, PLT

■ *Urine* ↑ alpha-aminonitrogen, ALT, Bil, Cu, DALA, fructose, G, galactose, **UBG**

hepatitis C (HCV)

↑ **ALT**, ✳ **anti-HCV, anti-LKM-1**, AST, Bil, HCV RNA, PT

hepatitis D (HDV)

↑ ALT, anti-HBc-IgG, anti-HBc-IgM, ✳ **anti-HDV**, ✳ **anti-HDV-IgM**, anti-
LKM-3, AST, HBsAg, ✳ **HDAg, HDV-RNA**

hepatitis E (HEV)

↑ ALT, ✳ **anti-HEV**, Bil, **HEV-RNA**

↓ WBC

hepatitis G (HGV)

↑ **anti-HGV, HGV-RNA**

infectious hepatitis (HAV)

↑ ADA, ADH, AFP, **aldolase, ALP, ALT**, AMA, ✳ **anti-HAV**, anti-HAV-IgA,
anti-HAV-IgG, ✳ **anti-HAV-IgM**, ASAL, ASMA, **AST**, beta globulins,
beta-glucuronidase, B2M, **Bil, conjugated Bil, unconjugated Bil**,

ceruloplasmin, CRP, **Fe**, phenylalanine, **ESR**, **gamma globulins**, **GMT**, ✱ **HAV-RNA**, IgA, IgG, IgM, ICD, complement – (C3), cryoglobulins, LDL-C, leucine, WBC, **lym**, mono, **PT**, PL, SD, syphilis Ab (false), T3, T4, **TBG**, thymidine kinase, TIBC, transferrin, VLDL-C

↓ **albumin**, **alpha-1-globulins**, alpha-2-globulins, beta globulins, beta-carotene, proteins, RBC, cholesterol, complement – (C3), WBC, mono, mucoproteins, **neu**, PL, T3, transferrin, UBBC, vitamin – (A), Zn, bile acids

- *Urine* ↑ albumin, alpha-aminonitrogen, ALT, **amino acids**, **conjugated Bil**, DALA, fructose, G, **galactose**, **porphyrins**, transferrin satur., T3, transferrin, **UBG**, **Zn**

  ↓ 17-KS, UBG
- *Stool* ↑ fat

  ↓ Bil, UBG
- *Cerebrospinal Fluid* ↑ proteins, lym
- *Synovial Fluid* ↑ WBC, PMN

lupus hepatitis

↑ ALP, ALT, AST, Bil, ASMA

neonatal hepatitis

↑ ALP, **ALT**, **AST**, **Bil**, **conjugated Bil**, **ESR**, GMT, lym (relat.), mono (relat.), PL

↓ Hb, HCT, lym, neu, PL, WBC

- *Urine* ↑ albumin, **conjugated Bil**, UBG

peliosis hepatitis

↑ ALP, ALT

- *Urine* ↑ proteins

postmedicamentous hepatitis

↑ ALP, ALT, ANA, anti-LKM-1, ASMA, AST, **Bil**, **conjugated Bil**, **unconjugated Bil**, ceruloplasmin, GMT, IgG

- *Urine* ↑ **conjugated Bil**, UBG

  ↓ UBG
- *Stool* ↓ Bil, UBG

toxic hepatitis

↑ AAP, AAT, aldolase, **ALP**, alpha-1-glycoprotein, **ALT**, AMA, A2MG, **ASAL**, **AST**, ATIII, **Bil**, **conjugated Bil**, unconjugated Bil, **beta-glucuronidase**, B2M, BSP retention, ceruloplasmin, CO_2, gamma globulins, G6PD, **GMT**, cholesterol, **ICD**, LAP, **LD**, **LD5**, Mn, 5-NT, PT, SD, TBG, VLDL-C

↓ AMS, G, cholesterol, proteins, Ni, urea

- *Urine* ↑ **Bil**, **UBG**
- *Stool* ↓ Bil, **UBG**

Hepatopathy

↑ ACE, ACP, AFP, ALP, ammonia, AST, beta globulins, proteins, Bil, conjugated Bil, unconjugated Bil, BSP, BT, gamma globulins, G, HDL-C, LD, LD5, LDL-C, WBC, RBC osmotic resistance, PT, serotonin

↓ albumin, alpha-1-globulins, alpha-2-globulins, proteins, Ca, Ca^{2+}, fibrinogen, G, Hb, HCT, cholesterol, CHS, IGFBP-3, K, cortisol, folic acid, WBC, Na, P, proconvertin, prothrombin, TIBC, PLT, urea

- *Urine* ↑ ALT
- *Stool* ↑ fat

Hepatosplenomegaly

↑ anti-toxocara Ab

Hernia

diaphragmatic hernia

- *Stool* ↑ blood
- *Amniotic Fluid* ↑ volume

hiatal hernia

↓ Fe
- *Urine* ↑ lactose, reducing sugars

Hirsutism

↑ androstenedione, **DHEA**, DHEAS, pregnenolone, SHBG, **testosterone**, free testosterone (F)

Histidinemia

↑ **alanine**, arginine, cystathionine, cysteine, cystine, * **histidine**, hydroxylysine, lysine, ornithine

↓ glutamic acid

- *Urine* ↑ alanine, arginine, cystathionine, cysteine, cystine, ethanolamine, * **histidine**, hydroxylysine, glutamic acid, **imidazole pyruvic acid**, imidazole acetic acid, imidazole lactic acid, lysine, ornithine, threonine
- *Cerebrospinal Fluid* ↑ glutamine

Histiocytosis X

↑ ALP, ALT, mono

↓ Hb, HCT, lym, WBC, PLT, pO_2

- *Urine* ↑ Ca, volume
- *Bronchoalveolar Lavage Fluid* ↑ eos, **Langerhans cells**, lym, macrophages, neu
- *Synovial Fluid* ↑ macrophages

Homocysteinuria

↑ PLT adhesion, * **homocysteine**, * **methionine**, valine

↓ cystine, folate

- *Urine* ↑ amino acids, asparagine, cystathionine, * **homocystine**, methionine
- *Cerebrospinal Fluid* ↑ **homocystine, methionine**

Hydrocephalus

non-obstructive hydrocephalus

↑ AFP

- *Cerebrospinal Fluid* ↑ eos, ependymal cells, glial fibrillary acidic protein, **CHS, LA, MBP**, pressure
- *Amniotic Fluid* ↑ AFP, volume

obstructive hydrocephalus

- *Cerebrospinal Fluid* ↑ prealbumin, pressure

Hydronephros

↑ RBC

- *Urine* ↑ **proteins, RBC, Hb, pus, blood**

Hydrops, Fetal

↑ hPL

- *Amniotic Fluid* ↑ volume

Hydrothorax

- *Urine* ↑ pH
- *Pleural Fluid* ↓ proteins, cholesterol, LD, lipids, lym

Hydroxyprolinemia, Hereditary

↑ * **hydroxyproline**

■ *Urine* ↑ ∗ hydroxyproline – (**total, free**)

Hyperadrenalism

↑ prealbumin
↓ **amino acids**
■ *Urine* ↑ G, K, 17-KS, **17-KGS**, pregnanediol
■ *Cerebrospinal Fluid* ↑ protein
■ *Sweat* ↑ K

Hyperalbuminemia

↑ **albumin**, Ca, **osmolality**
↓ ESR

Hyperaldosteronism

primary hyperaldosteronism (Conn's disease)

↑ ∗ **aldosterone, 18-OH DOC**, G, **HCO$_3$⁻, MAL, Na, volume**, pCO$_2$, **pH**
↓ angiotensin II, **chloride, ∗ K**, K (RBC), **Mg**, ∗ **PRA**
■ *Urine* ↑ **aldosterone**, ∗ **K**, pH, **volume**
↓ chloride, **Na**, pH, specific gravity
■ *Sweat* ↓ Na

secondary hyperaldosteronism (Bartter's sy)

↑ ∗ **aldosterone**, angiotensin, G, HCO$_3$⁻, kallikrein, **uric acid**, ∗ **MAL**,
∗ **PGE2**, PGF2, PGI2, pH, ∗ **PRA**
↓ ∗ **K, K** (RBC), **Mg, Mg** (WBC), **Na**, PLT aggregation, chloride, volume
(plasma)
■ *Urine* ↑ **aldosterone**, ∗ **chloride**, ∗ **K, Na**, kallikrein, ∗ **Mg**, volume, PG
↓ ∗ **osmolality**

Hyperammonemia, Congenital

↑ ∗ **ammonia**
↓ **urea**

Hyperbetaalaninemia

↑ ∗ **beta-alanine**, MAC
■ *Urine* ↑ beta-alanine, beta-aminobutyric acid, taurine

Hyperbilirubinemia, Familial in Infants

↑ Bil, TT
■ *Urine* ↑ **conjugated Bil**

Hypercalcemia

↑ ALP, ALT, AST, ∗ **Ca, Ca²⁺**, chloride, ESR, gastrin, cholesterol, calcitonin,
uric acid, creatinine, LD, MAC, **osmolality**, P, PTH, TAG, urea
↓ albumin, Hb, HCT, HCO$_3$⁻, WBC, **Mg**, P, pCO$_2$, **PTH**
■ *Urine* ↑ Ca, Ca²⁺, hydroxyproline, K, volume
↓ P
■ *Cerebrospinal Fluid* ↑ protein

familial hypocalciuric hypercalcemia

↑ ∗ **Ca, Ca²⁺**, Mg, ∗ **PTH**, vitamin – (D3)
↓ P
■ *Urine* ↑ cAMP
↓ **Ca**, Mg

hypercalcemia of malignancy

↑ ACE, **ALP**, ∗ **Ca, ESR**, HCO$_3$⁻, MAL, osteocalcin, P, **pH**, ∗ **PTHrP**, TAG,
vitamin – (**D3**)
↓ **albumin**, RBC, Hb, HCT, **chloride**, osteocalcin, P, ∗ **PTH**, vitamin – (D3)
■ *Urine* ↑ Ca, cAMP

Hypercalciuria, Renal Idiopathic
 ↑ PTH, vitamin – (D2, **D3**)
 ↓ P
 ■ *Urine* ↑ ✳ **Ca**, cAMP, creatinine, crystals – (Ca, P)

Hypercapnia
 ↑ pCO_2
 ■ *Cerebrospinal Fluid* ↑ proteins, glutamine

Hyperemesis Gravidarum
 ↑ FT4, MAL, **T4, urea**
 ↓ **proteins, chloride, K, Na**, TSH
 ■ *Urine* ↑ proteins, ketone bodies

Hyperfibrinogenemia
 ↑ PLT adhesion, **ESR, fibrinogen**, viscosity, von Willebrand's factor
 ↓ factor XIII, clot retraction

Hyperfibrinolysis
 ↑ APTT, PT, TT

Hypergammaglobulinemia
 ↑ CIC, **ESR**, ✳ **gamma globulins**, proteins
 ↓ complement – (C4)

Hyperglycemia, Chronic
 ↑ acetone, **G, glycated Hb, ketobodies, acetoacetic acid, osmolality**
 ↓ ESR, HCO_3^-, chloride, Mg, Na, GH
 ■ *Urine* ↑ acetone, **G**, creatinine
 ■ *Cerebrospinal Fluid* ↑ G

Hyperglycinemia
 ↑ ✳ **glycine**, ketones, MAC
 ↓ G, gamma globulins, neu, PLT
 ■ *Urine* ↑ ✳ **glycine**, ketones

Hyperhydratation
 ↑ MAC, Na, osmolality
 ↓ albumin, proteins, RBC, **Hb**, HCT, **chloride**, LD, Na, NBB, plasma volume, osmolality, urea
 ■ *Urine* ↑ specific gravity, volume
 ↓ K, specific gravity

 hypertonic hyperhydratation
 ↑ Na, osmolality
 ■ *Urine* ↑ specific gravity

 hypotonic hyperhydratation
 ↑ MAC
 ↓ **proteins, RBC, HCT**, chloride, **Na, osmolality**
 ■ *Urine* ↑ **volume**
 ↓ specific gravity

 isotonic hyperhydratation
 ↓ **proteins, RBC, HCT**
 ■ *Urine* ↑ Na, **volume**
 ↓ K, specific gravity

Hyperinsulinism
 ↑ C-peptide, ketobodies, acetoacetic acid, **insulin**
 ↓ **G**, isoleucine, leucine, P, SHBG, valine
 ■ *Urine* ↑ ketones

Hyperkalemia

    ↑ **aldosterone, K, MAC**

    ↓ PRA

    ■ *Urine* ↓ volume

Hyperlipidemia

    ↑ PLT adhesion, beta globulins, Ca, **GMT, lipids, TAG,** vitamin – (A, E), vWf

    ↓ Na, LCAT, lipase

Hyperlipoproteinemia

  chylomicron hyperlipoproteinemia

    ↑ apolipoprotein – (A-IV, B-48, C-II), cholesterol, chylomicrons, **TAG,** VLDL-C

    ↓ Apo C-II, HDL-C

  hyperlipoproteinemia I

    ↑ apolipoprotein – (A-I, A-II, A-IV, B-48, C-I, C-II, C-III, E), beta globulins, beta-carotene, glucagon, GHb, **cholesterol, chylomicrons,** plasminogen activator inhibitor, uric acid, LDL-C, WBC, LP lipase, **pre-beta-LP, TAG, VLDL-C,** viscosity

    ↓ alpha-1-LP, Apo – (A-I, B-100), beta-LPs, **HDL-C, LDL-C,** lipoprotein lipase

    ■ *Synovial Fluid* ↑ WBC, PMN

  hyperlipoproteinemia II

    ↑ PLT aggregation, apolipoprotein B-100, beta-carotene, **beta-LPs,** glucagon, GHb, HDL-C, **cholesterol,** IDL-C, uric acid, **LDL-C,** PL, TAG, viscosity, VLDL-C

    ↓ HDL-C

    ■ *Amniotic Fluid* ↑ LDL-C

    ■ *Synovial Fluid* ↑ WBC, PMN

  hyperlipoproteinemia III

    ↑ apolipoprotein – (B-100, C-I, C-II, C-III, E-II), beta-lipoproteins, **G,** GHb, **cholesterol,** chylomicrons, **IDL-C, uric acid,** LDL-C, pre-beta-lipoproteins, **TAG, VLDL-C**

    ↓ apolipoprotein – (A-I, E-III, E-IV), HDL-C, LDL-C

    ■ *Synovial Fluid* ↑ WBC, PMN

  hyperlipoproteinemia IV

    ↑ apolipoprotein – (B-48, B-100, C-I, C-II, C-III, E), beta-LPs, GIP, cholesterol, **uric acid, pre-beta-LPs, TAG, VLDL-C**

    ↓ alpha-1-LP, HDL-C

  hyperlipoproteinemia V

    ↑ apolipoprotein – (B-48, B-100, C-I, C-II, C-III, E), beta-LPs, G, **cholesterol, chylomicrons, uric acid,** pre-beta-LPs, **TAG, VLDL-C**

    ↓ alpha-1-LP, Apo A-I, beta-LPs, HDL-C, LDL-C

    ■ *Synovial Fluid* ↑ WBC, PMN

  HDL hyperlipoproteinemia

    ↑ Apo A-I, Apo A-II, HDL-C, cholesterol

  IDL hyperlipoproteinemia

    ↑ Apo E-II, cholesterol, TAG

    ↓ Apo E-III, Apo E-IV, HDL-C, LDL-C

  LDL hyperlipoproteinemia

    ↑ Apo B-100, cholesterol, LDL-C

    ↓ HDL-C

LDL, VLDL hyperlipoproteinemia

↑ Apo B-100, cholesterol, LDL-C, TAG

↓ HDL-C

VLDL hyperlipoproteinemia

↑ Apo B-100, Apo C-II, cholesterol, **TAG**

↓ Apo C-II, HDL-C

VLDL, chylomicron hyperlipoproteinemia

↑ apolipoprotein – (B-48, B-100, C-II), cholesterol, **TAG**

↓ Apo C-II, HDL-C

Hyperlordosis

■ *Urine* ↑ protein

Hyperlysinemia

↑ ammonia, **ethanolamine, GABA**, glutamine, ✳ **lysine**, saccharopine, **ornithine**

■ *Urine* ↑ ammonia, ethanolamine, alpha-aminoadipic acid, **lysine**, saccharopine

Hypermagnesemia

↑ Ca, K, Mg

Hypermethioninemia

↑ conjugated Bil, unconjugated Bil, ✳ **methionine**

Hypernatremia

essential hypernatremia

↑ **chloride, ✳ Na, ✳ osmolality**

↓ **aldosterone**

■ *Urine* ↑ osmolality

natrium overload hypernatremia

↑ Na,

■ *Urine* ↑ Na

water deficiency hypernatremia

↑ Na

Hyperornithinemia

↑ alanine, ammonia (after meals), glutamine, ✳ **ornithine**

↓ ammonia

■ *Urine* ↑ homocitrulline, ornithine

Hyperosmolality

↑ **osmolality**

■ *Cerebrospinal Fluid* ↓ **pressure**

Hyperostosis, Diffuse Idiopathic Skeletal (dish)

↑ G, cholesterol, IRI, retinol, urea

Hyperoxaluria

■ *Urine* ↑ ✳ **calcium oxalate**, RBC, **glycosaminoglycans**, Hb, crystals – (Ca-oxalate)

Hyperparathyroidism

primary hyperparathyroidism

↑ ACE, **ACP**, ACP (prostatic), **alpha-2-globulins, ALP**, beta globulins, ✳ **Ca**, ✳ **Ca²⁺**, citrate, Cu, **ESR**, G, **gastrin**, hydroxyproline, ✳ **chloride**, insulin, K, **calcitonin**, creatinine, **uric acid, MAC**, osteocalcin, P, ✳ **PTH**, N-telopeptides, urea, vitamin – (D2, **D3**), Zn

↓ **K**, HCO₃⁻, Hb, HCT, **cholesterol**, calcitonin, WBC, **Mg**, P, pCO₂, pH, RBP, T3, **TAG**

- **Urine** ↑ amino acids, Ca, Ca²⁺, cAMP, Cu, hydroxyproline – (**total, free**), chloride, K, crystals – (Ca, P, Ca-phosphate, Ca-oxalate), Na, **volume**, **P**, pH, Zn
  - ↓ Ca, **specific gravity, P**
- **Cerebrospinal Fluid** ↑ **Ca**
- **Gastric Fluid** ↑ basal acid secretion
- **Synovial Fluid** ↑ crystals – (hydroxyapatite, calcium pyrophosphate), pyrophosphate

secondary hyperparathyroidism
  ↑ ACP, **ALP**, Ca, Ca²⁺, **calcitonin**, MAC, P, * **PTH**
  ↓ **Ca**, Ca²⁺, P
- **Urine** ↑ Ca, hydroxyproline
  - ↓ Ca, P

Hyperphosphatasemia
benign familial hyperphosphatasemia
  ↑ ACP, **ALP**
benign transient hyperphosphatasemia
  ↑ **ALP**, ALT, AST, GMT, vitamin – (D3)

Hyperphosphatasia
  ↑ ACP, * **ALP**, ALP (WBC), uric acid, **P**
  ↓ **Ca**, vitamin – (D2)
- **Urine** ↑ uric acid
- **Synovial Fluid** ↑ crystals – (calcium pyrophosphate)

Hyperpituitarism
  ↑ G, **ILGF-I**, Mg, P, PRL, **GH**
- **Urine** ↑ **17-KS**

Hyperplasia
adrenal cortex hyperplasia
  ↑ ACTH, **aldosterone, androstenedione,** 11-deoxycortisol, **DHEA,** DHEAS, estrogens, HLA – (Bw47, Bw51, Bw53, Bw60, Dr7), **PRA,** progesterone, **17-OH progesterone, testosterone**
  ↓ **aldosterone,** cortisol, DHEA, 17-OH progesterone, **PRA**
- **Urine** ↑ aldosterone, estriol, estrogens, 17-KGS, **17-KS, cortisol, pregnanediol, pregnanetriol**
  ↑ aldosterone, 17-OHCS, 17-KS, pregnanetriol
- **Sweat** ↓ chloride, Na
- **Amniotic Fluid** ↑ * **androstenedione,** deoxycorticosterone, 11-deoxycortisol, HLA – (Bw47, Bw51, Bw53, Bw60, Dr7), * **17-OH-progesterone,** PRA, testosterone
benign prostate hyperplasia
  ↑ ACP, AMS, androgens, RBC, G, cholesterol, K, **creatinine, uric acid, WBC,** mono, Na, neu, PAP, PRL, progesterone, **PSA,** testosterone, **urea**
  ↓ **RBC, Hb, HCT,** LH
- **Urine** ↑ albumin, proteins, bacteria (+ culture), **RBC,** Hb, pus, blood, WBC

Hyperplasia of Thyroid C-Cells
  ↑ **calcitonin**

Hyperprolactinemia
  ↑ * **PRL**
  ↓ **estradiol,** FSH, LH, progesterone, SHBG

Hyperprolinemia

↑ * proline
- *Urine* ↑ glycine, hydroxyproline, proline

Hyperproteinemia

↑ proteins, Ca

Hypersplenism

↑ nucleated RBC, plasma volume, RTC, spherocytes, target cells
↓ eos, **RBC, Hb, HCT, WBC, MPV, neu, PLT**

Hypertension

arterial hypertension

↑ ACA, **aldosterone**, ANF, AST, beta-glucuronidase, Ca, Cd, CEA, Cu, 18-OH DOC, eos, epinephrine, ESR, **G**, globulins, **cholesterol**, CHS, insulin, K, **catecholamines, uric acid, creatinine**, LDL-C, WBC, **lipids, PRA, TAG**, PLT, **urea**
↓ **albumin**, aldolase, **proteins**, RBC, haptoglobin, **Hb**, HDL-C, HCT, hPL (F), **K**, lym, Na, Pb, PRA, prostacyclin, PG, TIBC, PLT, **Zn**
- *Urine* ↑ aldosterone, **proteins**, beta-glucuronidase, **RBC**, phosphoethanolamine, G, **haptoglobin**, hexosaminidase, 17-OHCS, catecholamines, WBC, Na, volume, casts – (granular, hyaline), VMA
  ↓ aldosterone, specific gravity

intracranial hypertension

- *Cerebrospinal Fluid* ↑ CK, CRP, LA
  ↓ protein

malignant hypertension

↑ **aldosterone**, HCT, **cholesterol**, pCO$_2$, pH, PL, **PRA**, schistocytes, **TAG, urea**
↓ ammonia, Hb, HCT, K, prostacyclin
- *Urine* ↑ albumin, aldosterone, **proteins**, RBC, Hb, **catecholamines**, hexosaminidase, **17-OHCS**, 17-KGS, **WBC**, blood, Mb, volume, casts – (**RBC**, granular, hyaline, fatty, **waxy**)
  ↓ **specific gravity**, volume

portal hypertension

↑ ALP, ALT, ammonia
↓ **AAT**, albumin, neu

pregnancy induced hypertension

↑ * alpha-aminonitrogen, ALP, amino acids, beta globulins, **chloride**, D-dimers, FDP, Hb, HCT, ICD, * **creatinine**, * **uric acid**, LA, WBC, neu, PAPP-A, PT, PTT, * **plasminogen**, TAG
↓ **albumin**, aldosterone, AMS, * **fibrinogen**, haptoglobin, * **Mg**, placental lactogen, plasminogen, **progesterone**, * **PLT**, * **urea**
- *Urine* ↑ * alpha-aminonitrogen, * **amino acids**, * **proteins**, ketones, uric acid, specific gravity, Na, casts – (**epithelial**)
  ↓ estriol, uric acid
- *Amniotic Fluid* ↑ **creatinine**, uric acid
  ↓ AFP, volume

pulmonary hypertension

↑ ANA, **RBC**
↓ pCO$_2$, pO$_2$ (later)

renovascular hypertension

↑ **aldosterone**, HCT, K, **creatinine**, uric acid, **Na, PRA, urea**
↓ K

■ *Urine* ↑ **proteins**, K, blood

Hyperthermia, Malignant

↑ **＊AST, ＊Ca** (early), **＊CK, ＊K** (early), **＊LD, WBC, ＊Mb**, P, **＊MAC-RAC**, pCO₂, pyruvate

↓ BE, Ca (later), K (later), pCO₂, pO₂, pH

■ *Urine* ↑ ketones, **＊Mb**
      ↓ volume (later)

Hyperthyroidism, Primary

↑ ACE, aldolase, aldosterone, alpha-aminonitrogen, **ALP, ALT**, amino acids, antimicrosomal Ab, anti-TSH-receptor Ab, antithyroidal Ab, anti-thyroglobulin Ab, **AST, Bil**, unconjugated Bil, BSP retention, ＊ Ca, Ca²⁺, cAMP, ceruloplasmin, CK-MB, **Cu**, 2,3-DPG (RBC), eos, **estradiol**, estrogens, **factor VIII, ferritin**, fibronectin, ＊ **FTI, FT₃**, ＊ **FT₄**, **ESR, G, gastrin, glycerol, GMT, G6PD** (RBC), HbA2, HbF, HLA – (A2, B8, B35, DR3), **hydroxyproline**, cholesterol, **CHS**, insulin, FT₄ index, iodine, carboanhydrase (RBC), ketones, 17-ketosteroids, **cortisol, creatinine, creatine, LATS**, LH, **lym**, mono, MPV, **Na, osteocalcin**, P, pH, **PL**, plasma volume, PRA, proinsulin, anti-intrinsic factor Ab, PTH, RF, **SHBG**, GH, ＊ **T₃**, T₃ uptake, ＊**T₄**, N-telopeptides, **testosterone, thyroglobulin**, triiodothyronine resin uptake, transketolase (RBC), TSH, **tyrosine, urea, FFA**

↓ albumin, **AMS**, Apo A-I, Apo B, bas, **proteins**, Bil, CBG, **CK**, G tolerance, **Hb, HCT, HDL-C, cholesterol**, immunoglobulins, K, catecholamines, carbonic anhydrase, ascorbic acid, **LDL-C, lipids, WBC**, LPs, MCH, MCHC, MCV, **Mg, neu**, O₂ satur., **pCO₂**, PL, **pO₂**, prealbumin, **PTH**, RBP, **TBG, TAG, TIBC**, PLT, ＊ **TSH**, vitamin – (B₁, B₂, B₁₂, C, **D₃, folate**), VLDL-C

■ *Urine* ↑ ALT, proteins, **Ca, G, total hydroxyproline**, ketones, **creatine**, creatinine, 17-OHCS, 17-KGS, Mg, **volume, P**, tyrosine, urea, **VMA**
      ↓ 17-OHCS, 17-KGS, hydroxyproline, creatinine

■ *Cerebrospinal Fluid* ↑ Na
      ↓ protein

■ *Stool* ↑ **Ca**, P, urobilin

Hypertriacylglycerolemia

↑ plasminogen activator inhibitor, LCAT, ＊ **TAG**, VLDL
↓ Apo C-II, **HDL-C**

familial hypertriacylglycerolemia

↑ TAG, VLDL-C

Hypertyrosinemia

↑ AFP, ALT, AST, **Bil**, MAC, methionine, **succinylacetate, succinylacetoacetate**, ＊ **tyrosine**

↓ RBC, Hb

■ *Urine* ↑ RBC, G, **methionine, succinylacetate, succinylacetoacetate, tyrosine**

Hyperuricemia

↑ cholesterol, **GPs**, ＊ **uric acid, IRI, LDL-C, MDA, SOD**, ＊ **TAG**
↓ HDL-C

■ *Urine* ↑ crystals – (urate)
■ *Synovial Fluid* ↑ crystals – (urate)

Hyperventilation

↑ **chloride**, LA, MAL, Na, osmolality, pH, **pO₂**

$\downarrow$ HCO$_3^-$, K, Na, P, **pCO$_2$**
- *Urine* $\uparrow$ HCO$_3^-$, K, Na
  $\downarrow$ chloride

Hypervitaminosis
nicotinic acid hypervitaminosis
$\uparrow$ G, uric acid

vitamin A hypervitaminosis
$\uparrow$ ALP, Bil, Ca, GMT, **carotene**, ESR, **PT**, vitamin – (**A**)
$\downarrow$ albumin, Hb, HCT, PTH
- *Urine* $\uparrow$ proteins, Ca

vitamin C hypervitaminosis
$\uparrow$ estrogens, **vitamin C**
- *Urine* $\uparrow$ uric acid, oxalate

vitamin D hypervitaminosis
$\uparrow$ ALP, **Ca**, Ca^{2+}, MAC, P, **vitamin D3**
$\downarrow$ ALP, PTH
- *Urine* $\uparrow$ proteins, Ca, RBC, Hb, crystals – (Ca-oxalate), P
- *Stool* $\downarrow$ Ca
- *Synovial Fluid* $\uparrow$ crystals – (hydroxyapatite)

vitamin E hypervitaminosis
$\uparrow$ PT, urea, **vitamin E**
$\downarrow$ PLT

Hypoadrenalism
$\uparrow$ **eos**, HCT, K, **creatinine**, **lym**, urea
$\downarrow$ **estrogens**, G, Hb, **cortisol**, Na, RTC
- *Urine* $\uparrow$ Ca, **chloride**
  $\downarrow$ estrogens, 17-OH corticosteroids, 17-ketosteroids
- *Sweat* $\downarrow$ Na, **chloride**

Hypoalbuminemia
$\downarrow$ **albumin**, Ca, Zn

hypoanabolic hypoalbuminemia
$\uparrow$ **cholesterol**
$\downarrow$ **albumin**

Hypoaldosteronism
primary hypoaldosteronism
$\uparrow$ **K**, chloride, MAC, PRA
$\downarrow$ **aldosterone**, Na, pH, **PRA**
- *Urine* $\uparrow$ **Na**
  $\downarrow$ Mg, K

secondary hypoaldosteronism
$\uparrow$ **K**, chloride, MAC, PRA
$\downarrow$ **aldosterone**, pH, PRA
- *Urine* $\uparrow$ **Na**

Hypocalcemia
$\uparrow$ PO$_4^-$, **PTH**, urea
$\downarrow$ albumin, **Ca**, Ca^{2+}, PTH
- *Urine* $\uparrow$ **Ca**

hereditary hypocalcemia
$\uparrow$ PO$_4^-$
$\downarrow$ albumin, proteins, **Ca**, Ca^{2+}, PTH

Hypocapnia

    ↑ LA

    ↓ pCO₂, pH

    ■ *Cerebrospinal Fluid* ↑ **LA**

Hypocorticism, Central

    ↑ Ca

    ↓ **ACTH, androgens,** EPO, **cortisol**

Hypofibrinogenemia

    ↑ **PLT aggregation, APTT,** BT, coagulation time, **FDP, PT, clot retraction, TT**

    ↓ **✳ fibrinogen,** ESR, PLT

Hypogammaglobulinemia

    ↓ albumin, **proteins,** B-lym, **✳ gamma globulins,** IgA, IgE, **✳ IgG,** IgM, complement – (C1q, C3), **lym**

    ■ *Sweat* ↓ chloride

Hypoglycemia

    ↑ ACTH, epinephrine, factor VIII, **✳ glucagon,** glycine, **✳ catecholamines,** cortisol, Mb, norepinephrine, **PRL, GH**

    ↓ alanine, **✳ G,** K, P

    ■ *Urine* ↑ glycine

      ↓ G

    ■ *Cerebrospinal Fluid* ↓ G

Hypogonadism

  central hypogonadism

    ↑ PRL, SHBG

    ↓ androstenedione, EPO, **estradiol,** estrogens, **FSH, ✳ GRH, LH, progesterone, ✳ testosterone,** free testosterone, **Zn**

    ■ *Urine* ↓ FSH, **17-KS**

  male hypogonadism

    ↑ FSH (early months), LH (early months), testosterone (early months)

    ↓ FSH (until puberty), LH (until puberty), testosterone (until puberty)

  peripheral hypogonadism

    ↑ FSH, **LH,** PRL, SHBG

    ↓ **estradiol,** estrogens, **progesterone, testosterone,** Zn

    ■ *Urine* ↑ FSH

Hypoinsulinism

    ↑ IGFBP-1, K

    ↓ **C-peptide, ✳ insulin**

Hypokalemia

    ↑ **CK,** HCO₃⁻, **MAL,** Mb, osmolality, pCO₂, pH, **PRA, RAL**

    ↓ **aldosterone,** insulin, proteins, **K,** P

    ■ *Urine* ↑ **K,** Mb, **volume**

Hypolipoproteinemia

    ↑ cholesterol, LDL-C, TAG

    ↓ apolipoprotein – (A-I, A-II, C-III), HDL-C, cholesterol, LDL-C, PL, TAG

  HDL hypolipoproteinemia

    ↑ cholesterol, LDL-C, TAG

    ↓ apolipoprotein – (A-I, A-II, C-III), HDL-C, cholesterol

  LDL hypolipoproteinemia

    ↓ Apo B-100, LDL-C, TAG

Hypomagnesemia

- ↓ Ca, **Ca²⁺**, K, **Mg**, **PO₄⁻**, **PTH**, vitamin – (D2)
- ■ *Urine* ↑ Mb
- ■ *Synovial Fluid* ↑ crystals – (calcium pyrophosphate)

Hyponatremia

hypervolemic hyponatremia
- ↑ aldosterone
- ↓ chloride, **Na**, TSH
- ■ *Urine* ↑ **osmolality**
- ↓ **Na**

hypervolemic hypotonic hyponatremia
- ■ *Urine* ↑ Na
- ↓ volume, **Na**

hypovolemic hyponatremia
– extrarenal hypovolemic hyponatremia
- ↓ Na
- ■ *Urine* ↑ osmolality
- ↓ **Na**

– renal hypovolemic hyponatremia
- ↑ urea
- ↓ Na
- ■ *Urine* ↑ Na

isovolemic hypotonic hyponatremia
- ↑ **ADH**
- ↓ uric acid, urea

normovolemic hyponatremia
- ↑ Ca
- ↓ chloride, **Na**, osmolality, urea
- ■ *Urine* ↑ **Na**, osmolality

Hypoosmolality Due to Hemodialysis
- ■ *Cerebrospinal Fluid* ↑ pressure

Hypoparathyroidism
- ↑ antiadrenal Ab, CK, CK-MB, **uric acid**, **MAL**, P, pH
- ↓ ALP, ✱ Ca, **Ca²⁺**, cAMP, **Mg**, osteocalcin, P, ✱ **PTH**, vitamin – (D2, **D3**)
- ■ *Urine* ↑ PO₄⁻
- ↓ Ca, **Ca²⁺**, cAMP, hydroxyproline, creatinine, **P**
- ■ *Cerebrospinal Fluid* ↑ proteins
- ■ *Sweat* ↓ Na, chloride

idiopathic hypoparathyroidism
- ↑ **anti-parathyroid Ab**

Hypophosphatasia
- ↑ Ca, ✱ **phosphoethanolamine**
- ↓ ✱ **ALP**
- ■ *Urine* ↑ ✱ **phosphoethanolamine**
- ↓ hydroxyproline

Hypophosphatemia
- ↑ aldolase, **ALP**, Ca, CK, megakaryocytes, spherocytes, vitamin – (**D3**)
- ↓ 2,3-DPG, **Mg**, ✱ **P**, **PTH**, PLT, uric acid, vitamin – (D)
- ■ *Urine* ↑ Mb, Mg
- ↓ **Ca**, osteocalcin, P
- ■ *Stool* ↑ **Ca**

Hypopituitarism

↑ ADH, conjugated Bil, **Cu**

↓ ACTH, Ca, **EPO**, estradiol, estriol, **estrogens**, FSH, FTI, **G**, Hb, HCT, **LH**, pepsinogen, PRL, **∗ ILGF-I**, IRI, **cortisol**, neu, **RTC**, **GH**, T4, testosterone, **TSH**

- *Urine* ↑ ketones
  ↓ **estriol**, estrogens, FSH, hydroxyproline, **17-OHCS**, 17-KGS, **17-KS**, **cortisol**, LH, tetrahydrodeoxycortisol
- *Amniotic Fluid* ↓ FSH
- *Seminal Fluid* ↑ **spermatozoa**

selective hypopituitarism

↓ ACTH, estradiol, FSH, G, Hb, HCT, ILGF-I, cortisol, LH, PRL, progesterone, **GH**, T4, testosterone, **TSH**

- *Urine* ↑ ketones
  ↓ FSH, 17-ketosteroids, 17-OHCS, cortisol
- *Amniotic Fluid* ↑ FSH

Hypoproteinemia

↑ cholesterol

↓ albumin, **alpha-1-globulins**, alpha-2-globulins, beta globulins, **proteins**, fructosamine, NBB, osmolality, **TBG**, **TIBC**

Hyposplenism

↑ **∗ RBC Howell–Jolly bodies, target cells**
↓ RBC osmotic fragility

Hypotension

↑ ADH, **ALP**, **epinephrine**, **LD**
↓ HCO_3^-, PRA, urea

- *Urine* ↑ specific gravity
- *Cerebrospinal Fluid* ↑ **LA**

fetal hypotension

- *Amniotic Fluid* ↑ meconium

Hypothermia

↑ ALT, AST, AMS, **∗ CK**, **∗ G**, Hb, HCT, **∗ K**, **LA**, LD, LD5, **MAC**, 11-OHCS, RAL (early), **pCO_2**, RAC (later), **∗ FFA**
↓ G, Mg, P, Na, O_2 satur., pCO_2, pO_2, pH, **tryptophan**, **tyrosine**, WBC

- *Urine* ↑ G, Na, norepinephrine
  ↓ **specific gravity**, volume
- *Pleural Fluid* ↑ CK

Hypothyroidism

central hypothyroidism

↓ **EPO**, FT3, **FT4**, **Hb**, cholesterol, TAG, **TSH**, T3, **T4**, vitamin B$_{12}$

hypothyroidism in children

↑ Bil, conjugated Bil, unconjugated Bil, FSH, LH, **TSH**
↓ **FT4**, **T3**, **T4**

primary hypothyroidism

↑ ADH, epinephrine, **albumin**, aldolase, alpha-aminonitrogen, **ALP**, **ALT**, anisocytes, **∗ anti-microsomal Ab**, antithyroglobulin Ab, **∗ antithyroperoxidase Ab**, **∗ anti-thyroid Ab** (early), anti-TSH-receptor Ab, **∗ thyroxine autoantibodies**, Apo A-I, Apo B, AST, bas, beta globulins, **beta-carotene**, beta-lipoprotein, Bil, conjugated Bil, Ca, CEA, **∗ CK**, CK-MB, **CK-MM**, Cu, EPO, estrogens, ESR, G, G tolerance, HCO_3^-, HLA – (DR3, DR5), 11-OHCS, **∗ cholesterol**, **chylomicrons**,

* IDL-C, immunoreactive proinsulin, ILGF-I, carotene, **catecholamines**, creatine, creatinine, **uric acid**, cryofibrinogen, LD, * **LDL-C**, LH, **lipids**, **macrocytes**, **Mb**, MCH, MCV, **Mg**, **norepinephrine**, pCO_2, PL, prealbumin, **PRL**, **TAG**, * **TBG**, testosterone, Tg, **TIBC**, * **TSH**, urea, VLDL-C

↓ ACE, * **ALP**, **EPO**, **RBC**, estradiol, factor – (**VIII**, IX), **Fe**, ferritin, fibronectin, **FT3**, * **FT4**, **G**, **gastrin**, GFR, GMT, G6PD (RBC), **Hb**, **HCT**, **HDL-C**, chloride, CHS, **ILGF-I**, **FT4 index**, **iodine**, 17-ketosteroids, cortisol, lipoprotein lipase, MCH, MCV, **Na**, neu, O_2 satur., osmolality, osteocalcin, P, pO_2, plasma volume, PRA, RTC, **SHBG**, somatomedin C, **GH**, **T3**, * **T4**, TAG, testosterone, TIBC, **T3 resin uptake**, transferrin satur., **TSH**, tyrosine, vitamin – (A, B_2, B_{12}, **folate**)

- *Urine* ↑ albumin, conjugated Bil, **proteins**, hydroxyproline, 17-OHCS, 17-KS, **catecholamines**, **creatinine**, Na
  - ↓ **Ca**, cAMP, Cu, 17-OHCS, hydroxyproline, 17-KGS, 17-KS, **creatine**, Mg, P, specific gravity
- *Cerebrospinal Fluid* ↑ **proteins**
- *Pericardial Fluid* ↑ cholesterol
- *Pleural Fluid* ↑ proteins, specific gravity
  - ↓ pH
- *Gastric Fluid* ↑ pH
- *Synovial Fluid* ↑ pyrophosphate
- *Sweat* ↓ chloride, Na

secondary hypothyroidism (pituitary h.)
↓ FT4, T3, T4, TSH
- *Urine* ↓ **17-ketosteroids**

tertiary hypothyroidism (hypothalamic h.)
↓ FT4, T3, T4, TSH

Hypoventilation
↑ RBC, **pCO_2**, **RAC**
↓ **pH**, **pO_2**

Hypoxia
↑ AST, FDP, uric acid, * **LA**, **LD**
↓ plasma volume, pH, pCO_2, pO_2
- *Urine* ↑ ALP, LAP
- *Cerebrospinal Fluid* ↑ LA

central nervous system hypoxia
- *Cerebrospinal Fluid* ↑ LA, MBP

Idiocy, Familial Amaurotic
- *Cerebrospinal Fluid* ↑ aldolase

Ileostomy
- *Stool* ↑ chloride, Na
  - ↓ K

Ileus

gallstone ileus
↑ **ALP**, **ALT**, **AMS**, **AST**, **Bil**, **ESR**, gamma globulins, **GMT**, cholesterol, **lipase**, WBC
↓ albumin, proteins

mechanic ileus
↑ creatinine, uric acid, urea
↓ proteins, cholesterol

meconium ileus

    ↑ unconjugated Bil

    ■ *Sweat* ↓ chloride, Na

postsurgery ileus

    ↑ creatinine, uric acid, serotonin, urea

Iminoglycinuria

    ■ *Urine* ↑ glycine, **proline, hydroxyproline**

familial iminoglycinuria

    ■ *Urine* ↑ glycine, hydroxyproline, proline

Immaturity, Pulmonary

    ■ *Amniotic Fluid* ↓ **phosphatidylglycerol**

Immobilization

    ↑ ALP, **Ca**, Ca²⁺, G, osteocalcin

    ↓ albumin, **HDL-C, PTH,** testosterone, **vitamin D3**

    ■ *Urine* ↑ **Ca,** Ca²⁺, PO₄⁻, hydroxyproline

Immunodeficiency

cellular immunodeficiency

    ↑ ∗ **eos, IgD, IgE**

    ↓ IgA, ∗ **lym,** ∗ **neu,** ∗ T-lym

common variable immunodeficiency

    ↓ B-lym, ∗ **IgA,** ∗ **IgG,** ∗ **IgM**

severe combined immunodeficiency (autosomal recessive)

    ↑ **eos, mono**

    ↓ **adenosine deaminase,** complement – (C1q), **B-lym, IgG, IgA,** purine nucleoside phosphorylase, **T-lym,** ∗ **lym**

Infarction

adrenal infarction

    ↓ cortisol

    ■ *Urine* ↓ **17-OHCS**

cerebral infarction

    ↑ Ab against beta-2 GP I, ACLA, A2MG, AST, CK, CK-BB, Cu

    ↓ **TAG**

    ■ *Cerebrospinal Fluid* ↑ CK, Cu, G, GMT, LA, **RBC, WBC,** macrophages, MBP

    ↓ pH

liver infarction

    ↑ ALT, AST, Bil, **WBC**

mesenterial infarction

    ↑ ALP, ALT, **AMS, AST, CK, LA, LD,** lipase, **WBC, MAC, P,** urea

    ■ *Urine* ↑ AMS

    ■ *Peritoneal Fluid* ↑ AMS

myocardial infarction

    ↑ **AAT,** Ab against beta-2 GP I, ACLA, **ACP,** epinephrine, AGP, **aldolase, alpha-1-globulins, alpha-2-globulins,** alpha-1-antichymotrypsin, alpha-HBD (12–24 hrs after, peak 24–48 hrs, decrease 3–14 d), **ALP,** ALT, **antimyocardial Ab,** Apo – ((a), B-100), **AST** (5x) (6–24 hrs after, peak 24–72 hrs, decrease 3–7 d), AT III, beta-glucuronidase, Bil, **BNP, CK** (6-12x) (2–12 hrs after, peak 12–48 hrs, decrease 2–4 d), ∗ **CK-MB** (16x) (3–12 hrs after, peak 12–24 hrs, decrease 24–72 hrs), CK-MM, **CRP, Cu, elastase,** enolase, epinephrine, estrogens, factor – (IV), **FDP, fibrinogen,** phosphohexoisomerase, phospholipase A2, fructose-1,6-diphosphate aldolase, **ESR** (12–48 hrs after, peak 4–5 d, decrease 1–4 months), **G**, glutathione reductase, **glycogen phosphorylase BB**, **GMT** (24 hrs after), G6PD (RBC), **haptoglobin**, **HBD** (6–12 hrs after, peak 2–6 d, decrease 4–14 d), **hexosaminidase**, HMWK, **HCT**, hypoxanthine, **cholesterol**, IgA, IgG, IgM, **plasminogen activator inhibitor**, **catecholamines**, complement – **(C3)**, **creatinine**, cortisol, cryofibrinogen, **uric acid**, LA, LD (3x) (6–48 hrs after, peak 24–72 hrs, decrease 4–14 d), **LD1** (6–24 hrs after, peak 24–144 hrs, decrease 4 d), LD2, LD1:LD2, **LP(a)**, LDL-C, **WBC** (6–12 hrs after, decrease 3–7 d), **mAST**, Mb, **MD**, **Mn**, mono (remission), **mucoproteins**, **myoglobin** (10x) (1–6 hrs after, peak 6–12 hrs, decrease 12–24 hrs), L-myosin (3–14 hrs after, peak 24–36 hrs, decrease 14 d), **neu**, **Ni**, **norepinephrine**, OCT, **PL**, plasma volume, PMN, pyruvate kinase, RF, ribonuclease, serotonin, **TAG**, **tropomyosin**, ✱ **troponin I** (2–12 hrs after, peak 10–24 hrs, decrease 4–14 d), ✱ **troponin T** (2–12 hrs after, peak 10–96 hrs, decrease 5 d – 3 months), TSH, **urea**, VLDL-C, viscosity, **FFA**

↓ **albumin**, platelet aggregation, AT III, bas, eos, epinephrine, factor – (XIII), **Fe**, G tolerance, HCT, HDL-C, **CHS**, K, LDL-C, lym, **Na**, Ni, O$_2$ satur., orosomucoid, **pH**, plasma volume, plasmocytes, **pO$_2$**, prealbumin, **transferrin satur.**, **T3**, vitamin – (B$_6$), **Zn**

■ *Urine* ↑ **G**, hexosaminidase, catecholamines, 17-KGS, 17-OHCS, crystals – (urate), LD, **Mb**, norepinephrine, VMA

■ *Cerebrospinal Fluid* ↑ G, K
    ↓ pH

■ *Pericardial Fluid* ↑ volume

pituitary infarction
    ↓ LH, GH

placental infarction
    ↑ antiphospholipid Ab

prostate infarction
    ↑ PAP, PSA

pulmonary infarction
    ↑ aldolase, ALP, ALT, **AMS**, AST, Bil, unconjugated Bil, CK, **CRP**, **ESR**, FDP, GMT, ICD, LD, LD – (2, 3, 4), pH, trypsin, **WBC**
    ↓ **pO$_2$**, pCO$_2$

■ *Urine* ↑ AMS, UBG

■ *Bronchoalveolar Lavage Fluid* ↑ RBC

■ *Pleural Fluid* ↑ ALP, AMS, blood, Hb, proteins, **RBC**, LD, WBC, **neu**, PMN

■ *Peritoneal Fluid* ↑ protein

■ *Sputum* ↑ blood

■ *Stool* ↑ UBG

renal infarction
    ↑ **ALP**, **ALT**, **AST**, **CRP**, eos, ESR, **LD**, LD1, LD1:LD2, **WBC**, **PRA**

■ *Urine* ↑ ALP, eos, **proteins**, RBC, Hb, **blood**, LD, lysozyme, pus, casts – (**RBC**)

pinal cord infarction

■ *Cerebrospinal Fluid* ↑ **proteins**, CK, eos, RBC, IgG, blood, LA, lym, WBC, **pressure**

spleen infarction
     ↑ ALP, **WBC**

Infertility
  male infertility
     ↑ ALT, **∗ anti-testicular Ab, ∗ antibodies against spermatozoa**, AST, eos, GMT, WBC
     ↓ Hb, HCT, testosterone
     ■ *Urine* ↓ 17-ketosteroids
     ■ *Seminal Fluid* ↑ antibodies against spermatozoa
       ↓ **alpha-glucosidase**, spermatozoa motility/count
  primary female infertility
     ↑ antispermatozoal Ab
     ↓ FSH

Injection
  intramuscular injection
     ↑ ALT, CK, CK-MM
  intrathecal injection
     ■ *Cerebrospinal Fluid* ↑ eos, WBC, macrophages

Injury, Endothelial
     ↑ **thrombomodulin, TPA, vWF**

Insufficiency
  adrenal insufficiency
  – **primary adrenal insufficiency (Addison's disease)**
     ↑ **∗ ACTH, ADH**, aldosterone, **AMA**, ANA, **∗ antiadrenal Ab**, anti-ovarian Ab, antithyroidal Ab, APA, proteins, **Ca, Ca²⁺**, Cu, DHEAS, **eos**, HLA – (**B8, DR3**, Dw3), **HCT**, chloride, **K**, ketones, creatinine, uric acid, **lym, WBC**, lym, MAC, **Mg**, osmolality, **P, PRA, PRL**, antiintrinsic factor Ab, **urea**
     ↓ **∗ aldosterone**, C-peptide, DHEA, DHEAS, **RBC, G, Hb, HCT, HCO₃⁻, chloride**, cholesterol, K, **∗ cortisol, WBC**, lym, mucoproteins, **Na, neu, osmolality**, P, pCO₂, pH, pepsinogen, PMNs, **pH**, 17-OH progesterone, RTC, TAG, urea, volume
     ■ *Urine* ↑ ammonia, aldosterone, ketones, 17-OHCS, 17-KS, **Na, osmolality**, pH
       ↓ aldosterone, ammonia, Cu, **chloride**, GFR, K, **17-OHCS, 17-KGS, 17-KS, cortisol**, tetrahydrodeoxycortisol, free cortisol, volume
     ■ *Cerebrospinal Fluid* ↓ chloride
     ■ *Sweat* ↓ chloride, Na
     ■ *Stool* ↑ fat
     ■ *Saliva* ↑ cortisol
     ■ *Gastric Fluid* ↑ pH
  – **secondary adrenal insufficiency**
     ↑ **ACTH**, Ca, K, WBC, PRL
     ↓ HCO₃⁻, chloride, cortisol, creatinine, K, Na, urea
     ■ *Urine* ↑ Na, pH
       ↓ K, 17-OHCS, volume, free cortisol
     ■ *Saliva* ↓ cortisol

cardiac insufficiency

↑ ACA, ADA, aldosterone, ALP, **ALT**, ANF, ASAL, **AST**, conjugated Bil, unconjugated Bil, **CK**, RBC, ESR, G, gamma globulins, GMT, Hb, HBD, chloride, cholesterol, CHS, ICD, K, creatine, creatinine, uric acid, **LA**, LD, MAC, mAST, MD, Mg, Na, pCO$_2$, PT, pH, PRA, prostacyclin, pyruvate, trypsin, urea

↓ albumin, **proteins**, eos, ESR, G, HCT, chloride, cholesterol, lym, Mg, Na, osmolality, pCO$_2$, pO$_2$, O$_2$ satur., PLT, vitamin – (B$_1$, folate)

■ *Urine* ↑ proteins, UBG, VMA

coronary insufficiency

↑ AAT, PLT adhesion, epinephrine, aldolase, ALT, **AST**, **CK**, **CK-MB**, elastase, FDP, fibrinogen, ESR, G, HBD, cholesterol, catecholamines, uric acid, **LA**, **LD**, LD1, **WBC**, LP(a), MD, Mb, neu, norepinephrine, pCO$_2$, PMN, pyruvate kinase, TAG, thrombomodulin, tropomyosin, troponin I, troponin T, urea, FFA, von Willebrand's factor

↓ HDL-C, CHS, K, Na, pH, **pO$_2$, satur. O$_2$,** Se, Zn

corpus luteum insufficiency

↑ PRL

↓ estradiol

gonadal insufficiency

↑ FSH, LH, PRL, SHBG

↓ androstenedione, EPO, estradiol, estrogens, FSH, LH, progesterone, testosterone, free testosterone, Zn

■ *Urine* ↑ FSH, LH

↓ estradiol, estrogens, FSH, 17-KS, pregnanediol, pregnanetriol

hepatic insufficiency

↑ alpha-aminonitrogen, ALP, **ALT**, **ammonia**, AST, Bil, **conjugated Bil**, **unconjugated Bil**, BT, factor – (**VIII**), **FDP**, **Fe** (early), **gamma globulins**, glucagon, insulin, citric acid, pyruvic acid, LA, **WBC**, MAC, MAL (early), PT, RAL, thrombomodulin, TT, **urea**, vitamin B$_{12}$ (early), FFA

↓ AFP, **albumin**, alpha-aminonitrogen, ALT, AST, **AT III**, beta-glucuronidase, **proteins**, Ca, euglobulin lysis time, RBC, factor – (**II**, **VII**, **IX**, **X**, **XIII**), fibrinogen, G, **cholesterol**, **CHS**, **ILGF-I**, K, complement – (C3), LD, Mg, Na, P, **PT**, testosterone, PLT, **urea**

■ *Urine* ↑ ALA, cystine, creatinine, crystals – (leucine, tyrosine), beta-hydroxybutyric acid, specific gravity, taurine

hypophysis insufficiency

↑ Ca, **eos**, G tolerance, cholesterol, chylomicrons, K, lym, WBC

↓ **ACTH**, **aldosterone**, angiotensin, Ca, estradiol, **FSH**, G, Hb, HCT, **hCG**, cortisol, **LH**, Na, P, **PRA**, **PRL**, progesterone, RTC, somatomedin C, **GH**, testosterone, TSH, **T4**, WBC

■ *Urine* ↑ chloride, volume

↓ aldosterone, hCG, 17-KGS, 17-OHCS, pregnanetriol

hypothalamus insufficiency

■ *Urine* ↓ FSH, LH

ovarian insufficiency

– primary ovarian insufficiency

↑ FSH, LH

↓ estradiol, **estrogens**, FSH, progesterone

■ *Urine* ↑ FSH

↓ **estrogens**, pregnanediol

- secondary ovarian insufficiency
    - ↓ FSH, ✻ LH
    - ■ *Urine* ↓ estrogens, FSH, ✻ **gonadotropins**, pregnanediol
pancreatic insufficiency
    - ↑ CCK-PZ, Fe, PP
    - ↓ **AMS**, proteins, **beta-carotene, cholesterol**, lipase, PT, vitamin – (**A**, B_{12}, D)
    - ■ *Urine* ↑ oxalate, porphyrins
        - ↓ AMS
    - ■ *Stool* ↑ **fat**
        - ↓ **chymotrypsin**, trypsin
placental insufficiency
    - ↑ Hb, HCT, IgA, IgM, viscosity
    - ↓ ALP, estriol, IgG, hPL, pregnancy-associated plasma protein – (A, B), pregnancy specific beta-1-glycoprotein
    - ■ *Urine* ↓ estriol
    - ■ *Amniotic Fluid* ↑ AFP, creatinine, uric acid, PL, urea
        - ↓ LAP
renal insufficiency
- acute renal insufficiency
    - ↑ ACP, AGBMA, Al, ALP, **AMS**, amylin, ANA, ANCA, ANF, Apo B, beta-endorphins, BHBA, **B2M**, proteins, Ca, CIC, CK, CK-MM, C-peptide, BT, enkephalins, eos, factor D, fructosamine, G, gastrin, GIP, glucagon, glycated albumin, haptoglobin, HCO_3^-, **chloride**, chymotrypsin, IDL-C, **K**, complement – (C3, C4), creatine, **creatinine, uric acid**, LD, LDL-C, lipase, WBC, MAC, MAL, **Mg**, myoglobin, Na, neu, neurotensin, plasma volume, osmolality, P, PT, PRL, PSA, PTH, PRL, thrombomodulin, trypsin, trypsinogen, **urea**
    - ↓ ALT, **proteins, Ca**, Ca^{2+}, EPO, RBC, G, **Hb, HCT**, HCO_3^-, chloride, K, cortisol, lipoprotein lipase, Lym, Mg, Na, volume, osmolality, P, **pH**, Se, serotonin, T4, **PLT**
    - ■ *Urine* ↑ AMS, proteins, RBC, Hb, pus, K, crystals – (urate, waxy), WBC, specific gravity, Na, volume, osmolality, tubular cells, casts – (RBC, granular, WBC, Mb)
        - ↓ Ca, chloride, K, **uric acid**, specific gravity, Mg, Na, volume, **P**, urea, UBG
- chronic renal insufficiency
    - ↑ ACP, Al, ALP, AMS, ANCA, c-ANCA, ANF, B2M, **Ca**, estriol, Fe, G, gastrin, glycated Hb, HCO_3^-, chloride, **K** (later), ✻ **creatinine**, creatine, **uric acid**, LDL-C, **lipase, MAC, Mg**, Na, plasma volume, osmolality, **P**, porphyrins, PTH, E selectin, trypsin, **urea**
    - ↓ amino acids, AST, **proteins, Ca, EPO, RBC, Fe, Hb, HCT**, HCO_3^-, **chloride**, K, Mg, **Na**, osmolality, P, **TIBC**, vitamin – (**D**), **Zn**
    - ■ *Urine* ↑ AMS, proteins, RBC, Hb, crystals – (urate), volume, casts – (**waxy**)
        - ↓ Ca, FDP, carnitine, uric acid, specific gravity, Mg, volume, **P**, pH, UBG, urea
respiratory insufficiency
    - ↑ AB, aldosterone, ammonia, BE, Ca, eos, EPO, RBC, ESR, Hb, HCT, HCO_3^-, K, LA, WBC, MAC, **pCO$_2$, RAC**
    - ↓ AAT, AB, ACE, **BE**, Hb, HCT, HCO_3^-, chloride, K, pH, **pO$_2$, satur. O$_2$**, PLT

testes insufficiency

   ↓ LH, **testosterone**

   ■ *Urine* ↓ 17-ketosteroids

Intestine, Blind Loop of

   ↑ neu

   ↓ RBC, Hb, HCT, vitamin – (B$_{12}$)

Intolerance

disaccharide intolerance

   ■ *Urine* ↑ galactose, lactose, saccharose

fructose intolerance

   ↑ amino acids, ALT, AST, Bil, **fructose**, IRI, uric acid

   ↓ aldolase, **G**, uric acid, **P**

   ■ *Urine* ↑ **amino acids**, proteins, conjugated Bil, **fructose**, reducing sugars

monosaccharide intolerance

   ■ *Urine* ↑ galactose, reducing sugars

   ■ *Stool* ↑ pH

Intoxication by

acetaminophen

   ↑ **ALT, AST**, Bil, PT, * **PTT**

   ↓ **G**

acetone

   ↑ creatinine, **MAC**, osmolar gap

   ↓ Hb, HCT, pH

   ■ *Urine* ↑ acetone, proteins, G, ketones, UBG

aflatoxin

   ↑ ALT, AST, GMT

alcohol, acute

   ↑ **acetone, AMS**, * **alcohol**, ALT, AST, ANF, beta-endorphins, **BHBA**, Ca, CK, GMT, **ketones**, uric acid, **LA**, LAP, LD, **MAC**, MAL, Ni, **osmolality, osmolal gap**, pCO$_2$, pH, urea

   ↓ BE, chloride, **G**, Mg, Na, pCO$_2$, pH, pO$_2$, PRL, uric acid, PLT

   ■ *Urine* ↑ **ketones**, volume

    ↓ aldosterone

   ■ *Cerebrospinal Fluid* ↑ protein

aluminum

   ↑ * **Al**, Ca, microcytes

   ↓ PTH, **Hb, HCT, microcytes**, RBC

   ■ *Urine* ↑ * **Al**

Amanita phalloides

   ↑ albumin, **ALT** (peak 72 hrs, decrease from 4th day), ammonia, **AST**, proteins, **Bil, conjugated Bil, Fe**, gamma globulins, GMD, **Hb**, HCT, K, **creatinine, LA, LD, WBC**, MAC (early), pyruvate, **urea**

   ↓ albumin (later), factors – (V, VII, X), fibrinogen, **G**, Hb, HCT, HCO$_3^-$, chloride, CHS, **K**, Na, pCO$_2$, PT, pH (early), plasminogen, prothrombin

   ■ *Urine* ↑ protein (later), G, urobilin, casts

    ↓ volume

   ■ *Cerebrospinal Fluid* ↑ pressure

ammonia

   ↑ uric acid

aniline

  ↑ anisocytes, Bil, **Heinz bodies** (RBC), **MHb**, poikilocytes, RTC
  ↓ RBC, Hb, HCT
  ■ *Urine* ↑ proteins, blood, MHb

antacids

  ↑ Ca, creatinine, MAL, Mg, urea

antimony

  ↑ ALT, AST, GMT, pyruvate, **Sb**

arsenic

  ↑ alpha-aminonitrogen, **ALT**, ✳ **As**, **AST**, BSP retention, Ca, **eos**, ESR, GMT,
      guanosine deaminase, cholesterol, ICD, creatinine, lym, **WBC**, MAC,
      neu, **RBC basophilic stippling**, **pyruvate**, RTC, urea
  ↓ ALP, CO_2, **RBC**, G, **Hb**, **HCT**, chloride, cholesterol, **WBC**, Na, pO_2, PLT
  ■ *Urine* ↑ albumin, ✳ **As**, **proteins**, **RBC**, **Hb** (acute), hemosiderin, blood,
      coproporphyrin III, casts
      ↓ phosphate, **volume**
  ■ *Cerebrospinal Fluid* ↑ proteins, WBC
  ■ *Stool* ↑ **As**
  ■ *Hair* ↑ ✳ **As**
  ■ *Bone* ↑ As
  ■ *Nails* ↑ ✳ **As**

baryum

  ↓ **K**
  ■ *Urine* ↓ volume

battery-industry environment

  ↑ Cd, Mn, Pb
  ■ *Urine* ↑ Cd, Mn, Pb

benzene

  ↑ CK, eos, WBC, neu, RTC
  ↓ proteins, RBC, gamma globulins, **Hb**, **HCT**, IgA, lym, **WBC**, neu, **PLT**
  ■ *Urine* ↑ Mb

– chronic intoxication by benzene

  ↑ **BT**, **eos**, **WBC** (early)
  ↓ RBC, Hb, HCT, IgA, **WBC** (later), **PLT**

beryllium

  ↑ Ca, WBC, uric acid
  ↓ ALP

bismuth

  ↑ amino acids
  ■ *Urine* ↑ **Bi**

botulotoxin

  ↓ ACH

bromide

  ↑ ✳ **bromide**
  ■ *Urine* ↑ ✳ **bromide**
      ↓ volume
  ■ *Cerebrospinal Fluid* ↑ proteins, pressure

cadmium

  ↑ ALT
  ■ *Urine* ↑ ✳ **Cd**

carbon dioxide
↑ CK

carbon disulfide
↑ ALT, AST, GMT

carbon monoxide
↑ AMS, anion gap, CK, CK-MB, RBC, **G**, ✱ **carboxy-Hb** (COHb), uric acid, LA, WBC, lym, **MAC**, neu, RAL (early)
↓ ESR, **pH**, pCO_2, pO_2
■ *Urine* ↑ Mb
↓ **volume**

carbon tetrachloride
↑ ALT, AST, WBC

chloroform
↑ alpha-aminonitrogen, lipids
↓ G, cholesterol
■ *Urine* ↑ UBG

chromium
↑ ALT, AST, **Cr**, GMT
↓ RBC, Hb, HCT
■ *Urine* ↑ proteins, **Cr**, blood
↓ volume

cobalt
↑ ✱ **Co**, lipids
■ *Urine* ↑ Co

cocaine
↑ CK, **ALT**, **AST**, **catecholamines**, eos, HBsAg, **lym**, PRL, RAL, tropomyosin
■ *Hair* ↑ ✱ **cocaine**

copper
– acute intoxication by copper
↑ ALT, AST, ✱ **Cu**, GMT
■ *Urine* ↑ Cu, Mb
– chronic intoxication by copper
↑ ALT, **ceruloplasmin, Cu**, GMT
↓ RBC, Hb
■ *Urine* ↑ **Cu**, RBC, Hb, Mb
↓ volume

coumarin
↓ ✱ **PT**, ✱ **PTT**

cyanide
↑ proteins, ✱ **cyanide**, G, LA, MAL (early), **MAC** (later), RAC (later)
↓ ALP, AST, HCO_3^-, uric acid, **pH**

drugs (chronic)
↑ **ALT**, AMS, **AST**, CK, **eos**, HBsAg, LD, **lym**, Mb, T4
↓ c-AMP, cholesterol, O_2 satur., pO_2

dyes/paint-industry
↑ Cd, Cr, Mn, Pb, Sb
■ *Urine* ↑ Cd, Cr, Mn, Pb, Sb

EDTA
↓ ALP

electro-industry
■ *Urine* ↓ Se

ether

    ↓ pH

ethylene glycol

    ↑ anion gap, **✱ ethylene glycol**, **✱ glycolic acid, glycol**, WBC, **✱ MAC**, MAC
      + RAC, neu, **osmolality, osmolal gap**

    ↓ Ca, HCO_3^-, Na, pH, pCO_2

    ■ *Urine* ↑ albumin, proteins, RBC, Hb, pus, blood, **hippurate, crystals,**
       oxalate, fat, casts – **(epithelial)**
      ↓ volume

    ■ *Cerebrospinal Fluid* ↑ proteins, PMN, pressure

    ■ *Synovial Fluid* ↑ crystals – (calcium oxalate)

fluoride

    ↑ CT, G
    ↓ Ca, ALP, AST, Ca

fluorine

    ↑ K, MAC
    ↓ Ca, Mg

food (staphylococci, clostridia, salmonella)

    ↑ MAC

formaldehyde

    ↑ MAC
    ↓ AST

    ■ *Urine* ↑ proteins, **RBC**, UBG, casts
      ↓ volume

fungicides

    ↑ Hg, Mn
    ■ *Urine* ↑ Hg, Mn

glass-industry

    ↑ Mn, Pb, Sb
    ■ *Urine* ↑ Mn, Pb, Sb, Se

glycerol

    ↑ osmolal gap

gold salts

    ↑ pyruvate

halothane

    ↑ GMD

heavy metals

    ↑ ALP, ALT, AST, B2M, BSP retention, Ca, eos, **ESR**, guanine deaminase,
      cholesterol, ICD, creatinine, lysozyme, **WBC**, MAC, neu, pyruvate,
      RTC, TAG, urea

    ↓ CO_2, RBC, Hb, HCT, CHS, ICD, uric acid, WBC, Na, vitamin – (C)

    ■ *Urine* ↑ albumin, As, **proteins, RBC**, Hb, hexosaminidase, coproporphyrin,
       phyrin, porphyrins, casts – **(epithelial)**
      ↓ phosphate

    ■ *Cerebrospinal Fluid* ↑ protein

heparin

    ↓ ✱ PT, ✱ PTT

herbicides

    ↑ aldolase, ALT, AST, Bil, CK, GMT, creatinine, LD, WBC, urea
    ↓ RBC, haptoglobin, Hb, HCT
    ■ *Urine* ↑ Mb

heroin

↑ AMS, **ALT**, **AST**, **eos**, HBsAg, **lym**, TBG
- *Urine* ↑ Hb

hexachloride

- *Urine* ↑ Mb

insecticides

↑ AMS, **G**, WBC
↓ ✶ **CHS**, ✶ **CHS** (RBC), CK, K
- *Urine* ↑ proteins, **G**

iron

↑ ALT, AST, ✶ **Fe**, **G**, GMT, **WBC**, MAC, TIBC, transferrin satur.
↓ **transferrin**
- *Urine* ↑ DALA
  ↓ volume

isopropanol (isopropyl alcohol)

↑ acetone, ✶ **isopropanol**, MAC, osmolal gap
- *Urine* ↑ acetone

lead

↑ **ALA**, aldolase, ALT, **anisocytes**, AST, **Bil**, Cu (RBC), **eos**, ESR, ✶ **RBC basophilic stippling**, **Fe**, GMT, HbA$_{1c}$, Hb (free), **uric acid**, ✶ **copro-porphyrin**, WBC, lym, mechanical fragility (RBC), MCV, microcytes, neu, ✶ **Pb**, PBG, **poikilocytes**, ✶ **porphyrins**, RTC, Sb, **siderocytes**, target cells, ✶ **free RBC protoporphyrin**, ✶ **zinc protoporphyrin**, **urea**
↓ **delta-aminolevulinic dehydratase**, RBC, factor XIII, glutathione (RBC), ✶ **Hb**, ✶ **HCT**, MCH, MCHC, MCV, **RBC osmotic fragility**, WBC, RBC osmotic resistance, pyrimidine-5 nucleotidase (RBC), PLT
- *Urine* ↑ ✶ **ALA**, **alanine**, albumin, **amino acids**, beta-amino-isobuty-ric acid, **proteins**, citrate, ✶ **DALA**, **G**, fructose, glutathione peroxi-dase (RBC), glycine, Hb (free), **coproporphyrin I**, **coproporphyrin III**, uric acid, ✶ **Pb**, phosphate, **porphobilinogen**, porphyrins, **proto-porphyrin**, Sb, **UBG**, uroporphyrin, casts – **(granular, hyaline)**
  ↓ **uric acid**, volume
- *Cerebrospinal Fluid* ↑ **proteins**, mono, pressure
- *Stool* ↑ **CP**, ✶ **Pb**, **protoporphyrins**
- *Hair* ↑ **Pb**
- *Synovial Fluid* ↑ crystals – (urate)

lipid-lowering drugs

↑ ALT, AST, G, chloride, MAC, uric acid
↓ TAG

lithium

↑ Ca, ✶ **Li**, WBC, Mg
↓ lym, Na
- *Urine* ↓ specific gravity

magnesium

↑ Ca, **Mg**

manganese

↑ ✶ **Mn**
↓ ALP
- *Urine* ↑ **Mn**
- *Stool* ↑ **Mn**

mannitol

↑ osmolal gap

marijuana

↑ **ALT, AST, eos**, HBsAg, **lym**, RAL

mercury

↑ * **Hg**, WBC, neu, pyruvate, urea

↓ chloride

■ *Urine* ↑ albumin, proteins, RBC, fructose, Hb, * **Hg**, coproporphyrin III, reducing sugars, fat, casts

    ↓ volume (later)

■ *Cerebrospinal Fluid* ↑ proteins, * **Hg**, WBC

methanol (methyl alcohol)

↑ AMS, anion gap, ketones, uric acid, formic acid, * **MAC, methanol, osmolality, osmolal gap**, urea

↓ Ca^{2+}, **HCO_3^-**, Na, pCO_2, pH

■ *Urine* ↑ acetone, proteins, RBC, Hb, ketones, **formic acid**, methanol

    ↓ volume

■ *Cerebrospinal Fluid* ↑ pressure

methyl bromide

↑ ALT, AST

■ *Cerebrospinal Fluid* ↑ pressure

mining-industry environment

↑ Hg, Mn, Pb

■ *Urine* ↑ Hg, Mn, Pb

mushroom

↑ ACH, albumin, **ALT**, ammonia, **AST**, proteins, **Bil**, conjugated Bil, Fe, gamma globulins, GMD, **GMT**, Hb, HCT, K, **creatinine, LA, LD, WBC, MAC, pyruvate**, urea

↓ albumin, factors – (V, VII, X), fibrinogen, G, Hb, HCT, HCO_3^-, chloride, CHS, K, Na, pCO_2, PT, pH, plasminogen, prothrombin, urea (later)

■ *Urine* ↑ **proteins**, Bil, G, urobilin, casts – (**hyaline**), UBG

    ↓ **volume**

■ *Cerebrospinal Fluid* ↑ pressure

naphthalene

↑ ALT, AST, GMT

■ *Urine* ↑ RBC, Hb

    ↓ volume

narcotics

↑ **ALT, AST, eos**, HBsAg, **lym**, MAC+RAC, Mb

nickel

↑ * **Ni**, WBC

nitrite/nitrate

↑ **Heinz bodies** (RBC)

■ *Urine* ↑ blood, **nitrates**

nitrobenzene

↑ ALT, AST, Bil, GMT, **Heinz bodies** (RBC), **MHb**, RTC

■ *Urine* ↑ Hb, MHb, urobilin

opiates

↑ ALT, HbA_{1c}, neu

■ *Urine* ↑ proteins, Mb

organophosphates

    ↑ ACH, AMS, **G**, WBC, MAC, PT
    ↓ G, ✳ **CHS**, ✳ **CHS** (RBC)
    ■ *Urine* ↑ proteins, RBC, G, Hb

oxalates

    ↑ **oxalate**
    ↓ ALP
    ■ *Urine* ↑ volume

paraldehyde

    ↑ osmolal gap

paraquat

    ↑ ACE
    ■ *Urine* ↓ volume

pesticides

    ↑ G, WBC
    ↓ **CHS**, CHS (RBC), K
    ■ *Urine* ↑ proteins, G

petrol

    ↑ lym
    ↓ WBC
    ■ *Urine* ↑ porphyrins

petrol-industry environment

    ↑ Mn
    ■ *Urine* ↑ Mn

phenacetine

    ↑ **Heinz bodies** (RBC), **MHb**, urea
    ↓ Hb, HCT
    ■ *Urine* ↑ **p-aminophenol**, proteins, blood, WBC

phenols

    ↑ MAC
    ■ *Urine* ↑ albumin, RBC, Hb, Mb, casts
      ↓ volume

phosphorus

    ↑ alpha-aminonitrogen, ALT, AST, Bil, GMT, lipids, WBC, MAC
    ↓ fibrinogen, ESR, G, cholesterol, prothrombin
    ■ *Urine* ↑ amino acids, ammonia, proteins, RBC, blood, P, urea
      ↓ volume

plastics-industry environment

    ↑ Pb
    ■ *Urine* ↑ Pb

rodenticides

    ↑ PT
    ↓ factors – (VII, X)

salicylates

    ↑ ALT, anion gap, AST, G (children), **chloride**, HCO$_3^-$, **MAC** (later), MAL,
        PT, pH, RAC, **RAL** (early), ✳ **salicylate**
    ↓ G, HCO$_3^-$, hydroxyproline, **K**, **Na**, P, **pCO$_2$**, pH, thrombin
    ■ *Urine* ↑ G, K, ketones, **Na**, pH, RBC, reducing substances
      ↓ pH, hydroxyproline, volume

selen

    ↑ **Se**

silver
- ↑ pH, urea
- ↓ chloride, Na
- ■ *Urine* ↑ proteins

smelting-industry environment
- ↑ Mn, Pb
- ■ *Urine* ↑ Mn, Pb

snake venom (snake bite)
- ↑ **ALT, APTT**, ACH, anti-ACHR, **AST**, CK, CT, **eos**, FDP, **LD, WBC, neu**, PT, **PTT, urea**
- ↓ **fibrinogen**, Hb, HCT, **PLT**
- ■ *Urine* ↑ albumin, proteins, RBC, Hb, **Mb**

spider venom (spider bite)
- ↑ **ALT, AST**, CK, CT, **eos, LD, WBC**, PT, **urea**
- ↓ Hb, HCT, **PLT**
- ■ *Urine* ↑ proteins, Hb, **Mb**

steel-industry environment
- ↑ Cd, Cr, Mn
- ■ *Urine* ↑ Cd, Cr, Mn

strychnine
- ↓ G
- ■ *Urine* ↑ Mb

styrene
- ■ *Urine* ↑ VMA

tetrachlorethane
- ↑ lym
- ↓ RBC, Hb, HCT

tetrachlormethane
- ↑ alpha-aminonitrogen, **ALT**, AST, **Bil, conjugated Bil**, lipids
- ↓ G, cholesterol
- ■ *Urine* ↑ **benzoic acid, hippuric acid, uric acid**, porphyrins
  - ↓ volume

thallium
- ↑ lym, WBC, urea
- ↓ WBC
- ■ *Urine* ↑ proteins, RBC, coproporphyrin, WBC, **thallium**, casts
  - ↓ volume
- ■ *Cerebrospinal Fluid* ↑ pressure

toluene
- ↑ MAC
- ↓ WBC
- ■ *Urine* ↑ hippuric acid, uric acid, Mb
  - ↓ volume
- ■ *Cerebrospinal Fluid* ↑ pressure

trichlorethylene
- ↑ ALT, AST, GMT
- ■ *Urine* ↑ * **trichloracetic acid**, * **trichlorethanol**

turpentine
- ↑ WBC, neu
- ■ *Urine* ↑ proteins, RBC, Hb, blood
  - ↓ volume

vinyl chloride
> ↑ ALP, ALT, AST
> ↓ albumin

water
> ↑ Mb
> ↓ albumin, chloride, Na, osmolality, proteins

weapons-industry environment
> ↑ Sb
> ■ *Urine* ↑ Sb

xylene
> ↑ CK

zinc
> ↑ Zn
> ■ *Urine* ↑ Mb

Ischemia

cerebral ischemia
> ↑ antiphospholipid Ab, CK
> ■ *Cerebrospinal Fluid* ↑ **CK, LA**, LD
> ↓ Mg

hepatic ischemia
> ↑ ALT, AST, LAP, WBC, **5-nucleotidase**

intestinal ischemia
> ↑ ALP, CK, WBC, **LD**

myocardial ischemia
> ↑ AAT, ACP, PLT adhesion, epinephrine, AGP, **aldolase, alpha-1-globulins, alpha-2-globulins**, AST, CEA, **CK, CK-MB, CRP**, Cu, elastase, enolase, FDP, **fibrinogen, ESR, G**, haptoglobin, **HBD, cholesterol**, plasminogen activator inhibitor, uric acid, **LD, LD1**, LD2, LDL-C, **LP(a), WBC**, mAST, MD, Mb, **mucoproteins**, neu, norepinephrine, OCT, PMN, pyruvate kinase, selectin, serotonin, TAG, thrombomodulin, tropomyosin, troponin I, urea, VLDL-C, FFA, vWf, Zn
> ↓ Cu, HDL-C, CHS, IDL-C, K, pH, pO$_2$, transferrin satur., Zn
> ■ *Urine* ↑ G, hexosaminidase, catecholamines, Mb, VMA

renal ischemia
> ↑ **aldosterone**, ammonia, urea
> ■ *Urine* ↑ K

Rh Isoimmunisation
> ↑ AFP
> ↓ estriol, PLT
> ■ *Urine* ↓ estriol
> ■ *Amniotic Fluid* ↑ AFP, **volume**, PRL

Jaundice

hemolytic jaundice
> ↑ ACP, ALP, ALT, **Bil, unconjugated Bil, Fe**, gamma globulins, **GMT**, uric acid, **LD**, MD, RBC osmotic fragility, urea
> ↓ conjugated Bil, Cu, **Hb**, cholesterol, RBC osmotic resistance
> ■ *Urine* ↑ ALT, conjugated Bil, **UBG**
> ■ *Stool* ↑ UBG
> ↓ UBG

– congenital hemolytic jaundice
> ↑ **Bil, conjugated Bil**, uric acid, urea
> ↓ ceruloplasmin, Cu

hepatocellular jaundice

↑ **ALP, ALT, AST, Bil, conjugated Bil,** unconjugated Bil, Cu, Fe, **GMT,** LAP, **LD, PT**

↓ cholesterol

■ *Urine* ↑ ALT, conjugated Bil, **UBG**
↓ UBG

mechanic jaundice

↑ ACP, ADA, aldolase, alpha-1-globulins, ALP, ALT, AST, **Bil,** unconjugated Bil, ceruloplasmin, Fe, gamma globulins, GMT, cholesterol, creatinine, uric acid, LD, MD, **PT,** TIBC, urea

↓ beta-carotene, proteins, conjugated Bil, Cu, Fe, fibrinogen, glucuronosyltransferase, Hb, cholesterol, CHS

■ *Urine* ↑ ALT, conjugated Bil, UBG
■ *Stool* ↑ UBG

neonatal jaundice

↑ Bil, **unconjugated Bil,** delta Bil

■ *Urine* ↑ conjugated bilirubin, galactose, reducing sugars

obstructive jaundice

↑ ACP, ADA, **aldolase,** alpha-1-globulins, **ALP, ALT,** aminotripeptidase, **AST,** ATPase, **beta globulins, Bil, conjugated Bil, unconjugated Bil, ceruloplasmin,** Cu, Fe, ferritin, phosphohexoisomerase, fructose-1,6-diphosphate aldolase, **gamma globulins, GMT,** guanine deaminase, **cholesterol,** CHS, ICD, IgA, IgG, complement – (C3), creatinine, LAP, **LD,** lipids, macrocytes, MD, **5-nucleotidase, OCT,** RBC osmotic resistance, PL, **TAG,** target cells, TIBC

↓ **AAT,** Apo A-IV, beta-carotene, proteins, Ca, Fe, fibrinogen, ESR, glucuronosyltransferase, CHS, uric acid, ligandin, TBG, vitamin – (A, **K**)

■ *Urine* ↑ ALT, conjugated Bil, **porphyrins**
↓ UBG

Kwashiorkor

↑ **alanine,** insulin, transferrin

↓ epinephrine, **albumin,** ALP, ALT, amino acids, AST, beta-carotene, **proteins,** C2, C3, Ca, **ceruloplasmin,** Cr, **Cu, RBC, Fe,** G, glycine, **Hb,** HCT, ICD, **ILGF-I,** isoleucine, K, cortisol, leucine, Mg, proconvertin, **RBP, transferrin satur.,** TIBC, **transferrin, transthyretin, tryptophan,** valine, vitamin – (A, B_1, B_2, B_6, B_{12})

■ *Urine* ↑ amino acids, ketones (early), volume
↓ Cu, hydroxyproline, osmolality

Lactation

↑ CA 15-3, Cu, DPD, osteocalcin, PTH, vitamin – (**D**)

↓ ACTH, **Ca,** Ca^{2+}, Fe, **Mg,** vitamin – (B_1, B_6, folate), Zn

■ *Urine* ↑ G, lactose, **reducing sugars**

vegane mother lactation

↑ **folate,** PTH

↓ Ca, Ca^{2+}, Mg, vitamin B_{12}

■ *Urine* ↑ pH

Lesion

choroid plexus lesion

■ *Cerebrospinal Fluid* ↑ albumin

CNS lesion

↑ LD, osmolality

■ *Cerebrospinal Fluid* ↑ CHS, IDH, MBP, somatostatin

hypothalamus lesion

↓ FSH
- *Urine* ↓ FSH

liver lesion

↑ **AAT, AD, ALT, A2MG,** amino acids, aminonitrogen, **AST, Bil, conjugated Bil,** clotting time, **Fe, ferritin, IgA,** IgG, LA, LD, mAST, **PT**

↓ **albumin,** alpha-1-globulins, alpha-2-globulins, AT III, factor II, haptoglobin, hemopexin, cholesterol, CHS, complement – (**C3,** C4), orosomucoid, P, **prealbumin, protein C,** TIBC, transferrin, urea
- *Urine* ↑ alpha-aminonitrogen, amino acids, **conjugated Bil,** G, galactose, P, reducing sugars, UBG
  ↓ UBG

– toxic liver lesion

↑ ALP, aminonitrogen, AST, Bil, **ESR,** GMT, IgA, LD

↓ albumin, proteins
- *Urine* ↑ Bil, G, UBG

minor myocardial lesion

↑ troponin T

pituitary gland lesion

↓ FSH, LH
- *Urine* ↓ FSH

renal lesion

↑ B2M, FDP, LA, LD, LDL-C

↓ aldosterone, EPO, PRA
- *Urine* ↑ RBC, G, LAP, casts – (RBC)
  ↓ creatinine, specific gravity

– toxic renal lesion

- *Urine* ↑ AST, G

skeletal muscle lesion

↑ ALT, **AST,** CK, creatinine, creatine, LD, LD – (1, 2, 3, 4, 5), tropomyosin, troponin I
- *Urine* ↑ creatine, creatinine

eucemia

↑ ACE, ACP, ACP (prostatic), ADA, ADH, Al, **aldolase,** alpha-aminonitrogen, alpha-1-globulins, alpha-2-globulins, ALP, ALP (tumor isoenzyme), ALP (WBC), ALT, ammonia, **ANA,** anisocytes, anti-ss-DNA, AST, bas, **RBC basophilic stippling,** B2M, Ca, CEA, ceruloplasmin, **CRP,** Cu, BT, euglobulin lysis time, elastase, eos, Fas-ligand, FDP, Fe, **ferritin,** fibrinogen, FPA, ESR, gamma globulins, glutathione peroxidase (RBC), HbF, HBsAg, cold agglutinins, ICD, IgG, sIL-2R, sIL-6R, K, creatinine, cryoglobulins, **uric acid, LA,** LAP (WBC), **LD,** LD – (1, 2, 3, 4), **WBC,** lipids, lym, lymphoblasts, lysozyme, macrocytes, MD, mono, MPV, myeloblasts, neu, TM – (ALP, ALP, beta-glucuronidase, B2M, c-abl/bcr-translocation, CEA, **ferritin, chromogranin A, B,** sialic acid, LD, lym, myeloperoxidase, N-ras-mutation, 5-nucleotidase, **glucocorticoid receptors,** terminal deoxytransferase, thymidine kinase), P, paraproteins, **PT,** poikilocytes, prothrombin fragment 1.2, **RF, RTC,** substance P, PLT, transcobalamin I, urea, vitamin B_{12} binding capacity, viscosity, vitamin – (B_1), hairy cells

  ↓ ACE, PLT aggregation, albumin, ALP, AT III, beta globulins, proteins, Ca, **RBC**, factor II, fibrinogen, FPA (remission), gamma globulins, Hb, **HCT**, IgA, **IgG**, IgM, K, folate, WBC, lym, lysozyme, Mg, mono, Na, neu, PTH, pyruvate kinase, PLT, vitamin – (B_6, B_{12}), Zn

 ■ *Urine* ↑ alpha-aminonitrogen, arylsulfatase A, Bence Jones protein, **proteins**, Ca, RBC, Hb, crystals – (urate), uric acid, lysozyme, porphyrins

  ↓ creatinine, lysozyme

 ■ *Cerebrospinal Fluid* ↑ bas, B2M, **proteins**, CK, eos, fibronectin, IgG, blood, LA, lym, **LD**, **WBC**, RBC, MBP, **pressure**

  ↓ **G**

 ■ *Gastric Fluid* ↑ BAO, blood

 ■ *Pleural Fluid* ↑ AMS, eos, lym, lysozyme

 ■ *Sputum* ↑ blood

 ■ *Synovial Fluid* ↑ PMN

  ↓ viscosity

acute leukemia

  ↑ ACE, CEA, ceruloplasmin, Cu, BT, **FDP**, Fe, **HbF**, creatinine, K, **uric acid**, LA, **LD**, P, **WBC**, urea

  ↓ ACE, PLT aggregation, albumin, Ca, RBC, fibrinogen, **Hb**, **HCT**, K, Mg, **PLT**

 ■ *Urine* ↑ lysozyme

 ■ *Cerebrospinal Fluid* ↑ B2M, LD, pressure, WBC

adult human T-cell leukemia/lymphoma sy

  ↑ ＊ **anti-HTLV-I antibodies**, ＊ **Ca**, ＊ **WBC**

  ↓ Hb, HCT, PLT

basophilic leukemia

  ↑ **bas**

 ■ *Gastric Fluid* ↑ BAO

chronic myelomonocytic leukemia

  ↑ WBC, **lysozyme, mono, neu**

  ↓ albumin, proteins, RBC, Hb, HCT, **PLT**, vitamin – (B_{12})

eosinophilic leukemia

  ↑ **eos**

erythroleukemia

  ↑ HbA2, HbF

  ↓ RBC

hairy cell leucemia

  ↑ **ALP** (WBC), ＊ **hairy cells**, ESR, HTLV I/II Ab, sIL-2R

  ↓ Hb, HCT, lym, **WBC**, lysozyme, mono, **PLT**

lymphatic leucemia
– acute lymphatic leucemia

  ↑ ACP, ALT, anti-ss-DNA Ab, CEA, glutathione peroxidase (RBC), cold agglutinins, sIL-2R, K, **uric acid**, LAP (WBC), **LD**, LD – (1, 2, 3), ＊ **WBC**, **lym**, lymphoblasts, TM – (beta-glucuronidase, 5-nucleotidase, terminal deoxytransferase, thymidine kinase), P, **terminal deoxynucleotidyl transferase**

  ↓ Ca, **RBC**, **Hb**, **HCT**, IgA, K, WBC, lysozyme, Na, **neu**, PTH, **PLT**

 ■ *Urine* ↓ lysozyme

 ■ *Cerebrospinal Fluid* ↑ **proteins**, fibronectin, B2M

  ↓ G

- **chronic lymphatic leucemia**
  - ↑ ACP, ammonia, anti-ss-DNA, B2M, CEA, **ESR**, gamma globulins, HbF, cold agglutinins, sIL-2R, **cryoglobulins, uric acid, LD,** LD – (2, 3, 4), **WBC, ∗ lym,** paraproteins, substance P
  - ↓ ACE, **albumin,** ALP, **beta globulins, RBC,** gamma globulins, **Hb, HCT, IgA, IgG, IgM,** lysozyme, neu, PTH, **PLT,** vitamin – (B$_{12}$)
  - ■ *Urine* ↑ **Bence Jones protein,** uric acid
  - ■ *Pleural Fluid* ↑ AMS, lym
  - ■ *Cerebrospinal Fluid* ↑ eos
- **megakarocyte leucemia**
  - ↑ PLT
- **monocytic leucemia**
  - ↑ **ALP,** ALP (WBC), APTT, **AST, proteins,** FDP, **Fe, gamma globulins,** globulins, IgA, IgG, IgM, creatinine, uric acid, **LD,** WBC, **lysozyme, mono,** PT, RTC, TT, **urea,** vitamin – (B$_{12}$)
  - ↓ **albumin, ALP** (WBC), beta globulins, **proteins,** factor – (V, VIII), fibrinogen, Hb, HCT, cholesterol, WBC, neu, **PLT,** Zn
  - ■ *Urine* ↑ proteins, **lysozyme**
  - ■ *Pleural Fluid* ↑ proteins
- **myelogenous leucemia**
- **– acute myelogenous leucemia**
  - ↑ ACP, ADA, **aldolase,** alpha-aminonitrogen, alpha-1-globulins, alpha-2-globulins, alpha-1-antichymotrypsin, alpha-1-glycoprotein, **ALP** (+ WBC), ALT, ANA, anisocytes, anti-ss-DNA, APTT, **arylsulfatase A, AST,** bas, beta globulins, Ca, Cu, eos, EPO, FDP, **Fe,** ferritin, gamma globulins, globulins, Hb (free), **ICD,** K, creatinine, **uric acid, LD, WBC, lysozyme, malate dehydrogenase,** MCH, MCV, Mg, mono, MPV, myeloblasts, Na, **neu,** TM – **(CEA,** myeloperoxidase), P, phosphoglu-comutase, poikilocytes, PLT, PT, RF, TT, UBBC, urea, vitamin – (B$_{12}$)
  - ↓ ACE, **ALP** (WBC), **albumin,** proteins, beta globulins, Ca, **RBC,** factor – (V, VIII), **fibrinogen, Hb, HCT,** cholesterol, **K, WBC,** lysozyme, Na, **neu,** PTH, **PLT,** RTC, Zn
  - ■ *Urine* ↑ alpha-aminonitrogen, Ca, creatine, K, uric acid, **lysozyme**
  - ■ *Cerebrospinal Fluid* ↑ **proteins**
    - ↓ **G**
  - ■ *Pleural Fluid* ↑ proteins, lysozyme
- **– chronic myelogenous leucemia**
  - ↑ ACE, **ACP,** aldolase, **alpha-1-globulins, alpha-2-globulins, ALP,** ALP (WBC), **ALT,** ammonia, anti-ss-DNA, APTT, arylsulfate, **AST, bas,** Ca, **CEA, eos,** ESR, FDP, ferritin, fibrinogen, G, **gamma globulins,** globu-lins, **granulocytes,** HbF, Hb, HCT, histamine, cholesterol, ICD, K, creatinine, **uric acid,** alpha-ketoglutaric acid, **LA, LD,** LD5, ∗ **WBC, lysozyme, malate dehydrogenase, megakaryocytes, metamyelo-cytes, mono,** MPV, myeloblasts, myelocytes, Na, **neu,** substance P, phosphoglucomutase, PT, RTC, **terminal deoxynucleotidyl trans-ferase,** transcobalamin I, **PLT,** TT, urea, **vitamin B$_{12}$ binding capac-ity,** vitamin – (B$_{12}$)
  - ↓ **albumin,** ALP, **ALP** (WBC), AT III, **beta globulins, proteins, RBC,** fac-tor – (II, V, VIII), fibrinogen, **G, Hb, HCT, IgA,** complement – (C4, total), LD5, lym, plasminogen, PTH, RTC, **PLT,** Zn
  - ■ *Urine* ↑ alpha-aminonitrogen, creatine, **uric acid, lysozyme**

- ■ *Cerebrospinal Fluid* ↑ bas, **WBC**
- ■ *Pleural Fluid* ↑ **proteins**
- – juvenile chronic myelogenous leucemia
  - ↑ ALP (WBC), **HbF, mono, WBC**
  - ↓ ALP (WBC)

Leukocytosis

- ↑ K, **WBC**, viscosity, vitamin – (B$_{12}$)
- ↓ ESR

Leukodystrophy, Metachromatic

- ↑ ALT
- ↓ ✳ **arylsulfatase A** (+ WBC)
- ■ *Urine* ↑ lipids
  - ↓ ✳ **arylsulfatase A**
- ■ *Cerebrospinal Fluid* ↑ **proteins**, ✳ MBP
- ■ *Tears* ↑ ✳ arylsulfatase A

Leukoencephalitis, Subacute Sclerosing

- ■ *Cerebrospinal Fluid* ↑ **proteins**, eos, gamma globulins, **IgG, lym**, MBP, **mono**, plasmocytes

Lipodystrophy

- ↑ C-3 nephritic factor, G, TAG, VLDL-C
- ↓ complement – (**C3**)

Lipoidosis

- ↑ beta globulins, **fibrinogen, cholesterol**, LDL-C, **lipids**
- ↓ albumin, Ca, gamma globulins, Mg
- ■ *Urine* ↑ **proteins, lipids, casts**

ceramide lactoside lipoidosis

- ↓ **beta-galactosidase** (+WBC)

Liver, Fatty (liver steatosis)

- ↑ **acanthocytes**, aldosterone, ✳ **ALP**, ✳ **ALT**, **ammonia**, ✳ **AST**, ✳ **Bil**, ✳ conjugated **Bil**, unconjugated Bil, C-peptide, factors – (II, VII, IX, X), **ferritin, G, globulins, GMT**, ✳ **cholesterol, CHS**, insulin, creatinine, uric acid, pre-beta LP, **WBC**, MDA, ✳ **PT**, RAL, ✳ **TAG, transferrin** satur., urea, VLDL-C
- ↓ **albumin**, ALT, AST, **RBC, Hb, HCT**, K, WBC, Mg, Na, P, PLT
- ■ *Urine* ↑ K, Mg, P

acute fatty liver in pregnancy

- ↑ **ammonia**, ✳ **AST**, ✳ **ALT**, ✳ **Bil**, FDP, creatinine, MAC, **uric acid, WBC**, PT, **PTT**, urea
- ↓ ✳ **fibrinogen, G**, ✳ **PLT, PT**
- ■ *Urine* ↑ ✳ **acetone**, specific gravity

Lupus

CNS lupus

- ■ *Cerebrospinal Fluid* ↑ proteins, IgG, MBP

discoid lupus

- ↑ ANA, anti-RNP Ab
- ↓ complement – (C3)

drug-induced lupus

- ↑ ✳ **ANA**, ANCA, anti-ds-DNA, **anti-ss-DNA**, ✳ **antihistone Ab**, anti-poly (ADP-ribose), anti-RNP, anti-Ro/SSA, anti-La/SSB, anti-Sm, HLA-DR4

systemic lupus erythematosus

↑ **AAT**, Ab against beta-2 GP I, ACE, **AGP**, albumin, aldolase, alpha-1-glo-
bulins, **alpha-2-globulins**, alpha-1-antichymotrypsin, **ALT**, A2MG,
AMA, ✳ **ANA**, ANCA, p-ANCA, ✳ **anti-ds-DNA**, **anti-ss-DNA**, **anti-
DNP**, antiendothelial Ab, antierythrocyte Ab, **antihistone Ab**, anti-
HSP 65, anti-HSP 90, **antiphospholipid Ab**, **anti-WBC**, **anticardio-
lipin Ab**, anti-Ku Ab, antilymphocyte Ab, **antimicrosomal Ab**, anti-
MPO, antimyocardial Ab, antineuronal Ab, anti-p16, anti-p 56, anti-
poly (ADP-ribose), antiribosomal-Po Ab, anti-RNA, **anti-PCNA**,
anti-RA33, **anti-RNP**, anti-Scl-70, ✳ **anti-Sm**, **anti-Ro/SSA**, anti-
La,Ha/SSB, **antiplatelet Ab**, antithyroglobulin Ab, **antithyroidal Ab**,
APTT, ASMA, **AST**, beta-2-glycoprotein I, proteins, **CIC**, CK, CK-MB,
C-3 nephritic factor, **CRP**, **Cu**, CT, factor D, ferritin, **ESR**, FDP, fibrinogen, **gamma globulins**, globulins, glycoproteins, hexosamine, histones, HLA – (**A1**, **B8**, C4A, DQ3, Dqw1, DR2, **DR3**, DR4), h-sICAM-1,
h-sVCAM-1, cold agglutinins, cholesterol, chylomicrons, IFN, **IgA**,
IgD, **IgG**, **IgM**, **K**, complement – (Ba, Bb, C3, C3a, C4d, C9, total), creatine, **creatinine**, cryofibrinogen, **cryoglobulins**, LCA, LD, LD – (3,
4), ✳ **LE cells**, lupus inhibitor, WBC, lym, MAC+RAL, Mb, Mg, **mono**,
MPV, mucoproteins, neopterin, 5-NT, **PT**, **anti-small nuclear RNP**,
anti-p56 annexin XI Ab, antinuclear antigen Ab, pyroglobulins, **RTC**,
RF, syphilis Ab (false), TAG, TT, thrombomodulin, UBBC, **urea**, VDRL
(false), **viscosity**, **VLDL-C**

↓ **albumin**, **proteins**, **CRP**, **RBC**, **factor B**, factors – (VIII, IX, XI, XII), beta-
galactosidase, **haptoglobin**, **Hb**, **HCT**, IL-1, IL-2, C1-esterase inhibitor,
complement – (**C1q**, **C1qINH**, **C1r**, **C1s**, **C2**, ✳ **C3**, ✳ **C4**, **C5**, C6, C7, **C8**,
✳ **CH50**), WBC, lipids, **lym**, **neu**, **T-lym**, **transferrin**, transferrin satur.,
PLT, Zn

■ *Urine* ↑ albumin, **proteins**, **RBC**, Hb, **LD**, creatine, **WBC**, volume, PG,
PT, casts – (**RBC**, cellular, **granular**, Hb, fatty, hyaline, tubular, miscellaneous, waxy)

↓ specific gravity, volume, Zn

■ *Cerebrospinal Fluid* ↑ anti-ds-DNA, **proteins**, IgA, **IgG**, IgM, WBC,
mono, antineuronal Ab

↓ G, complement – (C4, total)

■ *Synovial Fluid* ↑ **ANA**, proteins, **clot formation**, chylomicrons, crystals – (hydroxyapatite), **WBC**, **LE cells**, **lym**, macrophages, mono,
MPS, PMN, RF, viscosity, **volume**

↓ proteins, complement – (**C3**, C4, total), **G**, **WBC**, neu, RF, **viscosity**

■ *Pericardial Fluid* ↑ RBC, complement – (C4, total), volume

■ *Pleural Fluid* ↑ AMS, **ANA**, anti-DNA, proteins, CIC, **LE cells**, lym,
mononuclear cells, neu, PMN, specific gravity

↓ complement – (C3, C4, CH50, total), G, pH

Lymphadenitis, Mesenterial

↑ ESR, **WBC**, lym, neu

Lymphadenopathy, Angioimmunoblastic

↑ **gamma globulins**, WBC

↓ Hb, RBC, HCT, WBC, lym, PLT

Lymphangiectasis, Intestinal

↑ WBC

↓ lym

Lymphangitis

↑ ESR, neu, **WBC**

Lymphogranuloma inguinale

↑ B2M, proteins, eos, gamma globulins, mono

Macroamylasemia

↑ *** AMS**, AAT, lipase

■ *Urine* ↓ AMS

Malabsorption

↑ **ALP**, ALP (intestinal isoenzyme), **amino acids**, AMS, AST, proteins, ceruloplasmin, Cu, DPD, eos, ferritin, **ESR**, G, G tolerance, haptoglobin, HCT, HCO_3^-, K, folate, LD, lipids, **lym**, MAC, MCV, Na, P, **PT**, **PTH**, PLT, urea, TIBC

↓ AAT, **albumin**, ALP, Apo A-IV, *** proteins**, Bil, **Ca**, **ceruloplasmin**, CO_2, *** Cu**, factor – (II), *** Fe**, **RBC**, ferritin, **G**, GIP, haptoglobin, *** Hb**, *** HCT**, HDL-C, HCO_3^-, **cholesterol**, **CHS**, K, complement – (C3), ascorbic acid, **LDL-C**, lipids, **lym**, MAL, MCH, **Mg**, **Na**, P, plasma volume, *** PT**, prothrombin, T4, **TAG**, **TBG**, **trypsinogen**, **UBBC**, urea, vitamin – (A, B₁, B₂, B₆, B₁₂, C, D, E, **K**, *** beta-carotene**, folate), Zn

■ *Urine* ↑ Bence Jones protein, **chloride**, K, 5-HIAA, Na, **oxalate**, phosphate

↓ albumin, Ca, chloride, **K**, 5-HIAA, PABA, Mg, **Na**, **pH**, vitamin – (C)

■ *Stool* ↑ Ca, **volume**, *** fat**

↓ chymotrypsin

■ *Gastric Fluid* ↑ alpha-1-antichymotrypsin

Note: functional tests positive (xylose test, lactose test, lactulose-ramnose test, Schilling's test, beta-carotene test, alpha-1-antitrypsin intestinal clearance test)

folate malabsorption

↓ **folate**, Hb, HCT

intestinal malabsorption

↓ **albumin**, ALP, beta-carotene, **proteins**, **Ca**, **ceruloplasmin**, **Cu**, **Fe**, **G**, GIP, Hb, HDL-C, **cholesterol**, CHS, K, **LDL-C**, **Mg**, **PT**, **TAG**, TBG, urea, vitamin – (A, B₂, B₆, B₁₂, C, D, E, **carotene**, folate), **Zn**

■ *Stool* ↑ volume, fat

iron malabsorption

↓ RBC, **Fe**, Hb, HCT

methionine malabsorption

■ *Urine* ↑ phenylalanine, alpha-hydroxybutyric acid, **methionine**, tyrosine

Malnutrition

↑ **alpha-1-antichymotrypsin**, AST, beta-aminoisobutyric acid, epinephrine, globulins, ICD, **IgG**, immunoreactive trypsin (later), **uric acid**, plasma volume, PT, **GH**, **FFA**

↓ AAT, AGP, *** albumin**, **ALP**, alpha-aminonitrogen, ALT, A2MG, AMS, Apo B, AST, **beta globulins**, **proteins**, B-lym, **Ca**, carbohydrate-deficient transferrin (false), **ceruloplasmin**, CK, Cr, **Cu**, cystine, estradiol, estriol, RBC, factor VIII, *** Fe**, FSH, *** G**, globulins, **HDL-C**, **Hb**, HCT, **cholesterol**, **CHS**, *** IFN**, immunoglobulins, **IgA** (later), IgG (later), IgM (later), IL-1, ILGF-I, immunoreactive trypsin (early), C1-INH, insulin, **K**, complement – (**C1q**, C1s, **C2**, **C3**, C4, total), cortisol, **WBC**, LD, **LDL-C**, LH, lipase, **lym**, methionine, **Mg** (+RBC), *** P**, pH, plasmocytes, PL, plasma volume, ✱ **prealbumin**, PRL, RTC, **Se**, somatomedin C, **T3, T4, TAG, TBG, TIBC, T-lym**, ✱ **transferrin**, ✱ **transthyretin**, triiodothyronine resin uptake, tryptophan, tyrosine, ✱ **urea**, valine, vitamin – (A, B$_6$, B$_{12}$, folate), **Zn**

- *Urine* ↑ ammonia, beta-aminoisobutyric acid, N-formiminoglutamic acid, 3-methylhistidine, Na, volume
  - ↓ Cu, ESR, estriol, hydroxyproline, 17-OHCS, 17-KGS, creatinine, pH, volume, vitamin C
- *Sweat* ↓ chloride, Na
- *Stool* ↑ fat
- *Gastric Fluid* ↓ AMS, lipase, trypsin

Mastocytosis

↑ **bas**, histamine, **mastocytes**
↓ RBC, WBC
- *Gastric Fluid* ↑ BAO, HCl
  - ↓ pH
- *Urine* ↑ histamine
  - ↓ 5-HIAA

Megacolon, Toxic

↑ ESR, **WBC**, PMN
- *Stool* ↑ blood, RBC, Hb

Meningitis

↑ **ADH**, albumin, alpha-2-globulins, AST, proteins, **CK**, CRP, **ESR**, G, glutamine, creatinine, cryofibrinogen, lactoferrin, **LD, WBC**, neu, trypsin, urea
↓ fibrinogen, G, Hb, HCT, chloride, complement – (C3, C4), WBC, Na
- *Urine* ↑ albumin, RBC, G, GFR, volume, VMA
- *Cerebrospinal Fluid* ↑ AAT, adenylate kinase, AFP, albumin, A2MG, arginine, **bacteria** (+ culture), beta-glucuronidase, **proteins**, CRP, CK, eos, phenylalanine, **G**, globulins, glutamine, glycine, hCG, hydroxyproline, chloride, cholesterol, CHS, ICD, **IgG**, IgM, interferon, isoleucine, glutamic acid, **LA, LD**, LD – (4, 5), **WBC**, leucine, **lym**, lysine, **lysozyme**, macrophages, methionine, mono, **neu**, ornithine, P, PG, plasmocytes, PMN, proline, RF, taurine, **pressure**, tryptophan, tyrosine, valine, VMA
  - ↓ **G**, globulins, **chloride**, Mg, pH

acute purulent meningitis

- *Cerebrospinal Fluid* ↑ bacteria (+ culture), **proteins, WBC**, RBC, Na, **PMN, pressure**
  - ↓ **G**, chloride, pH

aseptic meningitis

↑ anti-enterovirus Ab, lym, WBC
- *Cerebrospinal Fluid* ↑ **proteins**, phenylalanine, glycine, leucine, **WBC, lym, mono**, PMN, proline, **pressure**, RBC, valine
  - *Cerebrospinal Fluid* ↓ G

bacterial meningitis

↑ ADH, alpha-2-globulins, **AST**, ✱ **bacteria** (culture), CK, **CRP, ESR**, G, **creatinine**, cryofibrinogen, **LD, WBC**, neu, urea
↓ **chloride**, Hb, **HCT**, complement – (C3, C4), WBC (infants, elderly), **Na**

- ***Cerebrospinal Fluid*** ↑ adenylate kinase, albumin, alpha-1-antichymotrypsin, A2MG, arginine, ✳ **bacteria** (+ culture), ✳ **proteins**, CRP, CK, defensin, eos, phenylalanine, G, globulins, **glutamine**, glycine, hydroxyproline, chloride, **ICD**, IgG, IgM, immunoglobulins, isoleucine, glutamic acid, **LA**, **LD**, LD4, **LD5**, lactoferrin, leucine, ✳ **WBC**, lym, lysine, **lysozyme**, methionine, **neu**, ornithine, **PMN**, proline, RF, taurine, **pressure**, tryptophan, tyrosine, valine
  - ↓ ✳ **G**, globulins, chloride
- ***Urine*** ↑ ✳ **bacteria** (+ culture), GFR, Na

carcinomatous meningitis
- ↑ albumin, proteins, WBC
- ↓ G
- ***Cerebrospinal Fluid*** ↑ AFP, beta-glucuronidase, proteins, phenylalanine, **glutamine**, glycine, hCG, isoleucine, glutamic acid, leucine, lysine, proline, taurine, pressure, RBC, tryptophan, tyrosine, valine
  - ↓ **G**

chemical meningitis
- ***Cerebrospinal Fluid*** ↑ lym, **proteins**, WBC

chronic meningitis
- ***Cerebrospinal Fluid*** ↑ bacteria (+ culture), **proteins**, **lym**, **pressure**, WBC
  - ↓ **G**

cryptococcal meningitis
- ↑ cryptococcal Ag
- ***Cerebrospinal Fluid*** ↑ **proteins**, **lym**, PMN, **WBC**
  - ↓ G

meningitis in amebiasis
- ***Cerebrospinal Fluid*** ↑ lym, **pressure**, WBC, PMN, **proteins**, RBC
  - ↓ G

meningitis in anthrax
- ***Cerebrospinal Fluid*** ↑ bacilli, **proteins**, RBC, PMN
  - ↓ G

meningitis in brucellosis
- ***Cerebrospinal Fluid*** ↑ proteins, lym
  - ↓ G, chloride

meningitis in coccidioidomycosis
- ***Cerebrospinal Fluid*** ↑ **proteins**, WBC, **pressure**

meningitis in cysticercosis
- ***Cerebrospinal Fluid*** ↑ proteins, WBC, pressure
  - ↓ G

meningitis in herpes simplex virus infection
- ***Cerebrospinal Fluid*** ↑ **proteins**, WBC, lym

meningitis in herpes zoster virus infection
- ***Cerebrospinal Fluid*** ↑ **proteins**, WBC

meningitis in leptospirosis
- ***Cerebrospinal Fluid*** ↑ **proteins**, WBC, **lym**, mono, PMN

meningitis in Lyme disease
- ***Cerebrospinal Fluid*** ↑ ✳ antibody against B. **burgdorferi**, **proteins**, IgG, lym, **WBC**

meningitis in measles
- *Cerebrospinal Fluid* ↑ **proteins**, WBC, lym, mono, pressure

meningitis in mumps
- *Cerebrospinal Fluid* ↑ **proteins**, G, IgG, IgM, WBC, **lym**, mono, PMN, pressure
  - ↓ G

meningitis in rabies
- *Cerebrospinal Fluid* ↑ **proteins**, lym, WBC, PMN

meningitis in sarcoidosis
- *Cerebrospinal Fluid* ↑ ACE, proteins, IgG, WBC, **lym**, lysozyme, mono, plasmocytes, pressure
  - ↓ G

meningitis in syphilis
- ↑ **syphilis antibodies**, * VDRL
- *Cerebrospinal Fluid* ↑ **proteins**, gamma globulin, lym, WBC, pressure, * **treponemal DNA (PCR)**, * **VDRL**
- ↓ G, lym

meningitis in toxoplasmosis
- *Cerebrospinal Fluid* ↑ **proteins**, eos, WBC, **mono**, **pressure**

meningococcal meningitis
- ↑ IL-8, **WBC**
- ↓ fibrinogen
- *Urine* ↑ albumin, RBC, G
- *Cerebrospinal Fluid* ↑ **proteins**, * WBC, PMN
  - ↓ G, chloride

Mollaret's meningitis
- ↑ WBC
- *Cerebrospinal Fluid* ↑ lym, * **PMN (early)**, * **proteins**
  - ↓ G

mycotic meningitis
- ↑ plasmocytes
- *Cerebrospinal Fluid* ↑ **proteins**, eos, LA, WBC, **lym**, lysozyme, macrophages, **mono**, plasmocytes, RBC, pressure
  - ↓ G

ricketsial meningitis
- *Cerebrospinal Fluid* ↑ eos, WBC

serous meningitis
- *Cerebrospinal Fluid* ↑ proteins, chloride, mono, Na, pressure

tuberculous meningitis
- ↑ ADH, ESR, **globulins**, **uric acid**, **lym**, WBC, **mono**, RF
- ↓ **proteins**, chloride, Na, * **mycobacterial antigen**, * **anti-mycobacteria Ab**
- *Urine* ↑ uric acid
- *Cerebrospinal Fluid* ↑ **proteins**, * **bacteria (+ culture)**, * **mycobacterial DNA (PCR)**, eos, uric acid, LA, LD, **WBC**, **lym**, lysozyme, macrophages, **mono**, P, plasmocytes, RBC, **tryptophan**, pressure
  - ↓ **G**, **chloride**, Mg

viral meningitis
- ↓ complement – (C4)
- *Cerebrospinal Fluid* ↑ **proteins**, eos, interferon, LD, LD2, LD3, **WBC**, **lym**, **mono**, plasmocytes, pressure

– acute anterior poliovirus meningitis
  - ■ *Cerebrospinal Fluid* ↑ AST, **proteins**, LD, LD2, LD3, **WBC**, **lym**, PMN
– acute viral meningitis
  - ■ *Cerebrospinal Fluid* ↑ ✳ anti-CMV, ✳ anti-EBV, ✳ anti-enterovirus antibody, ✳ anti-HSV, ✳ anti-St. Louis encephalitis virus Ab, ✳ anti-VZV, ✳ HSV antigen, ✳ IgM

Meningocele
  ↑ **AFP**
  - ■ *Amniotic Fluid* ↑ AFP

Meningoencephalitis
amebic meningoencephalitis
  ↑ ALT, **WBC**, **neu**
  - ■ *Cerebrospinal Fluid* ↑ ✳ amebas, **RBC**, **WBC**, lym, lysine, **neu**, PMN, proteins, pressure
  ↓ G
meningoencephalitis in mumps
  - ■ *Cerebrospinal Fluid* ↑ WBC
  ↓ G, WBC

Meningoradiculitis, Garin-Bujadoux-Bannwarth
  - ■ *Cerebrospinal Fluid* ↑ phenylalanine, **glutamine**, glycine, isoleucine, glutamic acid, leucine, lysine, ornithine, proline, valine

Meniscectomy
  - ■ *Synovial Fluid* ↑ crystals – (calcium pyrophosphate)

Menopause
  ↑ **FSH**, **LH**, MCV, P, N-telopeptides
  ↓ Apo B, ✳ **estradiol**, estriol, **estrogens**, HDL-C, **17-OH progesterone**
  - ■ *Urine* ↑ FSH
  ↓ **estriol, estrogens, 17-KS**

Menstruation
  ↑ aldosterone, CA 125, ESR, **fibrinogen**, cholesterol, WBC, Mg, osteocalcin
  ↓ **Fe**, ferritin, fibrinogen, osteocalcin, PLT, **transferrin satur.**
  - ■ *Urine* ↑ proteins (early), RBC (false), Hb (false), porphyrins
    ↓ estrogens (early), pregnanediol, chloride (early), Na (early), volume (early)

Metaplasia, Agnogenic Myeloid
  ↑ **ALP** (WBC), ✳ **anisocytes**, bas, eos, **teardrop RBC**, nucleated RBC, ✳ **PLT**, **poikilocytes**, **PT**, RTC, **uric acid**, vitamin B_{12}, WBC
  ↓ Hb, HCT, PLT, WBC

Methemoglobinemia
  ↑ RBC, RBC Heinz bodies, MAC, ✳ **MHb**

Microangiopathy
  ↓ PLT

Mole, Hydatidiform
  ↑ euglobulin lysis time, **ESR**, HbF, **WBC**, TM – (**hCG**), progesterone
  ↓ AFP, RBC, Hb, HCT, placental lactogen (hPL)
  - ■ *Urine* ↑ hCG
    ↓ pregnanediol

Mucopolysaccharidoses
mucopolysaccharidosis I (Hurler's sy)
  ↓ alpha-L-iduronidase
  - ■ *Urine* ↑ dermatan sulfate, heparan sulfate, ✳ **mucopolysaccharides**

mucopolysaccharidosis II (Hunter's sy)
- ↓ iduronate sulfatase
- ■ *Urine* ↑ dermatan sulfate, heparan sulfate, mucopolysaccharides

mucopolysaccharidosis III (Sanfilippo's sy)
- ↓ sulfamidase, alpha-hexosaminidase
- ■ *Urine* ↑ â **heparan sulfate**, mucopolysaccharides

mucopolysaccharidosis IV (Morquio's sy)
- ↓ beta-galactosidase, N-acetylgalactosamine-6-sulfatase
- ■ *Urine* ↑ ✳ **keratan sulfate**

mucopolysaccharidosis VI (Maroteaux–Lamy sy)
- ↓ arylsulfatase B
- ■ *Urine* ↑ ✳ **dermatan sulfate**

mucopolysaccharidosis VII (Sly's sy)
- ↓ beta-glucuronidase
- ■ *Urine* ↑ **dermatan sulfate**, heparan sulfate, chondroitin 4,6-sulfate

Myasthenia Gravis
- ↑ ACH, albumin, AMA, **ANA**, ✳ **anti-ACHR (binding, blocking, modulating)**, **anti-ds-DNA**, **anti-thymus Ab**, antithyroid Ab, **anti-thyroglobulin Ab**, APA, **ASMA**, CEA, CO_2, HLA – (A1, A3, B7, **B8**, DR2, DR3), **IgA, IgG**, creatinine, creatine, LE cells, MCH, MCV, norepinephrine, ✳ **anti-striational Ab to skeletal muscle**, pCO_2, RF, T3, T3 uptake, T4
- ↓ Hb, HCT, complement – (total), creatinine, **lym**, Mb, O_2 satur., pO_2
- ■ *Urine* ↑ **catecholamines**, creatinine

Myelitis, Acute
- ↑ **WBC**
- ■ *Cerebrospinal Fluid* ↑ **proteins, lym**
  ↓ WBC

Myelofibrosis
- ↑ ACP, **anisocytes**, ALP, ALP (WBC), **bas**, elliptocytes, **eos**, RBC, **glutathione** (RBC), HBD, cryofibrinogen, **uric acid, LD**, LD5, **WBC**, lysozyme, megakaryocytes, mono, myelocytes, **neu, PT, poikilocytes**, RTC, PLT, UBBC, **vitamin B**$_{12}$
- ↓ ALP (WBC), bas, **RBC** (later), **Hb, HCT, folate, WBC** (later), **neu**, osmotic fragility, **PLT** (later)
- ■ *Urine* ↑ uric acid

Myocarditis
- ↑ **ALT, ANA**, anti-enterovirus Ab, **antimyocardial Ab, antiviral Ab, ASLO, AST, CK, CK-MB, CRP, ESR, fibrinogen**, IgM, LD, WBC, lym, myosin
- ↓ cholesterol

bacterial myocarditis
- ↑ ALT, **AST**

rheumatic myocarditis
- ↑ ALT, **AST**

viral myocarditis
- ↑ ALT, **AST**, CK, CK-MB, CRP, **ESR**, IgM, LD, **WBC**, lym, **troponin T** (early)

Myoglobinuria, Paroxysmal
- ↑ aldolase, **aldosterone**, ALT, AMS, **AST**, CK, **CK-MB, K, LD**
- ■ *Urine* ↑ Hb, ✳ **Mb**, casts – (Hb, **Mb**)

Myopathy, Inflammatory

↑ aldolase, **anti-decorin Ab, anti-Sm Ab, anti-Ro,La/SS Ab, antithyroid Ab, B-lym**, CK, gamma globulins, **IL-2**, IL-2-alpha, **LD, mono**, uric acid, **T-lym**

↓ carnitine, gamma globulins

Myositis

↑ ALP, ALT, antisynthetase Ab, **AST, CK**, CK-MB, LD, WBC, **neu**

Myotonia

   atrophic myotonia

↑ ALT, AST

   congenital myotonia

↑ ALT, AST

Myxedema

↑ **ADH**, epinephrine, albumin, alpha-aminonitrogen, ALP, **ALT**, ✶ **anti-microsomal Ab**, ✶ **antithyroglobulin Ab, antithyroid Ab**, ✶ **antithyroperoxidase Ab, anti-TSH-receptor Ab**, AST, **Apo A-I**, Apo B, bas, **beta-carotene**, beta-lipoprotein, Bil, conjugated Bil, proteins, Ca, ✶ **CK, CK-MM, EPO**, ESR, G, HCO_3^-, HLA – (DR3, DR5), ✶ **cholesterol**, ✶ **IDL-C**, IL-6, catecholamines, creatine, creatinine, **uric acid**, LD, **macrocytes, Mb**, MCV, **Mg**, norepinephrine, **pCO₂**, prealbumin, PRL, **TAG**, ✶ **TBG**, ✶ **thyroxine autoantibodies**, ✶ **TSH**, urea, VLDL-C

↓ ALP, ACE, ALP, EPO, RBC, Fe, ferritin, fibronectin, FT3, ✶ **FT4**, ✶ **FTI**, G, **Hb, HCT, HDL-C**, chloride, CHS, iodine, Na, osmolality, osteo-calcin, **pepsinogen, SHBG, GH, T3**, ✶ **T4**, TIBC, tyrosine, vitamin – (A, B₂, B₁₂, folate)

▪ *Urine* ↑ proteins, conjugated Bil, 17-OHCS, 17-KS, catecholamines, creatinine, **Na**

  ↓ Ca, Cu, 17-OHCS, 17-KS, creatine, P

▪ *Cerebrospinal Fluid* ↑ **proteins**

▪ *Pericardial Fluid* ↑ volume

▪ *Peritoneal Fluid* ↓ proteins

▪ *Pleural Fluid* ↓ **proteins**

▪ *Synovial Fluid* ↑ crystals – (calcium pyrophosphate), WBC, viscosity, volume

▪ *Sweat* ↓ chloride, Na

Nanismus Hypophysalis

↓ ALP, **ILGF-I, GH**

Narcolepsy

↑ HLA – (DR2)

Necrosis

↑ AFP, alpha-1-antichymotrypsin, alpha-1-globulins, alpha-2-globulins, ALP, ALT, ammonia, AMS, AST, beta-glucuronidase, conjugated Bil, unconjugated Bil, ceruloplasmin, CK, CRP, Fe, **ESR**, gamma globulins, GMD, GMT, haptoglobin, hexosaminidase, K, creatinine, LD, LD1, LD2, WBC, Mg, Na, OCT, osmolality, TIBC, transferrin, urea

↓ albumin, AMS, proteins, Hb, cholesterol, Mg, pH, transferrin

▪ *Urine* ↑ amino acids, AMS, beta-2-glycoprotein I, proteins, RBC, Hb, hexosaminidase, WBC, volume, fat, casts – (epithelial, RBC)

  ↓ creatinine, specific gravity, volume, osmolality, urea

▪ *Pleural Fluid* ↑ LD

adrenal cortical necrosis
> ■ *Urine* ↑ RBC, Hb

intestine necrosis
> ↑ CK-BB, ESR
> ■ *Urine* ↑ **AMS**
> ■ *Pleural Fluid* ↑ LD

liver necrosis
> ↑ ACP, ADH, **AFP**, alpha-1-glycoprotein, aldolase, **ALP, ALT**, amino acids, **AST, ammonia, beta-glucuronidase, Bil, conjugated Bil, unconjugated Bil**, BSP retention, CEA, FDP, **Fe**, ferritin, **ESR** fibrinogen, gamma globulins, globulins, **GMD, GMT**, haptoglobin, Hb (free), HBsAg, **hexosaminidase**, cholesterol, ICD, IgA, IgM, complement – (C3), LAP, **LD**, LD – (3, 5), lecithin (RBC), **WBC**, lipids, lym, Mg, neu, 5-NT, **OCT**, P, phosphoglucomutase, PL (RBC), PT, pyruvate, RTC, TAG, **TIBC**, transferrin, vitamin B$_{12}$
> ↓ **albumin**, alpha-2-globulins, AMS, AT III, beta globulins, beta-glucuronidase, carotene, **proteins**, ESR, fibrinogen, G, G tolerance, globulins, haptoglobin, Hb, HCT, **cholesterol**, CHS, WBC, lipase, lym, neu, osmotic fragility (RBC), plasminogen, somatomedin C, transferrin, PLT, urea, vitamin – (A, folate), Zn
> ■ *Urine* ↑ **amino acids**, proteins, estrogens, coproporphyrin, N-form-iminoglutamic acid, tyrosine crystals, UBG
> ↓ sulphate
> ■ *Cerebrospinal Fluid* ↑ amino acids
> ■ *Stool* ↑ UBG

pancreas necrosis
> ■ *Urine* ↑ **AMS** (early stage), ESR
> ↓ AMS (later stage)

renal necrosis
– cortical renal necrosis
> ↑ **AST**, ESR, **LD**, LD1, LD2, **WBC**
> ↓ Hb, **HCO$_3^-$, pH**
> ■ *Urine* ↑ **proteins, RBC, WBC**, casts – (RBC)

– tubular renal necrosis
> ↑ K, CK, **creatinine**, Na, **osmolality, urea**
> ↓ Mg
> ■ *Urine* ↑ beta-2-glycoprotein I, **RBC**, Hb, hexosaminidase, Na, myoglobin, volume, fat, casts – (**epithelial**, granular)
> ↓ creatinine, **specific gravity**, volume, **osmolality, urea**

skeletal muscle necrosis
> ↑ carnitine, ESR, **LD**

tissue necrosis
> ↑ alpha-1-antichymotrypsin, alpha-1-globulins, ceruloplasmin, **CRP**, haptoglobin, Mg, Ni

Neonates, Premature
> ↓ Ca, **Cu**, euglobulin lysis time, **Fe**, phenylalanine, Se, vitamin – (E, **folate**)
> ■ *Urine* ↑ cystathionine, galactose, 17-KS

Nephrectomy
> ↓ angiotensin II, **aldosterone, PRA**

Nephritis

↑ AGBMA, alpha-aminonitrogen, alpha-1-globulins, beta-carotene, CEA, **CIC**, CRP, eos, Fe, **ESR**, G, **haptoglobin**, chloride, cholesterol, IgA, IgE, IgG, K, **creatinine**, creatine, **uric acid**, **WBC**, lipids, MAC (later stage), microcytes, mucoproteins, Na, neu, P, PRL, **urea**

↓ **albumin**, ALP, RBC, Hb, HCT, **HCO_3^-**, chloride, K, complement – (**C3**, C4, C6), LD, Mg, Na, neu, plasma volume, osmolality, pCO_2, pH, urea, PLT, vitamin – (A)

- *Urine* ↑ amino acids, **proteins**, eos, RBC, G, Hb, pus, HCO_3^-, K, blood, LD, **WBC**, volume, fat, casts – (RBC, **granular**, **hyaline**, WBC, lipid)
  ↓ Ca, GMT, chloride, **uric acid**, specific gravity, Na, volume, P, pH, urea

interstitial nephritis

– acute interstitial nephritis

↑ CRP, *** eos**, **ESR**, **chloride**, *** IgE**, IgG, K, **creatinine**, **WBC**, **MAC**, **neu**, **urea**

↓ **albumin**, RBC, **Hb**, HCT, **HCO_3^-**, chloride, K, complement – (C3, C6), Mg, **Na**, **pCO_2**, pH

- *Urine* ↑ amino acids, **proteins**, *** eos**, **RBC**, G, **Hb**, **pus**, HCO_3^-, **blood**, beta-2-glycoprotein I, hexosaminidase, Na, myoglobin, WBC, lym, volume, PO_4^-, fat, casts – (**RBC**, granular, epithelial, **WBC**, lipid)
  ↓ Ca, chloride, uric acid, **specific gravity**, Na, **volume**, **osmolality**, P, pH, **urea**

– chronic interstitial nephritis

↑ AGBMA, beta-carotene, CRP, cholesterol, IgE, K, MAC, **urea**

↓ albumin, Hb, HCT, K, Mg, vitamin – (A)

- *Urine* ↑ **proteins**, eos, **G**, pus, WBC, fat, casts – (**WBC**, lipid)
  ↓ Ca, GMT, chloride, specific gravity, volume, P, urea

lupus nephritis

↑ **anti-ss-DNA Ab**, antifibronectin, antilaminin, anti-nucleosome, anti-ribosome protein-P, anti-RNA-polymerase I, anti-Ro/SSA, anti-Sm Ab, CIC, WBC, **urea**

↓ albumin, complement – (C2, **C3**, C4), C1-INH, WBC

- *Urine* ↑ **amino acids**, **proteins**, G, RBC, Hb, **blood**, **WBC**, pus, casts – (epithelial, **RBC**, granular, hyaline, lipid, mixed)
  ↓ K, creatinine, **uric acid**, **volume**, urea

postradiation nephritis

↑ alpha-1-globulins, CEA, PRL, urea

↓ ALP, RBC, Hb, HCT, Mg, neu, plasma volume, **PLT**

- *Urine* ↑ proteins

salt-losing nephritis

↓ aldosterone, RBC, Hb, HCT, chloride, Na

- *Urine* ↑ albumin, chloride, Na
  ↓ specific gravity

Nephrocalcinosis

↑ **Ca**, **chloride**, **MAC**, urea

- *Urine* ↑ proteins, **Ca**, RBC, WBC, **volume**, **P**, casts – (WBC)

Nephrolithiasis

↑ Ca, creatinine, cystine, uric acid, PTH, urea

- *Urine* ↑ bacteria (+ culture), proteins, Ca, cystine, **RBC**, frequency, Hb, pus, **blood**, crystals, uric acid, **WBC**, specific gravity, oxalate, pH, casts, uromucoid, urea
  ↓ pH

Nephropathy

analgesic nephropathy
↑ creatinine, urea
↓ Hb, HCT
- *Urine* ↑ proteins, hexosaminidase, WBC

chronic lead nephropathy
↑ AMS, MAC, RTC, WBC
- *Urine* ↑ amino acids, proteins
- *Synovial Fluid* ↑ monosodium urate crystals

diabetic nephropathy
↑ amylin, G, chloride, K, creatinine, MAC, cystatine C, HbA$_{1c}$, urea
↓ albumin, renin, creatinine clearance
- *Urine* ↑ albumin, **proteins** (quantitatively, uricult), microalbumins, casts – (**granular, hyaline, waxy**)

hypercalcemic nephropathy
↑ Ca, urea
↑ proteins, **Ca**, RBC, WBC, casts – (RBC, WBC), volume (early)
- *Urine* ↑ GFR (later), volume (later)

salt-losing nephropathy
↑ **PRA**
↓ chloride, osmolality
- *Urine* ↑ volume

sickle cell nephropathy
↑ K
↓ K
- *Urine* ↑ **Hb, RBC, blood**
  ↓ **specific gravity, osmolality**

urate nephropathy
↑ creatinine, uric acid
- *Urine* ↑ proteins, blood

Nephrosclerosis, Malignant
↑ **aldosterone**, lipids, **PRA**, **urea**
↓ albumin, RBC, Hb, HCT, K
- *Urine* ↑ **proteins**, RBC, Hb, **blood**, LD, casts – (RBC, lipid, waxy)
  ↓ K, urea

Nephrosis
↑ AFP, aldosterone, alpha-1-globulins, A2MG, beta globulins, ceruloplasmin, Cu, fibrinogen, **ESR**, gamma globulins, GMT, haptoglobin, chloride, cholesterol, **CHS**, lipids, PRA, TAG, urea
↓ AAT, **albumin**, **alpha-2-globulins**, alpha-aminonitrogen, beta globulins, **proteins**, Ca, CBG, **ceruloplasmin**, Cu, Fe, fibrinogen, FT4, gamma globulins, HDL-C, HCO$_3^-$, mucoproteins, **pH**, T3, **T4**, **TBG**, thyroglobulin, TIBC, **transferrin**
- *Urine* ↑ alpha-aminonitrogen, ✳ **proteins**, lysozyme, specific gravity, casts – (**epithelial**, lipid, waxy)
  ↓ **Ca, 17-KS, P**
- *Cerebrospinal Fluid* ↑ chloride
- *Pleural Fluid* ↑ LA
- *Sweat* ↓ chloride, Na

Neuropathy

diabetic neuropathy

↑ GPs, HbA$_{1c}$
- *Urine* ↑ proteins
- *Cerebrospinal Fluid* ↑ proteins

motor neuropathy

↑ Ab against Ga1NAc-GD1a, anti-GM1 ganglioside Ab, anti-GD1a Ab, anti-MAG Ab

– multifocal motor neuropathy

↑ **anti-GM1 Ab** (IgM)
- *Cerebrospinal Fluid* ↑ proteins

sensory neuropathy

↑ Ab against Purkinje cells, anti-GD1b Ab, anti-MAG Ab

Neutropenia

idiopathic neutropenia

↑ **antineutrophil Ab**, mono
↓ WBC, **neu**

immune neutropenia

↑ **antineutrophil Ab**
↓ WBC, **neu**

periodic neutropenia

↑ eos, mono
↓ WBC, ✳ **neu**

Obesity

↑ ALT, androstenedione, AST, beta-endorphins, BHBA, cAMP, C-peptide, estrogens, estrone, **G**, glucagon, glycerol, GMT, **cholesterol**, **CHS**, **ILGF-I**, insulin, IRI, isoleucine, 17-KS, **uric acid**, ketobodies, cortisol, **LDL-C**, leucine, **lipids**, osteocalcin, PTH, **TAG**, VIP, vitamin – (D), **VLDL-C**, FFA

↓ AFP, euglobulin lysis time, fructosamine, FSH, G, HDL-C, IGFBP-1, LH, **SHBG**, **GH**, testosterone, vitamin – (C)

- *Urine* ↑ G, 17-OHCS, 17-KGS, 17-KS

Obstruction

biliary duct obstruction

↑ ACP, alpha-1-globulins, alpha-2-globulins, aldolase, **ALP**, ALP (biliary ways isoenzyme), **ALT**, AMS, ANA, Apo B-100, ASMA, **AST**, beta globulins, **Bil**, **conjugated Bil**, unconjugated Bil, BSP retention, CEA, CRP, clotting time, elastase, fibrinogen, GMD, **GMT**, **haptoglobin**, hexosaminidase, chenodeoxycholic acid, cholic acid, **cholesterol**, ICD, IgA, **LAP**, **LD**, LD5, lecithin (RBC), lipase, LPs, mucoproteins, **5-nucleotidase**, OCT, **PL**, **PT**, **TAG**

↓ factor II, lipase, osmotic fragility (RBC), vitamin – (A, B$_2$, K)

- *Urine* ↑ **conjugated Bil**, bile acids, LAP, pH, pregnanediol, **UBG** (infection)
  ↓ Na, volume, **UBG**
- *Stool* ↑ fat
  ↓ Bil, UBG

fetal intestinal obstruction

- *Amniotic Fluid* ↑ AFP

intestinal obstruction

    ↑ **ALP, AMS,** AMS (P), **AST,** unconjugated Bil, **CK, G, Hb** (later), **HCT** (later), HCO$_3^-$, chloride, **creatinine,** creatine, LD, **WBC,** lipase, **Na, neu, P,** pCO$_2$, **pH,** PMN, **urea**

    ↓ albumin, **cholesterol, chloride,** K, WBC, Na, pCO$_2$, pH, vitamin – (B$_2$)

    ■ *Urine* ↑ AMS, proteins, Na, **specific gravity**
        ↓ volume

    ■ *Peritoneal Fluid* ↑ AMS, bacteria, RBC, **proteins, TAG**

intracranial obstruction

    ■ *Cerebrospinal Fluid* ↑ **proteins,** pressure

intrahepatic obstruction

    ↑ **ALP,** ALP (WBC), ALT, Apo B, AST, **conjugated Bil,** unconjugated Bil, GMD, GMT, **cholesterol,** ICD, LDL-C, 5-nucleotidase, PT, **PL,** TAG

    ■ *Urine* ↑ **Bil**
        ↓ UBG

    ■ *Stool* ↓ Bil, UBG

lymphatic obstruction

    ■ *Peritoneal Fluid* ↑ **proteins,** TAG

pancreatic duct obstruction

    ↑ **AMS,** lipase, lipids

    ↓ AMS

    ■ *Stool* ↓ **chymotrypsin,** trypsin

pyloric obstruction

    ↑ **HCO$_3^-$, pH**

    ↓ **chloride, K, Na**

    ■ *Urine* ↑ pH
        ↓ Na

    ■ *Gastric Fluid* ↑ LA, **volume**

spinal cord channel obstruction

    ■ *Cerebrospinal Fluid* ↑ fibrinogen, pressure

superior vena cava obstruction

    ■ *Cerebrospinal Fluid* ↑ **pressure**

urinary tract obstruction

    ↑ EPO, RBC, K, **creatinine,** urea

    ↓ LD, osmolality

    ■ *Urine* ↑ bacteria (+ culture), **RBC, Hb, pus,** volume
        ↓ pus, **creatinine,** WBC, volume, osmolality, pH, casts

Occlusion, Renal Artery

    ■ *Urine* ↑ RBC, Hb, Mb
        ↓ **urea**

Omphalocele

    ↑ AFP

    ■ *Amniotic Fluid* ↑ **AFP**

Oophorectomy, Bilateral

    ↑ PRL

Orchidectomy

    ↑ LH

    ↓ **testosterone**

    ■ *Urine* ↑ hydroxyproline

Orchitis

    ↑ **FSH,** ESR, creatinine, **WBC**

    ■ *Urine* ↑ proteins, RBC, **FSH**

        ■ *Seminal Fluid* ↑ spermatozoa count

Osteitis Fibrosa Cystica
        ↑ ALP, CA, urea
        ↓ P, pCO$_2$

Osteoarthritis
        ↑ ESR, WBC, osteocalcin, RF
        ↓ osteocalcin
        ■ *Synovial Fluid* ↑ C3, clot formation, RBC, crystals – (hydroxyapatite,
            calcium pyrophosphate), WBC, mono, **viscosity**, volume

Osteoarthrosis
        ↑ CRP, hyaluronate, keratan sulfate
        ■ *Urine* ↑ deoxypyridinoline, glycosaminoglycans, pyridinoline
        ■ *Synovial Fluid* ↑ hydroxyapatite crystals, viscosity, **volume**

Osteochondritis Dissecans
        ■ *Synovial Fluid* ↑ **clot formation**, WBC, **viscosity**, **volume**

Osteochondromatosis
        ■ *Synovial Fluid* ↑ WBC, **viscosity**, volume

Osteodystrophy, Renal
        ↑ ALP, Ca, **osteocalcin**, **P**, PTH
        ↓ Ca, vitamin – (D)
        ■ *Urine* ↑ hydroxyproline
            ↓ **Ca**

Osteogenesis Imperfecta
        ↑ **ACP**, ALP, osteocalcin

Osteomalacia
        ↑ **ALP**, Ca, cAMP, osteocalcin, **PTH**, vitamin D
        ↓ **Ca**, Ca^{2+}, osteocalcin, P, vitamin – (**D**)
        ■ *Urine* ↑ **amino acids**, Ca, cAMP, G, hydroxyproline – (total, free), P
            ↓ Ca, Ca^{2+}, hydroxyproline, **P**

Osteomyelitis
        ↑ aldolase, alpha-2-globulins, **ALP**, **ALT**, ✳ **bacteria** (culture), **CRP**,
            elastase (PMN), ✳ **ESR**, ferritin, ✳ **WBC**, **mono**, ✳ **mucoproteins**, **neu**,
            RF, **PLT**
        ↓ albumin, **cholesterol**, **Hb**, **HCT**, immunoglobulins, P
        ■ *Urine* ↑ total hydroxyproline

    cranial osteomyelitis
        ■ *Cerebrospinal Fluid* ↑ WBC

Osteopetrosis
        ↑ **ACP**, lym, **nucleated RBC**
        ↓ Hb, HCT

Osteoporosis
        ↑ **ACP**, ACP (prostatic), ✳ **ALP**, ✳ ALP (bone isoenzyme), androstenedi-
            one (F), ✳ **deoxypyridinoline**, ESR, FSH, ✳ **hydroxyproline**, creati-
            nine, uric acid, **WBC**, ✳ **osteocalcin**, **PICP**, PT, PTH, pyridinoline,
            TSH, vitamin – (**D2**)
        ↓ albumin, **Ca**, fluoride, Hb, HCT, **osteocalcin**, P, vitamin – (D)
        ■ *Urine* ↑ ✳ **Ca**, **chloride**, hydroxyproline – (✳ **total**, ✳ **free**), ✳ **P**,
            telopeptide fragments

    primary postmenopausal osteoporosis
        ↑ ALP, **osteocalcin**
        ↓ osteocalcin, PTH, vitamin – (D)
        ■ *Urine* ↑ Ca, hydroxyproline – (total, free)

primary senile osteoporosis

   ↑ ALP, androstenedione (F), osteocalcin, PTH, vitamin – (D2)

   ■ *Urine* ↑ Ca²⁺, hydroxyproline – (total, free)

Otitis

   ↑ CRP, ESR, **WBC**, neu

   ■ *Cerebrospinal Fluid* ↑ WBC

Otorrhea, CSF

   ■ *Cerebrospinal Fluid* ↑ pressure

Ovulation

   ↑ FSH, LH, progesterone

   ↓ estrogen

   ■ *Urine* ↑ **pregnanediol**

Oxalosis, Primary

   ↑ ✻ oxalic acid, urea

   ■ *Urine* ↑ glycolic acid, glyoxylic acid, crystals – (calcium oxalate), ✻ oxalic acid

Pacemaker, Atrial

   ↑ **ANF**, cGMP, NT-pro-ANP

Pancreatectomy

   ↑ **G**

   ↓ **AMS, C-peptide, glucagon**, chymotrypsin

   ■ *Urine* ↑ AMS

Pancreatitis

acute pancreatitis

   ↑ AAT, ACA, **aldolase, ALP, ALT**, A2MG, ✻ **AMS** (3–6 hrs after, peak at 20–30 hrs, decrease 24–96 hrs), ✻ **AMS-P isoenzyme, AMS-S isoenzyme**, anti-Mycoplasma pneumoniae Ab, **AST, Bil**, unconjugated Bil, conjugated Bil, **Ca**, CA 15-3, CA 19-9, CA 125, **CEA, CK**, ✻ **CRP**, ✻ **elastase** (lasts 8 days), epinephrine, phospholipase A2, ✻ **ESR**, ✻ **G, globulins, glucagon**, glucocorticoids, alpha-glucosidase, ✻ **GMT, Hb**, ✻ **HCT**, cholesterol, chylomicrons, **chymotrypsin**, immunoreactive trypsin, calcitonin, catecholamines, ✻ **creatinine**, LA, **LAP, LD**, LD5, LDL-C, ✻ **lipase** (3–6 hrs after, peak at 18–24 hrs, decrease 7–14 days), lipids, LPs, ✻ **WBC**, MAC, MAL, **MD**, ✻ **methemalbumin**, neu, 5-NT, pancreatic polypeptide, PCT, PTH, ✻ **TAG**, ✻ **trypsin, trypsinogen, urea**, VLDL-C

   ↓ AAT, **albumin**, alpha-2-globulins, **A2MG**, amino acids, AMS, AT III, ✻ **Ca**, ✻ **Ca²⁺, Hb, HCT**, cholesterol, insulin, ✻ **K**, complement – (C3), lipoprotein lipase, **Mg, Na**, O₂ satur., osmolality, P, **pO₂**

   ■ *Urine* ↑ amino acids, ✻ **AMS**, Bil, **G, 17-OHCS**, 17-KGS, catecholamines, tetrahydrodeoxycortisol, **trypsinogen-2**

   ↓ Mg, volume

   ■ *Stool* ↑ fat

   ■ *Cerebrospinal Fluid* ↑ AMS

   ■ *Peritoneal Fluid* ↑ ACP, albumin, ✻ **AMS**, arylsulfatase, **proteins, RBC**, beta-glucuronidase, **lipase, WBC, methemalbumin**, volume

   ↓ AAT

   ■ *Pleural Fluid* ↑ albumin, AMS, **proteins**, eos, **RBC, LD, WBC, lipase, neu**, specific gravity, TM – (CEA)

   ↓ pH

   ■ *Saliva* ↑ GMT

acute hemorrhagic pancreatitis

↑ aldolase, AMS, G, WBC

↓ AMS

■ *Urine* ↑ ✱ AMS, G, 17-OHCS, tetrahydrodeoxycortisol, **trypsinogen-2**

chronic pancreatitis (relapsing)

↑ ACA, **ALP**, **ALT**, A2M, **AMS**, **AST**, beta-carotene, **Bil**, **CCK-PZ**, elastase, ESR, **G**, **GMT**, **cholesterol**, calcitonin, **lipase**, **WBC**, lipids, neu, **PL**, **TAG**, TM – (CA 15-3, CA 19-9, CA 125, CEA), PLT, **TAG**, trypsin, VLDL-C

↓ **albumin**, AMS (advanced), Apo A-IV, **proteins**, **Ca**, Ca²⁺, RBC, **elastase**, Fe, G, G tolerance, **glucagon**, Hb, immunoreactive trypsin, lipoprotein lipase, **Mg**, Na, osmolality, trypsin, ✱ **trypsinogen**, vitamin – (carotene, A, **B₁₂**, D, E)

■ *Urine* ↑ **AMS**, G

↓ AMS, Mg

■ *Stool* ↑ proteins, volume, FA, lipids, ✱ **fat**

↓ **chymotrypsin**, elastase-1

■ *Peritoneal Fluid* ↑ ✱ **AMS**, **proteins**

■ *Pleural Fluid* ↑ AMS, proteins, eos, RBC, LD, WBC, neu, specific gravity

↓ G, pH

■ *Duodenal Fluid* ↑ HCO₃⁻, AMS, trypsin

■ *Sweat* ↑ Na

■ *Saliva* ↓ HCO₃⁻

Pancytopenia

↑ LD, lym (relat)

↓ **Hb**, haptoglobin, **HCT**, lym, RBC, RTC, PLT, **WBC**

Panhypopituitarism

↑ conjugated Bil

↓ ✱ **ACTH**, ✱ **FSH**, **G**, cortisol, ✱ **LH**, Na, ✱ **osmolality**, PRL, progesterone, ✱ **GH**, T4, ✱ **TSH**

■ *Urine* ↓ FSH, 17-KGS, **17-KS**, LH

Panleukopenia, Autoimmune

↓ bas, lym, WBC, neu

Paralysis

familial periodic paralysis

↑ AST, **CK**, ketones, LA, **WBC**, Na, neu, pyruvate

↓ eos, ✱ **K** (attack), **P**, **uric acid**

■ *Urine* ↑ aldosterone, proteins, FSH, HCG, 17-KS, uric acid

↓ G, chloride, **K** (attack), Na

■ *Cerebrospinal Fluid* ↓ K

progressive paralysis

↑ **gamma globulins**, VDRL

■ *Urine* ↓ creatinine

■ *Cerebrospinal Fluid* ↑ proteins, **lym**, **PMN**

Paraproteinemia

↑ **beta globulins**, **proteins**, CIC, CMV, fibrinogen, ✱ **gamma globulins** (M-gradient, gamma/beta area), HIV, HLA – (B5), **IgG**, toxoplasma, viscosity

↓ TT

■ *Urine* ↑ proteins, Bence Jones protein

■ *Synovial Fluid* ↑ cryoprotein

Parotitis

↑ **AMS**, AMS (S-isoenzyme), **lipase**
- *Urine* ↑ **AMS**
- *Saliva* ↑ proteins, chloride, IgA, IgG, Na
  ↓ P

Pellagra

↑ Cu
↓ RBC, Hb, HCT, ✶ **niacin, tryptophan**, vitamin – (B$_6$)
- *Urine* ↑ **porphyrins**
  ↓ nicotinamide

Pemphigoid, Bullous

↑ **epidermal autoantibodies, eos, IgE,** ✶ **pemphigoid Ab,** WBC

Pemphigus, Vulgar

↑ alpha-1-globulins, alpha-2-globulins, ANA, **anti-skin Ab, eos, epidermal squamous cell autoantibodies,** eos, **ESR,** fibrinogen, **globulins,** HLA – (A10, DR4), **IgE,** IgM, **K,** cryoglobulins, **WBC,** ✶ **pemphigus Ab,** plasma volume, selectin E
↓ albumin, **proteins, Ca,** eos, **RBC, HCT, chloride,** IgG, complement – (total), **Na**
- *Urine* ↓ volume

Pentosuria

- *Urine* ↑ ✶ **L-Xylulose**

Perforation

   intestinal perforation

↑ ALP, **AMS,** elastase (PMN), **ESR, WBC, lipase**
- *Urine* ↑ AMS
- *Peritoneal Fluid* ↑ ammonia, AMS, proteins, LD, ✶ **WBC**

   peptic ulcer perforation

↑ ACE, alpha-1-globulins, alpha-2-globulins, **AMS,** Ca, CEA, ESR, gastrin, cryofibrinogen, WBC, pepsinogen, pH, TIBC, urea
↓ albumin, proteins, Fe, G, G tolerance, Hb, HCT, chloride, K, lipase, MCH, MCHC, MCV, Na, norepinephrine
- *Urine* ↑ AMS
- *Peritoneal Fluid* ↑ ammonia, **AMS,** proteins, **LD,** WBC
- *Gastric Fluid* ↑ lysolecithin, pH
  ↓ pH

   spontaneous esophagus perforation

   Pleural Fluid ↑ ✶ **gastric content**

Periarteritis, Cerebral

   Cerebrospinal Fluid ↑ proteins, eos, lym, mono

Pericarditis

↑ ammonia, ANA, anti-DNA, anti-Mycoplasma pneumoniae Ab, anti-myocardial Ab, anti-RNA, AST, **CK,** CK-MM, CRP, **ESR, WBC**
↓ albumin, lym
- *Pericardial Fluid* ↑ bacteria (+ culture), RBC, WBC, volume
  ↓ G
- *Urine* ↑ proteins

   bacterial pericarditis

↑ ammonia, ANA, anti-DNA, antimyocardial Ab, anti-RNA, AST, **CK,** CRP, **ESR, WBC**
↓ albumin, lym

- *Pericardial Fluid* ↑ RBC, WBC, volume
   ↓ G

constrictive pericarditis
   ↑ ALT
   ↓ albumin, lym
- *Urine* ↑ protein

idiopathic pericarditis
   ↑ ANA, anti-DNA, antimyocardial Ab, anti-RNA
- *Pericardial Fluid* ↑ RBC

purulent pericarditis
   ↑ ALT, **CRP, ESR, WBC**
- *Pericardial Fluid* ↑ RBC, WBC, volume

traumatic pericarditis
- *Pericardial Fluid* ↑ RBC, WBC, volume

tuberculous pericarditis
   ↑ lym
- *Pericardial Fluid* ↑ RBC, WBC, lym, volume

uremic pericarditis
- *Pericardial Fluid* ↑ RBC, volume

Peritonitis
   ↑ aldosterone, ALP, **AMS**, CA 125, CRP, **ESR, Hb, HCT**, catecholamines, lipase, **WBC, Na, neu, urea**
   ↓ **albumin**, proteins, osmolality, plasma volume, **K**, WBC, Na
- *Urine* ↑ aldosterone, AMS, catecholamines
   ↓ volume
- *Peritoneal Fluid* ↑ AMS, **bacteria** (+ culture), **proteins**, pus, eos, RBC, blood, LA, LD, ✳ **WBC, lym**, neu, PMN, **specific gravity**, volume
   ↓ **G, pH**
- *Pleural Fluid* ↑ RBC

bacterial peritonitis
   ↑ ALP, AMS, ✳ **bacteria** (culture), CA 125, **ESR, WBC**
- *Peritoneal Fluid* ↑ ✳ **bacteria** (+ culture), **LA, LD**, ✳ **WBC**, ✳ **neu**, ✳ **PMN**, ✳ **proteins**, specific gravity, volume
   ↓ **G**, ✳ **pH**

granulomatous peritonitis
- *Peritoneal Fluid* ↑ proteins

tuberculous peritonitis
- *Peritoneal Fluid* ↑ lym, specific gravity
   ↓ G

Pharyngitis, Acute
   ↑ ASLO, CRP, ESR, mucoproteins, WBC

Phenylketonuria
   ↑ ✳ **phenylalanine**, Mn
   ↓ Mn, Se, serotonin (untreated), tyrosine
- *Urine* ↑ amino acids, **phenylalanine**, acetic acid, **lactic acid**, phenylacetic acid, **phenylpyruvic acid**
   ↓ 5-HIAA, pH
- *Cerebrospinal Fluid* ↑ **phenylalanine**

Phlegmon
   ↑ alpha-1-globulins, proteins, **ESR, WBC**

Pityriasis Rosea

   ↑ eos, WBC

Plasmapheresis

   ↓ coagulation time, CHS, PLT, proteins

Pleuritis

   exudative pleuritis

   ↑ **CA 125**, **CRP**, **fibrinogen**, **ESR**, **WBC**, lym

   ↓ proteins

   ▪ *Pleural Fluid* ↑ adenosine deaminase, AMS, ANA, bacteria (+ culture), **proteins**, eos, RBC, G, blood, creatinine, **LD**, LE cells, **lipids**, lym, specific gravity, pH, **PMN**, RF

   ↓ G, cholesterol, WBC, pH

   lupus pleuritis

   ↑ ESR

   ▪ *Pleural Fluid* ↑ LD

   rheumatoid pleuritis

   ↑ ESR

   ↓ G

   ▪ *Pleural Fluid* ↑ adenosine deaminase, **proteins**, fibronectin, LD, lym, RF, turbidity

   ↓ **G**

Pneumoconiosis

   ↑ ACE, ANA, Ca, **RBC**, **gamma globulins**, Hb, pCO_2, RAC, RF, WBC

   ↓ Hb, HCT, pO_2, pCO_2, satur. O_2

   ▪ *Urine* ↑ beryllium, **Ca**

neumoencephalography

   ▪ *Cerebrospinal Fluid* ↑ WBC

Pneumonia

   ↑ AAT, **ADH**, albumin, aldolase, alpha-1-globulins, ALP, AMS, ANA, c-ANCA, ASLO, **AST**, **bacteria** (culture), Bil, CEA, ceruloplasmin, **CRP**, D-dimers, **fibrinogen**, phospholipase A2, **ESR**, haptoglobin, cold agglutinins, complement – (C3), **uric acid**, LA, lactoferrin, **LD**, LD3, **WBC**, lym, mucoproteins, **neu**, NSE, orosomucoid, pCO_2, **pH**, **RAL**, SCCA, TPA

   ↓ **albumin**, alpha-aminonitrogen, proteins, CO_2, **Hb**, **HCT**, **chloride**, cholesterol, IgA, complement – (C3, C4), WBC, Na, neu, O_2 satur., P, **pCO_2**, **pO_2**, prealbumin, transferrin, PLT

   ▪ *Sputum* ↑ bacteria (+ culture), pus, blood, * **WBC**, macrophages, volume, PMN, viscosity, color changes

   ▪ *Pleural Fluid* ↑ eos, **WBC**, PMN, RBC, **neu**, RF

   ↓ C3, C4, G, pH

   ▪ *Bronchoalveolar Lavage Fluid* ↑ mastocytes, PMN, T-lym

   ▪ *Urine* ↑ alpha-aminonitrogen, **proteins**, ketones, creatinine, uric acid, **WBC**, UBG, casts – (granular, hyaline)

   ↓ chloride

   ▪ *Cerebrospinal Fluid* ↓ chloride

   aspiration pneumonia

   ↑ **WBC**

   ↓ pCO_2

atypical pneumonia
> ↑ **Ab against Influenza virus**, ANA, **anti-Mycoplasma pneumoniae Ab**, **cold agglutinins**, **ESR**, LD, **WBC**, **mucoproteins**, syphilis Ab (false), VDRL (false)

bacterial pneumonia
> ↑ CEA, **CRP**, D-dimers, **fibrinogen**, phospholipase A2, **ESR**, LD, **WBC**, **mucoproteins, neu**
> ↓ complement – (C3), pCO_2
> ■ *Sputum* ↑ bacteria (+ culture), pus, blood, ✳ **WBC**, macrophages, volume, PMN, viscosity, color changes

eosinophilic pneumonia
> ↑ eos
> ■ *Bronchoalveolar Lavage Fluid* ↑ mastocytes, **PMN**, **T-lym** (CD4+, CD8+)

Mycoplasmal pneumonia
> ↑ ✳ **Ab against Mycoplasma pneumoniae** (IgG, IgM), ✳ **bacteria** (+ culture), CRP, **ESR**, WBC, **cold agglutinins**, ✳ **mycoplasma antigen**

pneumonia caused by Legionella
> ↑ ALT, AST, **ESR**, **WBC**, neu, urea
> ↓ Na, P
> ■ *Urine* ↑ proteins, blood
> ■ *Cerebrospinal Fluid* ↑ proteins, PMN

pneumonia caused by Pneumococci
> ↑ AST, complement – (C3), VDRL (false)
> ↓ pCO_2, WBC

pneumonia caused by Pneumocystis carinii
> ↑ RAL
> ↓ pCO_2, pO_2

pneumonia caused by Str. pneumoniae
> ↑ ✳ **bacteria** (culture), **ESR**, **WBC**
> ↓ pCO_2
> ■ *Sputum* ↑ ✳ **bacteria** (+ culture)

pneumonia caused by Staphylococci
> ↑ ✳ **bacteria** (culture), **ESR**, **WBC**
> ↓ WBC, pCO_2
> ■ *Sputum* ↑ ✳ **bacteria** (+ culture), ✳ **PMN**

viral pneumonia
> ↑ ADH, **ALP**, **AST**, CO_2, LD5, **lym**, WBC, neu, pCO_2
> ↓ Hb, HCT, pCO_2, pO_2, **WBC**, lym, neu, T-lym
> ■ *Pleural Fluid* ↑ proteins, CEA, eos, LD, specific gravity
> > ↓ G, pH

Pneumothorax
> ↑ ADH, **pCO_2**
> ↓ chloride, Na, pH, **pO_2**
> ■ *Bronchoalveolar Lavage Fluid* ↑ RBC
> ■ *Pleural Fluid* ↑ eos

Polyangiitis, Microscopic
> ↑ **ANCA, c-ANCA, p-ANCA**

Polyarteritis Nodosa

↑ AGBMA, albumin, alpha-1-globulins, **alpha-2-globulins**, **ALT**, **ANA**, ANCA, **c-ANCA**, p-ANCA, anti-ds-DNA Ab, anti-MPO, antineutrophil Ab, **beta globulins**, **CIC**, CK, **CRP**, **eos**, **ESR**, Fe, gamma globulins, globulins, **HBsAg**, **cholesterol**, **cold agglutinins**, IFN-alpha, IgD, IgE, IL-2, immunoglobulins, complement – (C3, C4, total), **creatinine**, **cryoglobulins**, LE cells, **WBC**, **lym**, MAC+RAL, **mono**, **neu**, RF, TIBC, TNF-alpha, **PLT**, **urea**

↓ **albumin**, RBC, Hb, HCT, complement – (**C3**, C4, total), MCH, MCHC, MCV, neu, transferrin satur.

■ *Urine* ↑ albumin, **proteins**, RBC, Hb, **blood**, creatinine, **fat bodies**, casts – (**RBC**, cellular, granular, hyaline)
↓ volume

■ *Pleural Fluid* ↑ eos

■ *Stool* ↑ blood

■ *Synovial Fluid* ↑ WBC, PMN, volume
↓ viscosity

Polychondritis

↑ alpha globulins, ANA, ANCA, c-ANCA, **ESR**, gamma globulins, WBC, RF

↓ RBC, Hb, HCT

■ *Urine* ↑ proteins, **RBC**, **Hb**

■ *Synovial Fluid* ↑ PMN
↓ viscosity

Polycythemia

chronic relative polycythemia

↑ ALP (WBC), EPO, ✳ RBC, ✳ Hb, ✳ HCT, cholesterol, ✳ uric acid, LD, ✳ WBC, ✳ RTC, ✳ PLT, transferrin, transferrin receptor, ✳ viscosity

↓ **ESR**, blood volume, plasma volume

■ *Urine* ↑ RBC, Hb

polycythemia vera

↑ ACP, PLT aggregation, aldolase, ✳ ALP (WBC), ✳ anisocytes, AST, bas, basophilic stippling (RBC), Bil, unconjugated Bil, Ca, elliptocytes, eos, FDP, ✳ RBC, ✳ Hb, ✳ HCT, histamine, nucleated RBC, cold agglutinins, IgG, IgM, K, **uric acid**, cryoglobulins, **LD**, ✳ WBC, lysozyme, macrocytes, MCV, ✳ microcytes, neu, blood volume, ✳ RBC mass, RBC osmotic resistance, plasma volume, PMN, pO₂, ✳ poikilocytes, pyroglobulins, RTC, O₂ satur, TT, TIBC, ✳ PLT, transferrin, transcobalamin I, III, UBBC, vitamin B₁₂ binding capacity, ✳ viscosity, vitamin – (B₁, B₁₂)

↓ AT III, ✳ **EPO**, factor – (V), Fe, ferritin, **fibrinogen**, ESR, MCH, MCHC, MCV, O₂ satur., plasma volume, PTT, **RBC osmotic fragility**, RTC, sideroblasts, siderocytes, transferrin satur.

■ *Urine* ↑ albumin, RBC, Hb, histamine, uric acid, lysozyme, UBG
↓ EPO

secondary polycythemia

↑ ALP (WBC), **Bil**, **EPO**, **RBC**, **Hb**, **histamine**, **HCT**, **cholesterol**, **uric acid**, LD, **MCH**, **MCV**, MHb, **blood volume**, pO₂, **RTC**, transferrin, viscosity

↓ **ESR**, Fe, MCH, MCHC, MCV, **pO₂**, **O₂ satur.**

■ *Urine* ↑ EPO, coproporphyrin

■ *Stool* ↑ urobilin

Polydipsia

↓ ADH, Na, osmolality

■ *Urine* ↑ **volume**
  ↓ **osmolality, specific gravity**

Polyglobulia

↑ **RBC, HCT, Hb,** NBB

↓ **ESR,** clot retraction

Polymyalgia, Rheumatic

↑ **alpha-1-globulins, alpha-2-globulins, ALP,** ALT, **AMA,** ANA, AST, **CRP, fibrinogen, ESR,** gamma globulins, IgM, cryoglobulins, **WBC,** 5-nucleotidase, RF, PLT

↓ **albumin, RBC, Hb, HCT,** complement – (C3)

■ *Synovial Fluid* ↑ WBC, PMN, volume
  ↓ viscosity

Polymyositis

↑ AHBD, **aldolase, alpha-2-globulins, ALT, ANA,** anti-ds-DNA, anti-ss-DNA, anti-aminoacyl-tRNA synthetase Ab – (anti-EJ, anti-OJ, ✶ **anti-PL-7,** anti-PL-12), ✶ **anti-histidyl-tRNA synthetase Ab,** ✶ **anti-Jo-1,** anti-Jo-2, anticardiolipin Ab, anti-Ku, anti-Mi-2, anti-p 56, **anti-PM-1, anti-RNP, anti-Scl 70,** anti-SRP, **anti-Ro/SSA, anti-La,Ha/SSB,** anti-SRP, **antisynthetase Ab,** ASMA, **AST,** beta globulins, **CK,** CK-MB, **CK-MM, eos,** ✶ **ESR, gamma globulins,** ✶ **HCV,** HLA – (B8, DQA1, **DR3,** DR5, DR7, DRw6, DRw52, DRw53), **LD,** LE cells, **WBC, Mb, non-histone ANA, pCO₂, PM-1 Ab, RF,** thymus ANA

↓ RBC, Hb, HCT

■ *Urine* ↑ **creatine,** Mb
  ↓ creatinine

■ *Synovial Fluid* ↑ WBC, PMN
  ↓ viscosity

Polyneuritis, Acute

↓ transketolase

■ *Cerebrospinal Fluid* ↑ proteins, eos, ✶ WBC, lym, mono

■ *Urine* ↑ VMA

Polyneuropathy

chronic immune demyelinating polyneuropathy

↑ Ab against Ga1NAc-GD1a, anti-GD1a Ab, **anti-heparan sulfate Ab** (IgM), anti-sulfatide Ab, **anti-tubulin Ab** (IgG, IgM)

■ *Cerebrospinal Fluid* ↑ **proteins**

peripheral polyneuropathy

↑ ANCA, c-ANCA, **Ab against Borrelia** (IgG, IgM), **anti-myelin Ab,** anti-sulfatide Ab, B-lym, HIV, E selectin

↓ vitamin – (B₁, E)

■ *Cerebrospinal Fluid* ↑ A2MG, **mono, MBP**

Polyp, Rectal

↑ CEA

↓ Fe

■ *Stool* ↑ blood

Polytrauma

↑ AAT, ADH, PLT adhesion, AGP, aldolase, alpha-1-antichymotrypsin, ALT, A2MG, AMS, **AST,** Bil, unconjugated Bil, CEA, ceruloplasmin, CK, CK-MM, **CRP,** Cu, D-dimers, **elastase,** FDP, fibrinogen, G, glucagon, haptoglobin, **HCT**, IL – (1, 6), K, complement – (Ba, Bb, C3, C3a, C5a, CH50), **creatinine**, creatine, LD, LD 5, lipase, **WBC**, Mb, MD, Mg, myosin, Na, **neu**, PCT, PGE, TNF, **PLT**, urea

↓ albumin, alpha-2-globulins, Cr, **eos**, **proteins**, RBC, **Fe**, **fibrinogen** (early), fibronectin, Hb, HDL-C, HCT, cholesterol, complement – (C1r, C1s, C2, C3, C5, C6, C7, C8, C9, **CH50**), LDL-C, LH, lym, Mn, T3, T-lym, Zn

- *Urine* ↑ AMS, proteins, Cr, RBC, Hb, hexosaminidase, catecholamines, ketones, creatine, creatinine, blood, WBC, Mb, 3-methylhistidine, casts – (lipid)
- *Peritoneal Fluid* ↑ AMS, proteins, RBC, blood, WBC, volume
- *Stool* ↑ blood
- *Synovial Fluid* ↑ clot formation, RBC, crystals – (calcium pyrophosphate), PMN, red colour, **volume**
- *Cerebrospinal Fluid* ↑ adenylate kinase, proteins, **CK**, G, **LA**, macrophages, **MBP**, PG, **pressure**
  ↓ cAMP, pH
- *Pericardial Fluid* ↑ RBC, blood, volume
- *Bronchoalveolar Lavage Fluid* ↑ RBC
- *Pleural Fluid* ↑ proteins, eos, RBC, LA, volume

abdominal polytrauma

↑ **AMS**, PCT, WBC
↓ RBC, HCT
- *Urine* ↑ AMS
- *Peritoneal Fluid* ↑ AMS, proteins, RBC, WBC
- *Stool* ↑ blood

chest polytrauma

↑ CK, PCT, PRL
- *Bronchoalveolar Lavage Fluid* ↑ RBC
- *Pleural Fluid* ↑ proteins, eos, RBC, LA, volume
- *Sputum* ↑ blood

CNS polytrauma

↑ ACE, ADH, AMS, Apo E, **CK**, **CK-MM**, IgM, NSE, pCO_2, prealbumin, protein S-100, transferrin
↓ pO_2, PLT
- *Urine* ↑ AMS, G
- *Cerebrospinal Fluid* ↑ adenylate kinase, proteins, **CK**, G, IgM, **LA**, macrophages, **MBP**, PG, prealbumin, **pressure**, protein S-100, transferrin
  ↓ cAMP, pH

electrical polytrauma

↑ AST, **CK**, CK-MB, LD 5, **WBC**
- *Urine* ↑ albumin, Hb, Mb
- *Cerebrospinal Fluid* ↑ blood

heart polytrauma

↑ myosin
- *Pericardial Fluid* ↑ RBC

joint polytrauma

- *Synovial Fluid* ↑ RBC, crystals – (calcium pyrophosphate), PMN, **volume**

kidney polytrauma

↑ FDP
- *Urine* ↑ proteins, **RBC, Hb**, hexosaminidase, blood, WBC

liver polytrauma

↑ ALT, AST, Bil, LD
- *Peritoneal Fluid* ↑ blood, volume

muscular polytrauma

↑ **aldolase, CK, creatine, creatinine, Mb, Mg**, myosin, **urea**
- *Urine* ↑ creatine, creatinine, Mb, casts – (lipid)

pancreas polytrauma

↑ AMS
- *Urine* ↑ AMS
- *Peritoneal Fluid* ↑ AMS, proteins, RBC, volume

thermic polytrauma

↑ **PLT adhesion**, albumin (early stage), **aldolase, alpha-1-globulins, alpha-2-globulins**, ALT, AMS, **AST**, proteins (early), **CK**, CRP, RBC, factor – (V, VIII), **FDP**, ferritin, fibrinogen (later), glucagon, **haptoglobin, Hb, HCT**, chloride, IgE, K, carboxy-Hb (inhalation), complement – (C3a, C5a), **creatinine**, LD 5, WBC, Na, **neu**, norepinephrine, osmolality, RBC osmotic fragility, P, pCO_2, PLT, schistocytes, **urea, viscosity**, VLDL-C

↓ **albumin** (later stage), **AMS, proteins** (later), **Ca**, Ca^{2+}, Cr, Cu, **eos, FDP**, fibrinogen (acute), G, Hb, HCT, **chloride**, cholesterol, CHS, **IgA, IgG, IgM**, K, complement – (C1r, C1s, C2, C3, C4, C5, C6, C7, C8, C9, CH50), LDL-C, lym, **Mg**, Mn, Na, osmolality, plasma volume, **RBC osmotic resistance**, pH, pO_2, TAG, **Zn**
- *Urine* ↑ amino acids, AMS, RBC, G, **Hb**, hemosiderin, hexosaminidase, total hydroxyproline, 17-KGS, WBC, lysozyme, **Mb**, 3-methylhistidine
  ↓ vitamin C

Porphyria

acquired porphyria

↑ Ca, protoporphyrin (RBC)
- *Urine* ↑ ALA, **PBG, porphyrins**
- *Stool* ↑ porphyrins

acute intermittent porphyria

↑ **ADH, ✻ ALA**, ALT, Apo B, Ca, **Fe**, ferritin, hexosaminidase, **cholesterol**, coproporphyrin I, **LDL-C**, WBC, **✻ PBG**, pre-beta-LP, porphyrins, T4, TAG, **TBG**, urea, uroporphyrinogen I synthase (RBC), **uroporphyrin I**

↓ AMS, chloride, complement – (C3), **uric acid**, Mg, Na, porphyrins, **✻ delta-ALA-dehydratase, ✻ PBG-deaminase** (RBC), triiodothyronine resin uptake
- *Urine* ↑ **✻ ALA**, coproporphyrin I, **✻ PBG, ✻ porphyrins**, uroporphyrin I, VMA
- *Stool* ↑ coproporphyrins, protoporphyrins, uroporphyrins

ALA-dehydratase deficiency

- *Urine* ↑ **✻ ALA, ✻ coproporphyrins**

congenital erythropoietic porphyria

↑ unconjugated Bil, Ca, HbF, **coproporphyrins** (RBC), RTC, **✻ uroporphyrins** (RBC)

↓ RBC, Hb, HCT, **uroporphyrinogen III cosynthetase** (RBC), triiodothyronine resin uptake

- ■ *Urine* ↑ coproporphyrin I, ✶ **porphyrins**, uroporphyrin I
- ■ *Stool* ↑ ✶ **coproporphyrin I**, ✶ **porphyrins**, protoporphyrin, uroporphyrin

erythropoietic protoporphyria

↑ ALP, AST, conjugated Bil, **coproporphyrins**, WBC, **porphyrins**, ✶ **protoporphyrin** (RBC), **uroporphyrins**, zinc protoporphyrin

↓ RBC, Hb, HCT

- ■ *Urine* ↑ coproporphyrins, protoporphyrin, uroporphyrin
- ■ *Stool* ↑ ✶ **coproporphyrin**, **protoporphyrin**

hepato-erythropoietic porphyria

↑ ALT, Apo B, AST, GMT, **protoporphyrin** (RBC)

↓ Hb, HCT, ✶ **uroporphyrinogen decarboxylase**

- ■ *Urine* ↑ **uroporphyrin I**, **uroporphyrin III**
- ■ *Stool* ↑ coproporphyrin I, coproporphyrin III

hereditary coproporphyria

↑ ✶ **ALA**, ✶ **coproporphyrin**, LDL-C, WBC, ✶ **PBG**

↓ ✶ **coproporphyrinogen III oxidase** (RBC), triiodothyronine resin uptake

- ■ *Urine* ↑ **ALA** (attack), ✶ **coproporphyrin III** (attack), **PBG** (attack), porphyrins, uroporphyrin
- ■ *Stool* ↑ ✶ **coproporphyrin III**, PBG, porphyrins, protoporphyrin, uroporphyrin

porphyria cutanea tarda

↑ ALA, ALT, Apo B, **Fe**, **coproporphyrin**, LDL-C, porphyrins, **protoporphyrins**, **transferrin satur.**, **uroporphyrin I, III**, uroporphyrinogen I synthase

↓ **uro-decarboxylase**

- ■ *Urine* ↑ ✶ **ALA**, ✶ **coproporphyrin III**, **porphyrins**, ✶ **uroporphyrin**, uroporphyrinogen, uroporphyrinogen decarboxylase II (RBC), VMA
- ■ *Stool* ↑ **coproporphyrin**, **uroporphyrin**

secondary coproporphyria

↑ ALT, AST, GMT, Fe, transferrin satur.

↓ CHS, Fe, sTfR

– hepatic secondary coproporphyria

↓ ALT, AST, GMT, CHS, Fe, sTfR

– secondary coproporphyria in anemia

↑ Bil, conjugated Bil, BSP

↓ CHS, Fe, RTC, sTfR

Note: positive functional tests (phenobarbital, nicotinic acid)

– secondary coproporphyria in malignant tumors

↑ AFP, B2M, PSA, thymidine kinase

variegate porphyria

↑ ALA, Apo B, LDL-C, PBG, uroporphyrinogen I synthase (RBC)

- ■ *Urine* ↑ ✶ **ALA** (attack), **coproporphyrin III**, ✶ **PBG** (attack), **porphyrins**, protoporphyrin, **uroporphyrin**
- ■ *Stool* ↑ ✶ **coproporphyrin III**, PBG, ✶ **protoporphyrin IX**, uroporphyrin

Postmaturity

↑ **squalene**

       ↓ estriol, hPL
       ■ *Amniotic Fluid* ↓ volume

Preeclampsia

       ↑ ✳ **alpha-aminonitrogen**, ✳ **ALP**, ✳ **ALT**, antiphospholipid Ab, antiplatelet Ab, ✳ **AST**, beta globulins, Bil, D-dimers, ✳ **FDP**, ✳ **fibronectin**, chloride, ICD, ✳ **creatinine**, ✳ **uric acid**, lupus anticoagulant, LA, LAP, ✳ **LD**, **WBC**, PT, PTT, ✳ **thromboxane A2**
       ↓ **albumin**, aldosterone, alpha-aminonitrogen, A2MG, **AMS**, AT III, **proteins**, DOC, RBC, estriol, haptoglobin, Hb, hPL, HCT, CHS, IgD, **IgG**, ketones, **uric acid**, **Mg**, plasma volume, plasminogen, **progesterone**, **PLT**
       ■ *Urine* ↑ alpha-aminonitrogen, **albumin**, ✳ **proteins** (+ quantitatively), RBC, ketones, uric acid, Na, casts – (RBC, granular, hyaline)
         ↓ Ca, **estriol**, GFR, Na, ✳ **volume**, pregnanediol
       ■ *Amniotic Fluid* ↑ creatinine
         ↓ AFP, volume
       ■ *Cerebrospinal Fluid* ↑ proteins, RBC
       ■ *Synovial Fluid* ↑ crystals – (urate)

Pregnancy

       ↑ AAT, ACP, ACTH, **AFP**, Al, **aldosterone**, alpha-aminonitrogen, alpha-1-globulins, alpha-2-globulins, alpha-2 pregnancy associated glycoprotein, **ALP**, ALP (WBC), ALT, **A2MG**, AMS, ANF, androstenedione, Apo – (A-I, (a), B, E), AST, beta-endorphins, **beta globulins**, **beta-carotene**, Bil, conjugated Bil, unconjugated Bil, CA 15-3, CA 27-29, CA 125, CA 549, carbohydrate-deficient transferrin, CBG, **ceruloplasmin**, **CK**, CK-MB, CRP, **Cu**, 11-deoxycortisol, DOC, DPD, **EPO**, estradiol, estrone, factor – (VIII, X), FDP, Fe, **fibrinogen**, **ESR**, osmotic fragility, G, glucagon, GMT, haptoglobin, HbF, ✳ **hCG**, hexosaminidase, hexosaminidase A, cold agglutinins, **cholesterol**, ICD, IGFBP-1, plasminogen activator inhibitor, C1-esterase inhibitor, insulin, **calcitonin**, carbonic anhydrase, ketobodies, complement – (C3), cortisol, creatinine, **acetoacetic acid**, LA, LAP, **LDL-C**, **WBC**, lipids, macrocytes, MAL+RAL, MCA, Mn, neu, **blood volume**, PT, pH, **PL**, plasminogen, PRA, PRL, **progesterone**, PTH, PRA, RTC, **SHBG**, somatostatin, syphilis Ab (false), pregnancy specific beta-1-glycoprotein, **T3**, **T4**, **TAG**, **TBG**, testosterone, TIBC, **transferrin**, PLT, TSH, TT, UBBC, VDRL (false posit.), vitamin – (A, **D2**, E), FFA
       ↓ ACE, **albumin**, ALT, **AST**, AT III, **proteins**, Ca, Ca²⁺, CK, CBG, Cr, enkephalins, **RBC**, factor – (XII, XIII), **Fe**, **ferritin**, fibrinogen, **FSH**, G, gamma globulins, glycated albumin, haptoglobin, **Hb**, **GHb**, HCT, HCO_3^-, IgA, IgE, creatinine, uric acid, LD, lipase, Mg, Mn, osmolality, P, pCO_2, pH, protein C, pseudocholinesterase, **Se**, **transferrin satur.**, triiodothyronine resin uptake, PLT, **urea**, vitamin – (A, **B₁**, B₂, B₆, B₁₂, beta-carotene), **C**, **folate**), **Zn**
       ■ *Urine* ↑ alpha-aminonitrogen, ALP, **proteins**, cystine, DALA, **estrogens**, **G**, glycine, Hb, ✳ **hCG**, histidine, hydroxyproline, 17-OHCS, 17-KGS, **17-KS**, **cortisol**, 5-HIAA, lactose, LD, WBC, porphyrins, **pregnanediol**, Se, T3, taurine, threonine, tyrosine, RBC casts, valine, volume
         ↓ FSH, P, Se
       ■ *Cerebrospinal Fluid* ↑ leucine

ectopic pregnancy
- ↑ ACTH, AMS, ✳ hCG, WBC
- ↓ hCG, ✳ **progesterone**
- ■ *Urine* ↑ AMS, ✳ hCG
  - ↓ hCG

1ˢᵗ trimester pregnancy
- ↑ angiotensin II, CA 125, fructosamine, FT4, hCG, IgG, PTH, **T4**, TSH
- ↓ AGP, albumin, CK, G, creatinine, uric acid, osmolality, osteocalcin, **proteins**, urea
- ■ *Urine* ↑ cystathionine, cystine, phenylalanine, creatinine, leucine, tyrosine, valine

3ʳᵈ trimester pregnancy
- ↑ AAP, **AAT, ALP,** ALT, AST, beta-glucuronidase, **Cu,** factor VIII, FDP, Fe, fibrinogen, fructosamine, ESR, gc-globulin, cholesterol, plasminogen activator inhibitor, LA, LAP, melatonin, 5-nucleotidase, plasma volume, oxytocin, **plasminogen,** 17-OH progesterone, PTH, TAG, **TIBC, transferrin,** thyroglobulin, urea, VLDL-C
- ↓ proteins, **Fe,** FT3, FT4, G, GMT, CHS, IgA, IgG, **ILGF-I,** vitamin – (B₁₂)
- ■ *Urine* ↑ estrogens, galactose, total hydroxyproline, **cortisol, volume,** reducing sugars

multiple pregnancy
- ↑ **AFP, estriol,** hCG, **hPL**
- ■ *Urine* ↑ **estriol,** hCG
- ■ *Amniotic Fluid* ↑ AFP, volume

Prematurity
- ↑ G
- ■ *Amniotic Fluid* ↑ **creatinine**

Proctitis
- ↑ CRP, ESR, WBC, mucoproteins
- ■ *Stool* ↑ blood

Proctocolitis, Idiopathic
- ■ *Stool* ↑ chloride, Na

Prostatectomy
- ↑ PSA

Prostatitis
- ↑ **ACP,** ✳ **CRP, ESR,** fibrinogen, ✳ **WBC,** mucoproteins, PAP, **PSA**
- ■ *Urine* ↑ ✳ **bacteria** (+ culture), RBC, Hb, **pus,** ✳ **WBC, blood**

Prostheses, Heart Valve
- ↑ **LD, RTC**
- ↓ **haptoglobin,** Hb, HCT, schistocytes, ✳ **PLT**
- ■ *Urine* ↑ **Hb,** hemosiderin

Proteinosis, Pulmonary Alveolar
- ↑ **CEA, RBC,** Hb, **LD,** WBC
- ↓ pO₂
- ■ *Bronchoalveolar Lavage Fluid* ↑ albumin, CEA, phospholipids, proteins, ✳ **surfactant protein A antibodies**
  - ↓ LD
- ■ *Sputum* ↑ macrophages, ✳ **surfactant protein A antibodies**

Proteinuria, Orthostatic
- ■ *Urine* ↑ **proteins,** WBC, casts – (granular, hyaline)

Pseudoaldosteronism Due to Ingestion of Licorice

↓ K, PRA
- *Urine* ↓ aldosterone, glycyrrhetinic acid

Pseudocyst of Pancreas

↑ **ALP, AMS**, Bil, **conjugated Bil**, G, **lipase**, TM – (CA 15-3, CA 72-4, CA 125, TPA)
- *Urine* ↑ AMS
- *Peritoneal Fluid* ↑ AMS
- *Pleural Fluid* ↑ AMS, **LD**

Pseudogout

↑ PTH, WBC
- *Synovial Fluid* ↑ **calcium pyrophosphate crystals, WBC**, volume

Pseudohypoaldosteronism

↓ P
- *Sweat* ↑ chloride, Na

Pseudohypoparathyroidism

↑ cAMP, calcitonin, **P, PTH**
↓ ALP, **Ca, Ca²⁺**, PRL, T4, vitamin – (**D3**)
- *Urine* ↑ cAMP
↓ Ca, cAMP, P

Pseudomyxoma Peritonei

- *Peritoneal Fluid* ↑ **proteins**

Psoriasis Vulgaris

↑ ANA, CIC, eos, phospholipase A2, HLA – (A13, B17, B27, Cw6), h-sICAM-1, IL – (6, 8), **uric acid**
↓ **folate**
- *Synovial Fluid* ↑ crystals – (urate)

Puberty

  delayed puberty

↓ ILGF-I

  male delayed puberty

↓ HDL-C, testosterone

  precocious puberty

  – male precocious puberty

↑ **ACTH, FSH, ILGF-I, LH**, PRL, **testosterone**
↓ ALP, SHBG
- *Urine* ↑ FSH, 17-KS, LH, PRL

  – female precocious puberty

↑ **androstenedione, estradiol**, FSH, **ILGF-I**, LH, PRL, progesterone
↓ ALP
- *Urine* ↑ estrogens, FSH, **17-ketosteroids**, LH, pregnanediol, PRL

Puncture, Lumbar

- *Cerebrospinal Fluid* ↑ **RBC, WBC**

Purpura

  allergic purpura

↑ ASLO, **eos, ESR**, capillary fragility, IgA, **creatinine, neu**, TIBC, **urea, WBC**
↓ albumin, Hb, HCT, RBC, MCH (RBC), MCHC (RBC), MCV (RBC), PLT, transferrin satur.
- *Urine* ↑ albumin, proteins, casts – (RBC c., granular c.), **RBC**
- *Stool* ↑ blood

autoimmune idiopathic thrombocytopenic purpura

↑ **antiplatelet Ab**, **BT**, euglobulin lysis time, G6PD (RBC), **WBC**, lym, mono, MPV, blood volume, **RTC**, PLT

↓ PLT aggregation, RBC, Fe, **Hb**, **HCT**, WBC, **✳ PLT**

Henoch-Schönlein purpura

↑ ANCA, p-ANCA, ASLO, CIC, **ESR**, fibronectin, IgA, cryoglobulins, WBC, RF

↓ eos, factor XIII, complement – (C2, C3, C4), WBC, neu

■ *Urine* ↑ **proteins**, eos, **RBC**, **Hb**, blood, LD, WBC, casts – (RBC, granular, hyaline, WBC)

   ↓ specific gravity, Na, volume, pH

■ *Stool* ↑ blood

■ *Synovial Fluid* ↑ WBC, PMN

thrombotic thrombocytopenic purpura

↑ ALT, **ANA**, APTT, AST, **RBC basophilic stippling**, Bil, **conjugated Bil**, unconjugated Bil, BT, euglobulin lysis time, FDP, fibrinogen, **nucleated RBC**, **Hb**, creatinine, **LD**, **WBC**, megakaryocytes, mono, **neu**, PT, **RTC**, spherocytes, **schistocytes**, TGT, thrombomodulin, **urea**

↓ **RBC**, **haptoglobin**, **Hb** (later), **HCT**, complement – (C3), WBC, **✳ PLT**

■ *Urine* ↑ **proteins**, RBC, **Hb**, **pus**, creatinine, **blood**, urea, casts – (**granular**)

   ↓ volume

Pyelitis

↑ CRP, **ESR**, kreatinín, **WBC**

↓ albumin

■ *Urine* ↑ bacteria (+ culture), proteins, RBC, G, Hb, pus, blood, WBC, specific gravity, casts – (epithelial, RBC, granular, hyaline, WBC)

Pyelonephritis

acute pyelonephritis

↑ alpha-1-globulins, alpha-2-globulins, conjugated Bil, **CRP**, **elastase**, **ESR**, gamma globulins, **haptoglobin**, chloride, IgA, IgM, **creatinine**, uric acid, LA, LD5, **WBC**, lysozyme, **MAC**, **Na**, procalcitonin, osmolality, **urea**

↓ albumin, estriol, **K**, osmolality, PT, PLT

■ *Urine* ↑ AAP, albumin, **bacteria** (+ culture), B2M, **proteins**, RBC, G, **Hb**, **pus**, K, **blood**, **WBC**, LD4, LD5, lysozyme, **specific gravity**, N-acetylglucosaminidase, nitrites, **pH**, casts – (epithelial, **RBC**, granular, hyaline, **WBC**)

   ↓ estriol, G, GFR, K, **creatinine**, specific gravity, volume, osmolality, **urea**

chronic pyelonephritis

↑ alpha-1-globulins, alpha-2-globulins, conjugated Bil, **CRP**, **elastase**, **ESR**, gamma globulins, **haptoglobin**, chloride, IgA, IgG, IgM, **creatinine**, uric acid, LA, **WBC**, lysozyme, **MAC**, osmolality, **urea**

↓ albumin, estriol, K, **Mg**, pH

■ *Urine* ↑ AAP, albumin, **bacteria** (+ culture), B2M, **proteins**, RBC, G, **Hb**, esterase (WBC), hexosaminidase, **pus**, **K**, **blood**, LD4, LD5, **WBC**, nitrites, volume, osmolality, fat, casts – (epithelial, RBC, **granular**, hyaline, **WBC**)

   ↓ estriol, G, GFR, K, **creatinine**, **specific gravity**, volume, osmolality, **urea**

Pylephlebitis, Septic

   ↑ ALT, AST, **Bil**, **PMN**, **WBC**

   ↓ Hb, HCT

Pylorostenosis

   ↑ unconjugated Bil, **gastrin**

   ■ *Gastric Fluid* ↑ **LA**

Pyoderma, Streptococcal

   ↑ ALT, **ASLO**, **ESR**, **WBC**

Pyometra

   ↑ ESR, WBC

Pyonephrosis

   ■ *Urine* ↑ **pus**

Pyopneumothorax

   ↑ ESR, uric acid, neu, **WBC**

   ■ *Sputum* ↑ ✳ **bacteria** (+ culture), ✳ **pus**, blood, **volume**, **viscosity**

   ■ *Pleural Fluid* ↑ proteins, **RBC**, LA, LD, **WBC**, **neu**, **PMN**

Pyosalpinx

   ↑ ESR, WBC

   ■ *Urine* ↑ **pus**

Pyoureter

   ↑ ESR, WBC

   ■ *Urine* ↑ **bacteria**, **protein**

Pyropoikilocytosis, Hereditary

   ↑ pyknocytes, RBC osmotic fragility

   ↓ **Hb**, **HCT**, **MCV**

Rachitis

   ↑ **ALP**, lipase, P, **PTH**

   ↓ **Ca**, Ca^{2+}, **P**, vitamin − (✳ **D2**, D3)

   ■ *Urine* ↑ alpha-aminonitrogen, **amino acids**, cAMP, G, glycine, hydroxy-proline − (total, free), chloride, P

     ↓ **Ca**, Ca^{2+}, **P**

   ■ *Gastric Fluid* ↓ pH

Reaction

  acute phase reaction

   ↑ AAT, alpha-1-antichymotrypsin, alpha-2-antiplasmin, alpha-1-globu-lins, alpha-2-globulins, A2MG, Apo E, AT III, ceruloplasmin, CRP, factor − (VII, VIII), fibrinogen, haptoglobin, hemopexin, C1-esterase inhibitor, complement − (C1, C2, C3, C4, C9, **CH50**), Lp(a), oroso-mucoid, plasminogen

  graft-versus-host reaction

   ↑ **B2M**, IL − (2, 6), 5-nucleotidase, TNF-alpha

   ↓ PLT

  leukemoid reaction

   ↑ **ALP** (WBC), nucleated RBC, ✳ **WBC**, PL

  posttransfusion reaction

   ↑ antineutrophil Ab, **Bil**, nucleated RBC, WBC, **leukocyte antibodies**, neu, spherocytes

   ↓ RBC, **haptoglobin**, HCT, methemalbumin, PLT

   ■ *Urine* ↑ Hb, hemosiderin

     ↓ volume

Rejection
   transplanted heart rejection
        ↑ ESR, LD, LD1, WBC
   transplanted kidney rejection
        ↑ B2M, Ca, **CRP**, **elastase**, EPO, **FDP**, **fibrinogen**, GMT, **GST**, h-sVCAM-1, **chloride**, IL – (2, 6), **creatinine**, LCA, **LD**, **WBC**, lym, lysozyme, **MAC**, Na, **PRA**, SAA, schistocytes, TNF-alpha, **urea**
        ↓ complement – (**C3**, C4), C1-INH, pH, PLT
        ■ *Urine* ↑ beta-alanine, **proteins**, IL – (2, 6), **lysozyme**, TNF-alpha, casts – (cellular, **epithelial**, granular, **hyaline**, **waxy**)
           ↓ FDP, hexosaminidase, **volume**, **osmolality**
   transplanted liver rejection
        ↑ ALP, **ALT**, **AST**, **Bil**, conjugated Bil, **GMT**, **GST**, creatinine, Na, WBC
        ■ *Urine* ↑ proteins

Resection
   small intestine resection
        ↑ gastrin
        ↓ Ca, **Mg**, vitamin – (B_2, B_{12}, folate)
        ■ *Urine* ↑ oxalate
           ↓ 5-HIAA
        ■ *Stool* ↑ fat
        ■ *Synovial Fluid* ↑ crystals – (calcium oxalate)
   stomach resection
        ↑ **gastrin**
        ↓ Ca, pepsinogen

Resistance, Antiinsulin
        ↑ antiinsulin Ab, insulin

Response, Allergic
   delayed allergic response
        ↑ C3, fibrinogen, gamma globulins, haptoglobin, alpha-1-proteinase inhibitor
        ↓ albumin, haptoglobin
        ■ *Cerebrospinal Fluid* ↑ plasmocytes
   immediate allergic response
        ↑ C3, fibrinogen, haptoglobin, alpha-1-proteinase inhibitor
        ↓ albumin, transferrin

Resuscitation, Cardio-Pulmo-Cerebral
        ↑ CK-MB, LA, MAC+RAC, Mb, pCO_2
        ↓ BE, pH, pO_2

Retardation
   growth retardation
        ↓ ALP, vitamin – (A), **Zn**
   intrauterine growth retardation
        ↓ estriol, hPL
        ■ *Amniotic Fluid* ↓ volume

Reticulocytosis
        ↑ anisocytes, RBC basophilic stippling, **RTC**

Rhabdomyolysis
        ↑ aldolase, AST, Ca, CK, **K**, creatinine, **Mb**, Mg, P
        ↓ **Ca**

Rhinitis, Allergic

    ↑ eos, **IgE**

Rhinorrhea, CSF

    ■ *Cerebrospinal Fluid* ↓ pressure

Rupture

aortic aneurysm rupture

    ↑ AMS

    ■ *Peritoneal Fluid* ↑ RBC

bladder rupture

    ■ *Peritoneal Fluid* ↑ creatinine, urea

esophageal rupture into pleural cavity

    ↑ AMS

    ■ *Pleural Fluid* ↑ **AMS**, LD, WBC, PMN

    ↓ G, **pH**

tubar pregnancy rupture

    ↑ AMS, **WBC**, lipase

    ■ *Urine* ↑ **AMS**

    ■ *Peritoneal Fluid* ↑ AMS

Salpingitis

    ↑ **ESR**, **WBC**, neu

    ■ *Urine* ↑ RBC, Hb

Sarcoidosis

    ↑ * **ACE**, albumin, **alpha-1-globulins, alpha-2-globulins, ALP**, ALP isoenzymes, **ALT**, AMS, ANA, anti-EBV, **AST, beta globulins, B2M, proteins,** * **Ca**, Ca²⁺, **CIC**, CO₂, **eos, ESR**, fibrinogen, * **gamma globulins**, globulins, **GMT**, hydroxyproline, **IgA**, IgD, IgE, **IgG, IgM**, immunoglobulins, complement – (C₃, total), **uric acid, creatinine**, cryoglobulins, **LAP, LD**, WBC, **lysozyme, mono**, 5-NT, P, pCO₂, pH, PRL, **RF**, vitamin – (**D2, D3**)

    ↓ ADH, **albumin, RBC, Hb, HCT, chloride**, LH, **WBC, lym**, O₂ satur., P, pCO₂, pO₂, **PTH, PLT**, T-lym (CD4+)

    ■ *Urine* ↑ proteins, Ca, Ca²⁺, **total hydroxyproline**, lysozyme, volume, oxalate

    ↓ P

    ■ *Sputum* ↑ **lym**

    ↓ alveolar macrophages

    ■ *Cerebrospinal Fluid* ↑ **ACE, proteins**, IgG, **WBC, lym**, lysozyme, mono, plasmocytes, pressure

    ↓ G

    ■ *Bronchoalveolar Lavage Fluid* ↑ **lym**, eos, neu, macrophages, **T-lym (CD4+)**

    ↓ macrophages

    ■ *Pleural Fluid* ↑ adenosine deaminase, eos, **lym**

    ↓ alveolar macrophages

    ■ *Synovial Fluid* ↑ crystals – (hydroxyapatite), WBC, PMN

    ↓ viscosity

    ■ *Stool* ↓ Ca

CNS sarcoidosis

    ■ *Cerebrospinal Fluid* ↑ proteins, eos, IgG, lym, lysozyme, mono, plasmocytes, pressure

    ↓ **G**

Schizophrenia

↑ aldolase, HLA – (A28), serotonin

Scleroderma

↑ **ACA, ACE,** AHA, AMA, **ANA,** ANCA, p-ANCA, ✱ **anticentromere Ab,**
anti-ds-DNA, anti-ss-DNA, anti-DNP, **antiendothelial Ab,** anti-HSP
90, antichromosomal Ab, anticardiolipin Ab, anticollagen Ab, anti-
Ku, anti-NOR 90, ✱ **antinucleolar Ab,** anti-p 56, anti-PM/Scl, **anti-
RNA-polymerase,** anti-RNP, ✱ **anti-Scl-70 (anti-DNA-topoisome-
rase I Ab),** anti-SSA, anti-SSB, CIC, **eos, ESR, gamma globulins,** HLA
– (DQ5, DQ7, **DR1, DR2, DR3, DR5, DR8, DRW52), cold agglutinins,**
IgG, IgM, cryofibrinogen, cryoglobulins, **LE cells,** lym, PRA, **anti-U1-**
nucleolar RNP, anti-U3-nucleolar RNP, RF, urea, VRDL (false)

↓ RBC, Hb, HCT, complement – (C3, C7), microcytes, neu, T-lym, vitamin –
(B₁₂, folate)

- *Urine* ↑ proteins, blood, casts
  ↓ volume
- *Stool* ↑ fat
- *Synovial Fluid* ↑ crystals – (hydroxyapatite), WBC, mono, PMN, viscosity, **volume**
  ↓ viscosity

Sclerosis

amyotrophic lateral sclerosis

↑ **antibodies against gangliozides, Ab against cytoskeleton,** CK, SOD, GPs

- *Urine* ↑ **polyamines**
- *Cerebrospinal Fluid* ↑ **proteins,** ✱ **neurofilaments**

Note: molecular biology – glutamate receptor polymorphism

multiple sclerosis

↑ PLT adhesion, ✱ **anti-MBP autoantibodies,** Apo-E, CRP, HLA – (A3, B7,
B18, B27, **DR2,** DR3, **Dw2),** h-sICAM-1, inositol, **oligoclonal proteins**
(immunoglobulins), pCO₂

↓ ceruloplasmin, Cu, PL

- *Cerebrospinal Fluid* ↑ **albumin** (CSF/serum), alpha-2-glycoprotein,
  B2M, **proteins,** CK, eos, **gamma globulins,** HLA – (DR2), cholesterol,
  CHS, IgA (index), ✱ **IgG** (index), IgA, ✱ **IgG,** ✱ **IgG/albumin,** IgM,
  acid proteinases, **LA, WBC, lym,** ✱ **MBP, mononuclears,** ✱ **oligoclo-**
  nal proteins (immunoglobulins), **plasmocytes,** somatostatin, tryptophan
  ↓ arginine, tryptophan
- *Stool* ↑ fat

Note: molecular biology – gene polymorphism CTLA4, TNF-alpha. MRZ
reaction (measles, rubeolla, zoster antibody index)

Scurvy

↑ **Bil,** haptoglobin, **RTC**

↓ **ALP,** RBC, Hb, HCT, PT, **vitamin C,** vitamin C (WBC)

- *Urine* ↑ RBC, Hb, casts – (RBC)
  ↓ vitamin C
- *Gastric Fluid* ↑ blood
- *Stool* ↑ blood
- *Synovial Fluid* ↑ **RBC**

Sepsis, Neonatal

↑ **✻ bacteria** (culture), Bil, conjugated Bil, unconjugated Bil, CRP, **ESR, WBC**

↓ Hb, HCT, RBC, WBC, **PLT**

■ *Urine* ↑ albumin, lactose, reducing sugars, casts

■ *Cerebrospinal Fluid* ↑ **✻ bacteria** (+ culture), **✻ WBC**

Shock

↑ ADH, epinephrine, albumin, **✻ alpha-1-globulins**, ALP, ALT, amino acids, anion gap, AST, beta globulins, BHBA, Bil, **CK**, CK-BB, CK-MM, D-dimers, **✻ elastase**, elastase (PMN), eos, RBC, FDP, **✻ phospholipase A2**, ESR, G, glycine, HCT, **HCO_3^-**, IFN-gamma, IgA, IgE, IgG, IgM, IL – (**✻ 1-beta, ✻ 2, ✻ 6**), plasminogen activator inhibitor, K, catecholamines, **ketobodies**, complement – (**✻ C3a**, C4a, C5a), **✻ uric acid, ✻ creatinine, ✻ LA**, lactoferrin, LD, **WBC**, **✻ MAC**, Mb, methionine, neu, norepinephrine, NSE, **✻ osmolality**, **✻ PAF**, pCO_2, **PCT**, PGE2, pH, **✻ PMN**, RAL, TT, tyrosine, **urea**

↓ **✻ albumin**, aldosterone, A2MG, arginine, AT III, bas, **✻ proteins**, Ca, Ca^{2+}, CBG, **eos** (later), RBC (later), factor B, factor – (XII), fibrinogen, ESR, G, gamma globulins, G6PD (RBC), Hb, HCT, HCO_3^- (later), **✻ cholesterol, ✻ CHS**, IgA (later), IgG (later), IgM (later), K, complement – (C3, C4), **WBC** (severe), LH, lym, **Na**, neu, P, **pH**, pCO_2, pO_2, protein C, RTC, PLT

■ *Urine* ↑ amino acids, AMS, **proteins**, RBC, G, Hb, pus, LD, Mb, specific gravity, metanephrines, osmolality, **VMA**

↓ creatinine, osmolality, **urea**, volume, specific gravity, VMA

anaphylactic shock

↑ **✻ eos**, RBC, **✻ IgE**, catecholamines, **✻ uric acid**, tryptase

↓ **bas**, eos, factor B, pO_2, ESR, **neu, PLT**

cardiogenic shock

↑ ALT, anion gap, ANP, **✻ CK, ✻ CK-MB, ✻ cTnT**, catecholamines, uric acid, MAC, **✻ Mb**, troponin I

↓ pH, pO_2

electrical shock

↑ catecholamines, CK, CK-MB, LD 5, WBC

■ *Urine* ↑ Mb

hypovolemic shock

↑ anion gap, K, catecholamines, creatinine, LD, Na

↓ **Hb, HCT**, pH, pO_2, RTC, PLT

■ *Urine* ↑ specific gravity, osmolality

↓ creatinine

renal shock

■ *Urine* ↑ G, casts – (lipid)

septic shock

↑ epinephrine, alanine, alpha-1-globulins, ALP, ALP (WBC), **ALT**, anion gap, ASLO, **AST, beta globulins**, Bil, CK, **CRP**, Cu, D-dimers, **✻ elastase, ✻ elastase** (PMN), **✻ FDP**, phospholipase A2, **✻ ESR, G, globulins**, glycine, IFN-gamma, **IgA**, IgD, IgG, IgM, IL – (**✻ 1-beta, ✻ 6, ✻ 8**), insulin, plasminogen activator inhibitor, **catecholamines**, complement – (C3a, C4a, C5a), **creatinine**, uric acid, LA, lactoferrin, **LD**, lipids, * **WBC**, lym, **MAC**, **methionine**, **mono**, **neu**, NSE, 5-NT, osmolality, PAF, **PCT**, **PGE2**, **pH** (early), phenylalanine, * **PMN**, PT, RAL (early), E selectin, **TAG**, taurine, tryptophan, TT, tyrosine, **urea**

↓ **albumin**, aldosterone, A2MG, Apo – (AI, B), arginine, AT III, Ca, Ca^{2+}, CBG, factor – (II, XII), **Fe**, **fibrinogen**, G, G tolerance, **gamma globulins**, **G6PD** (RBC), **Hb**, **HCT**, HCO_3^-, HDL-C, **cholesterol**, **CHS**, IgA, IgG, IgM, complement – (**C3**, C4, total), **WBC**, lipids, **lym**, Mg, Mg (PMN), neu, P, pCO_2 (early), **pO_2**, protein C, **PLT**, RTC, TBG, TIBC

■ *Urine* ↑ proteins, RBC, **G**, Hb, catecholamines, 17-OHCS, 17-KGS, casts – (RBC)

↓ osmolality

toxic shock

↑ **ALT**, **AST**, **CK**, catecholamines, **creatinine**, **WBC**, urea

↓ Ca, **PLT**

– toxic shock (gram-negative, coliform bacteria)

↑ ALP, **AMS**, * **AST**, Bil, CRP, elastase, G, **K**, catecholamines, * **WBC**, * **MAC**, pCO_2, * **urea**

↓ **eos**, G, MAL, **Na**, **pH**, pO_2

■ *Urine* ↑ proteins

↓ **volume**

– toxic shock (Staphylococcus aureus, streptococci, group A)

↑ ALT, * **AST**, * **Bil**, CK, CRP, * **ESR**, GMT, catecholamines, * **creatinine**, * **WBC**, * **LD**, * **MAC**, **PCT**, * **PT**, **PTT**, **SAA**, * **urea**

↓ albumin, **proteins**, Ca, Ca^{2+}, RBC, **Hb**, HCT, K, Na, P, **pH**, PLT

■ *Urine* ↑ proteins, RBC, **pus**

traumatic shock

↑ catecholamines, LA, LD 5

■ *Urine* ↑ AMS

Shunt, Portocaval

↑ unconjugated Bil, **FDP**

Sialoadenitis

↑ AMS, AMS (S)

Sialolithiasis

↑ AMS, AMS (S)

Silicosis

pulmonary silicosis

↑ **ACE**, **ANA**, gamma globulins, WBC, pCO_2, RAC, RF

↓ pO_2, satur. O_2

silicotuberculosis

↑ lym, WBC

Sinusitis

↑ **ESR**, bas, **WBC**

■ *Cerebrospinal Fluid* ↑ WBC

Smoking

↑ Apo B-100, PLT aggregation, **androstenedione**, * **CEA**, **ceruloplasmin**, * **COHb**, **Cu**, RBC, estradiol, estrone, G, **cholesterol**, cortisol, * **cotinine**, * **LDL-C**, WBC, macrocytes, MCV, MHb, Pb, PRL (M), P-selectin, SHBG, TSH, FFA, vWf

↓ ACE, Apo A-I, **HDL-C**, melatonin, plasma volume, PRL (F), Se, T3, thrombomodulin, vitamin – (B_6, B_{12}, beta-carotene, **C**, folate)

S

- *Urine* ↑ Cd, 17-KGS, **cotinine**, 5-HIAA, VMA
  ↓ 17-KS, **creatinine/thiocyanate index**, Se
- *Bronchoalveolar Lavage Fluid* ↑ neu
- *Pleural Fluid* ↑ neu
- *Seminal Fluid* ↓ volume
- *Sputum* ↑ volume
- *Saliva* ↑ **thiocyanate**

Spina Bifida

↑ *** AFP**, *** ACHE**, A2MG, Bil
- *Amniotic Fluid* ↑ *** AFP**, volume

Splenectomy

↑ acanthocytes, bas, **GHb**, RBC Heinz bodies, *** RBC Howell–Jolly bodies**, **WBC**, *** lym**, macrocytes, **mono**, *** RBC osmotic resistance**, *** RTC**, siderocytes, target cells, *** PLT**, **viscosity**
↓ IgM, Hb, RBC osmotic fragility

Splenomegaly

↑ plasma volume
↓ fibronectin, Hb, WBC, **neu**, **PLT**

Spondylitis
  ankylosing spondylitis

↑ alpha-2-globulins, **ALP**, *** ANA**, beta globulins, *** CIC**, *** CK**, *** CRP**, Cu, ESR, HLA – (*** B27**), *** IgA**, *** IgG**, *** IgM**, LE cells, **mucoproteins**, RF
↓ RBC, Hb, HCT, complement – (C3, C7)
- *Cerebrospinal Fluid* ↑ proteins
- *Synovial Fluid* ↑ **C3**, WBC, PMN
  ↓ **viscosity**

  psoriatic spondylitis

↑ HLA-B27

Sprue, Tropical

↑ ALT, MCV, motilin, PT
↓ **albumin**, **proteins**, **ceruloplasmin**, Cu, Hb, HCT, Mg, vitamin – (A, B_2, B_{12}, folate), **Zn**
- *Urine* ↑ **5-HIAA**
- *Stool* ↑ **fat**

Starvation

↑ **acetone**, **acetoacetate**, aldosterone, **amino acids**, ANF, beta globulins, BHBA, Bil, unconjugated Bil, Ca, gamma globulins, GIP, **glucagon**, glycine, isoleucine, K (early), **ketobodies**, **uric acid**, leucine, MAC, **fatty acids**, Na, rT3, secretin, **GH**, **urea**, FFA
↓ ACE, **albumin**, ALP, AMS, **proteins**, Ca, C-peptide, EPO, **Fe**, **folate**, G, Hb, HDL-C, HCT, HCO_3^-, cholesterol, **ILGF-I**, **insulin**, K (later), LDL-C, LH, **lipids**, **Mg**, osmolality, P, **pH**, T3, TAG, TIBC, **urea**
- *Urine* ↑ **acetone**, Ca, **chloride**, K, **ketones**, creatine, creatinine, uric acid, Mg, **Na**, volume, **VMA**
  ↓ chloride, K, **creatinine**, **uric acid**, osmolality, **pH**
- *Cerebrospinal Fluid* ↑ leucine
- *Synovial Fluid* ↑ crystals – (urate)

Status Epilepticus

↑ CK, K
- *Urine* ↑ Mb

Steatorrhea

↑ PT, somatostatin

↓ **proteins**, **∗ Ca**, **∗ Fe**, **cholesterol**, **∗ Mg**, vitamin – (**∗ beta-carotene**, C, D, **∗ E**, **∗ folate**), **∗ Zn**

- *Urine* ↑ **∗ oxalate**, reducing sugars

  ↓ **Ca**, lactose, **P**

- *Stool* ↑ volume, **∗ fat**

Stenosis, Renal Artery

↑ aldosterone, RBC, MAL, creatinine, **∗ PRA** (level sampling), urea

↓ **∗ K**

- *Urine* ↑ hexosaminidase, **proteins**, specific gravity, volume

  ↓ Na

Sterility, Male

↑ estradioltestosterone, vitamin – (A)

Stomatitis

angular stomatitis

↓ vitamin B$_2$

stomatitis aphtosa

↑ HLA – (B12)

Stomatocytosis, Hereditary

↑ **∗ stomatocytes**

Storm, thyroid

↑ ALT, AST, Ca, G, GMT, WBC

↓ K, pCO$_2$

Strangulation, Intestinal

↑ AMS, AST, CK, LD, lipase, P

- *Urine* ↑ **AMS**

- *Peritoneal Fluid* ↑ ammonia, AMS

Stress

↑ **AAT, ACTH, ADH**, **epinephrine**, aldosterone, **alpha-1-globulins**, **alpha-2-globulins**, ALP (WBC), beta-endorphins, proteins, **ceruloplasmin**, CRP, elastase, RBC, factor – (VIII), FDP, fibrinogen, **G**, **glucagon**, glucocorticoids, glycerol, haptoglobin, **GHb**, **cholesterol**, insulin, iodine, **catecholamines**, **acetoacetic acid**, **ketobodies**, **uric acid**, **cortisol**, LDL-C, LH, lipids, lym, **neu**, norepinephrine, **PRL**, secretin, **GH**, **TAG**, **PLT**, **TSH**, urea, VLDL-C, FFA

↓ **albumin**, aldosterone, Apo B, **Cr**, eos, G tolerance, **HDL-C**, K, LDL-C, LH, **lym**, Mb, Mn, Na, osmolality, oxytocin, pCO$_2$, **Se**, TBG, testosterone, vitamin – (B$_2$, C), **Zn**

- *Urine* ↑ ADH, epinephrine, proteins, G, **catecholamines**, **17-OHCS**, 17-KGS, 17-KS, catecholamines, **cortisol**, uric acid, **metanephrines**, norepinephrine, tetrahydrodeoxycortisol, casts – (**granular, hyaline**), **VMA**

  ↓ Na, Se, vitamin C

Stroke

heat stroke

↑ **albumin**, aldosterone, alpha-1-glycoprotein, ALT, **AST**, **Bil**, BSP retention, BT, clotting time, CK, CK-BB, CK-MM, factor VIII, FDP, G, **Hb**, HCT, **chloride**, **K**, ketones, **creatinine**, uric acid, LA, **LD**, **lym**, **WBC**, MDA, Na, neu, GH, MAC (later), Mb, mono, P, Pb, PT, RAL (early), urea

    ↓ **Ca**, * **Ca**$_{2+}$, proteins, carotene, * **chloride**, **fibrinogen**, G, K, * **Na**, P, plasma volume, **PLT**, PT

    ■ *Urine* ↑ **proteins**, ketones, **Mb**
      ↓ volume

sun stroke

    ↑ FDP

Strumectomy

    ↑ proteins, cholesterol, TSH
    ↓ Ca, Ca^{2+}

Suction, Gastrointestinal

    ↑ HCO$_3^-$
    ↓ **chloride**, K, MAL, Mg, Na, P

    ■ *Urine* ↑ pH
      ↓ **chloride**

Surgery

    ↑ epinephrine, AGP, aldolase, alpha-1-globulins, AMS, AST, beta-endorphins, CK, CK-MB, **CRP**, elastase, FDP, ESR, G, GIP, glucagon, HCT, plasminogen activator inhibitor, cortisol, LA, LD – (1, 5), WBC, lipase, norepinephrine, PCT, PRL, GH, taurine, **PLT**, urea

    ↓ **proteins**, **Cr**, **cystine**, Fe, **fibrinogen**, HDL-C, **K**, Mn, protein C, protein S, TBG, Zn

    ■ *Urine* ↑ 17-KGS, osmolality, Zn

abdominal surgery

    ↑ AMS, AST, CK, lipase, TSH, urea
    ↓ glycine, isoleucine, glutamic acid, leucine, lysine, ornithine, T3, T4, tryptophan

CNS surgery

    ↑ protein S-100
    ↓ ADH

    ■ *Cerebrospinal Fluid* ↑ MBP

heart surgery

    ↑ AMS, antimyocardial Ab, **AST**, CK, CK-MB, **FDP**, myosin, TSH
    ↓ ALP, T3, T4

lung surgery

    ↑ **FDP**, euglobulin lysis time, TSH
    ↓ T3, T4

prostate surgery

    ↑ CK, PAP
    ■ *Urine* ↑ Hb

spinal canal surgery

    ■ *Cerebrospinal Fluid* ↑ fibrinogen

Sweating

    ↑ chloride, Na, osmolality
    ↓ **chloride**, K, Mg, **Na**

    ■ *Urine* ↑ **specific gravity**
      ↓ chloride, Na

Syndrome

adrenogenital syndrome

    ↑ * **aldosterone**, * DHEA, DOC, * FSH, LH, * **testosterone**
    ↓ * **aldosterone**, Ca, **estradiol**, estriol, * **chloride**, * **Na**, osmolality, **progesterone**

- *Urine* ↑ 17-ketosteroids, 17-OH ketosteroids, pregnanetriol, 17-OH progesterone, pregnanetriol
  ↓ * aldosterone, estriol, * cortisol, 17-OH corticosteroids

Alagille syndrome
  ↑ ALP, ALT, AMS, AST, **Bil**, **Bil conjugated**, ESR, GMT, **cholic acid**, LAP, lipase, lipids, **PT**, PL, **TAG**, **bile acids**
  ↓ RBC, Hb, HCT, prothrombin
- *Urine* ↑ **conjugated Bil**, UBG

Alport's syndrome
  ↑ * **C3**, * **immunoglobulins**, cholesterol, proline, urea, creatinine
  ↓ PLT
- *Urine* ↑ * **proteins**, * **RBC**, Hb, * **blood**

autoimmune lymphoproliferative syndrome
  ↑ ANA, * **anticardiolipin Ab**, * **B-cells**, gamma globulins, IL-10, RF, * **T-cells**
  ↓ Hb, HCT, neu

Bassen-Kornzweig syndrome
  ↑ acanthocytes
  ↓ beta-carotene, beta-lipoprotein, cholesterol
- *Stool* ↑ fat

Beckwith-Wiedemann syndrome
  ↑ HCT, RBC
  ↓ Ca, G

Behcet's syndrome
  ↑ CIC, * **CRP**, * **ESR**, HLA – (**B5**, B51), * **IgA**, complement – (C3, C4), WBC, lymphocytotoxic Ab
  ↓ * **Hb**, * **HCT**
- *Cerebrospinal Fluid* ↑ proteins, WBC

Bernard-Soulier syndrome
  ↑ BT, MPV
  ↓ PLT adhesion, * **PLT**
  Note: molecular biology – GPIb/IX

Blackfan-Diamond syndrome
  ↓ neu

breast-milk jaundice syndrome
  ↑ Bil, **unconjugated Bil**
- *Urine* ↑ conjugated Bil

Buckley's syndrome
  ↑ IgE

carbohydrate deficient glycoprotein syndrome 1a
  ↓ **GPs**, sialic acid, galactose, N-acetylgalactosamine, N-**acetylglucos-aminyltransferase**

cerebellar syndrome
  ↑ **Ab against Purkinje cells**, anti-Hu Ab
- *Cerebrospinal Fluid* ↑ anti-Hu Ab

Chediak-Higashi syndrome
  ↑ BT
  ↓ * **WBC**, * **neu**, elastase (PMN), phagocytic activity, PCT, PLT

chronic fatigue syndrome
  ↑ ALT, lym

Churg-Strauss syndrome
> ↑ ANCA, p-ANCA, c-ANCA, anti-MPO, **＊ eos**, **＊ ESR**, IgA, **＊ IgE, WBC**, RF
> ↓ **＊ RBC**, **＊ Hb**, **＊ HCT**

chylomicron syndrome
> ↑ **chylomicrons**
> ↓ Apo C-II, lipoprotein lipase

CIDP-like syndrome (chronic inflammatory demyelinating polyneuropathy)
> ↑ **anti-tubulin Ab**

CREST syndrome
> ↑ **＊ ACA**, AMA, anti-ds-DNA Ab, anti-p16, **anti-Scl 70 Ab**, HLA-DR3, RF
> ■ *Synovial Fluid* ↑ crystals – (hydroxyapatite)

Crigler-Najjar syndrome
> ↑ ALT, **Bil**, conjugated Bil, **＊ unconjugated Bil**, delta Bil, GMT
> ↓ **＊ UDPGT**
> ■ *Urine* ↑ conjugated bilirubin
> ↓ UBG
> ■ *Stool* ↑ UBG

crush syndrome
> ↑ aldolase, ALT, AST, CK, **＊ K**, **＊ Mb, urea**
> ↓ **Na**
> ■ *Urine* ↑ **RBC, Hb, Mb**, casts – (Hb, Mb)
> ↓ volume

Cushing's syndrome
> ↑ **＊ ACTH, aldosterone, alpha-2-globulins**, alanine, **ALP, androstenedione**, Apo B, Apo B-100, **beta-LPs, Ca**, CO_2, DHEAS, DOC, 18-OH DOC, **RBC**, factor VIII, **＊ G**, glucagon, Hb, HbA_{1c}, HCO_3^-, HCT, HDL-C, **chloride, cholesterol**, IDL-C, **＊ insulin**, IRI, ketobodies, **＊ cortisol**, creatine, LDL-C, **WBC, MAC, MAL, Na**, neu, pCO_2, pH, PL, **PRA**, PRL, pregnenolone, progesterone, testosterone, TAG, **urea**, VLDL-C
> ↓ ACTH, **aldosterone**, amino acids, **angiotensin II, bas**, Ca, CK, **eos**, gamma globulins, glucose tolerance, Hb, HCT, HDL-C, IGFBP-1, chloride, **＊ K**, uric acid, **lym**, neu, P, PGE2, **pH, PRA**, GH, testosterone, **TBG**, volume, Zn
> ■ *Urine* ↑ **Ca, G, ＊ 17-OHCS, K**, 17-KGS, **＊ 17-KS, creatine, ＊ free cortisol**, pregnanetriol, volume
> ↓ **Na**
> ■ *Saliva* ↑ cortisol

– Cushing's syndrome due to ectopic ACTH production
> ↑ **＊ ACTH**, androstenedione, DHEA, **corticoids**, corticosterone, free cortisol, WBC, **MAL, pH**
> ↓ K
> ■ *Urine* ↑ **17-OHCS, 17-KS**, free cortisol, corticoids

– iatrogenic Cushing's syndrome
> ↑ **ACTH, cortisol**

defibrination syndrome
> ↓ fibrinogen

DiGeorge syndrome
> ↑ **B-lym**, lym, IgE
> ↓ **Ca**, gamma globulins, **IgA**, IgG, IgM, **lym, ＊ PTH**, thymuline, **＊ T-lym**

distress syndrome

– adult respiratory distress syndrome (ARDS)

↑ **elastase**, HCO$_3^-$, uric acid, LA, WBC, MAC, pH (early), RAC, **RAL** (early), TAG, thrombomodulin

↓ ACE, complement – (C4), **Hb**, **HCT**, K, pH, ✱ **pCO$_2$** (early), ✱ **pO$_2$**, protein C, protein S, selectin L, ✱ **PLT**

■ *Urine* ↓ volume

■ *Bronchoalveolar Lavage Fluid* ↑ eos, IL-8, neu, **PMN**, selectin – (E, L, P)

– fetal distress syndrome

↓ estriol, hPL

■ *Urine* ↓ **estriol**

■ *Amniotic Fluid* ↑ AFP, meconium

– neonatal respiratory distress syndrome

↑ HCO$_3^-$ (early), pH (early), **pCO$_2$** (later), **RAC**

↓ AAT, Ca, HCO$_3^-$ (later), Hb, HCT, G, ✱ **lecithin-phosphatidylcholine**, pCO$_2$ (early), pH (later), PL, plasminogen, RBC, **pO$_2$**

Down syndrome

↑ ALP (WBC), A2MG, antithyroglobulin Ab, globulins, HbF, **hCG**, **uric acid**, WBC, **neu**, TAG

↓ ACP, ✱ **AFP**, estriol, ILGF-I, serotonin, **testosterone**, free estriol

■ *Urine* ↑ beta-aminoisobutyric acid, cystine

↓ 5-HIAA

Dressler's syndrome

↑ antimyocardial Ab, ESR, CRP

Dubin-Johnson syndrome

↑ ✱ **ALP**, ALT, AST, ✱ **Bil**, ✱ **conjugated Bil**, unconjugated Bil, **PT**

■ *Urine* ↑ Bil, **conjugated Bil**, ✱ **coproporphyrin I**, leukotrienes, UBG

↓ coproporphyrin – (I, III), **coproporphyrin III/coproporphyrin I index**, UBG

■ *Stool* ↓ UBG

dumping syndrome

↑ AMS, ✱ **G** (early), glucagon, ✱ **serotonin**

↓ RBC, **Fe**, **G** (later), G tolerance, Hb, HCT, ✱ K, MCH, MCHC, MCV, **plasma volume**, **vitamin B$_{12}$**

■ *Urine* ↑ G, serotonin, 5-HIAA

■ *Stool* ↑ fat

empty sella syndrome

↑ ACTH, **PRL**

↓ ACTH, PRL

eosinophilia-myalgia syndrome

↑ **aldolase**, ALT, AST, CK, ✱ **eos**, ESR, GMT, WBC, **LD**

euthyroid sick syndrome

↑ FTI, **reverse T3**, **T3 uptake**

↓ FTI, T3, T4

Evans' syndrome

↓ PLT, **specific Ab**

Fanconi's syndrome

↑ aldosterone, ALP, ✱ **chloride**, ✱ **MAC**, MAL, P, PTH, PRA

↓ Ca, RBC, ✱ **HCO$_3^-$**, K, ✱ **uric acid**, Na, ✱ P, **PLT**, vitamin D3

- *Urine* ↑ albumin, ✳ amino acids, ammonia, ✳ proteins, B2M, ✳ Ca, ✳ G, HCO_3^-, ✳ K, uric acid, volume, ✳ P, ✳ pH

Felty's syndrome
↑ ✳ ANA, ANCA, p-ANCA, atypical-ANCA, B2M, C3, C4, ✳ CIC, LE cells, ✳ RF
↓ ✳ RBC, ✳ Hb, HCT, ✳ WBC, ✳ neu, PLT

Forbes-Albright syndrome
↑ PRL

galactorrhea-amenorrhea syndrome
↓ **progesterone, PRL**

GBS syndrome (gay bowel syndrome)
↑ **Ab against Ga1Nac-GD1a**

Goodpasture's syndrome
↑ ✳ AGBMA, ✳ ANCA, ✳ p-ANCA, ✳ CIC, eos, HLA – (DR2), ✳ creatinine, ✳ MAC+RAL, urea
↓ RBC, Fe, Hb, HCT
- *Urine* ↑ proteins, ✳ RBC (dysmorphous), Hb, hexosaminidase, casts – (cellular, ✳ RBC, granular)
- *Bronchoalveolar Lavage Fluid* ↑ RBC, ✳ hemosiderin, ✳ macrophages
- *Sputum* ↑ blood, macrophages, hemosiderin

gray-platelet syndrome
↑ BT
↓ PLT

Guillain-Barré syndrome
↑ ADH, anti-GQ1b Ab, anti-heparan sulfate Ab, **antibodies against Campylobacter jejuni, antibodies against neurofilamenta, anti-Mycoplasma pneumoniae Ab, myelin-specific Ab, anti-CMV Ab,** ✳ **CRP,** ✳ **IgE,** immunoglobulins, WBC, E selectin, pCO_2
- *Cerebrospinal Fluid* ↑ ✳ adenylate kinase, antibodies against Campylobacter jejuni, antibodies against neurofilamenta, anti-Mycoplasma pneumoniae Ab, myelin-specific Ab, anti-CMV Ab, ✳ proteins, CK, gamma globulins, ✳ CHS, ✳ IgG, lym, ✳ MBP, mono, plasmocytes, pressure
↓ WBC

Guillain-Barré like syndrome
↑ anti-GD1a Ab

Hamman-Rich syndrome
↑ ANA, ESR
↓ pCO_2, pO_2

Hand-Schueller-Christian syndrome
↑ ALT, **nucleated RBC**
↓ WBC

HELLP syndrome (hemolysis, elevated liver enzymes, low platelets)
↑ ALT, Bil, LD
↓ PLT

hemolytic-uremic syndrome
↑ anisocytes, Bil, ✳ **unconjugated Bil,** ✳ FDP, ESR, ✳ creatinine, LD, NSE, WBC, RTC, spherocytes, **schistocytes,** urea
↓ RBC, ✳ **haptoglobin,** ✳ Hb, HCT, complement – (✳ C3), ✳ PLT
- *Urine* ↑ ✳ proteins, ✳ RBC, Hb, pus, blood, casts – (RBC, ✳ granular)
↓ volume

hepatorenal syndrome

↑ ALT, K (later), **creatinine, urea**

↓ albumin, **K** (intracellular), **Na**

■ *Urine* ↑ **proteins**, osmolality, RBC, **specific gravity**, casts – (hyaline, granular)

↓ GFR, **Na, volume**, pH

Hermansky-Pudlak syndrome

↑ BT

↓ PLT

hypereosinophilic syndrome

↑ ALT, AST, ✳ **eos, eosinophil kationic protein**, WBC

↓ Hb, HCT, uric acid, PLT

hyper-IgE syndrome

↑ ✳ **eos**, ✳ **IgE**

■ *Sputum* ↑ **eos**

hyper-IgM syndrome

↑ IgD, ✳ **IgM**

↓ Hb, ✳ IgA, ✳ IgG, ✳ IgE, neu, PLT

insulin autoimmune syndrome

↑ ✳ **antiinsulin Ab, C-peptide, insulin**

↓ G

irritable bowel syndrome

↑ CCK-PZ, motilin, somatostatin

↓ vitamin – (B$_2$)

■ *Stool* ↑ mucus

Joseph's syndrome

■ *Urine* ↑ proline, hydroxyproline, glycine

Kawasaki syndrome

↑ **AAT**, ALT, atypical-ANCA, antiendothelial Ab, AST, C$_3$, **CRP, ESR, immunoglobulins**, IgE, WBC, lym, **PLT**

↓ RBC, **Hb, HCT**

■ *Urine* ↑ proteins, pus, mono

■ *Cerebrospinal Fluid* ↑ WBC, mono

■ *Synovial Fluid* ↑ WBC

Kimmelstiel-Wilson syndrome

↑ urea

↓ proteins

■ *Urine* ↑ **albumin**, ✳ **proteins**, blood, RBC, casts – (epithelial, fatty, granular, hyaline)

Klinefelter's syndrome

↑ ✳ **FSH**, ✳ **LH**

↓ estradiol, **testosterone**

■ *Urine* ↑ **FSH**, hydroxyproline – (total, free), **LH**

↓ **17-ketosteroids**

■ *Seminal Fluid* ↓ spermatozoa count

■ *Sweat* ↑ chloride, Na

Leigh's syndrome

■ *Cerebrospinal Fluid* ↑ enkephalins

Lesch-Nyhan syndrome

↑ ✳ **uric acid**

■ *Urine* ↑ RBC, Hb, blood, hypoxanthine, crystals – (urate), ✳ **uric acid**

Liddle's syndrome
>> ↑ Na, pH
>> ↓ ✶ aldosterone, K, MAL, PRA
>> ■ *Urine* ↑ K

lymphoproliferative syndrome linked to X-chromosome
>> ↑ lym

Marfan's syndrome
>> ↓ beta-glucuronidase, mucoproteins
>> ■ *Urine* ↑ homocystine, hydroxyproline – (total, free)

Meigs' syndrome
>> ■ *Peritoneal Fluid* ↑ proteins

MEN syndrome (type I)
>> ↑ ACTH, Ca, calcitonin, gastrin, glucagon, insulin, cortisol, PP, **PRL**, **PTH**, GH, serotonin, serotonin (PLT), somatostatin, VIP

MEN syndrome (type IIa)
>> ↑ ACTH, ✶ **epinephrine, Ca**, ✶ **dopamine**, ✶ **calcitonin**, ✶ **catecholamines**, **norepinephrine**, serotonin, serotonin (PLT), ✶ **PTH, PRA**
>> ■ *Urine* ↑ **G, HVA, catecholamines, metanephrine, VMA, free epinephrine**, free norepinephrine
>> **Note:** chromosome 10q13 mutation (ret proto-oncogene)

MEN syndrome (type IIb)
>> ↑ ACTH, ✶ **epinephrine, Ca**, ✶ **dopamine**, calcitonin, **catecholamines**, **norepinephrine, PRA**, serotonin, serotonin (PLT)
>> ■ *Urine* ↑ **G, catecholamines, HVA, metanephrine, VMA, free epinephrine**, free norepinephrine
>> **Note:** tyrosine-kinase domain mutation

Menkes' syndrome
>> ↓ **ceruloplasmin**, ✶ **Cu**
>> ■ *Urine* ↑ **Cu**
>> ■ *Amniotic Fluid* ↑ **Cu**

Mikulicz syndrome
>> ↑ AMS, WBC

milk-alkali syndrome
>> ↑ ✶ **Ca**, ✶ **MAL, P**, pH, urea
>> ↓ ALP, ✶ **chloride**, K, Na, ✶ **PTH**
>> ■ *Urine* ↓ Ca, P
>> ■ *Synovial Fluid* ↑ crystals – (hydroxyapatite)

Miller-Fisher syndrome
>> ↑ anti-GQ1b Ab

motor neuron syndrome
>> ↑ anti-GM1 ganglioside Ab, anti-GD1a Ab

Nelson's syndrome
>> ■ *Cerebrospinal Fluid* ↑ endorphins

neonatal thick blood syndrome
>> ↑ Bil, ✶ **HCT**
>> ↓ G, PLT

nephritic syndrome
– acute nephritic syndrome
>> ↑ AGBMA, **antideoxyribonuclease, antihyaluronidase, antistreptokinase, ASLO**, IgA, IgG, **WBC**, urea
>> ↓ **RBC, Hb, HCT**, complement – (C3, C4, CH50)

■ *Urine* ↑ **proteins**, **RBC**, Hb, pus, **WBC**, tubular cells, casts – (RBC, granular, Hb, WBC, waxy)

– chronic nephritic syndrome
> ↑ creatinine, MAC, P, urea
> ↓ RBC, Hb, HCT
> ■ *Urine* ↑ **proteins**, RBC, Hb, **blood**, casts – (**RBC**, **granular**, **hyalinic**, waxy)

nephrotic syndrome
> ↑ AAT, AFP, PLT aggregation, **aldosterone**, ALP, alpha-1-globulins, ✻ **alpha-2-globulins**, alpha-2-lipoproteins, **A2MG**, **Apo B**, **bas**, ✻ **beta globulins**, beta-carotene, **beta-lipoproteins**, ceruloplasmin, CK, CRP, elastase, eos, RBC, factor – (**V**, VII, **VIII**, **X**), FDP, Fe, **fibrinogen**, fibrinopeptide A, **ESR**, GMT, **haptoglobin**, HbA$_{1c}$, HBsAg, HDL-C, chloride, ✻ **cholesterol**, **CHS**, chylomicrons, IDL-C, IgA, IgE, IgG, IgM, complement – (**C3**), **creatinine**, cryoglobulins, **uric acid**, LAP, **LD**, LD5, ✻ **LDL-C**, **WBC**, ✻ **lipids**, beta-LP, LPs, MAL, Na, **neu**, P, ✻ **PL**, **protein C**, T3, T3 uptake, ✻ **TAG**, triiodothyronine resin uptake, **PLT**, **urea**, VDRL (false), **VLDL-C**

> ↓ AAT, ADH, AGP, ✻ **albumin**, **alpha-1-globulins**, alpha-2-antiplasmin, **amino acids**, Apo – (A-I, C-II), **AT III**, ASLO, AT III, ✻ **proteins**, B2M, Ca, **ceruloplasmin**, Cu, EPO, RBC, factors – (**IX**, **XI**, **XII**), Fe, ferritin, **FT4**, ✻ **gamma globulins**, globulins, **Hb**, HDL-C, hemopexin, HCT, chloride, cholesterol, **IgA**, **IgG**, **IgM**, immunoglobulins, K, complement – (**C3**, **C4**), cortisol, **lipoprotein lipase**, **lym**, Mg, Na, Ni, osmolality, plasma volume prealbumin, prekallikrein, protein C, protein S, SHBG, **T3**, **T4**, **TBG**, **TIBC**, **transferrin**, **urea**, **urokinase**, vitamin – (D2, **D3**), **Zn**

> ■ *Urine* ↑ albumin, aldosterone, alpha-1-globulin, ✻ **proteins**, beta globulins, B2M, Ca, **Cu**, **RBC**, Hb, hexosaminidase, IgA, immunoglobulins, **K**, **blood**, LD, WBC, lipids, lysozyme, Mg, specific gravity, transferrin, ✻ **fat bodies**, casts – (**epithelial**, RBC, **granular**, hyaline, **lipid**, WBC, **waxy**)
> ↓ Ca, GFR, 17-OHCS, 17-KGS, 17-KS, **Na**
> ■ *Peritoneal Fluid* ↑ RBC, WBC
> ↓ **proteins**
> ■ *Pleural Fluid* ↑ pH
> ↓ **proteins**, LD, specific gravity
> ■ *Stool* ↑ Ca
> ■ *Sweat* ↑ chloride, Na

KT3-induced cytokinerelated syndrome
> ↑ IFN-gamma, IL-2, TNF

paraneoplastic syndrome
> ↑ **Ab against Purkinje cells**, ✻ **ACTH**, ✻ **ADH**, ALP, ✻ **Ca**, EPO, RBC, FSH, ✻ **gastrin**, Hb, ✻ **hCG**, HCT, cholesterol, ✻ **calcitonin**, cryofibrinogen, LH, LPs, ✻ **MSH**, PRA, ✻ **PRL**, ✻ **PTH**, serotonin, ✻ **somatomedin**, STH, TSH
> ↓ G, osmolality

pickwickian syndrome
> ↑ RBC, Hb, **pCO$_2$**, **RAC**
> ↓ **pH**, **pO$_2$**

Plummer-Vinson syndrome

↓ **RBC**, **Fe**, **Hb**, **HCT**, MCH, MCHC, **MCV**

POEMS syndrome (polyneuropathy, organomegaly, endocrinopathy, M-protein, skin changes)

↑ IgA, IgG, IL – (1-beta, 6), MMP – (1, 2, 3, 9), TNF-alpha, VEGF, TIMP

■ *Cerebrospinal Fluid* ↑ proteins

postantrectomy syndrome

■ *Gastric Fluid* ↑ pH
  ↓ HCl

postcardiotomy syndrome

■ *Pleural Fluid* ↑ RBC, WBC

postcholecystectomy syndrome

↑ ALT, ASAL, AST, lipase

postcommissurotomy syndrome

↑ ∗ AST, â CRP, â ESR, **WBC**

posthepatectomy syndrome

↑ ammonia

postpericardectomy syndrome

■ *Pericardial Fluid* ↑ RBC

postradiation syndrome

↑ alpha-1-globulins, alpha-2-globulins, **ALT**, AMS, **AST**, beta-aminoiso-butyric acid, **Bil**, CEA, **eos**, factor – (VIII), ferritin, fibrinogen, **globulins**, uric acid, LAP, LD, WBC, lym, MHb, **neu**, OCT, properdin, PT, urea

↓ ALP, bas, DNA (free), **RBC**, **Hb**, **HCT**, CHS, uric acid, **WBC**, **lym**, Mg, neu, **PLT**, taurine

■ *Urine* ↑ proteins, Bil, creatine, LAP, lysozyme

– acute postradiation syndrome

↑ ∗ alpha-1-globulins, alpha-2-globulins

↓ RBC, ∗ **Hb**, WBC, ∗ **lym**, ∗ **PLT**

■ *Urine* ↑ Bil

– chronic postradiation syndrome (occupational)

↑ RBC, WBC, **lym**

↓ bas, Hb, HCT, Mg, **neu**, **PLT**

– mild postradiation syndrome

↑ neu (early)

↓ WBC, **lym**, Mg, PLT

primary antiphospholipid syndrome

↑ Ab against beta-2 GP I, ∗ **ACLA**, AHA, ANA, anti-DNA, ∗ **anticardiolipin Ab**, anti-nRNP, anti-Ro/SSA, APLA, ∗ **lupus anticoagulant factor**, PT, PTT, **VDRL** (false)

↓ PLT

Raynaud's syndrome

↑ ACA, PLT aggregation, ∗ **anticardiolipin Ab**, ∗ **cold agglutinins**, ∗ **cryoglobulins**, ∗ **viscosity**

Reaven's (metabolic) syndrome

↑ ∗ G, fibrinogen, **cholesterol**, insulin, ∗ **IRI**, ∗ uric acid, LPs, ∗ **TAG**, VLDL-C

↓ HDL-C

■ *Urine* ↑ albumin

Reiter's syndrome

↑ CIC, **✳ CRP**, **✳ ESR**, globulins, HLA – (**✳ B27**), **✳ IgA**, WBC, **neu**, **✳ RF**

↓ RBC, Hb, HCT

■ *Urine* ↑ bacteria (culture), WBC

■ *Synovial Fluid* ↑ **✳ proteins**, clot formation, **✳ C3 complement**, **pus**, WBC, **✳ PMN**, volume

↓ **viscosity**

Reye's syndrome

↑ **alanine**, ALP, **✳ ALT**, amino acids, **✳ ammonia**, **✳ AST**, Bil, **✳ CK**, CK-MB, GD, **glutamine**, LA, LD, **lysine**, **fatty acids**, Na, osmolality, P, **✳ PT**, pyruvate, **✳ RAL-MAC**, urea, FFA

↓ Apo B, CO_2, **✳ G**, K, LDL-C, **Na**, osmolality, P, pH, pCO_2, **PT**

■ *Urine* ↑ alpha-aminoadipic acid

■ *Cerebrospinal Fluid* ↑ **glutamine**, pressure

↓ **G**, proteins

Rotor's syndrome

↑ ALT, **✳ Bil**, **✳ conjugated Bil**, unconjugated Bil

■ *Urine* ↑ **conjugated Bil**, coproporphyrin – (**✳ I**, **✳ III**), **✳ UBG**

↓ UBG, **coproporphyrin III/coproporphyrin I index**

■ *Stool* ↓ UBG

Sezary's syndrome

↑ ALP, ALT

↓ albumin

Sheehan's syndrome

↓ **✳ ACTH**, RBC, estradiol, **✳ G**, FSH, LH, GH, Hb, HCT, WBC, TSH, **✳ PRL**

■ *Urine* ↓ 17-KS, 17-OHCS

SIADH (Syndrome of Inappropiate ADH Secretion)

↑ **ADH**, aldosterone, angiotensin, RBC, uric acid, MAL, Mg, PG, PRA

↓ **✳ albumin**, **✳ chloride**, K, creatinine, **uric acid**, LD, Mg, **✳Na**, **✳ osmolality**, PRA, proteins, urea

■ *Urine* ↑ **✳ ADH**, K, **kallikrein**, specific gravity, Mg, **✳ Na**, volume, **✳ osmolality**, PG

Sjögren's syndrome

↑ anticardiolipin Ab, alpha globulins, AMS, **✳ ANA**, **✳ ANCA**, **p-ANCA**, **✳ anti-ds-DNA**, anti-ss-DNA, **✳ antiphospholipid Ab**, antigamma globulin Ab, **antimicrosomal Ab**, anti-p 56, anti-poly(ADP-ribose), **anti-RNP**, anti-Scl 70, anti-Sm, **✳ anti-Ro/SSA**, **✳ anti-La,Ha/SSB**, **antithyroglobulin Ab**, antithyroid Ab, APA, CIC, CRP, eos, **✳ ESR**, **✳ gamma globulins**, HLA – (B8, DQ1, DR2, **✳ DR3**, DR4, DR52, Drw52, Dw3), IgA, IgG, IgM, **cryoglobulins**, LE cells, non-histone ANA, anti-Golgi complex Ab, antinuclear antigen Ab, **anti-salivary duct Ab**, **✳ RF**, **✳ viscosity**

↓ RBC, Hb, HCT, complement – (**C3**, C4, C6), **✳ WBC**, **✳ PLT**

■ *Urine* ↑ proteins, volume

■ *Saliva* ↑ B2M, chloride, IgA, **✳ IgG**, lysozyme, Na, **✳ RF**

↓ P

■ *Synovial Fluid* ↑ WBC, **✳ lym**, PMN

sleep apnea syndrome

↑ RBC, Hb, **✳ MAC**, **✳ pCO_2**, **✳ RAC**

↓ pH, pO_2

Stein-Leventhal syndrome

↑ *** androstenedione, * 3-alpha-androstanediol glucuronide, * DHEA, * estradiol**, estrone, FSH, **insulin, * LH, PRL, testosterone, * free testosterone**

↓ estradiol, estriol, *** FSH**, progesterone, SHBG

■ *Urine* ↑ estrogens, **17-ketosteroids**, LH, pregnanetriol, testosterone

   ↓ estriol, **FSH**

Stevens-Johnson syndrome

↑ anti-Mycoplasma pneumoniae Ab

systemic capillary leak syndrome

↑ **Hb**, light chains, **WBC**

↓ albumin

testicular feminization syndrome

↑ FSH, LH, SHBG, testosterone

■ *Urine* ↑ FSH, LH

Turner's syndrome

↑ antithyroglobulin Ab, *** FSH**, cholesterol, *** LH**

↓ aldosterone, *** estradiol**, estriol, *** estrogens**, progesterone

■ *Urine* ↑ Cr, **FSH, LH**

   ↓ aldosterone, **estriol**, 17-KS

■ *Amniotic Fluid* ↑ AFP

■ *Stool* ↑ blood

Waterhouse-Friederichsen syndrome

↑ K, WBC, urea

↓ G, *** chloride, * cortisol**, Na

WDHH syndrome (watery diarrhea, hypokalemia, hypochlorhydria)

↑ **VIP**

↓ K, Cl

Weil's syndrome

↑ ALP, ALT, AST, Bil, conjugated Bil, ESR,WBC, PLT, **urea**

↓ Hb, HCT, prothrombin, PLT

■ *Urine* ↑ proteins, RBC, pus, blood, WBC, casts – (hyaline, granular)

   ↓ volume

Werner's syndrome

↑ Apo B, cholesterol, LDL-C, TAG

Wiskott-Aldrich syndrome

↑ B-lym, BT, *** IgA, * IgE**, IgG, T-lym (CD4+, CD8+)

↓ B-lym, IgG, **IgM, * lym, * MPV, * PLT**, T-lym

Zollinger-Ellison syndrome

↑ ACTH, *** gastrin**, glucagon, GH-RH, insulin, *** calcitonin**, TM – (NSE), **pepsinogen**, PP, PTH, **secretin**, VIP

↓ albumin, K, vitamin – (B$_{12}$)

■ *Gastric Fluid* ↑ *** BAO, * basal secretion, HCl, MAO, volume, PAO**

   ↓ *** pH**

■ *Urine* ↑ gastrin

■ *Stool* ↑ fat, **volume**

   ↓ pH

Synovitis

crystal induced synovitis

■ *Synovial Fluid* ↑ clot formation, WBC, PMN, volume

   ↓ viscosity

idiopathic eosinophilic synovitis
> ■ *Synovial Fluid* ↑ eos, Charcot-Leyden crystals

villonodular synovitis
> ■ *Synovial Fluid* ↑ RBC, **clot formation**, WBC, lym, macrophages, viscosity, **volume**

Tachycardia, Atrial Paroxysmal
> ↑ ✱ **ANF**, cGMP, NT-pro-ANP, ✱ **WBC**

Tetany
> ↑ pH
>
> ↓ ✱ **Ca**, ✱ **Ca²⁺**, **chloride**, MAL, **Mg**, P, pO₂

Therapy
electroconvulsive therapy
> ↑ **epinephrine**, ALT, beta-endorphins, catecholamines
>
> ■ *Cerebrospinal Fluid* ↑ GMT

malignant tumor therapy
> ↑ uric acid

Thoracentesis
> ↓ albumin (repeated)

hrombasthenia, Hereditary Glanzmann's
> ↑ ✱ **BT**, **IL-6**, **PT**, TGT
>
> ↓ **PLT adhesion**, ✱ **PLT aggregation**, ✱ **clot retraction**, platelet factor 3

Thrombocytopenia
> ↑ Ab against beta-2 GP I, **antibodies against PLT** (autoimmune thrombocytopenia, idiopathic t., post-transfusion t.), **antibodies induced by drugs**, **antibodies induced by pregnancy**, ACLA, **heparin associated Ab**, BT, clot retraction
>
> ↓ **PLT**
>
> ■ *Urine* ↑ RBC, Hb
>
> ■ *Sputum* ↑ blood
>
> ■ *Synovial Fluid* ↑ RBC

Thrombocytosis
primary thrombocytosis
> ↑ ✱ **ACP**, ✱ **PLT aggregation**, ALP (WBC), Ca, K, **uric acid**, ✱ **LD**, ✱ **WBC**, ✱ **neu**, ✱ **PLT**, viscosity
>
> ↓ ✱ **ALP** (WBC), RBC, Hb, ✱ **HCT**, pO₂
>
> ■ *Synovial Fluid* ↑ RBC

secondary thrombocytosis
> ↑ ACP, bas, K, LD, PLT

Thrombophlebitis
cerebral thrombophlebitis
> ↑ ESR, WBC
>
> ■ *Cerebrospinal Fluid* ↑ WBC, pressure

septic thrombophlebitis
> ↑ ACP, ✱ **alpha-1-globulins**, AST, **bacteria** (culture), ✱ **CRP**, ✱ **ESR**, ✱ **fibrinogen**, ✱ **WBC**, MAC, neu, RAL, urea
>
> ↓ pH, **pO₂**
>
> ■ *Cerebrospinal Fluid* ↑ protein

Thrombosis
> ↑ Ab against beta-2 GP I, ACLA, ACP, ALT, APLA, D-dimers, **FDP**, **homocysteine**, **factor V Leiden**, WBC, prothrombinogen, neu

    ↓ **∗ AT III**, protein C, prostacyclin
    ■ *Urine* ↑ 5-HIT
acute thrombosis
    ↑ protein S, factor VIII, vWF, PAI
carotid thrombosis
    ■ *Urine* ↑ hexosaminidase
cerebral vein thrombosis
    ↑ Ab against beta-2 GP I, TAG
    ■ *Cerebrospinal Fluid* ↑ **proteins**, CK, WBC, lym, RBC, **pressure**
deep venous thrombosis (lower extremity)
    ↑ Ab against beta-2 GP I, factor VIII, fibrinopeptide A, **plasminogen acti-**
      vator inhibitor
    ↓ **protein C, protein S**
mesenteric vein thrombosis
    ↑ **AMS**, lipase
    ■ *Peritoneal Fluid* ↑ AMS
    ■ *Stool* ↑ blood
renal vein thrombosis
    ↑ **FDP, chloride, WBC**, lipids, **MAC**
    ↓ **albumin, RBC, G, Hb, HCT**, osmolality, **pH**, PLT
    ■ *Urine* ↑ **proteins**, RBC, G, Hb, pus, **blood**, osmolality, casts – **(RBC)**
      ↓ **volume**

Thyroidectomy

    ↓ T4, TSH, thyroglobulin

Thyroiditis

  autoimmune chronic thyroiditis (Hashimoto's thyroiditis)
    ↑ ANA, antiadrenal Ab, **∗ antimicrosomal Ab**, antithyroglobulin Ab,
      antithyroidal Ab, ∗ antithyroperoxidase Ab, thyroxine autoanti-
      bodies, APA, ESR, FT4, HLA – (Bw35, B37, DR5), IgA, IgM, LATS,
      WBC, antithyroid components Ab, anti-TSH receptor Ab, T3, **∗ T4**
      (early), TSH, thyroglobulin
    ↓ iodine, complement – (C3), FT4, T3, **T4** (later), **TSH**
  lymphocytic thyroiditis
    ↑ AAT, **AMA,** ANA, antiadrenal Ab, **antimicrosomal Ab, antithyroglobu-**
      lin Ab, antithyroid Ab (later), antithyroperoxidase Ab, APA, thyrox-
      ine autoantibodies, FT3, FT4, **ESR,** cholesterol, IgA, IgM, **calcitonin,**
      complement – (C3), LATS, WBC, **neu,** antibodies against thyroid
      components, anti-TSH-receptor Ab, **T3** (early), **T4** (early), TSH
      (later), **thyroglobulin**
    ↓ RBC, FT4, Hb, HCT, iodine, complement – (C3), WBC, T3, T4 (later),
      TSH (early)
  subacute thyroiditis (Quervain's t.)
    ↑ ALP, **antimicrosomal Ab, antithyroglobulin Ab**, antithyroidal Ab,
      antithyroperoxidase Ab, AST, beta-carotene, CK, FT3, **FT4** (early), **∗**
      ESR, glycoproteins, **GMT**, HLA – (**∗ B35**), **cholesterol**, IgD, IgM,
      complement – (C3), LATS, **LD, WBC, T3**, T3 uptake, **T4** (early), **TSH**
      (recovery phase), **thyroglobulin**
    ↓ AAT, **RBC, G, Hb, HCT**, IgA, complement – (C3), WBC, **Na**, T4, TSH
      (early)

Thyrotoxicosis

↑ ACE, epinephrine, **ALP**, ALT, AMA, anti-ds-DNA, antithyroglobulin Ab, ✻ **antithyroid Ab**, AST, Ca, Ca²⁺, **ceruloplasmin**, Cu, ferritin, ✻ **FTI**, ✻ **FT4**, G, CHS, iodine, catecholamines, creatine, **ketobodies, acetoacetic acid**, WBC, LATS, **lym**, neu, norepinephrine, plasma volume, SHBG, thyroglobulin, ✻ **T3**, ✻ **T4**

↓ albumin, **AMS**, proteins, **cholesterol**, Hb, IgA, K, WBC, neu, PICP, PTH, TBG, TIBC, ✻ **TSH**, vitamin – (D)

- ◾ *Urine* ↑ Ca, creatine, G, 17-OHCS
  - ↓ 17-KS
- ◾ *Gastric Fluid* ↑ pH
  - ↓ HCl
- ◾ *Stool* ↑ Ca, fat

Tonsillitis

↑ ASLO, CRP, ESR, WBC, mucoproteins

Transfusion

exchange blood transfusion

↑ Ca, folic acid, K, MAC, Na

↓ G, HbA₁c, PLT

fetal-maternal transfusion (maternal blood)

↑ ✻ fetal RBC, nucleated RBC, RTC

↓ Fe, **Hb**, **HCT**

incompatible blood transfusion

↑ ✻ **Bil**, euglobulin lysis time, ✻ **FDP**, WBC

↓ ✻ **Hb**, ✻ **HCT**

- ◾ *Urine* ↑ RBC, Hb, casts – (hemoglobin)

massive blood transfusion

↑ APTT, ✻ **BT**, ✻ **FDP**, Fe, folic acid, ✻ **K**, ✻ LD2, LD3, LD4, MAL, MAL+RAL, ✻ **PT**

↓ alpha-2-globulins, Ca, factor VIII, **fibrinogen**, HbA₁c, K, proaccelerin, **PLT**

- ◾ *Urine* ↑ RBC, casts – (hemoglobin)

maternal-fetal transfusion (fetal blood)

↑ unconjugated Bil, Hb, HCT

multiple blood transfusion

↑ APTT, **Fe**, **fibrinogen**, folic acid, lupus inhibitor, **PT**, VDRL (false posit.)

↓ alpha-2-globulins, HbA₁c, Mg, **PLT**

- ◾ *Urine* ↑ hemosiderin

old blood transfusion

↑ ✻ **unconjugated Bil**, ✻ **K**, ✻ **LD**, P

↓ haptoglobin

plasma transfusion

↑ **PT**

Transplantation

heart transplantation

↑ antimyocardial Ab, **ESR**, LD, LD1, WBC

kidney transplantation

↑ AMS, B2M, Ca, **RBC**, FDP, GMT, K, **LDL-C**, RF

↓ HDL-C, Mg

- ◾ *Urine* ↑ AAP, volume

liver transplantation
> ↑ ALP, ALT, AST, Bil, conjugated Bil, GMT

pancreas transplantation
> ↑ C-peptide

skin transplantation
> ↑ RF

Transudation
> ↑ aldosterone
> ↓ albumin

Trauma

blunt trauma of abdomen
> ■ *Peritoneal Fluid* ↑ * AMS, * RBC, * WBC
> ↓ RBC

penetrating trauma of abdomen
> ↑ PCT, WBC
> ■ *Peritoneal Fluid* ↑ ALP, AMS, **bacteria** (+ culture), **proteins**, * RBC, TAG, * WBC

trauma of aspiration
> ■ *Synovial Fluid* ↑ RBC
> ■ *Pleural Fluid* ↑ RBC
> ■ *Peritoneal Fluid* ↑ RBC
> ■ *Cerebrospinal Fluid* ↑ RBC

trauma of chest
> ↑ PCT
> ■ *Peritoneal Fluid* ↑ **proteins**, TAG

trauma of head
> ↑ NSE
> ■ *Cerebrospinal Fluid* ↑ **proteins**, * IgM, * **prealbumin**

Trisomy

13 (Patau's syndrome)
> ↑ AFP, HbF
> ↓ AFP

18
> ↑ conjugated Bil
> ↓ AFP, hCG, estriol

Tumor Lysis
> ↑ K, creatinine, **uric acid**, MAC, P, urea
> ↓ Ca
> ■ *Urine* ↑ LAP
> ↓ volume

Tumors
> ↑ AAT, ACA, AD, PLT adhesion, albumin, aldolase, **alpha-1- antichymotrypsin, alpha-1-globulins, alpha-2-globulins**, alpha-2 pregnancy associated glycoprotein, **ALP**, A2MG, AMA, ANA, anti-La/SSB, ASAL, **ASMA**, AST, beta globulins, proteins, **Bil, unconjugated Bil, Ca**, Ca²⁺, **ceruloplasmin**, Cu, CK, CK-MB, CK-MM, estradiol, FDP, ferritin, ESR, G, **gamma globulins**, glycated Hb, **haptoglobin**, Hb, hemopexin, h-sVCAM-1, IgG, IgM, **C1-INH**, plasminogen activator inhibitor, complement – (C3, C4), cortisol, cryofibrinogen, **cryoglobulins**, **uric acid, LA, LD**, LD – (2, 3, 4, 5), **WBC**, lupus inhibitor, MAC, mac-

rocytes, MD, microcytes, mucoproteins, Na, TM – (**AFP**, B2M, CEA, hCG, TPA), **orosomucoid**, osteocalcin, PAPP-A, **parathyroid hormone-related protein**, plasmocytes, PP, pyruvic acid, RF, TNF, PLT, UBBC, urea, VDRL (false posit.)

↓ **albumin**, ALT, **proteins**, Ca, ceruloplasmin, Cu, **RBC**, **Fe**, fibrinogen, G, globulins, **Hb**, **HCT**, cholesterol, CHS, IgA, IgE, IgG, IgM, inter-alpha-trypsin inhibitor, complement – (CH50), cortisol, uric acid, MCV, P, **PT**, pO_2, prealbumin, **transferrin satur.**, Se, GH, **TIBC**, transferrin, **PLT**, vitamin – (B$_1$, B$_2$, B$_{12}$, C, folate), Zn

- *Urine* ↑ alpha-aminonitrogen, G, Hb, coproporphyrin III, **17-OHCS**, crystals – (urate), beta-aminoisobutyric acid, PBG, porphyrins, **urea**, uroporphyrin, VMA, **Zn**
    ↓ vitamin C

- *Cerebrospinal Fluid* ↑ adenylate kinase, AFP, beta-glucuronidase, **proteins**, phenylalanine, **glutamine**, glycine, hCG, isoleucine, glutamic acid, leucine, lysine, MBP, P, proline, taurine, pressure, RBC, tryptophan, tyrosine, valine
    ↓ **G**

- *Pleural Fluid* ↑ albumin, A2MG, **blood**, proteins, CK, eos, **RBC**, FDP, haptoglobin, hemopexin, IgA, IgG, **LD**, **lym**, mononuclear cells, mucopolysaccharides, **neu**, volume, **WBC**
    ↓ alpha globulins, C3, C4, pH

- *Pericardial Fluid* ↑ lym
    ↓ G

- *Peritoneal Fluid* ↑ ALP, AMS, bacteria (+ culture), **proteins**, cholesterol, fibronectin, RBC, LA, specific gravity, TAG, TM – (**CEA**), WBC
    ↓ LA

- *Sputum* ↑ **blood**
- *Stool* ↑ **blood**
- *Synovial Fluid* ↑ volume

adenoma
– adenoma of hypophysis

↑ ACTH, G, GH, LH, TM – (PTH), **PRL**
↓ cortisol

– adrenocortical adenoma

↑ ADH, aldosterone, 11-deoxycortisol, EPO, GH-RH, G, Na, hCG, **ILGF-II**, **cortisol**, MAL, cholesterol
↓ **ACTH**, **PRA**, **K**, chloride

- *Urine* ↑ aldosterone, estrogens, 17-OHCS, **17-KGS**, 17-KS, 18-OH cortisol, **free cortisol**

– pancreatic adenoma

↑ ALP, Bil, **G**, TM – (CA 19-9, CA 50, CEA, DU-PAN-2, SPAN-1, PCAA), pancreatic oncofetal antigen

- *Peritoneal Fluid* ↑ **proteins**, TAG

– thyroid adenoma

↑ antimicrosomal Ab, **T3**, **T4**, **thyroglobulin**

- *Urine* ↑ 5-HIAA

adrenal tumors

↑ ADH, **aldosterone**, **androgens**, **androstenedione**, 11-deoxycortisol, DHEA, EPO, estriol, **estrogens**, RBC, G, GH-RH, **ILGF-II**, **cortisol**, MAL, cholesterol, TM – (ACTH, ADH, hCG, NSE, VIP), PRA, pregnenolone, 17-OH progesterone, progesterone, testosterone

    ↓ **ACTH**, G, **K**, chloride, **PRA**

    ■ *Urine* ↑ **aldosterone, estriol**, estrogens, **17-OHCS, 17-KGS, 17-KS,** cortisol, pregnanetriol, **free cortisol**

    ↓ FSH

– adrenal medulla tumors

    ↑ epinephrine

bladder tumors

    ↑ ADA, beta-lipotropin, Ca, CK, CK-MB, CK-MM, endorphins, enkephalins, TM – (ACTH, beta-lipotropin, ✳ **BTA, CEA**, CK-BB, galactosyl-transferase, Tennessee antigen, **TPA**)

    ■ *Urine* ↑ arylsulfatase A, **RBC**, FDP, fibrinogen, **frequency, Hb, pus, blood**, LAP, LD, NMP22,**WBC**

bone marrow tumors

    ↑ eos, neu, nucleated RBC, schistocytes, teardrop RBC, WBC

    ↓ fibrinogen, PLT, **WBC**

bone tumors

    ↑ **ACP, ALP,** ALP (bone isoenzyme), Ca, Cu, deoxypyridinoline, WBC, TM – (ALP, CEA), P, pyridinoline, N-telopeptides

    ■ *Urine* ↑ Ca, hydroxyproline

    ↓ Ca

    ■ *Synovial Fluid* ↑ RBC, **volume**

– osteosarcoma

    ↑ ACP, alpha-2-globulins, **ALP**, Zn

breast tumors

    ↑ ACP, **aldolase, ALP,** ALT, AMS, AMS (P), ANA, beta-glucuronidase, ✳ **Ca**, ceruloplasmin, CK, CK-BB, CK-MB, CK-MM, CRP, Cu, **EGF-R**, endorphins, enkephalins, ferritin, glycolipids, **HER-2 growth factor**, CHS, calcitonin, caseine, lym, mono, ✳ **nucleated RBC, WBC**, TM – (ACTH, AFP, alpha-lactalbumin, ALP, arylsulfatase B, AST, **BCM**, B2M, beta-lipotropin, ✳ **CA 15-3,** CA 19-5, CA 27.29, CA 50, CA 72-4, CA 125, CA 242, **CA 549,** ✳ **CEA**, c-erb-B-amplification, CK-BB, esterase, **estrogen**/glucocorticoid/**progesterone receptors**, ferritin, hCG, hPL, calcitonin, sialic acid, M2-PK, **MCA**, PSA, PTH, sialyl-transferase, **TPA**), PL, procathepsin D, prostacyclin

    ■ *Urine* ↑ beta-2-glycoprotein I, Ca, hCG

    ↓ **pregnanediol**

    ■ *Cerebrospinal Fluid* ↑ TM – (✳ **CEA**)

    ■ *Peritoneal Fluid* ↑ proteins, TM – (CEA)

    ■ *Pleural Fluid* ↑ TM – (CA 125), **CEA**, orosomucoid

carcinoid

    ↑ **ACTH,** ADH, ALT, bradykinin, **CRH, endorphins, enkephalins,** gastrin, GH-RH, glucagon, histamine, calcitonin, kallikrein, catecholamines, WBC, methionine, **neurophysin,** TM – (beta-lipotropin, CEA, hCG, ✳ **5-HIAA,** ✳ **NSE**), **oxytocin,** P, gastrin-releasing peptide, **PG,** PP, ✳ **serotonin, somatostatin,** GH, substance K, **substance P,** VIP

    ↓ albumin, amino acids, isoleucine, lysine, niacin, ornithine, tryptophan, tyrosine, valine, vitamin – (A)

    ■ *Urine* ↑ ✳ **5-HIAA,** 5-OH-tryptophan, proline, ✳ **serotonin,** VMA

    ↓ niacin

    ■ *Stool* ↑ fat

    ■ *Synovial Fluid* ↑ WBC, PMN

carcinomatosis

   ↑ albumin, CEA, LD

   ↓ G, Hb

   ■ *Cerebrospinal Fluid* ↑ AFP, * **proteins**

     ↓ G

   ■ *Peritoneal Fluid* ↑ WBC

     ↓ G

cerebral tumors

   ↑ **aldolase**, ALT, CK, TM – (NSE)

   ■ *Cerebrospinal Fluid* ↑ **proteins**, CK, IDH, IgG, IgM, **WBC**, lym, lysozyme, **MBP**, **tumor cells**, P, **pressure**

     ↓ G

cervix uteri tumors

   ↑ ALP, Cu, lym, TM – (beta-glucuronidase, CA 27-29, * **SCCA**)

   ■ *Urine* ↑ gonadotropin peptide

chorionepithelioma

   ↑ ALT, AST, **estrogens**, fibrinogen, ESR, GMT, WBC, TM – (**AFP**, CEA, * **hCG**), **progesterone**, T4

   ↓ RBC, Hb, HCT, **hPL**

   ■ *Urine* ↑ **hCG**, pregnanediol

   ■ *Cerebrospinal Fluid* ↑ hCG

CNS tumors

   ↑ ADH, **aldolase**, AST, CK, ICD, LD 5, TM – (NSE)

   ↓ Na

   ■ *Urine* ↑ G

   ■ *Cerebrospinal Fluid* ↑ **proteins**, CK, G, cholesterol, CHS, IDH, IgG, IgM, **LA**, **LD**, WBC, lym, lysozyme, **MBP**, mono, tumor cells, P, plasmocytes, **pressure**

     ↓ **G**, WBC

colorectum tumors

   ↑ ALP, aldolase, beta-glucuronidase, AMS, AMS (P, S), **arylsulfatase A**, B2M, CK, **CK-BB**, CK-MB, CK-MM, endorphins, enkephalins, **ESR**, hCG, **WBC**, TM – (ACTH, ADH, AFP, aldolase, AMS, arylsulfatase B, beta-glucosidase, beta-lipotropin, CA 15-3, * **CA 19-9**, **CA 27.29**, CA 50, CA 72-4, **CA 195**, **CA 242**, CA 549, * **CEA**, * **CASA**, CK-BB, galactosyltransferase, h-sICAM-1, LD, M2-PK, beta-oncofetal antigen, ribonuclease, sialyltransferase, Tennessee antigen, TAG 72, TPA, * **TPS**), PP

   ↓ RBC, Hb, HCT, **K**

   ■ *Urine* ↑ arylsulfatase A, hCG, pus

   ■ *Stool* ↑ **blood**, **Hb**, **RBC**, **mucus**

   ■ *Peritoneal Fluid* ↑ **proteins**, TAG, TM – (CEA)

   ■ *Pleural Fluid* ↑ AMS

embryonic tumors

   ↑ TM – (**AFP**, hCG)

   ■ *Urine* ↑ hCG

endometrium tumors

   ↑ GH-RH, TM – (CA 125)

   ■ *Urine* ↑ gonadotropin peptide

   ■ *Peritoneal Fluid* ↑ CA 125

esophagal tumors

↑ **AMS**, Ca, WBC, TM – (CEA, M2-PK, SCCA)

■ *Stool* ↑ blood

feminizing tumors

↑ estradiol

↓ FSH, LH, progesterone

gallbladder tumors

↑ alpha-1-globulins, **ALP**, **ALT**, **AST**, **Bil**, conjugated Bil, CK, CRP, clotting time, elastase, endorphins, enkephalins, fibrinogen, GMD, **GMT**, **haptoglobin**, **cholesterol**, IgA, LAP, 5-nucleotidase, **PL**, **PT**, TAG, TM – (ACTH, beta-lipotropin, CA 19-9, CA 27-29, CEA, TPA)

↓ RBC, Hb, HCT, factor II, vitamin – (B$_2$)

■ *Urine* ↑ **conjugated Bil**, pH

↓ Na, volume, **UBG**

■ *Stool* ↑ blood

↓ **Bil**, **UBG**

gastrointestinal tract tumors

↑ ADH, **aldolase**, ALP, CK, CK-BB, CRP, Cu, **IgA**, WBC, neu, TM – (ALP, CA 19-5, CA 19-9, CA 50, CA 72-4, CA 125, CA 242, ✱ **CEA**, c-erb-B-2-amplification, CK-BB, DU-PAN-2, galactosyltransferase, sialic acid, PSA, SCCA, Tennessee antigen)

↓ G, **Se**, transferrin satur.

■ *Urine* ↑ 5-HIAA

■ *Peritoneal Fluid* ↑ **proteins**, TAG, TM – (CEA)

■ *Pleural Fluid* ↑ TM – (CA 125, **CEA**)

■ *Stool* ↑ blood

hemangioma

↓ **PLT**

■ *Synovial Fluid* ↑ **RBC**

hypophysis tumors

↑ ACTH, CRH, GH-RH, PRL, **GH**

↓ ADH, ILGF-I

■ *Urine* ↑ **17-OH corticosteroids**, **cortisol**, 17-KS, specific gravity

intracranial tumors

– astrocytoma

■ *Cerebrospinal Fluid* ↑ enolase, fibronectin

– dysgerminoma

■ *Cerebrospinal Fluid* ↑ AFP, hCG, **MBP**

– ganglioblastoma

↑ epinephrine, CK, catecholamines, **norepinephrine**, VIP

■ *Urine* ↑ **catecholamines**, **HVA**, normetanephrine, VMA

– ganglioneuroma

↑ epinephrine, CK, dopamine, **catecholamines**, TM – (CEA, NSE, VIP), **norepinephrine**

■ *Urine* ↑ HVA, **catecholamines**, cystathionine, **norepinephrine**, **normetanephrine**, **VMA**

– neuroblastoma

↑ epinephrine, ILGF-II, LATS, ✱ **catecholamines**, ✱ **dopamine**, TM – (CEA, ferritin, ✱ **NSE**, VIP), protein S-100, norepinephrine

↓ RBC, Hb, HCT, WBC, PLT

■ *Urine* ↑ cystathionine, ✱ **HVA**, **catecholamines**, metanephrines, **norepinephrine**, **normetanephrine**, ✱ **VMA**

– paraganglioma

↑ epinephrine, catecholamines, **norepinephrine**

■ *Urine* ↑ catecholamines

Kaposi's sarcoma

↑ HLA – (DR5), IL-6

kidney tumors

↑ ALP, ALT, amylin, ANA, AST, Ca, **endorphins, enkephalins**, RBC, **EPO**, ESR, glucagon, IL-6, WBC, TM – (**ACTH, AFP, beta-lipotropin**, CA 27-29, CA 50, CEA, **✳ M2-PK**, NSE, PRL, PSA, PTH, GH), PGE, **PRA**, PLT, PT

↓ albumin

■ *Urine* ↑ ALP, proteins, **RBC, Hb, blood**, LAP, LD

– hypernephroma

↑ alpha-2-globulins, ALP, ALT, AST, Bil, **Ca, Ca²⁺, RBC**, EPO, **ESR**, HCT, **PT**, PGE, PRA, PRL, PSA, PLT, **PTH**

↓ albumin, RBC, Hb, HCT

■ *Urine* ↑ **RBC, Hb, blood**

– nephroblastoma

↑ **EPO**, ILGF-II

■ *Urine* ↑ RBC, Hb, LAP

larynx tumors

↑ ACTH, beta-lipotropin, endorphins, enkephalins, TM – (**✳ SCCA**)

■ *Urine* ↑ 5-HIAA

left heart atrium myxoma

↑ AST, CRP, **ESR, gamma globulins**, IgG, LD, WBC, **poikilocytes**, RTC

↓ **RBC, Hb, HCT**, PLT

leiomyoma

↑ EPO

liver tumors

↑ ACTH, **aldolase, ALP, ALT**, ASMA, **AST**, beta-glucuronidase, **Bil, conjugated Bil**, unconjugated Bil, B2M, Ca, CK-MB, CK-MM, **RBC, EPO**, estrogens, ferritin, **ESR, GMT**, hPL, cholesterol, ICD, IgA, **ILGF-II**, calcitonin, cryofibrinogen, **LAP, LD**, LDL-C, WBC, Na, neu, TM – (**✳ AFP**, aldolase, alcohol dehydrogenase, ALP, CA 15-3, **CA 19-9, CA 27-29**, CA 125, **CEA**, ferritin, GMT, hCG, hexokinase, LAP, LD, **5-nucleotidase**, placental lactogen, PTH, pyruvate kinase, TPA), **OCT**, prothrombin, SD, TAG, UBBC, vitamin B₁₂, bile acids

↓ AAT, AMS, **RBC**, fibrinogen, **G, Hb, HCT**, cholesterol, **IgM**, ILGF-I, Mg

■ *Urine* ↑ cystathionine, ethanolamine, hCG

■ *Peritoneal Fluid* ↑ ✳ **blood**, RBC, sTM – (CEA)

lung tumors

↑ **ACTH**, ACP, ADH, **aldolase, ALP**, ALT, AMS, **AMS** (S), ANA, proteins, **Ca**, CIC, CK, CK-BB, CK-MB, CK-MM, **CRH**, CRP, Cu, elastase, eos, RBC, ferritin, fibrinogen, **gastrin, GH-RH**, glucagon, **hPL**, insulin, **calcitonin**, LD, lipase, WBC, ✳ **nucleated RBC**, TM – (ACTH, ADH, AFP, aldolase, ALP, B2M, bombezin, CA 15-3, CA 19-9, **CA 27.29**, CA 50, CA 72-4, CA 125 – small-cell, epithelial, CA 549, ✳ **CEA – small-cell**, epithelial, CK-BB, c-myc-translocation, CYFRA 21-1, DU-PAN-2, ferritin, **hCG**, hPL, calcitonin, **chromogranin A, B** – small-cell, sialic acid, L-dopa-decarboxylase, M2-PK, MCA, MSH, **neurophysins, NSE** – small-cell, **oxytocin**, PRL, PSA, PTH, ribonuclease, **SCCA** epithelial, sialyltransferase, TPA – small-cell, thymidine kinase – small-cell, **VIP**), gastrin-releasing peptide, PTH, serotonin, **somatostatin**, GH

- ↓ **ACE, fibrinogen**, Hb, HCT, **Na**, RBC
- ■ *Urine* ↑ alpha-aminonitrogen, amino acids, AMS, Ca, G, hCG
- ■ *Pleural Fluid* ↑ albumin, A2MG, AMS, beta-glucuronidase, **blood**, **proteins**, TM – **(CA 125)**, **CEA**, eos, **RBC**, FDP, haptoglobin, hemopexin, IgA, IgG, **LD**, **lym**, **WBC**, mononuclear cells, mucopolysaccharides, **neu**, volume, orosomucoid
  - ↓ alpha globulins, C3, C4, G, **pH**
- ■ *Peritoneal Fluid* ↑ TM – (CEA)
- ■ *Sputum* ↑ **blood**, **✻ malignant cells**
- ■ *Bronchoalveolar Lavage Fluid* ↑ **✻ malignant cells**

– **non-small cell bronchogenic tumor**

↑ B2M, CEA

– **small cell bronchogenic tumor**

↑ ADH, CK-BB, **CRH**, **endorphins**, **enkephalins**, fibrinogen, **GH-RH**, TM – (**ACTH**, ADH, bombesin, **✻ CEA**, CRP, elastase, **hCG**, cortisol, neurophysins, **✻ NSE**, placental lactogen, thymidine kinase, VIP), **oxytocin**, PRL

- ↓ WBC
- ■ *Urine* ↑ 5-HIAA
- ■ *Pleural Fluid* ↑ proteins, eos
  - ↓ alpha globulins
- ■ *Sputum* ↑ **✻ malignant cells**
- ■ *Bronchoalveolar Lavage Fluid* ↑ **✻ malignant cells**

lymphosarcoma

↑ alpha-2-globulins, **IgM**, cryoglobulins, **lym**

- ■ *Urine* ↑ uric acid
- ■ *Cerebrospinal Fluid* ↑ LD

malignant lymphoma

↑ ADH, aldolase, ANA, conjugated Bil, unconjugated Bil, Ca, CK, CK-MB, CK-MM, CK-BB, **Cu**, eos, Fas-ligand, gamma globulins, hPL, **cold agglutinins**, chylomicrons, IDL-C, IgG, IgM, IL-6, creatinine, **cryoglobulins**, **uric acid**, sialic acid, LA, **LD**, LD – (2, 3, 4), WBC, **mono**, neu, TM – (AFP, ALP, **BCL-2, B2M, CD 30+**, CEA, CK-BB, c-myc-translocation, **ferritin**, **fibronectin**, immunoglobulins, LD, sialic acid, **thymidine kinase**), paraproteins, placental lactogen, PRL, pyroglobulins, **terminal deoxynucleotidyl transferase**, PLT, vitamin – (D2), VLDL-C

- ↓ ALP, Hb, C1-esterase inhibitor, folate, lym, **neu**, **PLT**, vitamin D2, Zn
- ■ *Urine* ↑ Bence Jones protein, **proteins**, Ca, RBC, casts
- ■ *Cerebrospinal Fluid* ↑ enolase, **LD**
  - ↓ G
- ■ *Pericardial Fluid* ↑ volume
- ■ *Peritoneal Fluid* ↑ eos, volume, **proteins**, **TAG**
- ■ *Pleural Fluid* ↑ B2M, **lym**

– **Burkitt's malignant lymphoma**

↑ ALT, anti-EBV, B2M, Ca, CRP, elastase, gamma globulins, IgG, **WBC**

↓ IgM, lym

- cutaneous T-cell malignant lymphoma
    ↑ ✶ lym, ✶ Sézary cells, WBC
- Hodgkin's malignant lymphoma
    ↑ ACE, Al, **alpha-1-globulins**, **alpha-2-globulins**, ALP, ALP (WBC), **ALT**, AST, baso, **Bil**, beta globulins, **B2M**, BSP retention, **Ca**, **ceruloplasmin**, CO_2, **CRP**, **Cu**, **eos**, **ferritin**, ESR, **nucleated RBC**, fibrinogen, fucose, gamma globulins, **globulins**, **GMT**, **haptoglobin**, hexokinase, HBsAg, HLA – (A1, DP3, DP4), h-sICAM-1, **hydroxyproline**, chylomicrons, IgA, IgE, IgG, IgM, uric acid, complement – (total), **creatinine**, cryofibrinogen, **cryoglobulins**, uric acid, **LA**, LAP (WBC), **LD**, LD – (2, 3, 4), **WBC**, **lym**, **lysozyme**, **mono**, mucoproteins, **neu**, 5-NT, TM – (**AFP**, ALP, CEA, ferritin), osmotic fragility (RBC), paraproteins, pCO_2, prealbumin, pyruvate, RF, RTC, **PLT**, vitamin B_{12} binding capacity, vitamin – (B_1), VLDL-C, Zn
    ↓ ACE, **albumin**, ALP, ALP (WBC), beta globulins, **proteins**, BT, EPO, **RBC**, **Fe**, gamma globulins, **Hb**, **HCT**, cholesterol (RBC), IgA, IgG, complement – (C3), **uric acid**, **WBC**, **lym**, **PLT**, **TIBC**, transferrin satur., T-cells, Zn
    ■ *Urine* ↑ hydroxyproline, lysozyme, PBG, **porphyrins**
    ■ *Cerebrospinal Fluid* ↑ B2M, enolase, eos
    ■ *Peritoneal Fluid* ↑ eos, volume, **proteins**, TAG
    ■ *Pleural Fluid* ↑ AMS, proteins, eos, lym
- lymphocytic malignant lymphoma
    ■ *Peritoneal Fluid* ↑ **proteins**
- non-Hodgkin's malignant lymphoma
    ↑ AAT, ACP, ACP (prostatic), aldolase, **ALP**, ALP (WBC), alpha-2-globulins, **ALT**, **AST**, **B2M**, **Bil**, BSP retention, Ca, Cu, ESR, ferritin, fucose, gamma globulins, GMT, haptoglobin, hexokinase, cold agglutinins, chylomicrons, immunoglobulins, IgG, IgM, creatinine, cryoglobulins, **uric acid**, **LA**, **LD**, WBC, **lym**, **mono**, **Na**, 5-NT, pyruvate, RF, TM – (ferritin, CA 125, CEA, LD), UBBC, **urea**, vitamin – (B_{12}, D3), VLDL-C
    ↓ ACE, ACP (WBC), albumin, ALP, ALP (WBC), beta globulins, proteins, RBC, Fe, **gamma globulins**, globulins, **Hb**, **HCT**, cholesterol, immunoglobulins, WBC, MCH, MCHC, MCV, RTC, **PLT**, TIBC, transferrin satur., vitamin – (D3), Zn
    ■ *Urine* ↑ Ca, uric acid, 5-HIAA
    ■ *Cerebrospinal Fluid* ↑ **B2M**
    ■ *Pleural Fluid* ↑ proteins
maskulinizing tumors
    ↑ estradiol, FSH, LH, progesterone
    ■ *Urine* ↑ 17-ketosteroids
mastocytosis, systemic
    ↑ APTT, eos, bas, ✶ **histamine**, **tryptase**, WBC
    ↓ Hb, HCT, PLT, WBC
    ■ *Urine* ↑ ✶ **histamine**, ✶ **histamine metabolites**
    ■ *Gastric Fluid* ↑ HCl
        ↓ pH
melanoma
    ↑ aldolase, ALT, ANA, eos, h-sICAM-1, MAC, WBC, neu, TM – (melanoma-associated Ag, **B2M**, CEA, hCG, sialic acid, NSE, ✶ **intracellular S-100 protein**, SCCA, thymidine kinase)

        ↓ IgD, **MIA**
- *Urine* ↑ hCG, melanin
- *Cerebrospinal Fluid* ↓ G

mesothelioma
- *Pleural Fluid* ↑ eos, hyaluronic acid
- *Bronchoalveolar Lavage Fluid* ↑ mesothelial cells
- *Peritoneal Fluid* ↑ **hyaluronic acid**, volume

myelodysplastic syndrome

↑ BT, EPO, WBC, **macrocytes**, MCV, **mono**, poikilocytes, schistocytes, transferrin receptor

↓ RBC, Hb, HCT, WBC, neu, pyruvate kinase, RTC, **PLT**

ovary tumors

↑ ALP, ALT, AMS, **AMS** (S), ANA, **androstenedione**, B2M, **Ca²⁺**, CK-BB, CK-MB, CK-MM, RBC, estriol, **estrogens**, gastrin, ILGF-II, mono, TM – (**AFP** – germinative cells, ALP-placental, antigen of ovarian carcinoma, CA 15-3 – epithelial cells, CA 19-5, **CA 19-9** – epithelial cells, **CA 27.29**, CA 50, CA 72-4 – epithelial cells, ✶ **CA 125** – epithelial cells, CA 549, ✶ **CASA**, **CEA**, CK-BB, c-erb-B-2-amplification, DU-PAN-2, galactosyltransferase, glycosyltransferase, **hCG** – germinative cells, hPL, MCA, PRL, procollagen, ribonuclease, TPA – epithelial cells), progesterone, 17-OH progesterone, **PTH**, testosterone

- *Urine* ↑ AMS, estriol, estrogens, gonadotropin peptide, **hCG**, **17-KS**, pregnanetriol

    ↓ FSH, **pregnanediol**

- *Peritoneal Fluid* ↑ AMS, ✶ **proteins** (adenocarcinoma), TM – (CA 125, CEA)
- *Pleural Fluid* ↑ AMS, TM – (CA 125), orosomucoid

– eminizing arrhenoblastoma

↓ **pregnanediol**

- *Urine* ↑ pregnanediol

    ↓ FSH

– masculinizing arrhenoblastoma

↑ ✶ **testosterone**

- *Urine* ↑ androsterone, **17-KS**, testosterone

    ↓ FSH

pancreatic tumors

↑ ADH, aldolase, **ALP**, ALT, AMS, **AMS** (P, S), beta-glucuronidase, Bil, conjugated Bil, Ca, **Ca²⁺**, CRP, euglobulin lysis time, elastase, **endorphins**, **enkephalins**, ferritin, fibrinogen, **GH-RH**, **GMT**, h-sICAM-1, cholesterol, chymotrypsin, ILGF-II, **calcitonin**, glutamic acid, LAP, **lipase**, WBC, TM – (**ACTH**, ADH, AFP, AMS, **beta-lipotropin**, CA 15-3, CA 19-5, **CA 19-9**, **CA 27.29**, CA 50, CA 72-4, CA 125, CA 195, **CA 242**, **CEA**, DU-PAN-2, ferritin, galactosyltransferase II-isoenzyme, **hCG**, calcitonin, chromogranin A, B, **LAP**, NSE, pancreatic oncofetal antigen, SPAN-1, TPA, VIP), pancreatic ribonuclease, **PTH**, somatostatin, GH, thrombomodulin

↓ AMS (later), **fibrinogen**, glucagon, immunoreactive trypsin, lipase (later), trypsin, vitamin – (E)

- *Urine* ↑ AMS, conjugated Bil, G, hCG, UBG
- *Stool* ↑ blood, fat
- *Peritoneal Fluid* ↑ AMS, **proteins**, TAG, TM – (CEA)
- *Pleural Fluid* ↑ AMS, orosomucoid

– glucagonoma

    ↑ G, ✱ glucagon, ✱ insulin, PP

    ↓ Hb, HCT

– insulinoma

    ↑ C-peptide, immunoreactive proinsulin, ✱ insulin, IRI, PP, ✱ proinsulin

    ↓ ✱ G

– pancreatic head tumors

    ↑ ✱ ALP, ✱ Bil, ✱ conjugated Bil, ✱ PT, ✱ cholesterol

    ■ *Urine* ↓ UBG

    ■ *Stool* ↓ UBG

pheochromocytoma

    ↑ epinephrine, aldosterone, Ca, dopamine, endorphins, enkephalins, RBC, EPO, G, gastrin, GH-RH, glucagon, HbA$_{1c}$, hPL, ✱ catecholamines, cholesterol, calcitonin, LDL-C, WBC, TM – (ACTH, beta-lipotropin, NSE, VIP), ✱ norepinephrine, PRA, somatostatin, FFA

    ↓ RBC, K, HCT, P

    ■ *Urine* ↑ proteins, G, ✱ catecholamines, HVA, ✱ metanephrines, urea, VMA, free epinephrine, free norepinephrine

placental tumors

    ↑ hCG

    ■ *Urine* ↑ hCG

pleural tumors

    ↑ CA 125

    ■ *Pleural Fluid* ↑ ALP, eos

prolactinoma

    ↑ ✱ PRL

    ↓ FSH, LH, testosterone

    ■ *Seminal Fluid* ↓ spermatozoa

prostate tumors

    ↑ ADA, ADH, aldolase, ALP, ALT, AMS, AMS (S), beta-lipotropin, CK, CK-BB, CK-MB, CK-MM, euglobulin lysis time, endorphins, enkephalins, cholesterol, IGFBP-2, LD 5, ✱ nucleated RBC, TM – (✱ ACP, ACTH, ALP, CA 15-3, CA 50, CA 549, CEA, CK-BB, GMT, sialic acid, ✱ prostatic ACP, ✱ PSA, TPA), PT, plasmin, prostacyclin, urea

    ↓ fibrinogen, Hb, HCT, testosterone

    ■ *Urine* ↑ RBC, Hb, pus, blood, LAP, LD, WBC

    ■ *Pleural Fluid* ↑ AMS

renin secreting tumors

    ↑ aldosterone, HCT, Na, PRA

    ↓ K

reticulosarcoma

    ↑ alpha-2-globulins, beta globulins, gamma globulins, cold agglutinins

retinoblastoma

    ↑ TM – (NSE)

sarcoma

    ↑ alpha-2-globulins, Ca, CK-MB, MAC, TM – (ALP)

    ■ *Urine* ↑ Bence Jones protein

seminoma

    ↑ ALP, FSH, LD1, TM – (AFP, ALP, CEA, ✱ hCG, hPL, NSE, LD)

    ■ *Urine* ↑ hCG

somatostatinoma

↑ ACTH, G, gastrin, glucagon, insulin, calcitonin, PG, **somatostatin**, substance P, VIP

↓ G, chloride

spinal cord tumors

↑ TM – (CA 125)

■ *Cerebrospinal Fluid* ↑ * proteins

stomach tumors

↑ aldolase, ALT, **APA**, CK-MB, CK-MM, Cu, echinocytes, ESR, **gastrin**, hCG, hexosaminidase, h-sICAM-1, chymotrypsin, insulin, WBC, lym, mono, TM – (AFP, aldolase, beta-glucuronidase, **CA 19-9, CA 27-29**, CA 50, **CA 72-4**, CA 125, CA 195, **CA 242, CEA, hCG**, chromogranin A, B, M2-PK, pancreas-associated antigen, **TPA**), PP

↓ albumin, RBC, G, Hb, HCT, **pepsinogen**, transferrin satur., vitamin – (B_{12})

■ *Urine* ↑ hCG, pepsinogen I

■ *Stool* ↑ Hb, **RBC, blood**

■ *Peritoneal Fluid* ↑ volume, **proteins**, TAG, TM – (CEA)

■ *Pleural Fluid* ↑ AMS

■ *Gastric Fluid* ↑ beta-glucuronidase, CEA, fetal sulfoglycoprotein antigen, mucus, **blood, LA, volume, pH**

↓ BAO, MAO, **HCl**

sympathoblastoma

■ *Urine* ↑ VMA

teratoma

↑ **LD1**, TM – (AFP, hCG)

■ *Urine* ↑ hCG

testis tumors

↑ aldolase, ALP, **ALP** (placental), androstenedione, anti-human papilloma virus Ab, beta-lipotropin, Ca, CK, endorphins, enkephalins, estriol, **estrogens**, ferritin, LD, TM – (ACTH, * **AFP**, ALP, **CEA**, CK-BB, ferritin, * **hCG**, hPL, **LD**, * M2-PK, SP-1, TPA), testosterone

↓ FSH, LH, testosterone

■ *Urine* ↑ **estriol, estrogens, 17-ketosteroids**

↓ FSH

thymus tumors

↑ ACTH, ADH, beta-lipotropin, endorphins, enkephalins

↓ WBC

thyroid gland tumors

↑ antimicrosomal Ab, antithyroglobulin Ab, antithyroidal Ab, thyroxine autoantibodies, **endorphins, enkephalins, histaminase**, iodine, nucleated RBC, LD, TM – (**ACTH**, AFP, **beta-lipotropin**, CA 50, CEA – follicular, medullar, hCG, * **calcitonin** – medullar, NSE, TPA – medullar, thyroglobulin – follicular), gastrin-releasing peptide, PP, somatostatin, substance P, T3, T4, TSH, * **thyroglobulin**, **VIP**

■ *Urine* ↑ 5-HIAA

uterus tumors

↑ beta-lipotropin, CK, endorphins, enkephalins, **EPO**, RBC, TM – (ACTH, CA 15-3, CA 27-29, CA 125, **CEA**, CK-BB, beta-glucuronidase, hPL, **SCCA, TPA**)

■ *Urine* ↑ pus, LAP

VIPoma

↑ Ca, G, MAC, PP, ✳ VIP
↓ chloride, K, P, pH
- *Gastric Fluid* ↓ HCl
- *Stool* ↑ HCO₃⁻, ✳ volume

Tumors, Malignant, Metastases Into

↑ ALP, ALT, Bil, ESR, GMT, uric acid, LA, LD, WBC
↓ CK, LH, osteocalcin, PT, GH
- *Urine* ↑ RBC

bone

↑ ACP, ALP, Ca, fibrinogen, HbF, TM – (ALP, PSA), osteocalcin, P
↓ gamma globulins, P, PTH
- *Urine* ↑ Bence Jones protein, Ca, free hydroxyproline, TM – (hydroxyproline), P
  ↓ Ca

– osteoblastic bone tumor metastases

↑ ACP, ALP, Ca, P
↓ Ca, P
- *Urine* ↓ Ca

– osteolytic bone tumor metastases

↑ ACP, ALP, Ca, P
- *Urine* ↑ Ca

central nervous system

- *Cerebrospinal Fluid* ↑ A2MG, CEA, CK, enolase, fibronectin, LA, LD, MBP, WBC
  ↓ G

gastrointestinal tract

↑ eos
- *Peritoneal Fluid* ↑ AMS, volume
  ↓ pH

liver

↑ aldolase, ALP, arylsulfatase, AST, conjugated Bil, unconjugated Bil, GMT, guanine deaminase, h-sICAM-1, LD, 5-nucleotidase, OCT
↓ pseudocholinesterase

lung

↑ Ca, CA 549, eos

pancreas

↑ Ca
- *Peritoneal Fluid* ↑ pH

prostate

↑ ACP, CA 549, LD 5, plasmin, plasminogen
↓ fibrinogen

Tyrosinemia

↑ AFP, conjugated Bil, unconjugated Bil, phenylalanine, methionine, ✳ tyrosine
↓ delta-aminolevulinic dehydratase, Hb, HCT, PLT, serotonin, WBC
- *Urine* ↑ tyramine, ✳ tyrosine, acetic acid, delta-aminolevulic acid, lactic acid, phenylalanine, p-OH-phenylpyruvic acid, p-OH-phenylacetic acid, ✳ succinylacetone
  ↓ 5-HIAA
- *Amniotic Fluid* ↑ succinylacetone

Undernutrition

↓ **albumin**, ALP, ESR, gamma globulins, Hb, cholesterol, CHS, **lym, trans-ferrin**, urea
- *Gastric Fluid* ↓ pH

Uremia

↑ ACTH, * Al, alpha-aminonitrogen, * **ALP, AMS,** * **ANA,** * **ANCA,** ANF, **ammonia**, Apo B, beta-endorphins, BHBA, * **B2M**, BNP, **BT**, Ca, * Ca$_{2+}$ (stage dependent), CA 19-9, **CEA, CK,** CK-MB, CK-BB, **C-pep-tide,** * **cystatine C**, echinocytes, estriol, Fe, fluoride, fructosamine, **gastrin**, fibrinogen, G, **glucagon**, glycerol, glycated albumin, cGMP, HbF, histamine, hydroxyproline, * **chloride, cholesterol, chymot-rypsin**, ILGF-I, IGFBP-3, **insulin**, * **K, calcitonin**, catecholamines, cortisol, * **creatinine**, * **uric acid**, LA, LD, **LDL-C**, LH, **LPs**, WBC, **MAC**, Mg, Na, neu, Ni, NT-pro-ANP, * **osteocalcin**, plasma volume, NSE, **osmolality, P, PP**, PT, **PRA, PRL**, * **PTH**, pyruvate, schistocytes, Se, secretin, somatostatin, **GH**, * **TAG**, thrombomodulin, **trypsin**, cTnT, **TT**, PLT, * **urea**, vitamin – (A, B$_{12}$, D, E), **VLDL-C**

↓ PLT adhesion, PLT aggregation, * **albumin**, aldosterone, AST, **proteins**, Ca, * **Ca^{2+}** (stage dependent), **RBC**, * **EPO**, factors – (II, VII, IX, X, XIII), * **Fe**, G, **haptoglobin, Hb, HCT, GHb, HDL-C, HCO$_3^-$**, choles-terol, K, complement – (C3, C5, C6, C7, C8), cortisol, glutamic acid, LCAT, WBC, lym, **Na, pH**, PRA, prekallikrein, progesterone, Se, sero-tonin, **T3**, T4, TAG, **testosterone**, transferrin, transferrin receptor, **PLT**, vitamin – (B$_1$, B$_6$, **D$_3$**, folate), **Zn**
- *Urine* ↑ AMS, * **proteins**, * **RBC**, G, **pus**, K, * **blood**, WBC, **Na**, casts – (cellular, granular, hyaline, **waxy**), VMA
  ↓ * **specific gravity**, Mg, * **volume** (later), oxalate, pH, Se urea, VMA
- *Cerebrospinal Fluid* ↑ proteins, G, **pressure**, WBC, urea
- *Pericardial Fluid* ↑ RBC, volume
- *Pleural Fluid* ↑ proteins, eos, RBC, lym
- *Gastric Fluid* ↑ pH
  ↓ HCl
- *Stool* ↑ blood
- *Seminal Fluid* ↓ spermatozoa count
- *Synovial Fluid* ↑ crystals – (hydroxyapatite, urate)
- *Sweat* ↑ chloride, Na

Urethritis

- *Urine* ↑ RBC, Hb, pus, WBC

Urolithiasis

↑ * **Ca**, * **uric acid**, * **PTH**
↓ Fe, * **P**
- *Urine* ↑ Ca, proteins, cystine, **RBC, Hb, pus, blood**, creatinine, crystals, oxalate, WBC, pH, urea
  ↓ volume, pH

calcium urolithiasis

↑ Ca, cAMP
- *Urine* ↑ cAMP

Urticaria

↑ **eos, eosinophilic cationic protein**, WBC
↓ **bas**
- *Synovial Fluid* ↑ eos

Uveitis, Acute Anterior
- ↑ HLA – (B27)
- **Note:** molecular biology – polymorphism CTLA-4

Vaccination
- ↑ VDRL (false)
- ■ *Cerebrospinal Fluid* ↑ eos

Vagotomy
- ↑ **gastrin**
- ↓ somatostatin
- ■ *Gastric Fluid* ↑ pH
  - ↓ HCl

Varicocele
- ■ *Seminal Fluid* ↓ alpha-glucosidase, spermatozoa count

Vasculitis
- ↑ AAT, **ALT**, ✳ **ANA**, ✳ **ANCA**, c-ANCA, **p-ANCA**, antiendothelial Ab, anti-MPO, APLA, **AST**, **B2M**, CIC, **CK**, **CRP**, **elastase, eos**, phospholipase A2, ✳ **ESR**, ✳ **gamma globulins**, **HBsAg**, h-sVCAM-1, ✳ **IFN-gamma**, IgA, IgG, **IL-1**, **creatinine**, ✳ **cryoglobulins**, **WBC**, lym, lymphocytotoxic Ab, **neu**, RF, schistocytes, ✳ **TNF-alpha, PLT**, urea
- ↓ ACE, albumin, **RBC**, **Hb**, **HCT**, complement – (**C3**, C4, CH50), WBC, PLT
- ■ *Urine* ↑ **proteins**, Hb, blood, RBC, casts – (**RBC**)
- ■ *Cerebrospinal Fluid* ↑ CK, WBC, MBP
- ■ *Peritoneal Fluid* ↑ eos
- ■ *Sputum* ↑ blood
- ■ *Synovial Fluid* ↑ clot formation, WBC, PMN, volume
  - ↓ viscosity

allergic vasculitis
- ↑ eos, ESR, cryoglobulins, WBC, RF
- ■ *Urine* ↑ protein

necrotizing vasculitis
- ↑ ANA, ANCA, CRP, eos, ESR, gamma globulins, HBsAg, immunoglobulins, WBC, neu, RF
- ↓ RBC, Hb, HCT, complement – (C3, C4, CH50)

urticarial vasculitis
- ↑ eos, ESR
- ↓ complement – (C3)

Vasculopathies
- ↑ BT, Rumpel–Leede test positive

Vasectomy
- ↑ ✳ **antispermatozoal Ab**
- ■ *Seminal Fluid* ↑ ✳ **antispermatozoal Ab**
  - ↓ alpha-glucosidase, spermatozoa count

Virilism
- ↑ DHEA, testosterone, free testosterone (F)
- ■ *Urine* ↑ 17-OHCS

Vitiligo
- ↑ ANA
- ■ *Gastric Fluid* ↑ pH
  - ↓ HCl

Vomiting

↑ ✳ **acetone, proteins,** Ca, CO_2, RBC, ✳ HCO_3^-, K, ✳ **acetoacetic acid, ketobodies, creatinine,** WBC, MAC, ✳ **MAL, Na, neu,** osmolality, pCO_2, PT, ✳ **pH,** RAC, ✳ **urea**

↓ ✳ **chloride,** K, Na, osmolality, **plasma volume, P**

■ *Urine* ↑ acetone, ammonia, **K, ketones,** specific gravity, **pH**

 ↓ **chloride,** K, Na, pH

Vulvovaginitis

↑ WBC, PMN

■ *Urine* ↑ **bacteria** (+ culture), **fungi, WBC, PMN, pH**

■ *Vaginal Fluid* ↑ ✳ **bacteria** (+ culture), ✳ **fungi, pH**

Xanthelasma

↑ cholesterol

Xanthinuria

↑ hypoxanthine, xanthine

↓ ✳ **uric acid**

■ *Urine* ↑ hypoxanthine, xanthine, xanthine calculi

 ↓ **uric acid**

Xanthochromatosis

■ *Synovial Fluid* ↑ macrophages

Xanthoma

↑ **cholesterol, LDL-C, lipids,** TAG

↓ HDL-C

Xerophthalmia

↓ vitamin – (**A**)

III

Medicaments – Interfering Factors

Medicaments – Interfering Factors

D. Mesko, G. Nosalova

Abacavir *(abacavirum, abacavir, abacavir)*
    antiretroviral agent
        ↑ ALT, AST, G, GMT, MAC, TAG, urea
        ↓ lym

Abciximab *(abciximabum, abciximab, abciximab)*
    antiplatelet
        ↑ K, WBC
        ↓ Hb, HCT, RBC, PLT
        ■ *Urine* ↑ blood, Hb, RBC

Acarbose *(acarbosum, acarbose, acarbose)*
    antidiabetic
        ↑ ALP, ALT, AST, eos, GMT
        ↓ G

Acebutolol *(acebutololum, acebutolol, acébutolol)*
    selective beta-1-adrenoceptor antagonist, antihypertensive, antiarrhythmic, antianginal
        ↑ ALP, ALT, ANA, ANF, AST, K, creatinine, LE cells, P, TAG
        ↓ G, granulocytes, HDL cholesterol, cholesterol, FFA, PLT

ACE Inhibitors
        ↑ Bil, G, K, creatinine, uric acid, PG, renin, urea
        ↓ aldosterone, ANF, angiotensin II, G, GFR
        ■ *Urine* ↑ Na, volume

Acetaminophen (USP) *(paracetamolum, paracetamol, paracétamol)*
    analgesic, antipyretic
        ↑ ALP, ALT, ammonia, AMS, AST, Bil, chloride, G, GMT, histamine, IgE, creatinine, LA, lipase, MHb, neu, 5-nucleotidase, OCT, PT, RTC, urea, uric acid
        ↓ Ca, blood, factors – (II, VII, X), G, Hb, HCT, Na, neu, P, PLT, WBC
        ■ *Urine* ↑ proteins, RBC, Hb, blood, 5-HIAA, metanephrines
           ↓ volume

Acetanilid *(acetanilidum, acetanilide, acétanilide)*
    antipyretic, analgesic
        ↑ MHb

Acetazolamide *(acetazolamidum, acetazolamide, acétazolamide)*
    carbonic anhydrase inhibitor, anticonvulsant, treatment of glaucoma
        ↑ ammonia, Bil, G, quinidine, chloride, uric acid, MAC, Mg
        ↓ Ca, Ca^{2+}, granulocytes, Hb, HCT, HCO_3^-, K, Li, WBC, Na, neu, P, pH, GFR, PLT
        ■ *Urine* ↑ blood, proteins, Ca, Ca^{2+}, estrogens, G, 17-OHCS, iodide, K, 5-HIAA, 17-KGS, 17-KS, crystals, Mg, Na, P, RBC, volume
           ↓ estrogens, Mg
        ■ *Gastric Fluid* ↓ HCl
        ■ *Stool* ↑ Hb

Acetohexamide (*acetohexamidum, acetohexamide, acétohexamide*)
oral hypoglycemic
↑ ALP, ALT, AST, Bil, eos, insulin, creatinine, urea
↓ factors – (II, VII, X), G, granulocytes, Hb, HCT, mono, lym, Na, uric acid, WBC, PLT

Acetophenazine (*acetophenazinum, acetophenazine, acétophénazine*)
antipsychotic, neuroleptic
↑ conjugated Bil

Acetylcholine Chloride (*acetylcholini chloridum, acetylcholine chloride, d´acetylcholine chlorure*)
cholinergic agonist
↑ neu

Acetylcysteine (*acetylcysteinum, acetylcysteine, acétylcystéine*)
mucolytic, antidote
↑ ALT
↓ LP(a)
■ *Sputum* ↑ blood

Acetylsalicylic Acid (*acidum acetylsalicylicum, acetylsalicylic acid, acide acetylsalicylique*)
antipyretic, non-steroid antiinflammatory
↑ ALP, ALT, APTT, AST, Bil, Bil unconjugated, CK, CK-MB, BT, eos, ethanol, Fe, phenytoin, fibrinogen, FT4, G, G6PD, HbA_{1c}, cholesterol, catecholamines, creatinine, uric acid, LA, LD, MAC, Mg, 5-nucleotidase, pCO_2, pH (early), PT, TAG, TBG, TT, urea
↓ PLT aggregation, factors – (II, VII, X), Fe, phenytoin, FT4, ESR, G, GFR, Hb, HCT, HCO3., cholesterol, uric acid, WBC, neu, P, pH (later), renin, T3, T4, TAG, PLT, TSH, vitamin – (C, folate), Zn
■ *Urine* ↑ albumin, ALP, amino acids, blood, Hb, HVA, RBC, G, ketones, acetoacetate, glucuronic acid, LD, VMA
↓ G, hydroxyproline, VMA
■ *Gastric Fluid* ↑ Hb
■ *Stool* ↑ Hb, blood

Aciclovir (*aciclovirum, aciclovir, aciclovir*)
antiviral, antiherpetic
↑ ALT, AST, factors – (II, VII, X), creatinine, GMT, MCV, urea
↓ K, PLT, WBC
■ *Urine* ↑ crystals, Hb
↓ volume

Acipimox (*acipimoxum, acipimox, acipimox*)
nicotinic acid analog, lipid-lowering agent
↑ HDL cholesterol, GH
↓ G, cholesterol, lipase (hepatic), TAG

Aclarubicin (*aclarubicinum, aclarubicin, aclarubicine*)
antineoplastic, antibiotic
↑ ALT

Acriflavine (*acriflavinum, acriflavine, acriflavine*)
parasiticide
■ *Urine* ↑ porphyrins

ACTH (*corticotropinum, corticotropin, corticotropine*)
adrenocorticotropic hormone
↑ aldosterone, AMS, proteins, DHEA, eos, euglobulin lysis time, G, HDL cholesterol, 17-OHCS, K, WBC, MAL, Na, neu, RTC, GH, free testosterone, Zn

    ↓ ALP, Apo B, Apo E, bas, Ca, eos, Fe, ESR, G, Hb, chloride, cholesterol, K, creatinine, uric acid, LDL cholesterol, LP(a), lym, T4, TAG, TBG, transferrin

    ■ *Urine* ↑ creatine, estriol, G, K, 17-KS

        ↓ estrogens, 5-HIAA, 17-KGS, 17-KS, volume

    ■ *Gastric Fluid* ↑ HCl

Adenosine *(adenosini phosphas, adenosine phosphate, phosphate d´adénosine)*

    purine nucleoside, antiarrhythmic

        ↑ epinephrine, norepinephrine

        ■ *Seminal Fluid* ↑ abnormal spermatozoa

        ↓ spermatozoa count

Adipiodone *(adipiodonum, adipiodone, adipiodone)*

    diagnostic aid (radiopaque medium)

        ↓ uric acid

Alpha-Adrenergic Blockers

        ↑ ADH

        ↓ Na, GH

Beta-Adrenergic Blockers

        ↑ ALT, ANA, PLT aggregation, ALP, ANP, AST, Bil, proteins, Ca, CK, CK-MB, BT, FT4, FT3, G, GMT, HbA$_{1c}$, HDL cholesterol, cholesterol, insulin, catecholamines, LDL cholesterol, K, LH (males), PRL (males), lipids, uric acid, GH, TAG, PLT, urea, VLDL cholesterol, epinephrine, cortisol, norepinephrine, theophylline, T4, FFA

        ↓ G, PLT aggregation, aldosterone, ALP, Ca, FT3, FT4, GFR, G tolerance, HDL cholesterol, insulin, K, cortisol, LH (females), neu, rT3, T3, T4, PLT, melatonin, renin, Apo A-I, C-peptide, glucagon, granulocytes, cholesterol, K, Mg, norepinephrine, PRL, PTH, WBC, apolipoprotein B, LDL cholesterol, neu, TBG, PTH, TAG

    ■ *Urine* ↑ 5-HIAA

        ↓ hydroxyproline

    ■ *Gastric Fluid* ↓ HCl

    ■ *Seminal Fluid* ↓ spermatozoa count

Ajmaline *(ajmalinum, ajmaline, ajmaline)*

    antiarrhythmic

        ↑ ALA, ALP, ALT, AST, Bil, eos, GMT, IgA, catecholamines, LD

        ↓ factors – (II, VII, X), WBC, neu, PLT

    ■ *Urine* ↑ vanilmandelic acid

    ■ *Gastric Fluid* ↑ HCl

        ↓ pH

Alanine *(alaninum, alanine, alanine)*

    amino acid

        ↑ G, insulin, P, GH

        ↓ K

Albendazole *(albendazolum, albendazole, albendazole)*

    anthelmintic, parasiticide

        ↑ ALT, AST

        ↓ neu

Albumin *(albuminum, albumin, albumin)*

    plasma protein

        ↑ ALP

Albuterol *(salbutamolum, salbutamol, salbutamol)*
beta-2-adrenoceptor agonist, bronchodilator
↑ HDL cholesterol, LA, MAC, renin
↓ aldosterone, Ca^{2+}, corticosteroids, Mg, P

Aldatense
diuretic
↑ uric acid
↓ ALP, GMT

Aldesleukin *(aldesleukinum, aldesleukin, aldesleukine)*
(interleukin 2) antineoplastic agent
↑ ALP, ALT, AST, Bil, Ca^{2+}, eos, G, GMT, K, creatinine, uric acid, MAC, MAL, Na, P, WBC, urea
↓ albumin, proteins, Ca, Ca^{2+}, G, cholesterol, K, lym, Mg, Na, P, PLT, WBC
■ *Urine* ↑ blood, Hb, RBC
↓ proteins, volume

Aldosterone *(aldosteronum, aldosterone, aldostérone)*
hormone, mineralocorticoid
↑ HCO_3, corticosteroids
↓ chloride, K, Mg
■ *Urine* ↑ K, Mg
↓ Na

Alemtuzumab *(alemtuzumabum, alemtuzumab, alemtuzumab)*
immunomodulator, monoclonal antibody
↑ neu
↓ lym, PLT

Alendronate *(acidum alendronicum, alendronic acid, acide alendronique)*
hormone, aminobisphosphonate
↓ Ca, P

Alkaline Diuretics
↓ chloride

Allopurinol *(allopurinolum, allopurinol, allopurinol)*
antiarthritic, uricostatic
↑ ALP, ALT, AST, Bil, BT, eos, phenytoin, ESR, GMT, creatinine, LD, WBC, theophylline, urea
↓ albumin, proteins, factors – (II, VII, X), Fe, ESR, chloride, uric acid, neu, PLT, WBC
■ *Urine* ↑ Bil, blood, RBC, Hb, WBC

Alosetron *(alosetronum, alosetron, alosétron)*
selective 5-HT_3 antagonist
↑ ALT, AST, GMT

Alprazolam *(alprazolamum, alprazolam, alprazolam)*
anxiolytic, hypnotic, anticonvulsant
↑ ALP, ALT, AST, GMT, LD
↓ granulocytes, Hb, HCT, neu, PLT, WBC

Alprenolol *(alprenololum, alprenolol, alprénolol)*
non-selective beta-adrenergic blocker
↓ neu, rT3, T3, PLT

Alteplase *(alteplasum, alteplase, altéplase)*
tissue plasminogen activator, thrombolytic, fibrinolytic
■ *Urine* ↑ blood, Hb, RBC
■ *Sputum* ↑ blood

Altretamine *(altretaminum, altretamine, altrétamine)*
    antineoplastic
             ↑ ALP, creatinine, neu, urea
             ↓ PLT

Aluminum Hydroxide *(algeldratum, algeldrate, algeldrate)*
    antacid
             ↑ Al, ALP, Ca, vitamin D3
             ↓ digoxin, phenytoin, salicylic acid, P, PTH, vitamin D
             ■ *Urine* ↑ Ca
                ↓ P

Amantadine *(amantadinum, amantadine, amantadine)*
    antiviral
             ↑ ALP, urea

Amidotrizoic Acid *(acidum amidotrizoicum, amidotrizoic acid, acide amidotrizoique)*
    diagnostic aid
             ↑ AMS, T3, T4, TSH
             ↓ uric acid

Amifostine *(amifostinum, amifostine, amifostine)*
    radioprotector, mucolytic
             ↓ Ca, pO$_2$

Amikacin *(amikacinum, amikacin, amikacine)*
    antibiotic
             ↑ creatinine, urea
             ↓ Ca, G, GFR, LD, Mg
             ■ *Urine* ↑ proteins, casts, RBC, WBC
                ↓ volume

Amiloride *(amiloridum, amiloride, amiloride)*
    potassium-sparing diuretic
             ↑ aldosterone, AMS, angiotensin II, K, creatinine, uric acid, MAC, Mg,
                neu, renin, urea
             ↓ chloride, Hb, HCT, Na, neu, osmolality, WBC
             ■ *Urine* ↑ Ca, volume
                ↓ Ca^{2+}

Amineptine *(amineptinum, amineptine, amineptine)*
    antidepressant
             ↑ ALT

Amino Acids
             ↑ phenylalanine, gastrin, glucagon, insulin
             ↓ P

Aminocaproic Acid *(acidum aminocaproicum, aminocaproic acid, acide aminocaproique)*
    antifibrinolytic
             ↑ CK, BT, K
             ↓ plasmin, PLT, WBC
             ■ *Urine* ↑ Mb

Aminoglutethimide *(aminoglutethimidum, aminoglutethimide, aminoglutéthimide)*
    anticonvulsant, antineoplastic
             ↑ ALP, ALT, ANA, androstenedione, AST, Bil, factors – (II, VII, X), FSH,
                GMT, cholesterol, LH, testosterone, theophylline, TSH
             ↓ aldosterone, androgens, digitoxin, estradiol, estrogens, estrone, gluco-
                corticoids, cortisol, WBC, Na, neu, T4, testosterone

Aminoglycosides
> ↑ ALP, Bil, B2M, creatinine, lysozyme, urea
> ↓ Ca, Ca²⁺, GFR, K, Mg, Na, pH, vitamin B₁₂
> ■ *Urine* ↑ B2M, proteins, Hb, hexosaminidase, casts
> ↓ volume

Aminohippuric Acid *(acidum aminohippuricum, aminohippuric acid, acide aminohippuric)*
renal diagnostic aid
> ↑ K

Aminophenazone *(aminophenazonum, aminophenazone, aminophénazone)*
analgesic, antipyretic, antineuralgic
> ↓ AST, proteins, Bil, G, GMT, neu, PLT
> ■ *Urine* ↑ PBG, porphyrins

Aminophylline *(aminophyllinum, aminophylline, aminophylline)*
xanthine derivative, bronchodilator, diuretic
> ↑ ADH, epinephrine, G, norepinephrine, FFA
> ↓ eos, K
> ■ *Urine* ↑ catecholamines, proteins, volume

Aminopyrine *(aminophenazonum, aminophenazone, aminophénasone)*
analgesic, antipyretic
> ↑ cholesterol

Aminosalicylic Acid *(acidum aminosalicylicum, aminosalicylic acid, acide aminosalicylique)*
tuberculostatic
> ↑ ALT, AMS, AST, Bil, conjugated Bil, eos, G, GMT, Heinz bodies (RBC), creatinine, lipase, lym, MCV, TSH, FFA
> ↓ factors – (II, VII, X), folate, FT4, G, granulocytes, haptoglobin, Hb, HCT, cholesterol, K, cobalamines, LDL cholesterol, neu, pH, T3, T4, TAG, WBC, PLT
> ■ *Urine* ↑ G, Hb, homogentisic acid, PBG, UBG, VMA
> ■ *Stool* ↑ Hb, fatty acids
> ■ *Synovial Fluid* ↑ proteins

Amiodarone *(amiodaronum, amiodarone, amiodarone)*
antiarrhythmic
> ↑ ALP, ALT, Apo B, AST, Bil, CK, digitoxin, digoxin, factors – (II, VII, X), phenytoin, flecainide, FT3, FT4, ESR, G, GMT, quinidine, cholesterol, creatinine, LD, LDL cholesterol, WBC, neu, OCT, procainamide, rT3, SHBG, T3, T4, TAG, TSH, thyroglobulin
> ↓ albumin, FT3, FT4, Hb, cholesterol, T3, T4, TAG, transthyretin, PLT, TSH, thyroglobulin, vitamin B₆

Amitriptyline *(amitriptylinum, amitriptyline, amitriptyline)*
antidepressant
> ↑ ADH, ALP, ALT, AST, Bil, eos, G, norepinephrine, PRL
> ↓ G, granulocytes, Hb, WBC, Na, neu, PLT
> ■ *Urine* ↑ greenish-blue color

Amlodipine *(amlodipinum, amlodipine, amlodipine)*
calcium channel blocker
> ↑ ALT, AST, GMT, K, urea
> ↓ PLT, WBC

Ammonium Chloride *(ammonii chloridum, ammonium chloride, chlorure de ammoniaque)*
expectorans
> ↑ chloride, G, MAC, urea

$\downarrow$ HCO$_3$-, K, Mg, Na, pH
- *Urine* $\uparrow$ Ca, G, Mg, P

Amobarbital (*amobarbitalum, amobarbital, amobarbital*)
  sedative, hypnotic
$\downarrow$ Bil, granulocytes, PLT

Amodiaquine (*amodiaquinum, amodiaquine, amodiaquine*)
  antimalarial
$\uparrow$ ALP, ALT, Bil, GMT
$\downarrow$ lym, neu

Amoxapine (*amoxapinum, amoxapine, amoxapine*)
  antidepressant
$\uparrow$ eos, G, creatinine, PRL
$\downarrow$ G, granulocytes, WBC, neu, PLT

Amoxicillin (*amoxicillinum, amoxicillin, amoxicilline*)
  antibiotic
$\uparrow$ ALP, ALT, AST, baso, BT, GMT, eos, creatinine, lym, mono, Na, PT, PLT
$\downarrow$ albumin, granulocytes, Hb, HCT, K, WBC, lym, neu, PLT, proteins, uric acid
- *Urine* $\uparrow$ Hb

Amphetamine (*amfetaminum, amphetamine, amfétamine*)
  sympathomimetic, central stimulant
$\uparrow$ CK, FT4, Hb, catecholamines, corticosteroids, cortisol, Mb, RAL, GH, T3, T4, TSH, FFA
$\downarrow$ G, Hb, PRL
- *Urine* $\uparrow$ epinephrine, amino acids, catecholamines, HVA, metanephrines, norepinephrine, VMA
- *Stool* $\uparrow$ Hb

Amphotericin B (*amphotericinum B, amphotericin B, amphotéricine B*)
  antifungal
$\uparrow$ ALP, ALT, AST, Bil, conjugated Bil, CK, eos, ESR, cholesterol, G, K, creatinine, LD, MAC, neu, urea, WBC
$\downarrow$ Ca, eos, EPO, ESR, G, granulocytes, GFR, K, Hb, HCT, WBC, Mg, Na, pH, PLT
- *Urine* $\uparrow$ blood, proteins, Hb, hexosaminidase, RBC, K, Mg, volume
  $\downarrow$ volume
- *Stool* $\uparrow$ fat, Hb

Ampicillin (*ampicillinum, ampicillin, ampicilline*)
  antibiotic
$\uparrow$ albumin, ALP, ALT, AST, baso, BT, eos, GMT, creatinine, LD, lym, mono, uric acid, WBC, urea, PLT
$\downarrow$ albumin, estriol, factors – (II, VII, X), folate, Hb, HCT, cholesterol, K, lym, neu, progesterone, PLT, proteins, WBC
- *Urine* $\uparrow$ proteins, estriol, catecholamines, WBC
  $\downarrow$ DHEA, DHEAS, estriol, estrogens, 17-KGS, 17-KS, crystals, pregnanediol

Ampicillin-Sulbactam (*ampicillinum-sulbactamum, ampicillin-sulbactam, ampicillin-sulbactam*)
  antibiotic, beta-lactamase inhibitor
$\uparrow$ ALP, creatinine, LD, urea
$\downarrow$ albumin, proteins

- **Urine** ↑ casts

Amprenavir (*amprenavirum, amprenavir, amprénavir*)

antiviral

↑ cholesterol, G, ketobodies, lipids, TAG

↓ Hb, HCT

Amrinone (*amrinonum, amrinone, amrinone*)

selective inhibitor PDE III

↑ ALP, ALT

↓ PLT

Amsacrine (*amsacrinum, amsacrine, amsacrine*)

antineoplastic

↑ ALP, ALT, AST, Bil

↓ Mg

Amylnitrite (*amylum nitrosum, amylnitrite, amylnitrite*)

coronary vasodilator, spasmolytic

↑ MHb

↓ Hb, HCT

Anabolic Steroids

↑ PLT aggregation, albumin, ALP, ALT, Apo B, AST, AT III, proteins, Bil, conjugated Bil, Ca, Ca²⁺, euglobulin lysis time, EPO, estradiol, estrogens, G (diabetics), GMT, haptoglobin, chloride, K, uric acid, LD, LDL cholesterol, MAL, Na, OCT, P, GH, testosterone, TSH, urea

↓ ACTH, AMS, Apo A-I, Apo (a), bas, factors – (II, VII, X), fibrinogen, FSH, FT4, G, HDL cholesterol, CHS, K, creatinine, LH, LP(a), P, progesterone, renin, SHBG, T3, T4, TAG, TBG, testosterone, TSH, urea

- **Urine** ↑ Ca
- **Seminal Fluid** ↓ azoospermia, spermatozoa count

Anagrelide (*anagrelidum, anagrelide, anagrélide*)

platelet-reducing agent

↑ ALT, AST, GMT

- **Urine** ↑ blood, Hb, RBC

Androgens

↑ AAT, ACP (female), ALP, ALT, AST, proteins, Ca, Ca²⁺, ceruloplasmin, cyclosporine, RBC, estradiol, HCT, chloride, HDL cholesterol, cholesterol, K, creatinine, uric acid, LD, LDL cholesterol, Na, 5-nucleotidase, OCT, P, SHBG, GH, TBG, TSH, urea

↓ DHT, factors – (II, V, VII, X), FSH, FT4, G, HDL cholesterol, cholesterol, uric acid, LH, P, SHBG, GH, T3, T4, TBG, testosterone, TAG, TSH, free testosterone

- **Urine** ↑ Ca, 17-KS, P

  ↓ Ca²⁺

- **Seminal Fluid** ↓ volume, spermatozoa count

Anesthetics

↑ eos, G

Anistreplase (*anistreplasum, anistreplase, anistreplase*)

thrombolytic, fibrinolytic

↑ APTT, PT, TT

↓ fibrinogen, plasminogen

- **Urine** ↑ blood, Hb, RBC
- **Sputum** ↑ blood, RBC

Antacids

↑ MAL, PT

↓ P

Antazoline *(antazolinum, antazoline, antazoline)*

antihistaminic, antiarrhythmic

↓ WBC, PLT

Antiarrhythmics

↑ ALA, ALP, ALT, ANA, antihistone Ab, AST, Bil, CK, digitoxin, digoxin, eos, ESR, GMT, cholesterol, IgA, insulin, catecholamines, K, creatinine, LA, LE cells, WBC, uric acid, LD, MAC, neu, RTC, TAG, urea, TSH

↓ Apo A-I, Apo A-II, Apo B, bas, Bil, eos, haptoglobin, Hb, factors – (II, VII, X), G, quinidine, cholesterol, CHS, K, WBC, neu, TAG, PLT

■ *Urine* ↑ Hb, 17-OHCS, catecholamines, 17-KS, corticosteroids, vanilmandelic acid

↓ VMA, volume

■ *Gastric Fluid* ↑ HCl

↓ pH

Anticoagulants

↑ ACTH, PLT aggregation, ALP, APTT, ALT, AST, AT III, Bil, proteins, Ca^{2+}, coagulation time, chloride, cholesterol, hexosaminidase, IgG, insulin, K, corticosteroids, creatinine, LD, neu, P, FDP, FT3, FT4, ESR, G, GMT, BT, clotting time, phenytoin, PT, renin, T3, T4, TAG, TT, TSH, FFA, uric acid

↓ ACP, ACTH, albumin, aldosterone, Apo A-I, Apo B, AT III, Ca^{2+}, factors – (II, VII, IX, X), fibrinogen, FT3, FT4, cholesterol, cortisol, insulin, LDL cholesterol, Na, pCO_2, T3, T4, TAG, TBG, PLT, TSH, G, protein C, prothrombin, uric acid, WBC

■ *Urine* ↑ blood, Hb, RBC, proteins, histamine, uric acid

↓ G, 5-HIAA

■ *Sputum* ↑ blood

■ *Cerebrospinal Fluid* ↑ eos

Anticonvulsants

↑ ALP, Apo A-I, SHBG

↓ Ca, Ca^{2+}, vitamin – (B_6, B_{12}, E, folate)

Antiepileptics

↑ ALP, ALT, amino acids, Apo A-I, AST, ceruloplasmin, cyclosporine, factors – (II, V, VII, X), FSH, GMT, haptoglobin, HDL cholesterol, cholesterol, LH, MCV, 5-nucleotidase, orosomucoid, PRL, PTH, RBP, SHBG, GH, testosterone, vitamin A

↓ albumin, amino acids, Bil, Ca, Ca^{2+}, Cu, fibrinogen, folate, FT3, FT4, GMT, Hb, quinidine, IgA, calcitonin, carbamazepine, cortisol, uric acid, WBC, P, GH, T3, T4, testosterone, PLT, vitamin – (B_6, B_{12}, biotin, D, E), free testosterone, Zn

■ *Cerebrospinal Fluid* ↓ 5-HIAA

Antihemophilic Factor (VIII)

↑ ALT, AST, GMT

↓ PLT

Antihistamines

↑ cholesterol, PT

↓ PLT

■ *Urine* ↑ G

Antihypertensives
       ↑ PRL, renin

Antimalarials
       ↑ Heinz bodies

Antineoplastics
       ↑ G, K
       ↓ hydroxyproline

Antipsychotics
       ↓ WBC

Antipyretics
       ↑ G

Antithymocyte Globulin
       ↑ eos
       ↓ PLT, WBC

Apomorphine Hydrochloride *(apomorphini chloridum, apomorphine hydrochloride, chlorure de apomorphine)*
emetic, dopamine agonist
       ↑ GH
       ↓ PRL, TSH

Aprindine *(aprindinum, aprindine, aprindine)*
antiarrhythmic
       ↑ ALP, ALT, AST, Bil, GMT
       ↓ neu

Apronal *(apronalum, apronal, apronal)*
sedative, hypnotic
       ↓ PLT

Arbekacin *(arbekacinum, arbekacin, arbékacine)*
antibiotic
       ↑ ALT

Ardeparin *(ardeparinum natricum, ardeparin sodium, ardéparine sodique)*
anticoagulant
       ↑ ALT, AST, GMT
       ↓ PLT
       ■ *Urine* ↑ blood, Hb, RBC

Argatroban *(argatrobanum, argatroban, argatroban)*
anticoagulant
       ↑ ALT, AST, GMT
       ■ *Urine* ↑ blood, Hb, RBC
       ■ *Sputum* ↑ blood

Arginine *(argininum, arginine, arginine)*
amino acid
       ↑ K, creatinine, PRL, GH, urea
       ↓ P, pH

Arnifostine *(arnifostinum, arnifostine, arnifostine)*
cytoprotective
       ↓ Ca

Arsenic *(arsenum trioxidatum, arsenic trioxide, trioxide de arseni)*
veterinary agent, heavy metal, poison
       ■ *Urine* ↑ proteins

Ascorbic Acid *(acidum ascorbicum, ascorbic acid, acide ascorbique)*
antiscorbutic vitamin, factor in resisting infection, antioxidant

↑ ALP, Apo A-I, Bil, conjugated Bil, G, HDL cholesterol, Heinz bodies (RBC), cholesterol, K, creatinine, uric acid, oxalate

↓ ALT, AST, Bil, fructosamine, G, GMT, cholesterol, K, uric acid, urea, vitamin B_{12}

- **Urine** ↑ blood, Ca, G, Hb, catecholamines, oxalate, crystals – (cystine, oxalate, urate), RBC

   ↓ G, Hb, hydroxyproline, nitrite
- **Stool** ↓ Hb

Asparaginase *(asparaginasum, asparaginase, asparaginase)*
antineoplastic

↑ ALP, ALT, ammonia, AMS, AST, Bil, BT, Ca, fibrinogen, G, GMT, cholesterol, ketobodies, lipase, lipids, 5-nucleotidase, P, TAG, PLT, urea, uric acid

↓ albumin, AT III, Ca, ceruloplasmin, C-peptide, factors – (II, V, VII, VIII, X), fibrinogen, haptoglobin, Hb, cholesterol, insulin, lipids, WBC, lym, neu, plasmin, SHBG, T3, T4, TAG, TBG, transferrin, FFA

- **Urine** ↑ proteins, G, volume

Aspartame *(aspartamum, aspartame, aspartam)*
sweetener

↑ phenylalanine

Aspoxicillin *(aspoxicillinum, aspoxicillin, aspoxicilline)*
antibiotic

↑ ALT, AST

Atenolol *(atenololum, atenolol, aténolol)*
selective beta-1-adrenergic receptor antagonist, antihypertensive

↑ ALT, ANA, ANP, AST, Bil, Ca, FT3, G, GMT, HbA_{1c}, HDL cholesterol, cholesterol, insulin, LDL cholesterol, uric acid, GH, lipids, TAG

↓ Apo A-I, C-peptide, G, glucagon, granulocytes, HDL cholesterol, cholesterol, K, Mg, rT3, T3, FFA, PLT, WBC

- **Urine** ↑ 5-HIAA

Atorvastatin *(atorvastatinum, atorvastatin, atorvastatin)*
antihyperlipidemic/HMG-co-enzyme A reductase inhibitor

↑ ALT, AST, GMT

Atovaquone *(atovaquonum, atovaquone, atovaquone)*
antiinfective, antiprotozoal

↑ ALT, AMS, AST, creatinine, G, GMT, urea

↓ Hb, HCT, Na, neu

Atrial Natriuretic Peptide
diuretic, hypotensive

↑ GFR

Atropine *(atropini sulfas, atropine sulfate, atropine sulfate)*
antimuscarinic spasmolytic, mydriatic

↑ HCT, WBC

↓ G, gastrin, volume (plasma)

- **Urine** ↓ volume
- **Gastric Fluid** ↓ pH

Auranofin *(auranofinum, auranofin, auranofine)*
analgesic, antirheumatic, gold compound

↑ ALT, AST, GMT

$\downarrow$ Hb, HCT, PLT, neu, WBC
- *Urine* $\uparrow$ blood, proteins, RBC

Aurothioglucose *(aurothioglucosum, aurothioglucose, aurothioglucose)*
non-steroid antiinflammatory
$\downarrow$ PLT

Azapropazone *(azapropazonum, azapropazone, azapropazone)*
analgesic, antiinflammatory
$\uparrow$ ALT, AST, Bil, phenytoin, GMT, creatinine, Li, urea
$\downarrow$ factors – (II, VII, X), Hb, uric acid, PLT
- *Stool* $\uparrow$ Hb

Azathioprine *(azathioprinum, azathioprine, azathioprine)*
immunosuppressant, antineoplastic
$\uparrow$ ALA, ALP, ALT, AMS, AST, Bil, factors – (II, VII, X), GMT, Hb, K, uric acid (tissue destruction), lipase, WBC, MCV, TAG
$\downarrow$ CRP, ESR, Hb, HCT, cholesterol, IgM, uric acid (gout), WBC, neu, P, PLT
- *Urine* $\downarrow$ uric acid, volume
- *Stool* $\uparrow$ FA
- *Seminal Fluid* $\downarrow$ spermatozoa count

Azlocillin *(azlocillinum, azlocillin, azlocilline)*
antibiotic, acylureido-penicillin
$\uparrow$ ALT, AST, BT, eos, Na, OCT
$\downarrow$ PLT aggregation, K, uric acid, WBC

Aztreonam *(aztreonamum, aztreonam, aztréonam)*
antibiotic, monobactam
$\uparrow$ ALP, ALT, AST, eos, GMT, creatinine, PLT

Bacillus Calmette-Guerin Vaccine *(vacc. tuberculosis lyophilisatum, BCG vaccine, BCG vaccin)*
antiprotozoal, immunizing agent, immunostimulant
$\uparrow$ ALT, AST, GMT
- *Urine* $\uparrow$ blood, Hb, RBC

Bacitracin *(bacitracinum, bacitracin, bacitracine)*
topical antibacterial
$\uparrow$ eos, urea
- *Urine* $\uparrow$ albumin, blood, proteins, Hb, RBC, casts

Baclofen *(baclofenum, baclofen, baclofène)*
muscle relaxant
$\uparrow$ ALP, ALT, AST, G, GH
- *Urine* $\uparrow$ RBC, Hb, blood

Barbiturates
$\uparrow$ ADH, ALP, ammonia, CK, dihydrotestosterone, factors – (II, VII, X), GMT, HDL cholesterol, creatinine, uric acid, RAC, testosterone, free testosterone
$\downarrow$ Bil, Ca, digoxin, folate, G, Hb, chloride, cortisol, ascorbic acid, uric acid, WBC, neu, pO_2, T4, theophylline, thiamine, PLT, vitamin D
- *Urine* $\uparrow$ Bil, ALA, estriol, coproporphyrin, PBG, porphyrins, uroporphyrin
$\downarrow$ 17-OHCS, volume
- *Gastric Fluid* $\downarrow$ HCl

Basiliximab *(basiliximabum, basiliximab, basiliximab)*
immunosuppressant
↑ cholestrol, G, K, lipids, MAC, proteins, RBC, uric acid
↓ Ca, G, Hb, HCT, K, Mg, P, PLT
■ *Urine* ↑ albumin, blood, RBC
↓ volume

Beclobrate *(beclobratum, beclobrate, beclobrate)*
lipid-lowering agent
↑ CK

Beclomethasone *(beclometasonum, beclomethasone, béclométasone)*
glucocorticoid, antiasthmatic, antiinflammatory, immunosuppressant
↑ cholesterol, eos, insulin, LA
↓ cortisol, osteocalcin
■ *Urine* ↓ 17-OHCS

Benazepril *(benazeprilum, benazepril, bénazépril)*
ACE inhibitor, antihypertensive, vasodilator
↑ ALT, AST, Bil, Ca, eos, G, GMT, cholesterol, K, LDL cholesterol, TAG, urea, uric acid
↓ Mg, Na, PLT, WBC
■ *Urine* ↑ proteins

Bendroflumethiazide *(bendroflumethiazidum, bendroflumethiazide, bendrofluméthiazide)*
salidiuretic, antihypertensive
↑ BE, Ca, HCO_3^-, creatinine, LD, LD isoenzymes, MAL, renin, urea, Zn
↓ K, Mg, Na, PLT

Benfluorex *(benfluorexum, benfluorex, benfluorex)*
antilipidemic, anorexic
↓ HbA_{1c}, uric acid

Benorilate *(benorilatum, benorilate, bénorilate)*
analgesic, antiinflammatory, antipyretic
↑ ALT

Benoxaprofen *(benoxaprofenum, benoxaprofen, benoxaprofén)*
non-steroid antiinflammatory
↑ ALP, ALT, ANA, AST, Bil
↓ PLT

Benserazide *(benserazidum, benserazide, bensérazide)*
decarboxylase inhibitor, antiparkinsonic
↑ PRL, TSH

Benziodarone *(benziodaronum, benziodarone, benziodarone)*
antiarrhythmic, coronary vasodilator
↑ TSH
↓ uric acid, T3, TSH

Benzocaine *(benzocainum, benzocaine, benzocaine)*
local anesthetic
↑ MHb

Benzodiazepines
↑ ALP

Benzphetamine Hydrochloride *(benzphetaminum hydrochloridum, benzphetamine hydrochloride, benzphétamine hydrochloride)*
CNS stimulant, anorexiant
↓ granulocytes, WBC

Benzylpenicillin *(benzylpenicillinum, benzylpenicillin, benzylpénicilline)*
    antibiotic
        ↑ BT, creatinine
        ↓ K, coagulation factors, WBC, neu
Benzylthiouracil *(benzylthiouracilum, benzylthiouracil, benzylthiouracil)*
    thyroid inhibitor
        ↑ ALP, ALT, AST, GMT
Bepridil *(bepridilum, bepridil, bépridil)*
    coronary vasodilator, antiarrhythmic
        ↑ digoxin
Beractant *(beractantum, beractant, béractant)*
    lung surfactant
        ↑ pO_2
Betamethasone *(betamethasonum, betamethasone, bétaméthasone)*
    corticosteroid
        ↑ C-peptide, G, cholesterol, insulin, MAL, Na, WBC, urea
        ↓ Ca, estriol, cortisol, K, PLT, T3, T4, TBG
        ■ *Urine* ↑ G
           ↓ 17-OHCS
        ■ *Seminal Fluid* ↑ spermatozoa
        ↓ spermatozoa
Betaxolol *(betaxololum, betaxolol, bétaxolol)*
    long-acting selective beta-1-adrenoceptor blocker
        ↑ ALT, AST, cholesterol, G, GMT, lipids, LD, MAC, TAG
        ↓ G, granulocytes, K, pH, PLT
Bethanechol Chloride *(bethanecholi chloridum, betanechol chloride, chlorure de betanechole)*
    cholinergic agonist
        ↑ AMS, lipase
Bevantolol *(bevantololum, bevantolol, bévantolol)*
    beta-adrenergic blocker, antiarrhythmic
        ↑ TAG
Bexarotene *(bexarotenum, bexarotene, bexarotene)*
    retinoid
        ↑ ALT, AST, G, GMT, cholesterol, lipids, TAG
        ↓ Na, WBC
Bezafibrate *(bezafibratum, bezafibrate, bézafibrate)*
    lipid-lowering agent
        ↑ ALP, ALT, CK, HDL cholesterol, creatinine
        ↓ Apo B, Apo E, fibrinogen, G, GMT, cholesterol, insulin, TAG, VLDL cholesterol
Bicalutamide *(bicalutamidum, bicalutamide, bicalutamide)*
    non-steroidal antiandrogen
        ↑ ALT, AST, GMT
Bicarbonates
        ↓ chloride, Na
Biguanides
        ↑ MAC
        ↓ Na
Bisacodyl *(bisacodylum, bisacodyl, bisacodyl)*
    laxative
        ↓ K
        ■ *Stool* ↑ FA

Bisantrene *(bisantrenum, bisantrene, bisantréne)*
    antineoplastic
          ↑ ALT

Bismuth Salts
          ↑ ALP, ALT, Bil, creatinine, LD, LD (isoenzymes)
          ↓ PLT
          ■ *Urine* ↑ proteins, G

Bisoprolol Fumarate *(bisoprololum, bisoprolol, bisoprolol)*
    selective beta-1-adrenoceptor blocker, antihypertensive, antiarrhythmic
          ↑ ALT, ANA, AST, Bil, Ca, G, GMT, cholesterol, K, creatinine, lipids, uric
            acid, P, TAG, urea
          ↓ Apo A-I, G, HDL cholesterol, granulocytes, K, Mg, PLT, WBC

Bitolterol *(bitolterolum, bitolterol, bitoltérol)*
    selective beta-2-adrenoceptor agonist, bronchodilator
          ↓ K

Bivalirudin *(bivalirudinum, bivalirudin, bivalirudin)*
    anticoagulant
          ■ *Urine* ↑ blood, Hb, RBC
          ■ *Sputum* ↑ blood

Bombesin *(bombesinum, bombesin, bombesin)*
    gastric acid secretion stimulant
          ↑ FSH, LH
          ↓ PRL, TSH

Bopindolol *(bopindololum, bopindolol, bopindolol)*
    beta-adrenergic blocker
          ↑ TAG
          ↓ cholesterol, renin

Boric Acid *(acidum boricum, boric acid, acide borique)*
    antiseptic
          ↑ chloride

Bretylium *(bretylii tosilas, bretylium tosilate, tosilate de brétylium)*
    antihypertensive, antiarrhythmic
          ↓ catecholamines
          ■ *Urine* ↓ VMA

Bromfenac Sodium *(bromfenacum, bromfenac, bromfénac)*
    analgesic, NSAID
          ↑ ALT, AST, BT, GMT, K, urea, uric acid
          ■ *Urine* ↑ blood, Hb, RBC

Bromides
          ↑ chloride
          ↓ chloride
          ■ *Urine* ↑ chloride, blood, Hb, RBC
          ■ *Stool* ↑ blood

Bromocriptine *(bromocriptinum, bromocriptine, bromocriptine)*
    dopaminergic agonist, prolactin inhibitor, antiparkinsonic
          ↑ ADH, ALP, ALT, AST, CK, CRP, ESR, pCO_2, GH, testosterone, urea
          ↓ HbA_{1c}, catecholamines, norepinephrine, PRL, T4, TSH
          ■ *Urine* ↓ VMA
          ■ *Pleural Fluid* ↑ eos, WBC

Bucindolol *(bucindololum, bucindolol, bucindolol)*
    beta-adrenoceptor antagonist, antihypertensive
          ↑ CK

Budesonide *(budesonidum, budesonide, budésonide)*
corticosteroid, antiasthmatic, antiinflammatory
↓ osteocalcin
Bumetanide *(bumetanidum, bumetanide, bumétanide)*
loop diuretic
↑ ALT, G, uric acid, pH, urea
↓ Ca, chloride, K, WBC, Na, neu, P, PLT
■ *Urine* ↑ chloride
Bunitrolol *(bunitrololum, bunitrolol, bunitrolol)*
beta-adrenergic blocker
↓ HDL cholesterol, cholesterol
Bupivacaine *(bupivacainum, bupivacaine, bupivacaine)*
local anesthetic
↑ epinephrine
Buprenorphine *(buprenorphinum, buprenorphine, buprénorphine)*
partial opiate agonist, analgesic
↑ PRL
↓ LH
Buserelin *(buserelinum, buserelin, buséréline)*
gonadorelin analogue
↑ cholesterol
↓ FSH, LH, testosterone
Buspirone *(buspironum, buspirone, buspirone)*
neuroleptic, anxiolytic
↑ GH, PRL
Busulfan *(busulfanum, busulfan, busulfan)*
antineoplastic
↑ ALP, ALT, Bil, Fe, GMT, uric acid
↓ Hb, WBC, neu, PLT
■ *Urine* ↑ blood, Hb, RBC
Butorphanol *(butorphanolum, butorphanol, butorphanol)*
analgesic, antitussive
↑ PRL
Butyrophenones
↑ PRL

Ca-EDTA *(natrii calcii edetas, sodium calcium edetate, calcium édétate de sodium)*
chelating agent, antidote
■ *Urine* ↑ proteins, RBC, Hb
Caffeine *(coffeinum, caffeine, caféine)*
stimulant, analeptic, diuretic
↑ epinephrine, ALT, Apo B, beta-endorphins, G, gastrin, chloride, choles-
terol, K, insulin, catecholamines, cortisol, uric acid, linoleic acid, LA,
LDL cholesterol, Na, norepinephrine, renin, TAG, theophylline, FFA
↓ ALP, AST, Bil, G, GMT, TAG
■ *Urine* ↑ Ca, epinephrine, dopamine, catecholamines, 5-HIAA, Mg,
Na, volume, VMA
■ *Gastric Fluid* ↑ HCl
Calcifediol *(calcifediolum, calcifediol, calcifédiol)*
vitamin D, calcium regulator
↑ Ca, P

Calcipotriene *(calcipotriolum, calcipotriol, calcipotriol)*
    vitamin D analog, antipsoriaticum
        ↑ Ca
        ■ *Urine* ↑ Ca

Calcitonin *(calcitoninum, calcitonin, calcitonine)*
    calcium regulating hormone
        ↑ G, glucagon, cortisol, PRL, TSH
        ↓ ALP, Ca, C-peptide, insulin, P, PRL, GH
        ■ *Urine* ↑ Ca^{2+}, hydroxyproline, K, Mg, Na, P
          ↓ hydroxyproline

Calcitriol *(calcitriolum, calcitriol, calcitriol)*
    vitamin D 3, calcium regulator
        ↑ Apo A-I, Ca, osteocalcin, P
        ↓ ALP, PTH, TAG, TSH
        ■ *Urine* ↑ Ca

Calcium Carbonate *(calcii carbonas, calcium carbonate, carbonate de calcium)*
    dietary supplement, antacid, phosphate binder
        ↑ Ca, gastrin
        ↓ P

Calcium-Channel Blockers
        ↑ ALT, AST, cyclosporine, digoxin, GFR, GMT, HbA_{1c}, HDL cholesterol, K,
          G, catecholamines, MAC, norepinephrine, renin, urea, TSH
        ↓ cholesterol, LDL cholesterol, PLT, T4, WBC
        ■ *Urine* ↑ Na, volume

Calcium Chloride *(calcium chloridum, calcii chloride, calcii chloride)*
    calcium salt
        ↑ gastrin

Calcium Dobesilate *(calcii dobesilas, calcium dobesilate, dobésilate de calcium)*
    hemostatic, vasotropic
        ↓ CK

Calcium Gluconate *(calcii gluconas, calcium gluconate, gluconate de calcium)*
    calcium replenisher
        ↑ gastrin, 17-OHCS, insulin, calcitonin
        ↓ Mg, PTH
        ■ *Urine* ↑ Na
          ↓ hydroxyproline
        ■ *Gastric Fluid* ↑ HCl

Calfactant *(calfactantum, calfactant, calfactant)*
    lung surfactant
        ↑ pO_2

Calusterone *(calusteronum, calusterone, calustérone)*
    antineoplastic
        ↑ Ca

Candesartan *(candesartanum, candesartan, candésartan)*
    angiotensin II receptor antagonist
        ↑ ALT, AST, GMT, K, urea
        ↓ neu, PLT, WBC

Capecitabine *(capecitabinum, capecitabine, capéticabine)*
    antineoplastic
        ↑ ALT, AST, Bil, GMT
        ↓ lym, neu, PLT, WBC

Capreomycin *(capreomycinum, capreomycin, capréomycine)*
    tuberculostatic
            ↑ eos, creatinine, uric acid, urea
            ↓ Ca, K, Mg
            ■ *Urine* ↑ Hb, proteins, WBC

Captopril *(captoprilum, captopril, captopril)*
    ACE inhibitor, antihypertensive, antianginal, cardiotonic
            ↑ aldosterone, ALP, ALT, AMS, ANA, ANP, Apo A-I, AST, Bil, Ca, CK, eos, G, GFR, GMT, chloride, cholesterol, K, creatinine, LD, Na, renin, RTC, TAG, urea, uric acid
            ↓ ACE, PLT aggregation, aldosterone, angiotensin II, factors – (XII), G, GFR, granulocytes, Hb, HCT, insulin, K, catecholamines, LDL cholesterol, lym, WBC, Mg, mono, Na, neu, pH, PLT, Zn
            ■ *Urine* ↑ acetone, AMS, proteins, G, Hb, acetoacetate, Na, volume
              ↓ volume

Carbamates
            ↓ PLT aggregation, CHS

Carbamazepine *(carbamazepinum, carbamazepine, carbamazépine)*
    anticonvulsant, antiepileptic, analgesic
            ↑ ADH, ALA, ALP, ALT, ammonia, ANA, Apo A-I, AST, Bil, conjugated Bil, ceruloplasmin, CK, Cu, eos, factors – (II, VII, X), phenytoin, G, GMT, HDL cholesterol, homocysteine, cholesterol, CHS, cortisol, LDL-C, LA, WBC, OCT, PRL, SHBG, TAG, TBG, TSH, urea, vasopressin, free cortisol
            ↓ ADH, androstenedione, Ca, Ca²⁺, cyclosporine, Cu, DHEA, DHEAS, phenobarbital, phenytoin, FT3, FT4, haloperidol, haptoglobin, Hb, chloride, 11-OHCS, IgA, IgG, IgM, K, carnitine, lym, WBC, Na, mono, neu, orosomucoid, osmolality, P, PRL, GH, T3, T4, TBG, testosterone, theophylline, PLT, TSH, urea, valproate, vitamin – (B6, biotin, D3, E, folate), free testosterone, Zn
            ■ *Urine* ↑ albumin, ALA, G, 17-OHCS, 17-KS, osmolality, PBG, porphyrins, uroporphyrin
              ↓ hCG, 17-KS, volume

Carbarsone *(carbarsonum, carbarsone, carbarsone)*
    antiamebic
            ↑ ALT

Carbenicillin *(carbenicillinum, carbenicillin, carbénicilline)*
    antibiotic
            ↑ ALP, ALT, AST, baso, BE, BT, creatinine, eos, GMT, lym, mono, Na, pH, PLT, PT, urea
            ↓ albumin, proteins, granulocytes, Hb, HCT, factors – (II, VII, X), K, lym, Mg, neu, PLT, PLT aggregation, uric acid, WBC
            ■ *Urine* ↑ proteins, RBC, blood, hyaline casts, pus
              ↓ volume

Carbenoxolone *(carbenoxolonum, carbenoxolone, carbénoxolone)*
    antiulcer agent
            ↑ CK, Na, 5-nucleotidase
            ↓ chloride, K

Carbidopa *(carbidopum, carbidopa, carbidopa)*
    amino acid decarboxylase inhibitor
            ↑ ALT, AST, Bil, GMT
            ↓ creatinine, PLT, uric acid, urea, WBC

Carbimazole *(carbimazolum, carbimazole, carbimazole)*
   thyroid inhibitor
        ↑ ALP, ALT, AST, Bil, CBG, CK, GMT
        ↓ Hb, WBC, neu, SHBG, PLT

Carbonic Anhydrase Inhibitors
        ↑ MAC, Zn
        ↓ HCO_3, K
        ■ *Urine* ↑ G, HCO_3, K, crystals, Na, volume, P, pH

Carboplatin *(carboplatinum, carboplatin, carboplatin)*
   antineoplastic
        ↑ ALP, ALT, Bil, creatinine, GMT, urea, uric acid
        ↓ Ca, Ca^{2+}, GFR, Hb, K, Mg, Na, neu, P, PLT, WBC

Carbutamide *(carbutamidum, carbutamide, carbutamide)*
   oral hypoglycemic
        ↑ ALP, ALT, AST, Bil, creatinine, urea
        ↓ G, cholesterol, WBC, PLT
        ■ *Urine* ↑ proteins

Carfenazine *(carfenazinum, carfenazine, carfenazine)*
   neuroleptic, antipsychotic
        ↑ ALP

Carisoprodol *(carisoprodolum, carisoprodol, carisoprodol)*
   skeletal muscle relaxant
        ↑ ALP, eos, GMT

Carmustine *(carmustinum, carmustine, carmustine)*
   antineoplastic
        ↑ ALT, AST, GMT, OCT, urea
        ↓ neu, PLT, WBC
        ■ *Urine* ↑ Hb

Carnitine *(carnitinum, carnitine, carnitine)*
   facilitator of aerobic metabolism of carbohydrates
        ↓ TAG

Carprazidil *(carprazidilum, carprazidil, carprazidil)*
   peripheral vasodilator, antihypertensive
        ↑ HDL cholesterol

Carprofen *(carprofenum, carprofen, carproféne)*
   non-steroid antiinflammatory, antipyretic, analgesic
        ↑ ALT

Carteolol *(carteololum, carteolol, cartéolol)*
   non-selective beta-adrenergic blocker
        ↑ ANA, CK, CK-MB, cholesterol, G, HbA_{1c}, lipids, LD, TAG
        ↓ G, granulocytes, PLT

Carvedilol *(carvedilolum, carvedilol, carvédilol)*
   beta-adrenergic blocker, vasodilator, antihypertensive
        ↑ ANP, G, TAG
        ↓ G, PLT

Catecholamines
        ↑ ANF, Apo B, gastrin, cholesterol, LA, LDL cholesterol, TAG
        ↓ P
        ■ *Urine* ↑ catecholamines, metanephrines, VMA

Cefaclor *(cefaclorum, cefaclor, céfaclor)*
antibiotic, 1st generation cephalosporin
↑ ALT, AST, eos, lym, WBC
↓ Hb, HCT, neu, PLT, WBC
■ *Urine* ↑ proteins (false positive), G (false positive), 17-KS (false positive), pus, Hb, RBC, blood

Cefadroxil *(cefadroxilum, cefadroxil, céfadroxil)*
antibiotic, 1st generation cephalosporin
↑ ALT, AST, eos, lym, WBC
↓ Hb, HCT, neu, PLT, WBC
■ *Urine* ↑ proteins (false positive), G (false positive), 17-KS (false positive), Hb, RBC, blood

Cefalexin *(cefalexinum, cefalexin, céfalexine)*
antibiotic, 1st generation cephalosporin
↑ ALP, ALT, AST, BE, Bil, eos, creatinine, lym, WBC
↓ Hb, HCT, K, WBC, neu, PLT
■ *Urine* ↑ proteins (false positive), G (false positive), creatinine, 17-KS (false positive), pus, Hb, RBC, blood

Cefaloridine *(cefaloridinum, cefaloridine, céfaloridine)*
antibiotic, 1st generation cephalosporin
↑ ALP, K, creatinine
■ *Urine* ↑ proteins, 17-OHCS

Cefalotin *(cefalotinum, cefalotin, céfalotine)*
antibiotic, 1st generation cephalosporin
↑ ALT, AST, eos, ESR, creatinine, GMT, LD, lym, WBC, urea
↓ ammonia, Hb, HCT, WBC, neu, PLT
■ *Urine* ↑ proteins (false positive), B2M, G, 17-OHCS, G (false positive), creatinine, 17-KS (false positive), pus, Hb, RBC, blood

Cefamandole *(cefamandolum, cefamandole, céfamandole)*
antibiotic, 2nd generation cephalosporin
↑ ALP, ALT, AST, Bil, eos, Hb, creatinine, lym, WBC
↓ factors – (II, VII, X), Hb, HCT, WBC, neu, PLT
■ *Urine* ↑ proteins (false positive), G (false positive), 17-KS (false positive), Hb, RBC, blood
■ *Stool* ↑ Hb

Cefapirin *(cefapirinum, cefapirin, céfapirine)*
antibiotic, 1st generation cephalosporin
↑ ALT, AST, eos, ESR, GMT, creatinine, LD, lym, WBC
↓ Hb, HCT, neu, PLT
■ *Urine* ↑ proteins (false positive), G (false positive), creatinine, 17-KS (false positive), pus, Hb, RBC, blood

Cefazolin *(cefazolinum, cefazolin, céfazoline)*
antibiotic, 1st generation cephalosporin
↑ ALP, ALT, AST, Bil, eos, creatinine, lym, WBC, PLT
↓ factors – (II, VII, X), Hb, HCT, neu, PLT, WBC
■ *Urine* ↑ proteins (false positive), G (false positive), 17-KS (false positive), Hb, RBC, blood

Cefdinir *(cefdinirum, cefdinir, cefdinir)*
antibiotic, cephalosporin
↑ ALT, AST, eos
↓ WBC

> - *Urine* ↑ proteins, G (false positive), 17-KS (false positive), Hb, RBC, blood, pH

Cefepime *(cefepimum, cefepime, céfépime)*
antibiotic, 4ᵗʰ generation cephalosporin
> ↑ ALT, AST, GMT

Cefixime *(cefiximum, cefixime, céfixime)*
antibiotic, 3ʳᵈ generation cephalosporin
> ↑ ALT, AST, eos, lym, WBC, PLT
> ↓ Hb, HCT, neu, PLT, WBC
> - *Urine* ↑ proteins (false positive), G (false positive), 17-KS (false positive)

Cefmenoxime *(cefmenoximum, cefmenoxime, cefménoxime)*
antibiotic, 3ʳᵈ generation cephalosporin
> ↑ ALT
> ↓ neu

Cefmetazole *(cefmetazolum, cefmetazole, cefmétazole)*
antibiotic, 2ⁿᵈ generation cephalosporin
> ↑ ALT, AST, eos, lym, WBC, creatinine, urea
> ↓ Hb, HCT, neu, PLT
> - *Urine* ↑ proteins (false positive), G (false positive), 17-KS (false positive)

Cefonicid *(cefonicidum, cefonicid, céfonicid)*
antibiotic, 2ⁿᵈ generation cephalosporin
> ↑ ALT, AST, eos, lym, WBC
> ↓ Hb, HCT, neu, PLT
> - *Urine* ↑ pus, proteins (false positive), G (false positive), 17-KS (false positive), Hb, RBC, blood

Cefoperazone *(cefoperazonum, cefoperazone, céfopérazone)*
antibiotic, 3ʳᵈ generation cephalosporin
> ↑ ALP, ALT, AST, Bil, BT, eos, GMT, creatinine, lym, PT, WBC
> ↓ factors – (II, VII, X), haptoglobin, Hb, HCT, WBC, neu, PLT
> - *Urine* ↑ proteins (false positive), G (false positive), 17-KS (false positive)

Ceforanide *(ceforanidum, ceforanide, céforanide)*
antibiotic, 2ⁿᵈ generation cephalosporin
> ↑ PLT

Cefotaxime *(cefotaximum, cefotaxime, céfotaxime)*
antibiotic, 3ʳᵈ generation cephalosporin
> ↑ ALT, eos, galactose, lym, P, urea, uric acid, WBC
> ↓ Hb, HCT, neu, PLT, WBC
> - *Urine* ↑ proteins (false positive), G (false positive), 17-KS (false positive), pus, Hb, RBC, blood

Cefotetan *(cefotetanum, cefotetan, céfotétan)*
antibiotic
> ↑ ALT, AST, eos, lym, PT, WBC
> ↓ factors – (II, VII, X), Hb, HCT, neu, PLT
> - *Urine* ↑ proteins (false positive), G (false positive), 17-KS (false positive), pus, Hb, RBC, blood

Cefoxitin *(cefoxitinum, cefoxitin, céfoxitine)*
antibiotic, 2ⁿᵈ generation cephalosporin
> ↑ ALP, ALT, AST, Bil, eos, GMT, creatinine, LD, lym, WBC

    ↓ factors – (II, VII, X), Hb, HCT, neu, WBC, PLT
    ■ ***Urine*** ↑ proteins (false positive), G (false positive), creatinine, 17-KS
       (false positive), pus, RBC, blood

Cefpodoxime *(cefpodoximum, cefpodoxime, cefpodoxime)*
antibiotic, 2nd generation cephalosporin
    ↑ ALT, AST, eos, GMT, creatinine, LD, lym, WBC
    ↓ Hb, HCT, neu, PLT
    ■ ***Urine*** ↑ proteins (false positive), G (false positive), creatinine, 17-KS
       (false positive), pus, Hb, RBC, blood

Cefprozil *(cefprozilum, cefprozil, cefprozil)*
antibiotic, 2nd generation cephalosporin
    ↑ ALT, AST, eos, GMT, creatinine, LD, lym, WBC
    ↓ Hb, HCT, neu, PLT, WBC
    ■ ***Urine*** ↑ proteins (false positive), G (false positive), creatinine, 17-KS
       (false positive), pus, Hb, RBC, blood

Cefradine *(cefradinum, cefradine, céfradine)*
antibiotic, 1st generation cephalosporin
    ↑ ALT, AST, GMT, eos, PT, urea
    ↓ neu, WBC

Ceftazidime *(ceftazidimum, ceftazidime, ceftazidime)*
antibiotic, 3rd generation cephalosporin
    ↑ ALT, AST, eos, creatinine, lym, WBC, PLT
    ↓ GFR, Hb, HCT, neu, PLT, WBC
    ■ ***Urine*** ↑ proteins (false positive), G (false positive), creatinine, 17-KS
       (false positive), pus, Hb, RBC, blood

Ceftibuten *(ceftibutenum, ceftibuten, ceftibuténe)*
antibiotic, 3rd generation cephalosporin
    ↑ ALT, AST, eos, GMT, creatinine, LD, lym, WBC
    ↓ Hb, HCT, neu, PLT
    ■ ***Urine*** ↑ proteins (false positive), G (false positive), creatinine, 17-KS
       (false positive), pus, Hb, RBC, blood
    ■ ***Stool*** ↑ blood

Ceftizoxime *(ceftizoximum, ceftizoxime, ceftizoxime)*
antibiotic, 3rd generation cephalosporin
    ↑ ALP, ALT, AST, BT, eos, GMT, creatinine, LD, lym, WBC, PLT, PT, urea
    ↓ Hb, HCT, neu, PLT, WBC
    ■ ***Urine*** ↑ proteins (false positive), G (false positive), creatinine, 17-KS
       (false positive), pus, Hb, RBC, blood

Ceftriaxone *(ceftriaxonum, ceftriaxone, ceftriaxone)*
antibiotic, 3rd generation cephalosporin
    ↑ ALT, AST, eos, phenytoin, creatinine, lym, PLT, PT, WBC
    ↓ factors – (II, VII), Hb, HCT, neu, PLT, WBC
    ■ ***Urine*** ↑ proteins (false positive), G (false positive), creatinine, 17-KS
       (false positive), pus, Hb, RBC, blood

Cefuroxime *(cefuroximum, cefuroxime, céfuroxime)*
antibiotic, 2nd generation cephalosporin
    ↑ ALT, AST, eos, creatinine, GMT, lym, WBC
    ↓ eos, GFR, Hb, HCT, neu, PLT, WBC
    ■ ***Urine*** ↑ proteins (false positive), G (false positive), creatinine, 17-KS
       (false positive), pus, Hb, RBC, blood

Celecoxib *(celecoxibum, celecoxib, celécoxib)*
   non-steroid antiinflammatory, COX-2 inhibitor
   ↑ ALT, AST, GMT, urea
Celiprolol *(celiprololum, celiprolol, céliprolol)*
   beta-adrenergic blocker, antihypertensive
   ↑ HDL cholesterol
   ↓ cholesterol, LDL cholesterol, TAG
Cephalosporins
   antibiotics
   ↑ ALP, ALT, antineutrophil Ab, AST, Bil, BT, eos, GMT, K, creatinine, LD, PLT, urea
   ↓ factors – (II, VII, X), GFR, Hb, WBC, neu, PLT
   ■ *Urine* ↑ proteins, G, 17-KS, creatinine, LD, pus, Hb, RBC, blood
Cerivastatin *(cerivastatinum, cerivastatin, cerivastatin)*
   lipid-lowering agent, antisclerotic
   ↑ ALT, AST, GMT
Ceruletide *(ceruletidum, ceruletide, cérulétide)*
   diagnostic aid
   ↓ amino acids
Cetirizine *(cetirizinum, cetirizine, cétirizine)*
   antihistamine
   ↑ ALT, AST
   ■ *Urine* ↑ RBC, blood, Hb, volume
Chenodeoxycholic Acid *(acidum chenodeoxycholicum, chenodeoxycholic acid, acide chéno-désoxycholique)*
   gallstone dissolving agent
   ↑ ALP, ALT, AST, Bil, HDL-C, cholesterol, LDL-C
   ↓ HDL-C, TAG, VLDL-C
Chenodiol *(acidum chenodeoxycholicum, chenodeoxycholic acid, acide chénodésoxy-cholique)*
   bile acid, gallstone dissolving agent
   ↑ ALT, AST, GMT
Chloral Hydrate *(chloralum hydratum, chloral hydrate, hydrate de chlorique)*
   hypnotic, sedative
   ↑ Bil, eos, factors – (II, VII, X), catecholamines, urea
   ↓ factors – (II, VII, X), WBC
   ■ *Urine* ↑ albumin, proteins, G, catecholamines, 17-OHCS, 17-KS (false), ketones, glucuronic acid
   ↓ G
Chlorambucil *(chlorambucilum, chlorambucil, chlorambucil)*
   antineoplastic
   ↑ ALP, ALT, AST, Bil, FSH, GMT, uric acid, WBC
   ↓ Hb, IgM, lym, neu, PLT, WBC
   ■ *Seminal Fluid* ↓ spermatozoa count
Chloramphenicol *(chloramphenicolum, chloramphenicol, chloramphénicol)*
   antibiotic
   ↑ ALP, ALT, AST, Bil, unconjugated Bil, eos, Fe, phenobarbital, phenytoin, GMT, creatinine, LD, 5-nucleotidase, urea
   ↓ factors – (II, VII, X), folate, G, granulocytes, Hb, HCT, uric acid, WBC, MAC, neu, pH, RTC, transferrin, PLT, urea

■ *Urine* ↑ G, 17-KS

Chlordiazepoxide *(chlordiazepoxidum, chlordiazepoxide, chlordiazépoxide)*
benzodiazepine tranquilizer
↑ ALP, ALT, AST, Bil, G
↓ granulocytes, Hb, WBC, neu, PLT
■ *Urine* ↓ 17-KS, 17-OHCS

Chlorhexidine *(chlorhexidinum, chlorhexidine, chlorhexidine)*
topical antiseptic
↑ AMS

Chloroquine *(chloroquinum, chloroquine, chloroquine)*
antimalaric, antiamebic, antirheumatic
↑ ALT, C-peptide, WBC, MHb
↓ PLT aggregation, G, granulocytes, Hb, HCT, WBC, Ly, neu, PLT, vitamin D3
■ *Urine* ↑ brown color

Chlorothiazide *(chlorothiazidum, chlorothiazide, chlorothiazide)*
salidiuretic, antihypertensive
↑ ALT, AST, Ca, G, quinidine, chloride, uric acid
↓ Ca, GFR, Hb, K, WBC, neu
■ *Urine* ↑ G, 17-KS

Chlorotrianisene *(chlorotrianisenum, chlorotrianisene, chlorotrianiséne)*
estrogen
↑ cholesterol, PL, PT, TAG, TBG
↓ folate

Chlorphenamine *(chlorphenaminum, chlorphenamine, chlorphénamine)*
histamine H₁ receptor antagonist
↑ lym, RTC
↓ granulocytes, Hb, HCT, WBC, PLT

Chlorpromazine *(chlorpromazinum, chlorpromazine, chlorpromazine)*
neuroleptic, antiemetic
↑ ALP, ALT, ANA, APTT, AST, Bil, conjugated Bil, CK, eos, estrogens, phenobarbital, phenytoin, G, GMT, cholesterol, IgM, LE cells, WBC, PRL, TAG, TSH
↓ PLT aggregation, granulocytes, haptoglobin, Hb, HDL cholesterol, chloride, insulin, uric acid, coagulation factors, Li, WBC, neu, T4, PLT, urea
■ *Urine* ↑ proteins, Bil, G, catecholamines, hCG, 17-OHCS, 17-KS, metanephrines, PBG, UBG, pink to red-brown color
↓ 5-HIAA, 17-OHCS, VMA
■ *Cerebrospinal Fluid* ↑ proteins
■ *Spermatic Fluid* ↑ spermatozoa count

Chlorpropamide *(chlorpropamidum, chlorpropamide, chlorpropamide)*
oral hypoglycemic
↑ ADH, albumin, ALP, ALT, AST, Bil, Ca, Ca²⁺, eos, cholesterol, GMT, insulin, creatinine, LD, neu, urea
↓ albumin, G, GFR, granulocytes, Hb, HCT, HDL cholesterol, cholesterol, coagulation factors, LDL cholesterol, lym, mono, WBC, Na, neu, osmolality, T4, TAG, PLT
■ *Urine* ↑ ADH, proteins, osmolality, uroporphyrin
↓ UBG

Chlorprothixene *(chlorprothixenum, chlorprothixene, chlorprothixéne)*
   neuroleptic, antipsychotic
   ↑ ALP, ANA, Bil, eos, G
   ↓ uric acid, WBC, PLT
   ■ *Urine* ↑ hCG

Chlortalidone *(chlortalidonum, chlortalidone, chlortalidone)*
   long-acting thiazide diuretic, antihypertensive
   ↑ aldosterone, ALP, ammonia, AMS, BE, Bil, Ca, CK, G, cholesterol, insulin, creatinine, uric acid, LDL cholesterol, Mg, renin, TAG, urea, Zn
   ↓ chloride, granulocytes, Hb, HCT, HDL cholesterol, K, Mg, Na, neu, osmolality, PLT, WBC
   ■ *Urine* ↑ proteins, G, norepinephrine

Chlortetracycline *(chlortetracyclinum, chlortetracycline, chlortétracycline)*
   antibiotic
   ↑ ALP, ALT, AST, Bil, eos, urea
   ↓ cholesterol, WBC, PLT
   ■ *Urine* ↑ G, catecholamines

Chlorzoxazone *(chlorzoxazonum, chlorzoxazone, chlorzoxazone)*
   skeletal muscle relaxant
   ↑ ALT, AST, GMT

Cholestyramine *(cholestyraminum, cholestyramine, cholestyramine)*
   lipid-lowering agent, antipruritic
   ↑ ALP, ALT, Apo A-I, factors – (II, VII, X), chloride, FA, MAC, Na, P, TAG, vitamin A, VLDL cholesterol
   ↓ Apo B, digitoxin, digoxin, Hb, HCO_3^-, cholesterol, K, LDL cholesterol, lipids, Na, pH, PL, T3, T4, TAG, vitamin – (A, B_{12}, D, E, folate, K), bile acids
   ■ *Urine* ↑ Ca, Ca^{2+}
   ■ *Stool* ↑ fatty acids

Chorionic Gonadotropin *(choriongonadotropinum, chorionic gonadotropin, chorionic gonadotropin)*
   mimics pituitary luteinising hormone
   ↑ androgens, progesterone
   ↓ FSH, LH

Chromium *(chromium, chromium, chromium)*
   dietary supplement
   ↓ G

Cibenzoline *(cibenzolinum, cibenzoline, cibenzoline)*
   antiarrhythmic
   ↑ insulin
   ↓ G

Cidofovir *(cidofovirum, cidofovir, cidofovir)*
   antiinfective, antiviral
   ↑ ALP, ALT, AST, G, creatinine, lipids, MAC, urea
   ↓ Ca, Hb, HCT, K, neu, PLT
   ■ *Urine* ↑ Hb, RBC, blood, G, P, proteins

Cilazapril *(cilazaprilum, cilazapril, cilazapril)*
   long-acting ACE inhibitor, antihypertensive
   ↑ K, renin
   ↓ aldosterone

Cilostazol *(cilostazolum, cilostazol, cilostazol)*
antithrombotic, cerebral vasodilator
- ***Sputum*** ↑ blood

Cimetidine *(cimetidinum, cimetidine, cimétidine)*
histamine H$_2$ receptor antagonist, antiulcer, antihistaminic
- ↑ ALP, ALT, AMS, androstenedione, AST, Bil, CK, cyclosporine, diazepam, digoxin, estradiol (M), ethanol, phenytoin, FSH, G, gastrin, GMT, HDL cholesterol, quinidine, IgA, IgG, imipramine, carbamazepine, creatinine, uric acid, salicylic acid, lipase, LH, WBC, LD, nortriptyline, PRL, procainamide, testosterone, theophylline, TSH, urea, valproate
- ↓ Ca, digoxin, estradiol, factors – (II, VII, X), G, Hb, CHS, insulin, LDL cholesterol, WBC, Mg, neu, PTH, SHBG, T$_3$, testosterone, PLT, vitamin B$_{12}$
- ***Urine*** ↑ G
  - ↓ vitamin B$_{12}$
- ***Gastric Fluid*** ↑ Hb
  - ↓ HCl
- ***Seminal Fluid*** ↓ spermatozoa count

Cimoxatone *(cimoxatonum, cimoxatone, cimoxatone)*
antidepressant
- ↓ PRL

Cinepazide *(cinepazidum, cinepazide, cinépazide)*
peripheral vasodilator
- ↓ neu

Cinoxacin *(cinoxacinum, cinoxacin, cinoxacine)*
antibacterial
- ↑ ALT

Ciprofibrate *(ciprofibratum, ciprofibrate, ciprofibrate)*
lipid-lowering agent
- ↑ AST, HDL cholesterol
- ↓ Hb

Ciprofloxacin *(ciprofloxacinum, ciprofloxacin, ciprofloxacine)*
antibacterial
- ↑ ALP, ALT, AST, AMS, Bil, cyclosporine, eos, G, cholesterol, K, creatinine, uric acid, LD, MAC, TAG, theophylline, urea
- ↓ factors – (II, VII, X), G, K
- ***Urine*** ↑ albumin, proteins, RBC, Hb, blood, crystals, volume

Cisplatin *(cisplatinum, cisplatin, cisplatine)*
antineoplastic
- ↑ ADH, ALT, AMS, AST, Bil, Fe, ferritin, GMT, creatinine, uric acid, lipase, RTC, urea
- ↓ albumin, aldosterone, Ca, Ca^{2+}, phenytoin, GFR, haptoglobin, Hb, K, WBC, Mg, Na, neu, osmolality, P, renin, PLT, Zn
- ***Urine*** ↑ B2M, Cu, haptoglobin, Hb, hexosaminidase, Mg, Na, volume, Zn
  - ↓ ALA, coproporphyrin, PBG, uroporphyrin

Citalopram *(citalopramum, citalopram, citalopram)*
antidepressant
- ↑ ALT
- ↓ Na, osmolality

Citrate Sodium (*natrii citras, sodium citrate, citrate de sodium*)

    antiaggregans

        ↑ Al, G, uric acid

        ↓ Ca^{2+}, cholesterol, uric acid, Mg, P, pH, Se, TAG, vitamin A, Zn

        ■ *Urine* ↑ K, volume

            ↓ uric acid

Cladribine (*cladribinum, cladribine, cladribine*)

    antineoplastic

        ↓ lym, neu, PLT, WBC

Clanidanol (*clanidanolum, clanidanol, clanidanol*)

        ↓ Hb

Clarithromycin (*clarithromycinum, clarithromycin, clarithromycine*)

    antibiotic

        ↑ ALT, AST, Bil, BT, GMT, TP, urea

        ↓ G

Clavulanic Acid (*acidum clavulanicum, clavulanic acid, acide clavulanique*)

    beta-lactamase inhibitor

        ↑ ALP, ALT, AST, Bil, eos, GMT

        ↓ neu

Clebopride (*clebopridum, clebopride, clébopride*)

    antiemetic, stomachic

        ↑ PRL

Clemastine (*clemastinum, clemastine, clémastine*)

    antihistamine

        ↓ granulocytes, Hb, HCT, PLT

Clindamycin (*clindamycinum, clindamycin, clindamycine*)

    antibiotic

        ↑ ALP, ALT, AST, Bil, CK, eos, K, creatinine, neu, urea

        ↓ Hb, coagulation factors, WBC, neu, PLT

        ■ *Urine* ↑ proteins

            ↓ volume

        ■ *Stool* ↑ Hb

Clinofibrate (*clinofibratum, clinofibrate, clinofibrate*)

    lipid-lowering agent

        ↑ HDL cholesterol

Clobazam (*clobazamum, clobazam, clobazam*)

    anxiolytic

        ↑ phenytoin, LH

Clobetasol (*clobetasolum, clobetasol, clobétasol*)

    topical steroid

        ↑ G

        ↓ cortisol

Clofazimine (*clofaziminum, clofazimine, clofazimine*)

    tuberculostatic, leprostatic

        ↑ albumin, ALT, AST, Bil, G, GMT, K

Clofibrate (*clofibratum, clofibrate, clofibrate*)

    lipid-lowering agent, antiatherosclerotic

        ↑ ADH, ALP, ALT, AMS, AST, Apo A-I, proteins, Bil, CK, HDL cholesterol, creatinine, eos, K, uric acid, T3, T4, TBG

↓ PLT aggregation, ALP, Apo B, Bil, factors – (II, VII, X), fibrinogen, FT4, G, GMT, granulocytes, chloride, cholesterol, Hb, HCT, insulin, uric acid, LD, LDL-C, lipids, Na, osmolality, T4, TAG, TSH, VLDL-C, FFA, WBC

■ *Urine* ↑ blood, Hb, RBC, proteins, uric acid
↓ VMA, volume

Clometacin *(clometacinum, clometacin, clométacine)*
non-steroid antiinflammatory agent, analgesic
↑ ALA, ALP, ALT, AST, Bil, eos, ESR, GMT, creatinine, urea
↓ factors – (II, VII, X), PLT

Clomiphene *(clomifenum, clomifene, clomiféne)*
antiestrogen
↑ ALT, AST, androstenedione, DHEA, DHEAS, DHT, estradiol, FSH, GMT, LH, progesterone, T4, TBG, testosterone, TSH, free testosterone
↓ cholesterol, T3, T4, TSH

■ *Urine* ↑ estrogens
■ *Seminal Fluid* ↑ spermatozoa count

Clomipramine *(clomipraminum, clomipramine, clomipramine)*
antidepressant
↑ ACTH, ALT, AST, eos, G, HDL cholesterol, cortisol, PRL, GH, TBG
↓ FT3, G, granulocytes, Hb, HCT, Na, neu, GH, PLT, T3, TSH, WBC

Clonazepam *(clonazepamum, clonazepam, clonazépam)*
anticonvulsant
↑ ALP, ALT, AST, LD
↓ granulocytes, Hb, HCT, neu, PLT, WBC

Clonidine *(clonidinum, clonidine, clonidine)*
central alpha-2-adrenoceptor stimulant, antihypertensive
↑ ALT, ANA, CK, G, GFR, ILGF-I, Na, GH
↓ ACTH, ADH, epinephrine, aldosterone, ANP, beta-endorphins, cholesterol, catecholamines, cortisol, Na, norepinephrine, PRL, renin

■ *Urine* ↓ aldosterone, epinephrine, catecholamines, norepinephrine, VMA

Clopamide *(clopamidum, clopamide, clopamide)*
salidiuretic, antihypertensive
↑ CK, Cu, HDL cholesterol
↓ Cu, K, PLT, Zn

■ *Urine* ↓ chloride, K, Mg, Na

Clorazepate *(dikalii clorazepas, clorazepate dipotassium, clorazépate dipotassique)*
anxiolytic, sedative, hypnotic
↑ ALP, ALT, AST, LD

Clotrimazole *(clotrimazolum, clotrimazole, clotrimazole)*
antifungal
↑ ALP, ALT, AST, Bil
↓ neu

Cloxacillin *(cloxacillinum, cloxacillin, cloxacilline)*
antibiotic
↑ ALP, ALT, AST, Bil, eos
↓ factors – (II, VII, X), WBC, neu

Clozapine *(clozapinum, clozapine, clozapine)*
    atypic neuroleptic
        ↑ ALP, ALT, AST, eos, ESR, G, HVA, WBC, PRL
        ↓ granulocytes, WBC, neu, PLT

Cocaine Hydrochloride *(cocaini hydrochloridum, cocaine hydrochloride, cocaine de hydrochloride)*
    opioid analgesic, local anesthetic
        ↑ PLT aggregation, ALT, CK, CK-MB
        ↓ MCV

Codeine *(codeini phosphas, codeine phosphate, codeine de phosphate)*
    opioid analgesic, antitussive
        ↑ ALT, AMS, AST, eos, LD, lipase, WBC, urea
        ↓ Na, PLT, WBC
        ■ *Urine* ↑ proteins
           ↓ volume

Colchicine *(colchicinum, colchicine, colchicine)*
    antiarthritic, antirheumatic
        ↑ albumin, ALP, ALT, AST, Bil, CK, Heinz bodies (RBC), WBC, lym, MAC+RAC, MCV, PT
        ↓ Ca, granulocytes, Hb, HCT, cholesterol, Mg, Na, neu, P, PTH, PLT, vitamin – (folate, B_{12}), WBC
        ■ *Urine* ↑ blood, Hb, RBC, 17-OHCS, corticosteroids
        ■ *Stool* ↑ blood, fatty acids
        ■ *Seminal Fluid* ↓ spermatozoa count

Colestipol *(colestipolum, colestipol, colestipol)*
    lipid-lowering agent
        ↑ ALP, ALT, AST, factors – (II, VII, X), PT, TAG, TSH, VLDL cholesterol
        ↓ Apo B, FT4, cholesterol, carotene, LDL cholesterol, T3, T4, TAG, TBG, vitamin – (A, D, K)
        ■ *Stool* ↑ fat

Colestyramine *(colestyraminum, colestyramine, colestyramine)*
    lipid-lowering agent, antipruritic
        ↑ factors – (II, VII, X)
        ↓ factors – (II, VII, X), folate, Hb, pH

Colfosceril Palmitate *(colfoscerili palmitas, colfosceril palmitate, palmitate de colfoscéril)*
    lung surfactant
        ↑ pO_2

Colistin *(colistinum, colistin, colistine)*
    antibacterial cationic cyclic polypeptide
        ↑ creatinine, urea
        ■ *Urine* ↑ proteins

Contraceptives
        ↑ AAT, angiotensin, APTT, conjugated Bil, Fe, G, GMT, cholesterol, insulin, cortisol, LDL cholesterol, PT, renin, SHBG, T4, TAG, TBG, TIBC, transferrin, vitamin A
        ↓ C4 complement, HDL cholesterol, Mn, vitamin – (pyridoxine, C, folic acid), Zn
        ■ *Urine* ↑ cortisol
           ↓ 17-OHCS, 17-KS

Corticoids

corticosteroids

↑ albumin, ALP (neu), ALT, AMS, AST, Bil, proteins, C-peptide, Cu, RBC, C3 complement, G, HDL cholesterol, HCO_3, chloride, cholesterol, insulin, uric acid, LDL cholesterol, WBC, MAL, Na, orosomucoid, osmolality, PTH, GH, TAG, urea

↓ aldosterone, ACE, ALP, Ca, CRP, eos, FSH, ESR, gamma globulins, HDL cholesterol, chloride, cholesterol, IgG, K, cortisol, uric acid, salicylic acid, WBC, lym, osteocalcin, P, GH, testosterone, T3, T4, TBG, TSH, Zn

■ *Urine* ↑ Ca, chloride, proteins, estriol, G, K, 17-KS, creatinine, Mg
   ↓ hydroxyproline, 17-KS
■ *Stool* ↑ blood, Hb
■ *Seminal Fluid* ↑ spermatozoa count/motility
   ↓ spermatozoa count/motility

Cortisone (*cortisonum, cortisone, cortisone*)

hormone, glucocorticoid

↑ G, chloride, cholesterol, MAL, Na, neu

↓ Ca, eos, Fe, ESR, haptoglobin, chloride, K, PLT, uric acid, T4

■ *Urine* ↑ creatine

Cotrimoxazole (*cotrimoxazolum, cotrimoxazole, cotrimoxazole*)

antibacterial

↑ ALP, ALT, AST, Bil, eos, phenytoin, G, GMT, K, creatinine

↓ cyclosporine, factors – (II, VII, X), G, Hb, WBC, neu, pH, PLT, TSH

■ *Urine* ↑ proteins
■ *Cerebrospinal Fluid* ↑ WBC

Coumarin (*coumarinum, coumarin, coumarin*)

anticoagulant

↑ ALP, ALT, AST, AT III, Bil, BT, phenytoin, GMT, PT

↓ G, uric acid, proconvertin, protein C, prothrombin

Cromolyn (*acidum cromoglicicum, cromoglycic acid, acide cromoglicique*)

antiallergic, antiasthmatic

↓ 17-OHCS

Cyanocobalamin (*cyanocobalaminum, cyanocobalamin, cyanocobalamine*)

hematopoietic vitamin

↓ K

Cyclobenzaprine (*cyclobenzaprinum, cyclobenzaprine, cyclobenzaprine*)

skeletal muscle relaxant, sedative, antimuscarinic

↑ eos, G

↓ G, PLT, WBC

Cyclofenil (*cyclofenilum, cyclofenil, cyclofénil*)

ovulation stimulant

↑ ALP, ALT, AST, Bil, HDL cholesterol

↓ Hb, PRL

■ *Urine* ↓ estriol, estrogens
■ *Seminal Fluid* ↓ spermatozoa count

Cyclopenthiazide (*cyclopenthiazidum, cyclopenthiazide, cyclopenthiazide*)

salidiuretic, antihypertensive

↓ Na

Cyclophosphamide (*cyclophosphamidum, cyclophosphamide, cyclophosphamide*)
  antineoplastic
   ↑ ADH, ALP, ALT, AST, Bil, factors – (II, VII, X), FSH, GFR, cholesterol, K, creatinine, LH (M), plasma volume, uric acid
   ↓ estrogens, FSH (F), ESR, Hb, CHE, WBC, Na, neu, osmolality, progesterone, testosterone, PLT
    ■ *Urine* ↑ blood, RBC, Hb, Na, osmolality
     ↓ estrogens, volume
    ■ *Stool* ↑ Hb
    ■ *Seminal Fluid* ↓ spermatozoa count

Cyclopropane (*cyclopropanum, cyclopropane, cyclopropane*)
  anesthetic
   ↑ ALP, Bil, G, catecholamines
   ↓ catecholamines, pH

Cycloserine (*cycloserinum, cycloserine, cyclosérine*)
  tuberculostatic
   ↑ ALP, Bil, MCV
   ↓ vitamin – (B_6, B_{12}, folate)

Cyclosporine (*ciclosporinum, cyclosporine, ciclosporine*)
  immunosuppressant
   ↑ ALP, ALT, AMS, Apo B, AST, Bil, B2M, CK, C-peptide, digoxin, ESR, G, GMT, chloride, cholesterol, insulin, K, creatinine, uric acid, LDL cholesterol, lipids, LP(a), MAC, PRL, PTH, TAG, urea, bile acids
   ↓ aldosterone, Apo A-I, Apo B, estradiol, GFR, Hb, HDL cholesterol, HCO_3^-, cholesterol, WBC, Mg, PRL, renin, SHBG, testosterone, PLT
    ■ *Urine* ↑ Hb, proteins, Mg
     ↓ volume, osmolality

Cyproheptadine (*cyproheptadinum, cyproheptadine, cyproheptadine*)
  histamine H_1 receptor antagonist, antihistaminic, antiallergic
   ↑ ALP, AMS, Bil, PRL
   ↓ PLT aggregation, G, PRL, TSH

Cyproterone (*cyproteronum, cyproterone, cyprotérone*)
  antiandrogen
   ↑ ALT, androstenedione, Apo A-I, Bil, HDL cholesterol, cholesterol, insulin, LDL cholesterol, PL, TAG
   ↓ aldosterone, DHEAS, estradiol, estrone, G, HDL-C, cholesterol, LDL cholesterol, LH, PL, progesterone, renin, SHBG, testosterone, free testosterone
    ■ *Seminal Fluid* ↓ spermatozoa count

Cysteamine (*mercaptaminum, mercaptamine, mercaptamine*)
  in radiation sickness, depigmenting agent, antidote to paracetamol poisoning
   ↓ WBC

Cytarabine (*cytarabinum, cytarabine, cytarabine*)
  antineoplastic, antiviral, antileukemic
   ↑ ALP, ALT, AST, Bil, conjugated Bil, CK, GMT, uric acid, LD, MCV
   ↓ Hb, WBC, neu, RTC, PLT

Cytosine Arabinoside (*cytarabinum, cytarabine, cytarabine*)
  antineoplastic, antiviral
   ↓ Ca

Cytostatics
   ↑ ammonia, Bil, conjugated Bil, G, GMT, K, uric acid, P
   ↓ IgA, IgG, IgM, neu

■ *Urine* ↑ RBC, Hb, crystals – (urate), LD
↓ hydroxyproline
■ *Seminal Fluid* ↓ spermatozoa count

Dacarbazine *(dacarbazinum, dacarbazine, dacarbazine)*
antineoplastic
↑ ALT, AST, Bil, eos, creatinine, urea
↓ WBC, neu, PLT
Dactinomycin *(dactinomycinum, dactinomycin, dactinomycine)*
antibiotic, antineoplastic
↑ ALP, ALT, AST, GMT
↓ Ca, Hb, neu, WBC, RTC, PLT
Dalcizumab *(dalcizumabum, dalcizumab, dalcizumab)*
monoclonal antibody
↑ G
Dalfopristin *(dalfopristinum, dalfopristin, dalfopristin)*
antibiotic
↑ Bil, MAC
↓ G, Na, pO$_2$
■ *Urine* ↑ blood, Hb, RBC
Dalteparin Sodium *(dalteparinum natricum, dalteparin sodium, daltéparine sodique)*
anticoagulant
↑ ALT, AST, Bil
↓ PLT
Danaparoid *(danaparoidum, danaparoid, danaparoid)*
anticoagulant
↓ PLT
■ *Urine* ↑ blood, Hb, RBC
Danazol *(danazolum, danazol, danazol)*
anterior pituitary suppressant
↑ ALP, ALT, ANA, androstenedione, AST, Bil, Ca, cyclosporine, CK, C-peptide, DHEA, DHEAS, FT4, glucagon, GMT, Hb, cholesterol, insulin, K, carbamazepine, cortisol, LDL cholesterol, LH, PRL, testosterone, TAG, PLT, free cortisol, free testosterone
↓ ALP, Apo A-I, Ca^{2+}, DHEA, estradiol, factors – (II, VII, X), FSH, FT4, HDL cholesterol, LH, LP(a), osmotic fragility (RBC), progesterone, SHBG, T3, T4, TBG, testosterone, TAG, TSH, free cortisol
■ *Urine* ↑ 17-KS
Dantrolene *(dantrolenum, dantrolene, dantroléne)*
treatment of malignant hyperthermia, skeletal muscle relaxant
↑ ALP, ALT, AST, Bil, GMT, OCT
■ *Urine* ↑ crystals, blood, RBC
■ *Pleural Fluid* ↑ eos
Dapsone *(dapsonum, dapsone, dapsone)*
antibacterial, dermatitis herpetiformis suppressant, antileprosy
↑ ALP, ALT, AST, Bil, eos, Heinz bodies (RBC), MHb, RTC
↓ albumin, haptoglobin, Hb, WBC, neu
■ *Urine* ↑ proteins, PBG, porphyrins
Daunorubicin *(daunorubicinum, daunorubicin, daunorubicine)*
antineoplastic, antileukemic
↓ neu, PLT

Delavirdine *(delavirdinum, delavirdine, délavirdine)*
  antiviral
   ↑ ALP, ALT, AMS, AST, CK, eos, GMT, granulocytes, K, lipase, uric acid, WBC, PTT
   ↓ Ca, Hb, HCT, Na, P, RBC, PLT
   ■ *Urine* ↑ blood, protein, sperm count, volume
Demeclocycline *(demeclocyclinum, demeclocycline, déméclocycline)*
  antibiotic
   ↑ ALT, AST, eos, GMT
   ↓ ADH, Hb, neu, PLT
   ■ *Urine* ↑ catecholamines
    ↓ osmolality
Denileukin *(denileukinum, denileukin, dénileukin)*
  antineoplastic
   ↑ ALT, AST, GMT, urea
   ↓ albumin, Ca, lym, PLT, WBC
   ■ *Urine* ↑ blood, Hb, RBC
Denzimol *(denzimolum, denzimol, denzimol)*
  anticonvulsant, antiepileptic
   ↑ phenytoin, carbamazepine
Desipramine *(desipraminum, desipramine, désipramine)*
  antidepressant
   ↑ ACTH, ALP, ALT, bas, Bil, eos, folate, G, norepinephrine, PRL, GH, FFA
   ↓ G, Hb, WBC, neu, PLT
   ■ *Urine* ↓ volume
   ■ *Cerebrospinal Fluid* ↓ 5-HIAA
Desmopressin *(desmopressinum, desmopressin, desmopressine)*
  antidiuretic peptide hormone
   ↑ ALT, AST, factor – (VIII), GMT, cortisol, plasminogen activator inhibitor, WBC, norepinephrine
   ↓ BT, Na, osmolality
Desogestrel *(desogestrelum, desogestrel, désogestrel)*
  progestin
   ↑ G, HDL cholesterol, insulin
   ↓ HDL cholesterol, LDL cholesterol, LP(a), SHBG
Desonide *(desonidum, desonide, désonide)*
  glucocorticoid
   ↑ G
   ■ *Urine* ↑ G
Desoximetasone *(desoximetasonum, desoximetasone, désoximétasone)*
  glucocorticoid, antiinflammatory, antiallergic
   ↑ G, insulin
   ↓ cortisol
Dexamethasone *(dexamethasonum, dexamethasone, dexaméthasone)*
  glucocorticosteroid, antiinflammatory, antiallergic
   ↑ AMS, Apo A-I, Apo E, Ca^{2+}, C-peptide, phenytoin, G, HDL cholesterol, cholesterol, insulin, lym, MAL, WBC, Na, neu, rT3, SHBG, GH, free testosterone
   ↓ ACTH, Ca, beta-endorphins, DHEAS, estriol, FSH, K, catecholamines, corticosteroids, cortisol, LH, LP(a), lym, PLT, PRL, T3, T4, testosterone, TSH
   ■ *Urine* ↑ G, K, 17-KS, corticosteroids, Na

          ↓ androsterone, DHEA, estrogens, 17-OHCS, 17-KGS, 17-KS, VMA
- ■ *Seminal Fluid* ↑ spermatozoa
          ↓ spermatozoa

Dexmedetomidine *(dexmedetomidinum, dexmedetomidine, dexmédétomidine)*
   alpha-2-adrenoceptor agonist
          ↑ ALT, AST, GMT, WBC
          ↓ pO$_2$

Dexpanthenol *(dexpanthenolum, dexpanthenol, dexpanthénol)*
   vitamin
          ↑ BT

Dexrazoxane *(dexrazoxanum, dexrazoxane, dexrazoxane)*
   chemoprotectant
          ↓ PLT, WBC

Dextran *(dextranum, dextran, dextran)*
   plasma volume expander
          ↑ proteins, Bil, conjugated Bil, BT, Fe, phenobarbital, phenytoin, ESR, G, cholesterol, creatinine, MAC, Na
          ↓ PLT aggregation, albumin, A2MG, proteins, factors – (V, VII, IX), fibrinogen, G, haptoglobin, IgA, IgG, IgM, Na

Dextromethorphan *(dextromethorphanum, dextromethorphan, dextrométhorphane)*
   cough suppressant
          ↓ PLT

Dextropropoxyphene *(dextropropoxyphenum, dextropropoxyphene, dextropropoxyphene)*
   analgesic, antipyretic
          ↑ ALP, ALT, AST, Bil, GMT, carbamazepine
          ↓ coagulation factors
- ■ *Urine* ↑ G
          ↓ 17-OHCS, 17-KS

Dextrose *(glucosum, glucose, glucose)*
   fluid and nutrient replenisher
          ↑ Bil, K, osmolality
          ↓ Ca, ESR, K, cortisol, creatinine, uric acid, Na, P, testosterone
- ■ *Urine* ↑ Mg, osmolalit y
          ↓ estriol, estrogens, K, 17-OHCS, 17-KS

Dextrothyroxine Sodium *(dextrothyroxinum natricum, dextrothyroxine sodium, dextrothyroxine sodique)*
   thyromimetic, anticholesteremic
          ↑ G, T4
          ↓ beta-LP, cholesterol, LDL cholesterol, lipids, TAG

Diamorphine *(diamorphinum, diamorphine, diamorphine)*
   narcotic analgesic
          ↑ AST, T3, T4
          ↓ HDL cholesterol, cholesterol, pO$_2$, PLT

Diazepam *(diazepamum, diazepam, diazépam)*
   anxiolytic, anticonvulsant, hypnotic
          ↑ ALP, ALT, AST, Bil, estradiol, GMT, pCO$_2$, PRL, GH, testosterone, TAG, TSH
          ↓ granulocytes, Hb, HCT, PLT, WBC, neu, pO$_2$, T3, T4
- ■ *Urine* ↑ 5-HIAA, Mb, porphyrins
- ■ *Gastric Fluid* ↓ HCl
- ■ *Seminal Fluid* ↓ spermatozoa count

Diaziquone *(diaziquonum, diaziquone, diaziquone)*
   antineoplastic, antileukemic
        ↑ ALT
Diazoxide *(diazoxidum, diazoxide, diazoxide)*
   antihypertensive, hyperglycemic
        ↑ ALP, AST, Bil (infants), eos, G, IgG, iodine, catecholamines, ketobodies,
          coagulation factors, cortisol, uric acid, MAC, Na, plasma volume, PT,
          renin, urea, FFA
        ↓ phenytoin, G, GFR, Hb, HCT, IgG, insulin, cortisol, Na, neu, testoster-
          one, PLT, WBC
        ■ *Urine* ↑ albumin, blood, RBC, G
          ↓ G, HCO_3^-, chloride, K, cortisol, uric acid, Na, volume
Dibekacin *(dibekacinum, dibekacin, dibékacine)*
   antibiotic
        ↑ creatinine
Dibenzepin *(dibenzepinum, dibenzepin, dibenzépine)*
   antidepressant
        ↑ PRL
Diclofenac *(diclofenacum, diclofenac, diclofénac)*
   non-steroid antiinflammatory, analgesic
        ↑ ALA, ALP, ALT, ANA, AST, Bil, BT, G, GMT, cholesterol, creatinine, Li,
          urea
        ↓ PLT aggregation, factor – (II), Hb, HCT, WBC, Na, neu, PLT, urea
        ■ *Urine* ↑ blood, Hb, RBC
        ■ *Stool* ↑ Hb
Diclofenamide *(diclofenamidum, diclofenamide, diclofénamide)*
   carbonic anhydrase inhibitor
        ↓ K
Dicloxacillin *(dicloxacillinum, dicloxacillin, dicloxacilline)*
   antibiotic
        ↑ ALP, ALT, AST, bas, Bil, BT, eos, factors – (II, VII, X), creatinine, GMT,
          lym, mono, Na, PT, PLT
        ↓ albumin, granulocytes, Hb, HCT, K, neu, PLT, proteins, uric acid, WBC
        ■ *Urine* ↑ proteins, blood, RBC, pus, hyaline casts
          ↓ volume
Dicoumarol *(dicoumarolum, dicoumarol, dicoumarol)*
   anticoagulant
        ↑ ALP, ALT, AST, phenytoin, GMT, LD
        ↓ uric acid
Didanosine *(didanosinum, didanosine, didanosine)*
   synthetic purine nucleoside analog against HIV-1, antiviral
        ↑ ALP, ALT, AMS, AST, Bil, G, GMT, uric acid, LA, MAC, lipase
        ↓ granulocytes, Hb, K, neu, WBC, PLT
        ■ *Urine* ↑ phenylpyruvic acid
Dienestrol *(dienestrolum, dienestrol, diénestrol)*
   synthetic estrogen
        ↑ Bil
Diethylpropion *(diethylpropionum, diethylpropion, diethylpropion)*
   CNS stimulant, anorectic
        ↓ granulocytes, WBC

Diethylstilbestrol *(diethylstilbestrolum, diethylstilbestrol, diéthylstilbestrol)*
antineoplastic, non-steroid estrogen
   ↑ ALT, AST, Bil, Ca, Ca²⁺, CBG, GMT, LH, PRL, SHBG, TBG
   ↓ FSH, uric acid, LH, WBC, testosterone, PLT, free testosterone
   ■ ***Urine*** ↑ coproporphyrin, uric acid, vitamin A
      ↓ estradiol, estriol, 17-OHCS

Diflunisal *(diflunisalum, diflunisal, diflunisal)*
antipyretic, analgesic, non-steroid antiinflammatory
   ↑ ALP, ALT, AST, BT, eos, GMT, indomethacin
   ↓ granulocytes, Hb, HCT, uric acid, PLT, WBC
   ■ ***Urine*** ↑ blood, Hb, RBC
   ■ ***Stool*** ↑ Hb

Digitalis *(digitalis, digitalis, digitalis)*
cardiotonic
   ↑ ALT, AST, eos, FSH, GMT, K, neu
   ↓ K (chronic), LH, Mg, testosterone, PLT

Digitoxin *(digitoxinum, digitoxin, digitoxine)*
cardiotonic
   ↑ proteins, eos, K
   ↓ Hb, K, WBC, PLT

Digoxin *(digoxinum, digoxin, digoxine)*
cardiotonic
   ↑ CK, estradiol, estrogens, estrone, K
   ↓ DHT, K, LD, LH, Mg, neu, renin, testosterone, free testosterone
   ■ ***Urine*** ↑ G, 17-OHCS, 17-KS

Dihydralazine *(dihydralazinum, dihydralazine, dihydralazine)*
antihypertensive
   ↑ ALP, ALT, AST, Bil, BT, GMT

Dihydrotachysterol *(dihydrotachysterolum, dihydrotachysterol, dihydrotachystérol)*
calcium regulator
   ↑ Ca, P
   ■ ***Urine*** ↑ Ca

Dilantin *(dilantinum, dilantin, dilantin)*
anticonvulsant, antiepileptic
   ↑ ANA

Dilevalol *(dilevalolum, dilevalol, dilevalol)*
vasodilator
   ↑ ALT, AST
   ↓ ANP, renin

Diltiazem *(diltiazemum, diltiazem, diltiazem)*
slow calcium channel antagonist, antihypertensive, coronary vasodilator
   ↑ aldosterone, ALP, ALT, AST, cyclosporine, CK, BT, digoxin, phenytoin,
      G, GFR, GMT, HDL cholesterol, K, carbamazepine, creatinine, WBC,
      norepinephrine, PGE2, PTH, renin, theophylline, urea
   ↓ carbamazepine, neu, PLT, PTH
   ■ ***Urine*** ↑ Na, volume

Dimenhydrinate *(dimenhydrinatum, dimenhydrinate, diménhydrinate)*
antihistaminic
   ↑ theophylline (false)

Dimercaprol *(dimercaprolum, dimercaprol, dimercaprol)*
  antidote to heavy metal poisoning, to stimulation therapy
  ↑ MAC
  ↓ pH

Dimeticone *(dimeticonum, dimeticone, diméticone)*
  antidotum, deflatulencium
  ↓ coagulation factors

Dinoprost *(dinoprostum, dinoprost, dinoprost)*
  PGF-2-alpha, oxytocic, abortifacient, vasodilator, smooth muscle stimulant
  ↑ PRL, T3, T4
  ↓ estriol, progesterone

Diodone *(diodonum, diodone, diodone)*
  diagnostic aid
  ↓ uric acid

Diphenhydramine *(diphenhydraminum, diphenhydramine, diphénhydramine)*
  histamine H₁ receptor antagonist
  ↑ CK, haptoglobin
  ↓ ammonia, granulocytes, Hb, HCT, PLT

Diphenoxylate *(diphenoxylatum, diphenoxylate, diphénoxylate)*
  antiperistaltic
  ↑ AMS

Diphenylhydantoin *(phenytoinum, phenytoin, phénytoin)*
  anticonvulsant, antiepileptic
  ↑ Bil, PT
  ↓ PLT

Dipyridamole *(dipyridamolum, dipyridamole, dipyridamole)*
  coronary vasodilator, antithrombotic
  ↑ ANP
  ↓ PLT aggregation, neu

Dirithromycin *(dirithromycini, dirithromycin, dirithromycin)*
  antibiotic, macrolide
  ↑ CK, eos, K, neu, PLT
  ↓ HCO₃⁻,

Disopyramide *(disopyramidum, disopyramide, disopyramide)*
  antiarrhythmic
  ↑ ALP, ALT, ANA, AST, Bil, digoxin, eos, GMT, cholesterol, insulin, K, creatinine, LA, uric acid, LD, MAC, TAG, urea
  ↓ Apo A-I, Apo A-II, Apo B, factors – (II, VII, X), G, quinidine, cholesterol, K, WBC, neu, TAG
  Urine ↓ VMA, volume

Disulfiram *(disulfiramum, disulfiram, disulfirame)*
  adjunct in the treatment of chronic alcoholism
  ↑ ALP, ALT, AST, Bil, eos, phenytoin, GMT, cholesterol, catecholamines, LD, OCT, theophylline
  ↓ factors – (II, VII, X), vitamin B₆, norepinephrine
  ■ *Urine* ↑ acetoacetate, acetone, BHBA, catecholamines, homogentisic acid
  ↓ VMA

Diuretics
  ↑ Apo B, Ca, RBC, G, HCO₃⁻, chloride, cholesterol, K, creatinine, uric acid, LDL cholesterol, Li, LP(a), MAL, osmolality, renin, TAG

    ↓ PLT aggregation, Ca, GFR, HDL cholesterol, chloride, K, WBC, Mg, Mn,
     Na, osmolality, P, PLT
    ■ *Urine* ↑ K, Mg, P
     ↓ chloride

Dobutamine *(dobutaminum, dobutamine, dobutamine)*
 synthetic catecholamine, cardiac inotropic agent
    ↑ GFR, K, norepinephrine, renin
    ↓ K

Docetaxel *(docetaxelum, docetaxel, docétaxel)*
 antineoplastic
    ↑ ALT, AST, Bil, GMT
    ↓ neu, WBC

Dofetilide *(dofetilidum, dofetilide, dofétilide)*
 antiarrhythmic
    ↑ ALT, AST, GMT

Dolasetron *(dolasetronum, dolasetron, dolasétron)*
 antagonist 5-HT$_3$ receptors, antiemetic in chemotherapy induced emesis
    ↑ ALT, AST, GMT

Domperidone *(domperidonum, domperidone, dompéridone)*
 antiemetic
    ↑ PRL, TSH

Donezepil *(donezepilum, donezepil, donezepil)*
 cholinesterase inhibitor
    ↑ eos
    ↓ Hb, HCT, PLT

Dopamine *(dopaminum, dopamine, dopamine)*
 endogenous catecholamine, cardiac inotropic agent, sympathomimetic, vasopressor
    ↑ Bil, G, catecholamines, uric acid, norepinephrine, PRL, PTH, GH, FFA
    ↓ ALT, AST, FT4, LH, PRL, T3, T4, TSH
    ■ *Urine* ↑ epinephrine, amino acids, Ca, dopamine, K, catecholamines,
     Na, volume

Doxapram *(doxapramum, doxapram, doxapram)*
 respiratory stimulant
    ↑ epinephrine, G, urea
    ■ *Urine* ↑ proteins

Doxazosin *(doxazosinum, doxazosin, doxazosine)*
 alpha-1-receptor antagonist, antihypertensive, vasodilator
    ↑ HDL cholesterol, norepinephrine, renin
    ↓ G, cholesterol, insulin, LDL cholesterol, TAG, VLDL cholesterol
    ■ *Urine* ↑ volume

Doxepin *(doxepinum, doxepin, doxépine)*
 antidepressant, antipruritic
    ↑ ALP, eos, norepinephrine
    ↓ granulocytes, Hb, PLT, WBC

Doxercalciferol *(doxercalciferolum, doxercalciferol, doxercalciferol)*
 synthetic vitamin D analog
    ↑ Ca, P
    ■ *Urine* ↑ Ca

Doxorubicin *(doxorubicinum, doxorubicin, doxorubicine)*
 antineoplastic, antileukemic
    ↑ ALT, ANP, AST, Bil, GMT, OCT
    ↓ neu, PLT, WBC

Doxycycline *(doxycyclinum, doxycycline, doxycycline)*
    antibiotic
        ↑ ALT, AST, eos, GMT
        ↓ Hb, HCT, carbamazepine, WBC, neu, P, PLT

Droperidol *(droperidolum, droperidol, dropéridol)*
    neuroleptic, antiemetic
        ↑ G

EDTA *(acidum edeticum, edetic acid, acide edetique)*
    chelating agent, antidote, calcium replenisher
        ↑ ACE, ALP, Ca, G, hexosaminidase, uric acid, Na, urea
        ↓ Ca, HCO_3^-, cholesterol, K, lipids
        ■ *Urine* ↑ G, K
          ↓ G

Efavirenz *(efavirenzum, efavirenz, éfavirenz)*
    antiviral
        ↑ ALT, AST, GMT, cholesterol
        ■ *Urine* ↑ blood, RBC

Enalapril *(enalaprilum, enalapril, énalapril)*
    ACE inhibitor, antihypertensive
        ↑ ACE, ALP, ALT, AT I, AST, Bil, Ca, eos, G, GFR, GMT, cholesterol, K, creatinine, lipase, renin, TAG, urea, uric acid
        ↓ ACE, albumin, aldosterone, angiotensin II, EPO, G, GFR, granulocytes, Hb, HCT, HbA_{1c}, cholesterol, uric acid, WBC, lym, Mg, mono, Na, neu, PLT
        ■ *Urine* ↑ proteins, G

Enaprilat *(enalaprilatum, enalaprilat, énalaprilate)*
    ACE inhibitor, antihypertensive
        ↑ ALT, AST, Bil, eos, G, GMT, K, uric acid
        ↓ granulocytes, Hb, HCT, lym, mono, neu, PLT, WBC

Endralazine *(endralazinum, endralazine, endralazine)*
    antihypertensive
        ↑ GFR

Enflurane *(enfluranum, enflurane, enflurane)*
    anesthetic
        ↑ ALT, AST, Bil, COHb, eos, creatinine, GMT, PRL, rT3, T4, urea
        ↓ T3
        ■ *Urine* ↑ volume

Enoxacin *(enoxacinum, enoxacin, énoxacine)*
    antibacterial
        ↑ ALT, theophylline
        ↓ factors – (II, VII, X)

Enoxaparin *(enoxaparinum natricum, enoxaparin sodium, énoxaparine sodique)*
    LMW heparin fraction, prophylaxis of deep venous thrombosis
        ↑ ALT, AST, lipids, PLT, TAG
        ↓ Hb, HCT, PLT
        ■ *Urine* ↑ blood, Hb, RBC

Enoxolone *(enoxolonum, enoxolone, énoxolone)*
    antibacterial, antiiflammatory, antipruritic
        ↑ ANP, Na
        ↓ aldosterone, K

Ephedrine *(ephedrinum, ephedrine, éphedrine)*
sympathomimetic, antiasthmatic
↑ G, T3
↓ cortisol
■ *Urine* ↑ epinephrine, G, 5-HIAA
Epinephrine *(epinephrinum, epinephrine, épinéphrine)*
alpha- and beta-adrenergic agent, sympathomimetic, vasoconstrictor
↑ conjugated Bil, proteins, cAMP, factor – (VIII), G, gastrin, glucagon, Hb, cholesterol, K, calcitonin, catecholamines, uric acid, LA, WBC, LP, lym, MAC, neu, norepinephrine, PL, TBG, PLT, FFA
↓ amino acids, Ca²⁺, eos, Fe, GFR, K, P, tyrosine
■ *Urine* ↑ amino acids, proteins, G, catecholamines, VMA
↓ K, Na, volume
Epirubicin *(epirubicinum, epirubicin, épirubicine)*
antineoplastic, anthracycline antibiotic
↓ neu, PLT, WBC
Epoietin *(epoietinum, epoietin, époiétine)*
hormone controlling hematopoiesis
↑ K
Eprosartan *(eprosartanum, eprosartan, éprosartan)*
angiotensin II antagonist
↑ ALT, AST, GMT, K
Eptifibatide *(eptifibatidum, eptifibatide, éptifibatide)*
platelet aggregation inhibitor
■ *Urine* ↑ blood, Hb, RBC
Ergocalciferol *(ergocalciferolum, ergocalciferol, ergocalciférol)*
antirachitis vitamin
↑ AMS, Ca, cholesterol, P
↓ PTH
Ergonovine *(ergometrinum, ergometrine, ergométrine)*
ergot alkaloid, oxytocic
↑ urea
■ *Urine* ↑ ALA, proteins, porphyrins
Ergosterol *(ergocalciferolum, ergocalciferol, ergocalciférol)*
vitamin D2
↑ ALP
Ergot Alkaloids
↑ ALT, urea
↓ PRL
■ *Urine* ↑ proteins, porphyrins
Erythromycin *(erythromycinum, erythromycin, érythromycine)*
antibiotic
↑ ALP, ALT, AST, Bil, cyclosporine, digoxin, eos, GMT, carbamazepine, catecholamines, creatinine, LD, neu, OCT, RTC, theophylline
↓ factors – (II, VII, X), G, Hb, cholesterol, folate, PLT, WBC
■ *Urine* ↑ amino acids, blood, Hb, 17-OHCS, catecholamines, 17-KS, crystals, RBC
↓ estriol
Erythropoietin *(epoietinum, epoietin, époiétine)*
hematopoietic growth factor
↑ PLT aggregation, ANP, Hb, K, P, renin, RTC, PLT
↓ BT, Fe, ferritin, PRL

Erythrosine *(erythrosinum, erythrosine, erythrosine)*
    diagnostic aid
        ↑ TSH

Estradiol *(estradiolum, estradiol, estradiol)*
    estrogen
        ↑ ALP, ALT, Apo A-I, Apo B, AST, estrone, G, GMT, HDL cholesterol, cholesterol, 5-nucleotidase, SHBG, T4, TAG, TBG, VLDL-C
        ↓ AT III, FSH, G, HDL cholesterol, homocysteine, 17-alpha-hydroxyprogesterone, cholesterol, LDL cholesterol, LH, TAG

Estramustine *(estramustinum, estramustine, estramustine)*
    antineoplastic
        ↑ ALT, AST, Bil, GMT, HDL
        ↓ Ca, Ca^{2+}, PLT, WBC

Estriol *(estrioli succinas, estriol succinate, succinate d´estriol)*
    estrogen
        ↑ ALP

Estrogens
        ↑ AAT, A2MG, aldosterone, ALP, ALT, AMS, angiotensin, Apo A-I, AST, bas, Ca, Ca^{2+}, CBG, ceruloplasmin, Cu, DHT, factors – (II, VII, VIII, IX, X), Fe, fibrinogen, FSH, G, GMT, haptoglobin, HDL cholesterol, chloride, cholesterol, chylomicrons, calcitonin, cortisol, LDL cholesterol, LH, lipase, Mg, Na, OCT, P, plasminogen, PL, PRL, PT, progesterone, renin, RBP, SHBG, somatomedin C, GH, T3, T4, TAG, TBG, testosterone, transferrin, PLT, vitamin A, VLDL cholesterol
        ↓ albumin, ALP, Apo B, AT III, proteins, Ca, Ca^{2+}, CK, FSH, G, GMT, haptoglobin, Hb, HCT, CHE, cholesterol, IgA, IgG, IgM, ILGF-I, insulin, K, LP(a), carotene, ascorbic acid, uric acid (M), LDL-C, LH, Mn, orosomucoid, P, PRL, RBP, somatomedin C, TAG, testosterone, transthyretin, PLT, vitamin – (B_{12}, C, folate), FFA, WBC, Zn
        ■ *Urine* ↑ estriol, G, 17-OHCS, hydroxyproline, 17-KGS, P, porphyrins, pregnanediol
          ↓ 17-OHCS, 17-KS
        ■ *Seminal Fluid* ↓ spermatozoa count

Estrone *(estronum, estrone, estrone)*
    estrogen
        ↑ HDL
        ↓ cholesterol, LDL cholesterol

Ethacrynic Acid *(acidum etacrynicum, etacrynic acid, acide étacrinique)*
    loop diuretic
        ↑ ALT, ammonia, AMS, AST, BE, Bil, Ca, G, GMT, uric acid, pH, PT, urea
        ↓ Ca, factors – (II, VII, X), chloride, insulin, K, uric acid, Mg, Na, neu, PLT
        ■ *Urine* ↑ G, chloride, K, Mg, Na
          ↓ cortisol

Ethambutol *(ethambutolum, ethambutol, éthambutol)*
    tuberculostatic
        ↑ ALP, ALT, AST, Bil, GMT, creatinine, uric acid, urea
        ↓ PLT
        ■ *Urine* ↓ uric acid

Ethanol *(aethanolum, ethanol, éthanol)*
excitant, analeptic, narcotic, disinfectant, solvent

↑ acetaldehyde, acetone, acetoacetate (RBC), ACTH, epinephrine, aldosterone, ALP, ALT, alpha-LP, ammonia, AMS, antiplatelet Ab, Apo A-I, Apo A-II, Apo B, Apo E, AST, beta-hexosaminidase, Bil, Ca^{2+}, CK, BT, DHEA, estradiol, estrogens, estrone, factors – (II, VII, X), Fe, ferritin, fructosamine, FSH, G, GDH, glutathione peroxidase, GMT, haptoglobin, HDL-C, cholesterol, IgA, IL – (1, 6), plasminogen activator inhibitor, insulin, K, calcitonin, carnitine, catecholamines, cortisol, 17-KS, uric acid, LA, LD, LD5, LDL cholesterol, LH, lipase, LP lipase, WBC, MAC, MCH, MCHC, MCV, macrocytes, Na, neopterin, norepinephrine, PLT volume, OCT, orosomucoid, osmolality, P, pH, plasminogen, PRL, progesterone (F), PTH, RBP, renin, RTC, Se, SHBG, TAG, TBG, free testosterone (F), transferrin, transthyretin, trypsin, TNF, TSH, VLDL cholesterol

↓ AAT, ADH, albumin, aldehyde dehydrogenase (RBC), aminolevulinate-5-dehydratase (RBC), ANP, Apo A-I, Apo B, AT III, beta-endorphins, Ca, Ca^{2+}, CK, dihydrotestosterone, factors – (II, VII, X), phenytoin, fibrinogen, FSH, FT3, FT4, G, haptoglobin, Hb, hemopexin, cholesterol, CHS (RBC), insulin, K, carotenoids, cortisol, LDL cholesterol, LH, WBC, LP(a), Ly, Mg, osteocalcin, P, pH, protein C, PTH, RBP, Se, SHBG, T3, T4, testosterone, transferrin, transthyretin, PLT, vitamin – (B_1, B_6, B_{12}, D, E, folate), FFA, free testosterone, Zn

■ *Urine* ↑ acetoacetate, Cu, catecholamines, metanephrines, Mg, volume, testosterone, Zn

↓ VMA

■ *Gastric Fluid* ↑ HCl

■ *Stool* ↑ Hb

Ether *(aetherum, ether, éther)*
anesthetic, solvent

↑ CK, G, cholesterol, catecholamines, cortisol, WBC, T4

↓ insulin, P, pH

■ *Urine* ↑ acetoacetate, G

Ethinylestradiol *(ethinylestradiolum, ethinylestradiol, éthinylestradiol)*
estrogen

↑ Apo A-I, ALT, AST, ceruloplasmin, C-peptide, factors – (VII, X), GMT, HDL-C, cholesterol, insulin, cortisol, LDL cholesterol, SHBG, GH, T4, TAG, TBG, urea, vitamin D3, VLDL cholesterol

↓ ALP, ALT, Apo B, AST, Ca, FSH, GMT, cholesterol, uric acid, LDL cholesterol, LH, P, progesterone

Ethionamide *(ethionamidum, ethionamide, éthionamide)*
tuberculostatic

↑ ALP, ALT, AST, Bil, GMT

↓ T4

Ethosuximide *(ethosuximidum, ethosuximide, éthosuximide)*
anticonvulsant, antiepileptic

↑ ALT, ANA, AST, eos, GMT, LE cells, urea

↓ Hb, WBC, neu, PLT

Ethotoin *(ethotoinum, ethotoin, éthotoine)*
anticonvulsant, antiepileptic
↑ ALP, ALT, AST, Bil, GMT

Ethoxazene *(ethoxazenum, ethoxazene, éthoxazéne)*
↑ conjugated Bil
■ *Urine* ↑ porphyrins

Ethylestrenol *(ethylestrenolum, ethylestrenol, éthylestrénol)*
anabolic
↑ haptoglobin

Etidronate *(acidum etidronicum, etidronic acid, acide etidronique)*
geminal biphosphonate, calcium modifier, bone resorption inhibitor
↑ creatinine, P, urea, vitamin D
↓ Ca, Ca²⁺, Mg, P, vitamin D, WBC
■ *Urine* ↑ Ca
↓ Ca

Etodolac *(etodolacum, etodolac, étodolac)*
non-steroid antiinflammatory
↑ ALT, AST, GMT, urea
↓ GFR
■ *Urine* ↑ blood, Hb, RBC
■ *Stool* ↑ Hb

Etofibrate *(etofibratum, etofibrate, étofibrate)*
lipid lowering agent
↑ CK

Etomidate *(etomidatum, etomidate, étomidate)*
hypnotic
↑ ACTH, cortisol, GH
↓ aldosterone, cortisol

Etoposide *(etoposidum, etoposide, étoposide)*
antineoplastic
↑ ALP, ALT, AST, Bil, GMT, uric acid
↓ WBC, neu, PLT

Etretinate *(etretinatum, etretinate, étrétinate)*
antipsoriatic, antineoplastic
↑ ALP, ALT, Apo B, AST, CK, eos, GMT, cholesterol, LD, LDL cholesterol, OCT, TAG
↓ HDL cholesterol

Etynodiol *(etynodiolum, etynodiol, étynodiol)*
progestin
↑ albumin, ALT, AST, proteins, Bil, Ca, G, cholesterol, uric acid, P, TAG, urea
↓ CK, cholesterol, creatinine, uric acid, LD

Fadrozole *(fadrozolum, fadrozole, fadrozole)*
non-steroidal aromatase inhibitor, antitumor agent
↓ estrogens

Famotidine *(famotidinum, famotidine, famotidine)*
histamine H₂ receptor antagonist
↑ factors – (II, VII, X)
↓ WBC, PTH, PLT

Fat Emulsions

    ↑ ESR, G, FFA
    ↓ PLT aggregation

Felbamate *(felbamatum, felbamate, felbamate)*
anticonvulsant, antiepileptic

    ↑ ALT, AST, GMT
    ↓ PLT, WBC

Felodipine *(felodipinum, felodipine, félodipine)*
slow calcium channel blocker, antihypertensive

    ↑ ALT, AST, digoxin, GFR, GMT, norepinephrine, renin
    ↓ theophylline
    ■ *Urine* ↑ aldosterone, norepinephrine, volume

Fenbufen *(fenbufenum, fenbufen, fenbuféne)*
non-steroid antiinflammatory, analgesic

    ↑ ALP, ALT, AST, eos

Fenclofenac *(fenclofenacum, fenclofenac, fenclofénac)*
non-steroid antiinflammatory

    ↑ FT3, FT4, creatinine
    ↓ FT3, FT4, T3, T4, TSH

Fenfluramine *(fenfluraminum, fenfluramine, fenfluramine)*
anorexic

    ↑ G, ketones, cortisol, PRL, GH
    ↓ beta-LP, G, cholesterol, ascorbic acid, TAG
    ■ *Urine* ↑ volume

Fenofibrate *(fenofibratum, fenofibrate, fénofibrate)*
lipid lowering agent

    ↑ ALT, Apo A-I, AST, CK, eos, GMT, HDL, creatinine
    ↓ Apo B, PLT aggregation, ALP, Bil, fibrinogen, GMT, cholesterol, uric acid, LDL cholesterol, PLT, TAG, VLDL cholesterol, WBC

Fenoldopam *(fenoldopamum, fenoldopam, fénoldopam)*
antihypertensive

    ↑ PRL
    ↓ K, testosterone, TSH

Fenoprofen *(fenoprofenum, fenoprofen, fénoproféne)*
non-steroid antiinflammatory, analgesic

    ↑ ALT, FT3, creatinine, T3
    ↓ PLT aggregation, FT4, Hb, uric acid, neu, PLT
    ■ *Urine* ↑ blood, proteins, Hb, RBC
    ■ *Stool* ↑ Hb

Fenoterol *(fenoterolum, fenoterol, fénotérol)*
beta-2-adrenergic stimulant, sympathomimetic, bronchodilator, uterine relaxant

    ↑ norepinephrine, renin
    ↓ K

Fentanyl *(fentanylum, fentanyl, fentanyl)*
synthetic opioid m-receptor agonist, narcotic analgesic

    ↑ PRL
    ↓ Na

Fentiazac *(fentiazacum, fentiazac, fentiazac)*
non-steroid antiinflammatory, antipyretic

    ↑ ALP, ALT, LD

Fenyramidol *(fenyramidolum, fenyramidol, fényramidol)*
   analgesic, skeletal muscle relaxant
        ↓ cholesterol

Feprazone *(feprazonum, feprazone, féprazone)*
   non-steroid antiinflammatory, analgesic
        ↑ Bil

Fibrinolytics
        ↑ fibrinogen
        ↓ A2MG

Filgrastim *(filgrastimum, filgrastim, filgrastim)*
   colony stimulating factor
        ↑ WBC

Finasteride *(finasteridum, finasteride, finastéride)*
   competitive inhibitor of 5-alpha-reductase
        ↑ FSH, LH, testosterone
        ↓ PSA
        ■ *Seminal Fluid* ↑ volume
        ↓ volume

Fipexide *(fipexidum, fipexide, fipexide)*
   antidepressant, psychotonic
        ↑ ALT

Flavoxate *(flavoxatum, flavoxate, flavoxate)*
   tertiary amine muscarinic receptor antagonist
        ↑ eos
        ↓ WBC

Flecainide *(flecainidum, flecainide, flécainide)*
   antiarrhythmic
        ↑ ALP, ALT, AST, CK, digoxin
        ■ *Urine* ↑ volume

Fleroxacin *(fleroxacinum, fleroxacin, fléroxacine)*
   antibiotic
        ↑ ALT

Floctafenine *(floctafeninum, floctafenine, floctafénine)*
   analgesic
        ↑ ALT

Floxuridine *(floxuridinum, floxuridine, floxuridine)*
   antiviral, antineoplastic
        ↑ ALP, ALT, AST, GMT
        ↓ neu, PLT, WBC

Flucloxacillin *(flucloxacillinum, flucloxacillin, flucloxacilline)*
   antibiotic
        ↑ ALP, ALT, AST, Bil, eos, GMT, LD
        ↓ factors – (II, VII, X)

Fluconazole *(fluconazolum, fluconazole, fluconazole)*
   antifungal
        ↑ ALP, ALT, AST, cyclosporine, eos, phenytoin, GMT
        ↓ factors – (II, VII, X), Hb, K, creatinine, PLT, WBC, neu, PLT

Flucytosine *(flucytosinum, flucytosine, flucytosine)*
   antifungal
        ↑ ALP, ALT, AST, Bil, creatinine, GMT, urea
        ↓ ALP, ALT, Bil, G, Hb, K, WBC, neu, PLT
        ■ *Urine* ↑ crystals

Fludarabine *(fludarabinum, fludarabine, fludarabine)*
    antineoplastic
        ↑ uric acid
        ↓ pO$_2$, neu, PLT, WBC
Fludrocortisone *(fludrocortisonum, fludrocortisone, fludrocortisone)*
    orally active mineralocorticotid
        ↑ AMS, ANP, G, HCO$_3$, MAL, Na
        ↓ ACTH, aldosterone, G tolerance, K, renin
        ■ *Urine* ↑ K
            ↓ aldosterone, pH
Flunarizine *(flunarizinum, flunarizine, flunarizine)*
    calcium antagonist, vasodilator
        ↑ LH, PRL
        ↓ TSH
Flunisolide *(flunisolidum, flunisolide, flunisolide)*
    corticosteroid
        ↑ eos
Fluocinolone Acetonide *(fluocinoloni acetonidum, fluocinolone acetonide, acétonide de fluocinolone)*
    glucocorticosteroid
        ↓ ACTH, cortisol
Fluorides
        ↑ ALP, eos, K (later), uric acid, Na, osteocalcin, PTH, urea
        ↓ ACP, ALP, Ca, Ca^{2+}, G, cholesterol, LD, P
5-Fluorocytosine *(5-fluorocytosinum, 5-fluorocytosine, 5-fluorocytosine)*
    antifungal
        ↑ creatinine
        ↓ WBC, neu
Fluoroprednisolone *(fluoroprednisolonum, fluoroprednisolone, fluoroprednisolone)*
    glucocorticoid, antiinflammatory, antiallergic
        ↓ K
Fluoroquinolones
        ↑ ALT, AST, GMT
5-Fluorouracil *(5-fluorouracilum, 5-fluorouracil, 5-fluorouracil)*
    antineoplastic
        ↑ ALP, ALT, ammonia, Bil, LD, MCV, T3, T4, WBC, TBG
        ↓ Hb, cholesterol, neu, PLT, WBC
        ■ *Urine* ↑ 5-HIAA
Fluoxetine *(fluoxetinum, fluoxetine, fluoxétine)*
    antidepressant, serotonin reuptake inhibitor
        ↑ ALT, BT, G, cholesterol, lipids
        ↓ G, chloride, K, Na, osmolality
        ■ *Urine* ↑ albumin, proteins, volume
Fluoxymesterone *(fluoxymesteronum, fluoxymesterone, fluoxymestérone)*
    androgen
        ↑ ALP, ALT, AST, Bil, G, GMT, haptoglobin
        ■ *Urine* ↓ 17-OHCS
        ■ *Seminal Fluid* ↓ spermatozoa count
Fluphenazine *(fluphenazinum, fluphenazine, fluphénazine)*
    neuroleptic
        ↑ ALP, ALT, AST, Bil, eos, GMT, WBC, PRL

     ↓ Na, neu, PLT, WBC
     ■ *Urine* ↑ hCG

Flurandrenolide *(fludroxycortidum, fludroxycortide, fludroxycortide)*
 corticosteroid
     ↑ G
     ■ *Urine* ↑ G

Flurazepam *(flurazepamum, flurazepam, flurazépam)*
 benzodiazepine hypnotic
     ↑ ALP, ALT, AST, Bil, GMT

Flurbiprofen *(flurbiprofenum, flurbiprofen, flurbiprofen)*
 non-steroid antiinflammatory, analgesic
     ↑ ALT, AST, eos, GMT, K, urea, uric acid
     ↓ PLT, WBC
     ■ *Urine* ↑ blood, Hb, RBC

Flutamide *(flutamidum, flutamide, flutamide)*
 non-steroidal "pure" antiandrogen
     ↑ ALP, ALT, AST, Bil, GMT, creatinine, MHb, testosterone

Fluticasone *(fluticasonum, fluticasone, fluticasone)*
 corticosteroid
     ↑ eos

Fluvastatin *(fluvastatinum, fluvastatin, fluvastatine)*
 lipid lowering agent
     ↑ ALT, AST, GMT

Fluvoxamine *(fluvoxaminum, fluvoxamine, fluvoxamine)*
 inhibitor of 5-HT, antidepressant
     ↑ ALT, AST, GMT, imipramin
     ↓ Na, osmolality

Folic Acid *(acidum folicum, folic acid, acide folique)*
 hematopoietic vitamin
     ↓ phenytoin, homocysteine

Follitropin *(follitropinum alfa, follitropin alfa, follitropine alfa)*
 follicle-stimulating hormone
     ↓ albumin

Fomepizole *(fomepizolum, fomepizole, fomépizole)*
 antidote
     ↑ eos

Fomivirsen *(fomivirsenum, fomivirsen, fomivirsen)*
 antiviral
     ↑ ALT, AST, GMT
     ↓ neu, PLT

Foscarnet Sodium *(foscarnetum natricum, foscarnet sodium, foscarnet sodique)*
 antiviral
     ↑ ALP, AMS, CK, creatinine, MAC, Na, neu, P, urea
     ↓ proteins, Ca, Ca^{2+}, chloride, K, Mg, Na, neu, P
     ■ *Urine* ↑ albumin, G, volume

Fosfomycin *(fosfomycinum, fosfomycin, fosfomycine)*
 antibiotic
     ↑ ALT, AST

Fosinopril *(fosinoprilum, fosinopril, fosinopril)*
 ACE inhibitor, antihypertensive
     ↑ ALT, AST, Bil, Ca, G, GMT, cholesterol, K, TAG, urea, uric acid
     ↓ cholesterol, K, LDL cholesterol, LP(a), Mg, WBC

Fosphenytoin *(fosphenytoinum, fosphenytoin, fosphénytoine)*
anticonvulsant, antiepileptic
↑ ALT, AST, eos, GMT, WBC
↓ neu, PLT, WBC

Fructose *(fructosum, fructose, fructose)*
natural carbohydrate, fluid and nutrient replenisher
↑ Bil, G, insulin, creatinine, uric acid, LA, TAG, VLDL cholesterol
↓ P
■ *Urine* ↑ G, creatinine, 17-KS
↓ estrogens

Furazolidine *(furazolidinum, furazolidine, furazolidine)*
topical antiprotozoal, antibacterial
↑ Bil, eos, Heinz bodies
↓ WBC

Furosemide *(furosemidum, furosemide, furosémide)*
loop diuretic
↑ ADH, albumin, aldosterone, ALT, ammonia, AMS, angiotensin II, AST, Bil, Ca, FT4, G, cholesterol, creatinine, uric acid, LDL cholesterol, lipase, MAL, norepinephrine, P, pH, PTH, PRL, renin, TAG, theophylline, urea, VLDL cholesterol
↓ Ca, Ca^{2+}, GFR, glucose tolerance, Hb, HDL cholesterol, chloride, insulin, K, uric acid, Mg, Na, neu, plasma volume, T3, T4, theophylline, PLT, WBC
■ *Urine* ↑ epinephrine, aldosterone, Ca, dopamine, G, Mg, norepinephrine, VMA

Fusidic Acid *(acidum fusidicum, fusidic acid, acide fusidique)*
antibiotic
↑ ALP, ALT, Bil
↓ WBC, neu

Gabapentin *(gabapentinum, gabapentin, gabapentine)*
anticonvulsant, antiepileptic
↓ WBC

Gallium Nitrate *(gallii nitras, gallium nitrate, nitrate de gallium)*
hypocalcemic agent
↑ creatinine, urea
↓ Ca^{2+}, HCO_3^-, P, PTH
■ *Urine* ↑ hydroxyproline

Gamma Globulin *(gamma globulinum, gamma globulin, gamma globulin)*
agent for immunization
↓ Hb

Ganciclovir *(ganciclovirum, ganciclovir, ganciclovir)*
antiviral
↑ ALT, AST, creatinine, GMT, urea
↓ G, Hb, neu, PLT
■ *Urine* ↑ RBC, Hb, blood

Gastrin Tetrapeptide *(gastrinum tetrapeptidum, gastrin tetrapeptide, gastrin de tetrapeptide)*
peptid hormone (gastric acid, pepsin, intrinsic factor, insulin, glucagon, somatostatin secretion stimulant)
↑ glucagon
↓ Ca^{2+}

Gatifloxacin *(gatifloxacinum, gatifloxacin, gatifloxacin)*
   antibacterial
   - ↑ G
   - ↓ G, PLT, WBC
   - ■ *Urine* ↑ blood, Hb, RBC

Gemcitabine *(gemcitabinum, gemcitabine, gemcitabine)*
   antineoplastic
   - ↑ ALT, AST, GMT
   - ↓ neu
   - ■ *Urine* ↑ blood, Hb, RBC

Gemfibrozil *(gemfibrozilum, gemfibrozil, gemfibrozil)*
   lipid lowering agent
   - ↑ ALP, ALT, Apo A-I, Apo A-II, AT III, CK, eos, fibrinogen, HDL cholesterol, LDL cholesterol, LP lipase
   - ↓ AAT, Apo B, factors – (II, VII, X), G, cholesterol, insulin, LDL cholesterol, TAG, VLDL cholesterol, FFA, WBC

Gemtuzumab *(gemtuzumabum, gemtuzumab, gemtuzumab)*
   imunomodulator
   - ↑ ALT, AST, Bil, G, GMT, uric acid
   - ↓ pO₂, K, lym, Mg, neu, WBC
   - ■ *Urine* ↑ blood, Hb, RBC

Gentamicin *(gentamycinum, gentamicin, gentamycine)*
   antibiotic
   - ↑ ALP, ALT, AST, Bil, creatinine, urea
   - ↓ Ca, factors – (II, VII, X), GFR, Hb, chloride, K, Mg, Na, neu, PLT
   - ■ *Urine* ↑ amino acids, B2M, proteins, K, LD, Mg
   - ■ *Cerebrospinal Fluid* ↑ WBC

Gestagens
   - ↑ ALP, ALT

Glafenine *(glafeninum, glafenine, glafénine)*
   non-steroid antiinflammatory, analgesic
   - ↑ ALP, ALT, AST, Bil, eos

Glibenclamide *(glibenclamidum, glibenclamide, glibenclamide)*
   oral hypoglycemic
   - ↑ ALP, ALT, AST, Bil, eos, GMT, HDL cholesterol
   - ↓ G, cholesterol, TAG, PLT
   - *Urine* ↓ osmolality

Glimepiride *(glimepiridum, glimepiride, glimépiride)*
   oral hypoglycemic
   - ↓ G, Na

Glipizide *(glipizidum, glipizide, glipizide)*
   oral hypoglycemic
   - ↑ ALT
   - ↓ G, WBC

Glucagon *(glucagonum, glucagon, glucagon)*
   hyperglycemic pancreatic polypeptide hormone
   - ↑ G, insulin, K, calcitonin, GH, LA, FFA
   - ↓ Ca, Ca²⁺, gastrin, glucose tolerance, cholesterol, K, coagulation factors, LDL cholesterol, lipids, Mg, P, T₃, TAG
   - ■ *Urine* ↑ AMS, G, VMA, norepinephrine
   - ↓ dopamine
   - ■ *Gastric Fluid* ↓ pH

Glucocorticoids

↑ AMS, ANH, Apo B, DHEA, DHEAS, G, glucagon, Hb, cholesterol, cortisol, LP, MAC, MAL, Na, neu, pregnanediol, progesterone, PTH, GH, TAG, PLT, Zn

↓ ACTH, Apo A-I, Ca, Ca²⁺, eos, FT4, glucose tolerance, HDL cholesterol, CHS, IgA, IgG, IL-1, K, LDL cholesterol, leukotrienes, lym, mono, neu, osteocalcin, PG, PRL, GH, T3, T4, TBG, testosterone, T-lym, TSH, vitamin D3, VLDL cholesterol

■ *Urine* ↑ Ca²⁺, G, 17-OHCS, K, 17-KGS
↓ estradiol, estriol, estrogen, hydroxyproline

■ *Seminal Fluid* ↓ spermatozoa count

D-Glucose *(d-glucosum, d-glucose, d-glucose)*
fluid and nutrient replenisher

↑ Bil, insulin, LA, osmolality

↓ aldosterone, epinephrine, Ca, K, cortisol, uric acid, Na, norepinephrine, P, GH, TAG, testosterone, vitamin B₆

Glucose Polymers

↑ Na

Glutethimide *(glutethimidum, glutethimide, glutéthimide)*
sedative, hypnotic

↑ factors – (II, VII, X), HDL cholesterol, cholesterol, LDL cholesterol, MCV, PT, VLDL cholesterol

↓ folate, PLT

■ *Urine* ↑ PBG, porphyrins

Glyburide *(glibenclamidum, glibenclamide, glibenclamide)*
oral hypoglycemic

↓ G, Na, WBC

Glycerol *(glycerolum, glycerol, glycérol)*
mild laxative, solvent, humectant, taste corrigent

↓ Na

Glyceryl Trinitrate *(nitroglycerolum, glyceryl trinitrate, glyceryl de trinitrate)*
coronary vasodilator, spasmolytic, explosive

↑ catecholamines

Glycopyrronium Bromide *(glycopyrronii bromidum, glycopyrronium bromide, bromure de glycopyrronium)*
muscarinic antagonist

↑ ALP, ALT, AST, Bil

Gold Salts

↑ ALP, ALT, ANA, AST, Bil, eos, GMT, cholesterol, IgE, creatinine, LD, 5-nucleotidase, OCT, urea

↓ eos, ESR, GFR, Hb, IgA, IgG, IgM, WBC, lym, neu, PLT

■ *Urine* ↑ ALA, blood, proteins, RBC, Hb, IgA, IgG, IgM, coproporphyrin, WBC, neu

■ *Stool* ↑ Hb

Gonadorelin *(gonadorelinum, gonadorelin, gonadoréline)*
synthetic analog of luteinizing hormone and follicle stimulating hormone releasing factor

↑ estriol, FSH, LH

Gonadotropins

↑ DHEA, FT4, T3, testosterone

■ *Urine* ↑ androsterone, estrogens, etiocholanolone, 17-OHCS, 17-KS, pregnanediol, pregnanetriol, testosterone

Goserelin *(goserelinum, goserelin, goséréline)*
    antineoplastic
             ↑ Ca, HDL, lipids

Granisetron *(granisetronum, granisetron, granisétron)*
    antiemetic
             ↑ ALT, AST, GMT

Grepafloxacin *(grepafloxacinum, grepafloxacin, grépafloxacine)*
    antimicrobial
             ↓ WBC

Griseofulvin *(griseofulvinum, griseofulvin, griséofulvine)*
    antifungal
             ↑ ALP, ALT, ANA, AST, factors – (II, VII, X), GMT, creatinine, lym, mono,
               porphyrins, PT, urea
             ↓ Hb, neu
           ■ ***Urine*** ↑ ALA, proteins, coproporphyrin, PBG, porphyrins
           ■ ***Stool*** ↑ Hb

Guaifenesin *(guaifenesinum, guaifenesin, guaifénésine)*
    muscle relaxant, expectorant
             ↓ uric acid
           ■ ***Urine*** ↑ 5-HIAA, VMA

Guanabenz *(guanabenzum, guanabenz, guanabenz)*
    alpha-2-adrenergic agonist, antihypertensive
             ↓ apolipoprotein E, glucagon, cholesterol, norepinephrine, renin, TAG
           ■ ***Urine*** ↑ Na

Guanethidine *(guanethidinum, guanethidine, guanéthidine)*
    antihypertensive
             ↑ glucose tolerance, chloride, creatinine, Na, urea
             ↓ G, coagulation factors, renin
           ■ ***Urine*** ↑ epinephrine, VMA (early)
              ↓ catecholamines, metanephrines, norepinephrine, volume, VMA
               (later)

Guanfacine *(guanfacinum, guanfacine, guanfacine)*
    alpha-2-adrenergic agonist, antihypertensive
             ↑ GH
             ↓ epinephrine, dopamine, G, cholesterol, catecholamines, norepineph-
               rine, renin, TAG

Guanoxan *(guanoxanum, guanoxan, guanoxan)*
    antihypertensive
             ↑ ALT, ANA

Halcinonide *(halcinonidum, halcinonide, halcinonide)*
    corticosteroid
             ↑ G
             ↓ cortisol

Halofenate *(halofenatum, halofenate, halofenate)*
    lipid lowering agent, uricosuric
             ↑ CK
             ↓ Bil, uric acid

Haloperidol *(haloperidolum, haloperidol, halopéridol)*
    neuroleptic
        ↑ ALP, ALT, AST, Bil, CK, G, GMT, Li, WBC, lym, mono, PRL, TSH, WBC
        ↓ factors – (II, VII, X), G, cholesterol, WBC, Na, neu

Halothane *(halothanum, halothane, halothane)*
    anesthetic
        ↑ ALA, ALP, ALT, antimicrosomal Ab, AST, Bil, BT, CK, CK-MB, COHb, eos, F, FT_4, G, GMT, creatinine, uric acid, WBC, norepinephrine, OCT, rT_3, GH, T_4, urea
        ↓ PLT aggregation, GFR, T_3, testosterone
        ■ *Stool* ↑ Hb

Heparin Sodium *(heparinum natricum, heparin sodium, héparine sodique)*
    anticoagulant
        ↑ ACTH, PLT aggregation, ALP, ALT, APTT, AST, Ca^{2+}, coagulation time, BT, FDP, FT_3, FT_4, ESR, G, GMT, chloride, cholesterol, hexosaminidase, IgG, insulin, K, corticosteroids, creatinine, LD, neu, P, PT, renin, T_3, T_4, TAG, TT, TSH, FFA
        ↓ ACP, ACTH, albumin, aldosterone, Apo A-I, Apo B, AT III, Ca^{2+}, factors – (II, VII, X), fibrinogen, FT_3, FT_4, cholesterol, cortisol, insulin, LDL cholesterol, Na, pCO_2, T_3, T_4, TAG, TBG, PLT, TSH, WBC
        ■ *Urine* ↑ blood, Hb, RBC
            ↓ 5-HIAA

Heptabarbital *(heptabarbum, heptabarb, heptabarbe)*
    hypnotic, sedative
        ↑ PT

Heroin *(heroinum, heroin, heroin)*
    narcotic analgesic
        ↑ ALP, FT_4, cholesterol, K, T_3, T_4, TBG
        ↓ pO_2
        ■ *Urine* ↑ proteins

Histamine *(histaminum, histamine, histamine)*
    autacoid, CNS neurotransmitter, mediator of hypersensitivity reaction, diagnostic aid
        ↑ epinephrine, AMS, K, neu, norepinephrine, GH
        ↓ eos, GFR, plasma volume
        ■ *Urine* ↑ 17-OHCS, VMA
            ↓ volume

Histidine *(histidinum, histidine, histidine)*
    amino acid
        ↑ Bil, conjugated Bil
        ↓ creatinine

Histrelin *(histrelinum, histrelin, histréline)*
    LHRH agonist
        ↑ FSH (early), LH (early), lipids
        ↓ estradiol, FSH (later), LH (later)
        ■ *Urine* ↑ G, volume

Hydantoins
        ↑ ALP, ALT, Bil, creatinine, G, urea
        ↓ FT_4, insulin, T_4, PLT
        ■ *Urine* ↑ PBG

Hydralazine *(hydralazinum, hydralazine, hydralazine)*
long-acting peripheral vasodilator, antihypertensive

↑ aldosterone, ALP, ALT, ANA, AST, Bil, Bil conjugated, Ca, Ca²⁺, ESR, G, GMT, Hb, creatinine, uric acid, LE cells, metoprolol, norepinephrine, renin, RTC, urea

↓ digoxin, G, Hb, HCT, cholesterol, LDL cholesterol, WBC, neu, norepinephrine, renin, PLT, vitamin B₆

- *Urine* ↑ proteins, Hb, catecholamines, 17-OHCS
  ↓ 17-OHCS

Hydrazines

↑ ALP, Bil

↓ G

- *Urine* ↑ metanephrines, normetanephrine
  ↓ 5-HIAA, VMA

Hydrochlorothiazide *(hydrochlorothiazidum, hydrochlorothiazide, hydrochlorothiazide)*
salidiuretic, antihypertensive

↑ ALT, AMS, AST, Bil, Ca, Ca²⁺, G, GMT, HbA₁c, HDL cholesterol, chloride, cholesterol, K, uric acid, LDL cholesterol, Li, P, renin, TAG, urea

↓ glucose tolerance, HDL cholesterol, chloride, K, K (RBC), Mg, Na, neu, osmolality, P, PLT, WBC

- *Urine* ↑ aldosterone, estrogens, G, Mg, Na, P
  ↓ cortisol

Hydrocodone *(hydrocodonum, hydrocodone, hydrocodone)*
narcotic analgesic

↑ ALT, AST, GMT, K, uric acid

↓ Na

- *Urine* ↑ blood, Hb, RBC

Hydrocortisone *(hydrocortisonum, hydrocortisone, hydrocortisone)*
natural corticosteroid, antiinflammatory, antiallergic, immunosuppressant

↑ G, cholesterol, cortisol, MAL, Na, neu

↓ Ca, eos, K, lym, TSH

- *Urine* ↑ amino acids

Hydromorphone *(hydromorphonum, hydromorphone, hydromorphone)*
semisynthetic m-receptor agonist, narcotic analgesic

↑ pCO₂

↓ Na

Hydroxycarbamide *(hydroxycarbamidum, hydroxycarbamide, hydroxycarbamide)*
antineoplastic

↑ ALT, uric acid

Hydroxychloroquine *(hydroxychloroquinum, hydroxychloroquine, hydroxychloroquine)*
antimalarial, LE suppressant, antiarthritic

↑ ALT, AST, digoxin

↓ PLT aggregation, neu, PLT

Hydroxycortisone *(hydrocortisonum, hydrocortisone, hydrocortisone)*
corticosteroid, antiinflammatory, antiallergic, immunosuppressant

↑ G, cortisol, neu

↓ eos, K, lym

Hydroxyurea *(hydroxyureum, hydroxyurea, hydroxyurea)*
antineoplastic

↑ ALP, ALT, GMT, creatinine, macrocytes, uric acid, urea

↓ neu, PLT, TAG, WBC

Hypnotics

      ↑ CK, MAC+RAC, RAC
- ***Urine*** ↑ Mb

Ibopamine *(ibopaminum, ibopamine, ibopamine)*
    sympathomimetic
        ↑ G, insulin
        ↓ norepinephrine
Ibuprofen *(ibuprofenum, ibuprofen, ibuproféne)*
    non-steroid antiinflammatory, antirheumatic
        ↑ ALP, ALT, ANA, AST, Bil, BT, digoxin, Fe, GMT, K, creatinine, Li, urea, uric acid
        ↓ PLT aggregation, albumin, GFR, Hb, HCT, creatinine, uric acid, WBC, Na, neu, PLT
- ***Urine*** ↑ blood, proteins, Hb, RBC
- ***Stool*** ↑ Hb
- ***Cerebrospinal Fluid*** ↑ proteins, IgG, WBC
Idarubicin *(idarubicinum, idarubicin, idarubicine)*
    antineoplastic
        ↑ ALT, AST, GMT
        ↓ neu, PLT, WBC
Idoxuridine *(idoxuridinum, idoxuridine, idoxuridine)*
    antiviral
        ↑ ALT
Ifosfamide *(ifosfamidum, ifosfamide, ifosfamide)*
    antineoplastic, immunosuppressive
        ↑ ALT, Bil, creatinine, MAC, urea
        ↓ GFR, K, neu, P, PLT, WBC
- ***Urine*** ↑ blood, Hb, RBC
Imipenem-Cilastatin *(imipenemum, imipenem, imipénem)*
    antibiotic, beta-lactamase inhibitor
        ↑ ALP, ALT, Bil, chloride, K, creatinine, urea
        ↓ Na, neu, PLT, WBC
- ***Urine*** ↑ proteins, volume, casts
        ↓ volume
Imipramine *(imipraminum, imipramine, imipramine)*
    antidepressant
        ↑ ALP, ALT, AST, Bil, eos, phenytoin, G, GMT, cholesterol, LD, norepi-nephrine, PRL
        ↓ Na, neu, PLT, WBC
- ***Urine*** ↑ ADH, metanephrines
        ↓ 5-HIAA, VMA
- ***Cerebrospinal Fluid*** ↑ proteins
Immunoglobulins
        ↑ creatinine
        ↓ neu
Immunosuppressives
        ↑ macrocytes
        ↓ gamma globulins, IgA, WBC, PLT
- ***Urine*** ↑ RBC

Inamrinone *(inamrinonum, inamrinone, inamrinone)*
cardiotonic, inhibitor PDE III
↑ ALT, AST, GMT
↓ PLT
Indapamide *(indapamidum, indapamide, indapamide)*
antihypertensive, diuretic
↑ Ca, G, HbA$_{1c}$, C-peptide, HDL cholesterol, cholesterol, uric acid, MAL, TAG
↓ chloride, K, Na, P
■ *Urine* ↑ G
↓ Ca
Indinavir *(indinavirum, indinavir, indinavir)*
antiviral
↑ cholesterol, G, ketobodies, lipids, TAG
■ *Urine* ↑ blood, Hb, RBC
Indomethacin *(indometacinum, indomethacin, indométacine)*
non-steroid antiinflammatory, antipyretic, analgesic
↑ ALP, ALT, AMS, AST, Bil, BT, digoxin, eos, G, GMT, K, creatinine, lipase, lithium, 5-nucleotidase, urea, uric acid
↓ PLT aggregation, aldosterone, ESR, G, GFR, Hb, coagulation factors, creatinine, uric acid, WBC, Na, neu, renin, PLT, Zn
■ *Urine* ↑ blood, proteins, RBC, Hb
↓ proteins, Na, volume
■ *Stool* ↑ blood, Hb
Infliximab *(infliximabum, infliximab, infliximab)*
monoclonal antibody
↑ ALT, AST, GMT
Inosiplex *(inosiplexum, inosiplex, inosiplex)*
antiviral, immunostimulant
↑ uric acid
■ *Urine* ↑ uric acid
Insulin *(insulinum, insulin, insulin)*
hypoglycemic pancreas hormone
↑ ACTH, epinephrine, proteins, Ca, gastrin, glucagon, HDL cholesterol, catecholamines, corticosteroids, cortisol, LA, LP(a), norepinephrine, osteocalcin, PRL, PTH, GH, T3, T4
↓ Ca^{2+}, estradiol, G, cholesterol, K, levodopa, Mg, P, TAG, PLT, vitamin D, FFA
■ *Urine* ↑ amino acids, catecholamines, ketones, acetoacetate, VMA
↓ Na
Interferon Alpha *(interferonum alpha, interferon alpha, interféron alpha)*
antiviral, antineoplastic, immunomodulator
↑ ALP, ALT, ANA, anti-TSH-receptor Ab, AST, Bil, eos, FT4, G, glucagon, GMT, insulin, K, 11-OHCS, cortisol, T3, T4, TAG, theophylline, TSH
↓ Ca, estradiol, FT4, HDL-C, cholesterol, LDL cholesterol, WBC, neu, osmolality, progesterone, T3, T4, PLT, TSH, Zn
■ *Urine* ↑ proteins
■ *Cerebrospinal Fluid* ↑ lym
Interferon Beta-1b *(interferonum beta-1b, interferon beta-1b, interféron beta-1b)*
antiviral, antineoplastic, immunomodulator
↑ ALP, Bil, Ca, ketones, urea

   ↓ G, neu, WBC
  ■ *Urine* ↑ proteins, G, volume
   ↓ volume

Interferon Alpha-2a *(interferonum alpha-2a, interferon alpha-2a, interféron alpha-2a)*
 antiviral, antineoplastic, immunomodulator
   ↑ ALP, G, creatinine, uric acid, P, urea
   ↓ Ca, Ca²⁺, estradiol, neu, progesterone, WBC
  ■ *Urine* ↑ proteins, volume

Interferon Alpha-2b *(interferonum alpha-2b, interferon alpha-2b, interféron alpha-2b)*
 antiviral, antineoplastic, immunomodulator
   ↑ ALP, uric acid
   ↓ Ca, Ca²⁺, estradiol, neu, progesterone, WBC
  ■ *Urine* ↑ proteins, volume

Interferon Alpha-n1 *(interferonum alpha-n1, interferon alpha-n1, interféron alpha-n1)*
 antiviral, antineoplastic, immunomodulator
   ↑ ALP
   ↓ neu, WBC

Interferon Alpha-n3 *(interferonum alpha-n3, interferon alpha-n3, interféron alpha-n3)*
 antiviral, antineoplastic, immunomodulator
   ↑ ALP, Bil
   ↓ estradiol, progesterone, WBC

Interferon Alfacon-1 *(interferonum alpha, interferon alpha, interféron alpha)*
 antiviral, antineoplastic, immunomodulator
   ↑ ALP, Bil, lym
   ↓ estradiol, progesterone, WBC

Interferon Gamma-1b *(interferonum gamma-1b, interferon gamma-1b, interféron gamma-1b)*
 antiviral, antineoplastic, immunomodulator
   ↓ neu

Interleukin 2 *(interleukinum 2, interleukin 2, interleukin 2)*
 antineoplastic
   ↑ ALP, ALT, antithyroidal Ab, AST, beta-endorphins, Bil, Bil conjugated,
    CRP, eos, fibrinogen, GMT, cortisol, creatinine, LD, renin, rT3, TSH,
    urea
   ↓ albumin, Hb, HDL cholesterol, cholesterol, ascorbic acid, LDL choles-
    terol, melatonin, P, T3, T4, PLT, TSH

Inulin *(inulinum, inulin, inulin)*
 diagnostic agent
   ↑ osmolality
  ■ *Urine* ↓ estrogens

Iodides
   ↑ ALT, anti-TSH receptor Ab, Ca²⁺, eos, FT4, chloride, cholesterol, LA,
    MAC, T3, T4, TBG, TSH
   ↓ FT4, rT3, T3, T4, TSH
  ■ *Urine* ↑ blood, Hb, 17-OHCS, RBC
   ↓ volume

Iodine-Containing Preparations
   ↑ Ca²⁺, FT4, chloride, cholesterol, K, LDL cholesterol, LP(a), T4, TSH
   ↓ T3, T4, TSH
  ■ *Urine* ↑ 17-OHCS
  ■ *Stool* ↑ blood, Hb

Iodothiouracil *(iodothiouracilum, iodothiouracil, iodothiouracil)*
thyroid inhibitor
↓ WBC

Iopanoic Acid *(acidum iopanoicum, iopanoic acid, acide iopanoique)*
diagnostic aid
↑ FT4, creatinine, TSH
↓ CHS, uric acid, T3, PLT

Ipodate *(natrii iopodas, sodium iopodate, iopodate de sodium)*
antithyroid
↑ TSH

Iprindole *(iprindolum, iprindole, iprindole)*
antidepressant
↑ ALT

Iproniazid *(iproniazidum, iproniazid, iproniazide)*
tuberculostatic, antidepressant
↑ Bil

Irbesartan *(irbesartanum, irbesartan, irbésartan)*
angiotensin II antagonist
↑ Bil, Ca, cholesterol, K, urea, uric acid
↓ K, Mg, PLT

Irinotecan *(irinotecanum, irinotecan, irinotécan)*
antineoplastic
↑ ALT, AST, G, GMT
↓ lym, neu, PLT, WBC

Iron Preparations
↑ ALT, Fe, ferritin, ESR, G, WBC, MAC, neu, porphyrins (RBC)
↓ ceruloplasmin, Cu, G, Mg, P, transferrin, PLT, Zn
■ *Urine* ↑ Mg
■ *Stool* ↑ blood, Hb

Isocarboxazid *(isocarboxazidum, isocarboxazid, izocarboxazide)*
MAO inhibitor, antidepressant
↑ ALT, AST, GMT
↓ PLT

Isoflurane *(isofluranum, isoflurane, isoflurane)*
anesthetic
↑ ALT, AST, COHb, GMT

Isoniazid *(isoniazidum, isoniazid, isoniazide)*
tuberculostatic
↑ ALP, ALT, ANA, AST, Bil, diazepam, eos, phenytoin, G, GMT, K, carbamazepine, uric acid, LA, LD, LE cells, WBC, MAC, MCV, MHb, OCT, theophylline, bile acids
↓ albumin, Ca, cyclosporine, factors – (II, VII, X), G, haptoglobin, Hb, HCO_3, cholesterol, MHb, neu, P, pCO_2, pH, PTH, theophylline, PLT, vitamin – (B_6, D, folate), WBC
■ *Urine* ↑ acetoacetate, proteins, G, ketones
↓ 5-HIAA, volume

Isopamin *(isopaminum, isopamin, isopamin)*
oral hypoglycemic
↑ ALT

Isoprenaline *(isoprenalinum, isoprenaline, isoprénaline)*
   non-selective beta-adrenoceptor agonist, bronchodilator
        ↑ CK-MB, G, lym, theophylline
        ↓ GFR, Na, theophylline, PLT
        ■ *Urine* ↑ catecholamines

Isopropanol *(alcoholum isopropylicum, isopropanol, isopropanol)*
   antiseptic
        ■ *Urine* ↑ ketones

Isoproterenol *(isoproterenolum, isoproterenol, isoprotérénol)*
   non-selective beta-adrenoceptor agonist, bronchodilator
        ↑ conjugated Bil, cAMP, G, catecholamines, FFA
        ↓ Ca^{2+}
        ■ *Urine* ↑ epinephrine, catecholamines, VMA
          ↓ volume

Isosorbide Dinitrate *(isosorbidi dinitras, isosorbide dinitrate, dinitrate d'isosorbide)*
   coronary vasodilator
        ↑ AST, MHb, Na, urea
        ↓ PLT aggregation
        ■ *Urine* ↑ chloride, K, Na, volume

Isosorbide Mononitrate *(isosorbidimononitratum, isosorbidemononitrate, d'isosorbide-mononitrate)*
   coronary vasodilator
        ↑ AST, MHb, Na, urea
        ↓ PLT aggregation
        ■ *Urine* ↑ chloride, K, Na, volume

Isotretinoin *(isotretinoinum, isotretinoin, isotrétinoine)*
   retinoid, acne-therapeutic
        ↑ ALP, ALT, apolipoprotein B, AST, Ca, CK, CRP, G, GMT, HDL cholesterol, cholesterol, uric acid, LD, LDL cholesterol, lym, TAG, PLT, VLDL cholesterol
        ↓ Bil, FT4, HDL cholesterol, WBC, neu, PLT, T3, T4, vitamin D3
        ■ *Urine* ↑ blood, Hb, proteins, RBC, WBC

Isradipine *(isradipinum, isradipine, isradipine)*
   slow calcium channel blocker, antihypertensive
        ↑ HDL cholesterol
        ↓ LDL cholesterol

Itraconazole *(itraconazolum, itraconazole, itraconazole)*
   antifungal
        ↑ ALP, ALT, AST, cholesterol, creatinine, GMT, neu, TAG
        ↓ K, neu
        ■ *Urine* ↑ albumin

Josamycin *(josamycinum, josamycin, josamycine)*
   antibiotic
        ↑ ALT, cyclosporine

Kalium Sparing Diuretics
        ↑ K, renin

Kanamycin *(kanamycinum, kanamycin, kanamycine)*
    antibiotic
        ↑ eos, urea
        ↓ ammonia, cholesterol, carotenoids
        ■ *Urine* ↑ proteins, LAP, WBC, casts – (granular)
        ■ *Stool* ↑ FA

Ketamine *(ketaminum, ketamine, kétamine)*
    general anesthetic, analgesic
        ↑ ALT, AST, GMT, LH

Ketanserin *(ketanserinum, ketanserin, kétansérine)*
    competitive 5-HT$_2$ receptor antagonist, antihypertensive
        ↑ HDL cholesterol
        ↓ Apo B, Apo E, cholesterol, LDL cholesterol

Ketoconazole *(ketoconazolum, ketoconazole, kétoconazole)*
    antifungal
        ↑ ALP, ALT, AST, Bil, cyclosporine, eos, estradiol, FSH, GMT, 17-OH progesterone, K, 11-OHCS, creatinine, LD, LH, OCT, TAG, TSH
        ↓ ACP, aldosterone, Apo B, Ca, DHT, estradiol, factors – (II, VII, X), GFR, cholesterol, cortisol, LDL cholesterol, Na, osmolality, testosterone, vitamin D3, free testosterone
        ■ *Urine* ↓ cortisol, free cortisol
        ■ *Seminal Fluid* ↓ spermatozoa count

Ketoprofen *(ketoprofenum, ketoprofen, kétoproféne)*
    non-steroid antiinflammatory, analgesic
        ↑ ALT, AST, BT, Fe, creatinine, GMT, urea
        ↓ PLT aggregation, factors – (II, VII, X), LD
        ■ *Urine* ↑ blood, Hb, RBC
        ■ *Stool* ↑ Hb

Ketorolac *(ketorolacum, ketorolac, kétorolac)*
    non-steroid antiinflammatory, platelet aggregation inhibitor, analgesic
        ↑ ALT, AST, BT, creatinine, GMT, urea
        ↓ PLT aggregation
        ■ *Urine* ↑ blood, Hb, RBC
        ■ *Stool* ↑ Hb

Labetalol *(labetalolum, labetalol, labétalol)*
    alpha- and beta-adrenoceptor blocker, antihypertensive, vasodilator
        ↑ epinephrine, ALP, ALT, ANA, AST, Bil, CK, G, GMT, HDL cholesterol, K, catecholamines, creatinine, LD, LDL cholesterol, LE cells, norepinephrine, PRL, renin, TAG, urea
        ↓ HDL cholesterol, renin
        ■ *Urine* ↑ epinephrine, aldosterone, catecholamines, metanephrines
          ↓ aldosterone

Lactulose *(lactulosum, lactulose, lactulose)*
    disaccharide, laxative, treatment of hepatic coma, culture medium
        ↑ acetoacetate, creatinine, Na
        ↓ K, ammonia, Na
        ■ *Stool* ↑ FA

Lamivudine *(lamivudinum, lamivudine, lamivudine)*
antiviral
↑ ALT, AST, Bil, GMT, MAC
↓ neu, PLT

Lamotrigine *(lamotriginum, lamotrigine, lamotrigine)*
anticonvulsant, antiepileptic
↑ carbamazepine, eos
↓ PLT, WBC

Lansoprazole *(lansoprazolum, lansoprazole, lansoprazole)*
inhibitor proton pump
↑ ALT, AST, Bil, BT, GMT
↓ neu, PLT, WBC

Latamoxef *(latamoxefum, latamoxef, latamoxef)*
antibiotic
↑ ALP, ALT, AST, BT, eos, GMT
↓ PLT aggregation, eos, factors – (II, VII, X), Hb, WBC, PLT

Laxatives
↑ aldosterone, HCO_3^-, P, pH, renin
↓ proteins, Ca, Ca^{2+}, factors – (II, VII, X), chloride, K, Mg, Na
■ *Urine* ↑ aldosterone
↓ K
■ *Stool* ↑ fat

Leflunomide *(leflunomidum, leflunomide, léflunomide)*
antirheumatic
↑ ALT, AST, GMT
↓ PLT, WBC

Lepirudin *(lepirudinum, lepirudin, lépirudine)*
inhibitor of thrombin
■ *Urine* ↑ blood, Hb, RBC

Letrozole *(letrozolum, letrozole, létrozole)*
non-steroidal aromatase activity inhibitor
↑ Ca, cholesterol

Leuprolide *(leuprorelinum, leuprorelin, leuproréline)*
LHRH agonist, antineoplastic
↑ ALP, Ca, Ca^{2+}, cholesterol, creatinine, uric acid, LDL cholesterol, TAG, urea
↓ proteins, G, HDL cholesterol, WBC

Levamisole *(levamisolum, levamisole, lévamisole)*
anthelmintic, immunostimulant
↑ ALP, AST, Bil, creatinine, GMT
↓ WBC, neu, PLT

Levetiracetam *(levetiracetamum, levetiracetam, lévétiracétam)*
anticonvulsant, antiepileptic
↓ neu, WBC

Levobetaxolol *(levobetaxololum, levobetaxolol, lévobétaxolol)*
selective beta-1-adrenoceptor antagonist
↑ cholesterol, lipids

Levobupivacaine *(levobupivacainum, levobupivacaine, lévobupivacaine)*
local anesthetic
↑ MAC

Levodopa *(levodopum, levodopa, lévodopa)*
(L-dopa), antiparkinsonian

    ↑ ACTH, ALP, ALT, ANA, AST, Bil, conjugated Bil, C-peptide, 11-DOC, estrogens, FSH, G, GMT, cholesterol, insulin, K, catecholamines, uric acid, LD, WBC, lym, GH, T4, urea, FFA

    ↓ ammonia, G, Hb, K, cortisol, uric acid, neu, PLT, PRL, renin, T4, TAG, TSH, urea, WBC, vitamin B_6

    ■ *Urine* ↑ acetoacetate, blood, dopamine, RBC, estrogens, G, Hb, K, catecholamines, ketones, homogentisic acid, HVA, uric acid, Na, norepinephrine, VMA

      ↓ G, 5-HIAA, 17-OHCS, metanephrines, normetanephrine, volume, VMA

    ■ *Cerebrospinal Fluid* ↑ vitamin E

Levofloxacin *(levofloxacinum, levofloxacin, lévofloxacine)*
antibiotic/fluoroquinolone

    ↑ eos

    ↓ G, WBC

Levomepromazine *(levomepromazinum, levomepromazine, lévomepromazine)*
neuroleptic, analgesic

    ↑ ALP, ALT, ANA, TAG

    ↓ HDL cholesterol, WBC

Levonorgestrel *(levonorgestrelum, levonorgestrel, lévonorgestrel)*
progestation agent

    ↑ albumin, ALT, AST, androstenedione, Apo B, proteins, Bil, cyclosporine, Cu, G, GMT, LDL cholesterol, testosterone, Zn

    ↓ androstenedione, ceruloplasmin, estradiol, HDL cholesterol, cholesterol, LDL cholesterol, P, SHBG, T4, TAG, testosterone

Levothyroxine *(levothyroxinum natricum, levothyroxine sodium, lévothyroxine sodique)*
natural hormone

    ↑ AST, HDL cholesterol, SHBG

    ↓ Apo B, CBG, factors – (II, VII, X), cholesterol, IgA, LDL cholesterol, TSH, thyroglobulin

Lidocaine *(lidocainum, lidocaine, lidocaine)*
local anesthetic, antiarrhythmic

    ↑ CK, creatinine, MAC, MHb

    ↓ G

    ■ *Cerebrospinal Fluid* ↑ proteins

Lincomycin *(lincomycinum, lincomycin, lincomycine)*
antibiotic

    ↑ ALP, ALT, AST, Bil, eos, GMT

    ↓ G, folate, cholesterol, neu

    ■ *Stool* ↑ Hb

Linezolid *(linezolidum, linezolid, linezolid)*
antibacterial agent

    ↑ ALT, AST, GMT

    ↓ PLT

Liothyronine *(liothyroninum, liothyronine, liothyronine)*
thyromimetic

    ↓ Apo B, HDL cholesterol, cholesterol, LDL cholesterol, LP(a), TSH

Liquorice

    ↑ ANP, Na, pH

    ↓ aldosterone, K, renin

Lisinopril *(lisinoprilum, lisinopril, lisinopril)*
    competitive ACE antagonist, antihypertensive
        ↑ cholesterol, K, creatinine, renin, urea
        ↓ ACE, aldosterone, AT II, GFR
Lisuride *(lisuridum, lisuride, lisuride)*
    serotonin inhibitor, prolactin inhibitor
        ↑ GH
        ↓ PRL
Lithium *(lithium, lithium, lithium)*
    antimanic, antidepressive
        ↑ ADH, ALP, AMS, ANA, antithyroid Ab, Ca, Ca²⁺, CK, CK-MB, eos, FT4,
          G, cholesterol, K, cortisol, creatinine, WBC, Mg, Mg (RBC), neu, P, PTH,
          T3, T4, PLT, TSH, urea
        ↓ ADH, FT4, G tolerance, GFR, HCO₃⁻, CHS, cortisol, uric acid, WBC, lym,
          Na, P, T3, T4, TBG, vitamin D
        ■ *Urine* ↑ aldosterone, proteins, B2M, G, Hb, HCO₃⁻, uric acid, Mg, Na,
          volume, VMA
            ↓ Ca, norepinephrine, osmolality, specific gravity
Lomefloxacin *(lomefloxacinum, lomefloxacin, loméfloxacine)*
    antibacterial agent
        ↑ ALT, eos
Lomustine *(lomustinum, lomustine, lomustine)*
    antineoplastic
        ↑ ALP, Bil, creatinine, urea
        ↓ neu, PLT, WBC
Loop Diuretics
        ↑ Cr, G, cholesterol, creatinine, uric acid, LDL cholesterol, MAL, P, TAG,
          urea
        ↓ Ca, G tolerance, HDL cholesterol, chloride, K, Mg, Na
        ■ *Urine* ↑ chloride, Mg, Na
Loperamide *(loperamidum, loperamide, lopéramide)*
    antidiarrhoeal
        ■ *Gastric Fluid* ↓ HCl
Loracarbef *(loracarbefum, loracarbef, loracarbef)*
    antibiotic
        ↑ ALT, AST, eos, GMT, PT
        ↓ PLT, WBC
Lorcainide *(lorcainidum, lorcainide, lorcainide)*
    antiarrhythmic, local anesthetic
        ↓ Na, osmolality
Losartan *(losartanum, losartan, losartan)*
    angiotensin II antagonist
        ↑ ALT, AST, GMT, cholesterol, K, TAG, urea
        ↓ Na
Lovastatin *(lovastatinum, lovastatin, lovastatine)*
    HMG-CoA reductase inhibitor, lipid lowering agent
        ↑ ALP, ALT, ANA, Apo A-I, AST, CK, GFR, GMT, HDL cholesterol, K, crea-
          tinine, Mb, LP(a), T4
        ↓ Apo B, factors – (II, VII, X), cholesterol, LDL cholesterol, TAG, VLDL
          cholesterol

Loxapine *(loxapinum, loxapine, loxapine)*
   antipsychotic
               ↓ PLT

Lynestrenol *(lynestrenolum, lynestrenol, lynestrénol)*
   progestin
               ↑ CBG, ceruloplasmin, LDL cholesterol
               ↓ Apo A-I, HDL cholesterol, cholesterol, PRL, SHBG, TAG

Lysergide *(lysergidum, lysergide, lysergide)*
   sympatholytic, psychomimetic
               ↑ CK

Magnesium *(magnesii ascorbas, magnesium ascorbate, ascorbate de magnésico)*
   Mg²⁺ replacement, laxative
               ↑ ALP, Ca, Mg
               ↓ ACE, Ca

Magnesium Salts
               ↑ Ca, Mg, Mg²⁺
               ↓ Apo B, Ca, digoxin, phenytoin, K, salicylic acid, P, TAG

Mannitol *(mannitoli hexanitras, mannitoli hexanitrate, hexanitrate de mannitol)*
   osmotic diuretic
               ↑ K, creatinine, MAC, Na, osmolality, P
               ↓ Ca, chloride, K, uric acid, Li, Na, P
               ■ *Urine* ↑ Ca, uric acid, Mg, Na

MAO Inhibitors
               ↑ epinephrine, ALP, ALT, AST, Bil, CK, dopamine, G tolerance, catecholamines, MAC, norepinephrine, PRL, PT, serotonin
               ↓ G, cholesterol
               ■ *Urine* ↑ catecholamines, HVA, Mb, metanephrines, VMA
                     ↓ 5-HIAA, VMA

Maprotiline *(maprotilinum, maprotiline, maprotiline)*
   antidepressant
               ↑ ALT

Measles/Mumps/Rubella Vaccines
               ↓ PLT

Mebendazole *(mebendazolum, mebendazole, mébendazole)*
   anthelmintic
               ↑ ALP, ALT, AST, eos, GMT, urea
               ↓ G, Hb, PLT, WBC, neu
               ■ *Urine* ↑ blood, Hb, RBC

Mechlorethamine *(mechlorethaminum, mechlorethamine, méchlorethamine)*
   antineoplastic
               ↑ uric acid
               ↓ neu, PLT, WBC

Meclofenamic Acid *(acidum meclofenamicum, meclofenamic acid, acide méclofénamique)*
   non-steroid antiinflammatory, antirheumatic
               ↑ ALT, AST, GMT, urea
               ■ *Urine* ↑ blood, Hb, RBC
               ■ *Stool* ↑ Hb

Medroxyprogesterone *(medroxyprogesteronum, medroxyprogesterone, médroxyprogestérone)*
progestogen
   ↑ albumin, ALT, AST, Apo B, G, GMT, HDL cholesterol, cholesterol, insulin, LDL cholesterol, Mg, P, PTH, TAG
   ↓ estradiol, factors – (II, VII, X), gonadotropins, G tolerance, HDL cholesterol, cholesterol, insulin, cortisol, LDL cholesterol, LP(a), progesterone, SHBG, TAG, testosterone
   ■ *Urine* ↓ 17-OHCS, pregnanediol

Mefenamic Acid *(acidum mefenamicum, mefenamic acid, acide méfénamique)*
non-steroid antiinflammatory, analgesic
   ↑ ALP, ALT, AMS, AST, Bil, creatinine, lipase, MCV, PT, urea
   ↓ PLT aggregation, folate, WBC, neu

Mefloquine *(mefloquinum, mefloquine, méfloquine)*
antiparasitic, antimalarial
   ↑ ALT, AST, GMT, WBC
   ↓ PLT

Mefruside *(mefrusidum, mefruside, méfruside)*
salidiuretic, antihypertensive
   ↑ uric acid
   ↓ K

Megestrol *(megestrolum, megestrol, mégestrol)*
progestogen, antineoplastic
   ↑ ALP, ALT, AST, Ca, estradiol, G, GMT, insulin, LDL cholesterol, PRL
   ↓ 11-deoxycortisol, DHEA, estradiol, estrone, FSH, G, LH, SHBG

Meloxicam *(meloxicamum, meloxicam, méloxicam)*
non-steroid antiinflammatory
   ↑ ALT, AST, Bil, GMT, urea
   ↓ PLT, WBC
   ■ *Stool* ↑ blood

Melperone *(melperonum, melperone, melpérone)*
neuroleptic
   ↑ PRL
   ↓ WBC

Melphalan *(melphalanum, melphalan, melphalan)*
antineoplastic
   ↑ Bil, creatinine, WBC, urea, uric acid
   ↓ neu, PLT, WBC
   ■ *Urine* ↑ 5-HIAA

Menotropins
   ↑ ALT, AST, GMT, K
   ↓ albumin

Mepacrine *(mepacrinum, mepacrine, mépacrine)*
antimalarial
   ↑ ALP, ALT, Bil, cortisol
   ↓ Hb, WBC
   ■ *Urine* ↑ cortisol

Meperidine *(pethidinum, pethidine, péthidine)*
narcotic, analgesic
   ↑ ADH, AMS, CK, G, histamine, LD, lipase, pCO_2
   ↓ ACTH, Na, PLT, pO_2

   ■ *Urine* ↑ volume
        ↓ 17-OHCS, 17-KS

Mephenazine *(mephenazinum, mephenazine, méphénazine)*
 skeletal muscle relaxant
       ↑ serotonin

Mephenesin *(mephenesinum, mephenesin, méphénésine)*
 skeletal muscle relaxant
       ↑ eos

Mephenytoin *(mephenytoinum, mephenytoin, méphénytoine)*
 anticonvulsant, antiepileptic
      ↑ ALP, ALT, ANA, AST, eos, GMT, lym, mono
      ↓ Hb, WBC, neu, PLT

Mepindolol *(mepindololum, mepindolol, mépindolol)*
 beta-adrenergic blocker, antihypertensive, antiarrhythmic
      ↑ HDL cholesterol, TAG
      ↓ cholesterol, LDL cholesterol

Meprobamate *(meprobamatum, meprobamate, méprobamate)*
 anxiolytic, muscle relaxant
      ↑ ALP, Bil, cholesterol, eos
      ↓ Hb, WBC, neu, PLT, PT
     ■ *Urine* ↑ ALA, estriol, estrogens, 17-OHCS, 17-KGS, 17-KS, PBG, por-
       phyrins
      ↓ 17-KGS, 17-KS, volume

Mercaptopurine *(mercaptopurinum, mercaptopurine, mercaptopurine)*
 antineoplastic
      ↑ ALP, ALT, AST, Bil, eos, G, GMT, OCT, uric acid, MCV, PT
      ↓ WBC, neu, PLT

Mercurial Diuretics
      ↑ HCO_3^-
      ↓ proteins, Ca, chloride, Na

Mercury Preparations
      ↑ HCO_3^-, pH
      ↓ proteins, Ca, HCO_3^-, K, uric acid, Mg, Na, pH, PLT, urea
     ■ *Urine* ↑ albumin, G, uric acid, P

Meropenem *(meropenemum, meropenem, méropénem)*
 beta-lactam antibiotic
      ↑ ALT, AST, BT, eos, GMT, PLT
      ↓ PLT, WBC

Mesalazine *(mesalazinum, mesalazine, mésalazine)*
 antiinflammatory, antibacterial
      ↑ ALT, creatinine

Mestranol *(mestranolum, mestranol, mestranol)*
 estrogen
      ↑ A2MG, ALT, AST, GMT, factors – (VII, X), T3, T4, TAG, transferrin, urea
      ↓ albumin

Mesuximide *(mesuximidum, mesuximide, mésuximide)*
 anticonvulsant, antiepileptic
      ↑ phenobarbital, phenytoin, mono

Metahexamide *(metahexamidum, metahexamide, metahexamide)*
 oral hypoglycemic
      ↑ ALT
      ↓ G

Metamizole *(metamizolum natricum, metamizole sodium, métamizole sodique)*
    analgesic, antipyretic, antirheumatic, spasmolytic
        ↑ ALT, Bil
        ↓ G, Hb, cholesterol, WBC, neu, TAG, PLT
Metandienone *(metandienonum, metandienone, métandiénone)*
    anabolic, androgen
        ↑ ALP, ALT, AMS, AST, Bil, GMT, haptoglobin
        ↓ factors – (II, VII, X), FSH, LH, TAG, TBG, testosterone
Metaxalone *(metaxalonum, metaxalone, métaxalone)*
    muscle relaxant
        ↑ ALT, AST, GMT
        ↓ WBC
Metergoline *(metergolinum, metergoline, métergoline)*
    serotonin antagonist, migraine prophylactic
        ↓ TSH
Metformin *(metforminum, metformin, metformine)*
    oral hypoglycemic
        ↑ HDL cholesterol, LA, MAC, MCV
        ↓ BE, C-peptide, Fe, fibrinogen, G, Hb, HCO_3^-, cholesterol, plasminogen
           activator inhibitor, insulin, carotene, LDL-C, pH, TAG, vitamin – (B_{12},
           folate), VLDL-C, FFA
        ■ *Urine* ↑ ketones, acetoacetate
Methacholine *(methacholini chloridum, methacholine chloride, chlorure de méthacholine)*
    parasympathomimetic
        ↑ AMS, Bil, lipase
        ■ *Urine* ↑ norepinephrine
Methadone *(methadonum, methadone, méthadone)*
    narcotic analgesic
        ↑ ceruloplasmin, IgG, cortisol, pCO_2, PLT, PRL, T3, T4, TBG
        ↓ FT4, Na, testosterone
        ■ *Urine* ↑ hCG
        ↓ volume
Methandriol *(methandriolum, methandriol, méthandriol)*
    anabolic
        ↑ ALP, ALT, AST, Bil, GMT
Methanol *(alcoholum methylicum, methyl alcohol, alcohol méthylique)*
    solvent, antifreeze fluid
        ↑ LA, MAC
Methapyrilene *(methapyrilenum, methapyrilene, méthapyriléne)*
    antihistaminic, sedative
        ↓ Hb
Methazolamide *(methazolamidum, methazolamide, méthazolamide)*
    carbonic anhydrase inhibitor, diuretic, treatment of glaucoma
        ↓ Hb, neu, PLT
Methenamine *(methenaminum, methenamine, méthénamine)*
    antibacterial, urinary tract antiseptic
        ↑ catecholamines
        ■ *Urine* ↑ proteins, estrogens, G, Hb, catecholamines, 17-OHCS, blood,
           crystals, RBC, UBG, VMA
        ↓ estrogens, 5-HIAA, pH

Methimazole *(methimazolum, methimazole, methimazole)*
  thyroid inhibitor
    ↑ ALP, ALT, AST, G, GMT, cholesterol, PT, T3, TSH
    ↓ neu, PLT, T3, T4, WBC

Methionine *(methioninum, methionine, méthionine)*
  essential amino acid
    ■ *Urine* ↑ ketones

Methocarbamol *(methocarbamolum, methocarbamol, méthocarbamol)*
  skeletal muscle relaxant, spasmolytic
    ↓ WBC
    ■ *Urine* ↑ blood, Hb, HVA, RBC, 5-HIAA, VMA

Methotrexate *(methotrexatum, methotrexate, méthotrexate)*
  antineoplastic, antileukemic, folic acid antagonist
    ↑ ALP, ALT, AST, Bil, conjugated Bil, eos, Fe, phenylalanine, folate, ESR, GMT, Hb, homocysteine, cholesterol, creatinine, uric acid, LD, MCV, OCT, P, urea, bile acids
    ↓ CRP, factors – (II, VII, X), GFR, folate, Hb, IL-6, uric acid, WBC, lym, neu, RTC, TAG, PLT
    ■ *Urine* ↑ blood, Hb, RBC, crystals
    ■ *Cerebrospinal Fluid* ↑ proteins
    ■ *Seminal Fluid* ↓ spermatozoa count
    ■ *Stool* ↑ Hb, fatty acids

Methoxsalen *(methoxsalenum, methoxsalen, méthoxsalen)*
  dermatologic
    ↑ ALT, AST

Methoxamine *(methoxaminum, methoxamine, méthoxamine)*
  alpha-adrenergic agonist, vasoconstrictor
    ↑ ACTH, cortisol

Methoxyflurane *(methoxyfluranum, methoxyflurane, méthoxyflurane)*
  anesthetic
    ↑ ALP, ALT, AST, Bil, fluoride, chloride, GMT, creatinine, uric acid, Na, osmolality, oxalate, urea
    ↓ PLT aggregation, BE, Ca, pH
    ■ *Urine* ↑ Hb
    ↓ volume, osmolality

Methyclothiazide *(methyclothiazidum, methyclothiazide, méthyclothiazide)*
  diuretic, antihypertensive
    ↑ BE, cholesterol, uric acid, LDL-C, TAG, VLDL cholesterol
    ↓ K, Na, osmolality

Methyldopa *(methyldopum, methyldopa, méthyldopa)*
  antihypertensive
    ↑ ALA, ALP, ALT, AMS, ANA, AST, apolipoprotein C III, Bil, conjugated Bil, eos, G, GMT, chloride, cholesterol, IgG, catecholamines, coagulation factors, creatinine, uric acid, LE cells, Na, OCT, plasma volume, porphyrins, PRL, RF, RTC, TAG, urea
    ↓ G, GFR, GMT, haptoglobin, Hb, HCT, HDL-C, cholesterol, uric acid, LDL-C, Na, neu, norepinephrine, osmolality, GH, TAG, PLT, VLDL-C
    ■ *Urine* ↑ acetoacetate, epinephrine, G, catecholamines, ketones, coproporphyrin, creatinine, metanephrines, norepinephrine, PBG, porphyrins, VMA
    ↓ 5-HIAA, catecholamines
    ■ *Stool* ↑ blood, Hb

Methylphenidate *(methylphenidatum, methylphenidate, méthylphenidate)*
   sympathomimetic, central stimulant
      ↑ ALT, GH
Methylprednisolone *(methylprednisolonum, methylprednisolone, méthylprednisolone)*
   corticosteroid
      ↑ AMS, cyclosporine, G, GFR, HCO_3^-, LA, lipase, MAL, Na, plasma volume, trypsin
      ↓ ACE, ACTH, Ca, glucose tolerance, GRH, IgA, IgG, IgM, K, cortisol, P, PLT, pO_2, testosterone
Methyltestosterone *(methyltestosteronum, methyltestosterone, méthyltestostérone)*
   androgen
      ↑ ALP, ALT, AST, Bil, Ca, cyclosporine, RBC, GMT, haptoglobin, cholesterol, 5-nucleotidase, bile acids
      ↓ factors – (V, VII, X), HDL cholesterol, SHBG, TBG
      ■ *Urine* ↓ UBG
      ■ *Seminal Fluid* ↓ spermatozoa count
Methylthiouracil *(methylthiouracilum, methylthiouracil, méthylthiouracil)*
   thyroid inhibitor
      ↑ ALP, ANA, Bil
      ↓ Hb, neu, T3, T4, PLT
Methylxanthines
      ↑ catecholamines
      ■ *Urine* ↑ VMA
Methyprylon *(methyprylonum, methyprylon, méthyprylone)*
   hypnotic, sedative
      ■ *Urine* ↑ ALA, G, 17-OHCS, 17-KGS, 17-KS, porphyrins
Methysergide *(methysergidum, methysergide, méthysergide)*
   serotonin antagonist, migraine prophylactic
      ↑ eos, ESR, urea
      ↓ lym, neu, serotonin, TSH
Meticillin *(meticillinum, meticillin, méticilline)*
   antibiotic (penicillinase resistant)
      ↑ ALP, ALT, AST, eos, K, creatinine, uric acid, P, urea
      ↓ albumin, proteins, Ca, GFR, Hb, HCO_3^-, K, uric acid, WBC, neu, P, TAG, PLT, urea
      ■ *Urine* ↑ proteins, Hb, 17-KS, blood, casts – (hyaline)
      ■ *Cerebrospinal Fluid* ↑ proteins
Metirosine *(metirosinum, metirosine, métirosine)*
   antihypertensive
      ↓ catecholamines
      ■ *Urine* ↑ catecholamines, crystals, metanephrines, VMA
Metoclopramide *(metoclopramidum, metoclopramide, métoclopramide)*
   competitive antagonist D2 receptor, antiemetic, prokinetic
      ↑ ACTH, aldosterone, ALP, 11-DOC, cortisol, LH, MHb, pregnenolone, PRL, GH, TSH
      ↓ digoxin, G, K, LH, WBC
Metolazone *(metolazonum, metolazone, métolazone)*
   diuretic, antihypertensive
      ↑ ALP, ALT, AST, G, GMT, cholesterol, MAL, HCO_3^-, TAG, uric acid
      ↓ chloride, K, Mg, Na, neu, WBC
      ■ *Urine* ↑ G

Metoprolol *(metoprololum, metoprolol, métoprolol)*
    beta-adrenergic blocker
        ↑ epinephrine, ALT, AST, CK, G, GMT, HbA$_{1c}$, cholesterol, K, cortisol, norepinephrine, GH, TAG, theophylline, PLT, VLDL-C, FFA
        ↓ G, HDL-C, cholesterol, LDL-C, rT3, T3, testosterone, FFA

Metrifonate *(metrifonatum, metrifonate, métrifonate)*
    insecticide, anthelmintic, antiparasitic
        ↓ CHS

Metronidazole *(metronidazolum, metronidazole, métronidazole)*
    antimicrobial, antiprotozoal
        ↑ ALT, AMS, phenytoin, G, 17-OHCS, lipase
        ↓ AST, factors – (II, VII, X), G, cholesterol, cortisol, LD, LDL cholesterol, WBC, neu, TAG
        ■ *Urine* ↑ brown color, volume
           ↓ 17-KS

Metyrapone *(metyraponum, metyrapone, métyrapone)*
    inhibitor of glucocorticosteroid biosynthesis, diagnostic aid
        ↑ ACTH, androstenedione, 11-deoxycorticosterone, K, GH
        ↓ aldosterone, chloride, cholesterol, corticosterone, cortisol, Na, testosterone, TAG
        ■ *Urine* ↑ 17-OHCS, 17-KGS, Na, porphyrins
           ↓ 17-KS

Metyrosine *(metyrosinum, metyrosine, métyrosine)*
    alpha-adrenoceptor antagonist
        ■ *Urine* ↑ crystals

Mexiletine *(mexiletinum, mexiletine, mexilétine)*
    antiarrhythmic, anticonvulsant
        ↑ ALT, AST, digoxin, GMT, theophylline
        ↓ WBC, neu, PLT

Mezlocillin *(mezlocillinum, mezlocillin, mézlocilline)*
    antibiotic
        ↑ ALT, AST, BT, eos, GMT, creatinine, OCT
        ↓ PLT aggregation, K, WBC, neu

Mianserin *(mianserinum, mianserin, miansérine)*
    serotonin inhibitor, antihistaminic, thymoleptic
        ↑ ALP, ALT, Bil
        ↓ Hb, WBC, neu, PLT

Miconazole *(miconazolum, miconazole, miconazole)*
    antifungal
        ↑ CK, phenytoin, cholesterol, lipids, TAG, PLT
        ↓ factors – (II, VII, X), Hb, Na, PLT

Midazolam *(midazolamum, midazolam, midazolam)*
    anesthetic
        ↑ pCO_2
        ↓ neu, pO_2

Mifepristone *(mifepristonum, mifepristone, mifépristone)*
    progesterone, glucocorticoid receptor antagonist
        ↓ K

Milrinone *(milrinonum, milrinone, milrinone)*
    inhibitor PDE III, cardiotonic
        ↑ ALT, AST
        ↓ K, PLT

Mineralocorticoids

 ↑ ANF, HCO_3, Na
 ↓ K

Minocycline *(minocyclinum, minocycline, minocycline)*
 antibiotic

 ↑ ALT, AST, Bil, eos, GMT, urea
 ↓ neu

Minoxidil *(minoxidilum, minoxidil, minoxidil)*
 antihypertensive

 ↑ ALP, ANA, CK, G, HDL cholesterol, creatinine, renin, urea
 ↓ LDL cholesterol, WBC, PLT

Mirtazapine *(mirtazapinum, mirtazapine, mirtazapine)*
 antidepressant

 ↑ ALT, AST, GMT
 ↓ neu

Misoprostol *(misoprostolum, misoprostol, misoprostol)*
 prostaglandin E1 analogue, antiulcer agent

 ↑ ALP, ALT, AST, Bil

Mithramycin *(mithramycinum, mithramycin, mithramycin)*
 antineoplastic

 ↑ ALP, Bil, creatinine, urea
 ↓ Ca, K, P
 ■ *Urine* ↑ proteins, Ca
  ↓ hydroxyproline
 ■ *Seminal Fluid* ↓ spermatozoa count

Mitomycin *(mitomycinum, mitomycin, mitomycine)*
 antineoplastic

 ↑ ALT, creatinine, uric acid, urea
 ↓ Hb, neu, PLT, WBC
 ■ *Urine* ↑ blood, Hb, proteins, RBC

Mitotane *(mitotanum, mitotane, mitotane)*
 antineoplastic, insecticide

 ↑ ALP, HDL cholesterol, cholesterol, LA, LDL cholesterol, MAC
 ↓ glucocorticoids, pH, T4
 ■ *Urine* ↑ proteins, blood
  ↓ 17-OHCS

Mitoxantrone *(mitoxantronum, mitoxantrone, mitoxantrone)*
 antineoplastic

 ↑ ALT, AST, GMT
 ↓ Hb, WBC, neu, PLT

Moclobemide *(moclobemidum, moclobemide, moclobémide)*
 selective MAO inhibitor (type A), antidepressant

 ↑ ALT, AST, CK, LD
 ↓ factors – (II, VII, X)

Modafinil *(modafinilum, modafinil, modafinil)*
 CNS stimulant

 ↑ ALT, AST, G, eos, GMT

Moexipril *(moexiprilatum, moexiprilat, moexiprilate)*
 ACE inhibitor, antihypertensive

 ↑ ALT, AST, G, GMT, cholesterol, K, TAG, urea, uric acid

Molindone *(molindonum, molindone, molindone)*
    antipsychotic, antiemetic, analgesic
              ↑ PRL, FFA
Montelukast *(montelukastum, montelukast, montélukast)*
    non-selective 5-lipoxygenase inhibitor, antileukotriene
              ↑ eos
Moricizine *(moricizinum, moricizine, moricizine)*
    antiarrhythmic
              ↑ ALT, AST, GMT
              ↓ PLT
Morphine *(morphinum, morphine, morphine)*
    narcotic analgesic
              ↑ epinephrine, ADH, ALP, ALT, AMS, Bil, CK, G, gastrin, HbA$_{1c}$, histamine, HCO$_3$, LD, lipase, pCO$_2$, PRL, TSH
              ↓ enteroglucagon, GIP, chloride, insulin, cortisol, LA, motilin, Na, norepinephrine, pO$_2$, PP
              ■ *Urine* ↑ G, AMS
                ↓ 17-OHCS, 17-KS, volume, VMA
              ■ *Cerebrospinal Fluid* ↑ proteins
Moxalactam *(latamoxefum, latamoxef, latamoxef)*
    cephalosporin (3rd generation)
              ↑ BT
Moxifloxacin *(moxifloxacinum, moxifloxacin, moxifloxacin)*
    antibiotic
              ↑ ALT, AST, G, eos, GMT, lipids
              ↓ PLT, WBC
Mycophenolate *(acidum mycophenolicum, mycophenolic acid, acide mycophénolique)*
    immunosuppressant
              ↑ cholesterol, G, K, WBC
              ↓ K, neu, P, PLT, WBC
              ■ *Urine* ↑ blood, Hb, RBC

Nabumetone *(nabumetonum, nabumetone, nabumétone)*
    non-steroid antiinflammatory
              ↑ ALT, AST, GMT, urea
              ■ *Urine* ↑ blood, Hb, RBC
Nadolol *(nadololum, nadolol, nadolol)*
    beta-adrenergic blocker, antiarrhythmic
              ↑ AMS, G, HbA$_{1c}$, uric acid, TAG
              ↓ G, HDL cholesterol
Nafarelin *(nafarelinum, nafarelin, nafaréline)*
    LHRH agonist
              ↑ ALP, FSH (early), HDL, cholesterol, LH (early), P, TAG
              ↓ androstenedione, Ca, estradiol, FSH (later), LH (later), progesterone, testosterone
Nafcillin *(nafcillinum, nafcillin, nafcilline)*
    antibiotic
              ↑ ALP, ALT, AST, BT, eos, factors – (II, VII, X), GMT
              ↓ cyclosporine, Hb, K, WBC, PLT, neu
              ■ *Urine* ↑ proteins, G, K

Nalidixic Acid *(acidum nalidixicum, nalidixic acid, acide nalidixique)*
   antibacterial
        ↑ ALP, ALT, ANA, Bil, eos, G, creatinine, Heinz bodies (RBC), LA, MAC, urea
        ↓ factors – (II, VII, X), haptoglobin, Hb, WBC, pH, PLT
        ■ *Urine* ↑ G, 17-OHCS, 17-KGS, 17-KS, VMA

Nalorphine *(nalorphinum, nalorphine, nalorphine)*
   opioid receptor antagonist
        ↑ PRL, GH
        ↓ cortisol

Naloxone *(naloxonum, naloxone, naloxone)*
   opioid receptor antagonist
        ↑ ACTH, FSH, G, hCG, cortisol, LH
        ↓ PRL

Naltrexone *(naltrexonum, naltrexone, naltrexone)*
   opioid receptor antagonist
        ↑ ACTH, ALT, AST, FSH, GMT, LH, OCT

Nandrolone *(nandrolonum, nandrolone, nandrolone)*
   anabolic steroid
        ↑ ALP, ALT, AST, Bil, BT, Ca, fibrinogen, GMT, haptoglobin, HCT, cholesterol, 5-nucleotidase
        ↓ HDL cholesterol, coagulation factors, TAG
        ■ *Seminal Fluid* ↑ volume
        ↓ spermatozoa count

Naproxen *(naproxenum, naproxen, naproxéne)*
   non-steroid antiinflammatory, analgesic, antipyretic
        ↑ ALP, ALT, AMS, AST, Bil, BT, eos, ESR, GMT, HCO_3^-, K, creatinine, WBC, P, urea
        ↓ PLT aggregation, Hb, neu, WBC, TAG, PLT
        ■ *Urine* ↑ blood, Hb, RBC, proteins, 5-HIAA, 17-KGS, Zn
        ↓ chloride, Na, volume
        ■ *Stool* ↑ Hb

Narcotics
   (narcotic analgesics)
        ↑ ALT, AMS, AST, CK, G, GMT, lipase, MAC+RAC
        ■ *Urine* ↓ 17-OHCS, volume

Nefazodone *(nefazodonum, nefazodone, néfazodone)*
   antidepressant
        ↑ ALT, AST, GMT

Nelfinavir *(nelfinavirum, nelfinavir, nélfinavir)*
   antiviral
        ↑ Bil, cholesterol, G, ketobodies, lipids, TAG

Neomycin *(neomycinum, neomycin, néomycine)*
   antibiotic
        ↑ MCV, urea
        ↓ ammonia, Apo B, Apo (a), digoxin, cholesterol, K, carotene, LDL cholesterol, coagulation factors, LP(a), Mg, T3, TAG, TBG, thyroglobulin, vitamin – (A, B_{12}, folate), FFA
        ■ *Urine* ↑ amino acids, Hb, proteins, LD, casts
        ↓ Ca, estriol, estrogens
        ■ *Stool* ↑ Ca, fatty acids
        ■ *Seminal Fluid* ↓ spermatozoa count

Netilmicin *(netilmicinum, netilmicin, nétilmicine)*
    antibiotic
        ↑ ALT, creatinine
Neuroleptics
        ↑ PRL
        ■ *Urine* ↓ volume
Nevirapine *(nevirapinum, nevirapine, névirapine)*
    antiviral
        ↑ ALT, AST, Bil, eos, GMT
        ↓ neu
Niacin *(acidum nicotinicum, nicotinic acid, acide nicotinique)*
    essential water-soluble vitamin, antilipemic, vasodilator
        ↑ ALP, ALT, Apo A-I, G, GMT, G tolerance, HDL cholesterol, histamine,
          insulin, catecholamines, uric acid, GH
        ↓ beta-LP, G tolerance, cholesterol, LDL cholesterol, P, PL, pre-beta-LP,
          TAG, VLDL cholesterol, FFA
        ■ *Urine* ↑ G, ketones, Na
             ↓ K
Nicardipine *(nicardipinum, nicardipine, nicardipine)*
    slow calcium-channel blocker
        ↑ ALT, cyclosporine, digoxin, GFR, HbA$_{1c}$, HDL cholesterol, norepineph-
          rine, TSH
        ↓ T4
        ■ *Urine* ↑ Na, volume
Niceritrol *(niceritrolum, niceritrol, nicéritrol)*
    lipid lowering agent
        ↑ HDL cholesterol
        ↓ fibrinogen, G, HbA$_{1c}$, HDL cholesterol, cholesterol, LDL cholesterol,
          LP(a)
Nicotinamide *(nicotinamidum, nicotinamide, nicotinamide)*
    vitamin enzyme co-factor
        ↑ carbamazepine, lym, neu, primidone
        ↓ eos
        ■ *Urine* ↑ K, Na
Nicotine *(nicotinum, nicotine, nicotine)*
    alkaloid from Nicotiana tabacum
        ↑ ADH, epinephrine, PLT aggregation, G, 11-OHCS, cortisol, norepineph-
          rine, FFA
        ■ *Urine* ↑ catecholamines, 5-HIAA
        ■ *Seminal Fluid* ↓ spermatozoa motility, spermatozoa count
Nicotinic Acid *(acidum nicotinicum, nicotinic acid, acide nicotinique)*
    vasodilator, vitamin enzyme co-factor
        ↑ acetoacetate, ALP, Apo A-I, AST, Bil, CK, G, GMT, HbA$_{1c}$, HDL choles-
          terol, insulin, catecholamines, uric acid, LDL cholesterol, neu, GH, FFA
        ↓ apolipoproteins – (Apo B, Apo C, Apo E), Apo (a), eos, factors – (II, VII,
          X), G, cholesterol, insulin, LDL cholesterol, LP(a), lym, TAG, VLDL
          cholesterol, FFA
        ■ *Urine* ↑ catecholamines, acetoacetate, G, K, Na
        ■ *Gastric Fluid* ↑ HCl

Nicotinyl Alcohol *(nicotinyl alcoholum, nicotinyl alcohol, alcohol nicotinyque)*
peripheral vasodilator, lipid lowering agent
↓ TAG

Nifedipine *(nifedipinum, nifedipine, nifédipine)*
coronary vasodilator, slow calcium-channel blocker
↑ aldosterone, ALP, ALT, ANP, Apo A-I, Apo A-II, AST, BT, digoxin, phenytoin, G, GFR, glucagon, GMT, HDL cholesterol, cholesterol, K, catecholamines, creatinine, renin
↓ PLT aggregation, Apo B, G, cholesterol, quinidine, insulin, K, creatinine,
Na, norepinephrine, PRL, TAG, theophylline, TSH, urea, VLDL cholesterol
■ *Urine* ↑ albumin, B2M, uric acid, Na
↓ Mg, oxalate, urea

Niflumic Acid *(acidum niflumicum, niflumic acid, acide niflumique)*
non-steroid antiinflammatory, analgesic
↑ ALT, CK, LD

Nilutamide *(nilutamidum, nilutamide, nilutamide)*
antiandrogen
↑ ALT, AST, G, GMT, LH, testosterone, urea

Nimodipine *(nimodipinum, nimodipine, nimodipine)*
slow calcium-channel blocker
↑ ALT
↓ PLT

Nisoldipine *(nisoldipinum, nisoldipine, nisoldipine)*
slow calcium-channel blocker, coronary vasodilator
↑ ALT, AST, GMT, digoxin, HDL cholesterol, urea
↓ Hb, TAG

Nitrates
↑ conjugated Bil, MAC, MHb
↓ cholesterol
■ *Urine* ↑ blood, RBC, Hb, catecholamines, volume

Nitrazepam *(nitrazepamum, nitrazepam, nitrazépam)*
sedative, hypnotic, anticonvulsant
↑ HCO_3^-
↓ G
■ *Urine* ↑ 5-HIAA

Nitrendipine *(nitrendipinum, nitrendipine, nitrendipine)*
antihypertensive, calcium channel antagonist
↑ digoxin, renin
↓ ANP

Nitrofurantoin *(nitrofurantoinum, nitrofurantoin, nitrofurantoine)*
antibacterial
↑ ALP, ALT, AMS, ANA, antithyroglobulin Ab, AST, Bil, conjugated Bil, BT,
eos, ESR, GMT, Hb, Heinz bodies (RBC), IgG, creatinine, LD, LE cells,
WBC, MHb, Na, OCT, urea
↓ PLT aggregation, albumin, folate, G tolerance, haptoglobin, Hb, HCO_3^-,
WBC, lym, neu, TAG, PLT
■ *Urine* ↑ AMS, brown color, G
■ *Seminal Fluid* ↓ spermatozoa count
■ *Pleural Fluid* ↑ eos

Nitroglycerin (*nitroglycerinum, nitroglycerin, nitroglycerin*)
coronary vasodilator, spasmolytic, explosive
↑ catecholamines, TAG
↓ PLT
- ***Urine*** ↑ epinephrine, norepinephrine, VMA

Nitroprusside Sodium (*natrii nitroprussidum, nitroprusside, nitroprusside sodique*)
antihypertensive, reagent
↑ FT4, MHb, norepinephrine, T4, TSH
↓ digoxin, TSH, vitamin B$_{12}$

Nizatidine (*nizatidinum, nizatidine, nizatidine*)
histamine H$_2$ receptor antagonist
↑ ALT, AST, GMT

Nocloprost (*nocloprostum, nocloprost, nocloprost*)
cytoprotective, gastric secretion inhibitor
- ***Gastric Fluid*** ↑ pH

Nomegestrol (*nomegestrolum, nomegestrol, nomégestrol*)
progestin
↓ Apo A-I, AT III, estradiol

Nomifensine (*nomifensinum, nomifensine, nomifensine*)
antidepressant
↑ ALP, ALT, ANA, AST, Bil, eos, ESR, GMT, LD
↓ Hb, coagulation factors, cortisol, TSH

Non-Steroid Antiphlogistics
(non-steroid antiinflammatory drugs, NSAIDS)
↑ ALP, ALT, AMS, AST, Bil, BT, eos, G, GMT, chloride, K, creatinine, LE cells, lithium, PT, RAL+MAC, urea
↓ PLT aggregation, aldosterone, G, GFR, Hb, K, WBC, Na, neu, PG, renin
- ***Urine*** ↑ proteins, RBC, G, blood
- ***Stool*** ↑ Hb

Norepinephrine (*norepinephrinum, norepinephrine, norépinéphrine*)
endogenous catecholamine, sympathomimetic, vasoconstrictor
↑ G, uric acid, LA, WBC, lym, neu, T4
↓ Ca^{2+}

Noretandrostenolon (*noretandrostenolonum, noretandrostenolon, noretandrostenolon*)
anabolic, androgen
↑ ALP, ALT, Bil

Norethindrone (*norethisteronum, norethisterone, noréthistérone*)
oral contraceptive
↑ ALT, AST, G, GMT

Norethisterone (*norethisteronum, norethisterone, noréthistérone*)
oral contraceptive
↑ ALP, ALT, Apo B, AST, Bil, GMT, HDL-C, cholesterol, LDL-C
↓ Ca, estradiol, FSH, HDL cholesterol, LH, LP(a), P, SHBG, TAG

Norethynodrel (*norethynodrelum, norethynodrel, noréthynodrel*)
progestin
↑ ALP, ALT, AST, Bil, GMT, TBG

Norfloxacin (*norfloxacinum, norfloxacin, norfloxacine*)
antibacterial
↑ ALT, AST, creatinine, theophylline
↓ eos, factors – (II, VII, X), WBC, neu, PLT

Norgestrel *(norgestrelum, norgestrel, norgestrel)*
  progestin
  ↑ ALT, AST, G, GMT
  ↓ factors – (II, VII, X), HDL-C, cholesterol, SHBG, TAG
Nortriptyline *(nortriptylinum, nortriptyline, nortriptyline)*
  antidepressant
  ↑ ALP, AMS, eos, G, PT
  ↓ factors – (II, VII, X), G, PLT, WBC
Novobiocin *(novobiocinum, novobiocin, novobiocine)*
  antibiotic
  ↑ ALP, ALT, Bil, unconjugated Bil, conjugated Bil
  ↓ neu, PLT
Nystatin *(nystatinum, nystatin, nystatine)*
  antifungal, antibiotic
  ↑ G
  ↓ PLT

Octreotide *(octreotidum, octreotide, octréotide)*
  long-acting analogue of somatostatin
  ↑ ALT, G
  ↓ cyclosporine, CK, G, gastrin, glucagon, insulin, motilin, pancreatic
    polypeptide, secretin, serotonin, GH, VIP
  ■ *Urine* ↑ osmolality
  ■ *Stool* ↑ fat
Ofloxacin *(ofloxacinum, ofloxacin, ofloxacine)*
  antibacterial
  ↑ ALT, GMT, creatinine
  ↓ factors – (II, VII, X)
Olanzapine *(olanzapinum, olanzapine, olanzapine)*
  antipsychotic
  ↑ ALT, AST, GMT, PRL
  ↓ neu
Oleic Acid *(acidum oleicum, oleic acid, acide oleique)*
  substance for ointments
  ↑ LP(a)
  ↓ cholesterol, LDL cholesterol
Olsalazine *(olsalazinum, olsalazine, olsalazine)*
  antiinflammatory (intestinal)
  ↑ ALT, AST, GMT
Omeprazole *(omeprazolum, omeprazole, oméprazol)*
  proton pump inhibitor, antiulcer agent
  ↑ ALT, AST, Bil, diazepam, digoxin, factors – (II, VII, X), GMT, phenytoin,
    gastrin, WBC
  ↓ factors – (II, VII, X), G, gastrin, neu, pepsin, PLT, vitamin B_{12}
  ■ *Urine* ↑ G
  ■ *Gastric Fluid* ↑ pH
Ondansetron *(ondansetronum, ondansetron, ondansetron)*
  antiemetic, 5-HT$_3$-antagonist
  ↑ ALT, AST, GMT

Opioids
(opiates)
> ↑ epinephrine, aldosterone, ALT, AST, AMS, CK, G, GMT, K, cortisol, lipase, norepinephrine, renin
> ↓ TSH
> ■ *Urine* ↓ volume

Oprelvekin *(oprelvekinum, oprelvekin, oprelvekine)*
thrombopoietic growth factor
> ↓ K

Oral Contraceptives
> ↑ AAT, N-acetyl-B-glucosamidase, PLT adhesion, aldosterone, ALP, ALP (neu), ALT, A2MG, AMS, ANA, angiotensin I, II, angiotensinogen, Apo A-I (high dose estrogen), Apo B, Apo E, APTT, AST, AT III, beta-1c-globulin, beta-glucuronidase, beta-1-LP, Bil, conjugated Bil, ceruloplasmin, CBG, C-peptide, CRP, Cu, DHT, diazepam, estrogens, factors – (II, V, VII, VIII, IX, X, XII), Fe, phenytoin, ferritin, fibrinogen, G, GFR, GMT, Hb, HCT, HDL cholesterol, cholesterol, chylomicrons, insulin, calcitonin, C_3 complement, coproporphyrin, corticosteroids, cortisol, creatinine, LA, LAP, LD, LDL cholesterol, LE cells, WBC, lipase, lipids, LP, MCHC, MCV, Na, OCT, orosomucoid, oxytocin, P, PL, plasmin, plasminogen, prealbumin, PRL, protein C, RBP, rT_3, renin, Se, SHBG, GH, T_3, T_4, TAG, TBG, testosterone, theophylline, TIBC, transcortin, transferrin, transthyretin, PLT, vitamin A, VLDL cholesterol, FFA, free cortisol
> ↓ plasminogen activator, albumin, ALP, androstenedione, Apo A-I (low dose estrogen), AT III, beta-endorphins, Ca, CK, CRP, DHEA, DHEAS, RBC, estradiol, factor – (XIII), fibrinogen, FSH, G, GMT, G tolerance, haptoglobin, Hb, HDL cholesterol (low dose estrogen), 17-OH progesterone, 17-OHCS, cholesterol, CHS, IgA, IgG, IgM, plasminogen activator inhibitor, carotenoids, 17-KS, LDL cholesterol, LH, WBC, LP(a), MAO, Mg, Mn, orosomucoid, P, PT, progesterone, protein S, renin, testosterone, PLT, vitamins – (B_1, B_2, B_6, B_{12}, C, folate), free testosterone, Zn
> ■ *Urine* ↑ ALA, coproporphyrin, PBG, uroporphyrin, free cortisol
> ↓ Ca, estradiol, estriol, estrogens, FSH, 17-KGS, 17-KS, 17-OHCS, LH, Mg, pregnanediol, UBG

Orlistat *(orlistatum, orlistat, orlistat)*
lipase inhibitor
> ■ *Stool* ↑ fat

Orotic Acid *(acidum oroticum, orotic acid, acide orotique)*
uricosuric, metabolic, treatment of liver disorders
> ↓ uric acid

Orphenadrine *(orphenadrinum, orphenadrine, orphénadrine)*
M receptor antagonist, skeletal muscle relaxant, antiparkinsonic
> ↑ T_4

Osmotic Diuretics
> ↑ K, MAC, Na, urea
> ↓ K, Na
> ■ *Urine* ↑ chloride, Na
> ↓ osmolality, specific gravity

Oxacillin *(oxacillinum, oxacillin, oxacilline)*
    antibiotic
        ↑ ALP, ALT, AST, proteins, Bil, eos, GMT, K, creatinine, LD, lym, urea
        ↓ PLT, WBC, neu
        ■ *Urine* ↑ proteins, Hb, 17-KS
Oxametacin *(oxametacinum, oxametacin, oxamétacine)*
    antibiotic
        ↓ factors – (II, VII, X)
Oxandrolone *(oxandrolonum, oxandrolone, oxandrolone)*
    anabolic, lipid lowering agent
        ↑ ALP, ALT
        ↓ T4, TBG
Oxaprozin *(oxaprozinum, oxaprozin, oxaprozine)*
    antiinflammatory
        ↑ ALP, AST, GMT, urea
        ↓ PLT, WBC
        ■ *Urine* ↑ blood, Hb, RBC
Oxazepam *(oxazepamum, oxazepam, oxazépam)*
    anxiolytic, sedative
        ↑ ALP, ALT, AST, Bil, G, GMT
        ↓ cortisol
        ■ *Urine* ↓ G
Oxcarbazepine *(oxcarbazepinum, oxcarbazepine, oxcarbazépine)*
    anticonvulsant
        ↑ eos
        ↓ Na, osmolality
Oxprenolol *(oxprenololum, oxprenolol, oxprénolol)*
    beta-adrenergic blocker
        ↑ P, GH, TAG
        ↓ GFR, HDL cholesterol, renin, PLT, FFA
        ■ *Urine* ↑ 5-HIAA
Oxycodone *(oxycodonum, oxycodone, oxycodone)*
    opioid analgesic
        ↓ Na
Oxymetholone *(oxymetholonum, oxymetholone, oxymétholone)*
    anabolic, androgen
        ↑ AAT, ALP, ALT, AST, Bil, fibrinogen, GMT, haptoglobin, cholesterol,
          orosomucoid, TAG, TBG
        ↓ Fe, G
        ■ *Urine* ↓ 17-OHCS, 17-KS
Oxyphenbutazone *(oxyphenbutazonum, oxyphenbutazone, oxyphenbutazone)*
    non-steroid antiinflammatory, antirheumatic
        ↑ ALP, ALT, AMS, AST, Bil, G, GMT, chloride, creatinine, uric acid, MAC,
          Na, plasma volume, RAL, urea
        ↓ factors – (II, VII, X), G, Hb, uric acid, WBC, neu, T4, PLT
        ■ *Urine* ↑ proteins, crystals – (uric acid)
          ↓ volume
        ■ *Stool* ↑ Hb

Oxyphencyclimine (*oxyphencyciliminum, oxyphencyclimine, oxyphencycline*)
    anticholinergic, spasmolytic
           ■ ***Gastric Fluid*** ↓ HCl
Oxyphenisatine (*oxyphenisatinum, oxyphenisatine, oxyphénisatine*)
    laxative
           ↑ ALP, ALT, AMA, ANA, AST, Bil, LE cells
           ↓ albumin, coagulation factors
Oxytetracycline (*oxytetracyclinum, oxytetracycline, oxytétracycline*)
    antibiotic
           ↑ catecholamines
           ↓ G, TAG, PLT
           ■ ***Urine*** ↑ G, catecholamines, porphyrins, VMA
             ↓ G
           ■ ***Cerebrospinal Fluid*** ↑ proteins
Oxytocin (*oxytocinum, oxytocin, oxytocine*)
    oxytocic
           ↑ plasma volume
           ↓ ACTH, Na, osmolality

Paclitaxel (*paclitaxelum, paclitaxel, paclitaxel*)
    antineoplastic
           ↑ ALT, AST, GMT
           ↓ neu, PLT, WBC
Palivizumab (*palivizumabum, palivizumab, palivizumab*)
    monoclonal antibody
           ↑ ALT, AST, GMT
Pamidronate (*pamicogrelum, pamicogrel, pamicogrel*)
    agent affecting calcium/bone metabolism
           ↑ PTH
           ↓ ALP, Ca, K, lym, Mg, P, WBC
Pancreozymin (*pancreozyminum, pancreozymin, pancreozymin*)
    diagnostic agent
           ↑ AMS, G, insulin, uric acid, lipase
           ■ ***Urine*** ↑ uric acid
Pancuronium (*pancuronii bromidum, pancuronium bromide, bromure de pancuronium*)
    long acting non-depolarizing muscle relaxant
           ↑ Bil
           ↓ CHS
Pantoprazole (*pantoprazolum, pantoprazole, pantoprazole*)
    proton pump inhibitor
           ↑ ALT, AST, Bil, G, GMT
           ↓ PLT, WBC
Papaverine (*papaverinum, papaverine, papaverine*)
    spasmolytic, vasodilator
           ↑ ALA, ALP, ALT, AST, Bil, eos, G, GMT, MAC
           ↓ K
Paraaminobenzoic Acid (*acidum paraaminobenzoicum, paraaminobenzoic acid, acide paraaminobenzoique*)
    growth factor, sunscreen agent, antirickettsial
           ↑ ALT
           ↓ neu

Paracetamol *(paracetamolum, paracetamol, paracétamol)*
analgesic, antipyretic

↑ ALP, ALT, AMS, AST, Bil, G, GMT, histamine, IgE, creatinine, uric acid, lipase, 5-nucleotidase, RTC, urea

↓ factors – (II, VII, X), G, GMT, Hb, Na, neu, P, PLT

■ *Urine* ↑ proteins, 5-HIAA

Paraldehyde *(paraldehydum, paraldehyde, paraldehyde)*
hypnotic, anticonvulsant

↑ ALP, Bil, G, MAC, urea

↓ HCO_3^-, pCO_2, pH

■ *Urine* ↑ proteins, 17-OHCS, ketones, 17-KGS, corticosteroids

Paramethadione *(paramethadionum, paramethadione, paraméthadione)*
anticonvulsant, antiepileptic

↑ ALP, ALT, AST, Bil, GMT, cholesterol, creatinine, urea

↓ Ca, WBC, PLT, vitamin D3

■ *Urine* ↑ proteins

Parathyroid Hormone

↑ Ca, Mg, PRL

↓ P

■ *Urine* ↑ HCO_3^-, hydroxyproline, chloride, volume, pH

Paricalcitol *(paricalcitolum, paricalcitol, paricalcitol)*
vitamin D2 analog

↑ Ca, P

Paromomycin *(paromomycinum, paromomycin, paromomycine)*
antiamebic (antibiotic)

↑ ALT, creatinine, urea

↓ cholesterol

■ *Urine* ↑ proteins

Paroxetine *(paroxetinum, paroxetine, paroxétine)*
antidepressant

↑ ALP, ALT, Bil, G, cholesterol

↓ Ca, G, Hb, K, WBC, Na

■ *Urine* ↑ blood, volume

↓ volume

■ *Seminal Fluid* ↓ spermatozoa count

Pefloxacin *(pefloxacinum, pefloxacin, péfloxacine)*
antibacterial

↓ neu, PLT

Pegaspargase *(pegaspargasum, pegaspargase, pégaspargase)*
antineoplastic

↓ insulin

Pemoline *(pemolinum, pemoline, pémoline)*
sympathomimetic

↑ ALT, AST, GMT

Penicillamine *(penicillaminum, penicillamine, pénicillamine)*
chelating agent

↑ ALP, ALT, AMS, ANA, anti-DNA Ab, antiinsulin Ab, AST, Bil, CK, eos, GMT, cholesterol, creatinine, LD, LE cells, WBC, pCO_2, PLT, 5-nucleotidase, urea, Zn

↓ ALP, Cu, cystine, digoxin, G, GFR, Hb, cholesterol, IgA, WBC, neu, pO_2, PLT, vitamin B6

■ *Urine* ↑ albumin, amino acids, Cu, proteins, Hb, blood, RBC

Penicillin G *(benzylpenicillinum, benzyl penicillin, benzylpénicilline)*
    antibiotic
        ↑ ALP, ALT, ANA, antineutrophil Ab, AST, Bil, CK, BT, eos, GMT, creatinine, uric acid, WBC, MAL, Na, 5-nucleotidase, PTT, urea
        ↓ PLT aggregation, albumin, proteins, Bil, estriol, factors – (II, VII, X), folate, GFR, Hb, IgA, K, WBC, neu, T3, T4, PLT
        ■ *Urine* ↑ blood, proteins, RBC, G, Hb, K, DALA, 17-OHCS, 17-KGS, 17-KS
         ↓ estrogens, pus, blood, casts – (hyaline), volume
        ■ *Cerebrospinal Fluid* ↑ proteins

Pentagastrin *(pentagastrinum, pentagastrin, pentagastrine)*
    diagnostic aid
        ↑ calcitonin, PRL, GH
        ■ *Urine* ↑ histamine
        ■ *Gastric Fluid* ↑ pepsin

Pentamidine *(pentamidinum, pentamidine, pentamidine)*
    antiprotozoal, antimicrobial
        ↑ ALT, AMS, AST, G, GMT, insulin, K, creatinine, lipase, MCV, urea
        ↓ Ca, C-peptide, G, insulin, WBC, Mg, PLT, vitamin – (B₁₂, folate)
        ■ *Urine* ↑ Hb

Pentazocine *(pentazocinum, pentazocine, pentazocine)*
    analgesic
        ↑ epinephrine, AMS, lipase, norepinephrine
        ↓ WBC, neu, pH
        ■ *Urine* ↑ PBG, porphyrins
         ↓ 17-OHCS

Pentetrazol *(pentetrazolum, pentetrazol, pentétrazol)*
    analeptic, central stimulant
        ↓ cholesterol

Pentobarbital *(pentobarbitalum, pentobarbital, pentobarbital)*
    hypnotic
        ↓ PLT, theophylline

Pentosan *(natrii pentosani polysulfas, pentosan polysulfate sodium, pentosane polysulfate sodique)*
    urinary analgesic
        ↑ ALT, AST, GMT
        ↓ PLT

Pentostatin *(pentostatinum, pentostatin, pentostatine)*
    antiviral
        ↑ ALT, AST, CK, eos, gamma globulins, GMT, creatinine, MAC, urea
        ↓ cholesterol, Na, neu, PLT, WBC
        ■ *Urine* ↑ albumin, G, volume
         ↓ volume

Pentoxifylline *(pentoxifyllinum, pentoxifylline, pentoxifylline)*
    vasodilator
        ↓ Hb, WBC

Perazine *(perazinum, perazine, perazine)*
    neuroleptic
        ↑ ALT, ANA, AST, GMT

Pergolide *(pergolidum, pergolide, pergolide)*
    dopamine agonist
        ↑ ALT, G, cholesterol, uric acid, MAC

     ↓ G, K, PRL
     ■ *Urine* ↑ pus, uric acid
Perhexiline *(perhexilinum, perhexiline, perhexiline)*
 coronary vasodilator
     ↑ ALT
     ↓ G

Perindopril *(perindoprilum, perindopril, périndopril)*
 ACE inhibitor, antihypertensive
     ↑ ACE, ALT, AST, AT I, GMT, K, renin, urea
     ↓ aldosterone, AT II, GFR, neu, WBC

Perphenazine *(perphenazinum, perphenazine, perphénazine)*
 neuroleptic, antiemetic
     ↑ ALP, ANA, CK, eos, G, catecholamines, PRL, T3, T4, TAG, TBG, WBC
     ↓ G tolerance, HDL cholesterol, PLT, TBG, WBC

Pethidine *(pethidinum, pethidine, péthidine)*
 narcotic analgesic, spasmolytic
     ↑ G, pCO$_2$
     ↓ pO$_2$, PLT
     ■ *Urine* ↓ 17-OHCS, 17-KS

Phenacemide *(phenacemidum, phenacemide, phénacémide)*
 anticonvulsant, antiepileptic
     ↑ ALP, ALT, Bil, creatinine
     ↓ creatinine, neu
     ■ *Urine* ↑ proteins

Phenacetin *(phenacetinum, phenacetin, phénacétine)*
 analgesic, antipyretic
     ↑ ALT, Heinz bodies (RBC), creatinine, MCV, MHb, urea
     ↓ folate, Hb, neu, PLT
     ■ *Urine* ↑ red color, G, Hb, 5-HIAA
       ↓ creatinine
     ■ *Cerebrospinal Fluid* ↑ proteins

Phenazone *(phenazonum, phenazone, phénazone)*
 analgesic, antipyretic, antirheumatic
     ↑ Bil, G, GMT, MHb, RTC
     ↓ Hb, WBC, neu, PLT
     ■ *Urine* ↑ redish brown color, G, Hb, WBC

Phenazopyridine *(phenazopyridinum, phenazopyridine, phénazopyridine)*
 urinary analgesic and antiseptic, diagnostic aid
     ↑ ALT, AST, Bil, conjugated Bil, eos, GMT, Heinz bodies (RBC), MHb
     ↓ GFR, Hb
     ■ *Urine* ↑ proteins, ketones

Phencyclidine *(phencyclidinum, phencyclidine, phencyclidine)*
 analgesic, anesthetic
     ↑ CK

Phenelzine *(phenelzinum, phenelzine, phénelzine)*
 MAO inhibitor, antidepressant
     ↑ ALP, ALT, ANA, AST, Bil, conjugated Bil, G, GMT
     ↓ CHS

Pheneturide *(pheneturidum, pheneturide, phénéturide)*
 anticonvulsant, antiepileptic
     ↓ Ca

Phenformin *(phenforminum, phenformin, phenformine)*
oral hypoglycemic

↑ AMS, folate, K, LA, lipase, MAC, TAG

↓ G, HCO_3^-, cholesterol, insulin, coagulation factors, pCO_2, pH, TAG, vitamin – (B_{12}, folate)

■ *Urine* ↑ ketones

Phenindione *(phenindionum, phenindione, phénindione)*
anticoagulant

↑ ALP, ALT

↓ neu

Phenmetrazine *(phenmetrazinum, phenmetrazine, phenmétrazine)*
anorexic

■ *Urine* ↑ epinephrine, 5-HIAA

Phenobarbital *(phenobarbitalum, phenobarbital, phénobarbital)*
anticonvulsant, antiepileptic, hypnotic, sedative

↑ ALA, ALP, ALT, Apo A-I, Apo B, AST, Bil, conjugated Bil, ceruloplasmin, Cu, factors – (II, VII, X), GMT, HDL cholesterol, cholesterol, LA, RBP, TSH

↓ Apo B, Bil, Ca, cyclosporine, Cu, digitoxin, phenytoin, FSH, FT4, cholesterol, quinidine, insulin, carbamazepine, carnitine, creatinine, LDL cholesterol, LH, WBC, P, T3, T4, theophylline, PLT, TSH, vitamin – (B_6, biotin, D3, E, folate), Zn, bile acids

■ *Urine* ↑ amino acids, 5-HIAA, hydroxyproline

↓ G, 17-OHCS

Phenolphthalein *(phenolphthaleinum, phenolphthalein, phénolphthaléine)*
laxative, indicator

↑ G, LE cells

↓ K, coagulation factors, PLT

■ *Urine* ↑ acetoacetate, proteins, estrogens, red color

↓ estriol, estrogens

Phenothiazines

↑ ADH, ALP, ALT, anti-La Ab, AST, Bil, conjugated Bil, unconjugated Bil, eos, FT4, G, GMT, cholesterol, catecholamines, uric acid, LD, OCT, PRL, T3, T4, TBG, TSH

↓ DHT, phenytoin, G, G tolerance, FSH, Hb, HDL cholesterol, CHS, K, uric acid, LH, WBC, Na, neu, P, SHBG, GH, testosterone, PLT, free testosterone, urea

■ *Urine* ↑ Bil, estriol, G, 17-OHCS, hCG, homogentisic acid, 5-HIAA, 17-KS, metanephrines, volume

↓ estrogens, gonadotropins, 5-HIAA, 17-OHCS, 17-KGS, 17-KS, pregnanediol, VMA

Phenoxybenzamine *(phenoxybenzaminum, phenoxybenzamine, phénoxybenzamine)*
vasodilator, antihypertensive alpha-adrenergic blocker

↑ ADH

↓ Na

Phentolamine *(phentolaminum, phentolamine, phentolamine)*
short-acting alpha-adrenoreceptor blocking agent, antihypertensive

↑ insulin, catecholamines

↓ G, TSH

■ *Urine* ↑ 5-HIAA

Phenylbutazone *(phenylbutazonum, phenylbutazone, phénylbutazone)*
antirheumatic, non-steroid antiinflammatory

↑ ALP, ALT, AMS, ANA, AST, Bil, eos, phenytoin, ESR, G, GMT, chloride, immunoglobulins, creatinine, uric acid, LD, MAC, Na, plasma volume, pH, RAL, TSH, urea

↓ PLT aggregation, digitoxin, digoxin, factors – (II, VII, X), FT4, G, Hb, uric acid, WBC, neu, T3, T4, PLT

■ *Urine* ↑ blood, Hb, proteins, RBC, LD, PBG, porphyrins
↓ 17-OHCS, volume

■ *Stool* ↑ Hb

Phenylephrine *(phenylephrinum, phenylephrine, phényléphrine)*
alpha-1-adrenoceptor agonist, vasoconstrictor

↑ G

■ *Urine* ↑ amino acids, metanephrines

Phenylhydrazine *(phenylhydrazinum, phenylhydrazine, phenylhydrazine)*
agent for destroying erythrocytes

↑ Heinz bodies (RBC)

↓ haptoglobin, Hb

Phenylpropanolamine *(phenylpropanolaminum, phenylpropanolamine, phénylpropano-lamine)*
indirectly acting sympathomimetic amine, vasoconstrictor, nasal decongestant

■ *Urine* ↑ amino acids

Phenytoin *(phenytoinum, phenytoin, phénytoine)*
anticonvulsant, antiepileptic

↑ ALA, ALP, ALT, ANA, Apo A-I, APTT, AST, Bil, ceruloplasmin, CK, Cu, eos, estradiol, factors – (II, VII, X), FSH, FT4, G, GMT, G tolerance, HDL cholesterol, homocysteine, cholesterol, CHS, IgE, IgG, corticosteroids, creatinine, uric acid, LD, LE cells, LH, WBC, lym, MCV, MHb, 5-nucleo-tidase, OCT, P, PRL, PTH, RBP, SHBG, GH, T3, T4, TAG, testosterone, transcortin, TSH, urea, vitamin A, free cortisol

↓ ADH, albumin, Apo B, beta-1c-globulin, Ca, Ca^{2+}, cyclosporine, Cu, 11-deoxycortisol, DHEA, DHEAS, digitoxin, digoxin, FT3, FT4, GMT, G tolerance, Hb, quinidine, IgA, IgE, IgG, IgM, insulin, calcitonin, carbamazepine, cortisol, LDL cholesterol, WBC, lym, Mg, neu, P, pO_2, GH, T3, T4, TBG, theophylline, PLT, vitamin – (B_6, B_{12}, biotin, D_3, E, folate), free testosterone, Zn

■ *Urine* ↑ acetoacetate, redish brown color
↓ Ca, 17-OHCS, 17-KS

■ *Cerebrospinal Fluid* ↑ 5-HIAA

Phosphates

↑ Na, P, PTH

↓ ALP, Ca, Ca^{2+}, K

■ *Urine* ↑ crystals
↓ Mg

Phytate *(phytatum, phytate, phytate)*
tonic, hypocalcemic

↓ Ca, Fe, P, Zn

Phytomenadione *(phytomenadionum, phytomenadione, phytoménadione)*
prothrombogenic vitamin

↑ factors – (II, VII, X)

Pilocarpine *(pilocarpinum, pilocarpine, pilocarpine)*
    parasympathomimetic, miotic
          ↑ Hb, WBC
          ■ *Gastric Fluid* ↑ HCl

Pimozide *(pimozidum, pimozide, pimozide)*
    neuroleptic, antipsychotic
          ↑ PRL, TSH
          ↓ FSH, LH

Pinacidil *(pinacidilum, pinacidil, pinacidil)*
    antihypertensive, peripheral vasodilator
          ↑ HDL cholesterol
          ↓ cholesterol, LDL cholesterol, TAG

Pindolol *(pindololum, pindolol, pindolol)*
    non-selective beta-adrenergic receptor antagonist
          ↑ ALT, AST, CK, CK-MB, GMT, HDL cholesterol, cholesterol, K, LE cells,
            P, TAG
          ↓ apolipoprotein B, G, glucagon, HDL-C, LDL cholesterol, neu, PTH,
            renin, TAG
          ■ *Urine* ↑ 5-HIAA

Pioglitazone *(pioglitazonum, pioglitazone, pioglitazone)*
    oral hypoglycemic
          ↑ G
          ↓ G

Pipecuronium *(pipecuronii bromidum, pipecuronium bromide, bromure de pipécuronium)*
    skeletal muscle relaxant
          ↑ G, K

Piperacillin *(piperacillinum, piperacillin, pipéracilline)*
    antibiotic
          ↑ ALT, AST, Bil, BT, eos, GMT, cholesterol, creatinine, LD, OCT
          ↓ PLT aggregation, K, uric acid, LD, WBC, neu

Piperidines
          ↓ Ca^{2+}
          ■ *Urine* ↑ 17-OHCS, 17-KS

Pirazolac *(pirazolacum, pirazolac, pirazolac)*
    anticonvulsant, tranquilizer
          ↓ ESR

Pirenzepine *(pirenzepinum, pirenzepine, pirenzépine)*
    treatment of peptic ulcer, antiemetic, M_1-receptor antagonist
          ↑ ALT, AST, GMT
          ↓ neu, GH, PLT

Piribedil *(piribedilum, piribedil, piribédil)*
    peripheral vasodilator
          ↓ PRL, TSH

Piromidic Acid *(acidum piromidicum, piromidic acid, acide piromidique)*
    antibacterial
          ↑ creatinine

Piroxicam *(piroxicamum, piroxicam, piroxicam)*
    non-steroid antiinflammatory
          ↑ ALP, ALT, AST, Bil, BT, GMT, K, creatinine, lithium, WBC, urea
          ↓ PLT aggregation, haptoglobin, Hb, PLT
          ■ *Urine* ↑ blood, Hb, RBC, proteins

- **Stool** ↑ Hb

Pirprofen *(pirprofenum, pirprofen, pirprofen)*
non-steroid antiinflammatory
↑ ALT, Bil

Pivampicillin *(pivampicillinum, pivampicillin, pivampicilline)*
antibiotic
↓ carnitine, G

Pivmecillinam *(pivmecillinamum, pivmecillinam, pivmécillinam)*
antibiotic
↓ carnitine, G

Plicamycin *(plicamycinum, plicamycin, plicamycine)*
antineoplastic
↑ ALA, ALP, ALT, AST, BT, GMT, LD, OCT, urea
↓ Ca, factor – (V), Mg, neu, P, PLT, WBC
- **Urine** ↑ Hb

Polyestradiol Phosphate *(polyestradioli phosphas, polyestradiol phosphate, phosphate de polyestradiol)*
estrogen
↑ HDL
↓ TAG

Polymethyl-Methacrylate *(polymethyl-methacrylatum, polymethyl-methacrylate, poly-methyl-methacrylate)*
stomatological agent
↑ GMT

Polymyxin B *(polymyxinum B, polymyxin B, polymyxine B)*
antibiotic
↑ ammonia, creatinine, urea
↓ Ca, K, Na
- **Urine** ↑ albumin, ALP, amino acids, blood, proteins, Hb, casts, RBC

Polythiazide *(polythiazidum, polythiazide, polythiazide)*
salidiuretic, antihypertensive
↑ BE, Ca, G, uric acid
↓ G tolerance, chloride, K, Na, osmolality
- **Urine** ↑ G

Potassium Chloride *(kalii chloridum, potassium chloride, chlorure de potassium)*
potassium deficiency, digitalis poisoning therapy
↑ aldosterone, chloride, K
↓ G, renin, vitamin B_{12}
- **Urine** ↑ blood, Hb, RBC

Potassium Citrate *(kalii citras, potassium citrate, citrate de potassium)*
purgative, mild diuretic
↑ aldosterone
↓ renin

Potassium Iodide *(kalii iodidum, potassium iodide, iodid de potassium)*
expectorans
↑ aldosterone, AMS, eos, TSH
↓ renin, T_3, T_4, PLT
- **Urine** ↑ 17-OHCS, corticosteroids

Practolol *(practololum, practolol, practolol)*
selective beta-1-adrenoceptor antagonist
↑ ALP, ANA, Bil, LE cells, TAG

Prasterone *(prasteronum, prasterone, prastérone)*
adrenocortical hormone with psychotonic and antidepressant action
- ↑ ALT, AST, GMT
- ↓ LDL cholesterol

Pravastatin *(pravastatinum, pravastatin, pravastatine)*
HMG-CoA reductase inhibitor, lipid lowering agent
- ↑ ALT, Apo A-I, AST, CK, GMT, HDL cholesterol, TAG
- ↓ Apo B, cholesterol, LDL cholesterol, TAG, VLDL cholesterol

Praziquantel *(praziquantelum, praziquantel, praziquantel)*
anthelmintic
- ↑ ALT

Prazosin *(prazosinum, prazosin, prazosine)*
alpha-adrenoceptor blocker, antihypertensive, vasodilator
- ↑ ANA, G, HDL cholesterol, insulin, uric acid, lipoprotein lipase, norepinephrine, renin, T4, TSH, FFA
- ↓ aldosterone, ANP, Apo B, G, G tolerance, cholesterol, insulin, K, LDL cholesterol, renin, TAG, VLDL cholesterol
- ■ *Urine* ↑ metanephrines, VMA

Prednisolone *(prednisolonum, prednisolone, prednisolone)*
glucocorticoid
- ↑ AMS, cyclosporine, Cu, G, cholesterol, insulin, cortisol, MAL, Na, TAG, transthyretin
- ↓ Ca, Ca²⁺, G tolerance, HDL cholesterol, chloride, K, P, PLT, T3, TBG, Zn
- ■ *Urine* ↓ G

Prednisone *(prednisonum, prednisone, prednisone)*
glucocorticoid
- ↑ AMS, Apo A-I, C-peptide, G, GFR, HDL cholesterol, HCO₃⁻, cholesterol, insulin, cortisol, uric acid, WBC, MAL, mono, Na, neu, PTH, TAG, TSH, vitamin D3
- ↓ ACE, albumin, ALP, androstenedione, Bil, Ca, CK, DHEA, eos, estradiol, FT3, G tolerance, K, cortisol, WBC, lym, osteocalcin, T3, TBG, testosterone, PLT
- ■ *Urine* ↑ proteins

Pregnanediol *(pregnanediolum, pregnanediol, pregnanediol)*
progesterone metabolite
- ↑ unconjugated Bil

Prilocaine *(prilocainum, prilocaine, prilocaine)*
local anesthetic
- ↑ MHb

Primaquine *(primaquinum, primaquine, primaquine)*
antimalarial
- ↑ Bil, WBC, MHb, Heinz bodies (RBC)
- ↓ haptoglobin, Hb, neu, WBC
- ■ *Urine* ↑ blood, Hb, RBC

Primidone *(primidonum, primidone, primidone)*
anticonvulsant, antiepileptic
- ↑ ANA, GMT, LE cells
- ↓ Ca, FT4, carbamazepine, WBC, neu, T4, PLT, vitamin – (B6, B12, biotin, folate, D, E), free testosterone
- ■ *Urine* ↑ amino acids, crystals

Probenecid *(probenecidum, probenecid, probénécide)*
uricosuric

 ↑ ALP, ALT, AST, Bil, GMT, paracetamol, urea
 ↓ G, Hb, coagulation factors, 17-KS, uric acid, WBC
 ■ *Urine* ↑ blood, RBC, proteins, G, Hb, uric acid
  ↓ estriol, 17-KS

Probucol *(probucolum, probucol, probucol)*
lipid lowering agent

 ↑ ALP, ALT, AST, CK, eos, G, GMT, HCO$_3$, uric acid, urea, vitamin A
 ↓ Apo A-I, Apo B, Ca, HDL-C, cholesterol, LDL-C, GH, PLT, TAG

Procainamide *(procainamidum, procainamide, procainamide)*
cardiac depressant, antiarrhythmic

 ↑ ALP, ALT, ANA, antihistone Ab, AST, Bil, CK, digoxin, eos, ESR, GMT, K, LE cells, neu, RTC
 ↓ Apo A-I, Apo A-II, Apo B, bas, Bil, eos, haptoglobin, Hb, cholesterol, CHS, WBC, neu, TAG, PLT

Procaine *(procainum, procaine, procaine)*
local anesthetic, analgesic, geriatric

 ■ *Urine* ↑ PBG, UBG
 ■ *Cerebrospinal Fluid* ↑ proteins

Procarbazine *(procarbazinum, procarbazine, procarbazine)*
antineoplastic

 ↑ ALP, ALT, Bil, eos, Heinz bodies (RBC)
 ↓ digoxin, Hb, neu, WBC, PLT
 ■ *Urine* ↑ blood
 ■ *Stool* ↑ Hb
 ■ *Seminal Fluid* ↓ spermatozoa count

Prochlorperazine *(prochlorperazinum, prochlorperazine, prochlorpérazine)*
antiemetic, neuroleptic

 ↑ ALP, ALT, AST, Bil, CK, eos, GMT, cholesterol, PRL, WBC
 ↓ WBC, neu, PLT
 ■ *Urine* ↑ 17-KS
  ↓ 5-HIAA

Progabide *(progabidum, progabide, progabide)*
anticonvulsant, antiepileptic, gabamimetic

 ↑ ALT, AST

Progesterone *(progesteronum, progesterone, progestérone)*
naturally-occurring progestogen

 ↑ albumin, ALP, ALT, Apo B, AST, proteins, Bil, Ca, cystine, factors – (VII), G, GMT, HDL cholesterol, cholesterol, immunoglobulins, corticosteroids, cortisol, melatonin, Mg, Na, progesterone, TBG
 ↓ AT III, bas, FSH, G, G tolerance, HDL cholesterol, cholesterol, LDL cholesterol, LH, PRL, TAG
 ■ *Urine* ↑ aldosterone
  ↓ 17-OHCS, pregnanediol

Progestogens

 ↑ ALP, ALT, AST, Bil
 ↓ Apo A-I, Apo B, HDL cholesterol, cholesterol, LP(a), TAG
 ■ *Urine* ↑ ALA, porphyrins

Promazine *(promazini chloridum, promazine chloride, chlorure d´ promazine)*
neuroleptic

    ↑ ALP, AST, Bil, GMT, cholesterol, PRL

    ↓ PLT aggregation, coagulation factors, WBC, neu, PLT

    ■ *Urine* ↑ proteins

       ↓ proteins, 5-HIAA, 17-OHCS, 17-KS

Promethazine *(promethazinum, promethazine, prométhazine)*
antihistaminic, antiemetic, sedative

    ↑ ALP, ANA, Bil, eos, G, catecholamines, PRL, WBC

    ↓ G, WBC, P

    ■ *Urine* ↑ hCG

       ↓ 5-HIAA, 17-OHCS, corticosteroids

Propafenone *(propafenonum, propafenone, propafénone)*
antiarrhythmic

    ↑ ALP, ALT, digoxin, G, theophylline

    ↓ factors – (II, VII, X), Na

Propanidid *(propanididum, propanidid, propanidide)*
anesthetic

    ↓ bas

    ■ *Gastric Fluid* ↑ HCl

Propantheline *(propanthelini bromidum, propantheline bromide, bromure de propanthé-line)*
anticholinergic, spasmolytic

    ↑ digoxin

    ↓ G, GH

Propionate Sodium *(natrii propionas, propionate sodium, propionate de sodium)*
antifungal

    ↓ G

Propofol *(propofolum, propofol, propofol)*
general anesthetic, very short-acting intravenous anesthetic

    ↑ G, K, creatinine, lipids, MAC, osmolality, TAG, urea

    ■ *Urine* ↓ volume

Propoxyphene *(dextropropoxyphenum, dextropropoxyphene, dextropropoxyphéne)*
analgesic

    ↑ ALP, ALT, AST, GMT, carbamazepine, LD

    ↓ G

    ■ *Urine* ↓ 17-OHCS, 17-KS

Propranolol *(propranololum, propranolol, propranolol)*
beta-adrenergic blocker

    ↑ PLT aggregation, ALP, ALT, AST, proteins, Bil, CK, BT, FT_4, G, GMT, HbA_{1c}, HDL-C, cholesterol, insulin, K, catecholamines, uric acid, LH (males), PRL (males), rT_3, GH, T_4, TAG, theophylline, PLT, urea, VLDL-C

    ↓ PLT aggregation, aldosterone, ALP, Ca, C-peptide, FT_3, FT_4, G, GFR, G tolerance, glucagon, Hb, HDL-C, cholesterol, insulin, K, cortisol, LDL-C, LH (females), neu, norepinephrine, PRL, PTH, renin, T_3, T_4, TAG, TBG, urea, FFA

    ■ *Urine* ↓ hydroxyproline

    ■ *Gastric Fluid* ↓ HCl

    ■ *Seminal Fluid* ↓ spermatozoa count

Propylthiouracil (*propylthiouracilum, propylthiouracil, propylthiouracil*)
thyroid-inhibitor
      ↑ ALP, ALT, AMS, ANA, AST, Bil, factors – (II, VII, X), G, GMT, IgA, IgG,
        IgM, uric acid, T4, TSH, urea
      ↓ Ca, factors – (II, VII, X), Hb, WBC, neu, T3, T4, PLT, TSH, FFA

Propyphenazone (*propyphenazonum, propyphenazone, propyphénazone*)
analgesic, antipyretic
      ↓ neu

Proquazone (*proquazonum, proquazone, proquazone*)
antiinflammatory, analgesic
      ↓ uric acid

Prostaglandin E2 (*prostaglandinum E2, prostaglandin E2, prostaglandin E2*)
oxytocic, abortifacient, vasodilator, smooth muscle stimulant
      ↑ T3, T4
      ↓ insulin, TAG
      ■ *Sweat* ↑   chloride

Protamine Sulfate (*protamini sulfas, protamine sulfate, sulfate de protamine*)
heparin antagonist
      ↑ catecholamines, lipids
      ↓ lipase, LP lipase

Protionamide (*protionamidum, protionamide, protionamide*)
tuberculostatic
      ↑ ALP, ALT, Bil
      ↓ G

Protirelin (*protirelinum, protirelin, protiréline*)
thyrotropin-releasing hormone, diagnostic
      ↑ epinephrine, norepinephrine, GH
      ↓ Ca

Protriptyline (*protriptylinum, protriptyline, protriptyline*)
antidepressant
      ↑ ALP, ALT, AST, eos, GMT
      ↓ WBC

Psychoactive Preparations
      ↑ G

Pyrazinamide (*pyrazinamidum, pyrazinamide, pyrazinamide*)
tuberculostatic
      ↑ ALP, ALT, AST, Bil, Fe, GMT, uric acid
      ↓ albumin, proteins, globulins, Hb, PLT
      ■ *Urine* ↑ ketones, 17-KS, crystals – (urate), PBG, porphyrins
        ↓ 17-KS

Pyrazinoic Acid (*acidum pyrazinoicum, pyrazinoic acid, acide pyrazinoique*)
antituberculotic
      ↓ vitamin B6

Pyricarbate (*pyricarbatum, pyricarbate, pyricarbate*)
antiarteriosclerotic
      ↑ ALT

Pyridostigmin (*pyridostigmini bromidum, pyridostigmine bromide, bromure de pyridostig-mine*)
acetylcholinesterase inhibitor, parasympathomimetic
      ↑ GH

Pyridoxine *(pyridoxinum, pyridoxine, pyridoxine)*
vitamin B$_6$
　　　↑ AST
　　　↓ folate, fructosamine, cholesterol, oxalate, TSH
Pyrimethamine *(pyrimethaminum, pyrimethamine, pyriméthamine)*
antimalarial, antibacterial
　　　↑ ALP, ALT, Bil
　　　↓ phenylalanine, folate, Hb, WBC, lym, neu, PLT

Quinacrine *(mepacrinum, mepacrine, mépacrine)*
antimalarial, anthelmintic
　　　↑ ALP, ALT, AST, Bil, GMT, 11-OHCS, cortisol
　　　■ *Urine* ↑ cortisol
Quinapril *(quinaprilum, quinapril, quinapril)*
antihypertensive, ACE inhibitor
　　　↑ ALT, ANA, AST, eos, ESR, K, creatinine, urea
　　　↓ granulocytes, neu, PLT
Quinethazone *(quinethazonum, quinethazone, quinéthazone)*
salidiuretic, antihypertensive
　　　↑ G, uric acid
Quinidine *(chinidinum, quinidine, quinidine)*
antiarrhythmic
　　　↑ ALP, ALT, ANA, AST, Bil, CK, digitoxin, digoxin, GMT, insulin, cat-
　　　echolamines (false), LD, LE cells, WBC, MAC, neu, RTC
　　　↓ Apo A-I, Apo A-II, Apo B, factors – (II, VII, X), G, haptoglobin, Hb, cho-
　　　lesterol, K, WBC, neu, TAG, PLT
　　　■ *Urine* ↑ Hb, 17-OHCS, catecholamines, 17-KS, corticosteroids
Quinine *(quininum, quinine, quinine)*
antimalarial, antipyretic, tonic bitter stomachic
　　　↑ ALP, ALT, AST, Bil, digoxin, GMT, insulin, catecholamines, creatinine
　　　↓ factors – (II, VII, X), ESR, G, neu, PLT
　　　■ *Urine* ↑ brown color, Hb, 17-OHCS, 17-KGS, corticosteroids

---

Rabeprazole *(rabeprazolum, rabeprazole, rabéprazole)*
gastric acid secretion inhibitor
　　　↑ ALT, AST, GMT
　　　↓ PLT, WBC
Ramipril *(ramiprilum, ramipril, ramipril)*
ACE inhibitor, antihypertensive
　　　↑ GFR, K, creatinine, renin, urea
　　　↓ ACE, AT II, G, Na
　　　■ *Urine* ↓ K, Na
Ranitidine *(ranitidinum, ranitidine, ranitidine)*
histamine H$_2$ receptor antagonist
　　　↑ ACTH, ALP, ALT, AST, Bil, eos, ethanol, phenytoin, gastrin, GMT, crea-
　　　tinine, PRL, procainamide, theophylline
　　　↓ aldosterone, FT4, HDL cholesterol, CHS, cortisol, creatinine, WBC, neu,
　　　PRL, PTH, serotonin, T4, theophylline, PLT, TSH, vitamin B$_{12}$
　　　■ *Urine* ↓ 5-HIAA
　　　■ *Gastric Fluid* ↑ Hb

Rauwolfia Derivatives

↑ Na, PRL
- ***Urine*** ↑ catecholamines
  ↓ 17-OHCS, catecholamines, 17-KS, VMA
- ***Stool*** ↑ blood

H2-Receptor Antagonists

↑ ACTH, ALP, ALT, AMS, androstenedione, AST, Bil, CK, cyclosporine, diazepam, digoxin, eos, estradiol (M), ethanol, factors – (II, VII, X), phenytoin, FSH, G, gastrin, GMT, HDL cholesterol, quinidine, IgA, IgG, imipramine, carbamazepine, creatinine, uric acid, salicylic acid, lipase, LH, WBC, LD, nortriptyline, PRL, procainamide, testosterone, theophylline, TSH, urea, valproate

↓ aldosterone, Ca, digoxin, estradiol, factors – (II, VII, X), FT4, G, Hb, HDL cholesterol, CHS, insulin, cortisol, creatinine, LDL cholesterol, WBC, Mg, neu, PRL, PTH, serotonin, T4, theophylline, SHBG, T3, testosterone, PLT, TSH, vitamin B_{12}

- ***Urine*** ↑ G
  ↓ 5-HIAA, vitamin B_{12}
- ***Gastric Fluid*** ↑ Hb
↓ HCl
- ***Seminal Fluid*** ↓ spermatozoa count

Remoxipride *(remoxipridum, remoxipride, rémoxipride)*
antipsychotic, neuroleptic
↑ ALT
↓ Hb

Repaglinide *(repaglinidum, repaglinide, répaglinide)*
oral hypoglycemic
↓ G

Reserpine *(reserpinum, reserpine, réserpine)*
antihypertensive, tranquilizer
↑ ALT, coagulation factors, Na, PRL
↓ G, coagulation factors (early), neu, renin, T4, PLT
- ***Urine*** ↑ 17-OHCS, 5-HIAA, HVA, VMA
  ↓ 5-HIAA, catecholamines, 17-OHCS, 17-KS, metanephrines, VMA
- ***Gastric Fluid*** ↑ HCl

Resorcinol *(resorcinolum, resorcinol, résorcinol)*
antiseptic, dermatic, keratolytic
↑ Heinz bodies (RBC), MHb
↓ haptoglobin

Reteplase *(reteplasum, reteplase, rétéplase)*
tissue plasminogen activator
- ***Urine*** ↑ blood, Hb, RBC

Retinoid *(retinoidum, retinoid, rétinoid)*
derivative of vitamin A
↑ ALP, ALT, AST, GMT, cholesterol, LD, LDL cholesterol, TAG
↓ HDL cholesterol

Retinol *(retinolum, retinol, rétinol)*
antixerophthalmic vitamin
↑ ALP, ALT, AST, Ca, ferritin, ESR, cholesterol, TAG, transthyretin
↓ coagulation factors, neu, T4

Ribavirin *(ribavirinum, ribavirin, ribavirine)*
    antiviral
            ↑ ALT, Bil
Riboflavin *(riboflavinum, riboflavin, riboflavine)*
    vitamin enzyme co-factor
            ↑ catecholamines
            ■ *Urine* ↑ catecholamines, urobilin
Rifabutin *(rifabutinum, rifabutin, rifabutine)*
    antibiotic
            ↑ ALT, GMT
            ↓ cyclosporine, neu, PLT
Rifampicin *(rifampicinum, rifampicin, rifampicine)*
    antituberculotic, antileprotic
            ↑ N-acetyl-B-glucosamidase, ALP, ALT, AMS, AST, Bil, C-peptide, eos, factors – (II, VII, X), G, GMT, insulin, creatinine, uric acid, P, PRL, PTH, T3, testosterone, PLT, TSH, urea, bile acids
            ↓ proteins, cyclosporine, cortisol, digitoxin, digoxin, phenytoin, FT4, G, GFR, Hb, hydrocortisone, quinidine, cholesterol, corticosteroids, cortisone, WBC, neu, T4, theophylline, PLT, vitamin D3
            ■ *Urine* ↑ proteins, orange color, Hb, blood, casts, RBC, porphyrins
Rifapentine *(rifapentinum, rifapentine, rifapentine)*
    antibiotic
            ↑ ALT, AST, GMT
            ↓ lym, neu, WBC
            ■ *Urine* ↑ blood, Hb, RBC
            ■ *Sputum* ↑ blood
Riluzole *(riluzolum, riluzole, riluzole)*
    neuroprotective
            ↑ ALT, AST, GMT
Rimiterol *(rimiterolum, rimiterol, rimitérol)*
    beta-2-adrenoceptor agonist, bronchodilator
            ↑ G
            ↓ Ca, K, corticosteroids, Mg, P
            ■ *Urine* ↑ acetoacetate
Risedronate *(acidum risedronicum, risedronic acid, acide risédronique)*
            ↓ Ca, P
Risperidone *(risperidonum, risperidone, rispéridone)*
    antipsychotic
            ↑ PRL
Ritodrine *(ritodrinum, ritodrine, ritodrine)*
    beta-adrenergic receptor stimulant, uterine smooth muscle relaxant
            ↑ ALT, AST, Bil, cAMP, G, GMT, insulin, LA, LD, WBC, MAC, placental lactogen, renin, T3, FFA
            ↓ Ca (neonates), estradiol, G (neonates), Hb, K, pH
Ritonavir *(ritonavirum, ritonavir, ritonavir)*
    antiviral
            ↑ ALT, AST, G, GMT, cholesterol, ketobodies, lipids, TAG
Rituximab *(rituximabum, rituximab, rituximab)*
    monoclonal antibody
            ↓ neu, pO_2, PLT, WBC

Rofexocib *(rofexocibum, rofexocib, roféxocib)*
   non-steroid antiinflammatory, analgesic
          ↑ ALT, AST, GMT
        ■ *Stool* ↑ blood
Rokitamycin *(rokitamycinum, rokitamycin, rokitamycine)*
   antibiotic
          ↑ ALT
Rosiglitazone *(rosiglitazonum, rosiglitazone, rosiglitazone)*
   oral hypoglycemic
          ↑ cholesterol, G
          ↓ G
Roxithromycin *(roxithromycinum, roxithromycin, roxithromycine)*
   antibiotic
          ↑ ALT

Salazosulfapyridine *(sulfasalazinum, sulfasalazine, sulfasalazine)*
   antibacterial (for colitis), antiarthritic
          ↑ ALP, ALT, AMS, ANA, AST, Bil, eos, GMT, Heinz bodies (RBC), LD, LE
           cells, WBC, lym, MCV, MHb, RTC, PLT
          ↓ digoxin, folate, haptoglobin, Hb, IgA, immunoglobulins, WBC, neu, PLT
Salbutamol *(salbutamolum, salbutamol, salbutamol)*
   beta-2-adrenoceptor agonist, bronchodilator, muscle relaxant
          ↑ G, HDL cholesterol, insulin, lym, norepinephrine, renin
          ↓ Ca, digoxin, estriol, K, corticosteroids, Mg, P, theophylline, PLT
        ■ *Urine* ↑ acetoacetate
Salicine *(salicinum, salicine, salicine)*
   antipyretic, antineuralgic
          ↑ ALT, AST
Salicylamide *(salicylamidum, salicylamide, salicylamide)*
   analgesic, antipyretic
          ↓ TSH
Salicylates
          ↑ ALP, ALT, AST, Bil, BT, Ca, FT4, G (early), chloride, cholesterol, ketones,
           creatinine, uric acid, LA, MAC (mainly children), MAL, PT, pyruvate,
           RAC, RAL, TBG, urea
          ↓ Ca^{2+}, G (later), HCO_3^-, K, uric acid, Na, pCO_2, pH, T3, T4, thrombin, PLT,
           TSH, vitamin – (folate, B_{12}), FFA
        ■ *Urine* ↑ amino acids, proteins, Hb, HCO_3^-, K, ketobodies, Na, reduc-
           ing substances, VMA
          ↓ estriol, G, 5-HIAA, hydroxyproline, catecholamines, 17-KS, pH, VMA
        ■ *Stool* ↑ blood
Salmeterol *(salmeterolum, salmeterol, salmétérol)*
   selective beta-2-adrenoceptor agonist
          ↑ G
          ↓ K
Salsalate *(salsalatum, salsalate, salsalate)*
   analgesic, antiinflammatory, antibacterial
          ↑ creatinine
          ↓ albumin, T3, T4
        ■ *Urine* ↑ proteins

Saquinavir *(saquinavirum, saquinavir, saquinavir)*
   antiviral
        ↑ cholesterol, G, ketobodies, lipids, TAG
        ↓ neu, PLT
Sargramostim *(sargramostimum, sargramostim, sargramostim)*
   immunomodulator
        ↑ Bil, creatinine, WBC
        ↓ pO_2
Secobarbital *(secobarbitalum, secobarbital, sécobarbital)*
   hypnotic, sedative
        ↑ CK, factors – (II, VII, X)
        ↓ PLT, theophylline
Secretin *(secretinum, secretin, sécrétine)*
   parasympathomimetic
        ↑ AMS, Ca, G, insulin, lipase, PRL
        ↓ amino acids, gastrin, glucagon
        ■ *Urine* ↑ HCO_3, Na
Sedatives
        ↑ GMT, HCO_3, MAC, MAC+RAC
Senna *(sennum, senna, senna)*
   laxative (glycosides from senna)
        ■ *Urine* ↑ estradiol, estrogens
           ↓ estrone
Sertraline *(sertralinum, sertraline, sertraline)*
   antidepressant
        ↑ ALT, AST, GMT, cholesterol, TAG
        ↓ G, Na, uric acid
        ■ *Urine* ↑ uric acid, volume
Sibutramine *(sibutraminum, sibutramine, sibutramine)*
   CNS stimulant/anorexiant
        ↑ ALT, AST, GMT
Simvastatin *(simvastatinum, simvastatin, simvastatine)*
   HMG-CoA-reductase inhibitor, hypolipidemic
        ↑ ACTH, ALP, ALT, Apo A-I, AST, CK, GFR, GMT, HDL-C
        ↓ Apo B, Apo E, cholesterol, LDL cholesterol, TAG, VLDL-C
Sinorphan *(sinorphanum, sinorphan, sinorphane)*
   enkephalinase inhibitor
        ↑ ANP
Sirolimus *(sirolimusum, sirolimus, sirolimus)*
   immunosuppressive, macrolide antibiotic
        ↑ cholesterol, lipids, TAG, urea
        ↓ K, PLT, WBC
Sodium Bicarbonate *(natrium hydrocarbonicum, sodium bicarbonate, bicarbonate de sodique)*
   antacid
        ↑ LA, MAC, MAL, Na, pH
        ↓ chloride, K
        ■ *Urine* ↑ proteins, pH, UBG
Sodium Chloride
        ↑ ANP, Ca^{2+}, plasma volume
        ↓ aldosterone, angiotensin II, Bil, G, insulin, K, uric acid, renin
        ■ *Urine* ↑ Ca, cortisol, Mg, Zn

Sodium Lactate

↑ MAL, Na

Sodium Polystyrene

↓ Ca, K

Sodium Salts

↑ Ca, Ca²⁺, HCO₃⁻, Na, pH

↓ aldosterone, chloride, K, renin

■ *Urine* ↑ Ca

↓ Ca

Somatostatin *(somatostatinum, somatostatin, somatostatine)*

growth hormone-release inhibiting factor

↑ G

↓ AMS, FT3, GFR, lipase, Na, T3, T4, TSH

■ *Urine* ↓ volume

■ *Stool* ↑ FA

Somatostatin Analogues

↓ somatomedin C, GH, TSH

Somatotropin *(somatotropinum, somatotropin, somatotropine)*

growth hormone

↑ ALP, proteins, Ca, C-peptide, G, HDL-C, cholesterol, insulin, K, LDL cholesterol, WBC, LP(a), Na, P, TAG, TSH, FFA, Zn

↓ Apo B, FT4, G, cholesterol, LDL-C, leucine, T3, T4, TAG, urea

■ *Urine* ↑ Ca²⁺, blood, RBC, Hb, G, hydroxyproline

Somatotropin *(somatotropinum, somatotropin, somatotropine)*

synthetic human growth hormone

↑ PRL, somatomedin C

Sorbitol *(sorbitolum, sorbitol, sorbitol)*

natural sugar

↑ Bil, G, LA, MAC

↓ Na, pyruvate

■ *Urine* ↑ volume

Sotalol *(sotalolum, sotalol, sotalol)*

non-selective beta-adrenoreceptor blocker

↑ ALT, AST, G, GMT, cholesterol, LDL cholesterol, TAG

↓ G, HDL cholesterol, K, FFA

■ *Urine* ↑ metanephrines

Sparfloxacin *(sparfloxacinum, sparfloxacin, sparfloxacine)*

DNA gyrase inhibitor

↑ urea

↓ PLT, WBC

Spectinomycin *(spectinomycinum, spectinomycin, spectinomycine)*

antibiotic

↑ ALP, urea

■ *Urine* ↓ volume

Spinal Anesthetics

■ *Urine* ↓ chloride, Na, volume, UBG

Spirapril *(spiraprilum, spirapril, spirapril)*

ACE inhibitor, antihypertensive

↑ K, urea

Spirogermanin *(spirogermaninum, spirogermanin, spirogermanin)*

antineoplastic, antimalarial

↑ ALT

Spironolactone *(spironolactonum, spironolactone, spironolactone)*
potassium sparing diuretic, antihypertensive, antiandrogen

↑ aldosterone, ANA, angiotensin II, Ca, digoxin, DOC, eos, estradiol, FSH, HCT, 11-OHCS, 18-OHCS, chloride, cholesterol, insulin, K, coagulation factors, corticosteroids, cortisol, uric acid, LDL cholesterol, LH, MAC, renin, TAG, urea

↓ G, G tolerance, HDL cholesterol, cholesterol, uric acid, WBC, Na, neu, plasma volume, pH, testosterone, TAG

■ *Urine* ↑ aldosterone, Ca, estradiol, chloride, 17-OHCS, 17-KGS, 17-KS, cortisol

Stanozolol *(stanozoloum, stanozolol, stanozolol)*
anabolic, androgen

↑ ALP, ALT, LDL cholesterol, protein C

↓ Apo A-I, factors – (II, VII, X), FSH, G, HDL cholesterol, LH, LP(a), SHBG, T3, T4, TBG, testosterone, vitamin D, free testosterone

Stavudine *(stavudinum, stavudine, stavudine)*
antiretroviral

↑ ALT, AST, GMT, MAC

↓ neu, PLT

Steroids

↑ GMT, urea

↓ chloride, CK, estriol, T3

■ *Stool* ↑ blood

Stibophen *(stibophenum, stibophen, stibophen)*
antischistosomal, anthelmintic, tonic

↓ PLT

Stilbol *(diethylstilbestrolum, diethylstilbestrol, diéthylstilbestrol)*
synthetic estrogen

↑ ALT, AST, Bil, Ca, TBG

↓ uric acid, PLT

■ *Urine* ↑ 17-OHCS

Streptodornase *(streptodornasum, streptodornase, streptodornase)*
enzyme, surface-acting drug

↑ BT

Streptokinase *(streptokinasum, streptokinase, streptokinase)*
fibrinolytic

↑ AAT, ALP, ALT, A2MG, AST, CK, coagulation time, BT, eos, FDP, GD, GMT, creatinine, LD, LD (isoenzymes), WBC, PT, TT, urea

↓ fibrinogen, Hb, CHS, plasmin

■ *Urine* ↑ proteins, Hb, RBC, blood

■ *Sputum* ↑ blood

Streptomycin *(streptomycinum, streptomycine, streptomycine)*
antibiotic

↑ ANA, Bil, eos, creatinine, urea

↓ factors – (II, VII, X), Hb, WBC, neu, PLT, urea

■ *Urine* ↑ ALP, proteins, G, LAP

■ *Cerebrospinal Fluid* ↑ proteins

Streptozocin *(streptozocinum, streptozocin, streptozocine)*
antineoplastic

↑ acetoacetate, ALP, ALT, AST, Bil, G, GMT, chloride, insulin, creatinine, LA, MAC, pyruvate, urea

    ↓ albumin, G, gastrin, HCO$_3$⁻, K, FFA, neu, P, PLT, WBC
    ■ *Urine* ↑ G, Hb, volume

Strychnine *(strychninum, strychnine, strychnine)*
   CNS-stimulant, convulsant
      ↑ WBC, MAC
      ↓ G

Succimer *(succimerum, succimer, succimer)*
   antidote, diagnostic aid
      ↑ ALP, cholesterol
      ↓ CK, uric acid
      ■ *Urine* ↑ proteins, ketones

Succinimides
      ■ *Urine* ↑ ALA, proteins, Hb, blood, porphyrins

Succinylcholine *(succinylcholinum, succinylcholine, succinylcholine)*
   short-acting depolarizing skeletal muscle relaxant
      ↑ Ca^{2+}, CK, histamine, K, MAC, Mb, acetylcholine receptor antibodies
      ↓ CHS
      ■ *Urine* ↑ Mb

Sucralfate *(sucralfatum, sucralfate, sucralfate)*
   antiulcerant
      ↑ ALP, Ca, factors – (II, VII, X), vitamin D3
      ↓ ALP, digoxin, phenytoin, quinidine, P

Sucrose *(saccharosum, sucrose, sucrose)*
   nutrient, sweetener
      ↑ insulin, LA

Sulfacetamide *(sulfacetamidum, sulfacetamide, sulfacétamide)*
   sulfonamide, antibacterial
      ↑ Heinz bodies (RBC)

Sulfadiazine *(sulfadiazinum, sulfadiazine, sulfadiazine)*
   antibacterial
      ↑ ALP, ALT, phenytoin, cholesterol, creatinine
      ↓ Ca, G, neu, PLT, WBC
      ■ *Urine* ↑ proteins, blood, crystals
         ↓ volume

Sulfadimethoxine *(sulfadimethoxinum, sulfadimethoxine, sulfadiméthoxine)*
   antibacterial
      ↑ ANA

Sulfadoxine *(sulfadoxinum, sulfadoxine, sulfadoxine)*
   antibacterial
      ↑ ALP, ALT, eos

Sulfafurazole *(sulfafurazolum, sulfafurazole, sulfafurazol)*
   antibacterial
      ↑ ALP, AST, eos
      ↓ Ca, Hb, coagulation factors, WBC, neu
      ■ *Urine* ↑ proteins

Sulfamethizole Ammonium *(sulfamethizolum, sulfamethizole, sulfaméthizol)*
   antibacterial
      ↑ ALP, ALT
      ↓ Hb, WBC, PLT

Sulfamethoxazole *(sulfamethoxazolum, sulfamethoxazole, sulfaméthoxazole)*
   antibacterial

- ↑ ALP, ALT, AMS, AST, Bil, eos, phenytoin, GMT, Heinz bodies (RBC), K, creatinine, MHb, T4
- ↓ ALT, factors – (II, VII, X), G, haptoglobin, Hb, WBC, neu, PLT
- ■ *Urine* ↑ blood, Hb, RBC, crystals, porphyrins
- ■ *Cerebrospinal Fluid* ↑ WBC

Sulfamethoxypyridazine   *(sulfamethoxypyridazinum,*   *sulfamethoxypyridazine,*
sulfaméthoxypyridazine)
   antibacterial

- ↑ ALP, ALT, ANA, AST
- ↓ Hb, WBC, neu

Sulfanilamide *(sulfanilamidum, sulfanilamide, sulfanilamide)*
   antibacterial

- ↑ ALT

Sulfapyridine *(sulfapyridinum, sulfapyridine, sulfapyridine)*
   antibacterial

- ↑ Heinz bodies (RBC), TSH
- ↓ haptoglobin, Hb, neu
- ■ *Urine* ↑ UBG

Sulfasalazine *(sulfasalazinum, sulfasalazine, sulfasalazine)*
   antibacterial (for colitis), antiinflammatory, antiarthritic

- ↑ ALP, ALT, AMS, ANA, AST, Bil, conjugated Bil, eos, GMT, Heinz bodies (RBC), creatinine, LD, LE cells, WBC, lym, MCV, MHb, RTC, PLT
- ↓ ALP, proteins, Bil, digoxin, folate, haptoglobin, Hb, IgA, immunoglobulins, WBC, neu, PLT
- ■ *Urine* ↑ orange color
- ■ *Seminal Fluid* ↓ spermatozoa count

Sulfate-Containing Preparations

- ↓ Ca, K, Na
- ■ *Urine* ↑ Ca, K, Na

Sulfathiazole *(sulfathiazolum, sulfathiazole, sulfathiazol)*
   antibacterial

- ↑ ALT, Bil
- ↓ G, neu
- ■ *Urine* ↑ G, UBG

Sulfinpyrazone *(sulfinpyrazonum, sulfinpyrazone, sulfinpyrazone)*
   uricosuric, antiarthritic, platelet aggregation inhibitor

- ↑ BT, creatinine
- ↓ factors – (II, VII, X)

Sulfizoxazole *(sulfizoxazolum, sulfizoxazole, sulfizoxazole)*
   antibacterial

- ↓ PLT
- ■ *Urine* ↑ proteins, blood, RBC, Hb, crystals

Sulfobromphthalein *(sulfobromphthaleinum, sulfobromphthalein, sulfobromphthalein)*
   diagnostic agent (hepatic function determination)

- ↑ proteins, creatinine
- ■ *Urine* ↑ acetoacetate, red color, VMA

Sulfonamides

    ↑ ALP, ALT, AMS, AST, Bil, Bil unconjugated, BT, eos, RBC, phenytoin, G, GMT, Hb, Heinz bodies (RBC), cholesterol, creatinine, LD, WBC, lipase, MAC, MHb, neu, OCT, PLT, TSH, urea

    ↓ Bil, Ca, factors – (II, VII, X), folate, FT4, G, Hb, uric acid, WBC, neu, T3, T4, PLT, TSH

    ■ *Urine* ↑ ALP, blood, proteins, RBC, Hb, glucuronic acid, uric acid, crystals, LAP, PBG, porphyrins

       ↓ G, volume

Sulfones

    ↑ ALT

    ↓ WBC

    ■ *Urine* ↑ proteins

Sulfonylurea *(sulfonylureum, sulfonylurea, sulfonylurea)*

oral hypoglycemic

    ↑ acetaldehyde, ALP, ALT, AST, Bil, C-peptide, phenytoin, insulin, creatinine, WBC, MAC, TSH, urea

    ↓ FT4, G, Hb, K, WBC, Na, T3, T4, TAG, PLT, vitamin D

    ■ *Urine* ↑ hydroxyproline, PBG, porphyrins

Sulindac *(sulindacum, sulindac, sulindac)*

non-steroid antiinflammatory, antipyretic, analgesic

    ↑ ALP, ALT, AMS, ANA, AST, Bil, BT, eos, GMT, K, creatinine, LD, lipase, lithium, urea

    ↓ PLT aggregation, albumin, factors – (II, VII, X), GFR, Hb, WBC, neu, PGF2-alpha, renin, thromboxane B2, PLT

    ■ *Urine* ↑ blood, Hb, RBC

       ↓ proteins, PGE2

    ■ *Cerebrospinal Fluid* ↑ proteins, WBC

    ■ *Stool* ↑ Hb

Suloctidil *(suloctidilum, suloctidil, suloctidil)*

peripheral vasodilator, platelet aggregation inhibitor

    ↑ ALP, ALT, AST, GMT, HDL cholesterol

    ↓ cholesterol, TAG

Sulodexide *(sulodexidum, sulodexide, sulodexide)*

anticoagulant

    ↑ Apo A-I, HDL cholesterol

    ↓ cholesterol, LDL cholesterol, TAG

Sulpiride *(sulpiridum, sulpiride, sulpiride)*

antidepressant, selective antagonist D_2 receptor, antiemetic

    ↑ ALT, PRL

Sultiame *(sultiamum, sultiame, sultiame)*

anticonvulsant, antiepileptic

    ↑ phenytoin

    ↓ WBC

Suprofen *(suprofenum, suprofen, suprofén)*

non-steroid antiinflammatory, analgesic, antipyretic

    ↑ creatinine

    ■ *Urine* ↑ proteins, Hb

Suramin *(suraminum natricum, suramin sodium, suramine sodique)*
trypanocide
↑ ALT

Suxamethonium *(suxamethonii chloridum, suxamethonium chloride, chlorure de suxaméthonium)*
neuromuscular blocking agent, skeletal muscle relaxant
↑ CK, K, Mb

Sympathomimetics
↑ G, catecholamines, RAL
↓ K

Tacrine *(tacrinum, tacrine, tacrine)*
cholinesterase inhibitor (centrally acting)
↑ ALP, ALT, AST, eos, GMT

Tacrolimus *(tacrolimusum, tacrolimus, tacrolimus)*
immunosuppressant
↑ G, K, urea
↓ Apo A-I, Apo B, HDL cholesterol, cholesterol

Tamoxifen *(tamoxifenum, tamoxifen, tamoxiféne)*
antiestrogen
↑ AAT, ALP, ALT, AST, Bil, Ca, ceruloplasmin, estradiol, FSH, FT4, GMT, LH, lipids, progesterone, SHBG, T3, T4, TAG, TBG, testosterone, VLDL cholesterol
↓ ALP, AT III, CK, estradiol, factors – (II, VII, X), fibrinogen, FSH, haptoglobin, Hb, cholesterol, IGF-I, LDL cholesterol, LH, WBC, LP(a), neu, orosomucoid, PRL, testosterone, PLT
■ *Seminal Fluid* ↑ spermatozoal motility
■ *Amniotic Fluid* ↓ LP(a)

Tannic Acid *(acidum tannicum, tannic acid, acide tannique)*
adstringent
↑ ALT

Teicoplanin *(teicoplaninum, teicoplanin, téicoplanine)*
glycopeptide antibiotic
↑ ALT

Telmisartan *(telmisartanum, telmisartan, telmisartan)*
angiotensin II antagonist
↑ K, urea

Temafloxacin *(temafloxacinum, temafloxacin, temafloxacine)*
antibacterial
↓ G

Temozolomide *(temozolomidum, temozolomide, témozolomide)*
antineoplastic
↓ neu, PLT, WBC

Tenecteplase *(tenecteplasum, tenecteplase, ténectéplase)*
tissue plasminogen activator
■ *Urine* ↑ blood, Hb, RBC
■ *Sputum* ↑ blood

Teniposide *(teniposidum, teniposide, téniposide)*
  antineoplastic
      ↓ neu, PLT, WBC
Tenoxicam *(tenoxicamum, tenoxicam, ténoxicam)*
  non-steroid antiinflammatory, analgesic
      ↑ ALT
Terazosin *(terazosinum, terazosin, térazosine)*
  alpha-1-adrenoceptor antagonist, antihypertensive
      ↑ HDL cholesterol
      ↓ cholesterol, LDL cholesterol, TAG, VLDL cholesterol
Terbinafine *(terbinafinum, terbinafine, terbinafine)*
  antifungal
      ↑ ALT, AST, GMT, eos
      ↓ factors – (II, VII, X), neu, PLT
Terbutaline *(terbutalinum, terbutaline, terbutaline)*
  selective beta-2-adrenoceptor agonist, bronchodilator, uterine relaxant
      ↑ G, HDL cholesterol, insulin, LA, T3
      ↓ K, osmolality, pH, T4, theophylline
Testolactone *(testolactonum, testolactone, testolactone)*
  antineoplastic
      ↑ Ca
      ↓ estradiol
      ■ *Urine* ↑ creatinine, 17-KS
Testosterone *(testosteronum, testosterone, testostérone)*
  androgen
      ↑ ALP, ALT, androstenedione, Apo B, Ca, estradiol, estriol, estrone, RBC,
        GMT, Hb, cholesterol, insulin, corticosteroids, creatine, LDL choles-
        terol, Na, PRL, PSA, TAG
      ↓ Apo A-I, CBG, DHEA, estradiol, fibrinogen, FSH, haptoglobin, HDL
        cholesterol, cholesterol, CHS, LDL cholesterol, LH, 17-OH preg-
        nenolone, 17-OH progesterone, progesterone, SHBG, TAG, TBG, trans-
        ferrin, vitamin D3
      ■ *Urine* ↑ aldosterone, 17-OHCS, 17-KS, volume
      ■ *Seminal Fluid* ↓ spermatozoa count
Tetracosactide *(tetracosactidum, tetracosactide, tétracosactide)*
  synthetic ACTH-preparation
      ↑ G, HDL cholesterol, insulin, LA
      ↓ estriol, cholesterol, LDL cholesterol, lipase (hepatic), TAG
Tetracycline *(tetracyclinum, tetracycline, tétracycline)*
  antibiotic
      ↑ ALP, ALT, AMS, ANA, AST, Bil, conjugated Bil, digoxin, eos, G, GMT, K,
        catecholamines, uric acid, LD, lipase, lithium, WBC, MAC, Na, OCT, P,
        urea
      ↓ ammonia, Ca, Ca²⁺, factors – (II, VII, X), folate, G, Hb, HCO₃⁻, choles-
        terol, K, uric acid, neu, P, pH, testosterone, PLT, free testosterone
      ■ *Urine* ↑ amino acids, Bence Jones protein, proteins, estrogens, G, cat-
        echolamines, Hb, porphyrins, volume
      ↓ G
      ■ *Cerebrospinal Fluid* ↑ proteins
      ■ *Stool* ↑ fatty acids

Tetrahydrocannabinol *(tetrahydrocannabinolum, tetrahydrocannabinol, tétrahydrocanna-binol)*

euphoric, hallucinogen

↑ C-peptide, insulin, K

↓ cAMP, G, uric acid, LH (females), testosterone

■ *Urine* ↑ epinephrine, norepinephrine

Thalidomide *(thalidomidum, thalidomide, thalidomide)*

sedative, hypnotic, immunosuppressant

↓ neu

Thenalidine *(thenalidinum, thenalidine, thénalidine)*

antihistaminic, antipruritic

↓ WBC, neu

Theophylline *(theophyllinum, theophylline, théophylline)*

diuretic, cardiac stimulant, smooth muscle relaxant, bronchodilator

↑ epinephrine, ALT, AST, Bil, conjugated Bil, Ca, cAMP, CK, G, catechola-mines, homocysteine, uric acid, MAC, norepinephrine, PT, somatosta-tin, TAG, FFA

↓ ALP, phenytoin, HCO_3^-, chloride, K, lithium, Na, P, somatostatin, vita-min B_6

■ *Urine* ↑ proteins, catecholamines, volume

Thiabendazole *(tiabendazolum, thiabendazole, tiabendazol)*

antiparasitic, anthelmintic

↑ ALP, ALT, AMS, AST, Bil, ESR, G, GMT, cholesterol, urea

■ *Urine* ↑ proteins, blood, crystals

Thiamazole *(thiamazolum, thiamazole, thiamazol)*

thyroid inhibitor

↑ ALP, ALT, ANA, AST, Bil, factors – (II, VII, X), GMT, HDL cholesterol, cholesterol, LD, LDL cholesterol, LP(a), TSH

↓ Hb, neu, T4, PLT, TSH

Thiamine *(thiaminum, thiamine, thiamine)*

vitamin B_1, antineuritic

↑ uric acid

■ *Urine* ↑ UBG

Thiamphenicol *(thiamphenicolum, thiamphenicol, thiamphénicol)*

antibiotic

↓ Hb, neu, PLT

Thiazides

↑ ADH, aldosterone, ALP, ammonia, AMS, ANA, BE, BT, Ca, Ca^{2+}, Cu, G, GMT, HDL cholesterol, quinidine, chloride, cholesterol, insulin, crea-tinine, uric acid, LDL cholesterol, lithium, alpha-lipoprotein, MAC, MAL, Mg, pH, TAG, urea, VLDL cholesterol, Zn

↓ C-peptide, Cu, G (neonates), Hb, HDL cholesterol, HCO_3^-, chloride, insulin, K, LDL cholesterol, WBC, Mg, Na, neu, osmolality, P, PTH, PLT, Zn

■ *Urine* ↑ aldosterone, Ca, G, Hb, HCO_3^-, chloride, K, 17-OHCS, uric acid, Mg, Na, volume, pH

↓ Ca, uric acid, 17-KS, volume, free cortisol

Thiethylperazine *(thiethylperazinum, thiethylperazine, thiethylpérazine)*

D receptor antagonist, antiemetic, antipsychotic

↑ PRL

↓ neu, PLT

Thioguanine *(tioguaninum, thioguanine, tioguanine)*
   antineoplastic
   ↑ ALP, ALT, AST, Bil, GMT, uric acid
   ↓ Hb, WBC, neu, PLT
Thiopental *(thiopentalum natricum, thiopental sodium, thiopental sodique)*
   hypnotic, rapidly acting intravenous anesthetic
   ↑ ALP, ALT, AST, Bil, GMT, histamine, LD
   ■ *Gastric Fluid* ↑ HCl
Thioridazine *(thioridazinum, thioridazine, thioridazine)*
   neuroleptic
   ↑ ALP, ALT, ANA, AST, Bil, eos, phenytoin, PRL, WBC
   ↓ Bil, phenobarbital, Hb, LH, WBC, Na, neu, testosterone, PLT
   ■ *Urine* ↑ hCG
Thiotepa *(thiotepum, thiotepa, thiotépa)*
   antineoplastic, immunosuppressant
   ↑ uric acid
   ↓ WBC, neu, PLT
Thiothixene *(tiotixenum, thiothixene, tiotixéne)*
   neuroleptic, antipsychotic
   ↑ ALP, ALT, AST, Bil, eos, G, WBC, PRL
   ↓ G, Na, PLT, WBC
Thiouracil *(thiouracilum, thiouracil, thiouracil)*
   thyroid inhibitor
   ↑ ALP, ALT, Bil, cholesterol, LE cells
   ↓ WBC, neu, T3, PLT
Thiourea
   antithyroid
   ↓ FT4, thyroxine
Thrombolytics
   ↓ fibrinogen
Thyroid Hormones
   ↑ ALP, ALT, AST, proteins, G, HDL cholesterol, creatinine, osteocalcin, SHBG, somatomedin C, T4, urea
   ↓ Apo B, CBG, factors – (II, VII, X), HDL cholesterol, cholesterol, LDL cholesterol, TAG, TSH
Thyrostatics
   ↑ GMT
   ↓ T4
Thyrotropin *(thyrotrophinum, thyrotrophin, thyrotrophine)*
   hormone
   ↑ epinephrine, norepinephrine, PRL, T3, T4, TSH
Thyroxine *(thyroxinum, thyroxine, thyroxine)*
   thyromimetic, anticholesteremic
   ↑ albumin, proteins, G, SHBG, T3, T4, urea
   ↓ eos, HDL-C, cholesterol, LDL-C, norepinephrine, TSH
   ■ *Urine* ↑ hydroxyproline
   ↓ estriol
Tiapamil *(tiapamilum, tiapamil, tiapamil)*
   coronary vasodilator, antiarrhythmic, calcium channel antagonist
   ↑ digoxin

Tibolone *(tibolonum, tibolone, tibolone)*
   anabolic, synthetic steroid
        ↓ HDL cholesterol, cholesterol, LP(a), TAG

Ticarcillin *(ticarcillinum, ticarcillin, ticarcilline)*
   antibiotic
        ↑ ALT, BT, GMT
        ↓ PLT aggregation, factors – (II, VII, X), K, Mg, PLT

Ticlopidine *(ticlopidinum, ticlopidine, ticlopidine)*
   antithrombotic
        ↑ ALP, ALT, Bil, eos, GMT, cholesterol, PLT, TAG
        ↓ Na, neu, PLT

Tienilic Acid *(acidum tienilicum, tienilic acid, acide tiénilique)*
   diuretic, antihypertensive, uricosuric
        ↑ ALT, creatinine
        ↓ K, uric acid, Na

Timolol *(timololum, timolol, timolol)*
   non-selective beta-adrenoceptor blocker, antiglaucoma agent
        ↑ AST, PLT aggregation, ANA, GMT, K, uric acid, TAG
        ↓ G, HDL cholesterol, renin
        ■ *Urine* ↓ aldosterone

Tiocarlide *(tiocarlidum, tiocarlide, tiocarlide)*
   tuberculostatic, leprostatic
        ↑ ALT
        ↓ WBC

Tiopronin *(tioproninum, tiopronin, tiopronine)*
   detoxicant, mucolytic
        ↑ ALT
        ↓ neu, vitamin B_6
        ■ *Urine* ↑ proteins

Tirofiban *(tirofibanum, tirofiban, tirofiban)*
   platelet aggregation inhibitor
        ↓ PLT
        ■ *Urine* ↑ blood, Hb, RBC

Tizanidine *(tizanidinum, tizanidine, tizanidine)*
   skeletal muscle relaxant, alpha-2-adrenoceptor agonist
        ↑ ALT, AST, GMT

Tobramycin *(tobramycinum, tobramycin, tobramycine)*
   antibiotic
        ↑ ALT, AST, creatinine, urea
        ↓ Ca, Hb, K, WBC, Mg, PLT
        ■ *Urine* ↑ B2M, proteins, casts

Tocainide *(tocainidum, tocainide, tocainide)*
   antiarrhythmic
        ↑ ALT, ANA, AST, Bil, eos, GMT
        ↓ WBC, neu, PLT
        ■ *Urine* ↑ volume

Tocopherol *(tocofersolanum, tocofersolan, tocofersolan)*
   antioxidant
        ↑ AST, Bil, HDL cholesterol, cholesterol, PLT
        ↓ factors – (II, VII, IX, X), LP(a), lym, TAG, PLT, FFA

Tolazamide *(tolazamidum, tolazamide, tolazamide)*
oral hypoglycemic
↑ ALP, ALT, ANA, AST, Bil, immunoglobulins, insulin, 5-nucleotidase, PLT
↓ factors – (II, VII, X), G, Na, PLT, WBC
■ *Urine* ↓ osmolality

Tolazoline *(tolazolinum, tolazoline, tolazoline)*
alpha-adrenoceptor antagonist, systemic and pulmonary vasodilator
↓ Hb, WBC, PLT
■ *Gastric Fluid* ↑ HCl

Tolbutamide *(tolbutamidum, tolbutamide, tolbutamide)*
oral hypoglycemic
↑ ADH, ALP, ALT, AST, Bil, GMT, Heinz bodies (RBC), insulin, 5-nucle-
otidase
↓ factors – (II, VII, X), G, gastrin, Hb, chloride, cholesterol, insulin, Na,
neu, T4, PLT, WBC
■ *Urine* ↑ proteins

Tolcapone *(tolcaponum, tolcapone, tolcapone)*
selective COMT inhibitor, antiparkinsonian
↑ ALT, AST, GMT
■ *Urine* ↑ blood, Hb, RBC

Tolfenamic Acid *(acidum tolfenamicum, tolfenamic acid, acide tolfénamique)*
analgesic, non-steroid antiinflammatory, antirheumatic
↑ ALP, ALT

Tolmetin *(tolmetinum, tolmetin, tolmétine)*
non-steroid antiinflammatory, analgesic
↑ ALT, ANA, AST, BT, GMT, urea
↓ PLT aggregation, Hb, WBC
■ *Urine* ↑ blood, Hb, RBC
■ *Cerebrospinal Fluid* ↑ WBC
■ *Stool* ↑ Hb

Toloxatone *(toloxatonum, toloxatone, toloxatone)*
muscle relaxant, sedative, antidepressant
↑ AST, Bil

Topiramate *(topiramatum, topiramate, topiramate)*
anticonvulsant, antiepileptic
↓ WBC
■ *Urine* ↑ blood, Hb, RBC

Topotecan *(topotecanum, topotecan, topotécane)*
antineoplastic
↓ neu, PLT, WBC

Toremifene *(toremifenum, toremifene, torémiféne)*
antiestrogen, antineoplastic
↑ ALT, AST, Ca, GMT, WBC, SHBG
↓ ALP, ALT, AST, FSH, IgA, IgG, IgM, LH

Torasemide *(torasemidum, torasemide, torasémide)*
loop diuretic
↑ cholesterol, G, TAG, urea, uric acid
↓ K

Trandolapril *(trandolaprilum, trandolapril, trandolapril)*
ACE inhibitor, antihypertensive
  ↑ ALT, AST, GMT, K, urea
  ↓ neu, PLT

Tranquilizers
  ↑ CK-MB, G

Tranylcypromine *(tranylcyprominum, tranylcypromine, tranylcypromine)*
antidepressant, non-hydrazine MAO inhibitor
  ↑ ALT, AST, GMT
  ↓ Na

Trazodone *(trazodonum, trazodone, trazodone)*
antidepressant, anxiolytic, adjuvant agent in preanesthesia
  ↑ ALP, ALT, Bil, MHb
  ↓ Hb, HCT
  ■ *Urine* ↑ RBC, blood

Tretinoin *(tretinoinum, tretinoin, trétinoine)*
vitamin A derivative, keratolytic
  ↑ ALT, AST, Bil, Ca, GMT, cholesterol, LA, TAG, WBC
  ↓ Ca

Triamcinolone *(triamcinolonum, triamcinolone, triamcinolone)*
synthetic glucocorticoid
  ↑ AMS, G, cholesterol, MAL, Na
  ↓ Ca, G tolerance, K, 17-OHCS, cortisol, PLT
  ■ *Urine* ↑ Ca, G, K, 17-OHCS, Na

Triamterene *(triamterenum, triamterene, triamtérène)*
potassium sparing diuretic
  ↑ aldosterone, ALT, digoxin, eos, G, chloride, cholesterol, K, creatinine, uric acid, MAC, MCV, Mg, Na, renin, urea
  ↓ folate, GFR, G tolerance, HCO_3, chloride, Mg, Na, PLT, vitamin B_{12}
  ■ *Urine* ↑ aldosterone, green color, G, crystals, Na
    ↓ catecholamines
  ■ *Gastric Fluid* ↑ HCl

Triazolam *(triazolamum, triazolam, triazolam)*
short-acting benzodiazepine, sedative, hypnotic
  ↑ ALP
  ■ *Urine* ↓ cortisol

Trichlormethiazide *(trichlormethiazidum, trichlormethiazide, trichlorméthiazide)*
salidiuretic, antihypertensive
  ↑ ALP, Ca, eos, G, uric acid, TAG
  ↓ HDL cholesterol, K

Tricyclic Antidepressants
  ↑ ADH, ALP, ALT, G, GMT, catecholamines, cortisol, norepinephrine, PRL
  ↓ G, chloride
  ■ *Urine* ↑ catecholamines
    ↓ 5-HIAA, volume

Trifluoperazine *(trifluoperazinum, trifluoperazine, trifluopérazine)*
neuroleptic
  ↑ ALT, AST, CK, cholesterol, eos, WBC, PRL
  ↓ ALP, Hb, WBC, PLT

Trifluperidol *(trifluperidolum, trifluperidol, triflupéridol)*
   neuroleptic
        ↑ eos, ESR
        ↓ cholesterol

Trilostane *(trilostanum, trilostane, trilostane)*
   inhibitor of glucocorticoid biosynthesis, adrenocortical suppressant
        ↑ ACTH, DHEA, estradiol, testosterone
        ↓ aldosterone, glucocorticoids, cortisol
        ■ *Urine* ↑ 17-KS
          ↓ cortisol

Trimetaphan *(trimetaphani camsilas, trimetaphan camsilate, camsilate de trimétaphan)*
   antihypertensive, ganglion blocking agent
        ↑ G, histamine, K

Trimethadione *(trimethadionum, trimethadione, triméthiadone)*
   anticonvulsant, antiepileptic
        ↑ ALP, ALT, ANA, Bil
        ↓ Hb, WBC, neu, pH, PLT

Trimethoprim *(trimethoprimum, trimethoprim, triméthoprim)*
   antibacterial
        ↑ ALT, AST, Bil, GMT, K, MHb, urea
        ↓ Na

Trimethoprim-Sulfamethoxazole *(trimethoprimum-sulfamethoxazolum, trimethoprim-sulfamethoxazole, triméthoprim-sulfaméthoxazole)*
   antibacterial
        ↑ ALP, ALT, AMS, Bil, digoxin, G, K, creatinine, LD, MCV, procainamide, TSH, urea
        ↓ factors – (II, VII, X), folate, FT4, GFR, Hb, WBC, Na, neu, T3, T4, PLT
        ■ *Urine* ↑ crystals
          ↓ Na, volume
        ■ *Cerebrospinal Fluid* ↑ WBC

Trimetrexate *(trimetrexatum, trimetrexate, trimétrexate)*
   antineoplastic
        ↑ ALT, AST, GMT
        ↓ Ca, Na, neu, PLT

Trimipramine *(trimipraminum, trimipramine, trimipramine)*
   antidepressant
        ↑ ALP, ALT, AST, PRL

Triptorelin *(triptorelinum, triptorelin, triptoréline)*
   immunomodulator
        ↑ ALP, Ca
        ↓ PTH

Troglitazone *(troglitazonum, troglitazone, troglitazone)*
   oral hypoglycemic
        ↑ ALT, AST, GMT, cholesterol

Troleandomycin *(troleandomycinum, troleandomycin, troléandomycine)*
   antibiotic
        ↑ ALP, ALT, AST, estradiol, GMT, cholesterol, carbamazepine, methyl-prednisolone, theophylline

Trometamol (*trometamolum, trometamol, trométamol*)
  alkalizer, osmotic diuretic, antidote
    ↑ Ca, K, T_3, T_4
    ↓ G, pCO_2
Trovafloxacin (*trovafloxacinum, trovafloxacin, trovafloxacine*)
  fluoroquinolon, DNA gyrase inhibitor
    ↑ ALT, AST, GMT
    ↓ PLT, WBC
Trypsin (*trypsinum, trypsin, trypsin*)
  proteolytic enzyme
    ↓ Ca^{2+}
Tryptophan (*tryptophanum, tryptophan, tryptophane*)
  essential amino acid
    ↑ amino acids, eos, cholesterol, uric acid, PRL
    ■ *Urine* ↑ P
    ■ *Cerebrospinal Fluid* ↑ proteins
Tuberculostatics
    ↑ conjugated Bil, GMT, uric acid
Tubocurarine (*tubocurarini chloridum, tubocurarine chloride, chlorure de tubocurarine*)
  skeletal muscle relaxant
    ↑ CK, histamine, pH, RAL
    ↓ pH
Tumor Necrosis Factor (*tumor necrosis factor, tumor necrosis factor, tumor necrosis factor*)
  cytokine
    ↑ ACTH, CRP, cortisol, neu
    ↓ eos, Fe, WBC, lym, mono, neu, P
Tyramine (*tyraminum, tyramine, tyramine*)
  sympathomimetic, vasoconstrictor
    ↑ amino acids, G, uric acid, tyrosine, UBG
Tyrosine (*tyrosinum, tyrosine, tyrosine*)
  essential amino acid, dietetic
    ↑ Bil, conjugated Bil, uric acid, UBG
    ■ *Urine* ↑ crystals
    ■ *Cerebrospinal Fluid* ↑ proteins

Ubidecarenone (*ubidecarenonum, ubidecarenone, ubidécarénone*)
  cardiovascular agent
    ↑ factors – (II, VII, X)
Uracil (*uracilum, uracil, uracil*)
  potentiator in tegafur
    ↑ ALP, Bil
    ■ *Seminal Fluid* ↓ spermatozoa count
Urapidil (*urapidilum, urapidil, urapidil*)
  antihypertensive
    ↓ ANP
Urea (*carbamidum, urea, urea*)
  diuretic, dermatologic, keratolytic, antiseptic, fertilizer
    ↑ aldosterone, AT II, Ca^{2+}, cholesterol, creatinine, osmolality, renin, urea
    ↓ Bil, K, Mg, Na

- ■ *Urine* ↑ creatinine, homogentisic acid, uric acid, Mg, volume, osmolality
  - ↓ PBG, UBG, VMA

Urokinase *(urokinasum, urokinase, urokinase)*
fibrinolytic, thrombolytic
- ↑ BT, coagulation time, PT, TT
- ↓ fibrinogen, plasmin
- ■ *Urine* ↑ blood, Hb, RBC
- ■ *Sputum* ↑ blood

Ursodeoxycholic Acid *(acidum ursodeoxycholicum, ursodeoxycholic acid, acide ursodéoxycholique)*
gallstone dissolving agent
- ↑ ALT
- ↓ ALP, ALT

Valproic Acid *(acidum valproicum, valproic acid, acide valproique)*
anticonvulsant, antiepileptic
- ↑ ALA, ALP, ALT, ammonia, AMS, antiplatelet Ab, APTT, AST, barbiturate, Bil, cyclosporine, Cu, BT, diazepam, phenobarbital, phenytoin, G, glutathione peroxidase, GMT, CHS, IgG, carbamazepine, LA, LD, lipase, OCT, pyruvate, GH, testosterone, TSH, FFA
- ↓ acetoacetate, albumin, BHBA, factors – (II, VII, X), phenytoin, fibrinogen, folate, FT3, FT4, G, Hb, cholesterol, IgA, carnitine, ketones, LDL cholesterol, WBC, lym, neu, PRL, Se, somatostatin, GH, T3, T4, TBG, PLT, urea, free testosterone, Zn
- ■ *Urine* ↑ acetoacetate, ketones
- ■ *Seminal Fluid* ↓ spermatozoa count

Valrubicin *(valrubicinum, valrubicin, valrubicin)*
antineoplastic
- ↓ neu, WBC
- ■ *Urine* ↑ blood, Hb, RBC

Valsartan *(valsartanum, valsartan, valsartan)*
angiotensin II antagonist, antihypertensive
- ↑ ALT, AST, GMT, cholesterol, K, urea

Vancomycin *(vancomycinum, vancomycin, vancomycine)*
antibiotic
- ↑ antineutrophil Ab, eos, creatinine, urea
- ↓ WBC, neu, PLT
- ■ *Urine* ↑ Hb, proteins, casts

Vasopressin *(vasopressini injectio, vasopressin injection, soluté injectable de vasopressine)*
antidiuretic, vasopressor
- ↑ ACTH, ADH, CK, G, corticosteroids, cortisol, creatinine, GH, urea
- ↓ Na, osmolality, renin
- ■ *Urine* ↑ MHb
  - ↓ volume

Velaciclovir *(velaciclovirum, velaciclovir, velaciclovir)*
antiviral
- ↓ PLT

Verapamil *(verapamilum, verapamil, vérapamil)*
calcium channel antagonist, antihypertensive, coronary vasodilator, antiarrhythmic
↑ ALP, ALT, AST, Bil, cyclosporine, digitoxin, digoxin, eos, ethanol, GMT, HDL-C, HVA, quinidine, carbamazepine, LD, norepinephrine, PRL, PTH, TAG, theophylline
↓ G, cholesterol, cortisol, LDL cholesterol, lithium, PLT

Verteporfin *(verteporfinum, verteporfin, vertéporfin)*
photosensitizer, light-activated drug
↑ ALT, AST, GMT, WBC
↓ WBC

Vidarabine *(vidarabinum, vidarabine, vidarabine)*
antiviral
↑ ADH, ALT

Vigabatrin *(vigabatrinum, vigabatrin, vigabatrine)*
antiepileptic
↓ phenytoin

Viloxazine *(viloxazinum, viloxazine, viloxazine)*
antidepressant
↑ carbamazepine, theophylline

Vinblastine *(vinblastinum, vinblastine, vinblastine)*
antineoplastic
↑ ADH, uric acid
↓ Hb, uric acid, WBC, Na, neu, PTH, RTC, PLT
■ *Seminal Fluid* ↓ spermatozoa count

Vincristine *(vincristinum, vincristine, vincristine)*
antineoplastic
↑ ADH, ALT, CK, K, uric acid, PLT
↓ WBC, Na, neu, osmolality, PLT
■ *Urine* ↑ Na, volume, osmolality
■ *Seminal Fluid* ↓ spermatozoa count

Vinorelbine *(vinorelbinum, vinorelbine, vinorelbine)*
antineoplastic
↓ Na, neu, pO$_2$, PLT, WBC

Viomycin *(viomycinum, viomycin, viomycine)*
tuberculostatic
↑ eos, creatinine, uric acid, urea
↓ Ca
■ *Urine* ↑ Ca, proteins, Hb

Vitamin A *(retinolum, retinol, rétinol)*
antixerophthalmic vitamin
↑ ALP, Bil, Ca, G, PT
↓ RBC, Hb, HCT, WBC, PTH
■ *Urine* ↑ volume

Vitamin B-Complex
↑ catecholamines
■ *Urine* ↑ catecholamines
↓ estrogens

Vitamin B12 *(cyanocobalaminum, cyanocobalamin, cyanocobalamine)*
hematopoietic vitamin
↓ K

Vitamin C *(acidum ascorbicum, ascorbic acid, acidé ascorbique)*
antiscorbutic vitamin, factor in resisting infection, antioxidant
↑ oxalate
↓ TAG, uric acid
- **Urine** ↑ G (false), Hb, uric acid, crystals – (cystine, oxalate, urate)
- **Stool** ↑ blood

Vitamin D *(cholecalciferolum, cholecalciferol, cholecalciferol)*
antirachitis vitamin
↑ ALP, Ca, Ca²⁺, cholesterol, creatinine, MAC, P, urea
↓ PTH
- **Urine** ↑ proteins, Ca, Ca²⁺, hydroxyproline, volume
↓ P

Vitamin E *(tocoferolum, tocopherol, tocoferol)*
antioxidant
- **Urine** ↓ ALA, uroporphyrin

Vitamin K *(phytomenadionum, phytomenadione, phytoménadione)*
prothrombogenic vitamin
↑ Bil (neonates), catecholamines, Heinz bodies (RBC)
- **Urine** ↑ proteins, 17-OHCS, porphyrins

Warfarin *(warfarinum, warfarin, warfarine)*
anticoagulant
↑ ALP, ALT, AST, AT III, BT, proteins, eos, GMT, creatinine, PT, uric acid, T4, TSH
↓ albumin, factor – (II, VII, IX, X), G, uric acid, T3, PLT, WBC
- **Urine** ↑ blood, Hb, RBC, proteins, histamine, uric acid
↓ G
- **Cerebrospinal Fluid** ↑ eos

Xanthine *(xanthinum, xanthine, xanthine)*
treatment of liver disorders
↑ proteins, coagulation factors
- **Urine** ↑ chloride, K, crystals, Na, volume

Xenazoic Acid *(acidum xenazoicum, xenazoic acid, acide xenazoique)*
antiviral
↑ ALP

Xipamide *(xipamidum, xipamide, xipamide)*
diuretic, antihypertensive
↑ aldosterone, renin
↓ ANP

Xylitol *(xylitolum, xylitol, xilitol)*
dietetic
↑ Bil, uric acid, LA, MAC

Yohimbine *(yohimbinum, yohimbine, yohimbine)*
sympatholytic, aphrodisiac
↑ norepinephrine

Zafirlukast *(zafirlukastum, zafirlukast, zafirlukast)*
   leukotriene receptor antagonist
         ↑ ALT, AST, Bil, GMT
         ↓ granulocytes

Zalcitabine *(zalcitabinum, zalcitabine, zalcitabine)*
   antiviral
         ↑ ALP, ALT, AMS, AST, G, GMT, MAC
         ↓ Ca, neu, WBC
         ■ *Urine* ↑ volume

Zaltidine *(zaltidinum, zaltidine, zaltidine)*
   histamine H₂ receptor antagonist
         ↑ ALT

Zidovudine *(zidovudinum, zidovudine, zidovudine)*
   antiviral
         ↑ ALP, ALT, AST, Bil, CK, GMT, MAC, macrocytes
         ↓ Hb, WBC, neu, PLT

Zileuton *(zileutonum, zileuton, zileuton)*
   5-lipoxygenase inhibitor, bronchodilator
         ↑ ALT, AST, GMT

Zimeldine *(zimeldine hydrochloride, zimeldine, zimeldine)*
   antidepressant
         ↑ ALP, ALT, AST, ESR, GMT, creatinine, PRL
         ↓ WBC, PLT
         ■ *Cerebrospinal Fluid* ↓ 5-HIAA

Zinc *(zincum, zinc, zinc)*
   topical antiherpetic
         ↑ ALP, AMS, Ca, lipase
         ↓ ALP, Cu, Hb, HDL cholesterol, neu, PRL, WBC

Zolpidem *(zolpidemum, zolpidem, zolpidem)*
   non-benzodiazepine sedative, hypnotic
         ↑ Bil, cholesterol, lipids, urea
         ■ *Urine* ↑ volume

Zomepirac *(zomepiracum, zomepirac, zomepirac)*
   analgesic, antiinflammatory
         ↑ ALT
         ↓ neu
         ■ *Stool* ↑ Hb

Zonisamide *(zonisamidum, zonisamide, zonisamide)*
   anticonvulsant, antiepileptic
         ↑ ALT, AST, GMT, urea

Zoxazolamine *(zoxazolaminum, zoxazolamine, zoxazolamine)*
   skeletal muscle relaxant, uricosuric
         ↑ ALT, creatinine
         ↓ uric acid

Zuclopenthixol *(zuclopenthixolum, zuclopenthixol, zuclopenthixol)*
   neuroleptic
         ↑ ALP

Reference Ranges

R. Pullmann

Blood – Plasma – Serum

A – native blood, B – blood sampling into heparin, C – blood sampling into chelatone, D – pre-cooled tube, E – special sampling. IFCC – International Federation of Clinical Chemistry. DGKC – Deutsche Gesellschaft für Klinische Chemie (Germany). If age/gender not stated – values are valid for adults.

Analyte	Age/ Gender	Reference Range	SI Units	Note
Acetoacetate		20–40	µmol/l	A
Acetoacetic Acid	0–3 y	0–310	µmol/l	
	4–15 y	0–270	µmol/l	
	Adults	5–75	µmol/l	
Acetone				
Semiquantitative		negat.		A, B
Quantitative		0.05–0.34	mmol/l	HPLC, GC, isotachophoresis
Acetylsalicylic Acid		1.1–2.2	mmol/l	Blood collection 1–3 hrs after oral dose.
Acid Phosphatase (ACP)				A, B
Total ACP	F	<92	nkat/l	Determine immediately or
	M	<108	nkat/l	use acid to pH 4.5.
Prostatic ACP	M	<43	nkat/l	Substrate: alpha-naphthyl phosphate, pentadiole activated
Total ACP	F + M	75–215	nkat/l	Values determined by experiment without temperature conversion factors
Prostatic ACP	M	<68	nkat/l	Substrate: alpha-naphthyl phosphate without pentadiole activation.
Adrenocortico-tropic Hormone (ACTH)	Umbilicus	130–160	µg/l	C, EDTA, + aprotinine 400 kU/ml
	1–7 d	100–140	µg/l	mercaptoethanol 2 µl/ml
	Adults			
	8 AM	4.4–22	pmol/l	
	6 PM	<11	pmol/l	
Alanine Amino-transferase (ALT)	1 d	<0.52	µkat/l	A
Glutamate	2–5 d	<0.87	µkat/l	37 °C, IFCC,

Analyte	Age/Gender	Reference Range	SI Units	Note
Pyruvate Transaminase (GPT)	6 d–6 m	<1.00	µkat/l	DGKC, optimized
	7–12 m	<0.95	µkat/l	
	1–3 y	<0.65	µkat/l	
	4–6 y	<0.48	µkat/l	
	7–12 y	<0.65	µkat/l	
	13–17 y F	<0.38	µkat/l	
	13–17 y M	<0.43	µkat/l	
	Adults F	<0.52	µkat/l	
	Adults M	<0.68	µkat/l	
Albumin	Neonates	38–42	g/l	A
	Adults	33–50	g/l	Bromocresol-green method
		37–53	g/l	IFCC, (EDTA and citrate ⁻)
Aldolase	10–24 m	3.4–11.8	U/l	A
	25 m–16 y	1.2–8.8	U/l	
	Adults	<135	nkat/l	
Alkaline Phosphatase (ALP)				
Total	1 d	<10.00	µkat/l	A
	2–5 d	<9.22	µkat/l	37 °C
	6 d–6 m	<17.94	µkat/l	DEA buffer
	7 m–1 y	<18.45	µkat/l	
	2–3 y	<11.22	µkat/l	
	4–6 y	<10.74	µkat/l	
	7–12 y	<12.00	µkat/l	
	13–17 y F	<7.47	µkat/l	
	13–17 y M	<15.60	µkat/l	
	Adults F	<4.00	µkat/l	
	Adults M	<4.50	µkat/l	
	Adults F	0.74–2.1	µkat/l	IFCC
	Adults M	0.9–2.29	µkat/l	
Bone	Adults F	<2.00	µkat/l	DGKC, optimized
	Adults M	<2.50	µkat/l	
	Adults F	<0.83	µkat/l	IFCC
	Adults M	<1.00	µkat/l	
Aluminium		<0.11	µmol/l	E Only use tubes specifically designed for determination of trace elements.
Amino Acids See Individual AA				
Ammonia	1 d	<144	µmol/l	C, E
	5–6 d	<134	µmol/l	UV-test. Plasma treated with EDTA or lithium heparinate, refrigerated. Add
	Children	<48	µmol/l	serine (5 mmol/l) and borate (2 mmol/l) to block in vitro ammonia production
	Adults F	6–48	µmol/l	Perform assay immediately after sampling.
	Adults M	10–55	µmol/l	Mild sweat contamination. Full tube sampling

Analyte	Age/ Gender	Reference Range	SI Units	Note
Amylase (AMS)				A 37 °C
Total	Adults	0.50–3.67	µkat/l	EPS method, G7 substrate
				Frequent saliva contamination
Pancreatic	1–5 d	<0.03	µkat/l	EPS method, G7 substrate
	6 d–6 m	<0.27	µkat/l	Reference values are dependent on method
	7 m–1 y	<0.75	µkat/l	
	2–3 y	<1.02	µkat/l	
	4–6 y	<1.10	µkat/l	
	7–12 y F	<1.22	µkat/l	
	7–12 y M	<1.08	µkat/l	
	13–17 y	<1.28	µkat/l	
	Adults	<1.92	µkat/l	
Amylin		2.90–3.40	pmol/l	E
Androstenedione		2.9–9.4	nmol/l	A
	F post-menopause	<6.3	nmol/l	
Angiotensin Converting Enzyme (ACE)	2–9 y	250–440	U/l	A Neels' method
	10–20 y	280–450	U/l	
	21–50 y	252–360	U/l	
	51–80 y	233–314	U/l	
	Adults	6.1–21.1	U/l	Liebermann's method
		133–867	nkat/l	Enzymatic photometry
Anti-Acetylcholine Receptor Ab		<0.5	nmol/l	A Immunoanalysis
Anti-Cardiolipin Ab				A ELISA
IgG		<8.5	*	*GPL U/ml
IgA		10.5–100	**	**APL U/ml
IgM		9.0–100	***	***MPL U/ml
Anti-Cytomegalovirus Antibodies				
IgM	negative	<0.80		A
	borderline	0.81–0.99		ELISA, MEIA
	positive	>1.00		
Antideoxyribonuclease B Titre		<170	U/l	
Antidiuretic Hormone (ADH) plasma osmolality				E refrigerated plasma, RIA
270–280 mOsm/kg		<1.38	pmol/l	Correlation with Posm and Uosm needed
281–285 mOsm/kg		<2.38	pmol/l	
286–290 mOsm/kg		0.92–4.81	pmol/l	
291–295 mOsm/kg		1.84–6.45	pmol/l	
296–300 mOsm/kg		3.7–11.1	pmol/l	
Anti-DS-DNA Ab		6.3–20.0	IU/ml	A ELISA

Analyte	Age/ Gender	Reference Range	SI Units	Note
Ki-1 Antigen (CD30)		<6	U/ml	E ELISA
Anti-Gliadin Ab				A ELISA
IgG		1.23–100	U/ml	
IgA		1.23–100	U/ml	
Anti-Glomerular Basement Membrane				
Ab (IgG)		<3	U/ml	A ELISA
Anti-Intrinsic				
Factor Antibodies	negative	<0.9		A, B ELISA
	borderline	0.9–1.1		
	positive	>1.1		
Anti-Mitochondrial				
Ab		<1:20		A Immunofluorescency
Anti-Myeloperoxi-				
dase Ab (IgG)		<9.0	U/ml	A ELISA
Anti-Nuclear Ab				
(ANA)	borderline	1:80		A
	positive	>1:160		Indirect immunofluores- cency (IFF) A, EIA
Anti-p53				
negative index		<0.9		
positive index		>1.1		
Anti-Pancreatic				
Islet Cell Ab (ICA)		<2.5	JDF	
			U/ml	A
Anti-Proteinase				
Ab (Anti-PR3 IgG)		<2	U/ml	A As a part of anti-neutro- phil antibodies (c-ANCA).
Antistreptolysin O				
(ASLO)	Children	<150.10³	U/ml	A Immunoturbidimetric method
	Adults	<200.10³	U/ml	
Anti-Thyroglo- bulin Ab (ATGA)		<150	U/ml	A IRMA
Anti-Thyro-Peroxi- dase Antibodies (TPOA)		<20	U/ml	A RIA
Anti-Thyrotropin Receptor Antibodies		<0.140	U/ml	A ELISA
Alpha-1-Anti- Trypsin (AAT)		0.90–2.0	g/l	A (EDTA + chelates ↓) Immunonephelometry
Trypsin-inhibitory capacity (Pi)		1.4–2.4	kIU/l	Citrate plasma
Phenotype		PiMM		ELPHO, IEF
Apolipoprotein				
A-I	Children	1.20–1.76	g/l	A Do not refrigerate

Analyte	Age/ Gender	Reference Range	SI Units	Note
	F	1.15–1.98	g/l	Turbidimetric method
	M	0.95–1.76	g/l	
	F	1.20–2.20	g/l	A IFCC method and standard.
	M	1.10–2.00	g/l	Follow NCEP guidelines
Apolipoprotein A-II		300–500	mg/l	A Turbidimetric method. ID
Apolipoprotein A-IV		130–230	mg/l	A Turbidimetric method. ID
Apolipoprotein B	F	0.63–1.47	g/l	A Turbidimetric method
	M	0.70–1.60	g/l	
	F	0.60–1.25	g/l	A IFCC method and standard.
	M	0.55–1.35	g/l	Follow NCEP guidelines
Apolipoprotein				A Turbidimetric method. ID
C		30–110	mg/l	
C		10–70	mg/l	
C		30–230	mg/l	
Apolipoprotein D		<100	mg/l	A
Apolipoprotein E		20–60	mg/l	A Turbidimetric method. ID
Aspartate Amino- transferase (AST). Glutamate Oxalo- acetic Transaminase (GOT)	1 d	<1.82	µkat/l	A DGKC, 37 °C, IFCC, optimized
	2–5 d	<1.62	µkat/l	
	6 d–6 m	<1.28	µkat/l	
	7–12 m	<1.37	µkat/l	
	1–3 y	<0.80	µkat/l	
	4–6 y	<0.60	µkat/l	
	7–12 y	<0.78	µkat/l	
	13–17 y F	<0.42	µkat/l	
	13–17 y M	<0.48	µkat/l	
	Adults F	<0.52	µkat/l	
	Adults M	<0.62	µkat/l	
Bile Acids, Total				Enzymatic
	fasting	0.3–2.3	mg/l	
	2 hrs after meals	1.8–3.2	mg/l	
Bilirubin				
Total Bilirubin	1 d	<85.5	µmol/l	A
	2 d	<154	µmol/l	DPD. Protect from light, perform assay immediately, mainly in neonates
	3–5 d	<205	µmol/l	
	Children	<25.7	µmol/l	
	Adults	<22.2	µmol/l	
Conjugated bilirubin		<5.1	µmol/l	A
Bladder Tumor Antigen (BTA)		0.6–6.7	U/ml	A Immunochromatography.
Brain Natriuretic Peptide (BNP)		1.5–9.0	pmol/l	C (ANP/BNP >1)

Analyte	Age/Gender	Reference Range	SI Units	Note
CA 15-3 (Breast Cancer Mucin)		<28	U/ml	A ELISA, IRMA, MEIA. Specificity: 95%. Sensitivity (breast cancer + mts) 70–80%.
CA 19-9		<37	U/ml	A ELISA, IRMA, MEIA. Specificity: 95%
CA 50		<25	U/ml	A RIA, IRMA
CA 72-4		<4	U/ml	A ELISA, IRMA, MEIA. Specificity: 95%
CA 125		<35	U/ml	A ELISA, IRMA, MEIA. Specificity: 95%
CA 242		16–20	U/ml	A IRMA, ELISA
CA 549	F	0–11	U/ml	A IRMA, ELISA
	M	1.1–6.7	U/ml	
Caffeine		26–103	μmol/l	Blood collection – in premature infants 1 hour after an i.v. dose
Calcitonin (hCT)	M	3–26	pg/ml	E, C (A, B) RIA, IRMA, EIA
	F	2–17	pg/ml	Stabilization with aprotinine 400 U/ml.
Calcium				A o-cresolphthalein complexone, without deproteinization
Total Calcium	1 d–4 w	1.8–2.8	mmol/l	
	2–12 m	2.1–2.7	mmol/l	
	>1 y	2.1–2.6	mmol/l	
	Adults	2.15–2.55	mmol/l	
Free Ionized Calcium	Children	1.15–1.45	mmol/l	E Anaerobic collection of sample treated with low-concentration heparin minimizes binding of ionized calcium.
	Adults	1.13–1.32	mmol/l	Perform assay immediately after sample collection and determine pH.
Carbamazepine		17–43	μmol/l	A Blood collection: maximum 6–18 hrs after final dose, minimum immediately before next dose
Carbon Dioxide, Total (tCO₂)	Umbilical blood	14–22	mmol/l	E (anaerobic sampling)
	Immature neon.	14–27	mmol/l	
	Neonates	13–22	mmol/l	
	Infants	20–28	mmol/l	
	Children	20–28	mmol/l	
	Adults	23–30	mmol/l	

Analyte	Age/Gender	Reference Range	SI Units	Note
Carcino-embryonic Antigen (CEA)	Non-smokers	<3.7	ng/ml	A
	Smokers	<10.0	ng/ml	ELISA, IRMA, MEIA
	Inductors	<40	ng/ml	Dependent on individual reference values
Carnitine				A, C
Free	Adults F	17–45	µmol/l	
	Adults M	24–51	µmol/l	
Total	Adults F	23–53	µmol/l	
	Adults M	29–59	µmol/l	
Beta-Carotene		0.95–3.7	µmol/l	E Store and transport in dark. Perform assay immediately.
Catecholamines				E
Norepinephrine				Glutathione 1.2 mg/ml + EDTA
– recumbency		591–2364	pmol/l	special tube
– standing		1773–5320	pmol/l	separate plasma for 15 min then refrigerate to –20 °C
Epinephrine				
– recumbency		<382	pmol/l	
– standing		<546	pmol/l	
Dopamine		<196	pmol/l	Without position influence
Ceruloplasmin		0.15–0.45	g/l	A Immunoturbidimetric method
Chloramphenicol		31–77	µmol/l	Blood collection: maximum 2–3 hrs after final dose (subject to wide variability), minimum: immediately before next dose.
Chloride	1 d–4 w	95–116	mmol/l	A
	2–12 m	93–112	mmol/l	
	>1 y	96–111	mmol/l	
	Adults	98–106	mmol/l	
Cholesterol				
Total	<4 w	1.3–4.4	mmol/l	A Recommended values
	2–12 m	1.6–4.5	mmol/l	CHOD-PAP method
	Adults	2.8–5.2	mmol/l	
HDL	F	>1.68	mmol/l	mild risk 1.15–1.67 mmol/l high risk <1.15 mmol/l
	M	>1.45	mmol/l	mild risk 1.05–1.44 mmol/l medium risk 0.90–1.04 mmol/l high risk <0.89 mmol/l
LDL	Adults	<3.2	mmol/l	
		<2.8	mmol/l	Secondary prevention after MI and in more than 2 risk factors
VLDL		0.1–0.5	mmol/l	

Analyte	Age/ Gender	Reference Range	SI Units	Note
Cholinesterase (CHE)	Children, adults (M, F >40y)	88–215	μkat/l	A 37 °C
	F 16–39 y	72–187	μkat/l	Pseudocholinesterase, butyrylthiocholine iodide
	F 18–39 y*	60–152	μkat/l	*Pregnant women or taking oral contraceptives
Chromogranin A and B		10–53	μg/l	A, RIA
Circulating Immune Complexes				A
		<8.8	%	1/ complement fixation test
		<0.035		2/ PEG precipitation
		<6.1	%	3/ PEG-CIC-IgM
		<12.8	%	4/ PEG-CIC-IgG
		<12	mg/l	5/ C3-CIC-ELISA
Cobalt		80–170	μmol/l	E Special tube.
Complement Classical Pathway Components				A Fresh serum. Immuno-turbidimetric method
C1r		0.025–0.038	g/l	
C1s		0.025–0.038	g/l	
C2	Umbilical blood	0.016–0.028	g/l	
	1 m	0.019–0.039	g/l	
	6 m	0.024–0.036	g/l	
	Adults	0.016–0.040	g/l	
C3	Umbilical blood	0.570–1.160	g/l	Fresh serum
	1–3 m	0.530–1.310	g/l	
	3 m–1 y	0.620–1.800	g/l	
	1–10 y	0.770–1.950	g/l	
	Adults	0.830–1.770	g/l	
C4	Umbilical blood	0.070–0.230	g/l	Fresh serum
	1–3 m	0.070–0.270	g/l	
	3 m–10 y	0.070–0.400	g/l	
	Adults	0.150–0.450	g/l	
C5	Umbilical blood	0.034–0.062	g/l	
	1 m	0.023–0.063	g/l	
	6 m	0.024–0.064	g/l	
	Adults	0.038–0.090	g/l	
C6	Umbilical blood	0.010–0.042	g/l	

Analyte	Age/ Gender	Reference Range	SI Units	Note
	1 m	0.022–0.052	g/l	
	6 m	0.037–0.071	g/l	
	Adults	0.040–0.072	g/l	
C7		0.049–0.070	g/l	
C8		0.043–0.063	g/l	
C9		0.047–0.069	g/l	
Complement				Alternative pathway components
C4-Binding Protein Factor B (C3 Proactivator)	Umbilical blood	0.18–0.320	g/l	
	1 m	0.078–0.158	g/l	RID Nephelometry
	6 m	0.062–0.286	g/l	
	Adults	0.169–0.293	g/l	
Properdin	Umbilical blood	0.147–0.335	g/l	
	1 m	0.013–0.017	g/l	
	6 m	0.006–0.022	g/l	
	Adults	0.013–0.025	g/l	
		0.020–0.036	g/l	
C1-Esterase Inhibitor		0.174–240	g/l	A, B Perform assay immediately with fresh serum or refrigerated plasma
C1-INH (functionally)		70–130	%	Activity determination
		0.7–1.3		
Complement Total Hemolytic Activity (CH50)		75–160	IU/ml	A CH50 activity determination
Copper	Neonates			E AAS
	– premature	2.7–7.7	µmol/l	Bathocuproin disulphonate.
	– mature	8.3–11.2	µmol/l	Freeze.
	Children	10.3–21.4	µmol/l	
	Adults F	12.4–20.6	µmol/l	
	Adults M	11.6–19.2	µmol/l	
Corticosteroid Binding Globulin (CBG, Transcortin)	M	15–20	mg/l	Saturation analysis.
	F			
	Follicular phase	17–20	mg/l	
	Luteal phase	16–21	mg/l	
	Menopause	17–25	mg/l	
	Pregnancy			
	– 21–28 w	47–54	mg/l	
	– 33–40 w	55–70	mg/l	

Analyte	Age/Gender	Reference Range	SI Units	Note
Cortisol	7–8 AM	0.14–0.60	µmol/l	A
	4–7 PM	0.08–0.46	µmol/l	Homogenous enzyme immunoassay
	Midnight	0.03–0.11	µmol/l	RIA
	Children–AM	0.14–0.40	µmol/l	
Creatine	1–14 w	16.8–95.4	µmol/l	A creatine/creatinine coeficient ↓
	Adults	12.2–30.5	µmol/l	(only in infants)
Creatine Kinase, total (CK)	1 d	<11.9	µkat/l	A
	2–5 d	<10.9	µkat/l	37 °C
	6 d–6 m	<4.92	µkat/l	store in darkness
	7–12 m	<3.38	µkat/l	CK-BB is unstable without stabilizer
	1–3 y	<3.80	µkat/l	
	4–6 y	<2.48	µkat/l	
	7–12 y F	<2.57	µkat/l	
	7–12 y M	<4.12	µkat/l	
	13–17 y F	<2.05	µkat/l	
	13–17 y M	<4.50	µkat/l	
	Adults F	<2.78	µkat/l	
	Adults M	<3.17	µkat/l	
Creatine Kinase MB Mass (CK-MB)		<5	µg/l	A, B
Creatine Kinase MB (CK-MB)		<0.40	µkat/l	A 37 °C. DGKC, optimized. Myocardial infarction is suspected if the CK-M activity is 6–25% of the elevated total CK activity (elevated total CK activity >100 U/l or >1.67 µkat/l at 25 °C, >240 U/l or >4.00 µkat/l at 37 °C).
Creatine Kinase Isoenzymes CK-MM		0.97–1.00		A ELPHO. Portion of total activity
– MB		<0.03		
– BB		0		In physiological conditions
Creatine Kinase Isoforms MB$_2$/MB$_1$		≤1.5		C
– MM$_3$/MM$_1$		≤0.7		
– MB$_2$		<2.0		
Creatinine	Neonates	<106	µmol/l	A
	<6 m	<80	µmol/l	PAP method
	<7 m	<88	µmol/l	
	Adults F	<80	µmol/l	
	Adults M	<97	µmol/l	

Medicaments – Interfering Factors

Analyte	Age/ Gender	Reference Range	SI Units	Note
	Neonates	<115	μmol/l	Jaffé's kinetic method
	<1 w	<88	μmol/l	
	2–4 w	<44	μmol/l	Interference at bilirubin concentrations
	Adults F	<97	μmol/l	>171 μmol/l (Jaffé's, PAP methods).
	<50 y M	<115	μmol/l	
	>50 y M	<124	μmol/l	
Cryofibrinogen		<60	mg/l	E
Cryoglobulins		<80	mg/l	E
Cyclic Adenosine Monophosphate (cAMP)	M	17–33	nmol/l	E
	F	11–27	nmol/l	RIA
CYFRA 21-1		<3.3	ng/ml	A ELISA, IRMA Enzymun-Test CYFRA 21-1. Specificity 95%
Cystatine C	0–50 y	0.63–1.33	ng/l	A
	>50 y	0.94–1.55	ng/l	
Dehydroepiandro-sterone (DHEA)	M			A, C
	<9.8 y	1.07–11.96	nmol/l	IRMA, ELISA
	9.8–14.5 y	3.81–17.16	nmol/l	
	10.7–15.4 y	5.89–20.28	nmol/l	
	11.8–16.2 y	5.55–22.19	nmol/l	
	12.8–17.3 y	8.67–31.21	nmol/l	
	Adults	5.55–27.74	nmol/l	
	F			
	<9.2 y	1.07–11.96	nmol/l	
	9.2–13.7 y	5.20–19.76	nmol/l	
	10.0–14.4 y	6.93–20.80	nmol/l	
	10.7–15.6 y	6.93–24.27	nmol/l	
	11.8–18.6 y	7.45–29.47	nmol/l	
	Adults F	5.55–27.74		
Dehydroepian-drosterone Sulphate (DHEA-S)	M			A, C
	<9.8 y	0.34–2.16	μmol/l	IRMA, ELISA
	9.8–14.5 y	1.09–2.83	μmol/l	
	10.7–15.4 y	1.25–5.20	μmol/l	
	11.8–16.2 y	2.65–10.01	μmol/l	
	12.8–17.3 y	3.12–9.62	μmol/l	
	Adults	4.68–11.70	μmol/l	
	F			
	<9.2 y	0.49–2.96	μmol/l	
	9.2–13.7 y	0.88–3.35	μmol/l	
	10.0–14.4 y	0.83–8.48	μmol/l	
	10.7–15.6 y	1.51–6.76	μmol/l	
	11.8–18.6 y	1.14–6.45	μmol/l	
	Adults	1.56–7.7	μmol/l	

Analyte	Age/ Gender	Reference Range	SI Units	Note
Deoxypyridinoline	M	2.3–5.4	*	*nmol DPD/mmol creatinine. Collect into dark tube.
	F	3.0–7.4	*	
Digitoxin		17–33	nmol/l	A Collect blood 8–24 hrs after last dose.
Digoxin		1.0–2.6	nmol/l	A Collect blood 8–24 hrs after last dose.
Dihydrotesto-sterone (DHT)	M			A
	<9.8 y	<0.10	nmol/l	
	9.8–14.5 y	0.10–0.59	nmol/l	
	10.7–15.4 y	0.28–1.14	nmol/l	
	11.8–16.2 y	0.76–1.79	nmol/l	
	12.8–17.3 y	0.83–2.24	nmol/l	
	Adults	1.03–2.93	nmol/l	
	F			
	<9.2 y	<0.10	nmol/l	
	9.2–13.7 y	0.17–0.41	nmol/l	
	10.0–14.4 y	0.24–0.65	nmol/l	
	10.7–15.6 y	0.14–0.45	nmol/l	
	11.8–18.6 y	0.10–0.62	nmol/l	
	Adults	0.14–0.76	nmol/l	
Disopyramide		6–15	µmol/l	A Sampling: max. 2–3 hrs after final dose, min. immediately before next dose.
Dopamine		196–553	pmol/l	B HPLC, RE
Elastase (PMN)	Neonates			B
	1–2 d	<75	µg/l	EIA, RIA
	3–28 d	<50	µg/l	
	Adults	29–86	µg/l	C
Elastase-1, Pancreatic		<3.5	ng/ml	A
Endothelin-1	M	0.38–0.44	pg/ml	A, B
	F	0.36–0.39	pg/ml	
	>60 y	0.41–0.43	pg/ml	
Epinephrine		165–468	pmol/l	B
C1-Esterase Inhibitor		0.15–0.35	g/l	A Fresh sample, frozen stabilized plasma. Turbidimetric method.
Estradiol	<10 y	22–140	pmol/l	A, B
	F			ELISA
	Follicular phase		37–550	pmol/l
	Pre-ovulation	400–1 400	pmol/l	
	Luteal phase	300–910	pmol/l	
Post-menopause	40–170	pmol/l		
	Oral contra-ceptives	15–120	pmol/l	

Analyte	Age/ Gender	Reference Range	SI Units	Note
	Pregnancy			
	1st trimester	400–5000	pmol/l	
	2nd trimester	2500–62500	pmol/l	
	3rd trimester	8800–99700	pmol/l	
	M	35–150	pmol/l	
Estriol, Total	pregnancy (week)			A, B
	24–28	104–590	nmol/l	ELISA, IRMA
	28–32	140–760	nmol/l	
	32–36	208–970	nmol/l	
	36–40	280–1210	nmol/l	
	Adult M and non-pregnant F	<7.0	nmol/l	
Estriol, Free	pregnancy (week)			A
	25	12.1–34.7	nmol/l	ELISA, IRMA
	28	13.9–43.4	nmol/l	
	30	15.6–48.6	nmol/l	
	32	17.4–55.5	nmol/l	
	34	19.1–64.2	nmol/l	
	36	24.3–86.8	nmol/l	
	37	27.8–97.2	nmol/l	
	38	31.2–111.0	nmol/l	
	39	34.7–118.0	nmol/l	
	40–41	36.4–86.8	nmol/l	
Estrogens, Total	Children	<30	ng/l	A
	M	40–115	ng/l	ELISA, IRMA
	F–cycle day			
	1–10 d	61–394	ng/l	
	11–20 d	122–437	ng/l	
	21–30 d	156–350	ng/l	
	before puberty	<40	ng/l	
Ethosuximide		283–708	µmol/l	A Blood collection: interval between doses.
Fatty Acids, Free	Neonates	694–1034		A
	Infants	1450–2018		Perform assay immediately after collection. Lipase activation with heparin
	1 y	1433–2075	mg/l	
	2–5 y	2268–3006	mg/l	
	6–10 y	3018–3018	mg/l	
	11–15 y	2200–2800	mg/l	
	Adults	2879–3253	mg/l	
		0.15–0.71	mmol/l	
	F–lactation	5315–6245	mg/l	

Analyte	Age/ Gender	Reference Range	SI Units	Note
Ferritin	1 d–1 w	145–458	µg/l	A ELISA, RIA
	Infants	52–421	µg/l	Values dependent on method, age, sex
	3 m–10 y	9.3–65	µg/l	
	11–16 y Adults	12–150	µg/l	
	<50 y F	8–156	µg/l	
	Adults M Adults	8–140	µg/l	
	>50 y F	20–400	µg/l	
	6 w–18 y Adults	15–120	µg/l	Immunoturbidimetrie method
	<50 y F Adults	10–160	µg/l	
	>50 y F	30–300	µg/l	
	Adults M	30–300	µg/l	
Alpha-1-Fetoprotein	1–30 d F	<18700	µg/l	A
	1–30 d M	<16400	µg/l	ELISA, RIA, IRMA, MEIA
	1 m–1 y F	<77	µg/l	
	1 m–1 y M	<28	µg/l	
	2–3 y F	<11	µg/l	
	2–3 y M	<7.9	µg/l	
	4–6 y F	<4.2	µg/l	
	4–6 y M	<5.6	µg/l	
	7–12 y F	<5.6	µg/l	
	7–12 y M	<3.7	µg/l	
	13–18 y F	<4.2	µg/l	
	13–18 y M	<3.9	µg/l	
	Adults F	0.8–9.1	µg/l	Non-pregnant
	Adults M	0.8–9.5	µg/l	
	Pregnancy			
	4–8 w	<8.4	µg/l	
	15 w	<34.0	µg/l	
	16 w	<38.0	µg/l	
	17 w	<44.0	µg/l	
	18 w	<49.0	µg/l	
	19 w	<56.5	µg/l	
	20 w	<66.0	µg/l	
Fibronectin		0.25–0.40	g/l	E EIA
Folic Acid	Neonates	15.9–72.4	nmol/l	E Hemolysate (0.5 ml of
	F + M	4.1–38	nmol/l	blood + 4.5 ml of ascorbic acid).
		>4.3	nmol/l	A
Follicle Stimulating Hormone (FSH)	<10 y F	0.5–2	IU/l	A ELISA, RIA
	Follicular phase	2–12	IU/l	
	Mid-cycle	10–20	IU/l	

Analyte	Age/Gender	Reference Range	SI Units	Note
	Postmenopause	>20	IU/l	
	Luteal phase	2–10	IU/l	
	M	<11	IU/l	
Fructosamine	0–3 y	1.56–2.27	mmol/l	A
	3–6 y	1.73–2.34	mmol/l	Calibration on reference standard with molar unit. Photometric colorimetric test
	6–9 y	1.82–2.56	mmol/l	If protein <65 g/l or >80 g/l use formula fructosamine
	9–15 y	2.02–2.63	mmol/l	= actual fructosamine : total protein x 72
	Adults	1.6–2.6	mmol/l	
Fructose		<0.56	mmol/l	B
		19–47	µmol/l	
Galactose	Children	0–0.46	mmol/l	A
	Adults	0–0.24	mmol/l	
	Umbilical blood	0.417–0.787	*	*Galactose-1-phosphate in RBC
	0–1 y	0.491–0.779	*	(µmol/min/g Hb)
	Adults	0.33–0.585	*	
Galactose-1-Phosphate	5 m–17 y	0–0.17	*	*µmol/g Hb
Gastric Inhibitory Polypeptide (GIP)		8–10	pmol/l	A
Gastrin	fasting	<48	pmol/l	A Add aprotinine (2000 kIU/ml) to stabilize.12 hrs fasting.
	post-prandial	46–100	pmol/l	Reference values are method dependent.
		40–210	pg/ml	Freeze immediately.
Gentamicin		11–22	µmol/l	A Blood collection: maximum 30 min post i.v. infusion, minimum: immediately before next dose.
Gc-Globulin		350–450	mg/l	A
Glucagon		25–250	ng/l	Diagnostic values >1000 ng/l. Stabilization with aprotinine.
Glucose	Neonates 6 hrs	0.33–3.3	mmol/l	Sample treated with glycolysis inhibitors.
capillary blood	>5 d	0.72–4.2	mmol/l	
	1–2 y	1.8–6.2	mmol/l	
	3–4 y	2.9–5.4	mmol/l	
	5–6 y	3.8–5.5	mmol/l	
	Adults	3.3–5.5	mmol/l	
venous plasma	Adults	3.5–6.4	mmol/l	B

Analyte	Age/ Gender	Reference Range	SI Units	Note
Glucose-6-Phosphate Dehydrogenase (RBC)		8–40	µkat/l	B, C
Glutamate Dehydrogenase (GLDH)	1–30 d	<163	nkat/l	A
	1–6 m	<107	nkat/l	37 °C, DGKC, optimized
	13–24 m	<87	nkat/l	
	2–3 y	<63	nkat/l	
	13–15 y	<80	nkat/l	
	Adults F	<88	nkat/l	
	Adults M	<123	nkat/l	
Glutamic Acid				A
Free	Neonates	0–900	µmol/l	
	1–3 y	<180	µmol/l	
	Adults	25–115	µmol/l	
Total	Adults	517–720	µmol/l	
Glutamic Acid Decarboxylase Ab		1–2	U/ml	A
Glutamine	Neonates	20–120	µmol/l	A
	Infants	<300	µmol/l	
	Adults	<50	µmol/l	
Gamma-Glutamyl-transferase (GMT) 37 °C	1 d	<2.52	µkat/l	A
	2–5 d	<3.08	µkat/l	Method according to Szasz
	6 d–6 m	<3.40	µkat/l	
	7–12 m	<0.57	µkat/l	
	1–3 y	<0.30	µkat/l	
	4–6 y	<0.38	µkat/l	
	7–12 y	<0.28	µkat/l	
	13–17 F	<0.55	µkat/l	
	13–17 M	<0.75	µkat/l	
	Adults F	<0.53	µkat/l	
	Adults M	<0.82	µkat/l	
	Adults F	<0.75	µkat/l	IFCC
	Adults M	<1.07	µkat/l	
Glycerol, Free	Children	10–110	µmol/l	A Perform assay immediately.
	Adults	60–180	µmol/l	
Glycine	Neonates	240–480	µmol/l	A
	Infants	100–300	µmol/l	
	Children	170–370	µmol/l	
	Adults	170–260	µmol/l	
Glycogenphosphorylase (BB-isoenzyme)		<7	µg/l	A, B
Histamine	plasma	<10	nmol/l	A, B
		<1	ng/ml	
	whole blood	200–2 000	nmol/l	
		20–200	ng/ml	

Analyte	Age/Gender	Reference Range	SI Units	Note
	cellular spontaneous release	0.10–1.00		of total histamine
		<0.05		of total histamine
Histidine	Neonates	70–120	µmol/l	A
	Infants	50–120	µmol/l	
	Children	50–120	µmol/l	
	Adults	60–100	µmol/l	
Homocysteine	M			A Stabilized blood (NaF 4 mg/ml). Follow sampling rules precisely. Only 1 hour stability in room temperature. Serum levels > plasma levels.
	<30 y	6–14	µmol/l	
	30–59 y	6–16	µmol/l	
	>60 y	6–17	µmol/l	
	F			
	<30 y	6–14	µmol/l	
	30–59 y	5–13	µmol/l	
	>60 y	7–14	µmol/l	
Human Chorionic Gonadotropin (hCG)	M + F	<5	U/l	A
	F-postmeno-pause	<10	U/l	ELISA, RIA, IRMA, MEIA
	Pregnancy after conception	>5	U/l	
	7–10 d	>100	U/l	
	30 d	>2000	U/l	
	40 d	50000–100000	U/l	
	10 w	1000–2000	U/l	
	trophoblast diseases	>100000	U/l	
Human Placental Lactogen (hPL)	Pregnancy			
	>6 w	25–100	µg/l	A
	36 w	4–11	mg/l	
Human Soluble Endothelial Cell Leukocyte Adhesion Molecule-1 (h-sELAM-1)		0.13–2.8	ng/ml	A, B ELISA
Human Soluble Intercellular Adhesive Molecule-1 (h-sICAM-1)		100–400	ng/ml	A, B ELISA
Human Soluble Vascular Cell Adhesion Mole-cule-1 (h-sVCAM-1)		400–500	ng/ml	A, B ELISA. Kit dependent reference values.
Hydroxybutyrate		30–120	µmol/l	Deproteinated blood.

Analyte	Age/ Gender	Reference Range	SI Units	Note
Alpha-Hydroxy-butyrate Dehydrogenase (a-HBDH)		<3.03	µkat/l	A 37 °C, DGKC, optimized
Beta-Hydroxy-butyric Acid	Adults	55–164	µmol/l	A ITF, HPLC
17-Hydroxy-progesterone	M	0.82–6.03	nmol/l	A
	F Prolifer. phase	0.66–1.98	nmol/l	
	Secretory phase	3.90–8.90	nmol/l	
	Pregnancy			
	5–20 w	9.5–16.5	µmol/l	
	6–30 w	9.6–35	µmol/l	
	31–40 w	16.1–75	µmol/l	
Hydroxyproline, Free	Neonates	4.4–14	µmol/l	A 48 hours after non-collagen meals.
	Boys	11–37	µmol/l	
	Girls	8–32	µmol/l	
	F	7–25	µmol/l	
	M	9–31	µmol/l	
Hydroxyproline, Total	F	<105.3	µmol/l	A Upper limit
				F = 105 + 0.316 x age
	M	<108.3	µmol/l	M = 108 + 0.316 x age
Hypoxanthine	Neonates			
	12–36 hrs	2.7–11.2	µmol/l	
	3 d	1.3–7.9	µmol/l	
	5 d	0.6–5.7	µmol/l	
Immunoglobulins				A
IgA	1–3 m	0.013–0.53	g/l	EDTA and citrate lead to ↓.Immunoturbidimetric method
	4–6 m	0.044–0.84	g/l	
	7–12 m	0.11–1.06	g/l	
	2–5 y	0.14–1.59	g/l	
	6–10 y	0.33–2.36	g/l	
	Adults	0.70–3.12	g/l	
IgD	Neonates	0	g/l	
	Other	0–0.08	g/l	
IgE	Neonates	<1.5	IU/ml	ELISA
	7–12 m	<25	IU/ml	
	6 y	<126	IU/ml	
	11 y	<210	IU/ml	
	Adults	<200	IU/ml	
IgG	1 m	2.51–9.06	g/l	
	2–4 m	1.76–6.01	g/l	
	5–12 m	1.72–10.69	g/l	

Analyte	Age/ Gender	Reference Range	SI Units	Note
	1–5 y	3.45–12.36	g/l	
	6–10 y	6.08–15.72	g/l	
	Adults	6.39–15.49	g/l	
Subclasses				
– IgG1		4.0–13.0	g/l	
– IgG2		1.2–8.0	g/l	
– IgG3		0.4–1.3	g/l	
– IgG4		0.01–3.0	g/l	
IgM	1–4 m	0.17–1.05	g/l	
	5–9 m	0.3–1.26	g/l	
	10–12 m	0.41–1.73	g/l	
	2–8 y	0.43–2.07	g/l	
	9–10 y	0.52–2.42	g/l	
	Adults	0.56–2.3	g/l	
Immunoglobulin				A
kappa chain		1.7–3.7	g/l	IFCC
lambda chain		1.1–2.4	g/l	IFCC
Inorganic Phosphate	Neonates	1.6–3.1	mmol/l	A Platelet number dependent.
	2–12 m	1.6–3.5	mmol/l	
	>1 y	1.1–2.0	mmol/l	
	Adults	0.87–1.45	mmol/l	
Insulin (IRI)	Neonates	3.8–13.6	mU/l	A ELISA, RIA. Non-heparin plasma. 12 hrs fasting patient
	Children	6.96–26.6	mU/l	
	Adults	8.0–34.5	mU/l	
		58–172	pmol/l	
		0.34–1.0	µg/l	
Specific Insulin		2–25	µIU/ml	A, B, C IRMA. Monoclonal antibody against 2 epitopes. High specificity. Not reacting with pro-insulin and C-peptide.
Insulin in oGTT	Basal	7–24	µIU/ml	A
	30'	25–231	µIU/ml	
	60'	18–276	µIU/ml	
	120'	16–166	µIU/ml	
	180'	4–38	µIU/ml	
Insulin-Like Growth Factor I (ILGF-I)	M			
	1–2 y	4.05–21.96	nmol/l	
	3–4 y	5.88–30.07	nmol/l	
	5–6 y	6.67–37.65	nmol/l	
	7–8 y	20.66–50.33	nmol/l	
	9–10 y	17.78–40.27	nmol/l	
	11–12 y	23.53–57.52	nmol/l	
	13–14 y	28.76–80.53	nmol/l	
	15–16 y	26.15–109.30	nmol/l	
	17–18 y	37.39–81.97	nmol/l	

Analyte	Age/Gender	Reference Range	SI Units	Note
	19–20 y	44.32–54.65	nmol/l	
	21–25 y	26.4–56.61	nmol/l	
	Adults	17.6–58.7	nmol/l	
	F			
	1–2 y	1.43–26.93	nmol/l	
	3–4 y	9.81–41.84	nmol/l	
	5–6 y	9.15–37.65	nmol/l	
	7–8 y	16.34–51.77	nmol/l	
	9–10 y	16.08–43.14	nmol/l	
	11–12 y	24.97–60.40	nmol/l	
	13–14 y	37.39–87.33	nmol/l	
	15–16 y	31.64–87.33	nmol/l	
	17–18 y	31.38–66.15	nmol/l	
	19–20 y	31.64–71.90	nmol/l	
	21–25 y	30.19–59.21	nmol/l	
Insulin-Like Growth Factor II (ILGF-II)	Children			E EIA
	– pre-puberty	44.5–85.6	nmol/l	
	– puberty	32.7–98.2	nmol/l	
	Adults	38.4–98.1	nmol/l	
Insulin-Like Growth Factor Binding Protein 1 (ILGFBP-1)		0.6–14.4	ng/ml	A, B
	sensitivity	0.2	ng/ml	
Gamma-Interferon		<0.08	IU/ml	E, EMA
Interleukin				A, B Heparin plasma preferably. Monocyte supernatant
Alpha		0–5	pg/ml	
Beta		1–10	ng/ml	
Interleukin 2		<5	pg/ml	B, A IEMA
s-Interleukin 2 Receptor (Sil-2)		25–105	pmol/l	B, A IEMA
	Sensitivity	5	pmol/l	
Interleukin 5		<10	pg/ml	B, A IEMA
Interleukin 6		<10	pg/ml	B, A IEMA
s-Interleukin 6 Receptor(sIL-6)		10–90	ng/l	B, A IEMA
Interleukin 8		<10	ng/l	B, A Separate blood cells immediately. Store in –70 °C
Interleukin 10		<5	pg/ml	B, A IEMA
Intracellular Protein S-100			<0.20	µg/l E RIA
Iodine				E
inorganic		0.78–23.6	nmol/l	
butanol-extractable	Neonates	567–1040	nmol/l	
	Children	335–575	nmol/l	
	Adults	232–504	nmol/l	
bounded to protein	1–2 d	760–1135	nmol/l	
	4–5 w	440–725	nmol/l	

Analyte	Age/ Gender	Reference Range	SI Units	Note
	12 w	400–686	nmol/l	
	52 w	417–575	nmol/l	
	Adults	315–521	nmol/l	
Iron	2 w	11–36	μmol/l	A Ferrozine method
	6 m	5–24	μmol/l	
	12 m	6–28	μmol/l	
	<12 y	4–24	μmol/l	
	F <25 y	6.6–29.5	μmol/l	
	40 y–60 y	4.1–24	μmol/l	
	>60 y	7.0–26.7	μmol/l	
	Pregnancy			
	0–12 w	7.6–31.6	μmol/l	
	36–40 w	4.5–24.5	μmol/l	
	6 w post-labor	2.9–26.9	μmol/l	
	M <25 y	7.2–27.7	μmol/l	
	40 y–60 y	6.3–30.1	μmol/l	
	>60 y	7.2–21.5	μmol/l	
Iron-binding capacity, Total (TIBC)	1 d	24–57	μmol/l	A
	1 w	34–58	μmol/l	Conversion factor:
	1 w–2 m	27–61	μmol/l	10 mg/l of transferrin corresponds to approximately 12.7 μg/l of iron (0.227 μmol/l)
	3–12 m	52–78	μmol/l	
	1–3 y	49–85	μmol/l	
	4–10 y	47–89	μmol/l	
	11–16 y	52–79	μmol/l	
	Adults F	49–89	μmol/l	Ferrozine method
	Adults M	52–77	μmol/l	
Isocitrate-Dehydrogenase	Neonates	33–146	nkat/l	A
	Children	0–85.5	nkat/l	
	Adults	13.3–73	nkat/l	
Isoleucine	Neonates	<50	μmol/l	A
	Children	20–80	μmol/l	
	Adults	30–60	μmol/l	
Ketobodies, Total	Neonates	40–180	μmol/l	A
	0 w–1 w	90–1900	μmol/l	
	Infants	30–890	μmol/l	
	1–6 y	30–1100	μmol/l	
	Adults	5–280	μmol/l	
Lactate (Lactic acid)	Neonates	<2.9	mmol/l	UV test, fully enzymatic.
	Adults	<2.4	mmol/l	Plasma treated with glycolysis inhibitor – mannose/fluoride – oxalate/iodoacetate
		<1.8	mmol/l	Fully enzymatic test
Capillary Blood		1.0–1.8	mmol/l	

Analyte	Age/Gender	Reference Range	SI Units	Note
Venous Blood		<1.8	mmol/l	Fasting blood after deproteinization, do not use serum
Arterial Blood		<1.5	mmol/l	
Venous Plasma		<2.2	mmol/l	
Arterial Plasma		<1.8	mmol/l	lactate/pyruvate index about 10
Umbilical Blood		<3.3	mmol/l	
Lactate Dehydrogenase (LD, LDH)				
37 °C	1 d	<22.1	µkat/l	E
	2–5 d	<28.9	µkat/l	do not freeze, store in 4–8 °C
	6 d–6 m	<16.3	µkat/l	DGKC, optimized
	6–12 m	<18.3	µkat/l	
	1–3 y	<14.2	µkat/l	
	4–6 y	<10.3	µkat/l	
	7–12 y F	<9.67	µkat/l	
	7–12 y M	<12.7	µkat/l	
	13–17 y F	<7.27	µkat/l	
	13–17 y M	<11.4	µkat/l	
	Adults	<7.5	µkat/l	Merck Co.
		<6.3	µkat/l	Bayer Co.
Lactate Dehydrogenase – Isoenzymes	Adults			A
	I (heart)	0.175–0.36		
	II	0.304–0.50		ELPHO
	III	0.192–0.25		
	IV	0.096–0.10		
	V (liver)	0.055–0.13		
Lactoferrin		170–440	µg/l	A
Lead	Neonates	<0.48	µmol/l	E Special tube.
Whole blood	Adults F	0.15–0.41	µmol/l	Reference values in whole blood.
	Adults M	0.14–0.48	µmol/l	
Lecithin–Cholesterol Acyltransferase		18.3–23.7	*	A RIA, *nmol ³H.CE/substr/hrs
Leptin	normosthenic	0.1–15	ng/ml	A
	obese	5–50	ng/ml	
Leucine	Neonates	46–109	µmol/l	A
	Infants	40–150	µmol/l	
	Children	50–200	µmol/l	
	Adults	80–150	µmol/l	
Leucine-Aminopeptidase	Neonates	10–50	U/l	A
	Adults F	10–32	U/l	
	Adults M	20–35	U/l	
Lidocaine		6–21	µmol/l	A Blood collection: during infusion.
Lipase		<3.17	µkat/l	A, B, C Turbidimetric method.

Analyte	Age/Gender	Reference Range	SI Units	Note
		<2.67	µkat/l	Titration according to Rick.
		7.7–56	U/l	EIA. Method dependent reference values. EDTA binds calcium (activator).
Lipoprotein a Lp (a)		<0.28	g/l	A Turbidimetric method. Borderline range (0.25–0.35 g/l). Patients with <0.28 are Lp(a) negative. Store in 4 °C.
Lipoprotein X		<30	mg/l	A ELPHO, immunoprecipitation
Lithium		0.3–1.3	mmol/l	A Blood collection: 12 hrs after final dose.
Luteinizing Hormone (LH)	<10 y	0.5–1.0	IU/l	A
	F			ELISA, RIA
	Follicular phase	0.5–18	IU/l	
	Mid-cycle	15–80	IU/l	
	Luteal phase	0.5–18	IU/l	
	Post-menopause	18–64	IU/l	
	M	0.5–10	IU/l	
Lysine		100–250	µmol/l	A
Lysozyme		2–9	mg/l	A immunoanalysis
Alpha-2-Macroglobulin	F	1.30–3.0	g/l	A
		1.10–2.50	g/l	Turbidimetric method. IFCC
Magnesium	Neonates	0.83–1.11	mmol/l	A Remove blood cells before analysis.
	Children	0.87–1.07	mmol/l	AAS, Xylidyl blue reaction, hemolysis interferes.
	Adults	0.79–1.09	mmol/l	Mg in granulocytes represents intracellular Mg.
Malate Dehydrogenase	Neonates	1.6–4.0	µkat/l	A
	Children	1.0–2.32	µkat/l	
	Adults	0.83–1.73	µkat/l	
Malone Dialdehyde		<6.5	µmol/l	A, B Fresh sample. Photometric evaluation. Values obtained through HPLC are substantially different.
Manganese				A, E
Whole Blood		115–119	nmol/l	
-Serum		8–14	nmol/l	
Melanocyte Stimulating Hormone	Adults			A RIA
	7–8 AM	0.8–18.3	µg/l	

Analyte	Age/ Gender	Reference Range	SI Units	Note
	12 AM	0–33	µg/l	
	12 PM	0–200	µg/l	
Mercury	Children	6.2–7.0	nmol/l	E AAS
	Adults	9.5–23.5	nmol/l	
Methionine		10–40	µmol/l	A
Methotrexate	24 hrs after infusion start <10		µmol/l	A After high dose methotrexate therapy (infusion over 4–6 hrs), the mentioned guidance values should not be exceeded. Blood collection: 24, 48, 72 hrs after start of infusion. If elimination is delayed, further samples are required until the concentration of methotrexate is 0.05–0.1 µmol/l.
	48 hrs after infusion start	0.5–1.0	µmol/l	
	72 hrs after infusion start	0.05–0.10	µmol/l	
Beta-2- Microglobulin	Adults <60 y	0.80–2.4	mg/l	A RIA, EIA, LIA
	Adults >60 y	1.00–3.00	mg/l	
Molybdenum		8–60.3	nmol/kg	E
Motilin	Neonates	28–36	pmol/l	A EIA
	1 m	100–147	pmol/l	
	Adults	16–28	pmol/l	
Mucin-Like Cancer Associated Antigen (MCA)		0–15	U/ml	A IRMA. Sensitivity (breast cancer + mts) 70–80%.
Mucoproteins		<386	µmol/l	A Expressed like tyrosine. Method dependent reference values.
Myoglobin	F	17.0–65.5	µg/l	A RIA
	M	16.5–76	µg/l	
Natrium (Sodium)	1 d–4 w	132–147	mmol/l	A Flame photometry.
	2–12 m	129–143	mmol/l	
	>1 y	132–145	mmol/l	ISE, indirect method and enzymatic
	Adults	135–145	mmol/l	colorimetric test.
Nerve Growth Factor Beta		5–10	pg/ml	E EIA
Neuron-Specific Enolase		0–12	ng/ml	A, B IRMA, RIA. Sensitivity (oat-cell lung cancer) 60–80%.
Niacin				A
Serum		2–12	µmol/l	
Whole Blood		16–73	µmol/l	

Analyte	Age/Gender	Reference Range	SI Units	Note
Nickel		0.13–0.76	µmol/l	E AAS
5-Nucleotidase		33–250	nkat/l	A
Oral Glucose Tolerance Test (oGTT)				H=healthy people. Healthy people after 3 hrs <5.6 mmol/l
capillary blood	fasting – H	<5.6	mmol/l	75 g of glucose orally
	– DGT	<7.0	mmol/l	DGT–disordered glucose tolerance.
	– DM	>7.0	mmol/l	WHO criteria (1998)
	after 1 hour			
	– H	<8.9	mmol/l	DM >7.0 mmol/l fasting
	– DGT	>11.0	mmol/l	→ oral glucose
	– DM	>11.1	mmol/l	>11.1 mmol/l after 2 hours
	after 2 hrs			
	– H	<6.7	mmol/l	
	– DGT	8.0–11.0	mmol/l	
	– DM	>11.0	mmol/l	
venous blood	fasting – H	<6.7	mmol/l	
	– DGT	<7.0	mmol/l	
	– DM	>7.0	mmol/l	
	after 1 hour			
	– H	<10.0	mmol/l	
	– DGT	>10.0	mmol/l	
	– DM	>11.1	mmol/l	
	after 2 hrs	<10.0	mmol/l	
	– DGT	7.0–10.0	mmol/l	
	– DM	>10.0	mmol/l	
venous plasma, serum	fasting – H	>7.0	mmol/l	
	– DGT	<8.0	mmol/l	
	– DM	>8.0	mmol/l	
	after 1 hour			
	– H	<11.0	mmol/l	
	– DGT	>11.0	mmol/l	
	– DM	>11.0	mmol/l	
	after 2 hrs			
	– H	<8.0	mmol/l	
	– PGT	8.0–11.0	mmol/l	
	– DM	>11.1	mmol/l	
Ornithine	Neonates	120–220	µmol/l	A
	Children	50–200	µmol/l	
	Adults	50–120	µmol/l	
Orosomucoid (Alpha-1-Acid Glycoprotein)	F	0.40–1.20	g/l	A, B Turbidimetric method. IFCC
	M	0.50–1.30	g/l	

Analyte	Age/ Gender	Reference Range	SI Units	Note
Osmolality	Neonates Adults	265–275	mmol/kg	A
	<60 y	275–295	mmol/kg	Osm (mosmol/kg) = 2 x (Na) + glucose + urea (mmol)
	Adults >60 y	280–300	mmol/kg	
Osteocalcin		3.0–5.4	µg/l	C, D RIA Add aprotinine (2500 kIU/ml) to stabilize. Reference values are method dependent.
Pancreatic Polypeptide (PP)		<150	pmol/l	A RIA
Parathormone	Children	55–195	ng/l	C RIA
	Adults M	67–135	ng/l	
	Adults F	50–88	ng/l	
		1.5–6.5	pmol/l	
	pregnancy	80–230	ng/l	
Parathyroid Hormone-Related Protein (PTHrP)	Antibodies 1-34	<2.5	pmol/l	E RIA
	Antibodies 53-84	<21	pmol/l	
Pepsin	Neonates	10–138	nkat/l	A
	Children	17–51	nkat/l	
	Adults	13–43	nkat/l	
C-Peptide		1.1–3.6	ng/ml	A IRMA
		206–934	pmol/l	
Phenobarbital		65–172	µmol/l	A CEDIA[R] Phenobarbital homogenous enzyme immunoassay. Blood collection: interval between doses. Therapeutic concentrations.
Phenytoin	Premature infants	24–56	µmol/l	A CEDIA[R] Phenytoin, homogenous enzyme immunoassay.
	Adults	20–80	µmol/l	Blood collection: interval between doses.
Phospho-hexose Isomerase (PHI)		2.25–11.4	µkat/l	A
		15–67	U/l	
Phospholipase		<1	ng/ml	A
	sensitivity	1.25	ng/ml	
Phospholipids, Total	Neonates	0.75–1.70	g/l	A
	Infants	1.00–2.75	g/l	
	Children	1.80–2.95	g/l	
	Adults	1.25–2.75	g/l	

Analyte	Age/ Gender	Reference Range	SI Units	Note
Potassium (Kalium)	1 d–4 w	3.6–6.1	mmol/l	A
	2–12 m	3.6–5.8	mmol/l	ISE, indirect method and enzymatic colorimetric test.
	>1 y	3.1–5.1	mmol/l	Kalium concentration are assessed with pH values:
	Adults	3.6–4.8	mmol/l	6.8 + 0.2 K: 7.0 + 1.0
				7.1 + 0.1 6.0 + 0.5
				7.2 + 0.5 5.2 + 0.5
				7.3 + 0.5 4.5 + 0.5
				7.4 + 0.5 3.8 + 0.5
				7.7 + 0.5 3.5 + 0.5
				Serum platelet number dependent
Prealbumin		0.1–0.4	g/l	A Turbidimetric method
Beta-1 Pregnancy Specific Glyco- protein		<3	ng/ml	A RIA
Primidone		23–69	μmol/l	A Sampling: max. 2–4 hrs after final dose, min. imme- diately before next dose.
Procainamide		15–42	μmol/l	A Sampling: max. 1–5 hrs after final dose, min. imme diately before next dose.
Procalcitonin		<0.5	μg/l	A, B Immunoanalysis.
Progesterone	F			A
	Follicular phase	0.95–3.5	nmol/l	ELISA, RIA
	Luteal phase	5.7–67	nmol/l	
	>60 y	<3.2	nmol/l	
	Pregnancy			
	1st trimester	29–121	nmol/l	
	2nd trimester	60–413	nmol/l	
	3rd trimester	165–776	nmol/l	
	M	<0.95	nmol/l	
Proinsulin		<25	ng/l	A, B 12 hrs starvation
		<3	pmol/l	
		<25	ng/l	Prolonged starvation.
		<3	pmol/l	
		77–102	ng/l	Maximum stimulation (glucose, glucagon)
		8.5–11.3	pmol/l	
Prolactin (PRL)	1–30 d F	8–2 620	U/l	A
	1–30 d M	102–2240	U/l	Conversion of ng/ml to
	<1 y F	6–825	U/l	U/l depends on the type
	<1 y M	8–800	U/l	of standard used.
	2–3 y F	28–470	U/l	ELISA, RIA, MEIA
	2–3 y M	63–365	U/l	Do not use EDTA, citrate.
	4–6 y F	44–360	U/l	

Analyte	Age/Gender	Reference Range	SI Units	Note
	4–6 y M	22–465	U/l	
	7–9 y F	8–355	U/l	
	7–9 y M	52–320	U/l	
	10–12 y F	52–265	U/l	
	10–12 y M	25–355	U/l	
	13–15 y F	83–400	U/l	
	13–15 y M	44–460	U/l	
	16–18 y F	58–510	U/l	
	16–18 y M	75–420	U/l	
	Adults F	3.8–23.2	µg/l	
	Adults M	3.0–14.7	µg/l	
	Adults F	91–557	mU/l	
	Adults M	72–353	mU/l	
Proline	Neonates	130–350	µmol/l	A
	Infants	100–300	µmol/l	
	Children	60–300	µmol/l	
	Adults	120–240	µmol/l	
Properdin	Umbilicus	190–320	µmol/l	A
	<3 m	285–545	µmol/l	
	<1 y	600–838	µmol/l	
	Adults	527–1167	µmol/l	
Prostate-Specific Antigen (PSA)		<4.0	ng/ml	A ELISA, EPIA, IRMA
Prostate-Specific Antigen, Free		2.4–3.5	ng/ml	A
				PSA index = free PSA ng/ml : total PSA ng/ml borderline value 0.18 positive values <0.18 negative value >0.18
Proteins, Total	Premature infants, 1 d	34–50	g/l	A
	1 d–4 w	46–68	g/l	Biuret method
	2–12 m	48–76	g/l	plasma >serum (fibrinogen)
	>1 y	60–80	g/l	
	Adults	66–87	g/l	
Electrophoresis	Adults	0.55–0.69	%	
Albumin		55.3–68.9	%	Ponceau red S
– alpha-1- globulins		0.02–0.06	%	
		1.6–5.8	%	
– alpha-2- globulins		0.06–0.11	%	
		5.9–11.1	%	
– beta globulins		0.08–0.14	%	
		7.9–13.9	%	
– gamma globulins		0.11–0.18	%	
		11.4–18.2	%	
Albumin	Neonates	32.7–45.3	g/l	
	<1 y	35.7–51.3	g/l	

Analyte	Age/ Gender	Reference Range	SI Units	Note
	1–5 y	33.1–52.2	g/l	
	6–15 y	40–52.2	g/l	
	Adults	35.2–50.4	g/l	
– alpha-1-globulins	Neonates	1.1–2.5	g/l	
	<1 y	1.3–2.5	g/l	
	1–5 y	0.9–2.9	g/l	
	6–15 y	1.2–2.5	g/l	
	Adults	1.3–3.9	g/l	
– alpha-2-globulins	Neonates	2.6–5.7	g/l	
	<1 y	3.8–10.8	g/l	
	1–5 y	4.3–9.5	g/l	
	6–15 y	4.3–8.6	g/l	
	Adults	5.4–9.3	g/l	
– beta globulins	Neonates	2.5–5.6	g/l	
	<1 y	3.5–7.1	g/l	
	1–5 y	3.5–7.6	g/l	
	6–15 y	4.1–7.9	g/l	
	Adults	5.9–11.4	g/l	
– gamma globulins	Neonates	3.9–11	g/l	
	<1 y	2.9–11	g/l	
	1–5 y	4.5–12.1	g/l	
	6–15 y	5.9–13.7	g/l	
	Adults	5.8–15.2	g/l	
Protoporphyrin (ZN, ZPP)		2–15	nmol/l	B
		19–38	µmol/mol heme	C
Pyruvate	Children	11–86	mmol/l	E UV test, deproteinized blood immediately using ice-cold perchloric acid (0.6 mol/l).
	Adults F	41–67	mmol/l	
	Adults M	34–102	nmol/l	
Quinidine		6–15	µmol/l	Blood collection: not later than 1 hour (SR medicaments after 8 hrs). Minimum: immediately before next dose.
C-Reactive Protein		0.07–8.2	mg/l	A, B
Renin (PRA)	rest	0.5–1.9	ng/ml/h	C, D
	exertion	1.9–6.0	ng/ml/h	RIA. Plasma renin activity (PRA) as angiotensin I released is measured.
Retinol Binding Protein (RBP)	0–5 d	8–45	mg/l	A Immunoanalysis
	1–9 y	10–78	mg/l	
	10–13 y	13–99	mg/l	
	14–19 y	30–92	mg/l	

Analyte	Age/Gender	Reference Range	SI Units	Note
Rheumatoid Factor (RF)		<14	kU/l *	A *Provisional. Immunoturbidimetric method.
		<79	U/l	
		<40	kU/l	Nephelometry. Reference values are method dependent.
P-Selectin		19–521	ng/ml	A EIA, RIA
Selenium		3–6.2	μmol/l	E (special tube)
Serine	Infants	23–172	μmol/l	A
	Adults	76–164	μmol/l	
Serotonin	F	500–900	nmol/l	A, B RIA, EIA, fluorometry. Stabilization with ascorbic acid (1 mg/ml).
	M	300–700	nmol/l	
	platelet plasma depleteled	1000–2500	nmol/l	
	plasma	4–15	nmol/l	
Serum Amyloid A (SAA)		0.17–10	mg/l	A, B Latex nephelometric method.
Sialic Acid	Umbilical blood	240–420	mg/l	DPA reaction.
(Lipid Associated Sialic Acid, LASA)	1 m	450–670	mg/l	
	3 m	540–660	mg/l	
	1 y	<970	mg/l	
	Adults	569–633	mg/l	
Soluble CD4		0–20	ng/ml	E
	sensitivity	0.25	ng/ml	
Soluble Fas ^ Ligand		<0.11	ng/ml	A
Soluble GM-CSF Receptor		16–50	pmol	A
	sensitivity	5	pmol	
Soluble Transferrin Receptor (sTfR)		10–30	nmol/l	A, B RIA, immunonephelometry
Somatostatin		0–20	ng/l	A
Specific Tissue Polypeptide Antigen (TPSA)		<95	U/l	A IRMA
Squamous Cell Carcinoma Antigen (SCCA)		0–1.5	mg/l	A closed tube, RIA, IRMA, EIA – after skin contamination
Taurine	Neonates	70–240	μmol/l	A
	Infants	70–180	μmol/l	
	Adults	40–140	μmol/l	
Telopeptide		1.8–5.0	mg/l	A IRMA

Analyte	Age/Gender	Reference Range	SI Units	Note
N-Terminal Atrial Natriuretic Peptide (NT-Pro-ANP)		0.11–0.60	nmol/l	C
Testosterone	F	<2.98	nmol/l	A ELISA, IRMA
	Oral contracept.	<0.35	nmol/l	
	M	7.0–29.5	nmol/l	
Thalium		<25	nmol/l	E
Theophylline		10–20	mg/l	A FPIA
Thymidine Kinase		<9	U/l	A IRMA
Thyroglobulin		0–50	µg/l	A, B ELISA, IRMA
Thyroid Stimulating Hormone (TSH)	Neonates	<20	mU/l	A
	Adults	0.23–4.0	mU/l	IRMA, MEIA
Thyroxine, Free (FT4)	1–2 d	21–49	pmol/l	A MEIA, ELISA
	3–30 d	19–39	pmol/l	
	2–12 m	14–23	pmol/l	
	1–13 y	12–22	pmol/l	
	14–18 y	12–23	pmol/l	
	Adults	12–25	pmol/l	
Thyroxine, Total (T4)	1–2 d	138–332	nmol/l	A RIA, FIA, EIA
	3–30 d	100–253	nmol/l	
	2–12 m	69.5–178	nmol/l	
	1–7 y	68.2–158	nmol/l	
	8–13 y	77.2–143	nmol/l	
	14–18 y	63.1–138	nmol/l	
	Adults	60–155	nmol/l	
Thyroxine Binding Globulin (TBG)	1 d–1 y F	18–34	mg/l	A
	1 d–1 y M	18–32	mg/l	T4/TBG4
	2–3 y F	19–34	mg/l	3 ± 1.2 euthyroidism
	2–3 y M	17–32	mg/l	1.1 ± 0.9 hypothyroidism
	4–6 y F	18–31	mg/l	11.2 ± 3.6 hyperthyroidism
	4–6 y M	17–30	mg/l	ELISA, RIA. Enzymun-test.
	7–12 y F	15–30	mg/l	
	7–12 y M	17–29	mg/l	
	13–18 y F	14–29	mg/l	
	13–18 y M	14–26	mg/l	
	Adults F	14–26	mg/l	
	Adults M	9.6–18.5	mg/l	
Thyroxine Uptake (free thyroxine-binding capacity, T4-uptake)		0.29–0.40		A
Tissue Polypeptide Antigen (TPA)		<80	U/l	A IRMA

Analyte	Age/ Gender	Reference Range	SI Units	Note
Tobramycin		9–21	µmol/l	A Blood collection: maximum: 30 min post infusion, minimum: immediately before next dose
Transferrin	1–3 y	2.18–3.47	g/l	A Immunoturbidimetric method. EDTA and citrate lead to ↓
	4–9 y 10–19 y	2.08–3.78	g/l	
	+ Adults	2.24–4.44	g/l	
Transferrin Saturation	2 w	30–99	%	A
	6 m	10–93	%	
	12 m	10–47	%	
	1–15 y	7–46	%	
	M	16–45	%	
	F Pregnan.	16–45	%	
	12–16 w	18–50	%	
	3rd trimester	2–30	%	
	1–2 m post-labor	9–49	%	
Triacyl-glycerols	Umbilicus	0.10–0.90	mmol/l	A
	1–6 y	0.32–0.95	mmol/l	Interference from bilirubin >10 mg/dl (>171 µmol/l)
	6–10 y	0.35–1.14	mmol/l	
	Puberty	0.40–1.33	mmol/l	
	Adults M	0.40–1.60	mmol/l	
	Adults F	0.35–1.40	mmol/l	
		<1.6	mmol/l	Without stratification. Screening method.
Triiodothyronine, Free (FT3)	1–2 d	5.2–14.3	pmol/l	A
	3–30 d	4.3–10.6	pmol/l	ELISA, RIA, FIA
	2–12 m	5.1–10.0	pmol/l	Method dependent reference values.
	1–7 y	5.2–10.0	pmol/l	
	8–13 y	6.1–9.5	pmol/l	
	14–18 y	5.2–8.6	pmol/l	
	Adults	5.4–12.4	pmol/l	ELISA, RIA, FIA
Triiodothyronine, Reverse (RT3)	1–5 y	0.23–1.1	nmol/l	A
	5–10 y	0.26–1.2	nmol/l	
	10–15 y	0.29–1.36	nmol/l	
Triiodothyronine, Total (T3)	1–2 d	1.2–4.0	nmol/l	A ELISA, RIA, FIA
	3–30 d	1.1–3.1	nmol/l	Method dependent reference values.

Analyte	Age/Gender	Reference Range	SI Units	Note
	2–12 m	1.7–3.5	nmol/l	
	1–7 y	1.8–3.1	nmol/l	
	8–13 y	1.7–3.1	nmol/l	
	14–18 y	1.5–2.8	nmol/l	
	Adults	1.2–2.7	nmol/l	
Troponin I		<0.1	µg/l	A, B
Troponin T		<0.1	µg/l*	A, B *Provisional. TROP T^R ELISA
Tryptophan	Infants	45–65	µmol/l	A
	Adults	45–75	µmol/l	
Tumor Necrosis Factor-2		<5	pg/ml	E RIA, EIA
Tyrosine	Premature neonates	<180	µmol/l	A
	1 w	90–180	µmol/l	
	Infants	60–140	µmol/l	
	Adults	40–100	µmol/l	
Urea	Neonates	<7.0	mmol/l	A
	<6 m	<7.0	mmol/l	
	>7 m	<8.0	mmol/l	
	Adults F	2.2–6.7	mmol/l	Enzymatic UV test.
	Adults M	3.8–7.3	mmol/l	
Uric Acid	1–2 d	<340	µmol/l	A
	6 d	<220	µmol/l	Higher bilirubin concentration may interfere. Individual reference values.
	Infants	<150	µmol/l	
	Children	<390	µmol/l	
	Adults F	180–340	µmol/l	
	Adults M	180–420	µmol/l	PAP method
Uroporphyrin		0–0.9	nmol/l	A, B Protect against light.
Valine	Neonates	100–250	µmol/l	A
	Infants	100–300	µmol/l	
	Children	150–300	µmol/l	
	Adults	150–250	µmol/l	
Valproic Acid		347–693	µmol/l	A Blood collection: maximum: 1–4 hrs (up to 8 hrs) after final dose, minimum: immediately before next dose.
Vancomycin		14–28	µmol/l	Sampling: max. 30 min post i.v. infusion, min. immediately before next dose.
Vasoactive Intestinal Polypeptide (Vip)		<20	pmol/l	B RIA
Viscosity				A, B
Venous Plasma		1.09–1.15	mPa.s	
Blood in 0.7/S		21.2–25.6	mPa.s	
Blood in 95/S		4.3–4.7	mPa.s	

Analyte	Age/ Gender	Reference Range	SI Units	Note
Vitamin A	Neonates	1.22–2.60	μmol/l	A HPLC
	Children	1.05–2.80	μmol/l	
	Adults F	0.85–1.75	μmol/l	
	Adults M	1.05–2.27	μmol/l	
Vitamin B1		<75	nmol/l	A
Vitamin B2				A Method dependent reference values.
Blood		361–1770	nmol/l	
Serum		133–478	nmol/l	
Vitamin B5				
(Pantothenic Acid)		4.7–8.4	μmol/l	A HPLC
Vitamin B6		30–144	nmol/l	C HPLC Store in darkness.
Vitamin B12				C RIA, immunoanalysis.
Total Cobalamins	Adults	244–730	pmol/l	Store in darkness.
Vitamin B$_{12}$	Neonates	118–959	pmol/l	
	Adults	162–694	pmol/l	
	Pregnancy	<125	pmol/l	
Vitamin C	Adults	34–114	μmol/l	E Photometry. Stabilization with metaphosphate (60 mg/l).
Vitamin D	Children	75–175	pmol/l	A Chromatography, immunoanalysis.
1,25-(OH)$_2$D3	Adults	50–200	pmol/l	
25-OH-D2	– summer	50–300	nmol/l	A Immunoanalysis
	– winter	25–125	nmol/l	
Vitamin E	0–1 m	8–28	μmol/l	C
	1–6 m	10–31	μmol/l	
	6 m–6 y	20–30	μmol/l	
	Adults	11–45	μmol/l	
Vitamin K	Adults	0.3–2.64	nmol/l	A Protect against light. UV-light causes ↓
Zinc	Neonates			E AAS
	– premature	6.8–11	μmol/l	special tube (be aware of cork contamination)
	– mature	9.4–13.7	μmol/l	
	Adults F	10.1–16.8	μmol/l	
	Adults M	10.6–17.9	μmol/l	

Acid-base Balance

Analyte	Age/ Gender	Reference Range	SI Unit	Note
pH		7.35–7.45		E (anaerobic sampling)
Carbon Dioxide Partial Pressure (pCO$_2$)	M	4.7–6.0	kPa	E (anaerobic sampling)
	F	4.3–6.4	kPa	
Oxygen Partial Pressure (pO$_2$) arterial	Neonates	1.1–3.2	kPa	E (anaerobic sampling)
	5–10 min	4.4–10.0	kPa	
	30 min	4.1–11.3	kPa	
	>1 hour	7.3–10.6	kPa	
	1 d	7.2–12.6	kPa	
	Others	11–14.4	kPa	decrease with age
Oxygen Saturation arterial blood	Neonates	0.85–0.90		E
	Others	0.95–0.99		
Base Excess	Neonates	(-10)–(-2)	mmol/l	E (anaerobic sampling)
	Infants	(-7)–(-1)	mmol/l	
	Children	(-4)–(+2)	mmol/l	
	Adults	(-3)–(+3)	mmol/l	
Bicarbonates				E (anaerobic sampling)
arterial blood		21–28	mmol/l	
venous blood		22–29	mmol/l	
Anion Gap		14.1–18.1	mmol/l	$(Na + K) - (Cl + HCO_3^-)$

Hematology

Analyte	Age/ Gender	Reference Range	SI Unit	Note
Activated Partial Thromboplastin Time (APTT)	Children	<90	s	E (0.5 ml 3.8% Na-citrate + 4.5 ml venous blood), to compare with control
	Adults	25–35	s	
Activated Platelets (determined as P-Selectin (CD 62p) CD 63		<0.04		E
Alpha-2-Anti-plasmin		0.8–1.2		
		80–120	%	
		50–70	mg/l	
Antithrombin III (AT III)		0.8–1.2		E (3.8% Na-citrate)
		80–120	%	
		180–300	mg/l	concentration
Autohemolysis		2.5–5	% relat.	
Bleeding Time				
Ivy's		4–8	min	
Duke's		2–5	min	
Capillary Fragility Test (Rumpel-Leede)		<10	*	*petechiae over 16 cm^2
Carboxyhemo-globin (COHB)	Non-smokers	<0.012		B
	Smokers	<0.085		Cigarette number, sort and smoking habit dependent.

Analyte	Age/Gender	Reference Range	SI Unit	Note
	Lethal	>0.5		
Coagulation Factors				E (citrate)
factor II		<100	mg/l	E (citrate)
		0.7–1.2		activity
		70–120	%	
		0.6–1.40	µmol/l	
		0.5–1.5	kU/l	
		60–150	AU	
factor V		<10	mg/l	centrifuge in 4 °C
		0.7–1.2		activity
		70–120	%	
		0.6–1.40	µmol/l	
		0.5–2.0	kU/l	
		60–150	AU	
factor VII		<0.5	mg/l	
		0.7–1.3		activity
		70–130	%	
		0.7–1.30	µmol/l	
		65–135	AU	
factor VIII		<0.15	mg/l	
		0.6–1.5		activity
		60–150	%	
		0.5–2.0	µmol/l	
		60–145	AU	
factor VIII antigen		0.7–1.5		activity
		50–200	AU	
factor IX		<4	mg/l	
		0.6–1.5		activity
		60–150	%	
		0.6–1.40	µmol/l	
		60–140	AU	
factor X		<10	mg/l	
		0.7–1.3		activity
		70–130	%	
		0.7–1.30	µmol/l	
		60–130	AU	
factor XI		2–7	mg/l	
		0.6–1.4		activity
		60–140	%	
		0.6–1.40	µmol/l	
		65–135	AU	
factor XII		27–45	mg/l	
		0.6–1.4		activity
		60–140	%	
		0.6–1.40	µmol/l	
		65–150	AU	
factor XIII (fibrin-stabilizing factor)		<10	mg/l	
		0.6–1.5		activity
		60–150	%	

Analyte	Age/ Gender	Reference Range	SI Unit	Note
		20–50	U/l	
		1–2	AU	
prekallikrein		<50	mg/l	
Clot Retraction		>0.88		
		>88	%	
Clotting Time	37 °C	6–10	min	
Lee-White	20 °C	6–12	min	
D-dimers		0.2–0.4	µg/ml	glass latex agglutination
Erythrocyte Sedi-	3 m–13 y	12–24	mm	3.8% Na-citrate + blood (1:4)
mentation Rate	Adults M	5–10	mm	
	Adults F	10–20	mm	
Erythrocytes	Neonates	4.5–5.6*		*x 10^{12}/l
	3 m–13 y	3.8–5.0*		
	Adults M	4.6–5.5*		
	Adults F	4.2–5.0*		
Erythropoietin (EPO)		6–20	mU/ml	A, B RIA Transport refrigerated.
		25–125	mU/ml	Hemagglutination
Euglobulin Lysis Time		10–18	hrs	
Ferritin	M	30–310	ng/ml	
	F	22–180	ng/ml	
Fibrin Degradation Products		<5	mg/ml	Special tube (very unstable). Add inhibitor: 10 IU thrombin and 150 IU kallikrein.
		<10	mg/ml	ThromboWellco agglutination test. Aprotinine/trypsin inhibitor from soya beans.
Fibrinogen (factor I)	Neonates	1.25–3.0	g/l	Clauss' method. Reference values valid for hemocoagulation. Values in cardiovascular indications are lower.
	Adults	1.5–3.5	g/l	
		4.0–10.0	µmol/l	
Fibrinopeptide A		<3	ng/ml	
Glucose-6-Phosphate Dehydrogenase in RBC		0.22–0.52	*	*mU/mol Hb
		0.10–0.23	**	**nU/10^6 RBC
Glycated Protein		122–236	µmol/l	A
Haptoglobin	Adults	0.5–3.3	g/l	A
	Hp 1–1	0.7–2.3	g/l	
	Hp 2–1	0.9–3.6	g/l	
	Hp 2–2	0.6–2.9	g/l	
Hematocrit	Neonates	0.44–0.62		
	3 m–13 y	0.31–0.43		
	Adults M	0.42–0.52		
	Adults F	0.37–0.47		
Hemoglobin	Neonates	145–225	g/l	
	2 m	90–140	g/l	
	6–18 y	115–155	g/l	
	Adults M	130–160	g/l	
	Adults F	120–160	g/l	

Analyte	Age/ Gender	Reference Range	SI Unit	Note
Hemoglobin Hb A		>0.95		B
Hb A2		0.015–0.035		Electrophoresis.
Hb F		0.005–0.01		
Hemoglobin F	1 d	0.62–0.92		B
	5 d	0.65–0.88		Alkaline denaturation.
	3 w	0.55–0.85		
	6–9 w	0.31–0.75		
	3–4 m	0.02–0.59		
	6 m	0.02–0.09		
	Adults	<0.02		
Hemoglobin, free		0.01–0.05	g/l	
Hemoglobin, Glycated (HbA$_{1c}$)	Normal			B, C. Values are method dependent.
		0.036–0.058		Immunoturbidimetry
		0.042–0.063		– polyclonal Ab
		0.050–0.080		– monoclonal Ab
		0.050–0.080		Afinity chromatography
		0.033–0.056		– HbA$_1$
		0.044–0.057		– glycated Hb (total)
	Good compensation	0.06–0.07		ELPHO HbA$_{1c}$
	Insufficient compens.	>0.08		HPLC (reference) HbA$_{1c}$
Hemopexin	total	0.50–3.3	g/l	
	fenotype 1–1	0.70–2.3	g/l	
	fenotype 2–1	0.90–3.6	g/l	
	fenotype 2–2	0.60–2.9	g/l	
Heparin Cofactor II		90–105	mg/l	
High-Molecular Weight Kininogen		<60	mg/ml	
Leiden Factor		<0.80		Screening: normalized APC ratio
Leukocytes	Neonates	15–20*		*x 10^9/l
	Adults	4.1–10.9*		
Leukogram Granulocytes				K$_2$EDTA Dependent on machine.
– neutrophilic sticks	Adults	3–5	%	
		0.03–0.05		
		0.6–1.2	x 10^9/l	
– neutrophilic g.	Neonates	<65	%	
	Infants	<25	%	
	Adults	47–79	%	
		0.47–0.79		
		2.5–5.6	x 10^9/l	
– eosinophilic g.	Neonates	<3	%	
	Infants	<3	%	
	Adults	1–7	%	
		0.01–0.07		
		0.03–0.25	x 10^9/l	

Analyte	Age/ Gender	Reference Range	SI Unit	Note
– basophilic g.	Neonates	<0.75	%	
	Infants	<0.25	%	
	Adults	0–2	%	
		0–0.02		
		0–0.03	x 10⁹/l	
Monocytes	Neonates	<8	%	
	Infants	<10	%	
	Adults	2–11	%	
		0.02–0.11		
		0.15–0.58	x 10⁹/l	
Lymphocytes	Neonates	<22	%	
	Infants	<60	%	
	Adults	12–40	%	
		0.12–0.40		
		1.2–3.1	x 10⁹/l	
Plasmocytes	Neonates	<0.25	%	
	Infants	<0.5	%	
Lymphocytic Surface Markers (T-cells)	CD3	0.84–3.06*		B, Flow cytometry *x 10⁹ cells/l
		0.57–0.85		
	CD4	0.49–1.74*		
		0.30–0.61		
	CD8	0.18–1.17*		
		0.12–0.42		
	CD4/CD8	0.86–5.00		
Mean Corpuscular Hemoglobin (MCH)	Neonates	0.48–0.57	fmol	
	<2m	0.40–0.53	fmol	
	2 m–2 y	0.35–0.48	fmol	
	2 y–6 y	0.37–0.47	fmol	
	6 y–12 y	0.39–0.51	fmol	
	12–18 y	0.39–0.54	fmol	
	Adults	0.40–0.53	fmol	
		27–34	pg	
Mean Corpuscular Hemoglobin Concentration (MCHC)	Neonates	4.65–5.58	*	*mmol Hb/l RBC
	<2m	4.50–5.74	*	
	2 m–2 y	4.65–5.58	*	
	2 y–18 y	4.81–5.74	*	
	Adults	4.84–5.74	*	
		30–35	g/dl	
Mean Corpuscular Volume (MCV)	1–3 d	95–121	fl	
	6 m–2 y	70–86	fl	
	6 y–12 y	77–95	fl	
	12 y–18 y	78–100	fl	
	Adults	80–94	fl	
Mean Platelet Volume		7.8–11.0	fl	
Methemoglobin		9.3–37.2	μmol/l	B
	Infants	0.0041–0.0115		total Hb fraction
	Children	<0.02		

Analyte	Age/ Gender	Reference Range	SI Unit	Note
	Adults	<0.008		
	Smokers	<0.02		
Neutrophil Alkaline		<0.02		in less than 2% cells
Phosphatase		0.16–0.83		in 16–83% of cells
Osmotic Resistance of Erythrocytes				
in 20 ºC	min	0.44–0.40		
	max	0.32–0.30		
in 37 ºC	min	0.75–0.70		
	max	0.40–0.30		
Partial Thrombo- plastin Time				A (citrate plasma 1:9)
standard		60–85	s	
Phagocytosis (NBT-test)	spontaneous phagocytosis	0.60–0.80		B oxygen radicals 40–60%
	stimulated phagocytosis	0.80–1.00		B oxygen radicals 80–100%
Plasminogen		0.8–1.50		activity
		80–150	%	
		0.06–0.25	g/l	
Plasminogen Acti- vator Inhibitor (tPAi)		<10	AU/ml	
		0.6–3.5	U/ml	
Platelet Adhesion		44.5–53.5		whole blood, platelet number
		27.4–36.6		adhered in 20 fields, PRP
Platelet Aggregation		>0.60		Inductors: ADP >0.50 collagen >0.50 dmax (>0.30 smax) ristocetin >0.50
Platelet Distribution Width (index)		15.5–17.1		
Platelet Factor 4		<15	µg/l	E
Platelets	Neonates	290–350*		*x 10⁹/l
	Adults	130–370*		
Protein C		70–130	%	Ag, activity
		0.70–1.30		
		3–6	mg/l	
Protein S		70–140	%	Ag, activity
		0.70–1.40		
		418–600	mg/l	
Prothrombin Fragment 1+2		0.4–1.1	nmol/l	E (citrate)
Prothrombin Time (Quick)		12–15	s	
		0.8–1.2	(INR)	
		80–120	%	
Red Cell Distribution Width (index)		12.8–15.2		
Reptilase Time		15–22	s	

Analyte	Age/Gender	Reference Range	SI Unit	Note
Reticulocytes	Neonates	0.02–0.06* 0.100–0.300		*x 10^{12}/l. Blood treated with K_2EDTA.
	Adults	0.025–0.075* 0.005–0.015		Method dependent reference values.
Sulfhemoglobin		negat.		
Thrombin-Anti-thrombin Complex (TAT)		1.0–4.1	μg/l	E (citrate)
Thrombin Time		18–22	s	E (0.5 ml 3.8% Na-citrate + 4.5 ml blood). Control time ± 2 s if control is 9–13 s. Method dependent reference values.
Thrombocrit		0.001– 0.0036		
		0.19–0.36	%	
Thrombomodulin		20–40	ng/ml	
Beta-Thrombo-globulin		10–35	μg/l	E
Thromboxane B2		18–91	pg/ml	
von Willebrand's Factor		<8 0.6–1.5	mg/l IU/ml	

Urine

Analyte	Age/Gender	Reference Range	SI Unit	Note
Acetone		negat.		semiquantitatively
N-Acetyl-Beta-D-Glucosaminidase		<6.3 <0.56	U/l *	*kU/mol creatinine
Albumin (MAU)		<20 <30 <2.26	mg/l mg/d g/mol*	24 hrs urine, immunoturbi-dimetric method, molecular weight 64 kD *g/mol creatinine, 2nd morning urine, immunoturbidimetric method
Aldosterone				Concentrations valid for 3 g Na/day intake.
free		130–810 70–450	pmol/d ng/d	
		50–230	nmol/d	Natrium output 25 mmol/d.
		15–71	nmol/d	Natrium output 75–125 mmol/d.
		5–35	nmol/d	Natrium output 200 mmol/d.
aldosterone glucuronide		6.3–32	nmol/d	Produced in kidney.
tetrahydro-aldosterone		18–120	nmol/d	Produced in liver
Aluminium		0–1.2	μmol/d	E special tube

Analyte	Age/ Gender	Reference Range	SI Unit	Note
Delta-Aminolevulic Acid		<49	µmol/d	
Alpha-Amino- nitrogen		13.5–20.3	mmol/l	
		0.98–1.5	*	*mmol/creatinine
		0.03–0.04	**	**fraction excretion
Alpha-Amylase				37 °C, EPS method, G7 sub-
total		<16.7	µkat/l	strate spontaneously voided urine
		<15.0	µkat/d	24 hrs urine
		<77	kU/mol*	*kU/mol creatinine, sponta- neously voided urine
		<11.3	µkat/g*	*µkat/g creatinine, spontane- ously voided urine
pancreatic		<13.3	µkat/l	
		<53	kU/mol*	*kU/mol creatinine, sponta- neously voided urine
		<7.8	µkat/g*	*µkat/g creatinine
Bacteria	Children	<10^9	l	Chambert count
	Adults	<10^{11}	l	
Cadmium	non-smokers	<9	µmol/l	E
	intoxication	88–180	µmol/l	
Calcium	M	<7.5	mmol/d	24 hrs urine required
average diet intake	F	<6.2	mmol/d	To add an acid to make pH <2
non-calcium diet		0.13–1.0	mmol/d	
lower calcium diet*		1.25–3.8	mmol/d	*(5–10 mmol/d)
Carnitine		60–600	µmol/d	
Catecholamines				To add an acid to make pH <2
Norepinephrine	0–1 y	0–59	nmol/d	or EDTA (250 mg/l) + natri-
	1–2 y	0–100	nmol/d	um meta-bisulfide (250 mg/l).
	2–4 y	24–171	nmol/d	
	4–7 y	47–266	nmol/d	
	7–10 y	77–384	nmol/d	
	Others	87–473	nmol/d	
Epinephrine	0–1 y	0–13.6	nmol/d	
	1–2 y	0–19.1	nmol/d	
	2–4 y	0–32.7	nmol/d	
	4–7 y	1.1–55	nmol/d	
	7–10 y	2.7–76	nmol/d	
	Others	2.7–109	nmol/d	
Dopamine	0–1 y	0–555	nmol/d	
	1–2 y	65–914	nmol/d	
	2–4 y	261–1697	nmol/d	
	Others	424–2611	nmol/d	
Catecholamines total, free	0–1 y	10–15	µg/d	
	1–5 y	15–40	µg/d	
	6–15 y	20–80	µg/d	
	Others	30–100	µg/d	

Analyte	Age/Gender	Reference Range	SI Unit	Note
Chloride		85–170	mmol/d	24 hrs urine
		46–168	mmol/l	1st morning urine
Chromium		<1	μg/d	E
Citrates	2–4		mmol/dU	
Copper		0.16–0.94	μmol/dU	E
Coproporphyrins		51–351	nmol/d	
Cortisol, free	1–14 y	<74	nmol/d	During sampling store urine
	Puberty	<138	nmol/d	in refrigerator
	Adults	27–276	nmol/d	
Creatinine	M	5–18	mmol/d	24 hrs urine
	F	8–27	mmol/d	1st morning urine, PAP method.
	M 20–29 y	190–230	*	*μmol/kg/d
	M 70–79 y	100–152	*	
	F 20–29 y	140–207	*	
	F 70–79 y	81–123	*	
Cyclic Adenosine Monophosphate		<1000	nmol/d	Special sampling into inhibitors (cold, EDTA, theophylline). <6000 nmol/g creatinine. *nmol/mmol creatinine
		330–660	*	
Cyclic Guanosine Monophosphate (cGMP)		30–200	*	*nmol/mmol creatinine
Cystatine C		<0.01	mg/l	M. w. 13.3 kD
Cysteine		<317	μmol/d	
Estriol, total	Pregnancy			
	30 w	21–62	μmol/d	More than 40% decrease indicates fetus threat.
	35 w	31–97	μmol/d	
	40 w	45–146	μmol/d	
Estrogens, total	Children	<10	μg/d	
	M	5–25	μg/d	
	F Follicul. phase	5–25	μg/d	
	Ovulatory phase	28–100	μg/d	
	Luteal phase	22–80	μg/d	
	Pregnancy	<45 000	μg/d	
	30 w	17.4–55.5	μmol/d	
	35 w	34.7–97.1	μmol/d	
	40 w	52–140	μmol/d	
	Menopause	<10	μg/d	
Galactose	Neonates	<3.33	mmol/l	
	Children	<0.08	mmol/dU	
Glucose		0.3–1.1	mmol/l	1st morning urine, bacteria cause value decrease
Glycosamino-glycans	0–1 y	10.0–27.2	*	*mg/mmol creatinine
	1–2 y	7.8–13.4	*	
	2–4 y	7.6–12.0	*	
	4–6 y	6.5–8.3	*	
	6–10 y	4.9–7.7	*	
	10–15 y	3.4–5.6	*	

Analyte	Age/ Gender	Reference Range	SI Unit	Note
	15–20 y	1.9–3.9	*	
	20–50 y	0–1.6	*	
Homovanilic Acid	0–1 y	<20	*	*mmol/mol creatinine
	2–4 y	<14	*	
	5–19 y	<8	*	
	Adults	<8	*	
		<45	µmol/d	
17-Hydroxycorti-costeroids		0.9–2.5	*	*mmol/mol creatinine
	F	9.5–28	µmol/d	
	M	12–35	µmol/d	
5-Hydroxindole-acetic Acid		3–47	µmol/d	24 hrs urine, FIA. Acidify an urine (pH 2). Special diet.
Hydroxyproline				24 hrs urine. OH-proline/
total		362–458	µmol/d	creatinine 0.006–0.016 mol.
free		36–190	*	*µmol/d x BSA. 2-day low-collagen diet.
IgG/Albumin Quotient		9.6–56.9 *		*x 10^{-2}
Immunoglobulin G		<0.01	g/l	<10 mg/g creatinine, 1.13 g/mol creatinine. Do not freeze. M. w. 150 kD
Inorganic		11–32	mmol/d	
Phosphorus		0.11–0.45	ml/s*	*clearance
		0.07–0.20	**	**fraction excretion
Iron		<1.8	µmol/d	
Ketobodies (as OH-Butyrate)		<50	mg/l	12 hrs starvation
17-Ketosteroids	F <55 y	21–44	µmol/d	
	M <60 y	28–55	µmol/d	
17-Ketogenic Steroids	F <55 y	10–52	µmol/d	
	M <60 y	17–80	µmol/d	
Lead		<0.39	µmol/d	E
Light Chains kappa and lambda		<10	mg/l	
Lysozyme		<0.3	mg/l	M. w. 14 kD
Macroalbuminuria		>200	µg/min	>200 mg/g creatinine
		>300	mg/d	
		>200	mg/l	
Alpha-2-Macro-globulin		<10	mg/l	M. w. 250 kD
		<7	*	*mg/g creatinine
		<0.8	**	**g/mol creatinine
Magnesium		2.5–8.5	mmol/d	24 hrs urine
		0.70–1.05	mmol/l	1st morning urine, acidify to pH <2
		0.93–0.98	*	*tubular resorption
		0.02–0.07	**	**fraction excretion
Methylmalonic Acid	6–12 w	0–55	*	*mmol/mol creatinine

Analyte	Age/ Gender	Reference Range	SI Unit	Note
Alpha-1-Micro- globulin		<12	mg/l	Method dependent reference values. 1st morning urine.
		<20	mg/d	
	<40 y	<20	*	*g/mol creatinine
	>40 y	<2.2	*	
Beta-2-Micro- globulin		<0.30	mg/l	<0.20 mg/g creatinine
		0.5–2.0	µl/s*	*clearance
Microalbuminuria		<20	µg/min	
		<30	mg/d	
		<20	mg/l	
		<24	*	*mg/g creatinine
Myoglobin		<0.3	mg/l	Semiquantitatively. Stripe sensitivity 0.3 mg/l.
Natrium		30–300	mmol/dU	Natrium intake dependent results.
Neopterin	<25 y F	<208	nmol/l	A HPLC, fluorometry
	<25 y M	<195	nmol/l	
	26–35 y F	<240	nmol/l	
	26–35 y M	<182	nmol/l	
	36–55 y F	<229	nmol/l	
	36–55 y M	<197	nmol/l	
	55–65 y F	<250	nmol/l	
	55–65 y M	<218	nmol/l	
	>65 y F	<250	nmol/l	
	>65 y M	<230	nmol/l	
Nicotinic Acid		2.43–12.17	µmol/d	
Organic Acids				
lactic a.		13–46	*	*mmol/mol creatinine
2-hydroxyiso- butyric a.		0		undetectable
glycolic a.		18–55	*	*mmol/mol creatinine
3-hydroxy- butyric a.		0–2.0	*	*mmol/mol creatinine
3-hydroxyiso- butyric a.		4.1–19	*	*mmol/mol creatinine
2-hydroxyiso- valeric a.		0		undetectable
3-hydroxyiso- valeric a.		6.9–25	*	*mmol/mol creatinine
methylmalo- nic a.		0		undetectable
4-hydroxy- butyric a.		0.3–5.8	*	*mmol/mol creatinine
ethylmalonic a.		0.4–4.2	*	*mmol/mol creatinine
succinyl a.		0.5–16	*	*mmol/mol creatinine
fumaric a.		0.2–0.8	*	*mmol/mol creatinine
glutaric a.		0.6–2.6	*	*mmol/mol creatinine
3-methyl- glutaric a.		0		undetectable
adipic a.		0.8–35	*	*mmol/mol creatinine
pyruvic a.		2.6–7.9	*	*mmol/mol creatinine

Analyte	Age/Gender	Reference Range	SI Unit	Note
pyroglutamic a.		0.9–63	*	*mmol/mol creatinine
2-oxoisovaleric a.		0		undetectable
acetoacetic a.		0		undetectable
mevalonic a.		0.06–0.22	*	*mmol/mol creatinine
2-hydroxy-glutaric a.		0.8–52	*	*mmol/mol creatinine
3-OH-3-methyl-glutaric a.		0–10	*	*mmol/mol creatinine
p-hydroxy-phenylacetic a.		3.5–22	*	*mmol/mol creatinine
2-oxoisoca-proic a.		0		undetectable
suberic a.		0–2.9	*	*mmol/mol creatinine
orotic a.		0		undetectable
cis-aconitic a.		2.7–44	*	*mmol/mol creatinine
homovanilic a.		0.9–5.5	*	*mmol/mol creatinine
azalenic a.		1.3–5.5	*	*mmol/mol creatinine
isocitric a.		36–84	*	*mmol/mol creatinine
citric a.		70–226	*	*mmol/mol creatinine
seboic A.		0		undetectable
4-hydroxyphenyl-lactic a.		0.2–2.6	*	*mmol/mol creatinine
2-oxoglutaric a.		4–74	*	*mmol/mol creatinine
5-hydroxyindole-acetic a.		0–7.2	*	*mmol/mol creatinine
succinylacetone		0		undetectable
Osmolality		>850	*	*mOsm/kg H_2O. After 12 hrs water intake restriction.
Oxalates		<4.4	μmol/d	Urine sampling: acidify to pH 2 (6N HCl) + thymol (5 ml). Interference with vitamin C.
Phenols		<210	μmol/l	Exposure limit exceeds 3.5-times reference limit.
Phosphate Clearance		0.09–0.27	ml/s	
Porphobilinogen		0–8.8 negat	μmol/d	quantitatively qualitatively, urine pH 6–7 Store in darkness. pH <5 causes value decrease.
Porphyrins				Store in darkness.
total		<120	nmol/dU	Urine pH about 6–7.
uroporphyrin		4–29	nmol/dU	
coproporphyrin		20–120	nmol/dU	
carboxyporphy-rin (penta-, hexa-, hepta-)		<12	nmol/dU	
porphyrin (dicar-boxy-, tricarboxy-)		<3	nmol/dU	
Potassium		35–80	mmol/d	

Analyte	Age/ Gender	Reference Range	SI Unit	Note
Pregnanetriol	Children			
	2 w–2 y	0.06–0.6	µmol/d	
	5 y	<1.5	µmol/d	
	15 y	<4.5	µmol/d	
	Adults	<5.9	µmol/d	
Proteins		<70	mg/l	= 7.9 g/mol creatinine or
		<80	mg/d	70 mg/g creatinine
Retinol Binding Protein		<0.5	mg/l	M. w. 21 kD
Specific Gravity	Neonates	1.012		Daily urine, normal.
	First few days	1.002–1.006		
	Adults	1.002–1.030		Spontaneously voided urine.
		>1.025		After 12 hrs water intake decrease.
		1.015–1.025		24-hrs urine sample
N-Terminal Telopeptide Fragment Type I (NTx)	M 20–79 y	<79	*	*nmol/mmol creatinine
	F 21–55 y	<79	*	
	49–79 y	<140	*	
Thiamine	Children			
	1–3 y	75–85	*	*µmol/mol creatinine
	Adults	28–55	*	
TmP/GFR		0.8–1.4	mmol/l	
Transferrin		<1.2	mg/l	
TRP%		82–90	%	
Urea		170–580	mmol/dU	
Uric Acid		1.2–6.0	mmol/d	Without diet preparation.
		<3.6	mmol/d	With diet preparation.
		<1.78	mmol/l	Before sampling add NaOH or
		0.07–0.72	ml/s*	LiOH (0.1 N) to pH 8.
		0.044–0.122	**	*clearance, **fraction excretion
Urine Sediment				
Erythrocytes		0–1	per field	magnification x 400
Leukocytes		1–4	per field	
Squamous epithelial cells		5–15	per field	
Renal epithelial cells		0		
Casts				
– hyaline		occas.		
– epithelial		0		
– erythrocyte		0		
– granular		0		
– leukocyte		0		
Bacteria		0		
Yeast		0		
Trichomonads		0		
Salts		0		

Analyte	Age/ Gender	Reference Range	SI Unit	Note
Urine volume	1–2 d	0.03–0.06	l/d	Normal fluid intake.
	3–10 d	0.10–0.30	l/d	
	11 d–2 m	0.25–0.45	l/d	
	3 m–1 y	0.40–0.50	l/d	
	2–3 y	0.50–0.60	l/d	
	4–5 y	0.60–0.70	l/d	
	6–8 y	0.65–1.00	l/d	
	9–14 y	0.80–1.40	l/d	
	Adults	1.00–1.60	l/d	
Vanilmandelic Acid		18–33	µmol/d	Sampling: dark tube + 10–15 ml 6N HCl (pH 2). Special diet + drug withdrawal (if possible).
Xylose		0.16–0.33	abs.	ingested fraction, children 0.5 g/kg
Zinc		0.77–23	µmol/l	
		0.15–1.47	*	*mmol/mol creatinine

Cerebrospinal Fluid

Analyte	Age/ Gender	Reference Range	SI Unit	Note
Acetylcholine		95–265	nmol/l	Radioenzyme analysis
Albumin				
suboccipital liquor		61–180	mg/l	
ventricular l.		110–350	mg/l	
spinal l.		112–354	mg/l	
Albumin CSF/ Serum Ratio		<0.007		
Gamma-Amino-Butyric Acid (GABA)		190–280	nmol/l	Radioreceptor assay
Cells	Neonates	<32	WBC/l	
	Adults	0	WBC/l	
leukocytes				
– spinal liquor		0–5		
– suboccipit. l.		0–3		
– ventricular l.		0–1		
lymphocytes				
– spinal l.		0.6–0.85		
– suboccipit. l.		0.8–0.95		
– ventricular l.		0.9–1.00		
granulocytes				
– spinal l.		0.15–0.40		
– suboccipit. l.		0.05–0.20		
– ventricular l.		0–0.10		
Choline		0.3–3.2	µmol/l	Radioenzyme analysis
Cyclic Adenosine Monophosphate (cAMP)		4–19	nmol/l	Radioreceptor assay, RIA

Analyte	Age/ Gender	Reference Range	SI Unit	Note
Cyclic Guanosine Monophosphate		1.6–6.9	nmol/l	C Radioreceptor assay (with extraction).
(cGMP)		3.0–9.4	nmol/l	C (without extraction)
Dopamine		0.2–0.6	nmol/l	HPLC, GC-MS
Beta-Endorphins		6–15	pmol/l	RIA
Glial Fibrillary Acidic Protein		<9.5	µg/l	
Glucose	Children			
	<16 y	1.8–4.6	mmol/l	
	Adults	2.7–4.2	mmol/l	Adults – approximately 60%
blood/liquor co-efficient	Adults	1.1–1.6		of blood glucose concentration.
Homovanilic Acid (HVA)		161–349	nmol/l	HPLC
5-Hydroxyindoleacetic Acid (5-HIAA)		145–205	nmol/l	HPLC, MS
Hypoxanthine	0–1 m	1.8–5.5	µmol/l	
Immunoglobulin A				
suboccipital liquor		0–1.8	mg/l	
ventricular l.		0–3.9	mg/l	
spinal l.		379–4250	mg/l	
Immunoglobulin G				
suboccipital l.		5.0–23	mg/l	
ventricular l.		13.9–37.5	mg/l	
spinal l.		284–860	mg/l	
Immunoglobulin M				
suboccipital l.		<350	µg/l	
ventricular l.		<450	µg/l	
spinal l.		2658–24800	µg/l	
Intrathecal Ig-Production				Ig production = IgG liquor
IgG		0.6–0.7	mg/d	– 0,43 x
IgA		0.3–0.4	mg/d	x {(liquor albumin: serum
IgM		<0.1	mg/d	albumin) + 0,001} x IgG (serum)
Lactate	6 m–15 y	1.1–1.8	mmol/l	Store sample for max. 3 hrs at
	16–50 y	1.5–2.1	mmol/l	room temperature, max.
	51–75 y	1.7–2.6	mmol/l	24 hrs at 2 to 8 °C
Leu-Enkephalin		124–369	pmol/l	RIA
Alpha-2-Macro-globulin				
suboccipital l.		0–2.2	mg/l	
ventricular l.		0–3.3	mg/l	
spinal l.		469–2957	mg/l	
Met-Enkephalin		19–108	pmol/l	RIA
Myelin Basic Protein (MBP)		<2.5	µg/l	
Neopterin		<3	nmol/l	
Protein S-100		<2.5	µg/l	

Analyte	Age/ Gender	Reference Range	SI Unit	Note
Proteins, total	Premature infants			
	27–32 w of preg.	0.68–2.40	g/l	
	33–36 w of preg.	0.67–2.30	g/l	
	37–40 w of preg.	0.58–1.50	g/l	
	1 d–1 m	0.25–0.72	g/l	
	2–3 m	0.20–0.72	g/l	
	4–6 m	0.15–0.50	g/l	
	7–12 m	0.10–0.45	g/l	
	2 y	0.10–0.40	g/l	
	3–4 y	0.10–0.38	g/l	
	5–8 y	0.10–0.43	g/l	
	Adults	<0.45	g/l	
Electrophoresis				
Prealbumin		0.054–0.090		
Albumin		0.553–0.659		
alpha-1-globulins		0.028–0.056		
alpha-2-globulins		0.028–0.048		
beta globulins		0.099–0.155		
gamma globulins		0.082–0.146		

Amniotic Fluid

Analyte	Age/ Gender	Reference Range	SI Unit	Note
Estriol, free	Pregnancy			
	16–20 w	3.5–11.1	nmol/l	
	20–24 w	7.3–27.1	nmol/l	
	24–28 w	7.3–27.1	nmol/l	
	28–32 w	13.9–47.2	nmol/l	
	32–36 w	12.5–53.8	nmol/l	
	36–38 w	16.0–62.5	nmol/l	
	38–40 w	18.7–68.7	nmol/l	
Alpha-1-Fetoprotein	Pregnancy			
	15 w	10.8–16.92	µg/ml	
	16 w	8.32–15.08	µg/ml	
	17 w	7.27–13.33	µg/ml	
	18 w	6.28–12.72	µg/ml	
	19 w	4.24–9.96	µg/ml	
	20 w	2.55–7.45	µg/ml	
Lecithin	Lung maturity expected	>64	µmol/l	UV test, fully enzymatic (Boehringer Mannheim)

Analyte	Age/ Gender	Reference Range	SI Unit	Note
	Lung maturity not expected	<59	μmol/l	
Lecithin/Sphingomyelin		2.0–5.0		Fetal lung maturity

Stool

Analyte	Age/ Gender	Reference Range	SI Unit	Note
Bile acids		120–225	mg/d	
Blood				Not detectable. No intake of fish, meat, radish, horseradish, iron or copper containing preparations 3 days prior to test.
Chymotrypsin		>220	nkat/g	37 °C
Composition	Dry substance	10–60	g/d	
	Water volume	100–180	ml/d	
	Neutral fats	<7	g/d	
	Bile acid	300–400	mg/d	
	Stercobilinogen + stercobilin	60–200	mg/d	
Coproporphyrins		600–1 800	nmol/d	<45 nmol/g of dry weight
Pancreatic Elastase-1		>200	*	*μg/g of stool, sensitivity is 97%, specificity 96%
Weight		100–250	g/d	

Synovial Fluid

Analyte	Age/ Gender	Reference Range	SI Unit	Note
Alkaline Phosphatase		<1.2	μkat/l	
Cells		<200	μl	
Glucose		3.3–5.3	mmol/l	
Granulocytes		<0.10		
Hyaluronate		<3.0	mg/ml	
Lactate Dehydrogenase (LD)		<5.3	μkat/l	
Mononuclear Cells		>0.90		
N-Acetyl-Glycosamine		<10	U/l	
Proteins, total		10–20	g/l	
Urates		180–385	μmol/l	
Viscosity		300	cP	25 °C

Appendix

Basic Pharmacokinetic Parameters in Frequently Monitored Medicaments I.

h – hour, d – day, w – week, min – minute, i.m. – intramuscular injection/administration, p.o. – oral administration, inf. – infusion, i.v. – intravenous administration, admin. – administration, SR – slow release, cps – capsule

	Dosage	Peak concentration	Steady state time	Biological half-time	Take sample	Therapeutic range
Acetaminophen	2–4 g/d (children according to age)	30–60 min		1–4 h	1 h after theoretical peak value	(66–132 µmol/l) 10–20 mg/l
Amikacin	onset 5–7.5 mg/kg maintain 10–20 mg/kg/d			adults <30 y 30–180 min adults >30 y 1.5–15 h children 0.5–2.5 h	start 0.5–1 h after infusion, maintain 1 h after i.m.	peak 20–30 mg/l, maintain continuous <5 mg/l
Amiodarone	onset i.v. adults 5 mg/kg/30 min to 1000 mg/d children 5 mg/kg/30 min to 1–2 mg/kg/d p.o. adults 2x200 mg children 3x30 mg/kg/d maintain adults 100–400 mg/d children 4–8 mg/kg/d	4–6 h	100–150 d	20–60 d	before next dose	0.5–2.5 mg/l
Amitriptylin	75–300 mg/d	2–6 h	3–8 d	17–40 h	before next dose	120–250 µg/l

	Dosage	Peak concentration	Steady state time	Biological half-time	Take sample	Therapeutic range
Cyclosporine A	onset monotherapy 10–15 mg/kg/d combined therapy 7–10 mg/kg/d maintain 2–6 mg/kg/d autoimmune diseases 2.5–5 mg/kg/d	3 h	3–5 d	adults 14 h (4–50) children 9 h (3–20)	12–24 h after last dose	start 150–350 µg/l ↑ maintain 100–250 µg/l
Digoxin	p.o. 12–20 µg/kg children <10 y 10–40 µg/kg children 1–2 y 20–40 µg/kg i.v. 0.8 of p.o. dose	i.v. during time of admin. p.o. 60–90 min	5–7 d in <renal functions >7 d	adults 20–50 h children 18–33 h	8–24 h after admin.	0.8–2.0 µg/l
Disopyramide	onset adults 300 mg p.o. maintain 300–800 mg/d	2–3 h	1–2 d after MI >2 d	4.5–9 h patients with renal diseases 8–43 h		2–5 mg/l
Etosuximide	adults 15–30 mg/kg/d children 15–40 mg/kg/d	2–6 h	5–15 d	adults 30–60 h children 20–55 h	freely	40–100 mg/l
Phenobarbital	adults 1–4 mg/kg/d children 2–5 mg/kg/d	1–3 h	adults 10–25 d children 8–20 d	adults 50–150 h children 40–130 h		10–40 mg/l
Phenytoin	adults 3–6 mg/kg/d children 5–9 mg/kg/d	2–6 h 9 h in SR	4–24 d dose dependence			10–20 mg/l 1–2 mg/l free phenytoin
Flecainide	onset i.v. adults 2–4 mg/kg/30 min later i.v. inf. 0.1–0.25 mg/kg/h children 2 mg/kg p.o. adults 200–400 mg children 6 mg/kg	2–3 h	4–5 d	14 h adults 8 h children 20 h adults cardiacs	before next dose	200–600 µg/l
Flucytosin				3–6 h	30 min after i.v. inf.	25–50–100 mg/l

	Dosage	Peak concentration	Steady state time	Biological half-time	Take sample	Therapeutic range
Gentamicin	onset children + adults 1–2 mg/kg maintain adults 3–6 mg/kg/d, children 4–10 mg/kg/d			adults <30 y 0.5–3 h >30 y 1.5–15 h children 0.5–2.5 h	start 0.5–1 h after inf., 1 h after i.m. maintain – just before next dose	peak 5–10 mg/l, maintain <2 mg/l
Quinidine	adults 14–30 mg/kg/d children 15–60 mg/kg/d	1–3 h SR >3 h	2 d	6–7 h	before next dose	2–5 mg/l
Imipramin	onset p.o. 25–75 mg/d maintain 50–300 mg/d	1–6 h	2–5 d	6–28 h	just before next dose	150–250 µg/l
Carbamazepin	adults 2.5–25 mg/kg/d (anticonvulsant) 3–20 mg/kg/d (antineuralgic) children 5–30 mg/kg/d	4–8 h 12 h micronized	2–6 d	6–25 h	just before next dose	4–11 mg/l
Caffeine				neonates 96 h cirrhosis 50 h	just before next dose	5–20 mg/l (neonates)
Acetylsalicylic Acid	45–60 mg/kg/d	1–2 h		15–30 min salicylates 20 h	1–3 h after admin.	150–300 mg/l
Valproic Acid	adults 10–45 mg/kg/d children 10–60 mg/kg/d	syrup 0.5–1 h cps. 0.2–2 h enteric cps. 3–8 h	2–4 d in chronic admin.	adults 6–17 h children 5–15 h infants 15–60 h	just before next dose	50–100 mg/l
Lidocain	onset adults 200–300 mg cardiac patients 100–160 mg cirrhosis 200–300 mg	i.v. infusion end 5–10 h		adults 70–200 min cardiac patients 200–400 min	2 h after starting dose 6–12 h after starting dose	1.5–5.0 mg/l

	Dosage	Peak concentration	Steady state time	Biological half-time	Take sample	Therapeutic range
	children 1–5 mg/kg maintain adults 1.5–3 mg/min cardiac patients 0.9–1.8 mg/min cirrhosis 0.9–1.8 mg/min children 1–2 mg/min			cirrhosis 300 min	monitor daily, in cardiac patients every 12 h	
Lithium	900–1500 mg/d	1–3 h 5–6 h in SR	3–7 d	14–33 h	12 h after evening dose	0.3–1.3 mmol/l
Marprotilin	75–225 mg/d	12 h	7 d	51 h (active metabolites 60–80 h)	before next dose	100–600 μg/l
Methotrexate	p.o. 20 mg/m² i.v. 1–12 g/m² (special protocol)		12–24 h	2–4 h initially 8–15 h terminally	dose/infusion/ duration and clinical condition dependent (special therapeutic protocol)	see table p. 995
Netilmicin	onset adults + children 1–2 mg/kg maintain adults 4–8 mg/kg/d, children 4–12 mg/kg/d			adults <30 y 0.5–3 h >30 y 1.5–15 h children 0.5–2.5 h	peak 0.5–1 h after inf. end, 1 h after i.m. continuously before next dose	peak 5–12 mg/l, continuous <3 mg/l
Nortriptyline	30–100 mg/d	2–6 h	4–20 d	18–56 h	before next dose	50–150 μg/l
Primidone	p.o. adults 7.5–20 mg/kg/d children 5–25 mg/kg/d	0.5–7 h	2–4 d primidone 10–14 d metabolite phenylethylmalo-amid (PEMA),	4–22 h primidone 24–60 h PEMA 50–150 h phenobarbital	before next dose	5–15 mg/l

	Dosage	Peak concentration	Steady state time	Biological half-time	Take sample	Therapeutic range
Procainamide	onset 10–15 mg/kg maintain 35–50 mg/kg/d	1–4 h	10–25 d metabolite phenobarbital 25–35 h ↑ in <renal functions> up to 70 h	3–5 h	before next dose	4–10 mg/l N-acetylprocainamide 6–22 mg/l
Streptomycin	adults 15–25 mg/kg/d i.m. children 20–40 mg/kg/d			2–3 h	peak 1–2 h after i.m. admin. continuously before next dose	peak 15–40 mg/l, maintain <5 mg/l
Theophylline	1st dose 5 mg/kg i.v. if concentration is known or urgent 2 mg/kg i.v. maintain adults 0.4 mg/kg/h adult smokers 0.6 mg/kg/h adult cardiac patients + patients with liver disease 0.2 mg/kg/h children >10 y 0.7 mg/kg/h children <10 y 0.8 mg/kg/h children <1 y 0.008 x age in weeks + 0.21 chronic dose mg/kg/d adults 10–15 adult smokers 15–18 adult cardiac patients + patients with liver disease 4–8 children 12–16 y 18		adults 2–3 d children 1–2d infants 1–5 d neonates 5 d	adults 9 h (3–12) adult smokers 4h adult cardiac or patients with liver disease 10–56 h children 2–10 h infants 3–14 h neonates 30 h	before i.v. inf. 30 min after starting dose 4–6 h after beginning of continuous inf. ↑ p.o. 2 h after usual dose ↑ 4–8 h after SR	asthma 8–20 mg/l neonate apnea 6–11 mg/l

Dosage	Peak concentration	Steady state time	Biological half-time	Take sample	Therapeutic range
children 9–12 y 20					
children 1–9 y 24					
infants 6–52 w					
0.3 x age in weeks + 8					
Tobramycin			onset adults	peak 0.5–1 h after inf. end, 1 h after i.m.	peak 5–10 mg/l, maintain <2 mg/l
adults + children 1–2 mg/kg/d maintain			<30 y 0.5–3 h >30 y 1.5–15 h children 0.5–2.5 h	maintain before next dose	
Vancomycin			adults 4–10 h children 2–3 h	peak 1 h after inf. end, continuously before next dose	peak 20–40 mg/l, continuously 5–10 mg/l
adults 3–6 mg/kg/d children 4–10 mg/kg/d					
adults 20–40 mg/kg/d children 40–60 mg/kg/d					

Basic Pharmacokinetic Parameters in Frequent Monitored Medicaments II.

	Elimination	Bound	Toxicology	Interference
Acetaminophen	20–30% to proteins		concentrations >1300 µmol/l 220 mg/l in chronic admin. (4 h) >50 mg/l (12 h after admin.) hepatotoxicity	
Amikacin	kidney 90%	<10%		↓ renal diseases, dehydration, obesity ↑ obesity, burns, surgery
Amiodarone	liver	96%		dicoumaroles have rapid (50%) metabolism by amiodarone, digoxin slowed (up to 100%)
Amitriptylin	liver 95% (active metabolites 10-hydroxylated, inactive glucuronids)	>90%		see nortriptyline

	Elimination	Bound	Toxicology	Interference
Cyclosporine A	bile >90% kidney <6%	98–99%		↓ rifampicin, isoniazid, phenytoin, phenobarbital, carbamazepine ↑ ketoconazole, erythromycin, diltiazem, verapamil, nicardipine
Digoxin	kidney 75–80% liver <30%	20%		↓ quinidine, amiodarone ↑ spironolactone, antacids
Disopyramide	kidney 36–60% liver 20–30%	10–65%		
Ethosuximide	liver 80%	0%		↓ isoniazide, valproate
Phenobarbital	liver 70%	50%		↑ barbiturates, carbamazepine, phenytoin ↑ liver diseases, renal diseases, pregnancy, urine alkalization
Phenytoin	liver 95%	92%		↓ dextropropoxyphene, dicoumarol, warfarin, furosemide, methosuximide, methylphenidate, phenytoin, valproate ↑ viral diseases, phenylbutazone, valproate, sulfonamides, carbenicillin, amiodarone, cimetidine, isoniazid, phenothiazines, phenobarbital ↓ rifampicin, folic acid
Flecainide	liver 75%	40%		
Flucytosine	kidney 80%	10%		
Gentamicin	kidney 90%			↑ renal diseases, dehydration ↑ obesity, burns, after surgery ↓ phenobarbital, phenytoin
Quinidine	liver 60–80% kidney 10–30%	80–90%		
Imipramine	liver (all metabolites are active), kidney (conjugates)	63–96%		↓ barbiturates, carbamazepine ↑ cimetidine, antidepressives, phenothiazines

	Elimination	Bound	Toxicology	Interference
Carbamazepine	liver 99%	65–80%		↓ liver diseases, macrolide antibiotics, cimetidine, danazol, diltiazem, fluoxetine, fluvoxamine, isoniazid, verapamil, viloxazine ↑ pregnancy, barbiturates, phenytoin, felbamet, valproic acid
Caffeine	liver 96% (metabolites theobromine, theophylline)			
Acetylsalicylic Acid		50–90%	administration contraindication in children <6 y	
Valproic acid	95% liver	90%		Liver diseases decrease bound. ↓ absorption. Salicylates, barbiturates, phenytoin, carbamazepine by ↑ clearance
Lidocain	kidney <10%	60–70%		↓ phenobarbital ↑ non-selective beta-blockers, cimetidine
Lithium	kidney 90%			↓ ACE inhibitors ↑ NSAID, diuretics
Marprotilin	stool 30% kidney 57%	88%		↓ carbamazepine, MAO inhibitors ↑ cimetidine, haloperidol, phenothiazines
Methotrexate	kidney 70–90%	50–60%	minimum toxic concentration 10 nmol/l serum concentration connected with ↑ risk after 6 h inf. with a high concentration (5 g/m²) 24 h >5 µmol/l 48 h >0.5 µmol/l 72 h >0.05 µmol/l	renal diseases and ↓ urine pH leads to clearance ↓; ascites and pleural exudates prolong biological half-time. Absorption is ↓ by antibiotics, salicylates, NSAID, sulfonamides.
Netilmicin	kidney 90%	<10%		

	Elimination	Bound	Toxicology	Interference
Nortriptyline	liver (hydroxy-nortriptyline) kidney (glucurone conjugates)	87–93%		↓ barbiturates, carbamazepine ↑ cimetidine, haloperidol, phenothiazines
Primidone	liver 60% (PEMA, phenobarbital) kidney 40% (primidone)	<35%		liver diseases, kidney disorders cause ↑ PEMA and primidone concentrations. Isoniazid nicotin-amide, valproic acid, ethosuximide cause ↑ of primidone and PEMA. Carbamazepine, phenytoin decrease conversion to phenobarbital.
Procainamide	liver 20–50% kidney 50%			
Streptomycin	kidney	30%		
Theophylline	kidney 10%	55–65% 36% in cirrhosis		smoking causes ↑ clearance ↓ erythromycin, cimetidine, ciprofloxacin, enoxacin, verapamil, allopurinol ↑ aminoglutethimide, carbamazepine, phenobarbital, phenytoin, rifampicin
Tobramycin	kidney	<10%		
Vancomycin	kidney 90%	30–55%		peak concentration delay in renal diseases

Methotrexate concentration and leukovorine dosage (methotrexate concentration >42 hrs from infusion start)

Methotrexate concentration	Leukovorine dose
20–50 µmol/l	500 mg/m^2 each 6 h i.v.
10–20 µmol/l	200 mg/m^2 each 6 h i.v.
5–10 µmol/l	100 mg/m^2 each 6 h i.v.
1–5 µmol/l	30 mg/m^2 each 6 h i.v.
0.6–1 µmol/l	15 mg/m^2 each 6 h p.o.
0.1–0.5 µmol/l	15 mg/m^2 each 12 h p.o.
0.05–0.1 µmol/l	5–10 mg/m^2 each 12 h p.o.

Appendix

Appendix

Conversion Factors Between Conventional Units And Systéme International (SI) Units
Blood (B), plasma (P), serum (S), urine (U), cerebrospinal fluid (CSF), synovial fluid (SF), amniotic fluid (AF). All reference values is to serum unless otherwise stated.

Analyte	Conventional Units	SI units	Conversion Factors Conventional to SI units	SI to Conventional units
Acetoacetate	mg/dl	µmol/l	97.95	0.0102
Acid phosphatase	U/l	nkat/l	16.67	0.06
ACTH	pg/ml	ng/l	1	1
	pg/ml	pmol/l	0.2202	4.541
Alanine aminotransferase	U/l	µkat/l	0.0167	59.88
Albumin				
(S)	g/dl	g/l	10	0.1
(CSF, AF)	mg/dl	mg/l	10	0.1
Aldolase	U/l	nkat/l	16.67	0.06
Aldosterone				
(S)	ng/dl	nmol/l	0.0277	36.1
(U)	mEq/24 hrs	mmol/day	1	1
(U)	µg/24 hrs	nmol/day	2.77	0.36
Alkaline phosphatase	U/l	µkat/l	0.0167	59.88
Aluminium	µg/l	nmol/l	37.06	0.027
delta-Aminolevulinate (as levulinic acid)	mg/24 hrs	µmol/d	7.63	0.131
Ammonia				
(S)	µg/dl	µmol/l	0.714	1.4
(P)	µg/dl	µmol/l	0.5872	1.703
(CSF)	µg/dl	µmol/l	0.5872	1.703
Amylase	U/l	µkat/l	0.0167	59.88
Androstenedione	ng/dl	pmol/l	34.92	0.0286
Angiotensin II	ng/dl	ng/l	10	0.1
Angiotensin-converting enzyme (ACE)	nmol/ml/min	U/l	1	1
Anion gap	mEq/l	mmol/l	1	1
Antidiuretic hormone (ADH)	pg/ml	ng/l	1	1
Alpha-1-antitrypsin	mg/dl	g/l	0.01	100
AFP	ng/ml	µg/l	1	1
	ng/dl	ng/l	10	0.1
	mg/dl	g/l	0.01	100
	mg/dl	mg/l	10	0.1
	µg/dl	µg/l	10	0.1

Analyte	Conventional Units	SI units	Conventional to SI units	SI to Conventional units
			Conversion Factors	
Apolipoprotein A-I or B	mg/dl	mg/l	10	0.1
Aspartate aminotransferase (AST)	U/l	µkat/l	0.0167	59.88
Base excess	mEq/l	mmol/l	1	1
Bicarbonate	mEq/l	mmol/l	1	1
Bilirubin	mg/dl	µmol/l	17.1	0.0584
Calcitonin	pg/ml	ng/l	1	1
Calcium				
(S)	mg/dl	mmol/l	0.25	4.0
(S)	mEq/l	mmol/l	0.5	2.0
(U)	mg/24 hrs	mmol/day	0.025	40
(CSF)	mEq/l	mmol/l	0.5	2.0
Carbon dioxide (B, P, S)	mEq/l	mmol/l	1	1
Catecholamines (P)				
Epinephrine	pg/ml	pmol/l	5.458	0.183
Norepinephrine	pg/ml	nmol/l	0.0059	169.49
(U) (as norepinephrine)	µg/24 hrs	nmol/d	5.911	0.169
CO$_2$ partial pressure (pCO$_2$)	mm Hg	kPa	0.133	7.52
Carotene	µg/dl	µmol/l	0.0186	53.76
CEA	ng/ml	µg/l	1	1
	µg/ml	mg/l	1	1
Ceruloplasmin	mg/dl	mg/l	10	0.1
Chloride	mEq/l or mg/dl	mmol/l	1	1
Cholesterol	mg/dl	mmol/l	0.0259	38.61
HDL-cholesterol	mg/dl	mmol/l	0.0259	38.61
LDL-cholesterol	mg/dl	mmol/l	0.0259	38.61
Cholinesterase	U/l	µkat/l	0.0167	59.88
Copper				
(S)	µg/dl	µmol/l	0.157	6.37
(U)	µg/24 hrs	µmol/day	0.0157	63.69
Coproporphyrins				
(I and III)	µg/dl	nmol/l	15	0.067
(U)	µg/24 hrs	nmol/day	1.5	0.67
(F)	µg/g	nmol/g	1.5	0.67
Cortisol				
(S)	µg/dl	µmol/l	0.028	35.7
(S)	ng/ml	nmol/l	2.76	0.362
(U) – free	µg/dl	nmol/day	2.76	0.362
Creatine (S)	mg/dl	µmol/l	76.3	0.0131
Creatine kinase	U/l	µkat/l	0.0167	59.88
Creatinine				
(S, AF)	mg/dl	µmol/l	88.4	0.0113
(U)	g/24 hrs	mmol/day	8.84	0.1131
(U)	mg/24 hrs	mmol/day	0.00884	113.1
(U)	mg/kg/24 hrs	µmol/kg/day	8.84	0.113

Analyte	Conventional Units	SI units	Conventional to SI units	SI to Conventional units
clearance	ml/min/ 1.73 m²	ml/s/m²	0.00963	104
(CSF)	mg/dl	μmol/l	88.4	0.0113
17-OHKS (cortisol)	mg/24 hrs	μmol/day	2.759	0.3625
(U)	μg/24 hrs	nmol/day	2.759	0.3625
Cyclic adenosine mono-phosphate (cAMP)				
(S)	μg/l	nmol/l	3.04	0.329
(B)	ng/ml	nmol/l	3.04	0.329
(U)	mg/24 hrs	μmol/day	3.04	0.329
(U)	mg/g creatinine	μmol/mol	344	0.00291
11-Deoxycorticosterone (DOC) (S)	pg/ml	pmol/l	3.03	0.33
Dehydroepiandrosterone (P)	μg/l	nmol/l	3.467	0.288
DHEA-S				
(S)	μg/ml	μmol/l	2.6	0.38
(P)	μg/l	μmol/l	0.002714	368.45
(AF)	ng/ml	nmol/l	2.6	0.38
Dopamine (U)	μg/24 hrs	nmol/day	6.53	0.153
(U)	μg/mg creatinine	μmol/mol creatinine	738	0.00136
Estradiol	pg/ml	pmol/l	3.671	0.272
Estriol	μg/24 hrs	nmol/d	3.468	0.288
Estrogens (U) (as estriol)	mg/24 hrs	μmol/d	3.468	0.288
Estrone (P), (S)	pg/ml	pmol/l	3.699	0.27
Ethanol (P)	mg/dl	mmol/l	0.217	4.608
Ethylene glycol (P)	mg/dl	mmol/l	0.161	6.21
Ferritin	ng/ml	μg/l	1	1
alpha-Fetoprotein	ng/ml	μg/l	1	1
Folate	ng/ml	nmol/l	2.266	2.74
Fructose (P)	mg/dl	mmol/l	0.556	1.799
FSH (P)	mIU/ml	IU/l	1	1
Gastrin	pg/ml	ng/l	1	1
Glucagon	pg/ml	ng/l	1	1
Glucose	mg/dl	mmol/l	0.0555	18.02
(CSF)	mg/dl	mmol/l	0.0555	18.02
GMT	U/l	μkat/l	0.0167	59.88
Growth hormone	ng/ml	μg/l	1	1
Haptoglobin	mg/dl	g/l	10	0.1
5-HIAA (U)	mg/24 hrs	μmol/day	5.2	0.19
Homovanilic acid				
(U)	mg/24 hrs	μmol/day	5.49	0.182
(U)	μg/24 hrs	μmol/day	0.00549	182
(U)	μg/mg creatinine	mmol/mol creatinine	0.621	1.61

Analyte	Conventional Units	SI units	Conversion Factors Conventional to SI units	Conversion Factors SI to Conventional units
beta-Hydroxybutyrate	mg/dl	µmol/l	96.05	0.0104
17-Hydroxycorticosteroids (17-OHCS)	mg/g creatinine	mg/mol	113.1	0.00884
(U)	mg/d	µmol/day	2.76	0.362
17-Hydroxyprogesterone (P)	µg/l	nmol/l	3.026	0.33
Immunoglobulin G (CSF)	mg/dl	mg/l	10	0.1
Insulin	µU/ml	pmol/l	7.175	0.139
Iron	µg/dl	µmol/l	0.0179	55.87
Iron-binding capacity	µg/dl	µmol/l	0.0179	55.87
Iron saturation	%	Fraction saturation	0.01	100
17-KGS (as dehydroepiandrosterone)				
(U)	mg/24 hrs	µmol/day	3.467	0.2904
17-KS (as dehydroepiandrosterone)				
(U)	mg/24 hrs	µmol/day	3.467	0.2904
Lactate	mg/dl	mmol/l	0.111	9.01
(CSF)	mg/dl	mmol/l	0.111	9.01
Lead				
(S)	µg/dl	µmol/l	0.0483	20.72
(S)	mg/dl	µmol/l	48.26	0.0207
(U)	µg/24 hrs	µmol/day	0.00483	207.03
Lipids (total)	mg/dl	g/l	0.01	100
Alpha-2-macroglobulin	mg/dl	g/l	0.01	100
Magnesium				
(S)	mEq/l	mmol/l	0.5	2
(S)	mg/dl	mmol/l	0.411	2.433
(U)	mg/24 hrs	mmol/day	0.411	2.433
(CSF)	mEq/l	mmol/l	0.5	2
Natrium				
(S)	mEq/l	mmol/l	1	1
(U)	mEq/24 hrs	mmol/day	1	1
(U)	mg/24 hrs	mmol/day	0.0435	22.99
Osmolality	mOsm/kg	mmol/kg	1	1
Osteocalcin	ng/ml	µg/l	1	1
O_2 partial pressure (pO_2)	mm Hg	kPa	0.133	7.5
Oxytocin	ng/l	pmol/l	0.80	1.25
pH	nEq/l	nmol/l	1	1
Phosphate (inorganic phosphorus)				
(S)	mg/dl	mmol/l	0.323	3.10
(U)	g/24 hrs	mmol/day	32.3	0.031
Porphobilinogen	mg/24 hrs	µmol/day	4.42	0.226
Potassium				
(S)	mEq/l	mmol/l	1	1
(U)	mEq/24 hrs	mmol/day	1	1

Analyte	Conventional Units	SI units	Conversion Factors Conventional to SI units	SI to Conventional units
(U)	mg/24 hrs	mmol/day	0.02558	39.1
Progesterone	ng/ml	nmol/l	3.18	0.314
Protein, total				
(S)	g/dl	g/l	10	0.1
(U)	mg/24 hrs	g/day	0.001	1000
(CSF)	mg/dl	mg/l	10	0.1
PTH				
(S)	pg/ml	ng/l	1	1
(P)	μlEq/ml	mlEq/l	1	1
Pyruvate (P)	mg/dl	μmol/l	113.6	0.0088
Renin (PRA)	ng/ml/hr	μg/l/hr	1	1
Reverse T_3 (rT_3)	ng/dl	nmol/l	0.0154	65.1
Serotonin (S)	ng/ml	μmol/l	0.00568	176
Standard bicarbonate (hydrogen carbonate)	mEq/l	mmol/l	1	1
TBG	mg/dl	mg/l	10	0.1
	μg/dl	μg/l	10	0.1
Testosterone (total) (S)	ng/dl	nmol/l	0.0347	28.8
TSH	μU/ml	mIU/l	1	1
Thyroglobulin	ng/ml	μg/l	1	1
T3				
total	ng/dl	nmol/l	0.0154	65.1
free	pg/dl	nmol/l	15.4	0.0649
T4				
total	μg/dl	nmol/l	12.9	0.0775
free	ng/dl	pmol/l	12.9	0.0775
Transferrin	mg/dl	g/l	0.01	100
TRH	pg/ml	ng/l	1	1
	pg/ml	pmol/l	2.759	0.362
Triacylglycerols	mg/dl	mmol/l	0.0113	88.5
Unsaturated Vitamin B_{12} binding capacity				
(S)	pg/ml	pmol/l	0.738	1.355
Urea				
(S)	mg/dl	mmol/l	0.357	2.8
(U)	g/24 hrs	mol/day	0.0357	28
(U)	ml/min	ml/s	0.0167	59.88
Uric acid				
(S)	mg/dl	mmol/l	0.05948	16.9
(U)	mg/24 hrs	mmol/day	0.0059	169
Urobilinogen (U)	mg/d	μmol/day	1.693	0.591
Uroporphyrin				
(U)	μg/24 hrs	nmol/day	1.204	0.831
(U)	μg/g creatinine	nmol/mmol creatinine	1.1362	0.88

			Conversion Factors	
Analyte	Conventional Units	SI units	Conventional to SI units	SI to Conventional units
Vanilmandelic acid				
(U)	mg/24 hrs	μmol/day	5.05	0.198
(U)	μg/g creatinine	mmol/mol creatinine	0.571	1.75
Viscosity (S)	Centipoise	Same		
Vitamin A	μg/dl	μmol/l	0.0349	28.65
Vitamin B$_6$	ng/ml	nmol/l	5.982	0.167
Vitamin B$_{12}$ (cyanocobalamin)	pg/ml	pmol/l	0.738	1.355
Vitamin C (ascorbic acid)	mg/dl	μmol/l	56.78	0.176
Vitamin D				
(calcitriol; 1,25-dihydroxy-)	pg/ml	pmol/l	2.4	0.417
(25-hydroxy-)	ng/ml	nmol/l	2.496	0.401
Vitamin E (alpha-tocopherol)	ng/ml	nmol/l	23.22	0.0431
Xylose				
(U)	mg/dl	mmol/l	0.0666	15.01
(U)	g/5 hrs	mmol/5 hrs	6.66	0.15
Zinc	μg/dl	μmol/l	0.153	6.54

Hematology

			Conversion Factors	
Analyte	Conventional Units	SI units	Conventional to SI units	SI to Conventional units
Carboxyhemoglobin	%		0.01	100
Fetal hemoglobin	%	mol/mol (may omit symbol)	0.01	100
Fibrinogen	mg/dl	g/l	0.01	100
Haptoglobin	mg/dl	mg/l	10	0.1
HCT (packed cell volume)	%	volume fraction	0.01	100
Hemoglobin	g/dl	g/l	10	0.1
(whole blood)	g/dl	mmol/l	0.155	6.45
(plasma)	mg/dl	μmol/l	0.155	6.45
MCH (color index)	pg (or μg)	pg	1	1
	pg	fmol	0.06206	16.11
MCHC (saturation index)	g/dl	g/l	10	0.1
MCV (volume index)	μ^3 (cubic microns)	fl	1	1
Platelet count	10^3/cu mm	10^9/l	1	1

Analyte	Conventional Units	SI units	Conversion Factors	
			Conventional to SI units	SI to Conventional units
RBC count (erythrocytes)				
(B)	$10^6/\mu l$ or /cu mm	$10^{12}/l$	1	1
(CSF)	or /mm³ /cu mm	$10^6/l$	1	1
Reticulocytes	/cu mm	$10^9/l$	0.001	1000
WBC count (leukocytes)	/μl or /cu mm or	cells x $10^9/l$	0.001	1000
(B)	/mm³			
(CSF)	/cu mm or	$10^6/l$	1	1
	/cu μl	$10^6/l$	10^6	10^{-6}
(SF)	/μl	/l	10^6	10^{-6}

Pharmacology

Analyte	Conventional Units	SI units	Conversion Factors	
			Conventional to SI units	SI to Conventional units
Acetaminophen	μg/l	μmol/l	6.62	0.151
Amikacin	μg/ml	μmol/l	1.71	0.585
Amitriptyline	ng/ml	nmol/l	3.61	0.277
Carbamazepine	mg/l	μmol/l	4.233	0.236
Chloramphenicol	μg/ml	μmol/l	3.09	0.323
Chlorpromazine	ng/ml	nmol/l	3.176	0.315
Desipramine	ng/ml	nmol/l	3.754	0.266
Diazepam	mg/l	nmol/l	3.512	0.285
Digoxin	ng/ml	nmol/l	1.28	0.781
Ethosuximide	μg/ml	μmol/l	7.08	0.141
Gentamicin	μg/ml	μmol/l	2.09	0.478
Imipramine	ng/ml	nmol/l	3.57	0.28
Lidocaine	μg/ml	μmol/l	4.27	0.234
Lithium	mEq/l	mmol/l	1	1
Methotrexate	ng/ml	nmol/l	2.2	0.454
Nortriptyline	ng/ml	nmol/l	3.8	0.263
Phenobarbital	μg/ml	μmol/l	4.31	0.232
Primidone	μg/ml	μmol/l	4.58	0.218
Procainamide	μg/ml	μmol/l	4.23	0.236
Theophylline (aminophylline, others)	μg/ml	μmol/l	5.55	0.180
Tobramycin	μg/ml	μmol/l	2.14	0.467
Valproic acid	μg/ml	μmol/l	6.93	0.144
Vancomycin	μg/ml	mg/l	1	1

Cluster of Differentiation (CD) Molecules

Cluster Designation	Synonym	Cellular Expression
CD1a	T6, Leu-6, R4	thymocytes, dendritic cells, Langerhans cells
CD1b	R1	thymocytes, dendritic cells, Langerhans cells
CD1c	M241, R7	thymocytes, dendritic cells, Langerhans cells
CD1d	R3	intestinal epithelium, thymocytes,dendritic cells, Langerhans cells
CD1e	R2	thymocytes, dendritic cells, Langerhans cells
CD2	CD2R, E-rosette receptor, T11, LFA-2 (CD58 receptor)	E-rosette receptor-associated T-cells, NK-cells, B-cells, thymocytes
CD2R		activated T-cells
CD3	T3, Leu-4	T-cells, thymocytes
CD3delta	CD3d	T-cells
CD3epsilon	CD3e	T-cells
CD3gamma	CD3g	T-cells
CD4	T4, L3T4, W3/25, Leu-3a	T-cells subset (helper/inducer), thymocyte subsets, peripheral blood monocytes, tissue macrophages, granulocytes
CD5	T1, Leu-1, Ly-1, Lyb-1, Lyt-1, Tp67	T-cells subset, B-cells, thymocytes
CD6	T12	T-cells subset, B-cells subset, immature/mature thymocytes, neurons subset
CD7	FcμR, gp40	T-cells subset, NK-cells, thymocytes, pluripotential hematopoietic cells
CD8	T8, Leu-2, Lyt-2	cytotoxic/supressor T-cells subset, thymocyte subsets
CD8alpha	Leu2, T-cell co-receptor, T8	T-cells subset
CD8beta	Leu2, Lyt3	cytotoxic T-cells
CD9	p24, DRAP-27, MRP-1	monocytes, pre-B-cells, platelets, activated T-cells, eosinophils, basophils, endothelial cells, brain and peripheral nerves, vascular smooth muscle, cardiac muscle, epithelia
CD10	CALLA, common acute lymphoblastic leukemia antigen, J5, neprilysin, enkephalinase, gp100, neutral endopeptidase, NEP	germinal center B-cells, lymphocyte progenitor cells, granulocytesT-cell precursors, bone marrow stromal cells
CD11a	LFA-1 (alpha chain)	all leukocytes, macrophages, lymphocytes, granulocytes, monocytes
CD11b	Mac-1 (alpha chain of CR3), Mo1, alpha-M-beta2, C3biR,	monocytes, macrophages, granulocytes, NK-cells, some T-cells, subsets of B-cells, myeloid cells
CD11c	p150,95 (alpha chain), Leu-M5, Axb2, CR4, leukocyte surface antigen p150,95	monocytes, macrophages, granulocytes, B-cells subset, NK-cells, subset of T-cells

Cluster Designation	Synonym	Cellular Expression
CDw12	myeloid antigen, p90-120	granulocytes, monocytes, NK-cells, platelets
CD13	MY7, aminopeptidase N, APN, gp150	granulocytes, monocytes, endothelial cells, epithelial cells (renal proximal tubules, intestinal brush border), bone marrow stromal cells, osteoclasts, cells lining bile duct canaliculi, large granular lymphocytes
CD14	Leu-M3, Mo2, LPS receptor, LPS-R	monocytes, macrophages, granulocytes, epidermal cells
CD15	3-FAL, 3-FL, LNFP III, Lacto-N-neo-fucopentaose III, Lewis X, Lex, SSEA-1, X-hapten	monocytes, neutrophils, eosinophils
CD15s	sLE, sialyl Lewis X, sLex, sialylated Lewis X, SLe-x	monocytes, neutrophils, eosinophils
CD16a	Fc, RIII, FCRIIIA	macrophages, NK-cells, granulocytes
CD16b	FCRIIIB	macrophages, NK-cells
CDw17	lactosylceramide, LacCer	granulocytes, monocytes, platelets, basophils, peripheral B-cells subset, tonsillar dendritic cells
CD18	beta chain of CD11a, b, c, beta-2 integrin, beta2, beta-2 integrin chain	all leukocytes
CD19	Leu-12, B4	B-cells, follicular dendritic cells, malignant B-cells
CD20	Leu-16, B1, Bp35	B-cells
CD21	C3d receptor (CR2), B2, Epstein-Barr virus receptor, EBV-R	mature B-cells, follicular dendritic cells, subset of immature thymocytes
CD22	Leu-14, B3, MAG, BL-CAM, Lyb8	B-cells
CD23	FcRII (IgE receptor), B6, BLAST-2, FceRII, Leu-20, low affinity IgE receptor	activated B-cells, macrophages, NK-cells, monocytes, FDC apical light zone (T-cells, platelets, eosinohpils, neutrophils, Langerhans cells)
CD24	BA-1, heat stable antigen, HSA	B-cells, granulocytes, epithelial cells
CD25	Tac, beta chain of IL-2, IL-2 receptor alpha chain, IL-2R, Tac antigen	activated T-cells, B-cells, macrophages, monocytes, HTLV-I-transformed T-cell lines
CD26	Ta1, dipeptidylpeptidase IV, DPP IV ectoenzyme, adenosine deaminase-binding protein, ADA-binding protein	activated T-cells, B-cells, macrophages, thymocytes, NK-cells, renal proximal tubular epithelial cells, small intestinal epithelium, biliary canaliculi, splenic sinus lining cells
CD27	S152, T14	mature T-cells, activated T-cells, B-cells subset, NK-cells, medullary thymocytes

Cluster Designation	Synonym	Cellular Expression
CD28	p44(9.3), Tp44, T44	T-cells, thymocytes, plasma cells, activated B-cells
CD29	4B4, beta chain of VLA-4, platelet GPIIA, beta-1 integrin, beta-1 integrin chain	activated T-cells
CD30	Ki-1 antigen, Ber-H2 antigen	activated T-cells and B-cells, activated NK-cells, monocytes, large lymphoid cells in lymph node, tonsil, thymus, decidua and endometrial cells, Hodgkin's lymphoma, Reed–Sternberg cells, Hodgkin cells, anaplastic large cells lymphoma, pleomorphic and immunoblastic lymphoma, embryonal carcinoma, mixed germ cell tumor
CD31	PECAM-1, platelet endothelial cell adhesion molecule, endocam, platelet gpII	granulocytes, monocytes, macrophages, B-cells, platelets, endothelial cells, leukocytes and precursors, NK-cells, subsets of T-cells
CD32	Fc receptor (Fc-gamma-RII), FCR II	granulocytes, macrophages, B-cells, eosinophils, monocytes, platelets
CD33	MY9, gp67, p67	granulocyte/monocyte precursors, monocytes, macrophages
CD34	MY10, gp 105-120	lymphohematopoietic stem and progenitor cells, small-vessel endothelial cells, embryonic fibroblasts, some cells in fetal and adult nervous tissue, embryonic liver, aorta-associated hematopoietic progenitors
CD35	CR1, C3b receptor, C3bR, C4bR, complement receptor type one, immune adherence receptor	granulocytes, monocytes, B-cells, erythrocytes, eosinophils, T-cells, glomerular podocytes, follicular-dendritic cells, some astrocytes
CD36	platelet gpIIIb, GP IIIb, OKM5-antigen, PASIV	monocytes, platelets, macrophages, microvascular endothelial cells, mammary endothelial cells
CD37	gp52-40	B-cells, some T-cells, neutrophils, granulocytes, monocytes, myeloid cells
CD38	T10, Leu-17, ADP-ribosyl cyclase/cyclic ADP-ribose hydrolase	lymphocytes, progenitor cells, early B-cells, activated T-cells, plasma cells, brain, muscle, kidney
CD39	gp80	mature B-cells, endothelial cells, activated NK-cells, macrophages, dendritic cells
CD40	gp50, Bp50	B-cells, plasma cells, basal epithelial cells, epithelial cell carcinomas, macrophages, monocytes, follicular dendritic cells, endothelial cells, fibroblasts, keratinocytes, interdigitating cells, hemopoietic cell progenitors

Cluster Designation	Synonym	Cellular Expression
CD40-L	T-BAM, gp39	activated CD4, T-cells
CD41	gpIIb/IIIa complex, glyco-protein IIb, GPIIb, alpha IIb integrin chain	platelets, megakaryocytes, isoform 3 is expressed by leukemia, prostate adenocarcinoma and melanoma cells
CD42a	platelet gpIX, GPIX	platelets, megakaryocytes
CD42b	platelet gpIB, alpha, GPIb-alpha, glycocalicin	platelets, megakaryocytes
CD42c	GP1b-beta, GPIb-beta, GPIbb	platelets, megakaryocytes
CD42d	GPV	platelets, megakaryocytes
CD43	sialophorin, leukosialin	leukocytes (except circulating B-cells)
CD44	Pgp-1, ECMR III, H-CAM, HUTCH-1, Hermes, Lu, gp85	leukocytes, brain, erythrocytes, most cell types, (not at platelets, hepatocytes, cardiac muscle, kidney tubular epithelium, testis, portions of the skin)
CD44R	restricted epitope on CD44, CD44v, CD44v9	leukocytes, epithelial cells, monocyte lineage cells
CD45	T200, leukocyte common antigen (LCA), B220, Ly5	all hematopoietic cells, lymphocytes, leukocytes
CD45RA	Leu-18, restricted T200	T-cells, B-cells, granulocytes, monocytes
CD45RB	restricted T200	T-cells subset, B-cells, granulocytes, macrophages, monocytes
CD45RO	restricted T200, UCHL1, gp180	memory T-cells, B-cells, granulocytes, macrophages, monocytes
CD46	membrane cofactor protein, MCP	leukocytes, epithelial cells, fibroblasts, salivary gland ducts, kidney ducts, lymphocytes, endothelium, interstitial tissues, muscle cells, tumor cells
CD47	Rh-associated protein, gp42, integrin-associated protein, IAP, neurophilin, ovarian carcinoma antigen 3, OA3, MEM-133	broad tissue distribution, hematopoietic cells, epithelial/endothelial cells, fibroblasts, brain, mesenchymal cells, tumor cell lines
CD48	BCM1, Blast-1, Hu Lym3, OX-45	leukocytes
CD49a	VLA-alpha-1 integrin chain, very late antigen alpha-1 chain, VLA-1 alpha chain	T-cells, monocytes
CD49b	VLA-alpha-2 integrin chain, platelet gpIa	activated T-cells, platelets, monocytes, some B-cells, fibroblasts
CD49c	VLA-alpha-3 integrin chain	T-cells, some B-cells, monocytes, brain, heart, endothelial vein cells
CD49d	VLA-alpha-4 integrin chain	monocytes, T-cells, B-cells, eosinophils, basophils, mast cells, thymocytes, NK-cells, dendritic cells, embryo myeloblasts, myelomonocytic cells, melanoma cells, Kupffer cells, muscle cells, erythroblastic precursor cells, sickle reticulocytes

Cluster Designation	Synonym	Cellular Expression
CD49e	VLA-alpha-5 integrin chain, FNR alpha chain	T-cells, some B-cells and monocytes, platelets
CD49f	VLA-alpha-6 integrin chain, platelet gpI	platelets, megakaryocytes, activated T-cells, heart, kidney, placenta, colon, duodenum, myoblasts, myotubes
CD50	ICAM-3, intercellular molecule-3	leukocytes, monocytes, granulocytes, epidermal Langerhans cells, endothelial cells, thymocytes, T-cells, B-cells
CD51	alpha chain of vitronectin receptor, VNR-alpha chain, alpha-V integrin chain	platelets, megakaryocytes
CD52	CAMPATH-1	leukocytes, thymocytes, T-cells, B-cells, granulocytes, lymphocytes, monocytes, macrophages, epithelial cells lining the male reproductive tract
CD53	MRC OX44	leukocytes, plasma cells
CD54	ICAM-1, intercellular adhesion molecule-1	broad, B-cells, T-cells, myeloid cells, endothelial cells, monocytes, epithelial cells
CD55	decay accelerating factor, DAF	leukocytes, cells throughout the body, erythrocytes
CD56	Leu-19, NKH-1, isoform of N-CAM, neural cell adhesion molecule	NK-cells, subsets of T-cells, cerebellum, cortex, neuromuscular junctions, certain LGL leukemia, small cell lung carcinomas, neural-derived tumors, myelomas, myeloid leukemias
CD57	HNK-1, Leu-7	NK-cells, T-cells subset, B-cells, monocytes
CD58	LFA-3, lymphocyte function-associated antigen 3	broad spectrum of tissues and cells, hematopoietic cells, non-hematopoietic cells, leukocytes, erythrocytes, endothelial cells, epithelial cells, fibroblasts
CD59	Ly6c, membrane inhibitor of reactive lysis, MIRL, 1F-5Ag, H19, HRF20, MACIF, P-18, protectin	broad spectrum of tissues and cells
CDw60	9-o-acetyl-GD3	subset of T-cells, platelets, monocytes, thymic epithelium, activated keratinocytes, synovial fibroblasts, glomeruli, smooth muscle cells, astrocytes
CD61	integrin beta-3, GPIIb/IIIa, beta3, ITGB3	platelets, megakaryocytes, macrophages
CD62E	E-selectin, ELAM-1, LECAM-2	platelets, endothelial cells, endothelium in chronic inflammatory lesions of the skin and synovium, skin, placenta, bone marrow
CD62L	L-selectin, LECAM-1, Leu-8, MEL-14, TQ1, LAM-1, TQ-1	B-cells, monocytes, T-cells, granulocytes, platelets, endothelial cells, NK-cells, spleen lymphocytes, bone marrow lymphocytes, bone marrow myeloid cells, thymocytes

Cluster Designation	Synonym	Cellular Expression
CD62P	P-selectin, granule membrane protein-140, GMP-140, platelet activation dependent granule-external membrane protein, PADGEM	platelets, endothelial cells, megakaryocytes
CD63	platelet activation antigen, LIMP, MLA1, PTLGP40, gp55, granulophysin, lysosomal-membrane-associated glycoprotein 3, LAMP-3, melanoma-associated antigen, ME491, neuroglandular antigen, NGA	platelets, monocytes, macrophages, dysplastic nevi, radial growth phase primary melanomas, hematopoietic cells, endothelial cells, degranulated neutrophils, fibroblasts, osteoclasts, smooth muscle, neural tissue
CD64	Fc receptor (Fc-gamma-RI), FCR I	monocytes, macrophages, blood dendritic cell subset, germinal center dendritic cells, early myeloid lineage cells
CD65	ceramide-dodecasaccharide, VIM-2	granulocytes, myeloid cells
CD65s	sialylated-CD65, VIM-2	granulocytes, monocytes, myeloid leukemia cells, acute lymphatic leukemias
CD66a	BGP, NCA-160, biliary glycoprotein	granulocytes, epithelial cells
CD66b	CD67, p100, CGM6, NCA-95, carcinoembryonic antigen-related cell adhesion molecule 6, CEACAM6	granulocytes, myeloid cells
CD66c	NCA, NCA-50/90	myeloid cells, granulocytes, epithelial cells, neutrophils, colon carcinoma
CD66d	CGM1	myeloid cells, granulocytes, neutrophils
CD66e	CEA, carcinoembryonic antigen, carcinoembryonic antigen-related cell adhesion molecule 5, CEACAM5	myeloid cells, epithelial cells, adult colon epithelium, colon carcinoma
CD66f	pregnancy specific b1 glycoprotein, SP-1, PSG	placental syncytiotrophoblasts, fetal liver, myeloid cell lines
CD67	now CD 66b	monocytes, macrophages
CD68	macrosialin, gp 110	monocytes, macrophages, dendritic cells, neutrophils, basophils, mast cells, myeloid progenitor cells, subset of CD34+ hematopoietic bone marrow progenitor cells, activated T-cells, B-cells, liver, glomeruli, renal tubules, soluble form in serum and urine
CD69	activation inducer molecule, AIM, EA 1, MLR3, gp 34/28, very early activation, VEA	activated T-cells, B-cells, macrophages, NK-cells, thymocytes, neutrophils, eosinophils

Cluster Designation	Synonym	Cellular Expression
CD70	CD27-ligand, Ki-24 antigen	activated T-cells, activated B-cells, macrophages
CD71	T9, transferrin receptor	proliferating cells, macrophages, leukocytes, capillary endothelium in brain, reticulocytes, erythroid precursors
CD72	Lyb-2, Ly 32.2, Ly-19.2	B-cells
CD73	ecto 5-nucleotidase	T-cells subset, B-cells subset, dendritic cells, epithelial cells, endothelial cells
CD74	class II MHC, invariant gamma chain, Ii, class II-specific chaperone	B-cells, monocytes, macrophages, activated T-cells, activated endothelial and epithelial cells
CDw75		mature B-cells, subpopulation of peripheral blood T-cells, erythrocytes
CDw76		mature B-cells, T-cells subset, endothelial and epithelial cells subsets
CD77	Pk blood group antigen, Burkitt's lymphoma antigen, BLA, ceramide trihexoside, CTH, globotriaosylceramide, Gb3	follicular B-cells, Burkitt's lymphoma cells, follicular center lymphomas
CDw78	Ba	B-cells
CD79a	mb-1, Ig-alpha, MB1	B-cells
CD79b	B29, Ig-beta	B-cells
CD80	B7, BB1, B7-1	activated B-cells, activated T-cells, macrophages
CD81	TAPA-1	B-cells, hemopoietic cells, endothelial and epithelial cells, lymphocytes
CD82	R2, IA4, 4F9, C33, KAI1	B-cells, activated/differentiated hematopoietic cells, leukocytes
CD83	HB15	B-cells, activated T-cells, non-follicular dendritic cells, circulating dendritic cells, Langerhans' cells, thymic dendritic cells, lymphoblastoid cell lines, germinal center B-cells
CD84	GRb	mature B-cells, thymocytes, T-cells subset, monocytes, platelets, tissue macrophages
CD85	VMP-55, CH1/75	B-cells, plasma cells, germinal center cells, hairy cell leukemia, tissue macrophages, subpopulation of NK-cells in peripheral blood
CD86	FUN-1, BU63, B7-2, B70	B-cells, interdigitating dendritic cells, Langerhans' cells, peripheral blood dendritic cells, memory B-cells, germinal center B-cells, centrocytes, monocytes, T-cells subset
CD87	UPA-R, urokinase plasminogen activator receptor	myeloid cells, T-cells, NK-cells, monocytes, neutrophils, vascular endothelial cells, macrophages, fibroblasts, smooth muscle cells, keratinocytes, placental trophoblasts, hepatocytes, tumor cells (breast, colon, prostate carcinoma, melanoma)

Cluster Designation	Synonym	Cellular Expression
CD88	C5aR, C5a receptor	myeloid cells, granulocytes, monocytes, dendritic cells, macrophages, mast cells, hepatoma-derived cell line HepG2, astrocytes, microglia
CD89	Fc-alpha-R, IgA Fc receptor, IgA receptor	myeloid cells, activated eosinophils, alveolar and splenic macrophages, monocytes, granulocytes, B-cell subsets, T-cell subsets
CD90	Thy-1	myeloid cells, hematopoietic stem cells, neurons, connective tissue, fibroblast lines, stromal cells lines, thymocytes, peripheral T-cell, CD34+ cells in bone marrow, lymph node HEV endothelium, lymphoblastoid and leukemic cell lines
CD91	alpha-M-R, alpha-2-macroglobulin receptor, low density lipoprotein receptor-related protein, LRP	myeloid cells, monocytes
CDw92	GR9	myeloid cells, monocytes, granulocytes, peripheral blood lymphocytes, fibroblasts, endothelial cells, epithelial cells, platelets
CD93	GR11	myeloid cells, monocytes, granulocytes, AML blasts, myeloid cell lines, endothelial cells
CD94	KP43	NK-cells, in vitro activated NK-cells, T-cell subsets
CD95	APO-1, Fas, fas antigen, tumor necrosis factor receptor superfamily, member, TNFRSF6, apoptosis antigen 1, APT1	activated T- and B-cells
CD96	TACTILE, T-cell activation increased late expression	activated T-cells
CD97	GR1	activated T- and B-cells, monocytes, macrophages, dendritic cells, granulocytes
CD98	4F2, 2F3, FRP-1, RL-388	T-cells, B-cells, NK-cells, granulocytes, activated and transformed cells, all human cell lines
CD99	E2, MIC2, CD99R, MIC2 gene product	T-cells, lymphocytes, thymocytes
CD100	BB18, A8, GR3	T-cells, most of hematopoietic cells, germinal center B-cells
CD101	BB27, BA27, IGSF2, P126, V7	monocytes, macrophages, granulocytes, dendritic cells, activated T-cells
CD102	ICAM-2, intercellular adhesion molecule 2	leukocytes, vascular endothelial cells, resting lymphocytes, monocytes, platelets
CD103	HML-1, ITGAE, human mucosal lymphocyte	antigen 1, HML-1, integrin-alpha E chain leukocytes, intestinal intraepithelial lymphocytes, lamina propria T-lymphocytes in the intestine, intraepithelial lymphocytes in bron-

Cluster Designation	Synonym	Cellular Expression
		chi, inflammatory skin/breast/salivary glands, tumoral epithelium, peripheral lymphoid organs, enteropathy-associated T-cell lymphomas, hairy B-cell leukemia, adult T-cell leukemias associated with HTLV-1
CD104	beta-4 integrin chain, tumor specific protein 180 antigen, TSP-180, beta-4 integrin	leukocytes, epithelial cells, Schwann cells, colon, placenta, epidermis, lung, duodenum, heart, spleen, stomach, tumour cells
CD105	endoglin	endothelial cells, small/large vessels, activated monocytes, tissue macrophages, stromal cells of certain tissues, pre-B-cells in fetal marrow, erythroid precursors in fetal/adult bone marrow, syncytiotrophoblast throughout pregnancy, cytotrophoblasts during first trimester
CD106	VCAM-1, vascular cell adhesion molecule-1, INCAM-110	endothelial cells, macrophages, dendritic cells
CD107a	LAMP-1, lysosome-associated membrane protein 1	lysosomal membrane, degranulated platelets
CD107b	LAMP-2, lysosome-associated membrane protein 2	lysosomal membrane, degranulated platelets
CDw108	GR2, John–Milton–Hagen, JMH human blood group antigen	erythrocytes, leukocytes, circulating lymphocytes, lymphoblasts/lymphoblastic cell lines, some stromal cells
CD109	8A3, 7D1, E123, GR56	endothelial cells, activated T-cells, platelets
CD110	thrombopoietin receptor, TPO-R, myeloproliferative leukemia virus oncogene, MPL, C-MPL	hematopoietic stem and progenitor cells, megakaryocyte progenitors, megakaryocytic lineage cells, platelets
CD111	poliovirus receptor related 1, PRR1, HevC, nectin-1, herpesvirus Ig-like receptor, HIgR	hematopoietic cells, neuronal cells, endothelial cells, epithelial cells, brain, spinal cord, trachea, prostate, placenta, skin, kidney, lung, pancreas, thyroid, liver, erythroid lineages, fibroblastic cells
CD112	poliovirus related receptor 2, PRR2, herpesvirus entry mediator B, HVeB, herpesvirus entry protein B, poliovirus receptor-like 2, PVRL2, nectin 2	hematopoietic cells, neuronal cells, endothelial and epithelial cells, prostate, placenta, kidney, lung, pancreas, thyroid, liver, fibroblastic cells
CD114	CSF3R, HG-CSFR, granulocyte colony-stimulating factor receptor, G-CSFR	granulocytes, monocytes, mature platelets, endothelial cells, placenta, trophoblastic cells, cultured tumor cells

Cluster Designation	Synonym	Cellular Expression
CD115	CSF-1R, colony-stimulating factor 1R, M-CSF R, c-fms, M-CSFR	myeloid cells, osteoclasts, placental trophoblastic cells, breast during normal development and lactation, microglia, neurons, astrocytes, myeloid leukemic blast cells, breast and ovarian cancers, vascular smooth muscle cells in atheroma
CD116	GM-CSF R-alpha	monocytes, macrophages, neutrophils, eosinophils, endothelium, dendritic cells/precursors
CD117	c-KIT, stem cell factor receptor, SCFR	hematopoietic progenitors, acute myeloid leukemia cells, tissue mast cells, melanocytes, reproductive system, embryonic brain
CD118	IFN-alpha, beta R	broad cellular expression
CDw119	IFN-gamma R, IFNgR, IFNgRa	monocytes, macrophages, B-cells, endothelium
CD120a	TNF R type I, type I tumor necrosis factor receptor, p55, TNF-R55, TNFAR, TNFR60, p55-R, FPF	non/hematopoietic cells, epithelial cells
CD120b	TNF T type 2, TNF-R-II, TNF-R75, TNFBR, TNFR80, TNFR2, p75TNFR, TNFRII, p75, TNFR p80	non/hematopoietic cells, myeloid cells, stimulated T-cells, stimulated B-cells
CD121a	IL-1R type 1, type1IL-1R, interleukin 1 receptor type I, IL1RA, D2S1473, IL1R	thymocytes, T-cells
CD121b	IL-1R type 2, type2IL-1R, IL1R2, interleukin 1 receptor type II	monocytes, macrophages, B-cells
CD122	IL-2R beta, interleukin 2 receptor beta chain	NK-cells, resting T-cell subpopulation, B-cells, monocytes, macrophages
CD123	IL-3R alpha, IL-3 receptor alpha subunit	bone marrow stem cells, granulocytes, monocytes, megakaryocytes
CD124	IL-4R	mature B-cells and T-cells, hematopoietic precursor cells
CDw125	IL-5R-alpha	basophils, eosinophils, activated B-cells
CD126	IL-6R-alpha, interleukin-6 receptor	activated B-cells, T-cells, monocytes, plasma cells, most leukocytes, hepatocytes
CD127	IL-7R, interleukin-7 receptor, IL-7R alpha, p90	bone marrow lymphoid precursors, monocytes, pro-B-cells, mature T-cells
CDw128a	IL-8R, IL8RA, CXCR1, interleukin-8 receptor A, CMKAR1	basophils, neutrophils, T-cells subset
CDw128b	IL8RB, CXCR2, interleukin-8 receptor B	neutrophils, T-cells subset
CD130	IL-6R-beta, gp130	activated B-cells, plasma cells, most leukocytes, endothelial cells, almost all cell types

Cluster Designation	Synonym	Cellular Expression
CDw131	common beta subunit	most myeloid cells, early B-cells, monocytes, granulocytes, eosinophils
CD132	IL2RG, common cytokine receptor gamma chain	T-cells, B-cells, NK-cells, monocytes, macrophages, neutrophils, fibroblasts, hematopoietic precursors
CD133	PROML1, AC133, hematopoietic stem cell antigen, prominin	primitive cell populations (hematopoietic stem and progenitor cells, neural and endothelial stem cells), retina, retinoblastoma, developing epithelium (neuroepithelium, kidney, gut), fetal liver, bone marrow, teratocarcinoma cells line, retinoblastoma cells lines
CD134	OX40, TNFRSF4, tumor necrosis factor receptor superfamily member 4, ACT35, TXGP1L	lymphocytes, activated T-cells
CD135	FMS-like tyrosine kinase 3, flt3, Flk-2, STK-1	multipotential, myelomonocytic and primitive B-cell progenitors, carcinoma cells
CDw136	macrophage stimulating protein receptor, msp receptor, ron, p158-ron	epithelial tissues (skin, kidney, lung, liver, intestine, colon), hematopoietic cells, certain established neuroendocrine cells
CDw137	4-1BB, induced by lymphocyte activation, ILA	T-cells, B-cells, monocytes, epithelial cells, hepatoma cells
CD138	heparan sulfate proteoglycan, syndecan-1, SDC1	plasma cells
CD139	BU30	B-cells, monocytes, granulocytes, erythrocytes, some myeloid cell lines, smooth muscle of selective vessels, follicular dendritic cells
CD140a	PDGF receptor, PDGF-R, alpha platelet-derived growth factor receptor, PDGFRA	fibroblasts, osteoblasts, chondroblasts, smooth muscle cells, glial cells, endothelial cells
CD140b	PDGFRB, PDGFR, JTK 12, beta platelet-derived growth factor receptor	fibroblasts, osteoblasts, chondroblasts, smooth muscle cells, glial cells, endothelial cells
CD141	fetomodulin, thrombomodulin, TM	endothelial cells, keratinocytes, megakaryocytes, platelets, monocytes, neutrophils, smooth muscle cells, synovial lining cells, myeloid cells
CD142	F3, coagulation factor III, thromboplastin, tissue factor, TF	epidermal keratinocytes, monocytes, endothelial cells, glomerular epithelial cells, adventitial cells of blood vessels, astrocytes, myocardium, Schwann cells of peripheral nerves, stromal cells of liver, pancreas, spleen, thyroid
CD143	angiotensin-converting enzyme, ACE, kininase II, peptidyl dipeptidase A	endothelial cells, epithelial cells (proximal renal tubules, small intestine, ductuli efferentia of epididymis), cutaneous adnexes, breast, salivary/adrenal glands, neuronal cells, Leydig cells, fibroblasts, activated macrophages/histiocytes
CD144	VE-cadherin	endothelial cells

Cluster Designation	Synonym	Cellular Expression
CDw145		endothelial cells
CD146	MCAM, A32, MUC18, Mel-CAM, melanoma-CAM, S-endo	endothelial cells, melanoma, smooth muscle, intermediate trophoblast, activated T-cells, follicular dendritic cells
CD147	5A11, basigin, CE9, HT7, M6, neurothelin, OX-47, extracellular matrix metalloproteinase inducer, EMMPRIN, gp42	leukocytes, erythrocytes, platelets, endothelial cells, lymphocytes, myeloid cells
CD148	HPTP-eta, high cell density-enhanced PTP 1, DEP-1, p260	granulocytes, monocytes, resting T-cells, dendritic cells, platelets, fibroblasts, nerve cells, Kupffer cells
CDw150	SLAM, IPO-3 signaling lymphocyte activation molecule	thymocytes, T-cells subset, B-cell subset, dendritic cells, endothelial cells
CD151	PETA-3, SFA-1	endothelial cells, platelets, megakaryocytes, immature hematopoietic cells, epithelial cells
CD152	cytotoxic T-lymphocyte-associated protein-4, CTLA-4	activated T-cells, activated B-cells
CD153	CD30 ligand, CD30L	T-cells
CD154	CD40 ligand, CD40L, T-BAM, TNF-related activation protein, TRAP, gp39	activated T-cells
CD155	polio virus receptor, PVR	myeloid cells
CD156	ADAM8, MS2 human	neutrophils, monocytes
CD156b	ADAM17, a disintegrin and metalloproteinase domain 17, tumor necrosis factor alpha converting enzyme, TACE, snake venom-like protease, cSVP	all cells
CD157	BP-3/IF-7, BST-1, Mo5	granulocytes, monocytes, macrophages, B-cell progenitors, bone marrow stromal cell lines, myelomonocytic leukemia, human umbilical vein endothelial cells, rheumatoid arthritis-derived synovial cell lines, follicular dendritic cell lines, reticular cells of peripheral lymphoid tissues (spleen, lymph nodes, Peyers' patches)
CD158a	EB6, MHC class-I specific receptors, p50.1, p58.1	NK-cells, T-cells
CD158b	GL183, MHC class-I specific receptors, p50.2, p58.2	NK-cells, T-cells
CD160	BY55 antigen, NK1, NK28	peripheral NK-cells, T-lymphocytes with cytolytic effector activity

Cluster Designation	Synonym	Cellular Expression
CD161	KLRB1, NKR-P1A, killer cell, lectin-like receptor subfamily B member 1	NK-cells, T-cells subsets, subset of thymocytes, fetal liver T-cells
CD162	PSGL-1, PSGL	T-cells, monocytes, granulocytes, B-cells, bone marrow cells
CD163	GHI/61, M130, RM3/1	myeloid cells
CD164	MUC-24, multi-glycosylated core protein 24, MGC-24v	myeloid cells, T-cells, epithelial cells, bone marrow stroma cells, small intestine, colon, lung, thyroid, colorectal adenocarcinoma, pancreatic adenocarcinoma
CD165	AD2, gp37	subset of peripheral lymphocytes, immature thymocytes, monocytes, platelets, T-cell type acute lymphoblastic leukemia cells, central nervous system, islet cells of pancreas, Bowman's capsule of the kidney
CD166	BEN, DM-GRASP, KG-CAM, neurolin, SC-1, activated leukocyte cells adhesion molecule, ALCAM	neurons, activated T-cells, activated monocytes, epithelial cells, fibroblasts, NK-cells, platelets, thymocytes, activated B-cells, eosinophils, endothelial cells, keratinocytes
CD167a	DDR1, tyrosine kinase receptor E, TRKE, cell adhesion kinase, CAK, epithelial discoidin domain receptor precursor 1, EDDR-1, discoidin domain receptor family	epithelial cells, mammary gland, kidney, lung, colon, thyroid, brain islets of Langerhans, tumors (breast, ovary, esophagus)
CD169	sialoadhesin, Sn, Siglec-1, sialic acid-binding immunoglobulin-like lectin 1	resident and inflammatory macrophages (spleen, lymph node, bone marrow, liver, gut, lung)
CD171	L1CAM, N-CAM L1, CAML1, L1 cell adhesion molecule	epithelial cells, cells of lymphoid and myelomonocytic origin, T-cells subset, B-cells, monocytes, monocyte-derived dendritic cells, human post-mitotic neurons, glial cells, Schwann cells of the peripheral nervous system
CD178	fas L, fas-L, tumor necrosis factor superfamily, member 6, TNFSF6, apoptosis antigen ligand 1, APT1LG1	T-lymphocytes, non-activated NK-cells, parenchymal cells of the retina and cornea, retinal pigment epithelial cells, neutrophils, autoimmune thyrocytes, keratinocytes, astrocytes, microglia, mature erythroblasts, breast epithelial cells, vascular endothelial cells, placenta, various tumors
CD179a	VpreB, pre-B lymphocyte gene 1, VPREB1, immunoglobulin iota chain, IGVPB, immunoglobulin iota polypeptide chain, IGI	early pre-B-cells, pro-B-cells

Cluster Designation	Synonym	Cellular Expression
CD179b	lambda5, IGL5, immunoglobulin omega chain, immunoglobulin lambda-like polypeptide 1, IGLL1, IGVPB	pro-B-cells, early pre-B-cells
CD180	RP105	mantle zone B-cells, marginal zone B-cells, monocytes, dendritic cells
CD183	chemokine CXC receptor 3, CXCR3, G protein-coupled receptor 9, GPR9, CKR-L2, IP10 receptor, IP10-R, Mig receptor, Mig-R	T-cells, B-cells subset, NK-cells subset, malignant B-cells from chronic lymphoproliferative disorders, plasmacytoid dendritic cells, eosinophils, GM-CSF activated CD34 hematopoietic progenitors
CD184	chemokine C-X-C receptor 4, CXCR4, fusin, leukocyte-derived seven transmembrane domain receptor, LESTR, neuropeptide Y receptor Y3, NPY3R, HM89, FB22, LCR1	blood cells, B-cells, T-cells, monocytes, macrophages, dendritic cells, granulocytes, megakaryocytes, platelets, lymphoid and myeloid precursor cells, endothelial and epithelial cells, astrocytes, neurons
CD203c	neucleotide pyrophosphatase 3, NPP3, phosphodiesterase I nucleotide pyrophosphatase 3, PDNP3, B10, gp130RB13-6, ecto-nucleotide	basophils, mast cells, uterus, prostate, glioma cells
CD206	mannose receptor, C-type lectin	subsets of mononuclear phagocytes, hepatic/lymphatic endothelial cells, immature dendritic cells, retinal pigment epithelium, mesangial cells
CD222	cation-independent mannose-6 phosphate receptor, man-6p receptor, CIMPR, insulin-like growth factor 2 receptor, IGF2R, IGFII, mannose-6 phosphate receptor, M6P-R	ubiquitously
CD226	platelet and T-cell activation antigen 1, PTA1, DNAX accessory molecule-1, DNAM-1, T-lineage-specific activation antigen 1, TLiSA1	NK-cells, platelets, monocytes, T-cells subset, thymocytes
CD227	MUC1, mucin 1, episialin, PUM, PEM, EMA, DF3 antigen, H23 antigen	apical surface of all glandular and ductal epithelial cells, all circulating monocytes, bone marrow hematopoietic mononuclear cells
CD231	A15, T-cell acute lymphoblastic leukemia associa-	T-cell acute lymphoblastic leukemia, neuroblastoma cells, normal brain neuron, acute lym-

Cluster Designation	Synonym	Cellular Expression
	ted antigen 1, TALLA-1, transmembrane 4 super-family member 2, mem-brane component, X chro-mosome, surface marker 1, MXS1, CCG-B7	phoblastic leukemia cells, neuroblastoma cells
CD233	erythrocyte band 3, anion exchange protein 1, AE1, anion transport protein, solute carrier family 4, Diego blood group, EPB3	erythrocyte plasma membrane, basolateral membrane of a-intercalated cells of the distal tubules and collecting ducts of the kidney
CD234	GPFY, Fy glycophorin, FY glycoprotein	erythrocytes, endothelial cells, epithelial cells of kidney collecting duct, lung and thyroid, neurons
CD244	2B4 NK cell activation-inducing ligand, NAIL, p38	NK-cells, gamma/delta T-cells, CD8+ T-cells, monocytes, basophils

Some Important Polymorphism Frequency in Slovak Population

DNA polymorphism	Control group				
	Genotypes			Alleles	
	+/+	+/-	-/-	+	-
CTLA-4/BbvI	0.025	0.475	0.500	0.2625	0.7375
CTLA-4/TruI	0.05	0.125	0.825	0.113	0.887
HSP70-2/PstI	0.27	0.330	0.400	0.439	0.561
ACE ins./del.	0.247	0.460	0.293	0.477	0.523
Apo B/XbaI	0.262	0.510	0.228	0.517	0.483
Apo B/EcoRI	0.262	0.510	0.228	0.900	0.100
Apo B/MspI	0.810	0.190	0.000	0.910	0.090
Fibrinogen/HaeIII	0.670	0.260	0.070	0.798	0.202
FV-Leiden/Mval	0.960	0.040	0.000	0.980	0.020
GIIIA/NciI	0.670	0.310	0.020	0.830	0.170
	Allele frequency – name/frequency				
Apo E/Hin6	E2	E3	E4	E – non-3	
	0.047	0.862	0.091	0.138	
IL-1RA VNTR	2	4	5		
	0.191	0.796			

Inflammation Mediators

Function	Mediators
Increased small vessels permeability	Histamine, serotonin, bradykinin, C3a, C5a, PGD2, PGE2, LTC4, activated Hageman's factor, high-molecular weight kininogen fragments, fibrinopeptides

Function	Mediators
Vasoconstriction	N-formylmethionyl peptides, C5a, TXA2, LTB4, LTC4, LTD4
Smooth muscle contraction	C3a, C5a, histamine, LTB4, LTC4, LTD4, TXA2, serotonin, PAF
Increased endothelial cell adhesivness	IL-1, TNF-alpha, MCP-1, LTB4, LPS
Mastocyte degranulation	C3a, C5a, MCP-1, IL-8
Phagocytes	IL-3, G-CSF, GM-CSF, M-CSF
proliferation	G-CSF, GM-CSF, M-CSF, IL-1
mobilization from bone marrow	iC3b, IgG, fibronectin, lectins
adherence and aggregation	C5a, LTB4, IL-8 and other chemokines, PAF, his-
chemotaxia	tamine, laminine, N-formylmethionyl peptides, collagen fragments, chemotactic factors produced by lymphocytes, fibinopeptides
lysosome enzyme release	C5a, IL-8, PAF, most of chemotactic factors, phagocytosis
oxygen reactive intermediate products	C5a, TNF-alpha, PAF, IL-8, phagocytable particles, many chemotactic factors
phagocytosis	C3b, iC3b, IgG (Fc-part), fibronectin, IFN-gamma increases Fc-receptor expression
granuloma creation	IFN-gamma, TNF-alpha, IL-1
Pyrogens	IL-1, TNF-alpha, IL-6, PGE2
Pain	PGE2, bradykinin

(Ferenčík M, Štvrtinová V, Hulín I. Inflammation. With kind permission Rovenský J. Reumatológia v teórii a praxi V [Rheumatology in theory and practice V]. Martin: Osveta 1998, p. 146, in Slovak).

Efficient and Regulatory Macrophage Products

Agent groups	Single products
Microbicide and cytotoxic	Superoxide, hydrogenperoxide, hydroxyl radical, hypochlorite, chloramines
Reactive intermediates of oxygen	Nitric oxid, nitrites, nitrates
Reactive intermediates of nitrogen	Neutral proteases, acid hydrolases, lysozyme, defensins
Tumoricide	H_2O_2, NO^-, TNF-alpha, C3a, proteases, arginase, thymidine
Tissue damaging	H_2O_2, NO^-, TNF-alpha, neutral proteases
Endogenous pyrogens	IL-1, IL-6, TNF-alpha, MIP-1
Inflammation regulators	
Bioactive lipids	Prostaglandins, prostacyclin, thromboxanes, leukotrienes
Bioactive oligopeptides	Glutathione
Complement components and factors	C1, CC4, C2, C3, C5, factors B, D, P, I, H
Hemocoagulation factors	V, VII, IX, X, prothrombin, plasminogen activator, plasminogen activator inhibitor
Cytokines	IL-1, IL-6, TNF-alpha, IFN-gamma, macrophage inflammatory proteins (MIP-1, MIP-2, MIP-3), regulatory growth factors (M-CSF, GM-CSF, G-CSF, PDGF)

Agent groups	Single products
Neutral proteases	Elastase, collagenase, angiotensin convertase, stromelysin
Protease inhibitors	alpha-2-macroglobulin, alpha-1-protease inhibitor, plasmin and collagenase inhibitor, plasminogen activator inhibitor
Acid hydrolases	Acid proteases (cathepsin D a L), peptidases, lipases, lysozyme and other glycosidases, ribonucleases, phosphatases, sulfatases
Stress proteins	Heat-shock proteases
Involved in tissue reorganization	Elastase, collagenase, hyaluronidase, regulatory growth factors, fibroblast growth factor, (FGF), transforming growth factors (TGF-alpha, TGF-beta), angiogenesis factors
Others	Apolipoprotein E, inhibitors IL-1, purine and pyrimidine derivatives (thymidine, uracil, neopterin)

(Ferenčík M, Štvrtinová V, Hulín I. Inflammation. With kind permission Rovenský J. Reumatológia v teórii a praxi V [Rheumatology in theory and practice V]. Martin: Osveta 1998, p. 134, in Slovak).

Serum – Plasma – Whole Blood – Sampling Rules

(Guder WG, Ehret W, da Fonseca-Wollheim F, Heil W, Müller-Plathe O, Töpfer G, Wisser H, Zawta B. Serum, Plasma oder Volblut. Welche Antikoagulantien? DG Klin. Chem Mitteilungen, 29,1998;3:81–103)

Citr – citrate, Hep – heparin

Analyte	Serum	Plasma Hep	Plasma EDTA	Plasma Citr	Whole blood Hep	Whole blood EDTA	Whole blood Citr	Notes
Acetaminophen	+	+α, β	+α					
Acetylsalicylic acid	+	+β	+β	(+)β				
Adrenocorticotropic hormone (ACTH)		+	*					Add aprotinine 400 U/ml, mercaptoethanol 2 μl/ml to stabilize
Alanine aminotransferase (ALT, GPT)	+	+	+	(+)				
Albumin	+	+!	+	(+)				! suggested biochromatic tests for colorimetric methods
Aldosterone	+	+	*					
Alkaline phosphatase	+↑	*	–	(+)				EDTA complexes essential zinc
Aluminium	–	–	–	–				special probe

Analyte	Serum	Plasma Hep	Plasma EDTA	Plasma Citr	Whole blood Hep	Whole blood EDTA	Whole blood Citr	Notes
Amikacin	+	+	+β	(+)β				
Amiodarone	+	+	+					HPLC
Amitriptyline	+	+						HPLC
Ammonia	–↑	(+)↑	*	–	+			add serine (5 mmol/l) and borate (2 mmol/l) for in vitro ammonia production blockage, do not use NH$_4$-heparinate
Amphetamine	+	+	+					
Amylase – total	+	+	+	(+)				
Amylase – pancreatic	+	+	+	(+)				
Androstenedione	+							
Angiotensin converting enzyme (ACE)	+		–	–				
CD34 antigen			+					
Antibodies against Rickettsia	+							
Antibodies against rotaviruses	+							
Anticonvulsants	+							see phenobarbital, phenytoin, valproic acid
Antidiuretic hormone (ADH)			+					Freeze plasma.
Antithrombin III	–			*			+!	! Pharmacia Co. test
Antithrombin III, imunochemically			+δ	(+)δ				
Alpha-1-antitrypsin	+	+γ	+γ					
APC resistance (screening – functional test)				*				in high heparin concentrations add heparin-binding agents
APC resistance (factor V Leiden, genotypization)					*		*	
Apolipoprotein A1	+↑	+γ, δ	*γ, δ	(+)				see NCEP recomm.
Apolipoprotein B	+↑	+γ, δ	*γ, δ	(+)				see NCEP recomm.
Aspartate aminotransferase (AST)	+↑	*	+	(+)				
Aspergillus antigen evidence	+							

Analyte	Serum	Plasma Hep	EDTA	Citr	Whole blood Hep	EDTA	Citr	Notes
Aspergillus spp.					+?			hemoculture
Barbiturates (see also Pheno-barbital)	+	+						
Benzodiazepins	+	+						
Bicarbonate	+	+						see also blood gases
Bilirubin (direct, total)	+	+	+	(+)				
Blood gases (CO$_2$, O$_2$)					*			use titred heparin
CA 125	+	+γ	+γ	(+)γ				
CA 15-3	+	+γ	+βγ	(+)γ				
CA 19-9	+	+γ	+γ	(+)γ				
CA 72-4	+	+γ	+γ	(+)γ				
Cadmium	–		*	–				special tubes
Calcitonin	+	+						stabilized with aprotinine 400 U/ml
Calcium	+	+	–↓	–↓	+			
Calcium – ionized (free)	–	(+)	–	–	+			use calcium titrating heparin
Candida antigen evidence	+							
Candida spp.					+?			hemoculture method dependent
Carbohydrate-deficient transferrin (CDT)	+	+						
Carcinoembryonic antigen (CEA)	+	+βγ	+βγ	+γ				
Carbamazepine	+	+βγδ	+βγ	(+)βγ				
Catecholamines (adrenaline, noradrenaline)	–	*	(+)	–				stabilized with EGTA and/or gluta-thioner 1.2 mg/ml
Ceruloplasmin	+	+	+					
Chloramphenicol	+	+β	+β					
Chlorides	+	+	–	–	+			
Cholesterol	+	+	+	(+)				
HDL-cholesterol	+	+	+δ	–				
LDL-cholesterol	+	–	+	–				
Cholinesterase	+	+	+					
Coagulation factors II – XIII	–	–	–	*				
Cocaine	+	+			+			NaF recommended to stabilize
Complement C3	+	+	+γ	(+)γ				
Complement C4	+	+	+	(+)				
Copper	+	+	–	–				use special pipes

Analyte	Serum	Plasma Hep	Plasma EDTA	Plasma Citr	Whole blood Hep	Whole blood EDTA	Whole blood Citr	Notes
Cortisol	+	+	+γ					
C-peptide	+							
C-reactive protein (CRP)	+	(+)!! +αε	(+)! +αε	(+)				!method dependent !! lower results dependent on patient
Creatinine	+	+	+	(+)				
Creatine kinase	+	+βδ	+βδ	(+)				
Creatine kinase MB, enzymatic	+	+	−↓	(+)δ				
Creatine kinase MB, immuno-analysis	+	+βγ	+βγδ	+γ				
Cryptococcus neoformans					+			hemoculture
Cyclosporine A	−	−	−	−	*	*β		
CYFRA 21-1	+	+γ	+γ	(+)γ				
Cystatine C	+	+						
Cytomegalovirus – DNA amplification	−					*		
Dehydroepiandro-sterone sulfate	+							
Diazepam	+	+	+					
Digitoxin	+	+βγ	+γ					
Digoxin	+	+αβγ	+αβγ	(+)β				
D-dimers	−	+	−	*				
Disopyramide	+	+	+	(+)				
DNA and RNA analysis – after amplification					−	*	+	heparin inhibits Taq-polymerase and restriction enzymes; LiCl 1.8 mol/l eliminates this inhibition
Dopamine			+					
Elastase						+		
Elastase – pancreatic	+							
Erythrocyte sedimentation rate (ESR)							*	1 citrate portion, 4 blood portions
Erythrocyte count					(+)	*	(+)	
Erythropoietin	*	+	+					
C1-esterase inhibitor	+		+ε	(+)				Plasma stabilized by refrigeration.
Estradiol (E2)	+	(+)γ	(+)γ	(+)γ				
Estriol (E3)	(+)	+						
Ethanol	+	*β	+β	(+)βδ		+!		!10 g/l NaF recommended to stabilize
Ethosuximide	+	+	+					

Analyte	Serum	Plasma Hep	EDTA	Citr	Whole blood Hep	EDTA	Citr	Notes
Ferritin	+	+βγδ	(+)!γ	(+)γ				!method dependent
Alpha-1-feto-protein (AFP)	+	+βγ	+βγ	(+)βγ				
Fibrin degra-dation products	(+)!	–	–	(+)!!				! special tube stabilized with 10 U thrombin and 150 U kallikrein/ml blood !!aprotinine or tryp-sin inhibitor from syoabean, special tube
Fibrin monomers	–	–	–	*				
Fibrinogen, imunochemically	–	–	–	*				
Fibrinogen	–	–	–	*				Clauss' method
Fibrinopeptide A	–	–	–	*				
Folic acid	+	+	+β	(+)β	+β			hemolysate, created from 0.5 ml blood + 4.5 ml ascorbic acid (2 g/l). Na-he-parinate interferes with Axsym test (β)
Follicle stimu-lating hormone (FSH)	+	+βγ	+βγ	(+)γ				
Free fatty acids	+	(+)↑!	(+)↓					! lipase activation with heparin
Free triiodothyro-nine (fT3)	+	+βγ	+βγ	(+)γ				method dependent plasma differences
Free thyroxine	+	+βγ	+γ	(+)γ				
Free thyroxine capacity (T4-uptake)	+	+βγ	+βγ	(+)γ				
Galactose-1-P-uridyltransferase						+		RBC (Beutler's test)
Gamma-glutamyl-transferase	+	+	+	(+)				IFCC (Szasz)
Gastrin	+	*!	+	(+)				! add aprotinin (2000 KIU/ml) to stabilize
Gentamicin	+	+βγδ	+βγδ	(+)β				
Glucagon			+					add aprotinine to stabilize
Glucose	–↓	+↓	+↓		(+)			use whole blood with universal gly-colysis inhibitor (manose, fluoride)
Glucose, capillary	–				(+)			
Glutamate dehydrogenase	+	+	+					
Gold	+							

Analyte	Serum	Plasma			Whole blood			Notes
		Hep	EDTA	Citr	Hep	EDTA	Citr	
Hantavirus – DNA-amplification					–	*	+	
Haptoglobin	+	+	+					
HBsAg	+	+δ	+δ	(+)δ				
HbeAg	+	+β	+β	(+)β				
Hematocrit					+	*		
Hemoglobin A$_{1c}$						*		hemolysate
Hemoglobin F (HbF)						+		
Hemoglobin – blood						*		
Hemoglobin – plasma	(+)↑	*	+					hemolysis during coagulation
Hemogram						*		
Heparin (anti Xa)				*				
Heparin-associated thrombocytopenia	+							HIPA-test
Hepatitis B – virus; DNA determination	+		+					
Hepatitis C – viral genome typization (RNA)	+		+					
Hepatitis C – virus; RNA amplification, qualitative, quantitative	+		+					
Hepatitis D – viral RNA amplification	+		+					
Hepatitis D –anti-viral antibodies	+							
Hepatitis E – amplification RNA	+		+					(after stay in Asia)
HHV 6-, 7-, 8- DNA amplification						*		
HIV 1 (provirus) – DNA amplification						*		
HIV 1 – RNA amplification, qualitative, quantitative			+					
HIV-1, 2 antibodies	+	+β	+β	(+)β				MEIA, ELISA, immunoblotting
HLA-B27					*	*		NH_4-heparinate – (blood)
HLA DR – typization					*			
HLA ABC – typization						*		NH_4-heparinate – (blood)

Analyte	Serum	Plasma			Whole blood			Notes
		Hep	EDTA	Citr	Hep	EDTA	Citr	
Homocysteine	+↑	+	+	(+)		*		probe with EDTA/citrate (0.5 mol/l). Store in 0–4 °C. Avoid hemolysis if possible.
HTLV-I antibodies (T-cell leukemia)	+							
HTLV-I (provirus) – DNA amplification						*		
HTLV-I – RNA amplification	+		+					
Human chorio-gonadotropic hormone (beta-hCG)	+	+βγ	+βγ	(+)γ				
Human growth hormone (hGH)	+	+						
Hydroxybutyrate					+			Deproteinized blood
Immuno-complex C (in blood circulation)	+							
Immuno-globulin A	+	+γδ	+γδ					
Immuno-globulin D	*		−↓γ					
Immuno-globulin E	*	αδε	−↓+δ	(+)ε				
antigen specific IgE	+		ε					
Immuno-globulin G	+	+γδ	−↓	−				
IgG subclasses	+							
Immuno-globulin M	+	+γδ	↓γ +δ					
Insulin	(+)↓	+	+					
Iron (Fe)	+	+	−	−↓				
JS viruses – DNA amplification (PML)						*		
Kalium	(+)↑	*	−	−	+			dependent on serum platelet count
Lactate	−↑	−↑	−↑	−	(+)			use tubes with inhibitor (fluoride/oxalate) if deproteinization of whole blood was not performed

Analyte	Serum	Plasma Hep	Plasma EDTA	Plasma Citr	Whole blood Hep	Whole blood EDTA	Whole blood Citr	Notes
Lactate dehydrogenase (LDH)	(+)↑	*	+	(+)				be aware of also on platelets LD activity dependence during separation. Store at about 8 °C.
Lead (Pb)	–	–	+	–	(+)			use special tubes
Leukocyte count					+	*	(+)	
Leukocytes – differentiation						*		K₃ or K₂EDTA, machine dependent
Lidocaine	+	+β	+β					
Light chains kappa, lambda	+	+γ	+γ					
Lipase	+	+	–↓	–				EDTA binds calcium (activator)
Lipoprotein (a)	+	+γ	+γ	–γ				
Lipoproteins – electrophoresis	*	–	–	–				
Lithium	+	+!	–	–				! no Li-heparinate
Lupus inhibitor (lupus anticoagulant)	–	–	–	*				
Luteinizing hormone (LH)	+	+β	+β					
Lymphocytes – subtypes					(+)			special stabilizer recommended (Cyfix II)
Lymphocytic choriomeningitis –viral DNA amplification						*		
Magnesium	+↑	+	–	–↓	*			separate blood cells before analysis
Malaria Plasmodium spp.						*		whole blood microscopic examination
Measles, virus – RNA amplification						*		
Mercury					+			special tubes
Methadone	+	+						
Methotrexate	+							
Microfilariasis					+	+		concentrated sample, microcartridge
Alpha-1-Microglobulin	+							
Beta-2-Microglobulin	+	+γ	+γ	(+)γ				
Mycobacterium spp. DNA amplification						*		(M. tuberculosis and atypic mycobacteria)
Myoglobin	+	+γε	+δε	(+)γε				

Analyte	Serum	Plasma			Whole blood			Notes
		Hep	EDTA	Citr	Hep	EDTA	Citr	
N-acetylpro-cainamide	+	+β	+β	(+)β				
Natrium	+	+	–	–	+!			! use heparin (8–12 IU/ml blood) stabilized with 140 mmol/l Na
Netilmicin	+							
Neuron-specific enolase (NSE)	+↑	*						↑ in thrombocytosis
Nitrazepam	+	+β	+β	(+)β				
Opiates	+	+						
Orosomukoid	+	+γ	+γ	(+)				
Osmolality	+	+						
Osteocalcin			*					use 2500 kU/ml aprotinine to stabilize
Paracetamol	+	+β	+β	(+)β				
Parathyroid hormone (PTH)			*					
Partial thrombo-plastin time	–	–	–	*				
Parvovirus B19, DNA amplification						*		
Phencyclidine	+							
Phenobarbital	+	+βγδ	+βγδ	+βγδ				
Phenytoin	+	+βγδ	+βγδ	(+)βγ				
Phosphate – in-organic	(+)↑	*	+					depends on serum platelet count
Plasma renin activity	–	–	+	–				
Platelets, function							*	special tubes set
Platelet count					(+)↓	*	(+)	heparinized/citrate blood in EDTA-pseudothrombo-cytopenia
Pneumococci								hemoculture
Prealbumin	+		+γ					
Primidone	+	+	+	(+)				
Procainamide	+	+β	+β	(+)β				
Procalcitonin	+	δ						
Progesteron	+	+β	+β					
Prolactin	+	+βδ	+β					
Propafenone	+	+						
Propoxyphene	+	+						
Prostate specific antigen – free (PSA)	+	+γ	+γ					
Prostate specific antigen – total (PSA)	+	+γ	+γ	(+)γ				

Analyte	Serum	Plasma Hep	Plasma EDTA	Plasma Citr	Whole blood Hep	Whole blood EDTA	Whole blood Citr	Notes
Protein C	–	–	–	*				
Protein S	–	–	–	*				
Protein S100	+							
Prothrombin time (fast)	–	–	–	*				
Pyruvic acid	–↓	–↓			+			deproteinized blood
Quinidine	+	+β	+β	(+)β				
Reptilase time				*				
Reticulocytes count					(+)	*		K$_2$ or K$_3$EDTA, method dependent
Rheumatoid factors (RF),	+		+γ	(+)γ				
subfractions IgA, IgG	+							
Rubella – virus; DNA amplification						*		
Salicylate	+	+βδ	+βδ	(+)βδ				
Selen	–	–	–	–			+	special tube set
Serum amyloid A (SAA)	+							
Squamous cell carcinoma antigen (SCCA)	+							
Surface blood cells markers (immuno-cytometry)					+	+		special stabilizer recommended (Cyfix II)
Tacrolimus (FK 506)			–	–	*			
Teophylline	+	+βγ	+βγδ	(+)βγ				
Testosterone	+	+γ	+γ	(+)γ				
Tetrahydrocanabinol acid (THCA)	+	+						
Thrombin – kinetics	–	–	–	*				
Thyroglobulin	+							
Thyrotropic hormone (TSH)	+	+βγ	+βγ	(+)γ				
Thyroxine (T4)	*	+βγ	+βγ	(+)γ				method dependent plasma differences
Thyroxine-binding globulin (TBG)	+	+						
Tobramycin	+	+βδ	+βδ	(+)β				
Total proteins	+↓	*	+δ	(+)				higher in plasma (fibrinogen)
Total serum proteins – electrophoresis	*	(+)						in heparinized plasma processing a fibrinogen must be taken into account, can be abolished

Analyte	Serum	Hep	EDTA	Citr	Hep	EDTA	Citr	Notes
Transferrin	+	+	+γ					
Treponema pallidum – DNA amplification					*			
Triacylglycerols	+	+	*	(+)				
Tricyclic anti-depressants	+	+β	+β	(+)β				
Triiodothyronine (T3)	+	(+)↑βγδ						method dependent plasma differences
Troponin I	+	+	+			+		method dependent
Troponin T	+	+γ	(+)γ					
Trypanosoma gondii						(+)		ideal: blood stain from capillary sampling
Urates	+	+	+↓	(+)				
Urea	+	+	+					NH₄-heparinate cannot be used
Valproate	+	+βγδ	+βγδ	(+)βγ				
Vancomycin	+	+β	+β	(+)β				
Varicella–zoster, viral DNA amplification					*			
Vitamin A (retinol)	+							
Vitamin B₁ (thiamine)		+	+					
Vitamin B₂ (riboflavin)		+	+					
Vitamín B₆ (pyridoxal phosphate)			*					
Vitamin B₁₂ (cobalamin)	+	+β	*β					
Vitamin C (ascorbic acid)		+						stabilization with 60 mg/l m-phosphate
Vitamin D 1,25-dihydroxy-cholecalciferol	+							
25-hydroxy-cholecalciferol	+							
Vitamin E (tocopherol)	+		*					
Zinc	–	+	–	–				special tube set, prevent cork material contamination

Part II

Analyte	Serum	Plasma			Whole blood			Notes
		Hep	EDTA	Citr	Hep	EDTA	Citr	
Antibodies and DNA amplification in HSV 1.2 (and + for serum)								
Antibodies:								
anti-HAV	+	+β	+β	(+)β				
anti-HBsAG	+	+βδ	+βδ	(+)βδ				
anti-HBc	+	+β	+β	+β				
anti-HBe	+	+β	+β	(+)β				
anti-HCV	+	+β	+β	(+)β				
anti-HEV	+							
Antibodies: Pappataci fever	+							
Antibodies: Q-fever	+							
Antibodies against adenoviruses	+							complement fixation test, ELISA, IgG, IgM
Antibodies against Aspergillus spp.	+							
Antibodies against Bartonella spp.	+							(cat cry disease)
Antibodies against Bordetella pertussis	+							
Antibodies against Borrelia burgdorferi	+							ELISA, Western blot
Antibodies against brucellae	+							
Antibodies against Campylobacter jejuni	+							
Antibodies against Candida albicans	+							
Antibodies against Clostridium tetani, toxin	+							
Antibodies against Corynebacterium diphtheriae, toxin	+							
Antibodies against Coxiella burnetii	+							(Q-fever)
Antibodies against Cytomegalovirus	+	+β	+β	(+)β				
Antibodies against Echinococcus spp.	+							
Antibodies against ECHO viruses	+							
Antibodies against Entamoeba histolytica	+							
Antibodies against enteroviruses	+							

Analyte	Serum	Plasma			Whole blood			Notes
		Hep	EDTA	Citr	Hep	EDTA	Citr	
Antibodies against Francisella tularensis	+							
Antibodies against hantaviruses	+							(hemorrhagic fever + renal diseases)
Antibodies against Helicobacter pylori	+							ELISA, virulence factors ↑ immuno-blotting examination (cag A and others)
Antibodies against Herpesvirus 6	+							(HHV 6)
Antibodies against chlamydia (C. trachomatis, C. pneumoniae)	+							
Antibodies against Legionella spp.	+							
Antibodies against Leishmania spp.	+							visceral leishmaniasis
Antibodies against Leptospira spp.	+							
Antibodies against Listeria monocytogenes	+							
Antibodies against Mycoplasma pneumoniae	+							
Antibodies against Neisseria gonorrhoeae	+							
Antibodies against Parvovirus B19 – (Erythema infectiosum)	+							
Antibodies against Plasmodium malariae	+							
Antibodies against polioviruses 1-, 2-, 3-	+							
Antibodies against reoviruses	+							
Antibodies against respiratory syncytial virus (RSV)	+							
Antibodies against Toxoplasma gondii (IgA, IgG, IgM)	+	+β	+β	+β				
Antibodies against Treponema pallidum	+							TPHA, IFT, FTA – abs., VDRL, immunoblotting
Antibodies against thyrotropin receptors	+							
Antibodies against Coxsackie viruses	+							

Analyte	Serum	Plasma			Whole blood			Notes
		Hep	EDTA	Citr	Hep	EDTA	Citr	
Antibodies against JC viruses	+							(progressive multifocal leukoencephalopathy, PML)
Antibodies against encephalitis viruses	+							
Antibodies against Dengue virus	+							
Antibodies against Epstein–Barr virus (anti-EBNA, -VCA, -EA), IgG, IgM, IgA	+							
Antibodies against FSME virus	+							encephalitis viruses
Antibodies against influenza virus A, B, C	+							
Antibodies against parotitis virus	+							
Antibodies against measles virus	+							
Antibodies against measles virus – RNA amplification						*		
Antibodies against rubella virus	+		+β	+β	(+)β			
Antibodies against Varicella–zoster virus	+							
Antibodies against Yersinia enterocolitica	+							
Anticardiolipin antibodies	+							
Anti-DNA antibodies	+							
Antimitochondrial antibodies (AMA)	+							
Antineutrophil cytoplasm antibodies (ANCA)	+							
Antinuclear antibodies (ANA)	+							
Antistaphylococcal antibodies (anti-staphylolysin)	+							
Antistaphylolysin	+		+γ	+γ				
Antistreptococcal antibodies (anti-hyaluronidase)	+							
Antistreptococcal antibodies (anti-DNase B)	+							

Analyte	Serum	Plasma			Whole blood			Notes
		Hep	EDTA	Citr	Hep	EDTA	Citr	
Antistreptococcal antibodies (antistreptolysin O, antistreptokinase)	+							
Antistreptodornase B	+							
Antistreptokinase	+							
Antistreptolysin	+	+βγδ	+βγδ					
Antithrombocytic antibodies				+	+			
Antithyroidal antibodies	+							
Autoantibodies								
Cold autoantibodies						+?		blood incubated in 37 °C, water thermostat
Cytomegalovirus antigen (PP65)						*		
Heterophil antibodies against Epstein–Barr virus	+							
LCM antibodies	+							Lymphocytic choriomeningitis
Listeria monocytogenes –DNA amplification						*		

Notes

*	recommended material
+	can be used without analytic result influence
(+)	restricted use (see notes), in citrate plasma the restriction is needed for citrate solution volume
–	not recommended
↓ ↑	lower (↓) or higher (↑) results can be awaited in comparison to recommended material
NCEP	National cholesterol program (USA)

Company sources

α	Ortho: Vitros
β	Abbott: Axsym
γ	Roche–Boehringer: Elecsys
δ	Beckman: Synchron(s)
ε	Dade-Behring: Nephelometer analyzer

English Synonymous Vocabulary

A

Achalasis
cardiospasm, esophageal aperistalsis, megaesophagus

Acoustic neurinoma
vestibular Schwannoma, acoustic neuroma, 8th nerve tumour

Acute bacterial pyelonephritis
acute infective tubulointerstitial nephritis

Acute epiglottitis
supraglottitis

Acute intermittent porphyria
AIP, Swedish porphyria, pyrroloporphyria

Acute necrotizing ulcerative gingivitis
trench mouth, Vincent's infection, Fusospirochetosis

Acute nephritic syndrome
acute glomerulonephritis, postinfectious glomerulonephritis

Acute stress gastritis
acute erosive gastritis, acute stress erosion, acute gastric ulcer, acute hemorrhagic gastritis

Adams-Stokes syndrome
Adams-Stokes syncope, Stokes-Adams syncope, Morgagni-Adams-Stokes sy

Addisonian syndrome
Addison's disease, primary/chronic adronocortical insufficiency, bronzed disease

Adrenal virilism
adrenogenital sy

Adult respiratory distress syndrome
ARDS, shock lung

Adult rumination
merycism

Alopecia
baldness

Amebiasis
entamebiasis

Amnestic syndrome
amnesic sy, amnestic-confabulatory sy, dysmnesic sy

Anal fissure
fissure in ano, anal ulcer

Angioedema
giant urticaria, angioneurotic edema

Ankylosing spondylitis
Marie-Strümpell disease

Anorectal fistula
fistula in ano

Anthrax
malignant pustule, Woolsorter's disease

Anxiety neurosis
generalized anxiety disorder, anxiety reaction

Aortic arch syndrome
Takayasu's arteritis

Aortic dissection
dissecting aneurysm, dissecting hematoma

Arteriolar nephrosclerosis
intercapillary nephrosclerosis, glomerulosclerosis

Arthrogryposis multiplex congenita
multiple congenital contractures

Atopic dermatitis
infantile eczema, atopic eczema

Atrial septal defect
ostium secundum, sinus venosus

B

Banti's disease
congestive splenomegaly, Klemperer's disease, splenic anemia

Barret's syndrome
Barret's esophagus

Bartter's syndrome
juxtaglomerular cell hyperplasia

Basal cell carcinoma
rodent carcinoma

Basedow's disease
Graves' disease
Beef tapeworm infection
Taenia saginata infection, Taeniasis saginata
Bekhterev's disease
ankylosing spondylitis
Benign giant hypertrophic gastritis
Ménétrier's disease
Benign prostate hyperplasia
benign prostate hypertrophy
Benign nephrosclerosis
hyaline arteriolar nephrosclerosis
Benign paroxysmal positional vertigo
postural/positional vertigo, cupulolithiasis
Bernard-Soulier disease
Bernard-Soulier syndrome, giant platelet disease
Berylliosis
beryllium disease/poisoning/granulomatosis
Besnier-Boeck disease
sarcoidosis
Biliary calculi
gallstones
Blastomycosis
North American blastomcyosis, Gilchrist's disease
Blue disease
Rocky Mountain spotted fever
Bornholm disease
epidemic pleurodynia
Bronzed disease
Addison's disease
Brucellosis
undulant Malta-Mediterranean-Gibraltar fever
Budd-Chiari syndrome
Budd-Chiari disease, Chiari's disease, endophlebitis hepatis obliterans
Buerger's disease
thrombangiitis obliterans
Bulbar syndrome
Dejerine's syndrome

C

Cacchi-Ricci disease
sponge kidney
Callus
tyloma

Calve-Perthes disease
osteochondrosis of the capitular epiphysis of the femur
Candidosis
candidiasis, moniliasis
Caplan's syndrome
rheumatoid pneumoconiosis
Carbohydrate intolerance
lactose intolerance, lactase deficiency, disaccharidase deficiency, glucose-galactose malabsorption, alactasia
Carcinoma of the kidney
hypernephroma
Carotid sinus syndrome
carotid sinus syncope, Charcot-Weiss-Baker syndrome
Cat-scratch disease
benign lymphoreticulosis, cat-scratch fever, regional lymphadenitis
Celiac disease
gluten enteropathy, nontropical sprue, celiac sprue
Cerebrovascular disease
stroke, cerebrovascular accident
Chagas' disease
American trypanosomiasis
Charcot's disease
neuropathic arthropathy
Charcot-Marie-Tooth disease
Charcot-Marie atrophy (syndrome), peroneal muscular atrophy, Marie-Tooth disease, Tooth's disease
Chédiak-Higashi syndrome
Beguez César disease, Chédiak-Higashi anomaly
Chlamydial pneumonia
Taiwan acute respiratory agent pneumonia
Chorionepithelioma
choriocarcinoma
Chromomycetoma
chromoblastoma, verrucous dermatitis
Chronic bacterial pyelonephritis
chronic infective tubulointerstitial nephritis
Chronic fatigue syndrome
Iceland disease, benign myalgic encephalomyelitis, chronic Epstein-Barr virus infection, chronic mononucleosis, epidemic neuromyasthenia
Chronic lymphocytic leukemia
CLL, chronic lymphatic leukemia

Chronic myelocytic leukemia
CML, chronic myeloid leukemia, chronic myelogenous/myelogenic leukemia, chronic granulocytic leukemia

Chronic nephritic/proteinuric syndrome
chronic glomerulonephritis, slowly progressive glomerular disease

Circling disease
Listeriosis

Claude's syndrome
inferior syndrome of red nucleus, rubrospinal cerebellar peduncle sy

Coal workers' pneumoconiosis
coal miners' pneumoconiosis, black lung disease, anthracosis

Coccidioidomycosis
San Joaquin Fever, valley fever, desert rheumatism, California disease

Cold injury
frostnip, frostbite, accidental hypothermia, Trench foot, chilblains, pernio

Colonic inertia
atonic constipation, colon stasis, inactive colon

Common variable immunodeficiency
acquired agammaglobulinemia

Congenital erythropoietic porphyria
CEP, Günther's disease, erythropoietic porphyria, congenital porphyria, congenital hematoporphyria, erythropoietic uroporphyria

Congenital glaucoma
infantile glaucoma, buphthalmos, hydrophthalmus

Cooley's disease
beta-thalassemia

Cori's disease
glycogen storage disease, type III

Corrigan's disease
aortic regurgitation

Creeping eruption
cutaneous larva migrans

Creutzfeldt-Jakob disease
Jakob's disease, subacute spongiform encephalopathy

Cri di chat syndrome
cat's cry syndrome

Crigler-Najjar syndrome
congenital hyperbilirubinemia, congenital nonhemolytic jaundice

Crohn's disease
regional enteritis, regional ileitis, granulomatous ileitis/ileocolitis

Croup
acute laryngotracheobronchitis

Cryptococcosis
Buschke's disease, torulosis, European blastomycosis

Cryptogenic fibrosing alveolitis
fibrosing alveolitis, idiopathic pulmonary fibrosis, diffuse interstitial pulmonary fibrosis

Cushing's disease
Cushing's syndrome, secondary hyperadrenocorticism (pituitary)

Cystic disease of breast
chronic cystic mastitis, fibrocystic disease, fibrocystic disease of breast, Schimmelbusch's disease

Cystic disease of lung
pseudocysts of lung, pulmonary pseudocysts

Cystic fibrosis
mucoviscidosis, fibrocystic disease of the pancreas, pancreatic cystic fibrosis

Cystine disease
cystinosis

D

Decompression sickness
Caisson disease, the bands

Dengue
breakbone fever, Dandy fever

Diabetes insipidus
DI, central diabetes insipidus, vasopressin-sensitive diabetes insipidus

DiGeorge anomaly
DGA, DiGeorge syndrome, thymic hypoplasia, 3rd and 4th pharyngeal pouch sy

Di Guglielmo's disease
erythroleukemia

Discoid lupus erythematosus
DLE, cutaneous lupus erythematosus, chronic DLE

Disseminated intravascular coagulation
consumption coagulopathy, defibrination sy

Döhle disease
syphilitic aortitis

Down syndrome
trisomy G
Dracunculiasis
dracontiasis, fiery serpent, guinea worm disease
Drug dependence
substance use disorders, drug addiction, drug abuse, drug habituation
Drug eruptions
dermatitis medicamentosa
Duhring's disease
dermatitis herpetiformis
Duchenne's disease
spinal muscular dystrophy, bulbar paralysis, tabes dorsalis, Duchenne's muscular dystrophy
Duke's disease
Filatov-Dukes disease, scarlatinella
Dyschezia
disordered evacuation, dysfunction of pelvic floor/anal sphincters

E

Echinococcosis
Echinococcus granulosus infection, hydatid disease
Engel-Recklinghausen disease
osteitis fibrosa cystica
English disease
rickets
Eosinophilic endomyocardial disease
Löffler's endocarditis
Epistaxis
nosebleed
Epstein's disease
pseudodiphtheria
Erb-Goldflam disease
myasthenia gravis
Erythema infectiosum
fifth disease, Parvovirus B19 infection
Erythema multiforme
erythema multiforme exudativum/bullosum
Erythroblastosis fetalis
hemolytic disease of newborn
Erythropoietic protoporphyria
EPP, protoporphyria, erythrohepatic protoporphyria

Esophageal webs
Plummer-Vinson sy, Paterson-Kelly sy, sideropenic dysphagia
Euthyroid goiter
simple goiter, endemic goiter, nontoxic diffuse goiter, nontoxic nodular goiter
Exanthema subitum
roseola infantum
Exogenous/exogenic allergic alveolitis
allergic alveolitis, extrinsic allergic alveolitis, hypersensitivity pneumonitis, allergic pneumonitis
Exophthalmos
proptosis

F

Fabry's disease
angiokeratoma corporis diffusum, diffuse angiokeratoma
Fahr-Volhard disease
malignant nephrosclerosis
Familial Mediterranean fever
familial paroxysmal peritonitis
Farber's disease
Farber's lipogranulomatosis, ceramidase deficiency
Fibromyalgia
myofascial pain sy, fibromyositis
Fiedler's disease
Weil's syndrome
Fifth disease
erythema infectiosum
Filatov's disease
infectious mononucleosis
Fish tapeworm infection
diphyllobothriasis
Focal scratch dermatitis
lichen simplex, neurodermatitis
Fölling disease
phenylketonuria
Forbes'disease
glycogen storage disease, type III
Fourth disease
Dukes'disease
Fourth venereal disease
specific gangrenous and ulcerative balanoposthitis, granuloma inguinale
Francis'disease
tularemia

Frei's disease
  lymphogranuloma venereum
Friedländer's disease
  endarteritis obliterans
Friedreich's disease
  paramyoclonus multiplex
Frommel's disease
  Chiari-Frommel syndrome
Functional cardiovascular disease
  neurocirculatory asthenia

G

Gas embolism
  air embolism
Genital warts
  condylomata acuminata, moist/venereal
  warts
Gerhardt's disease
  erythromelalgia
German measles
  rubella, three day measles
Giant cell arteritis
  temporal arteritis, cranial arteritis
Giant platelet disease
  Bernard-Soulier disease
Globus sensation
  lump in the throat, globus hystericus
Glycogen storage disease
  glycogenosis
Goldstein's disease
  hereditary hemorrhagic teleangiectasia
Gonadal dysgenesis
  Turner's sy, Bonnevie-Ullrich sy
Graft-versus-host disease
  GVH, graft-versus-host reaction
Graves's disease
  cachexia exophthalmica, diffuse toxic
  goiter, exophthalmic goiter, Flajani's dis-
  ease, tachycardia strumosa exophthal-
  mica
Guillain-Barré syndrome
  GBS, acute polyneuropathy, acute poly-
  radiculitis, infectious acute idiopathic
  polyneuropathy, Landry's ascending
  paralysis, acute segmentally demyelinating polyradiculoneuropathy
Guinea worm disease
  dracunculiasis
Gumboro disease
  infectious bursal disease

Günther's disease
  congenital erythropoietic porphyria

H

Hagner's disease
  hypertrophic pulmonary osteoarthropathy
Hamman's disease
  pneumomediastinum
Hammond's disease
  athetosis
Hand-Schüller-Christian disease
  chronic idiopathic xanthomatosis,
  cholesterol thesaurismosis
Hansen's disease
  leprosy
Hashimoto's disease
  autoimmune thyroiditis, Hashimoto's
  thyroiditis/struma, struma lymphoma-
  tosa, chronic lymphocytic thyroiditis
Hay fever
  allergic rhinitis, pollinosis
Headache
  cephalalgia
Heat stroke
  sunstroke, hyperpyrexia, thermic fever,
  siriasis
Heine-Medin disease
  poliomyelitis
Hemochromatosis
  iron storage disease, iron overload,
  hemosiderosis
Hemolytic disease of the newborn
  erythroblastosis fetalis
Hemorrhagic fever with renal syndrome
  Korean hemorrhagic fever, epidemic
  nephrosonephritis, nephropathia epidemica
Hemorrhagic shock and encephalopathy
  Newcastle sy
Hemorrhoids
  piles
Henoch-Schönlein purpura
  Henoch-Schönlein vasculitis, anaphylac-
  toid purpura, allergic purpura
Hepatolenticular disease
  Wilson's disease, hepatolenticular dege-
  neration
Hepatorenal glycogen storage disease
  glycogen storage disease, type I

Hereditary hemorrhagic teleangiectasia
Rendu-Osler-Weber disease
Hereditary nephritis
Alport's syndrome
Herniated nucleus pulposus
herniated/ruptured/prolapsed intervertebral disk, disk sy
Herpes zoster
shingles, zona, acute posterior ganglionitis
Herpes zoster oticus
Ramsay Hunt's sy, viral neuronitis and ganglionitis, geniculate herpes
Hers' disease
glycogen storage disease, type I
Hiccup
hiccough, singultus
Hirschsprung's disease
congenital megacolon
Histiocytosis X
Letterer-Siwe disease, Hand-Schüller-Christian disease, eosinophilic granuloma
Hodgkin's disease
Reed-Hodgkin disease, Hodgkin's lymphoma
Hookworm disease
ancylostomiasis
Hordeolum
stye
Human Immunodeficiency Virus Infection
HIV infection, acquired immunodeficiency syndrome, AIDS
Hyaline membrane disease
HMD, Respiratory Distress Syndrome, RDS
Hydaticmole, Hydatidiform mole
cystic mole, vesicular mole
Hyper-IgE syndrome
Job-Buckley sy
Hypernephroma
renal cell carcinoma
Hyperlipoproteinemia I
exogenous hypertriglyceridemia, familial fat-induced lipemia, hyperchylomicronemia
Hypersensitivity pneumonitis
extrinsic allergic alveolitis, diffuse hypersensitivity pneumonia, allergic interstitial pneumonitis, organic dust pneumoconiosis

Hypertrichosis
hirsutism
Hypochondriacal neurosis
hypochondriasis, atypical somatoform disorder
Hypophosphatemic rickets
vitamin D-resistant rickets
Hypopituitarism in children
pituitary dwarfism
Hypothyroidism
myxedema
Hysterical neurosis
conversion reaction, conversion disorder, dissociative reaction/disorder

I

Ichtyosis
dry skin, xeroderma
Icterus
jaundice
Idiopathic hypereosinophilic syndrome
disseminated eosinophilic collagen disease, eosinophlic leukemia, Löffler's fibroplastic endocarditis with eosinophilia
Idiopathic primary renal hematuric proteinuric syndrome
IgA nephropathy, Berger's disease
Immunodeficiency disease
immunodeficiency disorder, immunodeficiency syndrome
Immunologically mediated renal diseases
immune renal diseases
Inclusion conjunctivits
inclusion blenorrhea, swimming pool conjunctivitis
Infectious gastroenteritis of uncertain etiology
traveler's diarrhea, intestinal flu
Infectious mononucleosis
glandular fever
Influenza
grippe, grip, flu
Inhibited orgasm
retarded ejaculation
Intestinal lymphangiectasia
idiopathic hypoproteinemia
Iron-deficiency anemia
anemia of chronic blood loss, hypochromic-microcytic anemia, chlorosis,

hypochromic anemia of pregnancy/infancy and childhood
Iron-transport-deficiency anemia
atransferrinemia
Iron-reutilization anemia
anemia of chronic disease
Iron-utilization anemia
sideroblastic anemia
Iron storage disease
hemochromatosis
Irritable bowel syndrome
spastic colon, mucous colitis

K

Kala-azar
visceral leishmaniasis, dumdum fever
Kaposi's sarcoma
multiple idiopathic hemorrhagic sarcoma
Kawasaki disease/syndrome
mucocutaneous lymph node syndrome, infantile polyarteritis
Keratinous cyst
wen, sebaceous cyst, steatoma
Keratomalacia
xerotic keratitis, xerophthalmia
Keratoconjunctivitis sicca
keratitis sicca, dry eyes
Kinky hair disease
Menkes' syndrome
Kussmaul's disease
polyarteritis nodosa

L

Laughing disease
kuru
Lead poisoning
plumbism
Legionellosis
legionnaires' disease, pontiac fever
Leigh disease
subacute necrotizing encephalomyelopathy
Leprosy
Hansen's disease
Leptospirosis
Weil's disease/syndrome, infectious jaundice, canicola fever

Letterer-Siwe disease
acute disseminated histiocytosis x
Lipedema
painful fat syndrome
Lipid storage disorder
lipidosis
Lobstein disease
osteogenesis imperfecta
Lunger disease
pulmonary adenomatosis, atypical interstitial pneumonia
Lyme disease
Lyme borreliosis
Lymphogranuloma venereum
lymphogranuloma inguinale, lymphopathia venereum

M

Macroglobulinemia
primary macroglobulinemia, Waldenström's macroglobulinemia
Maduromycosis
Madura foot, mycetoma
Malignant nephrosclerosis
hyperplastic arteriolar nephrosclerosis, Fahr-Volhard disease, malignant nephroangiosclerosis
Maple syrup urine disease
MSUD, branched-chain ketoaciduria
Marasmus
infantile atrophy, inanition, athrepsia
Marchiafava-Micheli disease
paroxysmal nocturnal hemoglobinuria
Marie-Bamberger disease
hypertrophic pulmonary osteoarthropathy
Marie-Strümpell disease
ankylosing spondylitis
McArdle's disease
glycogen storage disease, type V
Measles
morbilli, rubeola, nine-day measles
Ménétrier's disease
giant hypertrophic gastritis
Meniere's disease
recurrent aural vertigo
Mental retardation
mental handicap, mental subnormality

Meyer-Betz disease
idiopathic myoglobinuria, familial myoglobinuria
Miller's disease
osteomalacia
Milroy's disease
Meige's disease, congenital lymphedema
Minimal change disease
foot process disease, minimal change
glomerulopathy, lipid nephrosis, lipoid
nephrosis
Mitchell's disease
erythromelalgia
Möbius' disease
ophthalmoplegic migraine
Mood disorders
affective disorders
Morbilli
measles, rubeola
Moschcowitz' disease
thrombotic thrombocytopenic purpura
Mucha's disease
acute lichenoid pityriasis
Multiple endocrine neoplasia
multiple adenomatosis, familial endocrine adenomatosis, type I (Werner's sy),
type II (Sipple's syndrome), type III
(mucosal neuroma syndrome)
Multiple myeloma
plasma cell myeloma, myelomatosis
Multiple sclerosis
disseminated sclerosis
Mumps
epidemic parotitis
Murine/endemic typhus
rat-flea typhus, urban fever of Malaya
Myasthenia gravis
myasthenia gravis pseudoparalytica,
Erb-Goldflam disease, Goldflam's disease, Goldflam-Erb disease
Mycoplasmal pneumonia
primary atypic pneumonia, Eaton agent
pneumonia
Myelodysplastic syndrome
preleukemia, refractory anemia, Ph-chro-
mosome-negative chronic myelocytic
leukemia, chronic myelomonocytic leukemia, agnogenic myeloid metaplasia
Myelofibrosis
myelosclerosis, agnogenic myeloid
metaplasia

N

Nail-patella syndrome
osteoonychodysplasia, arthroonychodys-
plasia, onychoosteodysplasia
Nanism
dwarfism
Neonatal conjunctivits
conjunctivitis neonatorum, ophthalmia
neonatorum
Neonatal sepsis
sepsis neonatorum
Neurogenic arthropathy
neuropathic arthropathy, Charcot's joints
Niacin deficiency
pellagra
Niemann's disease
Niemann-Pick disease, sphingolipidosis,
sphingomyelin lipidosis, sphingomyelinase deficiency

O

Obsessive-compulsive neurosis
obsessive-compulsive disorder, obsessio-
nal neurosis
Oid-oid disease
exudative discoid + lichenoid dermatitis
Onchocerciasis
river blindness
Orchidectomy
orchiectomy
Osgood-Schlatter disease
apophysitis tibialis adolescentium,
Schlatter's disease
Osler's disease
polycythemia vera, hereditary
hemorrhagic teleangiectasia, Osler-
Vaquez disease
Osler-Weber-Rendu disease
hereditary hemorrhagic teleangiectasia
Osteoarthritis
OA, degenerative joint disease, DJD,
osteoarthrosis, hypertrophic osteoarthritis
Osteodystrophia cystica
osteitis fibrosa cystica
Osteodystrophia fibrosa
osteitis fibrosa cystica
Osteodystrophy
osteodystrophia

P

Paget's disease of bone
osteitis deformans
Papilledema
choked disk
Papillitis
optic neuritis
Paracoccidioidomycosis
South American blastomycosis
Parkinson's disease
paralysis agitans, shaking palsy
Parrot disease
psittacosis
Partial trisomy 22
the cat-eye sy
Periapical abscess
dentoalveolar abscess
Peripheral atherosclerotic disease
arteriosclerosis obliterans
Peripheral ulcerative keratitis
marginal keratolysis, peripheral rheuma-
toid ulceration
Pernicious anemia
anemia due to vitamin B_{12}deficiency
Peroneal muscular atrophy
hypertrophic interstitial neuropathy,
Charcot-Marie-Tooth disease, Dejerine-
Sottas disease
Persistent pulmonary hypertension
persistent fetal circulation
Pertussis
whooping cough
Pfeiffer's disease
infectious mononucleosis, glandular
fever
Phenylketonuria
PKU, phenylalaninemia, phenylpyruvic
oligophrenia
Phobic neurosis
phobic disorders, phobic reactions
Phycomycosis
mucormycosis zygomaticus
Pinworm infestation
enterobiasis, oxyuriasis
Pituitary nanism
hypophysial infantilism
Plummer's disease
toxic nodular goiter

Poliomyelitis
infantile paralysis, acute anterior poliomyelitis
Polyarteritis nodosa
periarteritis nodosa
Polycystic disease of the kidneys
polycystic kidneys, polycystic renal
disease
Polycystic ovary disease
Stein-Leventhal syndrome
Polycythemia vera
erythremia, erythrocytemia, polycythemia rubra, splenomegalic polycythemia,
myelopathic polycythemia, erythrocytosis megalosplenica, Osler's disease,
Vaquez's disease, Vaquez-Osler disease,
primary polycythemia
Pompe's disease
glycogen storage disease, type II
Pork tapeworm infection
Taenia solium infection, cysticercosis
Porphyria cutanea tarda
PCT, symptomatic porphyria, porphyria
cutanea symptomatica, idiosyncratic
porphyria
Portal-systemic encephalopathy
hepatic encephalopathy, hepatic coma
Posadas-Wernicke disease
coccidioidomycosis
Premature ovarian failure
premature menopause
Premenstrual syndrome
premenstrual tension
Pressure sores
bedsore, decubitus ulcer, trophic ulcer
Primary dysmenorrhea
functional dysmenorrhea
Primary thrombocythemia
essential thrombocythemia
Progressive supranuclear palsy
Steele-Richardson-Olszewski syndrome
Progressive systemic sclerosis
scleroderma
Protein malnutrition
protein-calorie malnutrition, PMC, kwashiorkor, protein-energy malnutrition
Pruritus
itching
Pseudogout
calcium pyrophosphate dihydrate crystal
deposition

Pseudotumor cerebri
benign intracranial hypertension
Psittacosis
ornithosis, parrot fever
Pulmonary air-block syndrome
pulmonary interstitial emphysema,
pneumomediastinum, pneumothorax,
pneumopericardium
Pulmonary embolism
pulmonary thromboembolism
Pulseless disease
Takayasu's arteritis
Purpura simplex
easy bruising
Pyogenic granuloma
granuloma teleangiectaticum

Q

Quincke's disease
angioedema

R

Rabies
hydrophobia
Rapidly progressive nephritic syndrome
rapidly progressive glomerulonephritis,
crescentic glomerulonephritis
Recklinghausen's disease
neurofibromatosis
Recklinghausen's disease of bone
osteitis fibrosa cystica
Regional enteritis
Crohn's disease
Relapsing
tick-recurrent-favine fever
Remnant removal disease
familial dysbetalipoproteinemia
Renal glucosuria
renal glycosuria
Renal nanism
infantile renal osteodystrophy
Respiratory distress syndrome
hyaline membrane disease
Retinopathy of prematurity
retrolental fibroplasia
Riboflavin deficiency
ariboflavinosis

Rice disease
beriberi
Rickettsial pox
vesicular ricketsiosis
Rocky Mountain spotted fever
spotted fever, tick fever, tick typhus
Roseola infantum
exanthema subitum, pseudorubella
Rubella
German measles, three-day measles,
rubeola in French and Spanish
Rubeola
measles, morbilli

S

Salivary gland disease
cytomegalic inclusion disease
Sander's disease
epidemic keratoconjunctivitis
Sandhoff's disease
gangliosidosis, type GM2
Scabies
itch
Schaumann's disease
sarcoidosis
Schistosomiasis
bilharziasis
Scrub typhus
Tsutsugamushi disease, mite-borne
typhus, tropical typhus
Seborrheic keratoses
seborrheic warts
Secondary dysmenorrhea
acquired dysmenorrhea
Secondary polycythemia
secondary erythrocytosis
Secretory otitis media
serous otitis media
Senile nanism
progeria
Sexual arousal disorder
erectile dysfunction, impotence
Shigellosis
bacillary dysentery
Sickle cell disease
HbS disease, drepanocytic anemia,
meniscocytosis
Small-for-gestational-age infant
dysmaturity, intrauterine growth
retardation

Smallpox
variola
Spontaneous abortion
miscarriage
Staphylococcal scalded skin syndrome
Ritter-Lyell sy
Still's disease
juvenile rheumatoid disease
Strabismus
squint, cross-eyes, heterotropia
Strongyloidiasis
threadworm infection
Subacute sclerosing panencephalitis
SSPE, Dawson encephalitis
Subacute thyroiditis
granulomatous thyroiditis, giant cell/de
Quervain's thyroiditis
Sydenham's chorea
chorea minor, rheumatic chorea, St.
Vitus' dance
Syncope
fainting
Syphilis
lues
Systemic fungal disease
systemic mycosis
Systemic lupus erythematosus
SLE, disseminated lupus erythematosus

T

Takayasu arteritis
pulseless disease, arteritis brachiocepha-
lica, brachiocephalic ischemia, Marto-
rell's sy, reversed coarctation, Takayasu's
disease/sy, aortic arch arteritis/syn-
drome, young oriental female arteritis,
occlusive thromboarthropathy
Temporal arteritis
giant cell arteritis, cranial arteritis,
Horton's arteritis
Tetanus
lockjaw
Tetany of vitamin D deficiency
infantile tetany
The eosinophilic pneumonia
pulmonary infiltrate with eosinophilic
sy, Löffler's sy
The common cold
acute coryza, upper respiratory infection

Thiamine deficiency
beriberi
Thyrocardiac disease
thyrotoxic heart disease
Toxocariasis
visceral larva migrans
Trachoma
granular conjunctivits, Egyptian ophthalmia
Transient tachypnea of the newborn
neonatal wet lung syndrome
Traumatic hemolytic anemia
microangiopathic hemolytic anemia
Trench fever
Wolhynia fever, shin bone fever, quintan
fever
Trichinosis
trichiniasis
Trichuriasis
whipworm infection, trichocephaliasis
Trigeminal neuralgia
tic douloureux
21-Trisomy
Down syndrome, mongolism
Trypanosomiasis
African sleeping sickness, Chagas'
disease
Tularemia
rabbit-deer fly fever
Tunnel disease
decompression sickness
Typhoid Fever
enteric fever, abdominal typhus, Salmonella typhi fever
Typhus Fever
epidemic/exanthematic/exanthematous
typhus, Ricketsia prowazekiityphus,
European/classic/louse-borne typhus,
jail/prison/ship/war fever
Tyrosinemia
tyrosinosis, hereditary tyrosinemia,
hepatorenal tyrosinemia

U

Uremic bone disease
renal osteodystrophy
Urinary calculi
nephrolithiasis, urolithiasis
Urticaria
angioedema, hives

V

Vacuolar nephrosis
hydropic nephrosis, hypokalemic nephrosis, osmotic nephrosis
Varicella
chickenpox
Variegate porphyria
porphyria variegata, protoporphyria, South African genetic porphyria, Royal Malady variegate porphyria
Venous thrombosis
thrombophlebitis, phlebitis
Vertigo
dizziness
VIPoma
diarrheogenic tumor, Verner-Morrison sy, WDHA, WDHH (watery diarrhea, hypokalemia, a/hypo/chlorhydria), pancreatic cholera
Vitamin A deficiency
night blindness, xerophthalmia, keratomalacia, retinol deficiency
Vitamin B$_1$ deficiency
thiamine deficiency, beriberi
Vitamin C deficiency
scurvy
Vitamin D deficiency
rickets
von Gierke's disease
glycogen storage disease, type I
von Recklinghausen's disease
neurofibromatosis
von Willebrand's disease
angiohemophilia, vascular hemophilia

W

Wards
verrucae
Wegener's granulomatosis
lethal midline granuloma
Werlhof's disease
idiopathic thrombocytopenic purpura
Werner-Schultz disease
agranulocytosis
Whipple's disease
intestinal lipodystrophy
Wilms' tumor
nephroblastoma

Wilson's disease
hepatolenticular degeneration, familial hepatitis, pseudosclerosis
Winiwarter-Buerger disease
thrombangitis obliterans
Wiskott-Aldrich syndrome
Aldrich's sy

X

X-linked agammaglobulinemia
Bruton's a., congenital a.

Z

Zollinger-Ellison syndrome
gastrinoma

Literature Used

Abbas AK, Lichtman AH, Pober JS (2000) Cellular and Molecular Immunology. 4th edn. WB Saunders Co. – A Harcourt Health Sciences Company, Philadelphia

Abeloff MD, Marshall EK, Armitage JO, Lichter AS, Niederhuber JE (1999) Clinical Oncology. Churchill-Livingstone, New York

Adams RD, Victor M, Ropper AH (1997) Principles of Neurology. 6th edn. McGraw-Hill, New York

Albert RK, Spiro SG, Jett JR (1999) Comprehensive Respiratory Medicine. Mosby-Wolfe, London

Americal Hospital Formulary Service. Drug information (1997) American Society of Health System Pharmacists, Bethesda

Andreani D, Lefebvre PJ, Marks V, Tamburrano G (1992) Recent Advances on Hypoglycemia. Raven Press, New York

Andreoli TE, Bennett JC, Carpenter ChJ, Plum F (1997) Cecil's Essentials of Medicine. 4th edn. WB Saunders, Philadelphia

Armstrong D, Cohen J (1999) Infectious Diseases. vol. I, II. Mosby-Wolfe, London

Bacon BR, Di Bisceglie AM (1999) Liver Disease. Diagnosis and Management. Churchill Livingstone, New York

Bakerman S (1994) Bakerman's ABC's of Interpretive Laboratory Data. 3rd edn. Interpretive Laboratory Data Inc, Myrtle Beach

Balint G, Földes K, Szebenyi B, Balint P (1997) Prakticka reumatologia (Practical Rheumatology). Osveta, Martin

Ballinger A, Patchett S (1999) Saunder's Pocket Essentials of Clinical Medicine. 2nd edn. WB Saunders, Philadelphia

Bannister B, Begg N, Gillespie S (2000) Infectious Disease. 2nd edn. Blackwell Science, Oxford

Barker LR, Burton JR, Zieve PD (1995) Principles of Ambulatory Medicine. 4th edn. Williams–Wilkins, Baltimore

Barkin RM (1997) Pediatric Emergency Medicine. 2nd edn. Mosby, St. Louis

Bast RC, Kufe DW, Pollock RE, et al. (2000) Cancer Medicine. 5th edn. BC Decker, Hamilton

Becker D (1987) Vademecum Labordiagnostik. VEB Verlag Volk und Gesundheit, Berlin

Becker KL, Bilezikian JP, Bremner WJ, et al. (2000) Principles and Practice of Endocrinology and Metabolism. 3rd edn. Lippincott Williams and Wilkins, Philadelphia

Bednar M, Frankova V, Schindler J, Soucek A, Vavra J (1996) Lekarska mikrobiologie (Medical Microbiology). Marvil, Prague

Behrman RE, Kliegman RM (1998) Nelson Essentials of Pediatrics. 3rd edn. WB Saunders, Philadelphia

Behrman RE, Kliegman RM, Jenson HB (1999) Nelson Textbook of Pediatrics. 16th edn. WB Saunders Co., Philadelphia

Berg DD (1998) Primary Care Medicine. 2nd edn. Lippincott–Raven, Philadelphia

Berkowitz CD (1996) Pediatrics. WB Saunders, Philadelphia

Berzinec P, Plutinsky J, Zrubcova O, Vondrak V, Letkovicova H (1994) Carcinoembryonic antigen (CEA) levels in pleural effusion and serum in differentiation of malignant and benign pleural effusion. Radiol Oncol 28:316-319

Besa EC, Catalano PM, Kant JA, Jefferies LC (1992) Hematology. The National Medical Series for Independent Study. Harwal Publishing, Malvern

Bezkorovainy A, Rafelson ME (1996) Concise Biochemistry. Marcel Dekker Inc, New York

Bishop ML, Duben–Engelkirk JL, Fody EP (1999) Clinical Chemistry. 4th edn. Lippincott Williams & Wilkins, Philadelphia

Blann AD, Dobrotova M, Kubisz P, McCollum CN (1995) Von Willebrand factor, soluble P-selectin, tissue plasminogen activator and plasminogen activator inhibitor in atherosclerosis. Thrombosis and Hemostasis 74,2:623–630

Blann AD, Lanza F, Galajda P, Guerney D, Moog S, Cazenave JP, Lip GYH (2001) Increased platelet glycoprotein V levels in patients with coronary and peripheral atherosclerosis. The influence of aspirin and cigarette smoking. Thromb Haemost 86:777–783

Bone RC, Rosenn RL (1994) Quick Reference to Internal Medicine. Igaku–Shoin, New York

Borgsdorf LR, Tatro DS (2000) A to Z Drug Facts. 2nd edn. Lippincott Williams & Wilkins, Philadelphia

Bosmansky K, Pullmann R, Hybenova J, Skerenova M, Melus V, Pullman R Jr (2000) Frequency of genetic polymorphisms of apolipoprotein E, apolipoprotein B, apolipoprotein AI, angiotensin-converting enzyme in primary gout. Ann Rheum Dis 59:64

Bouchier IA, Ellis H, Flemin PR (1996) French's Index of Differential Diagnosis. 13th edn. Butterworth–Heinemann, Oxford

Bradley WG, Daroff RB, Fenichel GM, Marsden CD (1996) Neurology in Clinical Practice. 2nd edn. Butterworth–Heinemann, Boston

Braunwald E, Zipes DP, Lippy B (2001) Heart Disease. 6th edn. WB Saunders, Philadelphia

Braverman LE, Utiger RD (2000) Werner-Ingbars' – The Thyroid. 8th edn. Lippincott Williams & Wilkins, Philadelphia

Brenner GM (2000) Pharmacology. WB Saunders, Philadelphia

Brewis RAL, Corrin B, Geddes DM, Gibson GJ (1998) Respiratory Medicine. WB Saunders, London

Briggs GG, Freeman RK, Yaffe SJ (1998) Drugs in pregnancy and lactation. Williams and Wilkins, Baltimore

Buc M, Ferencik M (1994) Imunogenetika (Immunogenetics). Alfa plus, Bratislava

Buc M (2001) Imunologia (Immunology). Veda, Bratislava

Buchancova J (1993) Profesionalne otravy (Professional Intoxication) In: Kvetensky J, ed. Vybrane kapitoly z vnutorneho lekarstva (Internal Medicine Chapters). Comenius University Press, Bratislava

Buchancova J, Knizkova M, Vrlik M, Mesko D (1992) Sucasny pohlad na biochemicke ucinky a kinetiku chromu v organizme a na hodnoty chromu v biologickom materiali neexponovanych dospelych (AAS metody) (Biochemical effects and kinetics of chromium in human body and chromium levels in unexposed adults). Pracov Lek 44,4:165–169

Buchancova J, Vrlik M, Knizkova M, Mesko D, Holko L (1993) Obsah vybranych prvkov (Fe, As, Cd, Pb, Zn, Mn) v biologickom materiali u pracovnikov vyroby ferochromovych zliatin (Content of elements in biological material in ferrochromium-alloy workers). Bratisl lek Listy 94:373–386

Buchancova J, Knizkova D, Hyllova D, Vrlik M, Mesko D, Klimentova G, Galikova E (1994) Obsah vybranych prvkov v krvi, moci a vo vlasoch u darcov krvi bez profesionalnej expozicie kovom (Blood, urine and hair metal concentrations in unexposed blood donors). Central European Journal of Public Health 2:82–87

Buchancova J, Knizkova M, Hyllova D, Fabianova E, Musak L, Mesko D, Drga J, Hazlingerova M, Horvathova E, Vrlik M, Klimentova G, Galikova E, Papayova A (1994) Expozicia chromu vo vztahu ku vybranym imunologickym a cytogenetickym parametrom u hutnikov pri vyrobe ferochromovych zliatin (Chromium exposure in relation to some immunological and cytogenetical parameters in ferrochromium-alloy workers). Pracov Lek 46:167–175

Buchancova J, Knizkova M, Hyllova D, Mesko D, Kubisz P, Klimentova G, Galikova E, Zigova A, Karaffova A (1995) Hodnoty kovov v krvi, v moci a vo vlasoch u muzov z okresov Martin, Orava a Prievidza

(Blood, urine and hair metal concentrations in men from district Martin, Orava and Prievidza). Slov Lekar 5,8:9-13

Buchancova J, Klimentova G, Knizkova M, Hyllova D, Mesko D, Musak L, Zigova A, Tomikova K, Luptakova M, Galikova E, Kubisz P, Hazlingerova M, Cap J, Sevcovicova D (1995) Prierez imunologickymi hodnotami a cytogeneticke vysetrenia u hutnikov pri vyrobe oceloliatiny a sivej liatiny po dlhorocnej pracovnej expozicii (Immunological parameters and cytological examination in ferro-alloy workers after long-term professional exposure). Pracov Lek 47:153-160

Buchancova J, Vrlik M, Galikova E, Musak L (1992) Sucasny pohlad na toxicitu chromu u cloveka a posudzovanie neskorych ucinkov vo vztahu k expozicii chromu (Chromium toxicity in man and evaluation of late effects in chromium exposure). Pracov Lek 44,5:190–193

Buchancova J, Klimentova G, Knizkova M, Mesko D, Galikova E, Kubik J, Fabianova E, Jakubis M (1998) Health status of workers of thermal power station exposed for prolonged periods to arsenic and other elements from fuel. Centr eur J publ Hlth 6,1:29–36.

Buchanec J, et al. (1994) Repetitorium pediatra (Vademecum of Pediatrics). Osveta, Martin

Buchanec J, et al. (2001) Vademekum pediatra (Vademecum of Pediatrician). Osveta, Martin

Burnett AF, Songster GS (2000) Clinical Obstetrics and Gynecology. Blackwell Science, Oxford

Burtis CA, Ashwood ER (2001) Tietz Fundamentals of Clinical Chemistry. 5th edn. WB Saunders Co, Philadelphia

Cahill M, Foley M, et al. (1995) Professional Handbook of Diagnostic Tests. Springhouse Corp, Springhouse

Cameron P, Jelinek G, Kelly AM (2000) Textbook of Adult Emergency Medicine. Churchill-Livingstone, New York

Campbell AG, McIntosh A (1998) Forfar and Armeils's Textbook of Pediatrics. 5th edn. Churchill-Livingstone, New York

Cantor T (2001) CAP and the CAP/CIP Ratio: The 3rd Generation of PTH Assays for the Prediction of Parathyroid Function and Bone Status. Revised 3rd Generation book. SCANTIBODIES Clinical Laboratory, Inc., Santee

Carey ChF, Lee HH, Woeltje KF (1998) The Washington Manual of Medical Therapeutics. 29th edn. Lippincott–Raven, Philadelphia

Carpenter DO, ed. (1998) Professional Guide to Diseases. Springhouse Corp, Springhouse

Cavanaugh BM (1999) Nurse's Manual of Laboratory and Diagnostic Test Handbook. 3rd edn. F. A. Davis Co, Philadelphia

Champe PC, Harvey RA (1994) Biochemistry. 2nd edn. JB Lippincott, Philadelphia

Chernecky CC, Berger BJ (2001) Laboratory Tests and Diagnostic Procedures. 3rd edn. WB Saunders, Philadelphia

Civetta JM, Taylor RW, Kirby RR (1997) Critical Care. 3rd edn. Lippincott–Raven, Philadelphia

Clinical Laboratory Tests: Values and Implications (2001) 3rd edn. Lippincott Williams & Wilkins, Philadelphia

Cohn RM, Roth KS (1996) Biochemistry and Disease. Williams–Wilkins, Baltimore

Collier JAB, Longmore JM, Hodgetts TJ (1995) Oxford Handbook of Clinical Specialties. 4th edn. Oxford University Press, Oxford

Collins RD (1993) Diferencialni diagnostika prvniho kontaktu (Differential Diagnosis in Primary Care). Grada Avicenum, Prague

Collins RD (1998) Algorithmic Selection and Interpretation of Diagnostic Tests. Lippincott Williams & Wilkins, Philadelphia

Committee on Drugs. American Academy of Pedatrics (1994) The transfer of drugs and other chemicals into human milk. Pediatrics 93:137-150.

Concise Medical Dictionary. Oxford Reference (1992) 3rd edn. Oxford University Press, Oxford

Corbett J V (2000) Laboratory Tests and Diagnostic Procedures with Nursing Diagnoses. 5th edn. Prentice-Hall International, New Jersey

Corrin B (1997) Pathology of Lung Tumors. Churchill-Livingstone, New York

Cowan DF, Olano JP (1997) A Practical Guide to Clinical Laboratory Testing. Blackwell Science, Malden

Dambro MR (2001) Griffith's 5-minute Clinical Consult. 9th edn. Lippincott Williams & Wilkins, Philadelphia

Dart RC, Hurlbut KM, Kuffner EK, Yip L (2000) The 5-minute Toxicology. Lippincott Williams & Wilkins, Philadelphia

Davis NM (1997) Medical abbreviations: 12 000 conveniences at the expense of communications and safety. 8th edn. M Davis Associates, Neil Huntington Valley

Dawson DM, Sabin TD (1993) Chronic fatigue syndrome. Little, Brown and Co, Boston

DeGowin RL (2000) Diagnostic Examination. 7th edn. McGraw Hill, New York

DeVita VT, Hellman S, Rosenberg SA (2000) Cancer. Lippincott Williams & Wilkins, Philadelphia

Devlin TM (1997) Textbook of Biochemistry with Clinical Correlations. John Wiley and Sons, New York

Dienstbier Z, Skala E (1995) Nadorova diagnostika pro lekare v praxi (Tumour Diagnostics for Practice). Avicenum–Grada, Prague

Dieska D, et al (1995) Vademecum medici. Osveta, Martin

Dirix A, Knuttgen HG, Tittel K (1988) The Olympic Book of Sports Medicine. Vol. 1. Blackwell Scientific Publications, Oxford

Dobrota D, Tkac I, Mlynarik V, Liptaj T, Boldyrev AA, Stvolinsky SL (1997) Carnosine protective effect on ischemic brain in vivo study using proton magnetic resonance spectroscopy. In: Teelken A, Korf J eds. Neurochemistry – Cellular, Molecular and Clinical Aspects 29,284:177–182

Dobrota D, Matejovicova M, Kurella E, Boldyrev AA (1999) Na/K-ATPase under oxidative stress: Molecular mechanisms of injury. Cellular and Molecular Neurobiology 19:141–149

Dollery C (1999) Therapeutic Drugs. 2nd edn. Churchill-Livingstone, London

Dorland's Illustrated Medical Dictionary (1994) 28th edn. WB Saunders, Philadelphia

Dornbrand L, Hode AJ, Fletcher RH (1997) Manual of Clinical Problems in Adult Ambulatory Care. 3rd edn. Lippincott–Raven, Philadelphia

Dreisbach RH (2001) Dreisbach's Handbook of Poisoning. 13th edn. The Parthenon Publishing Group, New York

Drobny M, Annamarie (1998) Neurology Lectures, Reference Text and Study Guide. 2nd edn. Matica Slovenska Press, Martin

Droste C, von Planta M (1997) Memorix – Clinical Medicine. Chapman and Hall Medical, London

Dufour DR (1998) Clinical Use of Laboratory Data. Williams–Wilkins, Baltimore

Dugdale DC, Eisenborg MS (1992) Medical Diagnostics. WB Saunders, Philadelphia

Duris I, Payer J, Huorka M (1995) Gastrointestinalne hormony v klinickej praxi (Gastrointestinal Hormones in Clinical Practice). Slovak Academic Press, Bratislava

Duris I, Hulin I, Bernadic M (eds.) (2000) Principy internej mediciny (Principles of Internal Medicine). Slovak Academic Press, Bratislava

Dzurik R, et al. (1996) Standardna klinicko-biochemicka diagnostika. (Standard Clinical-biochemical Diagnostics) 2nd edn. Osveta, Martin

Eddleston M, Pierini S (1999) Oxford Handbook of Tropical Medicine. Oxford University Press, Oxford

Edwards CRW, Bouchier IAD, Haslett C, Chilvers ER (1995) Davidson's Principles and Practice of Medicine. 17th edn. Churchill–Livingstone, Edinburgh

Eichenauer RH, Vanherpe H (1996) Urologie – klinika a praxe (Urology and Practice). Scientia Medica, Prague

Einer G, Zawta B (1991) Präanalytikfibel. 2. Aufl. JA Barth Verlag, Leipzig

Elgert KD (1996) Immunology. Understanding the Immune System. Willey–Liss, New York

Ellenhorn MJ (1997) Ellenhorn's Medical Toxicology. 2nd edn. Williams–Wilkins, Baltimore

Fauci AS, et al. (1998) Harrison's Principles of Internal Medicine. 14th edn. McGraw Hill, New York

Feldman M, Scharschmidt BF, Sleisenger MH (1997) Sleisenger and Fordtran's Gastrointestinal and Liver Diseases. vol. 1-2, 6th edn. WB Saunders, Philadelphia

Ferencik M (1993) Handbook of Immunochemistry. Alfa, Bratislava

Ferencik M, Stvrtinova V, Bernadic M, Jakubovsky J, Hulin I (1997) Zapal – horucka – bolest (Inflammation – Fever – Pain). Slovak Academic Press, Bratislava

Ferencik M. et al. (2000) Biochemia (Biochemistry). Slovak Academic Press, Bratislava

Ferri FF (2001) Ferri's Clinical Advisor. Mosby, St. Louis

Fischbach F (1998) Common Laboratory and Diagnostic Tests. 2nd edn. JB Lippincott, Philadelphia

Fischbach, F (1999) A Manual of Laboratory and Diagnostic Tests. 6th edn. Lippincott Williams & Wilkins Publishers, Philadelphia

Fishman RA (1992) Cerebrospinal Fluid in Diseases of the Nervous System. 2nd edn. WB Saunders, Philadelphia

Fishman AP, Elias JA, Fishman JA, Grippi MA, Kaiser LR, Senior RM (1998) Fishman's Pulmonary Diseases and Disorders. 3rd edn. vol. 1–2. McGraw Hill, New York

Folds JD, Normansell DE (1999) Pocket Guide to Clinical Immunology. ASM Press, Washington

Forbes ChD, Jacskon WF (1997) Color Atlas and Text of Clinical Medicine. 2nd edn. Mosby–Wolfe, London

Ford MD, Delaney KA, Ling LJ, et al (2000) Clinical Toxicology. WB Saunders, Philadelphia

Fowler NO (1985) The Pericardium in Health and Disease. Futura Publishing, Mount Kisco

Foye WO, Lemke TL, Williams DA (1995) Principles of Medicinal Chemistry. 4th edn. Williams–Wilkins, Baltimore

Frank MM, Austen KF, Claman HN, Unanue ER (1995) Samter's Immunological Diseases. 5th edn. vol. 1,2. Little, Brown and Co, Boston

Franova S (2001) The Influence of Inhaled Furosemide on Adverse Effects of ACE-inhibitors in Airways. Bratisl Lek Listy 102:309–313

Franova S, Nosalova G (1998) ACE inhibitors and defence reflexes of the airways. Acta Physiol Hungarica 84:359–366

Friedmann B (1994) Hematologie v praxi (Hematology in Practice). Galen, Prague

Fry DE (1993) Peritonitis. Futura Publishing, Mount Kisco

Galajda P, Balaz D, Martinka E, Mokan M, Kubisz P (1998) Insulin treatment inhibits PAI-1 production in NIDDM patients with endothelial dysfunction. Clin Appl Thromb Hemost 4:250–252

Galikova E, Buchancova J, Zigova A, Vrlik M, Mesko D, Holla G, Knizkova M (1993) Retrospektivna studia u exponovanych pracovnikov ortuti z Chemickych zavodov Novaky (Retrospective Study in Mercury-exposed Workers). Prac Lek 45:3–7

Gallin JI, Snyderman R (1999) Inflammation. 3rd edn. Lippincott Williams & Wilkins, Philadelphia

Gao P, Scheibel S, D'Amour P, Cantor T (1999) Measuring the biologically active or authentic whole parathyroid hormone (PTH) with a novel immunoradiometric assay without cross-reaction to the PTH (7–84) fragment. J Bone Miner Res 14, Sept.

Gao P, Scheibel S, D'Amour P, John MR, Rao SD, Schmidt-Gayk H, Cantor T (2001) Development of a Novel Immunoradiometric Assay Excluvisely for Biologically Active Whole Parathyroid Hormone 1–84: Implications for Improvement of Accurate Assessment of Parathyroid Function. J Bone Miner Res 16:605–614

Gatter RA, Schumacher HR (1991) A Practical Handbook of Joint Fluid Analysis. 2nd edn. Lea & Febiger, Philadelphia

Gaw A, Cowan RA, et al. (1999) Clinical Biochemistry. 2nd edn. Churchill Livingstone, Edinburgh

Gazdik F, Sausa M (2001) Non-steroid anti-inflammatory therapy of asthma bronchiale. Slovakofarma Revue 11:16–19

Gibson J, Potparic O (1996) Memorix medical and biochemical abbreviations. 1st edn, Chapman and Hall, London

Giuliani ER, Gersh BJ, McCoon MD, Hayes DL, Schaff HV (1996) Mayo Clinic Practice of Cardiology. 3rd edn. Mosby, St. Louis

Goldfrank LR, Flomenbaum NE, Lewin NA, et al. (1998) Goldfrank's Toxicologic Emergencies. 6th edn. McGraw Hill, New York

Goldman L, Krevans J, Bennett J (1999) Cecil's Essentials of Medicine. 21st edn. WB Saunders, Philadelphia

Goljan EF (1999) Most Commons in Pathology and Laboratory Medicine. WB Saunders, London

Gomella LG (1993) Clinician's Pocket Reference. 7th edn. Appleton–Lange, Norwalk

Gomella LG (2000) The 5-minute Urology Consult. Lippincott Williams & Wilkins, Philadelphia

Grahame-Smith DG, Aronson JK (1992) Oxford textbook of clinical pharmacology and drug therapy. Oxford Univesrity Press, Oxford

Greaves I, Dyer P, Porter K (1995) Handbook of Immediate Care. WB Saunders, London

Green A, Morgan I (1993) Neonatology and clinical biochemistry. ACB Venture Publications, London

Greenberg A (1994) Primer on Kidney Diseases. Academic Press, San Diego

Greenberger NJ, Berntsen MS, Jones DK, Velakaturi VN (1998) Handbook of Differential Diagnosis in Internal Medicine. 5th edn. Mosby, St. Louis

Greene HL, Johnson WP, Maricic MJ (1993) Decision Making in Medicine. Mosby, St. Louis

Greenspan FS, Strewler GJ (1997) Basic and Clinical Endocrinology. 5th edn. Prentice-Hall International, London

Greenspan F, Gardner DG (2000) Basic and Clinical Endocrinology. 6th edn. McGraw Hill, New York

Gross S, Roath S (1996) Hematology. Williams–Wilkins, Baltimore

Grossman A (1998) Clinical Endocrinology. 2nd edn. Blackwell Science, Oxford

Guder WG, Ehret W, da Fonseca–Wollheim F, Heil W, Müller–Plathe O, Töpfer G, Wisser H, Zawta B (1998) Serum, Plasma oder Volblut. Welche Antikoagulantien? DG Klin Chem Mitteilungen 29:81–103

Guder WG, Narayanan S, Wisser H, Zawta B (1996) Samples from the patient to the laboratory. GIT Verlag, Darmstadt

Gvozdjak J, et al. (1995) Interna medicina (Internal Medicine). Osveta, Martin

Hallworth M, Capps A (1993) Therapeutic drug monitoring and clinical biochemistry. ACB Venture Publications, London

Hanno PM, Wein AJ (2000) Clinical Manual of Urology. 3rd edn. McGraw Hill, New York

Hardman JG, Limbird LE, Molinoff PB, Ruddon RW, Gilman AG (1996) The pharmacological basis of therapeutics. McGraw-Hill, New York

Harr RR (1999) Clinical Laboratory Science Review. 2nd edn. F. A. Davis Co, Philadelphia

Harries M, Williams C, Stanish WD, Micheli LJ (1994) Oxford Textbook of Sports Medicine. Oxford University Press, New York

Harwood-Nuss AL, Shepherd SM, Linden ChH, et al. (2000) The Clinical Practice of Emergency Medicine. 3rd edn. Lippincott Williams & Wilkins, Philadelphia

Haslett Ch, Chilvers ER, Hunter JAA, Bond NA (1999) Davidson's Principles and Practice of Medicine. 18th edn. Churchill-Livingstone, Edinburgh

Hay WW, Hayward AR, Levin MJ, Sondheimer JM (2000) Current Pediatric Diagnosis and Treatment. 15th edn. Appleton-Lange, Stamford

Hayes PC, Mackay TW, Forrest EH (1996) Churchill's Pocket Book of Medicine. 2nd edn. Churchill–Livingstone, Edinburgh

Heine W, Plenert W (1985) Labordiagnostik. 3rd edn. Volk und Gesundheit Verlag, Berlin

Heine W, Plenert W (1985) Normalwerte. 6th edn. Volk und Gesundheit Verlag, Berlin

Heintz R, Rahn KH (1984) Erkrankungen durch Arzneimittel – Diagnostik, Klinik, Pathogenese, Therapie. 3rd edn. Georg Thieme Verlag, Stuttgart

Henry JB (2001) Clinical Diagnosis Management by Laboratory Methods. 20th edn. WB Saunders Co, Philadelphia

Henry JB, Mathur SC (2000) On Call: Laboratory Medicine and Pathology. WB Saunders Co, Philadelphia

Herbert WJ, Wilkinson PC, Stott DI (1995) The Dictionary of Immunology. 4th edn. Academic Press, London

Herndon RM, Brumback RA (1989) The Cerebrospinal Fluid. Kluwer Academic Publishers, Boston

Hillman RS, Ault KA (1998) Hematology in Clinical Practice. 2nd edn. McGraw Hill, New York

Hodgson E, Levi PE (1997) A Textbook of Modern Toxicology. Appleton–Lange, Stamford

Hoffbrand AV, Pettit JE (2000) Essential Hematology. 4th edn. Blackwell Science, Oxford

Hoffman R, Benz EJ, Shattil SJ, et al. (1999) Hematology. 3rd edn. Churchill-Livingstone, New York

Hope RA, Longmore JM, Hodgetts TJ, Ramrakha PS (2001) Oxford Handbook of Clinical Medicine. 5th edn. Oxford University Press, Oxford

Horejsi V, Bartunkova J (1998) Zaklady imunologie (Basic Immunology). Triton, Prague

Horwich A (1995) Oncology – a multidisciplinary textbook. Chapman–Hall, London

Howanitz JH, Howanitz PJ (1991) Laboratory medicine. Churchill-Livingstone, New York

Howell JM, Jolly BT (1999) Pocket Companion to accompany Emergency Medicine. WB Saunders, Philadelphia

Hubbard JD (1997) A concise Review of Clinical Laboratory Science. Williams–Wilkins, Baltimore

Hughes RAC (1997) Neurological Investigations. BMJ Publishing Group, London

Hull D, Johnston DI (1999) Essential Pediatrics. 4th edn. Churchill Livingstone, London

Humes HD, DuPont HL, Gardner LB, et al. (2000) Kelley's Textbook of Internal Medicine. 4th edn. Lippincott Williams & Wilkins, Philadelphia

Hyanek J. et al. (1991) Dedicne metabolicke poruchy – zakladni biochemicke, klinicke a geneticke aspekty. (Inherited metabolic disorders) Avicenum, Praha

Hyrdel R (2001) Klinicky vyznam seroveho gastrinu (Clinical Importance of Serum Gastrin). CentroMedian, Banska Bystrica

Inglis TJ (1996) Microbiology and Infection. Churchill-Livingstone, New York

International nonproprietary names (INN) for pharmaceutical substances (1996), World Health Organization, Geneva

Isbister JP, Harmening Pittiglio D (1988) Clinical Hematology. Williams–Wilkins, Baltimore

Isselbacher KJ, Braunwald E, et al. (1994) Harrison's Principles of Internal Medicine. 13th edn. McGraw Hill, New York

Itatani CA (1998) An Introduction to Clinical Immunology and Serology. 2nd edn. F. A. Davis Co, Philadelphia

Jacobs DS, Demott WR, et al. (1996) Laboratory Test Handbook. 4th edn. Lexi & Co., Hudson

Jaffe MS, McVan BF (1997) Davis's Laboratory and Diagnostic Test Handbook. F. A. Davis Co, Philadelphia

Jamison JJ (1999) Differential Diagnosis for Primary Practice. Churchill-Livingstone, New York

Janeway CA, Travers P, Walport M, Capra JD (1999) Immunobiology. 4th edn. Churchill-Livingstone, New York

Javorka K, et al. (1996) Klinicka fyziologia pre pediatrov (Clinical Physiology for Pediatricians). Osveta, Martin

Jelinek G, Rogers I (1999) Emergency Medicine, Topics and Problems. Blackwell Science, Oxford

John MR, Goodman WG, Gao P, Cantor T, Salusky IB, Juppner H (1999) A Novel Immunoradiometric Assay Detects Full-Length Human PTH but not Amino-Terminally Truncated Fragments: Implications for PTH Measurements in Renal Failure. J Clin Endocrinol Metab 84:4287-4290

Johnson R, Feehally MJR (1999) Comprehensive Clinical Nephrology. Mosby, Philadelphia

Jones R, Payne B (1997) Clinical investigation and statistics in laboratory medicine. ACB Venture Publications, London

Jurko A Jr, Javorkova J, Jurko A, Buchanec J, Sparcova A, Farska Z (2000) Perikardialny vypotok pri hypotyreoze v detskom veku. (Pericardial effusion in child hypothyroidism) Cs Pediat 55:320-322

Kane RL, Ouslander JG, Abrass I (1999) Essentials of Clinical Geriatrics. 4th edn. McGraw Hill, New York

Kaplan A, Jack R, Opheim KE, Toivola B, Lyon AW (1995) Clinical Chemistry. 4th edn. Williams–Wilkins, Baltimore

Katzung BG (2000) Basic and Clinical Pharmacology. 8th edn. McGraw-Hill Professional Publishing, New York

Kee J (2001) Laboratory and Diagnostic Tests with Nursing Implications. 4th edn. Prentice-Hall International, New Jersey

Keller H (1986) Klinisch-chemische Labordiagnostik für die Praxis. G Thieme Verlag, Stuttgart – New York

Kelley WN (ed) (1997) Textbook of Internal Medicine. JB Lippincott, Philadelphia

Khan MG, Lynch III JP (1997) Pulmonary Diseases. Diagnosis and Therapy. Williams–Wilkins, Baltimore

Kirby RR, Taylor RW, Livetta JM (1997) Handbook of Critical Care. 2nd edn. Lippincott–Raven, Philadelphia

Klapdor R (1994) Current Tumor Diagnosis: Applications, Clinical Relevance, Research. W Zuckschwerdt Verlag, Munchen

Klein J, Horejsi V (1997) Immunology. 2nd edn. Blackwell Science, Oxford

Klener P, et al. (1997) Cytokiny ve vnitrnim lekarstvi (Cytokines in Internal Medicine). Grada Publishing, Prague

Kliment J, Hornak M, Beseda A, Svihra J (1996) Benigna hyperplazia prostaty (Benign Prostate Hyperplasia). Osveta, Martin

Klippel JH, Dieppe PA (1998) Rheumatology. vol. 1, 2. 2nd edn. Mosby, London

Kokko JP, Tannen RL (1996) Fluids and Electrolytes. 3rd edn. WB Saunders, Philadelphia

Komadel L, et al. (1997) Telovychovnolekarske vademecum (Vademecum of Sports Medicine). 2nd edn. Berlin–Chemie, Menarinni Group, Bratislava

Koopman WJ, (ed) (1997) Arthritis and Allied Conditions. A textbook of Rheumatology. vol. 1-2, 13th edn. Williams–Wilkins, Baltimore

Kruty F, Buchancova J (1995) Klinicka toxikologia (Clinical Toxicology). In: Gvozdjak J, ed. Interna medicina (Internal Medicine). 2nd edn. Osveta, Martin

Kubisz P, Seghier F, Dobrotova M, Stasko J, Cronberg S (1995) Influence of Teniposide on platelet functions in vitro. Thrombosis Research 77:145–147

Kuby J (1997) Immunology. 3rd edn. WH Freeman and Co, New York

Kumar PJ, Clark ML (1998) Clinical Medicine. 4th edn. WB Saunders, Philadelphia

Lacy ChF, Armstrong LL, Goldman MP, Lance LL (2001) Drug Information Handbook 2001–2002. 9th edn. Lexi Comp, Hudson

Lahita RG, Chiorazzi N, Reeves WH (2000) Textbook of the Autoimmune Diseases. Lippincott Williams & Wilkins, Philadelphia

Laker MF (1995) Clinical Biochemistry for Medical Students. WB Saunders, London

Lanken PN, Hansen CW, Manaker S (2000) The Intensive Care Manual. WB Saunders, Philadelphia

Lavin A (1994) Manual of Endocrinology and Metabolism. 2nd edn. Little, Brown and Co, Boston

Ledingham JGG, Warrell DA (2000) Concise Oxford Textbook of Medicine. Oxford University Press, Oxford

Lee WM, Williams R (1997) Acute Liver Failure. Cambridge University Press, Cambridge

Lehmann OA (1998) Saunders Manual of Clinical Laboratory Science. WB Saunders, Philadelphia

Lehotsky J, Dobrota D, Kaplan P, Racay P (1998) Medical Chemistry and Biochemistry. Comenius University Press, Bratislava.

Lenhard Jr RE, Osteen RT, Gansler T (2000) Clinical Oncology. 3rd edn. Blackwell Science, Oxford

Levin DL, Morriss FC (1997) Essentials of Pediatric Intensive Care. 2nd edn. Churchill-Livingstone, New York

Lilleyman JS, Hann I (1999) Pediatric Hematology. 2nd edn. Churchill-Livingstone, New York

Ling FW, Duff P (2000) Obstetrics and Gynecology. McGraw Hill, New York

Lukac J (1998) Systemova skleroza – sklerodermia. (Systemic sclerosis – sclerodermia). Lubor Seba, Puchov

Maddison PJ, Isenberg DA, Woo P, Glass DN (1998) Oxford Textbook of Rheumatology. Vol. 1, 2. Oxford University Press, Oxford

Mahon C, Smith LA, Burns Ch (1998) An Introductory to Clinical Laboratory Science. WB Saunders, Philadelphia

Mandach U, Böni R, Danko J, Huch R, Huch A (1995) Pharmacokinetics of fenoterol in pregnant women. Arzneim Forch Drug Resp 45:186–188

Marcek T, Horvatovicova V (1992) Vplyv exhaustivnej telesnej zataze na stav imunobiologickej rezistencie (Exhaustive Exertion and Immunobiology Resistance). Med Sport Bohemoslovaca, 1:7--10

Marcek T, Bohus B, Mesko D, et al. (1995) Sports Medicine. Comenius University Press, Bratislava

Marks V (1997) Insulinomas and Hypoglycemia. In: Grossman AB, ed. Clinical Endocrinology. Blackwell, Oxford

Marks V. C-peptide (2001) In: Creighton TE, John Wiley and sons, eds. Encyclopedia of Molecular Medicine. Wiley and sons, New York

Marks V, Williams CM (1990) Nutrition and Metabolism. In: Scurr C, Feldman S, Soni N eds. Scientific Foundations of Anaesthesia 4th edn. Heinemann, Oxford

Marks V, Teale JD (1993) Hypoglycaemia in the adult. In: Gregory JW, Aynsley-Green A eds. Clinical Endocrinology and Metabolism. Bailliere Tindall, London

Marshall WJ (2000) Clinical Chemistry. 4th edn. Mosby, St. Louis

Marshall WJ, Bangert SK (1995) Clinical Biochemistry. Churchill-Livingstone, New York

Martinka E, Strakova J, Shawkatova I, Buc M (1998) Latent autoimmune (type-1) diabetes mellitus in patients classified initially as having type-2 diabetes. In: Talwar GP, Nath I, Ganguly NK, Rao KV eds. Proceedings of 10th International Congress of Immunology. New Delhi, India. Monduzi Editore, 1211–1216

Masopust J (1990) Pozadovani a hodnoceni biochemickych vysetreni – I. (Ordering and evaluation of biochemical examination I.). Avicenum, Prague

Masopust J. Pozadovani a hodnoceni biochemickych vysetreni – II. (1990) (Ordering and evaluation of biochemical examination II.). Avicenum, Prague

Mayne PD (1996) Clinical Biochemistry in Diagnosis and Treatment. 6th edn. Arnold, London

Mazza JJ (1995) Manual of Clinical Hematology. 2nd edn. Little, Brown and Co, Boston

McBride LJ (1997) Textbook of Urinalysis and Body Fluids. JB Lippincott, Philadelphia

McClatchey KD, Alkan S, Hackel E, et al. (2001) Clinical Laboratory Medicine. 2nd edn. Lippincott Williams & Wilkins, Philadelphia

McMorrow ME, Malarkey L (1998) Laboratory and Diagnostic Tests. WB Saunders, Philadelphia

Melloni B, Dox ID (1997) Melloni's illustrated dictionary of medical abbreviations. The Parthenon Publishing Group, Carnforth

Melmon KL, Hoffman BB, Carruthers G, Nierenberg DW (2000) Melmon and Morreli's Clinical Pharmacology. 4th edn. McGraw Hill, New York

Mirossay L, Mirossay A, Kocisova E, Radvakova I, Miskovsky J (1999) Hypericin-Induced Phototoxicity of Human Leukemic Cell Line HL-60 is Potentiated by Omeprazole, an Inhibitor of $H+K+$-ATPase and 5´-(N,N-dimethyl)-amiloride, an Inhibitor of $Na+/H+$ Exchanger. Physiol. Res 48:135–141

Mitrakou A, Vuorinen-Markkola H, Raptis G, Toft I, Mokan M, Strumph P, et al. (1992) Simultaneous Assessment of Insulin Secretion and Insulin Sensitivity Using a Hyperglycemic Clamp. J Clin Endocrinol Metab 75:379–382.

Mokan M, et al. (1997) Metabolicky syndrom a metabolizmus tukov (Metabolic Syndrome and Lipid Metabolism). Media Group, Michalovce

Müller S (1997) Memorix – Emergency Medicine. Chapman–Hall Medical, London

Munson PL, Muller RA, Breese GR (1996) Principles of pharmacology. Chapman–Hall, New York

Murray RK, et al. (1988) Harpers Biochemistry. Appleton and Lange, Norwalk

Myers AR (1994) Medicine. 2nd edn. The National Medical Series for Independent Study. Harwal Publishing, Philadelphia

Nicoll D, McPhee SJ, Chou TM, Pignone M, Detmer WM (2000) Pocket Guide to Diagnostic Tests. 3rd edn. Appleton–Lange, Stamford

Niessen KH, et al. (1999) Paediatrie. 5th edn. Georg Thieme Verlag, Stutgart–New York

Noji EK, Kelen GD (1989) Manual of Toxicologic Emergencies. Year Medical Publishers, Chicago

Nosal S (1999) New possibilities of diagnosis chronic obstructive diseases of the airways in infant. In: The chapters of pediatrics. Jessenius Faculty of Medicine, Martin

Nosalova G (2000) New opinions on the mechanism of action of xanthine derivatives. Slovakofarma Revue 10,1–2:51–55.

Nyhan WL (1984) Abnormalities in amino acid metabolism in clinical medicine. Appleton-Century-Crofts, Norwalk

O'Grady J, Lake J, Howdle P (2000) Comprehensive Clinical Hepatology. Mosby, St. Louis

Okuda K, Tabor E (1997) Liver Cancer. Churchill-Livingstone, New York

Oski FA (1994) Principles and Practice of Pediatrics. JB Lippincott, Philadelphia

Pagana KD, Pagana TJ (1998) Mosby's Manual of Diagnostic Laboratory Tests. Mosby, St. Louis

Pagana KD, Pagana TJ (1998) Mosby's Diagnostic and Laboratory Test Reference. 3rd edn. Mosby, St. Louis

Pannal P, Kotasek D (1997) Cancer and clinical biochemistry. ACB Venture Publications, London

Pec J, Fetisovova Z, Frlickova Z, et al. (1997) Scleredema diabeticorum in a patient with latent autoimmune diabetes in adults. Eur J Dermatol 7:596–598

Pec M, Plank L, Szepe P, Belej K, Zubrikova L, Halakova E, Pec J (1998) A case of systemic mastocytosis – an ultrastructural and immunohistochemical study of the dermal mast cells in relation to activation of the epidermal melanin unit. J Eur Acad Dermatol Venereol 11:258–261

Pestana C (1999) Fluids and Electrolytes in the Surgical Patient. Lippincott Williams & Wilkins, Philadelphia

Pflederer A, Breckwoldt M, Martius G (2000) Gynäkologie und Geburtshilfe. 3rd edn. Georg Thieme-Verlag, Stuttgart–New York

Pinchera A, Bertagna X, Fischer J, et al. (2000) Endocrinology an Metabolism. McGraw Hill, New York

Planta M, Benedict M, Hartman G (1996) Differix. Internal Medicine. Chapman–Hall Medical, London

Polansky V (1999) Quick Review Cards for Clinical Laboratory Science Examinations. F. A. Davis Co, Philadelphia

Poole–Wilson PA, Colucci WS, Massie BM, Chatterjee K, Coats AJS (1997) Heart Failure. Churchill-Livingstone, New York

Porsova–Dutoit I (1996) Endokrinologie v praxi (Endocrinology for Practice). Grada–Avicenum, Prague

Potparic O, Gibson J (1993) A Dictionary of Clinical Tests. The Parthenon Publishing Group, Carnforth

Pounder R, Hamilton M (1995) Handbook of Current Diagnosis and Treatment. Churchill Livingstone, Edinburgh

Prakash UBS, ed (1998) Mayo Internal Medicine Board Review 1998-99. Lippincott–Raven, Philadelphia

Product information. (1995) Ansaid. The Upjohn Company

Product information. (1996) Activase. Genentech

Product information. (1997) Precose. Bayer Corporation

Professional Guide to Diseases (2001) 7th edn. Lippincott Williams & Wilkins, Philadelphia

Provan D, Duncombe AS, Chisholm M, Smith A (1998) Oxford Handbook of Clinical Hematology. Oxford University Press, Oxford

Pullmann R, Koskova E, Sokolik L, Jamriska P, Bacmanak S, Moric R (1983) Blood Carboxyhemoglobin, plasma and salivary thiocyanate in smokers. Bull Eur Physiopath Resp 35,Suppl.1:35

Pullmann R, Hybenova J, Skerenova M, Celec S, Pullmann R Jr (1996) Polymorphism of apolipoproteins B and E in different clinical pictures of premature atherosclerosis. Infor Listy, Gen Spol G Mendla 18:19-20

Pullmann R, Melus V, Hybenova J, Pullmann R Jr, Skerenova M, Celec S, Kubisz P (1999) Relation of the −455 G/A polymorphism of the beta-fibrinogen gene to the myocardial infarction. Blood Coagulat Fibrinol 1:101

Pullmann R Jr, Lukac J, Skerenova M, Rovensky J, Hybenova J, Melus V, Celec S, Pullmann R, Hyrdel R (1999) Association between systemic lupus erythematosus and insertion/deletion polymorphism of the angiotensin converting enzyme gene. Clin Exp Rheumatol 17:593–596

Pullman R Jr, Lukac J, Skerenova M, Rovensky J, Hybenova J, Melus V, Celec S, Pullmann R, Hyrdel R (1999) Cytotoxic T-lymphocyte antigen 4 (CTLA-4) dimorphism in patients with systemic lupus erythematosus. Clin Exp Rheumatol 17: 725–729

Pullmann R, Hybenova J, Skerenova M, Melus V, Pullmann R Jr (2000) Assessment of insertion/deletion polymorphisms of angiotensin-converting enzyme gene and its clinical importance. Bratisl lek Listy 101:177–178

Rakel RE (2000) Saunders Manual of Medical Practice 2nd edn. WB Saunders, Philadelphia

Ramzakha P, Moore K (1997) Oxford Handbook of Acute Medicine. Oxford University Press, Oxford

Rapid Acces Guide to Internal Medicine (1997) 3rd edn. Lippincott–Raven, Philadelphia

Ravel R (1995) Clinical Laboratory Medicine. 6th edn. Mosby, St. Louis

Reed GB, Claireaux AE, Bain AD (1989) Diseases of the fetus and newborn – pathology, radiology and genetics. Chapman and Hall Ltd., London

Rees PJ, Williams DG (1995) Principles of Clinical Medicine. Arnold, London

Rich RR, Fleisher TA, Shearer WT, Kotzin BL, Scroeder HW (2001) Clinical Immunology. Principles and Practice. 2nd edn. Mosby, St. Louis

Richterich, R (1969) Clinical Chemistry. S. Karger, Basel, New York

Riedl O, Vondracek V, et al. (1980) Klinicka toxikologie (Clinical Toxicology). Avicenum, Prague

Ritter JM, Lewis LD, Mant TGK (1995) A textbook of clinical pharmacology. 3rd edn. Arnold, London

Roitt I, Brostoff J, Male D (1997) Immunology. 5th edn. Mosby, London

Rose NR, de Macario EC, Folds JD, Lanc HC, Nakamura RM (1997) Manual of Clinical Laboratory Immunology. 5th edn. ASM Press, Washington

Rosen P, Barkin RM, Hayden SR, et al. (1999) The 5-minute Emergency Medicine Consult. Lippincott Williams & Wilkins, Philadelphia

Roskoski R (1996) Biochemistry. WB Saunders, Philadelphia

Rossoff IS (2001) Encyclopedia of Clinical Toxicology. The Parthenon Publishing Group, New York

Rovensky J, et al. (1998) Reumatologia v teorii a praxi V (Rheumatology in Theory and Practice). Osveta, Martin

Rovensky J, Pavelka K, et al. (2000) Klinicka reumatologia (Clinical Rheumatology) Osveta, Martin

Rucker LM (1997) . Essentials of Adult Ambulatory Care. Williams–Wilkins, Baltimore

Ruddy S, Harris ED, Sledge CB (2000) Kelley's Textbook of Rheumatology. 6th edn. WB Saunders, Philadelphia

Rudolf MCJ, Levene MI (1999) Pediatrics and Child Health. Blackwell Science, Oxford

Rudy DR, Kurowski K (1997) Family Medicine. Williams–Wilkins, Baltimore

Sacher RA, McPherson RA (2000) Widmann's Clinical Interpretation of Laboratory Tests. 11th edn. F. A. Davis Co, Philadelphia

Slatopolsky E, Finch J, Clay P, Martin D, Sicard G, Singer G, Gao P, Cantor T, Dusso A (2000) A novel mechanism for skeletal resistance in uremia. Kidney Int 58:753–61

Souberbielle JC, Cormier C, Kindermans C, Gao P, Cantor T, Forette F, Baulier E (2001) Vitamin D. Status and Redefining Serum Parathyroid Hormone Reference Range in the Elderly. J Clin Endocrinol Metab 86: 3086–3090

Sasinka M, Sagat T, et al. (1998) Pediatria (Pediatrics). Satus, Kosice

Saultz JW (2000) Textbook of Family Medicine. McGraw Hill, New York

Schäffler A, Braun J, Ulrich R (1994) Vademecum lekare (Physician Vademecum). Galen, Prague

Schettler G, Usadel KH, et al. (1995) Repetitorium praktickeho lekare (GP Vademecum). Galen, Prague

Schlager SI (1998) Clinical Management of Infectious Diseases. Williams–Wilkins, Baltimore

Schull PD, ed. (1998) Illustrated Guide to Diagnostic Tests. 2nd edn. Springhouse Corp, Springhouse

Schumacher HR, Reginato AJ (1991) Atlas of Synovial Fluid Analysis and Crystal Identification. Lea & Febiger, Philadelphia

Schwarz MI, King TE, Jr (1993) Interstitial Lung Disease. Mosby, St. Louis

Schwartz MW, Curry TA, Sargent AJ (1997) Pediatric Primary Care. 3rd edn. Mosby, St. Louis

Schwartz MW, Bell LM, Bingham PM, et al. (2000)The 5-minute Pediatric Consult. Lippincott Williams & Wilkins, Philadelphia

Shearman DJC, Finlayson NDC, Camilleri M (1997) Diseases of the Gastrointestinal Tract and Liver. 3rd edn. Churchill-Livingstone, New York

Shoemaker WC, Ayres SM, Grenvik A, Holbrook PR (1999) Textbook of Critical Care. 4th edn. WB Saunders, Philadelphia

Siegenthaler W (1999) Differentialdiagnose innerer Krankheiten. 18th edn. Georg Thieme-Verlag, Stuttgart – New York

Sigal LH, Ron Y (1994) Immunology and Inflammation. McGraw Hill, New York

Sinclair J, ed. (1994) Collins Cobuild English Language Dictionary. Harper Collins Publishers, London

Singer M, Webb AR (1994) Acute Medicine Algorithms. Oxford University Press, Oxford

Sirtori C, Kuhlmann J, Tillement JP, et al. (2000) Clinical Pharmacology. McGraw Hill, New York

Smith AF, Becket GJ, Walker S, Rae P (1998) Lecture Notes on Clinical Biochemistry. 6th edn. Blackwell Science, Oxford

Souhami RL, Moxham J (1997) Textbook of Medicine. 3rd edn. Churchill Livingstone, Edinburgh

Speicher CE (1993) The Right Test. A Physician's Guide to Laboratory Medicine. 2nd edn. WB Saunders, Philadelphia

Srsen S, Srsnova K (2000) Zaklady klinickej genetiky a jej molekularna podstata (Principles of Clinical Genetics and its Molecular basis). 3rd edn. Osveta, Martin

Starka L, et al. (1997) Endokrinologie (Endocrinology). Maxdorf–Jessenius, Prague

Steele RV (2000) The Clinical Handbook of Pediatric Infectious Diseases. The Parthenon Publishing Group, New York

Stein JH, ed. (1998) Internal Medicine, 5th edn. Mosby, St. Louis

Stein SF, Kokko JP (1999) Emory University Comprehensive Board Review in Internal Medicine. McGraw Hill, New York

Stiene-Martin EA, Lotspeich–Steininger ChA, Koepke JA (1998) Clinical Hematology. 2nd edn. JB Lippincott, Philadelphia

Stites DP, Terr AI, Parslow TG (1997) Medical Immunology. 9th edn. Prentice–Hall International, London

Strakova J, Tatarova A, Rozborilova E, Cap J, Raffajova J, Martinka E (1998) Activated T-cells and cytokines in bronchoalveolar lavage fluid (BAL) from patients with interstitial lung diseases. In: Talwar GP, Nath I, Ganguly NK, Rao KV, eds. Proceedings of 10th International Congress of Immunology. New Delhi, India. Monduzi Editore, 1011–1015

Strapkova A, Nosalova G, Franova S (1999) Mucolytics and antioxidant activity. Life Sci 65:1923–1925

Strasinger SK (1994) Urinalysis and Body Fluids. 3rd edn. F. A. Davis Co, Philadelphia

Swash M (1995) Hutchinson's Clinical Methods. 20th edn. WB Saunders, London

Tamparo CD, Lewis MA (2000) Diseases of Human Body. 3rd edn. F. A. Davis Co, Philadelphia

Taylor RB (2000) The 10-minute Diagnosis Manual. Lippincott Williams & Wilkins, Philadelphia

Teplan V (1998) Prakticka nefrologie (Practical Nephrology). Grada–Avicenum, Prague

The Merck Manual of Diagnosis and Therapy (1999). 17th edn. Merck Res Lab, Rahway

Thomas L, ed. (1992) Labor und Diagnose. 4th edn. MWM Verlag, Nearburg

Tierney LM, McPhee SJ, Papadakis MA (2001) Current Medical Diagnosis and Treatment. 40th edn. Lange Medical Books/McGraw-Hill

Tietz NW (1995) Clinical Guide to Laboratory Tests. 3rd edn. WB Saunders Co, Philadelphia

Tintinalli JE, Kelen GD, Stapczynski JS (1999) Emergency Medicine. 5th edn. McGraw Hill, New York

Trnovec T, Dzurik R (1998) Standardne diagnosticke postupy (Standard Diagnostic Procedures). Osveta, Martin

Tryding N (1996) Drug Effects in Clinical Chemistry. (Software). Polydata Ltd, PharmaSoft SWEDIS AB

Tryding N, Roos KA (1989) Drug Interferences and Drug Effects in Clinical Chemistry. 5th edn. Apoteksbogalet AB, Stockholm

Varsik P, Bielekova B, Brezny I, Traubner P et al. (1999) Neurologia. (Neurology) Lufema, Bratislava

Vaughn G (1999) Understanding and Evaluating Common Laboratory Tests. 1st edn. Prentice-Hall International, New Jersey

Viccellio P (1993) Handbook of Medical Toxicology. Little, Brown and Co, Boston

Vladutiu AO (1986) Pleural Effusion. Futura Publishing, Mount Kisco

Voet D, Voet JG (1995) Biochemistry. 2nd edn. John Wiley and Sons, New York

Volk W, Benjamin D, Kadner R, Parsons T (1991) Essentials of Medical Microbiology. 4th edn. JB Lippincott, Philadelphia

Wallach J (1998) Handbook of Interpretation of Diagnostic Tests. Lippincott–Raven, Philadelphia

Wallach J (2000) Interpretation of Diagnostic Tests. 7th edn. Lippincott Williams & Wilkins, Philadelphia

Weatherall DJ, Ledingham JCG, Warrel DA (1995) Oxford Textbook of Medicine, 3rd edn. (vol. 1, 2). Oxford University Press, Oxford

Wedding ME, Toenjes SA (1998) Medical Laboratory Procedures. 2nd edn. F. A. Davis Co, Philadelphia

Weir DM, Stewart J (1997) Immunology. 8th edn. Churchill-Livingstone, New York

Weiss RM, George NJR, O'Reilly PH (2000) Comprehensive Urology. Mosby, St. Louis

Wexler P, ed. (1998) Encyclopedia of Toxicology. vol. 1-3. Academic Press, San Diego

Whitlock SA (1997) Delmar's Clinical Laboratory Manual Series – Immunohematology. Delmar Publishers, Albane

Widmann FK, Itatani CA (1998) An Introduction to Clinical Immunology and Serology. 2nd edn. F. A. Davis Co, Philadelphia

Williams D, Marks V (1994) Scientific Foundations of Biochemistry in Clinical Practice. 2nd edn. Butterworth–Heineman, Oxford

Wilson JD, Foster DW, Kronenberg HM, Larsen PR (1998) Williams Textbook of Endocrinology. 9th edn. WB Saunders, Philadelphia

Wolfson AB, Paris PM (1996) Diagnostic Testing in Emergency Medicine. WB Saunders, Philadelphia

Woolliscroft JO, ed. (1998) Current Diagnosis and Treatment. 2nd edn. Mosby, St. Louis

Wyllie R, Hyams JS (1993) Pediatric Gastrointestinal Disease. WB Saunders, Philadelphia

Yamada T, Alpers DH, Owyang Ch, Powell DW, Silverstein FE (1995) Textbook of Gastroenterology. 2nd edn. vol. 1, 2. JB Lippincott, Philadelphia

Young DS (1997) Effect of preanalytical variables on clinical laboratory tests. 2nd edn. American Association for clinical chemistry press, Washington

Zibolen M, Zbojan J, Dluholucky S (2001) Prakticka neonatologia (Practical Neonatology). Neografia, Martin

Zilva JF, Pannall PR, Mayne PD (1988) Clinical Chemistry in Diagnosis and Treatment. 5th edn. Year Book Medical Publishers, Chicago

List of www sources

The Internet Drug Index, RxList Monographs, August 2001, http://www.rxlist.com/cgi/generic/index.html

Horst Ibelgauft: Cytokines Online Pathfinder Encyclopaedia, August 2001, http://www.copewithcytokines.de/cope.cgi?930

National Library of Medicine, Medline Plus Drug Information, August 2001, http://www.nlm.nih.gov/medlineplus/druginfo/drug_Aa.html

Infomed-Verlags AG, Bergliweg 17, CH-9500 Wil, Switzerland, Infomed Drug Guide, August 2001, http://www.infomed.org/100drugs/index.html

Complete Pharmaceutical Monographs, Rxmed, August 2001, http://www.rxmed.com/rxmed/b.main/b2.pharmaceutical/b2.prescribe.html

Drug Interactions Guide, August 2001, http://www.drugs.com/data/channel/md/drkoop.cfm?int=0

Drug Information Technologies, Full text Drug Monograph, August 2001, http://www.dispace.com/ditonline/start_neu.html

A to Z Durg Facts, August 2001, http://www.drugfacts.com

Register

lipodystrophy 753
lipoidosis 753
– ceramide lactoside l. 753
lipoprotein (a)
– blood 254
lipoprotein lipase
– blood 255
lipoprotein X
– blood 254
lipoxins
– blood (H) 456
liquorice (Ph) 882
lisinopril (Ph) 883
lisuride (Ph) 883
lithium
– blood 255
lithium (Ph) 883
liver, fatty 753
– acute fatty liver in pregnancy 753
lomefloxacin (Ph) 883
lomustine (Ph) 883
long-acting thyroid stimulator
– blood 255
loop diuretics (Ph) 883
loperamide (Ph) 883
loracarbef (Ph) 883
lorcainide (Ph) 883
losartan (Ph) 883
lovastatin (Ph) 883
low-molecular weight B-cell growth factor
– blood 256
loxapine (Ph) 884
lupus 753
– CNS l. 753
– discoid l. 753
– drug-induced l. 753
– systemic l. erythematosus 754
lupus inhibitor
– blood 256
luteinizing hormone
– blood 256
– urine 569
lymphadenitis, mesenterial 754
lymphadenopathy, angioimmunoblastic 754
lymphangiectasis, intestinal 754
lymphangitis 755
lymphocytes
– blood (H) 457
– cerebrospinal fluid 406

– pericardial fluid 496
– peritoneal fluid 502
– pleural fluid 511
– synovial fluid 538
lymphocytotoxic antibodies
– blood 257
lymphogranuloma inguinale 755
lynestrenol (Ph) 884
lysergide (Ph) 884
lysine
– blood 257
– cerebrospinal fluid 407
– urine 582
lysozyme
– blood 258
– cerebrospinal fluid 407
– pleural fluid 511
– saliva 514
– urine 582

M

macroamylasemia 755
macrophage inflammatory protein
– blood 259
macrophages
– cerebrospinal fluid 407
– synovial fluid 538
magnesium
– blood 259
– cerebrospinal fluid 407
– stool 527
– urine 582
magnesium (Ph) 884
magnesium salts (Ph) 884
malabsorption 755
– folate m. 755
– intestinal m. 755
– iron m. 755
– methionine m. 755
malate dehydrogenase
– amniotic fluid 386
– blood 261
malignant cells
– cerebrospinal fluid 407
malnutrition 755
malone dialdehyde
– blood 261
mammary-derived growth inhibitor
– blood 262
manganese
– blood 262

– hair 419
– urine 583
mannitol (Ph) 884
MAO
– gastric fluid 417
MAO inhibitors (Ph) 884
maprotiline (Ph) 884
mastocytes
– blood (H) 459
mastocytosis 756
matrix metalloproteinases
– blood 263
mean corpuscular hemoglobin
– blood (H) 460
mean corpuscular hemoglobin concentration
– blood (H) 460
mean corpuscular volume
– blood (H) 461
mean platelet volume
– blood (H) 462
measles/mumps/rubella vaccines (Ph) 884
mebendazole (Ph) 884
mechlorethamine (Ph) 884
meclofenamic acid (Ph) 884
meconium
– amniotic fluid 386
medroxyprogesterone (Ph) 885
mefenamic acid (Ph) 885
mefloquine (Ph) 885
mefruside (Ph) 885
megacolon, toxic 756
megestrol (Ph) 885
melanocyte stimulating hormone
– blood 266
melanogens
– urine 583
melanoma growth stimulating activity
– blood 271
meloxicam (Ph) 885
melperone (Ph) 885
melphalan (Ph) 885
meningitis 756
– acute purulent m. 756
– aseptic m. 756
– bacterial m. 756
– carcinomatous m. 757
– chemical m. 757
– chronic m. 757
– cryptococcal m. 757
– m. in amebiasis 757